MEDICAL RADIOLOGY
Diagnostic Imaging

Editors:
A. L. Baert, Leuven
K. Sartor, Heidelberg

Springer
Berlin
Heidelberg
New York
Hong Kong
London
Milan
Paris
Tokyo

R. F. Dondelinger (Ed.)

Imaging and Intervention in Abdominal Trauma

With Contributions by

G. M. Allen · C. Andreoli · G. Andreoli · M. Bezzi · W. A. Bhatti · J. H. Boverie
K. Breitschaft · N. Bulakbasi · H. Carty · O. Cornet · P. Damas · P. Deleuse · A. Denys
R. F. Dondelinger · A. K. Dixon · B. Ghaye · P. Goffette · A. Graham · H. Häuser
G. Hartstein · P. Huppert · J. Hillier · J. E. Jackson · P.-F. Laterre · S. Ledbetter · M. Lewin
B. Martin · E. Mayr · V. Miele · E. Mouhsine · A. Nchimi · D. B. Nunez, Jr. · G. Ponghis
F. Portier · D. Rickards · P. A. Schnyder · S. J. A. Sclafani · S. Sheeran · D. Szapiro
N. Theumann · G. Trotteur · J. P. Verdon · V. Willems · D. J. Wilson · N. Zügel

Foreword by

A. L. Baert

With 402 Figures in 808 Separate Illustrations, 20 in Color and 169 Tables

Springer

Robert F. Dondelinger, MD
Professor and Chairman
Department of Medical Imaging
University Hospital Sart Tilman
Domaine du Sart Tilman B35
4000 Liège
Belgium

Medical Radiology · Diagnostic Imaging and Radiation Oncology
Series Editors: A. L. Baert · L. W. Brady · H.-P. Heilmann · F. Molls · K. Sartor

Continuation of
Handbuch der medizinischen Radiologie
Encyclopedia of Medical Radiology

ISBN 3-540-65212-4 Springer-Verlag Berlin Heidelberg New York

Library of Congress Cataloging-in-Publication Data applied for

Bibliographic information published by Die Deutsche Bibliothek
Die Deutsche Bibliothek lists this publication in the Deutsche Nationalbibliographie; detailed bibliographic data is available in the Internet at <http://dnb.ddb.de>.

Springer-Verlag is a part of Springer Science+Business Media

http//www. springeronline.com

Printed in Germany

Cover-Design and Typesetting: Verlagsservice Teichmann, 69256 Mauer

21/3150xq – 5 4 3 2 1 0 – Printed on acid-free paper

To

Quenotte and Rambo du Site du Belvédère
Achilles-Boris and
Adonis-Ivan da Prada Rossa

For a lifetime of joy and love

Foreword

Most radiologists are frequently confronted with trauma patients in their everyday practice. It is of vital importance that the radiologist should assume full responsibility within the trauma team responsible for managing the patient to ensure that a rapid and optimal diagnosis is made. This can only be done if the radiologist is well informed about the latest treatment concepts for trauma victims.

This book is unique in that it provides a very comprehensive and integrated overview of the pathophysiology, clinical symptomatology, diagnosis, and treatment of abdominal trauma. Special emphasis is placed on diagnostic tests, modern imaging protocols, and minimally invasive, percutaneous treatment options.

I would like to congratulate Professor Dr. R.F. Dondelinger on his superb work as editor of this remarkable volume and commend the authors, all well-known international experts in the field, for their fine, up-to-date chapters on individual topics.

I highly recommend this volume to all radiologists involved in the management of abdominal trauma patients and to trauma surgeons and intensive care physicians. I am confident that readers will be as impressed by this outstanding volume as they have been by previous volumes published in this series.

Leuven

Albert L. Baert

Preface

Trauma kills or disables men and women, individuals young and old, unexpectedly, who up until a moment before the acute injury had been leading normal lives. Increasing civil urban violence either in the street or in private, high-speed traffic collisions, leisure activities, labour and sports accidents, and suicide attempts, associated with consumption of alcohol or other drugs, account for the diverse trauma scenes encountered across the Atlantic and in Europe.

Trauma predominantly kills young people, which, apart from the human suffering involved, has enormous social and economical implications. Trauma accounts for more lost years of life than do cancer and cardiovascular diseases combined. Each year, roughly eight to twelve thousand individuals are killed and several hundreds of thousand are temporarily or permanently disabled by road traffic accidents alone, in each of the largest European countries.

However trauma prevention and care does not attract the attention that it deserves. Research expenditures on trauma in Europe and the United States are ridiculously low in comparison with those of cancer or cardiovascular diseases. Medical teaching programmes only rarely reflect an integrated approach to the management of the most severe trauma patients, leading to the unpreparedness of physicians in smaller hospitals with limited caseloads.

Over the years modern medical imaging has become a cornerstone of management of trauma victims. Multislice computed tomography is well established as an optimal screening modality for polytrauma patients, provided the equipment is installed in emergency admissions and permanently operational. Trauma is a dynamic state that kills by means of predictable mechanisms and in predictable time frames. Although instantaneous imaging is able to detect the extent and severity of injuries, clinical symptoms and findings always take precedence in decision making on patient management. After reviewing the examination on the console, the radiologist should be able to formulate precisely the findings and should take part in the discussion on the clinical significance of the injuries observed and on management options, in so far as arteriographic hemostatic embolization or other interventional procedures are considered options.

The concept of the present book on imaging and intervention of abdominal trauma deviates from the usual format of books on "imaging". Pathophysiology of abdominal injuries, clinical symptoms and signs, and management options are discussed in detail together with the clinical significance of the relevant imaging findings. The book is written entirely by radiologists, who have devoted much time to the care of trauma victims, for radiologists and particularly for the new generation of "console radiologists", who do not necessarily have the same interest in clinical management as the older generation has.

I express the hope that residents and practicing radiologists who are taking care of trauma victims will find here a comprehensive insight into all aspects of imaging that are relevant to clinical management of abdominal injuries.

Liège

Robert F. Dondelinger

Contents

1 Organization of Imaging in the Emergency Environment

R. F. Dondelinger

CONTENTS

Key factors in organization of trauma imaging are: permanent access to state of the art CT, US and angiography, immediate reporting, permanent access to the complete image folder and reliable communication between all members of the trauma team.

R. F. Dondelinger, MD
Professor and Chairman, Department of Medical Imaging, University Hospital Sart Tilman, Domaine Universitaire du Sart Tilman B35, 4000 Liège, Belgium

1.1 General Principles of Trauma Care

Radiologists participating in care of trauma patients should be aware of the general principles governing trauma management. In no other radiological subspecialty will they have to be so intimately integrated into an interdisciplinary team. Upon completion of the examination, they must be able to formulate a reliable interpretation of the imaging findings and understand their correlation with the clinical observations.

- Trauma kills the young. More years of life are lost by trauma than by cardiovascular disease and cancer together. Hundreds of thousands of trauma victims remain temporarily or permanently disabled, and many cannot return to their previous work, despite intense and prolonged rehabilitation. Radiologists should be aware of the enormous social and economic implications of trauma care.

- Trauma kills by predictable mechanisms. Injuries to the central nervous system and large vessels are responsible for most immediate deaths at the site of accident. Trauma victims who have reached the hospital alive risk succumbing to internal hemorrhage during the first hours after admission. As Yoram Ben-Menachem, a superb trauma radiologist, has put it: "superficial is irrelevant." The primary objective of imaging is the detection of "ongoing internal hemorrhage" and of any other immediately life-threatening condition. The second objective is to recognize at once all injuries present and classify them according to their clinical significance for an appropriate hierarchy of treatment and reduction of morbidity and mortality. Radiologists should also be aware that posttraumatic mortality reaches a peak around the 3rd week, similar to the mortality peak of the first hours following admission. Causes of late mortality are mainly infection and multiorgan failure. More selective imaging than at admission plays a considerable role in timely diagnosis of late complications.

- Trauma kills in predictable time frames. As already mentioned, complete diagnosis of all injuries must be established during the "golden hour" after admission. In the past, when efficient cross-section imaging was not yet available, Ben-Menachem warned radiologists against wasting time in imaging of non-life-threatening injuries, before ongoing bleeding from internal injury was ruled out: "Imaging at admission should be inversely proportional to the severity of trauma"; "Do not diagnose the trauma patient to death." This warning remains valid today.

- Trauma is a dynamic state. Posttraumatic injuries that have stopped bleeding at the time of imaging may bleed again. Occult, unrecognized injuries may declare themselves hours, days or weeks after injury; other complications may develop during the healing process. Radiologists have to be aware that instantaneous imaging alone, despite the exquisite precision of internal anatomical display, cannot safely predict the clinical evolution of the trauma victim. The implication for radiologists is that all imaging equipment and expertise must be permanently available around the clock, not only for admissions, but also for inpatients whenever their condition deteriorates or any clinical observation suggests presence of missed injury or a posttraumatic complication.

- Trauma care cannot be improvised. Trauma care must be standardized, according to established protocols that are known by all physicians and paramedical personnel concerned with trauma management. Adherence to the general principles is more important than sticking strictly to complicated algorithms or decision trees. All efforts must be made to save time during imaging, avoid patient transfer out of the resuscitation environment and offer the best available combination of imaging equipment and front-line radiological expertise. The way ultrasound, computed tomography, angiography and conventional X-ray examinations are requested and obtained in a trauma victim, and how the radiological report is formulated, must be standardized and constant quality should be assured at any time. Resuscitation, primary and secondary survey and imaging are interwoven standardized processes, but must remain flexible. When indicated, imaging must be shortened, or aborted to be replaced by immediate surgery or angiographic hemostatic embolization.

- There is no untransportable patient. The dogma of the patient untransportable to the angiography suite is no longer tenable. Radiologists have to be aware that intractable retroperitoneal or pelvic bleeding associated with pelvic fractures is best treated by emergent arterial embolization, which requires transportation even of the hemodynamically unstable patient to the angiographic suite, if angiography is not available in the emergency room.

- Full cooperation between all members of the trauma team and free circulation of all information concerning the trauma victim is the key to success of trauma care. Radiologists should know the mechanism of trauma, the degree of severity of the accident, and the clinical observations made at admission. They must have access to all patient records, at the time of initial imaging and later. On the other hand, all imaging findings must be made immediately available, not only to all the members of the trauma team, but also to other consultant specialists who may be involved with trauma care.

- The trauma room is not the place where conflicts among hospital staff members or political struggles between different departments should take place. Complete confidence and reliance are absolutely necessary for efficient team work. Solo management guided by one's own inspiration is not applicable to trauma care. The full potential of the imaging department must be made available to trauma care. The most powerful imaging equipment, adapted to trauma management, must be available in the emergency environment. It is improper policy to install the newest computed tomography or ultrasound equipment in the main imaging department and take the old equipment to the emergency room. Full digitization, radiological information system (RIS) and picture archiving and communication system (PACS) should preferentially operate in the emergency environment. No separation should be made between diagnostic imaging and intervention. An interventional radiologist should be a front-line member of the trauma team.

1.2 Organization of Trauma Imaging

1.2.1 Imaging Modalities

1.2.1.1 Conventional Radiography

Conventional films were the cornerstone of imaging the trauma patient before the advent of cross-section imaging. Imaging protocols at admission still include frontal chest, frontal pelvis and lumbar spine, and lateral cervical spine films after primary survey of vital functions. But in the future, should all these films systematically obtained or should some be replaced by immediate CT imaging? A ceiling-mounted X-ray tube or a C-arm should be able to move freely around the patient support and resuscitation equipment. Imaging in the trauma environment should be fully digitized. Lead aprons must be available in sufficient number for all members of the trauma team, and must remain permanently in the trauma room.

1.2.1.2 Computed Tomography

State-of-the-art CT should be installed directly in the emergency environment and should be accessible without delay for trauma cases and other medical or surgical nontraumatic emergencies. Multislice CT will soon be the standard in all departments. Standardization of acquisition protocols (spirals, slice thickness, timing of contrast injection, viewing, archiving and reporting), are mandatory and should be formulated in detail. Fluoro-CT and a slave monitor should be available in the examination room and ceiling mounted. CT equipment should be installed to allow free access to the patient's head and body at any time during examination. The patient must be entirely seen from the operating console and the anesthesiologist should not be limited in monitoring the patient during patient installation and examination.

1.2.1.3 Ultrasound

State-of-the-art US equipment should be accessible in the emergency environment. A color-Doppler module and several probes, including a probe for small parts for diagnosis of peripheral musculoskeletal injuries, are mandatory. The selected US images should be integrated into the local imaging network and PACS and stored together will all other images of the patient.

1.2.1.4 Angiography

Angiographic procedures that are carried out in emergency conditions are almost exclusively therapeutic in the visceral area. Diagnostic angiographies may be required predominantly in penetrating injuries. In an optimal setting, only state-of-the-art angiographic equipment should be made available in the trauma environment. As an alternative, a state-of-the-art angiographic room can be installed close to the emergency environment and operated with scheduled procedures. A digitized X-ray table can serve for simple angiographic procedures only. Patient access from all sides is not optimal with this type of equipment. An angiographic C-arm can be brought or pivoted to the CT table, or the CT-patient support can be pivoted to the C-arm or moved on rails to the angiographic equipment installed in an adjacent room, separated by a movable wall.

1.2.2 Patient Support

The patient is generally moved several times from one support to another, during resuscitation, immediate surgery, and imaging. Patient transfer from one modality to another should be undertaken while preserving maximum patient safety and a minimum loss of time, so that the injury is not worsened or an additional injury created, without discontinuity of mechanical ventilation and without interruption of monitoring.

Unfortunately, neither interventional radiologists nor emergency or trauma radiologists have sufficient influenced major imaging equipment designers and obtained an adequate response to their specific needs. The concept of a universal patient support that fits several imaging procedures and serves as an operating table as well has been developed, but no mature solution is available yet. This patient support should fit digitized radiography, US, CT and angiography and include display of monitoring parameters integrated into the table. The patient support should be movable free hand like a floating table and also function for spiral CT acquisition.

1.2.3 Room Design

When planning an emergency and trauma admittance room, dedicated trauma radiologists should be consulted for optimal imaging design, including viewing, storage and communication facilities, with a sufficiently large area for case review and comparison of images and an adequate number of viewing consoles.

Room planning should be centered on installation of the CT equipment, preferably on a combination of CT and angiographic equipment. Recent changes in patient management attitudes in the US and Europe have contributed to wide implementation of CT: for instance, patients with penetrating abdominal injuries undergo more systematically thorough imaging than in the past. Peritoneal violation can be excluded by CT with great certainty; conservative management can be applied to some of the stab wounds to plain abdominal viscera, based on CT findings, etc. The fact that in some countries emergency physicians and trauma surgeons tend to use US for trauma and nontraumatic emergencies should not be an argument against installation of CT equipment in the emergency environment.

1.2.4 Communication

Complete and reliable communication and permanent access to the updated patient data to all members of the trauma team and other consulting specialists is a key issue of successful trauma management. Availability of electronic patient recording system (EPR), PACS and immediate reporting by voice recognition are of utmost importance in the emergency environment. If a full PACS-RIS system is not yet operating in the hospital, a mini PACS with a local network and sufficient online image storage capacity should be installed in the emergency department. Easy and permanent access for case review, without interference with new cases in a busy department is necessary, with the complete folder of all images and written reports permanently available. Radiologists should not rely on verbal transmission only, but should write a report mentioning all positive findings and any doubtful injury and specifying if repeated or additional investigation is required. This facilitates early recognition of worsening of injuries, detection of initially missed injuries and early detection of posttraumatic complications.

Teleradiology will be implemented in trauma care in large hospitals, transmitting patient data and images obtained before patient transfer from another hospital, where the patient was initially rescued. Patient data collected at the trauma scene can also reach the trauma center before the patient, to optimize management, particularly when several patients are severely injured simultaneously.

1.3 Standardization of Trauma Management

Although considerable efforts have been made, particularly in the larger European countries, standardization of trauma imaging remains suboptimal at present. National guidelines do not consider in detail design, equipment, medical qualification and functional organization of trauma imaging. Ironically, some national recommendations put more emphasis on the presence of a radiographer than a radiologist. Specific trauma centers are rare in European countries. Principles of initial patient rescue are not unequivocal throughout Europe. In the UK, more emphasis is put on rapid patient transfer to the hospital ("load and go"), whereas on the continent, full medical assistance is brought to the trauma scene before patient transfer ("stay and play"). Great discrepancies also exist in the attitude of radiologists toward basic situations in trauma management, as shown in a recent survey: 36% of unstable patients with blunt abdominal trauma will be directed to the operating room in the US and 22% in Europe. Diagnostic peritoneal lavage is used in 28% in the US, and in 10% outside the US. Ultrasound as the only imaging modality is used in 10% in the US and in 23% outside the US. Ultrasound followed by CT if normal (!) is used in almost 50% outside the US and in 17% by American radiologists. The diagnostic protocol for imaging of trauma victims who are hemodynamically stable following blunt abdominal trauma also shows large variations in the same survey: 57% of radiologists advocate CT with IV and oral contrast, 22% CT without oral contrast, 11% ultrasound only and 10% ultrasound followed by CT, if normal (Blackmore et al. 2000)!.

The diversity of trauma management protocols is explained by the variety of influencing factors, including hospital and emergency department design, availability of medical equipment, national or local guidelines, personal interest and local medical culture. Established protocols for trauma management such as Advanced Trauma Life Support only briefly mention imaging, without giving details on requirements. The training guidelines formulated by the European Association of Radiology for general and subspecialty training do not consider emergency or trauma imaging as a coherent subspecialty. Recommendations on general and specialized training are formulated by each of the European organ-specific radiological societies. However, a consistent body of more or less evidence-based knowledge on trauma imaging has built up in the literature, and is in constant movement, due to technological advances: reduction of examination time, which for CT and US is far below patient room transit time, is of paramount importance. Angiography remains generally underutilized: indications lack standardization, expertise is not widespread, and controlled trials are difficult to design for ethical limitations.

1.4 Staff

There are no detailed guidelines on functional organization of trauma imaging in Europe. Dedicated trauma or emergency radiologists are rare and their practice is limited to large hospitals and specialized trauma centers. In many academic hospitals, senior residents are in-house and supervised by a staff radiologist, who may be subspecialized. A radiologist, specialized in angiographic procedures, is usually on call and not directly involved in diagnostic trauma imaging. Practice has shown that senior residents with adequate training in cross-section imaging do not miss significant post-traumatic injury that requires immediate repair, in comparison with staff or trauma-dedicated radiologists. The integration of nurses in the team of radiographers or technicians is of great value for emergency imaging. Regular case review together with all members of the trauma team is crucial for quality assurance.

Reference

Blackmore CC, Mann FA, Nunez DB Jr (2000) Variability in the practice of emergency radiology: a survey of the members of the American Society of Emergency Radiology. Emerg Radiol 7:142–148

2 Resuscitation and Monitoring after Abdominal Trauma

P. Damas and G. Hartstein

CONTENTS

P. Damas, MD
General Intensive Care Unit, University Hospital of Liège, Department of Anaesthesia and Intensive Care, Domaine Universitaire du Sart-Tilman, 4000 Liège, Belgium
G. Hartstein, MD
Emergency Unit, University Hospital of Liège, Department of Anaesthesia and Intensive Care, Domaine Universitaire du Sart-Tilman, 4000 Liège, Belgium

- Trauma is primarily a disease of the young. It kills in reproducible time frames.
- Trauma is a surgical disease. Regardless of the exact division of labor existing in a given hospital center, both emergency physicians, including anesthesiologists *and* surgeons, must be involved with the care of *every* trauma patient as soon as he or she is admitted to the emergency department.
- Trauma is a dynamic disease. Any unexplained deterioration in patient status must prompt a rapid and effective reappraisal of the ABCs.
- Trauma care cannot be improvised. Established standards, based on quality research, should be followed, with adaptation to local situations as necessary.
- Prevention of trauma is vastly more effective than treatment.

2.1 Introduction

Trauma is a disease of the young. Abdominal injury may present alone or in conjunction with other lesions. Standardization of care is a major advance and should ideally follow the recommendations protocols that are accepted worldwide such as Advanced Trauma Life Support (American College of Surgeons 1997).

The initial management of these patients is not based on specific diagnoses, but rather on the rapid identification and treatment of immediately life-threatening problems, within minutes of the patient's admission to the emergency department (ED, the primary survey), followed by a more detailed secondary survey, which aims at revealing all injured body areas. These are then explored in detail as the clinical situation permits (Trunkey 1991). The physician caring for trauma victims constantly monitors the patient for deterioration, which could suggest the presence of as yet unidentified injuries. The principles of Advanced Trauma Life Support (ATLS), a system for management of multiply injured patients developed and licensed by the American College of Surgeons, has been accepted worldwide as a major advance in the standardization of such care (Jaffe and Wesson 1991). ATLS uses algorithms to facilitate the clinician's tasks when confronted with these often complicated patients.

2.2 Primary Survey

The first moments of trauma care, whether pre-hospital or in the ED itself, are devoted to identifying and treating immediately life threatening problems. The primary survey follows the classical ABC approach developed for cardiorespiratory arrest and should take only 5–10 min. As the trauma physicians proceed through the sequence, they correct each problem identified before moving on to the next step in the protocol. In the case of trauma, it is applied as follows:

- A (Airway):
  Loss of airway patency will cause death within minutes and is the greatest threat to life in the early phase after injury. The patency of the patient's airway is assessed, and, if required, stabilized. This is carried out with manual maneuvers, e.g., jaw thrust, but may require endotracheal intubation. Intubation is required, among other indications, for patients with diminished level of consciousness, shock states, or for upper airway obstruction. At the same time, the cervical spine is stabilized using a rigid cervical collar. Lesions of the cervical spine occur in 2–3% of major trauma cases, and must be assumed to exist in the presence of pain in the cervical area, decreased consciousness, due to head injury, drugs, alcohol, etc., painful lesions elsewhere, which could mask subtle findings in the neck, suggestive neurological findings, or any signs of trauma above the clavicles (Hoffman et al. 2000).

- B (Breathing):
  All trauma patients must receive 100% oxygen. For the patient breathing spontaneously, this means use of a nonrebreathing reservoir mask with a high flow of oxygen. Life-threatening problems revealed at this stage include tension pneumothorax, which requires immediate needle decompression followed by definitive chest-tube placement, massive hemothorax, open pneumothorax, and flail chest.

- C (Circulation):
  Initial evaluation of the circulation aims at identifying the patient in shock. This is usually identified by the presence of signs of inadequate tissue perfusion, such as thready pulses, cold, pale skin, diminished mental status, oliguria, or signs of the body's reaction to low cardiac output such as tachycardia, piloerection, moist skin, agitation and/or anxiety. Simultaneously, external hemorrhage is controlled using direct compression. Because the trauma patient is assumed to be suffering from hypovolemia until proven otherwise, venous access is obtained with at least two large-bore peripheral cannulae, and fluid resuscitation is begun (Landers and Dullye 1999). Blood is drawn at this point for laboratory studies, and sufficient quantities of red cell concentrates are ordered from the blood bank, either as type-specific units or as O negative. This ensures that blood is available for transfusion, should fluid resuscitation with up to 2 l of crystalloid and/or colloid prove inadequate to establish hemodynamic stability (McCunn and Karlin 1999).

During the primary survey, all victims of blunt trauma have three standard roentgenograms taken: lateral cross-table cervical spine views, making sure that the C7-T1 interspace is visualized, AP chest, and pelvis. It is becoming routine in centers which manage a large volume of trauma patients to perform a rapid bedside ultrasonographic examination of the chest to identify hemopericardium and hemothorax, and of the abdomen, to reveal free peritoneal blood. This approach is used because of favorable sensitivity and specificity, and especially because it does not require moving the patient and does not interfere with ongoing clinical care (Scalea et al. 1999). The primary survey continues with evaluation of the neurological status, details of which are not relevant to this chapter. It must be emphasized that throughout the clinical pathway of the trauma victim, the body temperature must be maintained. This avoids the numerous complications of hypothermia, including coagulopathy (Johnston et al. 1994), increased susceptibility to infection, and an increased incidence of myocardial ischemia. At the end of the primary survey, all immediately life-threatening problems will have been diagnosed and corrected. It is at this stage that a critical decision must be made: whether the patient requires immediate interventional stabilization or management can proceed in the ED. This decision is based on several criteria, among which are the patient's response to resuscitative measures. In general, failure to stabilize the patient with rapid infusion of 2 l of intravenous fluids implies that hemorrhage has not been controlled, that transfusion of red blood cells should begin, and that the patient will require more aggressive treatment. In these cases, the relative advantages of immediate surgery as compared to interventional radiological techniques must be considered. Radiological embolization to arrest hemorrhage can help to avoid surgery. No data are currently available in the literature which compare the risks and benefits of these techniques scientifically. While awaiting evidence-based criteria for choosing between surgery and interventional radiology, use of the latter must be considered investigational and proposed only in close collaboration with the trauma team. However, nonoperative management of blunt abdominal trauma in a patient who is hemodynamically stable has become the standard. It has been reported that the appropriate nonoperative management of injured children reduces the risk of receiving blood transfusion and decreased the length of hospitalized stay compared with aggressive operative intervention (Partrick et al. 1999).

Recent data suggests that unstable victims of penetrating thoracoabdominal trauma should not be fluid loaded in an attempt to normalize hemodynamic parameters, but rather brought directly to the operating room (Bickell et al. 1994). Overaggressive resuscitation may be deleterious by raising blood pressure, thus permitting dislodgment of vascular thrombi and by dilution of clotting factors, reducing the victim's capacity for hemostasis. It should be kept in mind that penetrating wounds of the abdominal cavity are absolute indications for laparotomy or laparoscopic exploration in certain cases (Townsend and Peitzman 2000); thus, aggressive fluid resuscitation is not abandoned, but rather postponed until surgical hemostasis has been ensured (Whinney et al. 2000). Throughout the management of the trauma victim, several principles must constantly be followed:

- Trauma is a surgical disease; regardless of the exact division of labor existing in a given hospital center, both emergency physicians, including anesthesiologists, and surgeons must be involved with the care of every trauma patient as soon as he or she is admitted to the ED.
- Trauma is a dynamic disease. Any unexplained deterioration in patient status must prompt a rapid and effective reappraisal of the ABCs.
- Trauma care cannot be improvised. Established standards, based on quality research, should be followed, with adaptation to local situations as necessary. These adaptations must reflect a consensus among all those who are responsible for the care of these patients, including emergency physicians, surgeons, anesthesiologists, and intensive care specialists (Mackenzie and Lippert 1999).
- As with any other disease, the quality of trauma care improves as the number of patients treated in a given center increases (Nathens et al. 2001).

2.3 Secondary Survey

The secondary survey consists of a detailed, anatomical examination of the patient, from head to foot. The goal is to finish with a complete picture of the exact injuries present. As mentioned above, but worthy of repetition, any deterioration in patient status requires rapid and effective reassessment and correction of the ABCs.

The secondary survey also involves collection of historical information concerning the mechanism of injury. This information helps to guide further treatment, because traumatic syndromes often result from specific mechanisms, e.g., pedestrians hit by cars. This information is frequently not available from the patient, but must be obtained from ambulance crews, police, or witnesses. As concerns abdominal trauma, one must bear in mind that unsuspected injuries are frequent. This is not surprising, given that subtle signs are often masked by other, more painful conditions or by altered levels of consciousness. The major goal in managing the acutely injured patient is not the exact definition of the injury itself, but rather the fact that injury is indeed present. This is obviously also true when considering the abdominal contents. Only when the presence of injury has been confirmed can rational treatment decisions be made.

The physical examination of the abdomen follows the classic sequence. *Inspection* reveals abrasions, contusions, lacerations, and entrance and exit wounds. The patient should be carefully turned onto his or her side to allow inspection of the back also. *Percussion* is used to determine the presence of peritoneal irritation by eliciting rebound tenderness. *Palpation* helps to determine the presence or absence of peritoneal signs and may help to localize the pathological process. Finally, *auscultation* allows the clinician to determine if bowel sounds and vascular bruits are present. Rectal examination, often ignored, should be carried out. Blood, bony fragments indicating pelvic fractures, sphincter tone (important in cases of spinal cord injury), and prostate position are useful elements in the work-up of the trauma victim.

Following the physical examination, the stomach should be intubated, via the mouth in cases of suspected basal skull fractures. The bladder should also be catheterized, via the urethra, unless injury to this structure is suspected. Clinical findings indicating urethral disruption include blood at the meatus, a high-riding prostate on rectal examination, and perineal ecchymoses and/or hematoma. Careful urethrography should be performed at the bedside if this injury is suspected. At this point in the management of the trauma victim, special diagnostic examinations, if appropriate, are called for. In fact, in our center, the most frequently used radiological examination for assessment of the abdominal cavity as well as the thorax is computed tomography (CT) with injection of contrast agent. This examination has replaced diagnostic peritoneal lavage because of its specificity, sensitivity, and repeatability. It is important to clearly understand the indications for, as well as the sequencing of this examination (Wilson et al. 1999). Based on a consensus established in our region, involving anesthesiologists, surgeons, intensivists, and emergency physicians, total body CT scanning is indicated in all cases of blunt trauma involving:

- Pedestrians hit by vehicles
- Falls from a height of 6 m or more
- Frontal vehicular collisions
- Passengers thrown from vehicles, including all bicycle and motorcycle victims
- Passengers in a vehicular accident with one occupant killed
- Passengers in a vehicular accident with one occupant severely injured
- Any clinical suspicion warranting further investigation

All the above mechanisms of injury imply transfer of large amounts of energy and are statistically associated with significant probability of injury of major intrathoracic and/or intra-abdominal structures. In terms of the sequencing of radiological investigations into the flow of care of the victim of blunt trauma, three situations can be envisaged:

- The patient was stable at the accident scene, and has remained so throughout care. In this case, the primary survey is completed, including cross-table lateral cervical spine, chest, and pelvis roentgenograms. The trauma team then proceeds to a full clinical secondary survey. Following this, standard imaging of the entire vertebral axis, as well as of any other suspected bone injuries, is carried out. After these films, body CT, if indicated, is performed.
- The patient was unstable at the accident scene, but has been fully stabilized or the patient arrives at the ED intubated, sedated, undergoing mechanical ventilation. These patients undergo a primary survey with, in addition to the three baseline roentgenograms, a sonographic examination of the chest and abdomen in the resuscitation area. They are then brought to the CT suite for body scanning. Care for any injuries revealed by this examination is undertaken if appropriate. After this, standard studies of the vertebral column and any other suspected orthopedic lesions are performed.
- The patient remains unstable despite adequate resuscitation. A primary survey, including three baseline films is carried out. In addition, rapid ultrasonographic assessment of the chest and abdomen is performed in the resuscitation area. This is useful in determining further treatment, as these patients will likely require urgent transport to the operating theater. After operative stabilization, the remainder of the secondary survey is undertaken.

2.4 Trauma Scores

Because numerous factors influence outcome after trauma, including patient factors, the anatomical areas and structures injured, the severity of the injuries, and the number of systems involved, standardization of data concerning trauma is extremely important. Various systems of trauma scoring have been created, in an attempt to help clinicians and researchers evaluate and quantify aspects of the care of these patients. Three principle goals are sought: standardization of the determination of severity, in order to facilitate triage to tiered systems of trauma care; use in clinical studies of various treatment modalities; epidemiology and quality assurance. Over the years, many different trauma scoring systems have been developed. Table 2.1 provides a reasonably comprehensive summary of existing scores.

Table 2.1. Summary of trauma scores

Name	Abbreviation	Reference
SIMBOL	SIMBOL	Williams and Schamadan (1969)
Trauma index		Kirkpatrick and Youmans (1971)
Abbreviated injury scale	AIS	American Medical Association (1971) American Association for Automotive Medicine (1985) Association for the Advancement of Automotive Medicine (1990)
Comprehensive injury scale	CRIS	American Medical Association (1972)
Prognostic index for severe trauma		Cowley et al. (1974)
Glasgow coma scale	GCS	Teasdale and Jennett (1974)
Renal index		Champion et al. (1974)
Therapeutic intervention scoring system	TISS	Cullen et al. (1974) Keene and Cullen (1983)
Injury severity score	ISS	Baker and O'Neill (1976) Copes et al. (1988)
Respiratory index	RI	Goldfarb et al. (1975)
CHOP index		Sacco et al. (1977)
Illness-injury severity index	IISI	Bever and Veenker (1979)
Triage index		Champion et al. (1980a)
Modified injury severity scale	MISS	Mayer et al. (1980, 1984)
Anatomical index	AI	Champion et al. (1980b)
Hospital trauma index		American College of Surgeons (1980)
Acute physiology and chronic health evaluation	APACHE	Knaus et al. (1981)
Trauma score	TS	Champion et al. (1981)
Penetrating abdominal trauma index		Moore et al. (1981)
Probability of death score	PODS	Somers (1982)
Circulation-respiration-abdomen-motor-speech scale	CRAMS	Gormican (1982)
Preliminary method	PRE	Champion et al. (1983)
State transition screen	STS	Champion et al. (1983)
Definitive methodology	DEF	Champion et al. (1983)
Mangled extremity syndrome	MES	Gregory et al. (1985)
Acute physiology and chronic health II	APACHE II	Knaus et al. (1985)
Prehospital index		Koehler et al. (1986)
Revised trauma score	RTS	Champion et al. (1989)
Acute physiology and chronic health III	APACHE III	Knaus et al. (1989)
Trauma score-injury severity score	TRISS	Boyd et al. (1987)
Pediatric trauma score	PTS	Tepas et al. (1987)
Outcome predictive score	OPS	Hershman et al. (1988)
Riyadh intensive care program	RIP	Chang et al. (1988)
Organ injury scaling	OIS	Moore et al. (1989)
Anatomical profile	AP	Copes et al. (1990)
A severity characterization of trauma	ASCOT	Champion et al. (1990)
Injury impairment scale	IIS	Association for the Advancement of Automotive Medicine (1994)
An ICD-9-based injury severity score	ICISS	Osler et al. (1996)
New injury severity score	NISS	Osler et al. (1997)

2.4.1 Physiological Scores

Trauma scoring can be based on a quantification of the disturbance of normal physiological systems. Ideally, the measured parameters should be objective and should demonstrate low inter- and intraobserver variability. Scoring should be possible by both medical as well as paramedical personnel.

2.4.1.1 Glasgow Coma Score

The Glasgow Coma Score (GCS), created in 1974 by Teasdale and Jennett, evaluates the depth of coma according to three indicators (Teasdale and Jennett 1974) (Table 2.2). These are assessed by stimulating the patient and recording the best response given as concerns eye opening, motor

Table 2.2. Glasgow Coma Score

Eye opening	Verbal response	Motor response	Score
		Obeys commands	6
	Oriented	Localizes pain	5
Spontaneously	Confused	Withdraws	4
To voice	Inappropriate	Flexion	3
To pain	Incomprehensible	Extension	2
None	None	None	1

response, and verbal response. The minimum score for each category is 1; the lowest score is thus 3, with the highest 15. The GCS has low variability, permits tracking of patient evolution over time, and is well correlated with morbidity as well as mortality.

2.4.1.2
Revised Trauma Score

The Triage Index was one of the first scoring systems useful for the prediction of outcome after trauma (Champion et al. 1980a). This index used statistical techniques to define a series of five physiological variables (the GCS, as well as respiratory expansion and capillary refill time) whose values were weighted to calculate the index. Two subsequent modifications (Champion et al. 1981), and the Revised Trauma Score (RTS) (Champion et al. 1989) have led to what is currently considered to be one of the most useful physiological scores (Table 2.3). This score is simple to calculate, objective, and has excellent predictive value if abnormal.

The RTS involves three parameters: the respiratory rate, the systolic blood pressure, and the GCS. Each is measured, and a score from 0 to 4 is assigned according to the value of each variable.

Table 2.3. Revised Trauma Score

Parameter	Value	Score
Respiratory rate (per minute)	10–29	4
	>29	3
	6–9	2
	1–5	1
	0	0
Systolic blood pressure (mmHg)	>89	4
	76–89	3
	50–75	2
	1–49	1
	0	0
Glasgow coma scale	13–15	4
	9–12	3
	6–8	2
	4–5	1
	3	0

2.4.2
Anatomical Scores

Because the severity of traumatic injury is related to the extent of anatomical damage, it would appear reasonable to assume that scoring systems based on assessment of the anatomy of the lesions produced should have prognostic value. However, because they are based on objective anatomical data, including protocols of radiological studies, operative reports and findings, and autopsy results (which obviously are only complete *after* complete diagnosis!), these systems are of no use for triaging trauma victims. They constitute *post hoc* scores which allow a posteriori stratification of victims into groups of relatively homogeneous severity.

2.4.2.1
Abbreviated Injury Scale

This score is calculated by dividing the body into nine regions: head, neck, face, thorax, abdomen, spine, upper extremity, lower extremity, and surface. For each region, the injuries present are scored from 1 (minor) to 6 (uniformly lethal). It has been continually revised to improve its power and to remedy perceived weaknesses. This scale is not an interval scale; that is, the gradation in severity in passing from a score of 1 to 2 is not at all the same as when passing from, for example, 3 to 4. In addition, the effects of multiple injuries in the same patient are not accounted for. Finally, the score represents a point in time, with no possibility to score dynamic characteristics of certain injuries. The AIS is a component of more complex scores.

2.4.2.2
Injury Severity Score

This score was devised to remedy some of the weaknesses of the AIS and makes use of some of the same principles. Scores range from 0 (no injury) to 75 (fatal injury). The body is divided into six regions: head and neck, face, thorax, abdomen, extremities, and external. Any patient with an AIS in any area is assigned an ISS of 75. The AIS code of the three regions with the most severe injuries are squared and added to calculate the ISS. This score reflects the additional morbidity caused by multiple injuries in the same patient. Unfortunately, it is also a noninterval scale. In addition, equal scores in different body regions are assumed to reflect equal severity. The effects of more minor injuries are also not considered.

2.5 Intrahospital Transport

As can be understood from the above, at some point in the management of all trauma patients, internal transfers become necessary. The danger and complexity of this phase of care must never be underestimated. Three aspects must be considered: personnel, material, and organization (Guidelines Committee of the American College of Critical Care Medicine, Society of Critical Care Medicine and American Association of Critical Care Nurses 1993).

2.5.1 Personnel

Sufficient personnel, with sufficient levels of training and experience, must be used when transporting these patients. At a minimum, a physician skilled in airway management and an emergency department or intensive care nurse must accompany the patient. Ideally, a porter should be available to help with the physical movement of the patient gurney. Because these people will devote their entire attention to the patient during the entire duration of the transfer, this should not detract from levels of care in other areas of the hospital.

2.5.2 Material

During the transfer, levels of monitoring must not be reduced, with respect to that applied in the resuscitation area of the ED, the operating theater, and the intensive care unit (ICU). Patient security must never be compromised during a transfer. For the patient receiving mechanical ventilation, transport respirators are available that, while lacking the sophistication of full critical care ventilators, nonetheless allow the clinician to control crucial parameters. The ability to apply positive end-expiratory pressure (PEEP) during the transfer can be life-saving. Continuous electrocardiographic display and pulse oximetry are mandatory, while monitoring of expired CO_2 for intubated patients provides crucial information about the integrity of the breathing circuit, tube dislodgment, and the state of the circulation. Blood pressure must be followed closely, using an automated noninvasive cuff or, when appropriate, by monitoring a previously inserted arterial cannula. Measures should be taken to maintain body temperature and avoid hypothermia: for transfers this usually means use of a Mylar space blanket to wrap the patient. The patient's temperature should also be measured before and after the transfer, because of the adverse effects of hypothermia mentioned above (Baron 2001).

Prior to leaving the ED, the clinical team must be certain that they have sufficient supplies of intravenous fluids, resuscitation drugs, oxygen, and airway management equipment. Tube position should be reassessed and the methods used to secure the tube confirmed. It is usually recommended to ventilate the patient with 100% oxygen during transfers. All intravenous lines should be checked, and organized on the gurney to avoid fumbling if rapid access becomes necessary. The patency and function of thoracostomy tubes, gastric tubes, and urinary catheters should also be verified. Finally, unless cervical spinal injury has already been ruled out, immobilization of the head and neck must be maintained during transfer.

2.5.3 Organization

The logistic details of the transfer must be attended to. This includes having elevators waiting and ready for the patient, and prearrival preparation of required equipment, supplies, and personnel at the destination. In addition, the transfer team must be able to summon additional help; this implies that all potential participants are available and that the means of communication are established.

2.6 The Radiology Suite

The same principles of management apply to the patient on arrival at the radiology suite for diagnostic or therapeutic procedures. All material usually present in an operating theater must be present, functional, and ready for use. This includes, of course, ventilators, monitors, suction apparatus, blood and fluid warmers, as well as devices to maintain body temperature. A full anesthesia cart, with fluids, drugs, and airway equipment must also be present in the suite. This implies that someone be charged with regular verification and restocking of this cart, so that it remains fully functional at all hours. A critical element during radiological investigations of potentially unstable patients is the presence of adequate personnel. It is imperative that the radiologist have adequate support, usually by a nurse from the radiology service; this must *not* be the same person upon whom the physician responsible for clinical care of the patient relies for help. Therefore, additional personnel must be available to assist the primary physician during the procedure. Investigation and treatment in the radiology suite may be lengthy; indeed, surgical intervention for these patients usually lasts several hours. What is important is not the absolute duration of the procedure(s), but rather the fact that communication is maintained between the clinician directly responsible for the patient, the radiologist performing the procedure, and the surgeon working with the trauma team. Inasmuch as the patient's condition remains constant, without serious deterioration in respiratory, hemodynamic, or neurological status, and with adequate maintenance of body temperature, the procedure can be continued. Any such deterioration should be communicated (preferably before serious physiological compromise has occurred) to the radiologist, in order to best decide on a course of action. On the other hand, unexpected findings, technical difficulties, or complications encountered by the radiologist must be immediately brought to the attention of the responsible clinician. The surgeon should be apprised of the progress of the procedure, in order to plan for subsequent management. As a corollary, any member of the trauma team, including the radiologist, should be able to decide when interventional procedures should be aborted. This should, ideally, represent a consensus, but must in no case require lengthy discussion, negotiations, or bargaining. Ultimate authority for such decisions must lie with the attending surgeon. Unbridled optimism, territorial disputes, and political intrigues have no role when making critical, often vital, decisions for trauma patients!

The decision to resort to radiological hemostasis, either in place of or in addition to subsequent operative management, cannot at this time be based on a set of anatomical or physiological criteria. It can only be made after discussion between the radiologist and the clinical trauma team members, based on the individual patient's condition, response to treatment, and the training, material, and experience of the radiologist. This type of decision-making should ultimately become easier, as the results of well-planned and properly executed clinical trials become available.

Nonoperative, noninterventional management is also an option for selected patients with hepatosplenic injury. This alternative does not represent passive therapeutic abstinence, but rather an active process. Several criteria determine if this choice is available to the trauma team.

- The patient must be hemodynamically normal. This means that there are no signs of ongoing bleeding, and that vital signs remain stable without significant fluid infusion. Base excess must be minimal, while blood pressure and heart rate must be appropriate for the patient's age.
- The patient must have frequent, ongoing abdominal examination, by experienced personnel. The patient must be alert and oriented. Any factors which would interfere with the results of this examination, such as altered level of consciousness, the presence of drugs and/or alcohol, or spinal cord injury make nonoperative management impossible.
- The patient must be cared for in a high-dependency area.

2.7 Subsequent Care

The vast majority of patients with abdominal trauma will be admitted to intensive care units after workup is complete and after any necessary surgical or radiological interventions are carried out. The procedures used to effect hemostasis (surgery or radiological intervention) do not determine the extent and intensity of monitoring of these patients; rather, their physiological status and the pattern of injuries are the crucial factors. Close attention to neurological status is required when head injury is associated with other trauma. Intracranial pressure monitoring may be instituted, as well as transcranial Doppler evaluation of the cerebral circulation. Clinical assessment is the key to the follow-up of the head-injured patient. Respiratory function and gas exchange are monitored using, again, clinical examination, pulse oximetry, and measurement of end-tidal CO_2 in the intubated patient. More sophisticated analysis of pulmonary mechanics can be applied, if necessary, especially when posttraumatic respiratory insufficiency develops. Circulatory status is evaluated clinically, with measurement of hemodynamic parameters (including invasive monitoring when necessary) a routine procedure in the modern ICU.

The quality of the hemostatic intervention is continually assessed. Clinical examination may reveal increasing abdominal girth, a loss of bowel sounds, or signs of hypovolemia or shock (see "Primary Survey"). Laboratory analysis may show a rising base deficit, decreasing hematocrit, or other signs of visceral hypoperfusion. Measurement of the pressure in the abdominal cavity is used increasingly often in severely traumatized patients to determine when and if secondary surgical intervention is necessary. Despite meticulous attention to all the above principles, the ICU physicians must always keep in mind the possibility that not all lesions have been diagnosed. This eventuality should be invoked whenever untoward or unexpected deterioration occurs. There should be no hesitation to resort to repeat imaging studies, followed if necessary by radiological or surgical intervention, when such lesions are revealed.

2.8 Conclusion

Care of the trauma patient is always challenging, but the rewards are great for the clinical team. Trauma is a disease of the young and effective management clearly contributes to reducing morbidity and mortality. Great strides have been made in applying the principles of evidence-based medicine to the care of these patients. Nonetheless, demands on the personnel involved with trauma care are very high; trauma care constitutes an extremely resource-intensive branch of emergency medicine and intensive care. The most acceptable modality to apply to the early management of these patients is based on use of protocols, which must be adapted to each hospital's specific situation. Application of nonstandard treatments must always be the result of a consensus among the physicians responsible for the clinical care of these complex patients, preferably supported by well-designed, statistically robust studies. It is only by keeping these principles in mind that progress can be made.

References

American Association for Automotive Medicine (now Association for the Advancement of Automotive Medicine; AAAM) (1985) Abbreviated injury scale, rev edn. AAAM, Des Plaines, Ill

American College of Surgeons (1997) Advanced trauma life support program for physicians, 6th edn. American College of Surgeons, Chicago

American College of Surgeons Committee on Trauma (1980) Field categorization of trauma patients and hospital trauma index. Bull Am Coll Surg 2:28–33

American Medical Association Committee on Medical Aspects of Automotive Safety (AMACMAAS) (1971) Rating the severity of tissue damage. I. The abbreviated scale. JAMA 215:277–280

American Medical Association Committee on Medical Aspects of Automotive Safety (AMACMAAS) (1972) Rating the severity of tissue damage. II. The comprehensive injury scale. JAMA 220:717–720

Association for the Advancement of Automotive Medicine (AAAM) (1990) Abbreviated injury scale, rev edn. AAAM, Des Plaines, Ill

Association for the Advancement of Automotive Medicine (AAAM) (1994) Injury impairment scale. AAAM, Des Plaines, Ill

Baker SP, O'Neill B (1976) The injury severity score: an update. J Trauma 16:822–885

Baron D (2001) Transports intrahospitaliers. In: Réanimation médicale. Collège des Enseignants de Réanimation Médicale, Masson, Paris, pp 645–647

Bever DL, Veenker CH (1979) An illness severity index for nonphysician emergency medical personnel. EMT J 3:45–49

Bickell W, Wall M, Pepe P et al (1994) Immediate versus delayed fluid resuscitation for hypotensive patients with penetrating torso injuries. N Engl J Med 331:1105–1109

Boyd CR, Tolson MA, Copes WS (1987) Evaluating trauma care: the TRISS method. J Trauma 27:370–378

Champion HR, Sacco WJ, Long W et al (1974) Indicators for early haemodialysis in multiple trauma. Lancet 1:1125–1127

Champion HR, Sacco WJ, Hannan DS (1980a) Assessment of injury severity: the triage index. Crit Care Med 8:201–208

Champion HR, Sacco WJ, Lepper RL (1980b) An anatomic index injury severity. J Trauma 20:197–202

Champion HR, Sacco WJ, Carnazzo AJ et al (1981) Trauma score. Crit Care Med 9:672–676

Champion HR, Sacco WJ, Hunt TK (1983) Trauma severity scoring to predict mortality. World J Surg 7:4–11

Champion HR, Sacco WJ, Copes WS et al (1989) A revision of the trauma score. J Trauma 29:623–629

Champion HR, Copes WS, Sacco WJ et al (1990) A new characterization of injury severity. J Trauma 30:539–546

Chang RWS, Jacobs S, Lee E (1988) Predicting outcome among intensive care unit patients using computerised trend analysis of daily APACHE II scores corrected for organ system failure. Intensive Care Med 14:558–566

Copes WP, Champion HR, Sacco WJ et al (1988) The injury severity score revised. J Trauma 28:69–77

Copes WS, Champion HR, Sacco WJ et al (1990) Progress in characterizing anatomic injury. J Trauma 20:1200–1207

Cowley RA, Sacco WJ, Gill W et al (1974) A prognostic index for severe trauma. J Trauma 14:1029–1035

Cullen DJ, Civetta J, Briggs BA et al (1974) Therapeutic intervention scoring system: a method for quantitative comparison of patient care. Crit Care Med 2:57–60

Goldfarb MA, Ciurej TH, McAslan TC et al (1975) Tracking respiratory therapy in trauma patients. Am J Surg 129:255–258

Gormican SP (1982) CRAMS scale: field triage of trauma victims. Ann Emerg Med 11:132–135

Gregory RT, Gould RJ, Peclet M et al (1985) The mangled extremity syndrome (MES): a severity grading system for multisystem injury of the extremity. J Trauma 25: 1147–1150

Guidelines Committee of the American College of Critical Care Medicine, Society of Critical Care Medicine and American Association of Critical Care Nurses (1993) Guidelines for the transfer of critically ill patients. Crit Care Med 21: 913–937

Hershman MJ, Cheadle WG, Kuftinec D et al (1988) An outcome predictive score for sepsis and death following injury. Injury 19:263–266

Hoffman J, Mower W, Wolfson A et al (2000) Validity of a set of clinical criteria to rule out injury to the critical spine in patients with blunt trauma. N Engl J Med 7:1164–1171

Jaffe D, Wesson D (1991) Emergency management of blunt trauma in children. N Engl J Med 324:1477–1482

Johnston TD, Chen Y, Reed RL (1994) Functional equivalence of hypothermia to specific clotting factor deficiencies. J Trauma 37:4313

Keene AR, Cullen D (1983) Therapeutic intervention scoring system: update 1983. Crit Care Med 11:1–3

Kirkpatrick JR, Youmans RL (1971) Trauma index: an aid in evaluation of injury victims. J Trauma 11:711–714

Knaus WA, Zimmerman JB, Wagner DP et al (1981) APACHE – acute physiology and chronic health evaluation: a physiologically based classification system. Crit Care Med 9: 591–597

Knaus WA, Draper EA, Wagner DP et al (1985) APACHE II: a severity of disease classification system. Crit Care Med 13: 818–829

Knaus W, Wagner D, Zimmerman JE et al (1989) APACHE III study design: analytic plan for evaluation of severity and outcome in intensive care unit patients. Crit Care Med 17: S169–S221

Koehler JJ, Baer LJ, Malafa SA et al (1986) Prehospital index: a scoring system for field triage of trauma victims. Ann Emerg Med 15:178–182

Landers D, Dullye K (1999) Vascular access and fluid resuscitation in trauma. Anesthesiol Clin North Am 17:125–139

Mackenzie C, Lippert F (1999) Emergency department management of trauma. Anesthesiol Clin North Am 17:45–61

Mayer T, Matlak ME, Johnson DG et al (1980) The modified injury severity scale in pediatric multiple trauma patients. J Pediatr Surg 5:719–726

Mayer T, Walker MI, Clark P (1984) Further experience with the modified abbreviated injury severity scale. J Trauma 24:31–34

McCunn M, Karlin A (1999) Nonblood fluid resuscitation. Anesth Clin North Am 17:107–123

Moore EE, Dun EL, Moore JB et al (1981) Penetrating abdominal trauma index. J Trauma 21:399–444

Moore EE, Schackford SR, Pachter HL et al (1989) Organ injury scaling: spleen, liver, kidney. J Trauma 29:1664–1666

Nathens AB, Jurkovich G, Maier R et al (2001) Relationship between trauma center volume and outcomes. JAMA 7: 1164–1171

Osler T, Rutledge R, Deis J et al (1996) ICISS: an international classification of disease-9 based injury severity score. J Trauma 41:380–388

Osler T, Baker SP, Long W (1997) A modification of the injury severity score that both improves accuracy and simplifies scoring. J Trauma 43:922–926

Partrick D, Bensard D, Moore E et al (1999) Nonoperative management of solid organ injuries in children results in decreased blood utilization. J Pediatr Surg 34:1695–1699

Sacco WJ, Milholland AV, Ashman et al (1977) Trauma indices. Comput Biol Med 7:9–20

Scalea TM, Rodriguez A, Chiu WC et al (1999) Focused assessment with sonography for trauma (FAST): results from an international consensus conference. J Trauma 46:466–472

Somers RL (1982) New ways to use the 1980 Abbreviated Injury Scale – the Probability of Death Score (PODS). Internal report University of Odense Denmark, Odense Laboratory for Public Health and Health Economics

Teasdale G, Jennett B (1974) Assessment of coma and impaired consciousness: a practical scale. Lancet 2:21–83

Tepas JJ, Mollitt DL, Talbert JL et al (1987) The pediatric trauma score as a predictor of injury severity. J Pediatr Surg 22:14–18

Townsend R, Peitzman A (2000) Penetrating thoraco-abdominal injury. Curr Opin Crit Care 6:390–394

Trunkey D (1991) Initial treatment of patients with extensive trauma. N Engl J Med 324:1259–1263

Whinney R, Cohn S, Zacur S (2000) Fluid resuscitation for trauma patients in the 21st century. Curr Opin Crit Care 6:395–400

William RE, Schamadan JL (1969) The SIMBOL rating and evaluating system: a measurement tool for injury persons. Ariz Med 16:886–887

Wilson W, Patel N, Hoyt D et al (1999) Perioperative anesthetic management of patients with abdominal trauma. Anesthesiol Clin North Am 17:211–236

3 CT Examination Protocols in Abdominal Trauma

P. Huppert

CONTENTS

- To examine patients with abdominal trauma, spiral CT scanning should be preferred using thin collimation and tailored i.v. contrast injection.
- Use of oral contrast material is not mandatory; however, if possible water-soluble contrast should be given without waiting for passage before scanning.
- Detection and grading of lesions to liver and spleen demand scanning during maximum enhancement of portal venous phase and delayed scans improve visualization of urinary tract lesions.
- True positive prediction of bowel wall perforations and pancreatic injuries strongly depend on thin collimation, overlapping reconstruction, subtle image reviewing, and follow-up studies in clinically selected cases.

P. Huppert, MD
Department of Diagnostic Radiology, Municipal Hospital Darmstadt, Grafenstrasse 9, 64283 Darmstadt, Germany

3.1 CT Technologies, Management, and Staffing

Since the first reports in the early 1980s, CT has proved to be a very effective technique for diagnosing traumatic abdominal injuries (Federle et al. 1981). Advantages of scanner hardware and software have provided faster scanning, improved spatial resolution and enhanced intravenous (i.v.) contrast opacification. Dynamic incremental CT allows abdominal imaging during build-up and maintenance of i.v. enhancement (Foley et al. 1987). Spiral (helical) CT provides volume scanning and was the most important development of the last decade in this context. Today multislice CT has further improved technical conditions for imaging work-up of trauma patients.

Accurate CT assessment of trauma patients requires routine use of optimized protocols. Mostly custom-tailored protocols are used, focused on types of injuries and anatomical regions clinically suspected. In patients with abdominal trauma, several methodical aspects have to be considered: selection of acquisition parameters, use of i.v., oral and rectal contrast material, scanning during different time intervals after i.v. contrast material administration, including delayed scanning, window settings during review and filming and optional postprocessing.

Though following abdominal trauma CT is generally performed only in hemodynamically stable patients, assessment should be as fast as possible. Blow et al. (1998) showed that the time interval to laparotomy was significantly longer in patients studied by (conventional incremental) CT compared to diagnostic peritoneal lavage (mean values 213 min vs 65 min). In emergency departments, CT protocols for trauma studies should be clearly defined and available at all times. Protocols must define all relevant methodical details concerning acquisition (collimation, table feed/pitch factor, image reconstruction intervals), use of contrast material (i.v., oral, and rectal), viewing, and postprocessing. If CT scanners are used capable of spiral acquisition or multislice scanning, appropriate protocols should be configured and available for selection at the desk.

Effective staffing is crucial in emergency CT. Two technologists should be scheduled together, one preparing the patient and setting up the technique for contrast material administration, while the other is programming the scanner. If possible, the patient's arms should be positioned above the head; monitor leads have to be removed from the gantry and the nasogastric tube should be withdrawn into the distal esophagus to obviate artifacts from metallic markers. The management of critically ill patients requires that emergency department nurses and physicians also be present. The CT technologists and radiologist are too occupied by scanning tasks and reviewing images.

3.2 Acquisition Protocols and Intravenous Contrast Material Use

Acquisition parameters depend on the CT technology available. To cover a sufficient length of interest within an appropriate time window, collimations differ during dynamic incremental CT, spiral CT, and multislice CT. Parameters of i.v. contrast material administration are matched with the time duration needed for acquisition (Table 3.1).

In dynamic incremental CT, the scan time is 2 s with a 6-s interscan delay (Foley et al. 1987). The slice thickness is 8–10 mm and equals table feed. Biphasic injection of 150–180 ml of 60% contrast material (50 ml, 5 ml/s; 100–130 ml, 1 ml/s) is recommended (Federle et al. 1987; Foley et al. 1987; Foley 1989; Mirvis et al. 1989a,b). Depending on the hemodynamic situation of the patient, a 45- to 60-s delay between the start of injection and the beginning of dynamic scanning is mandatory to obtain maximum parenchymal enhancement of the liver and spleen. Especially if craniocaudal scanning is performed, sufficient delay is important. The majority of liver lacerations are located in the upper segments of the right lobe. Furthermore, early phase inhomogeneous splenic contrasting can be confused with traumatic injuries. If dynamic incremental scanning appears impossible due to the patient's condition, stepwise incremental CT is the alternative during which contrast material is infused with 0.5 ml/s (Gay and Sistrom 1992). For routine scanning of the pelvis, 10 mm collimation and 15–20 mm/s table feed is useful (Richards and Derlet 1998).

Spiral CT technology offers several substantial advantages for trauma patients. Respiratory misregistrations are eliminated, volume data acquisition allows overlapping image reconstruction, thin slice collimation improves spatial resolution and facilitates multiplanar reformations (MPR), and shorter scanning times permit peak enhancement scanning of several regions. For routine protocols in patients with abdominal trauma, 10 mm collimation and a pitch factor of 1.0–1.5 is recommended (Löw et al. 1997; Soto et al. 2001); however, if scanner performance (tube heat capacity, reconstruction modes) allows, diagnostic quality will be improved if collimation is

Table 3.1. CT scanning protocols for imaging in abdominal trauma depending on CT technology

	Dynamic incremental CT	Single-slice Spiral CT[a]	Multi-slice CT Spiral CT[b]	
Collimation	10 mm	5 mm	4×1 mm	4×2 mm
Table feed per rotation	10 mm	7.5 mm	5.5 mm	11 mm
Helical pitch	–	1.5	5.5	5.5
Table feed per second	(1.25 mm)	7.5 mm	11 mm	22 mm
Covered length	300 mm	300 mm	300 mm	300 mm
Total scan time	240 s	40 s	27.3 s	13.6 s
Contrast volume (60% iodine)	150–180 ml	130 ml	130 ml	
Contrast flow	5 ml/s bolus (50 ml) 1 ml/s infusion	2 ml/s	3 ml/s	
		(100–130 ml)		
Delay	45–60 s	60–70 s	Bolus triggering: 170 HU+40 s[c]	

[a]Time per rotation 1.0 s.
[b]Time per rotation 0.5 s.
[c]Bolus triggering, 170 HU density level within aortic region of interest + 40 s delay

reduced to 7–5 mm. Collimation of 5 mm and 50% overlapping reconstructions should generally be used for imaging abdominal trauma in children, if pancreatic injury is suspected and if questionable lesions have been suspected during the routine CT assessment. For i.v. contrast material, administration volumes of 100–150 ml are recommended (NOVELINE et al. 1999; SOTO et al. 2001). A delay of 60–70 s is necessary to obtain sufficient enhancement including all parts of liver and spleen. The first volume scan should cover the region between the dome of the liver and the lower pole of the kidneys. A second volume scan should start after another delay with a minimum of 70 s to visualize the contrast-filled renal pelvis and lower urinary tract.

Using multislice CT, further reduction of collimation is possible and will significantly improve spatial resolution. If 4×1 mm collimation is selected and proper reconstruction algorithms are used isotropic voxels will be permitted. Partial volume effects are minimized and the quality of MPR images is improved. During reconstruction of axial images as well as during generation of MPR images, slabs 4–8 mm thick provide excellent diagnostic quality without exceeding the number of pictures to be reviewed. Multislice technology allows a number various scan parameters to be combined, resulting in similar scan times and volume coverage. Combining thinner collimations with higher pitch factors seems to be the best option, because this will result in improved image quality in terms of spatial resolution in the z-direction and reduced partial volume artifacts. Compared to single-section CT, multislice CT has about equal dose efficiency (RYDBERG et al. 2000).

Patients with abdominal trauma are often hemodynamically unstable to a variable degree. To optimize i.v. contrast enhancement, the use of the bolus triggering technique is recommended. In our experience, sufficient enhancement results if the cut-off level of density for an aortic region of interest is set to 170 HU followed by an additional fixed delay of 40 s.

3.3 Oral and Rectal Contrast Material Use

The use of oral contrast material during CT in patients with abdominal trauma has been hotly debated and is not generally an accepted standard (FOLEY et al. 1987; MIRVIS et al. 1989a,b; SHANKAR et al. 1999). Diagnosing bowel wall perforation by demonstration of intraperitoneal contrast leakage is seldom successful. In 16% of patients with surgically proven bowel perforations, leakage was seen, whereas other typical findings were present in the majority of cases (DONOHUE et al. 1987; RIZZO et al. 1989; KUNIN et al. 1993). Bowel wall thickening is one of these important findings and oral contrast material may improve delineation of bowel wall and lumen. From a practical standpoint, it is recommended that oral contrast material should be given if possible; however, one should not wait for passage. This strategy is supported by the fact that most gastrointestinal perforations involve the proximal tract including the jejunum and duodenum (ROTHROCK et al. 2000).

Water-soluble contrast material (1%–2%) should be administered orally or via the nasogastric tube. Administration of two portions will improve filling of the proximal parts of the tract. About 400 ml are given 20–30 min prior to CT examination and another 400 ml just before scanning. In children, the administration of 60–400 ml was recommended depending on the patient's size (STROUSE et al. 1999). However, in another study, the benefit of oral contrast material use in children was very low (SHANKAR et al. 1999). On the other hand it was proven that the risk of symptomatic aspiration of oral contrast material is very low. This holds true in adults (FEDERLE et al. 1995) as well as in children (LIM-DUNHAM et al. 1997). Artifacts to the liver and spleen may result from the contrast-filled stomach if concentrations of more than 3% are used.

Rectal contrast material application is recommended if colon injury is suspected. Especially in patients with penetrating trauma, the triple contrast technique (i.v., oral, and rectal contrast material) was advocated; however, the diagnostic benefit was low (MCALLISTER et al. 1994; GINZBURG et al. 1998; SOTO et al. 2001). Depending on the suspected location of injuries, 250–1000 ml of water-soluble contrast material (2%–3%) is used.

3.4 Contrast Phases, Delayed Scans, and Follow-up Studies

Native scans are of minor benefit in patients with abdominal trauma. Detection of the sentinel clot sign in patients with splenic trauma may be improved in some cases (SCATAMACCHIA et al. 1989). Other potential advantages are the differentiation of hematoma and incidentally detected neoplasms and the demonstration of hemoperitoneum. During arterial phase scanning, visualization of lesions to arteries and active arterial bleeding is optimized (Jeffrey et al. 1991). However, in the majority of cases, active bleeding can also be localized based on other typical findings. The sentinel clot sign helps to identify the site of bleeding in up to 84% of cases (Gay and Sistrom 1992).

Detection and grading of hepatic and splenic injuries is optimized during the maximal enhancement of the portal venous phase. If splenic enhancement is inhomogeneous (mottled) during earlier phases, delayed scans, after another contrast material injection, should be performed. If injuries to the renal pelvis or the lower urinary tract are suspected, delayed scans 70–120 s following the end of the first scan are recommended to detect urinary leakage. In patients with questionable clinical signs of pancreatic injury a second CT study 2–3 days following the injury is valuable (Dondelinger et al. 2000; Rothrock et al. 2000). Visualization of fluid collections, pancreatic edema and mesenteric infiltration is improved, especially if peak contrast scanning, thin collimation, and overlapping reconstructions are used.

Follow-up studies are recommended only if complications (rebleeding, abscess, biloma, urinoma) are suspected clinically or sonographically. Routine follow-up CT studies in patients with conservatively managed hepatic and splenic injuries have been advocated; however, several studies showed that there is no benefit in terms of altering treatment decisions (Allins et al. 1996; Ciraulo et al. 1996).

3.5 Viewing and Postprocessing

Images should be reviewed and major diagnoses defined while the patient is on the CT table. A decision has to be made as to the necessity of delayed scans, subtle reassessment of suspected lesions, and second contrast material administration. Abdominal and pelvic images must be reviewed using soft tissue window settings (width/center: 300 HU/30 HU) and lung window settings (1500 HU/–500 HU). If liver injury is suspected liver window settings (350 HU/150 HU) are mandatory.

Image reconstructions with 30%–50% overlap improve the detection of subtle traumatic lesions, especially of the pancreatic parenchyma and bowel wall. Multiplanar reformations and 3D reconstructions have been advocated for demonstration of diaphragmatic ruptures (Israel et al. 1996) and renal fractures (Michel et al. 1996); however, data demonstrating a substantial benefit are still lacking.

3.6 Special Methodological Aspects

3.6.1 Liver and Spleen

If liver injury is suspected an adequate delay between the beginning of contrast material injection and the start of scanning is necessary to obtain appropriate enhancement including all parts of the liver. Detection of lacerations, hematomas, periportal tracking and liver fractures is clearly improved during peak contrast scanning. Timing of contrast injection has taken into account that most of the lesions are located in the upper part of the right lobe, both in children (Stalker et al. 1986) and in adults (Foley et al. 1987). Craniocaudal scanning of the abdomen and pelvis is usually performed. Delay depends on the acquisition mode used. During dynamic incremental CT, 45–60 s is recommended and during spiral CT, 60–70 s. Using the bolus triggering technique, optimized enhancement is obtained, especially in multislice CT.

An adequate delay following i.v. contrast injection is also important to permit homogenous splenic enhancement. A minimal time delay of 60 s is also usually necessary in non-spiral CT (Federle et al. 1987). A second contrast injection is necessary in cases with questionable lesions seen during too early phases (Scatamacchia et al. 1989). Grading systems based on initial CT findings are unreliable to predict outcome (Mirvis et al. 1989b; Scatamacchia et al. 1989) and follow-up CT in conservatively managed patients should be indicated only if complications are suspected clinically (Umlas and Cronan 1991; Allins et al. 1996).

3.6.2 Bowel, Mesentery, and Perforating Injuries

CT is used by 77% of the surgical community in most cases to assess traumatic bowel and mesenteric injuries (Brownstein et al. 2000). Although CT does not reliably exclude traumatic bowel injuries, subtle scanning decreases the rate of false negative studies and is crucial. Collimation of 8 mm is not appropriate to detect minor lesions (Sherck et al. 1984; Strouse et al. 1999). Collimation of 5 mm using spiral CT and collimation of 4×1 mm to 4×2 mm using multislice CT with 50% overlapping image reconstruction improves detection of peritoneal fluid collections, bowel wall thickening, and free intraperitoneal air. Application of oral contrast material may facilitate diagnostic probability in some cases; however, demonstration of contrast leakage is very rare. In four studies collecting 31 patients with surgically proven traumatic bowel perforations, peritoneal fluid collections were seen in 100%, bowel wall thickening in 80%, free air in 55%, but contrast leakage only in 16% (Glazer et al. 1981; Donohue et al. 1987; Rizzo et al. 1989; Kunin et al. 1993). Similar figures are reported in a review by Brody et al. (2000). To detect free air within the intraperitoneal, retroperitoneal, and intramural spaces, a review of images using lung window settings is mandatory.

For CT assessment of patients with penetrating abdominal trauma, the triple contrast technique has been recommended (Phillips et al. 1986; Hauser et al. 1987; Rehm et al. 1989; McAllister et al. 1994; Ginzburg et al. 1998; Soto et al. 2001). This technique combines the oral, rectal, and i.v. application of contrast material. Nevertheless, detection of contrast leaks is rare and was described in these studies only in 3 of 292 patients. If bowel perforation is suspected, diagnostic peritoneal lavage should not be performed prior to CT because residual fluid collections may cause false positive CT findings.

3.6.3 Pancreas

Traumatic injuries to the pancreas are difficult to detect using routine CT scanning. Normal CT findings obtained with standard spiral CT collimation of 8–10 mm does not rule out pancreatic lesions. Thin collimation of 4–5 mm in spiral CT or 4×1 mm to 4×2 mm in multislice CT with 30%–50% overlapping reconstructions are necessary to visualize subtle changes (Dondelinger et al. 2000). The use of oral contrast material may be of value to demonstrate associated duodenal injuries; however, this is still being debated. Intravenous contrast administration is optimized by using power injectors and the bolus triggering technique. Follow-up CT studies are recommended if suspicion of pancreatic injury increases during follow-up. From 12 h to 7 days following traumatic ictus, findings of traumatic pancreatitis and main duct injury can be seen even if the initial CT study was normal (Dondelinger et al. 2000; Rothrock et al. 2000).

3.6.4 Kidney, Ureter, and Urinary Bladder

If major renal injury is suspected and spiral CT technology is available triple-phase scanning should be performed. During the arterial phase (20–30 s delay), vascular lesions can be detected clearly, during the parenchymal phase (60 s delay), grading of parenchymal injuries is optimized, and during the excretory phase (2–5 min delay), lesions of the collecting system and urinomas are demonstrable. Imaging during the parenchymal phase and the excretory phase are more important than the arterial phase. However, the arterial phase can replace native scanning for hematoma detection. Using spiral CT, 2- to 3-mm collimation and 4- to 6-mm table feed is recommended. Using multislice CT collimation of 4×1 mm and a pitch factor of 3–5 is useful. Multiplanar reformations in sagittal and coronal planes may improve visualization of lesions involving the upper or lower pole (Fig. 3.1).

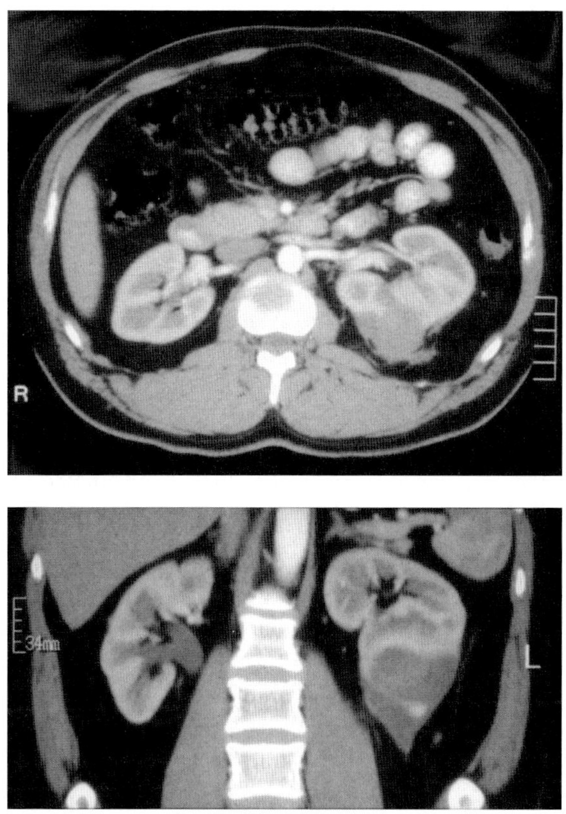

a
b

Fig. 3.1a, b. Blunt trauma to the left flank. Intraparenchymal, subcapsular, and perirenal hematoma. **a** Multislice spiral CT (4×1 mm collimation). **b** Active bleeding originating from the lower pole was visualized best in coronal MPR images

If injury to the ureter or urinary bladder is suspected delayed scans (5 min) are mandatory, although normal findings of the urinary bladder under these conditions do not rule out bladder injury. For definitive diagnosis, CT cystography (or X-ray cystography) is necessary. For this purpose, the bladder is filled with 300–400 ml of diluted contrast material (40 ml 60% contrast in 1000 ml saline) via a Foley catheter.

3.7 Conclusion

Accurate CT assessment of trauma patients requires routine use of optimized protocols considering acquisition parameters, contrast material administration, and postprocessing. Parameters of acquisition and of i.v. contrast material injection depend on the CT technology available. Compared to incremental scanning, spiral CT allows thinner collimation and faster acquisition, resulting in improved spatial resolution, peak contrast scanning, and improved lesion detection. Use of oral contrast material may improve detection of duodenal and small bowel wall injuries; however, this is contested. Rectal contrast material application is an option to facilitate visualization of large bowel wall perforation following penetrating trauma in highly selected patients. Detection and grading of lesions to the liver and spleen is optimized during maximal enhancement of the portal venous phase. Scanning during the arterial phase may improve visualization of lesions to arteries and delayed scans demonstrate urinary tract leaks. True positive prediction of bowel wall perforations is improved by using thin collimation, overlapping reconstruction, and thorough image review. This also holds true for pancreatic lesions, which take further advantage of follow-up studies in clinically selected cases.

References

Allins A, Ho T, Nguyen TH et al (1996) Limited value of routine follow-up CT scans in nonoperative management of blunt liver and splenic injuries. Am Surg 62:883–886

Blow O, Bassam D, Butler K et al (1998) Speed and efficiency in the resuscitation of blunt trauma patients with multiple injuries: the advantage of diagnostic peritoneal lavage over abdominal computerized tomography. J Trauma 44:287–290

Brody JM, Leighton DB, Murphy BL et al (2000) CT of blunt trauma bowel and mesenteric injury: typical findings and pitfalls in diagnosis. Radiographics 20:1525–1536

Brownstein MR, Bunting T, Meyer AA et al (2000) Diagnosis and management of blunt small bowel injury: a survey of the membership of the American Association for the Surgery of Trauma. J Trauma 48:402–407

Ciraulo DL, Nikkanen HE, Palter M et al (1996) Clinical analysis of the utility of repeat computed tomographic scan before discharge in blunt hepatic injury. J Trauma 41:821–824

Dondelinger RF, Boverie JH, Cornet O (2000) Diagnosis of pancreatic injury: a need to improve performance. JBR-BTR 83:160–166

Donohue JH, Federle MP, Griffiths BG et al (1987) Computed tomography in the diagnosis of blunt intestinal and mesenteric injuries. J Trauma 27:11–17

Federle MP, Goldberg HI, Kaiser JA, Moss AA, Jeffrey RB Jr, Mall JC (1981) Evaluation of abdominal trauma by computed tomography. Radiology 138:637–644

Federle MP, Griffiths B, Minagi H et al (1987) Splenic trauma: evaluation with CT. Radiology 162:69–71

Federle MP, Peitzman A, Krugh J (1995) Use of oral contrast material in abdominal trauma CT scans: is it dangerous? J Trauma 38:51–53

Foley WD (1989) Dynamic hepatic CT. Radiology 170:617–622

Foley WD, Cates JD, Kellman GM et al (1987) Treatment of blunt hepatic injuries: role of CT. Radiology 164:635–638

Gay SB, Sistrom CL (1992) Computed tomographic evaluation of blunt abdominal trauma. Radiol Clin North Am 30: 367–388

Ginzburg E, Carillo EH, Kopelman T et al (1998) The role of computed tomography in selective management of gunshot wounds to the abdomen and flank. J Trauma 45:1005–1009

Glazer GM, Buy JN, Moss AA et al (1981) CT detection of duodenal perforation. AJR 137:333–336

Hauser CJ, Huprich JE, Bosco P et al (1987) Triple-contrast computed tomography in the evaluation of penetrating posterior abdominal injuries. Arch Surg 122:1112–1115

Israel RS, Mayberry JC, Primack SL (1996) Diaphragmatic rupture: use of helical CT scanning with multiplanar reformations. AJR 167:1201–1203

Jeffrey RB, Cardoza JD, Olcott EW (1991) Detection of active intraabdominal arterial hemorrhage: value of dynamic contrast-enhanced CT. AJR 156:725–729

Kunin JR, Korobkin M, Ellis JH (1993) Duodenal injuries caused by blunt abdominal trauma: value of CT in differentiating perforation from hematoma. AJR 160:1221–1223

Lim-Dunham JE, Narra J, Benya EC et al (1997) Aspiration after administration of oral contrast material in children undergoing abdominal CT for trauma. AJR 169:1015–1018

Löw R, Düber C, Schweden F et al (1997) Ganzkörper-Spiral-CT zur Primärdiagnostik polytraumatisierter Patienten unter Notfallbedingungen. Fortschr Röntgenstr 166:382–388

McAllister E, Perez M, Albrink MH, Olsen SM, Rosemurgy AS (1994) Is triple contrast computed tomographic scanning useful in the selective management of stab wounds to the back? J Trauma 37:401–403

Michel LA, Lacrosse M, Decanniere L et al (1996) Blunt renal traumas: contribution of spiral CT with three-dimensional reconstruction to the surgical decision process? Int Surg 81:377–381

Mirvis SE, Whitley NO, Vainwright JR et al (1989a) Blunt hepatic trauma in adults: CT-based classification and correlation with prognosis and treatment. Radiology 171: 27–32

Mirvis SE, Whitley NO, Gens DR (1989b) Blunt splenic trauma

in adults: CT-based classification and correlation with prognosis and treatment. Radiology 171:33–39
Novelline RA, Rhea JT, Rao PM et al (1999) Helical CT in emergency radiology. Radiology 213:321–339
Phillips T, Sclafani SJA, Goldstein A et al (1986) Use of contrast-enhanced CT enema in the management of penetrating trauma to the flank and back. J Trauma 26:593–601
Rehm CG, Sherman R, Hinz TW (1989) The role of CT scan in evaluation for laparotomy in patients with stab wounds of the abdomen. J Trauma 29:446–450
Richards JR, Derlet RW (1998) Computed tomography for blunt abdominal trauma in the ED: a prospective study. Am J Emerg Med 16:338–342
Rizzo MJ, Federle MP, Griffiths BG (1989) Bowel and mesenteric injury following blunt abdominal trauma: evaluation with CT. Radiology 173:143–148
Rothrock SG, Green SM, Morgan R (2000) Abdominal trauma in infants and children: prompt identification and early management of serious and life-threatening injuries, part II. Specific injuries and ED management. Pediatr Emerg Care 16:189–195
Rydberg J, Buckwalter KA, Caldemeyer KS et al (2000) Multisection CT: scanning techniques and clinical applications. Radiographics 20:1787–1806
Scatamacchia SA, Raptopoulos V, Fink MP et al (1989) Splenic trauma in adults: impact of CT grading on management. Radiology 171:725–729
Shankar KR, Lloyd DA, Kitteringham L et al (1999) Oral contrast with computed tomography in the evaluation of blunt abdominal trauma in children. Br J Surg 86:1073–1077
Sherck JP, McCort JJ, Oakes DD (1984) Computed tomography in thoracoabdominal trauma. J Trauma 24:1015–1021
Soto JA, Morales C, Munera F et al (2001) Penetrating stab wounds to the abdomen: use of serial US and contrast-enhanced CT in stable patients. Radiology 220:365–371
Stalker HP, Kaufman RA, Towbin R (1986) Patterns of liver injury in childhood: CT analysis. AJR 147:1199–1205
Strouse PJ, Close BJ, Marshall KW et al (1999) CT of bowel and mesenteric trauma in children. Radiographics 19:1237–1250
Umlas SL, Cronan JJ (1991) Splenic trauma: can CT grading systems enable prediction of successful nonsurgical treatment? Radiology 178:481–487

4 Injuries of the Spleen

R. F. Dondelinger, O. Cornet, J. H. Boverie

CONTENTS

- An injection-to-scan delay of 60–90 s should be applied for optimal demonstration of splenic injury on CT.
- Despite the formulation of many splenic injury grading systems based on CT findings, inclusion of a patient in a trial of nonoperative conservative management should not be based solely on imaging.
- Contrast extravasation or an intrasplenic blush on CT suggests persistent hemorrhage and in most cases requires either arteriography and selective embolization or surgical intervention.
- Conservative management of splenic injury, including low grades, carries the risk of delayed bleeding and necessitates close observation and repeated imaging.

R. F. Dondelinger, MD
Professor and Chairman, Department of Medical Imaging, University Hospital Sart Tilman, Domaine Universitaire du Sart Tilman B35, 4000 Liège, Belgium
O. Cornet, MD
Resident, Department of Medical Imaging, University Hospital Sart Tilman, Domaine du Sart Tilman B35, 4000 Liège, Belgium
J. H. Boverie, MD
Chef de Clinique, Department of Medical Imaging, University Hospital Sart Tilman, Domaine du Sart Tilman B35, 4000 Liège, Belgium

4.1 History

The fragility of the spleen has been known since ancient times. Sharp blows to the left upper abdomen were reputed to be an effective means of assassination without the visibility of an external wound. The first medical description of posttraumatic splenic rupture was given by Paracelsus in the fifteenth century and the first splenectomy performed in human is attributed to Zaccavelli in 1549 (Griswold and Collier 1961). During the Renaissance period, the vital function of the spleen was questioned, and during the seventeenth and eighteenth centuries, complete recovery from occasional partial splenectomy for trauma was noted. In modern times, surgical resection of the entire spleen as a treatment for splenic injury was first reported by Riegner in 1892 (Lucas 1991). The spleen's important role of protection from infection was postulated as early as the beginning of the twentieth century without stringent clinical evidence, but the surgical dogma that "injuries to the spleen demand excision of the gland" remained prevalent and was based upon the permanent threat of delayed posttraumatic splenic rupture (Morris and Bullock 1919). This fearful complication has been recognized since the 1930s and reinforced the need for splenectomy, despite the suggestion of non-operative salvage of the injured spleen by Billroth (McIndoe 1931; Lucas 1991). The concept of overwhelming postsplenectomy infection (OPSI) with fatal outcome put pressure on the dogma of systematic splenectomy and fueled the development of surgical spleen-preserving surgical techniques and eventually conservative nonoperative management in children (King and Shumacker 1952). Despite resistance to nonsurgical management of splenic injuries, due to the unacceptable risk of rebleeding, simple observation of splenic injury became increasingly popular in properly selected pediatric and adult groups of patients, parallel to the advent of powerful cross-section imaging of the abdomen, and today is part of the accepted armamentarium of clinical management of splenic injury.

4.2 Incidence

In early reports, the spleen and the kidney were the most frequently contused abdominal organs. Later, splenic injury was believed to be much more common than renal and hepatic trauma, probably because minor hepatic injury was overlooked before the era of cross-section imaging (Benjamin et al. 1976; Federle 1983; Gay and Sistrom 1992; Haller et al. 1994). Actual observations show that injury to the spleen has a similar incidence to hepatic trauma, and the spleen may be less frequently involved in some reports (34% vs 30%), particularly in the pediatric age group (Sayers et al. 1992). Splenic injury, as do abdominal contusions at large, results from traffic accidents in 50%–84% of cases, and the remaining cases from sports injuries, falls, work-related trauma, or assaults (Watkins 1960; Griswold and Collier 1961; Fabri et al. 1974; Delany and Janson 1981; Resciniti et al. 1988; Black et al. 1992; Kluger et al. 1994a). In abdominal contusion, children and young males are predominantly involved. In the pediatric age group, motor vehicle accidents are the most frequent cause of splenic trauma, but the young victim is a pedestrian in 80% of cases (Lakhoo et al. 1991).

Blunt trauma accounts for 46%–100% of all splenic injury in large series and remains largely predominant in the European literature. Blunt splenic injury may occur alone in about one-third of cases, but due to complex impact forces, association with other abdominal and thoracic lesions is frequent (Steeke and Lim 1975). Associated abdominal injuries, mainly left renal, hepatic, aortic, duodenopancreatic and diaphragmatic, are observed in 36%–89% of cases (Traub and Perry 1981; Livingston et al. 1982; Chadwick et al. 1985; Feliciano et al. 1985; Wiig et al. 1987; Buntain et al. 1988; Buckman et al. 1988). In fact, left renal injury is described as the most frequently associated injury in some reports (Lannergren et al. 1990). An incidence of 18% of associated hepatic or renal contusions was observed and about 7% of children have associated liver-spleen injury (Stivelman et al. 1963; Saladino et al. 1991). In 40% of cases, left-sided rib fractures are associated (Roberts et al. 1993).

Penetrating injury of the spleen is much more frequent among admissions to American hospitals than in Europe, and accounts for 12%–51% of splenic trauma in the USA. Firearms or knives are mainly responsible for penetrating splenic injury (Fisher et al. 1978). Injuries caused by knife wounds may concern only the spleen in the abdominal cavity. Thoracoabdominal anatomy accounts for the frequently associated pulmonary, pleural, and phrenic injuries.

All splenic ruptures do not occur immediately after trauma. Posttraumatic splenic rupture is acute in 85%–99%, delayed in 1%–20% and occult in less than 1% of patients (Drapanas et al. 1969; Olsen and Pooley 1977). Delayed rupture of the spleen is defined as hemorrhage occurring more than 48 h following trauma and emphasizes the need for proper imaging at admission and during follow-up (McIndoe 1931).

4.3
Mechanism

4.3.1
Internal Structure of the Spleen

The spleen can be described as a lymph node that is traversed by blood instead of lymph. It is a particularly fragile plain abdominal organ, due to its loose internal lymphoid architecture and rich vascularization. The splenic capsule ruptures easily and the "open" intrasplenic blood circulation without endothelialized vessels favors profuse bleeding from the pulp through a capsular tear. Blood rarely accumulates within the splenic mesenchyma itself, because of the absence of intrasplenic tissular barriers, thus allowing immediate spread of hematoma to the subcapsular space and through a tear of the capsule in the perisplenic space. The spleen, due to its intrinsic vulnerability to contusion, is not effectively protected from blunt abdominal injury, despite its location in the left diaphragmatic concavity and the overlying lower rib cage.

4.3.2
Common Mechanisms of Trauma

Blunt splenic trauma is most frequently caused by a direct upper abdominal impact. In some cases, rapid deceleration is responsible for splenic rupture and is classically associated with thoracic aortic rupture or pelvic fractures. Lateral compression injuries during motor vehicle accidents carry significantly more upper abdominal visceral injuries with fatal outcome than accidents with a frontal crash force (Siegel et al. 1990). Stiff armrests were also shown experimentally to produce more abdominal compression and upper abdominal injury, including splenic injury, than soft ones due to decreased deformation and velocity energy absorption (Viano and Andrzejak 1993). Among the mechanisms of blunt splenic injury, the increasing importance of stick sports such as skiing and hockey was emphasized, which are responsible for a pinpointed blunt or an almost penetrating injury without a penetrating wound (Sartorelli et al. 1995). In handlebar injuries in children, the spleen is the most frequently involved organ, followed by the pancreas (Clarnette and Beasley 1997). Due to its reduced size or surface and its posterior location, the spleen is not often injured during localized penetrating trauma (Slate et al. 1969).

4.3.3
Uncommon Mechanisms of Trauma

4.3.3.1
Iatrogenic Injury

Surgery

Surgical mobilization accounts for iatrogenic splenic injury that may occur during caudal pancreatectomy, gastric surgery (gastrectomy, vagotomy, cure of hiatal hernia), left colon, left renal, or adrenal surgery, and more generally, during complex abdominal surgery or re-intervention. In some reports in the past, iatrogenic splenic injury accounted for 19%–50% of all splenectomies performed (Devlin et al. 1969; Slater 1973; Langevin et al. 1984; Kremer et al. 1995). More recent figures show a rate of 0.6% intraoperative splenic injury during major abdominal interventions or a rate of 4% splenectomies of either iatrogenic or undefined cause (Feliciano et al. 1990; Kremer et al. 1995).

Interventional Radiology

In the past, direct percutaneous splenoportography carried a definite risk of splenic hemorrhage and was therefore performed in the immediate preoperative period. Today, the spleen can still be injured during percutaneous splenic biopsy or catheter drainage procedures of splenic, perisplenic, pancreatic, lesser sac, or left thoracic fluid collections. When the patient is placed in a prone position, the spleen may shift into a partially retrorenal location in 15% of patients, particularly in the elderly population, probably due to an increased ligamentous laxity (Hopper and Chantelois 1989). This abnormal position may account for unintentional splenic puncture during percutaneous interventions in the left kidney, since the retrorenal position of the spleen is not present on imaging in dorsal decubitus. Splenic rupture was also reported following arterial splenic embolization or after fibrinolytic therapy (Eklof et al. 1978; Wholey et al. 1978).

Endoscopy

Diagnostic or therapeutic colonoscopy is occasionally responsible for splenic injury with or without colon perforation. True incidence is unknown and estimated at 0.015%. About 20 cases were reported in the literature (Teniere et al. 1985; Colarian et al. 1991; Ong et al. 1991; Viamonte et al. 1992;

Heath et al. 1994; Espinal et al. 1997). The endoscope hurts the spleen during difficult passage of an elongated splenic flexure of the colon. Excessive traction on the splenocolic ligament or on preexisting adhesions is the hypothesized mechanism of splenic injury in this setting. The injury is often not immediately recognized by the endoscopist, causing diagnostic delay, sometimes for several days. The diagnosis is made during urgent laparotomy, when the clinical condition of the patient suddenly deteriorates, without plausible explanation (Gores and Simso 1989; Coughlin and Aanning 1997). The diagnostic uncertainty, the delay, and the risk of possible associated perforation of the colon, makes surgical revision and splenectomy unavoidable in most cases.

Endoscopic retrograde cholangiopancreatography (ERCP) and endoscopic ultrasonography (EUS) may also be occasionally responsible for splenic and hepatic injury because of maneuvering the patient on the table or excessive movement of the endoscope inside the upper gastrointestinal tract. ERCP-related splenic injury is estimated at 0.006% (Ong et al. 1991; Lewis et al. 1991; Wu and Katon 1993). The diagnosis may not be established until splenic abscess develops on top of a subcapsular hematoma (Furman and Morgenstern 1993).

External Cardiac Massage

Prolonged and intense cardiopulmonary resuscitation with external cardiac massage may be encountered with increasing frequency as a cause of splenic rupture, although most reported cases in the literature are published as individual cases (Vitello and Hartung 1991; Bernard et al. 1993; Stallard et al. 1997). The spleen and the liver can be contused together by external cardiac massage (Johanet et al. 1989). However, resuscitative action was not found to cause an increased rate of lethal outcome by splenic rupture (Vock 1992).

In an animal experiment, it was shown that vigorous infusion of saline after massive splenic injury increased intra-abdominal hemorrhage and decreased survival time (Solomonov et al. 2000).

4.3.3.2 Spontaneous Rupture

Pseudospontaneous Rupture

Splenic rupture following unnoticed or neglected minor trauma to a normal or an enlarged and diseased spleen can be described as pseudospontaneous. Many conditions such as infectious mononucleosis, autoimmune, or hematologic disorders, lymphoma or leukemia, portal hypertension, and focal splenic solid tumor (sarcoma) or cysts (epidermoid, parasitic, pseudocyst) weaken the spleen and favor rupture following a minor impact (Gauderer et al. 1989; Spencer et al. 1996; Su et al. 1997). The battered child syndrome may also present as apparently spontaneous splenic rupture (Kirks 1983).

True Spontaneous Rupture

Isolated cases of true spontaneous rupture of the spleen without any recognized history of trauma are reported in the literature. Twenty proven cases were collected in the late 1950s (Orloff and Peskin 1958). The mechanism of rupture is explained by splenic enlargement caused by blood stasis such as splenic congestion resulting from splenic vein occlusion with or without infection; one or several space-occupying lesions or diffuse tumor infiltration or infection, eroding the splenic capsule, leading either to rupture or perforation in the gastrointestinal tract; or weakening of the splenic capsule, through infection or by chemical therapeutic agents or other processes. A selection of published causes of spontaneous splenic rupture are listed in Table 4.1.

Most reported patients present with sudden upper abdominal pain, hemoperitoneum, hypotension or shock and require immediate laparotomy. Preoperative cross-section imaging is not always obtained in such enigmatic emergency conditions, but imaging would be able to establish the diagnosis preoperatively, similarly to acute trauma patients. Splenectomy is most often performed due to diagnostic uncertainty. However, spleen-preserving procedures are advised in these fragile patients, with splenic tumor, infection or pregnancy, or more generally in any patient when splenectomy is not required for a definite diagnosis (Fletcher et al. 1989; Marin Leon et al. 1990; Martinez Ruiz et al. 1990; Zingman and Viner 1993; Paar et al. 1995). Fatal spontaneous splenic rupture was observed in some patients, such as in lymphoma or leukemia after initiation of chemotherapy, or in patients with an infectious spleen, or in hemophilia (Borgeat et al. 1989; Lippstone et al. 1998; Stout et al. 1973; Schiodt et al. 2000). Cases of combined spontaneous splenic and hepatic rupture with immunopathological reaction were described (Huttunen et al. 1975).

Table 4.1. Principal causes of apparently spontaneous or nontraumatic splenic rupture

Causative agent or underlying disease	Uncommon	Rare
Infection	Infectious mononucleosis Acute malaria Abscess	Hydatid cyst *Campylobacter jejuni* Salmonella Dublin Acute brucellosis Rubella Typhoid fever Influenza Chickenpox Viral hepatitis Tuberculosis Actinomycosis Tularemia Aspergillosis Syphilis Kala-Azar Meningococcal septicemia Virus-associated hematophagocytic syndrome Yaws Q fever
Asopa and Elhence (1965); Tapp (1969); Rawsthorne et al. (1970); Vizer and Weiland (1979); Rest et al. (1985); Marin Leon et al. (1990) (review); Baumbach et al. (1992); Zingman and Viner (1993) (review); Frizelle and Rietveld (1994); Broholm and Jans (1995); Nishida et al. (1995); Paar et al. (1995); Guleria et al. (1996); Lippstone et al. (1998) (review); Gunay et al. (1999); Vanhoenacker and de Schepper (2000).		
Tumor	Acute leukemia in general Lymphoma in general (Hem)angiosarcoma	Hodgkin's disease Plasma cell leukemia Acute myeloid leukemia Hairy cell leukemia Chronic lymphatic leukemia Histiocytic lymphoma (diffuse) T-cell lymphoma Chronic myelogenous leukemia Mycosis fungoides Angioma Angiomyolipoma Splenoma Metastatic (melanoma, hepatocellular carcinoma) Leukemic reticuloendotheliosis Hepatocellular carcinoma (without splenic metastasis) Pancreatic cystadenocarcinoma Choriocarcinoma
Cooray (1952); Hoagland and Henson (1957); Flood and Carpenter (1961); Hynes et al. (1964); Cafferata et al. (1966); Papp and Penner (1971); Heading et al. (1972); Gillet et al. (1973); Kubota et al. (1974); Autry and Weitzner (1975); Martinazzi et al. (1975); Dobrow (1977); Yam and Crosby (1979); Rogers and Shah (1980); Nieto Jimenez et al. (1981); von der Walde et al. (1981); Horie et al. (1982); Al-Obaidi (1989); Winde et al. (1991) (review); Brissette and Dhru (1992) (review); Buzbee and Legha (1992); Foiada et al. (1993); Gorg et al. (1994); Baradaran et al. (1995); Challis et al. (1996); Stites and Ultmann (1996); Asayama et al. (1998); Haj et al. (1999) (review); Sugahara et al. (1999); Patrinou et al. (2000); Schiodt et al. (2000) (review); Vanhoenacker and de Schepper (2000).		

▷▷

Table 4.1. Continued

Causative agent or underlying disease	Common	Uncommon
Hematological disease		Congenital afibrinogenemia Hemophilia and Kasabach-Merritt syndrome Idiopathic thrombocytopenic purpura Hemolytic disease of the newborn Autoimmune hemolytic anemia Congenital hemolytic anemia
Stout et al. (1973); Levy (1994); Vanhoenacker and de Schepper (2000).		
Vascular disease	Congestive splenomegaly Splenic vein thrombosis (chronic pancreatitis)	Peliosis Arterial splenic embolization Mycotic aneurysm Endocarditis Hepatic vein occlusion and portal vein thrombosis Acute pancreatitis
Saavedra (1965); Gautier-Benoit et al. (1973); Philipp et al. (1977); Wholey et al. (1978); Taxy (1978); Diebold and Audouin (1983); Welk et al. (1991); Kohr et al. (1993) (review); Nincheri Kunz et al. (1994); Garre Sanchez et al. (1996); Celebrezze et al. (1998); Rege et al. (1998); Shimono et al. (1998); Vanhoenacker and de Schepper (2000); Habib et al. (2000).		
Systemic disease	Amyloidosis	Histiocytosis Cohn's disease Rheumatoid arthritis Felty's syndrome Systemic lupus erythematosus Polyarteritis nodosa Wegener's granulomatosis Sarcoidosis Gaucher's disease
Becker and Brill (1949); Wiley et al. (1951); Drapiewski et al. (1955); Bonucci and Piegaja (1964); Okazaki et al. (1986) (review); Festa et al. (1989) (review); Hurd and Katholi (1980); Sandberg-Gertzen et al. (1998); de Lajarte-Thirouard et al. (1999); Vanhoenacker and de Schepper (2000).		
Other		Pregnancy Vomiting Defecation Chemotherapy (leukemia) Delayed posttraumatic splenic rupture Conservative splenic injury management (>5 years) Normal spleen Normal accessory spleen Intrasplenic pregnancy Birth (neonate) Liver cirrhosis (portal hypertension) Portal triad clamping Neonate (mother under anticonvulsant drug) Streptokinase Intra-abdominal foreign body Pancreatic pseudocyst
Druit (1947); Orloff and Peskin (1958); Cohen and Pearlman (1967); Texeira and Hardin (1974); Clark et al. (1975); Shafiroff et al. (1977); Eklof et al. (1978); Vas and Friend (1981); Thijs et al. (1983); Caruso and Hall (1984); Traggis et al. (1984); Cuckow (1991); Jeffrey (1991); Chien and Liaw (1993); Baradaran et al. (1995); Douzdjian and Broughan (1995); Molina et al. (1995); Deva and Thompson (1996); Katz et al. (1998) (review); Ashlock et al. (1998a); Coote et al. (1999); Longobardi et al. (2000).		

4.3.3.3
Nonacute Splenic Rupture

Secondary Splenic Rupture or Missed Diagnosis

Delayed or so-called secondary splenic rupture is a potential cause of mortality after blunt abdominal trauma and in the past prompted systematic splenectomy. Extended splenic lacerations were found at surgery in 5%–15% of the cases versus 1% in acute rupture (Emery 1997; Kluger et al. 1994a; Pappas et al. 1987; Taylor and Rosenfield 1984; Schultz and Froelich 1985). In the early literature, 15%–30% of splenic injuries were reported to be secondary ruptures, but the literature concurrent to the use of cross section imaging in trauma patients reported a drop in secondary splenic rupture to 1% (Zabinski and Harkins 1943; Cole et al. 1949; Bollinger and Fowler 1956; Orloff and Peskin 1958). In the past, scintigraphy and arteriography had shown that the so-called delayed splenic rupture was merely a missed diagnosis in most patients (Benjamin et al. 1976; Olsen and Pooley 1977; Kluger et al. 1994a). Delayed bleeding from a ruptured spleen occurs within 1 week in half of the patients. In 75% of the patients, the latent period described by Baudet was less than 2 weeks (Baudet 1907; Foster 1970). Presence of a subcapsular hematoma is not an accurate predictor per se for secondary rupture, but rather the increase in volume of a splenic hematoma (Blocker et al. 1998). True secondary splenic rupture with an initially intact capsule is a rare posttraumatic occurrence, secondary bleeding from a preexisting capsular tear being a more frequent event. The spleen may rebleed when massively revascularized after an initial period of arterial vasoconstriction or as a result of hemostatic clot lysis by endogenous fibrinolysis, after decompression of a subcapsular hematoma by catheter drainage or in situ injection of thrombolytic drugs in a hematoma, or rupture may be caused by infectious perisplenitis. Delayed splenic rupture has a worse prognosis than immediately recognized injury and carries a higher mortality rate than repair of a primary splenic rupture (Gay and Sistrom 1992; Kluger et al. 1994a). Delayed rupture is treated more often with splenectomy than primary rupture with similar severity (Mucha et al. 1986; Buntain et al. 1988; Resciniti et al. 1988).

Tertiary or Late Splenic Rupture

In some patients who had sustained secondary or delayed splenic rupture and who are still included in a conservative trial without surgery, a persistent subcapsular hematoma may rupture during follow-up, when it has increased in volume due to osmotic changes, or when lysis of a hemostatic clot at the splenic capsular tear takes place. We have observed two patients with a tertiary splenic rupture, occurring 1 month after the initial splenic injury.

Occult Rupture

Truly occult splenic rupture is observed in a small number of patients. A subcapsular hematoma remains contained by the intact capsule, reinforced by adhesions. The injury can remain undiagnosed and untreated, sometimes for years (Drapanas et al. 1969; Lorimer 1964; Bundy et al. 1985). About 1%–3% of all splenectomies are performed for occult posttraumatic splenic rupture. Usually the history is difficult to elicit in these circumstances, particularly in alcoholic patients or individuals in a low socio-economic environment, or victims with an erratic lifestyle.

4.3.4
Pathology of the Injured Spleen

Pathological studies have suggested that the weight of the spleen (208 g, standard deviation:76 g) can be independently associated to rupture after blunt trauma. Ruptured spleens seem to be larger than normal spleens in one study (Drachenberg and Papadimitriou 1996). Ruptured spleens also seem to exhibit evidence of preexisting immune stimulation. Pathology of the injured spleen suggests that splenic rupture after trauma may be related to prior immunological stimulation, but this observation certainly does not apply to all cases (Farhi and Ashfaq 1996).

4.4
Clinical Symptoms and Findings

Various clinical signs are suggestive of splenic injury, but specific signs are often absent or misleading:

- Classically the patient reports abdominal pain located in the left upper quadrant. Pain localized at palpation and caused by low rib fracture should not obscure splenic injury. Patients with apparently isolated left lower rib fractures should also be imaged, even when trauma seems benign. In fact, splenic injury is associated with fractures of the left lower ribs in up to 40% of cases (Roberts et al. 1993). The presence of three or more rib fractures significantly increases the relative risk of splenic and hepatic injury and is an indicator for thorough imaging (Lee et al. 1990).

- Difficulties in respiration caused by a limited diaphragmatic excursion due to pain or phrenic irritation is another suggestive symptom.
- Pain at the tip of the left shoulder or both (Kehr's sign), without evidence of scapular bone and joint injury should be correctly related to possible splenic trauma (Rao and Novelline 1996; Lowenfels 1966).
- Palpation of an enlarged spleen or hematoma as a left subcostal or abdominal mass of fixed dullness to percussion (Balance's sign).
- Signs of peritoneal irritation.
- Skin ecchymosis over the splenic area.
- A patient with splenic rupture may be stable or hypotensive or in shock. Delayed rupture of the spleen presents more often than acute injury as an acute abdomen with peritoneal irritation or shock.
- Hemoperitoneum is difficult to evaluate clinically but is easily detected with cross-section imaging. In occult splenic rupture, hemoperitoneum may simulate a groin hernia or fill an inguinal hernia sac (Sherman 1989). Acute uni- or bilateral scrotal swelling caused by hemoperitoneum due to occult splenic laceration was reported, the hematocele being produced by incomplete obliteration of the vaginalis. US shows scrotal hematocele with normal testes (Henry 1978; Sujka et al. 1986; Skoog and Belman 1986; Roback et al. 1996; Koumanidou et al. 2000).
- Occasionally a left hemothorax reveals a splenic rupture, when a lacerated spleen has herniated through a phrenic tear and bled in the thorax (Lansiaux et al. 1998; De Waele and Vermassen 1999).
- Finally, progressive enlargement of an occult splenic hematoma following a minor trauma may cause fever for several weeks and can suggest a malignant hemopathy (Shafran et al. 1992).
- A further misleading clinical presentation is a biphasic course, described in pediatric patients submitted to conservative treatment with bed rest. These patients showed an accelerated pulse, increased body temperature, abdominal pain and tenderness, without evidence of delayed bleeding 1 or 2 days after the accident (Lannergren et al. 1990).

Physical examination is accurate in the diagnosis of blunt splenic injury in 65% of the cases (Powell et al. 1982). Neither clinical symptoms, nor signs at admission, nor a pediatric or adult trauma score are able to predict with confidence the presence of splenic injury (Saladino et al. 1991).

4.5 Imaging

4.5.1 Computed Tomography

4.5.1.1 Technique

Computed tomography (CT) is the most effective and efficient means of diagnosis of splenic trauma. Adequate CT technique is of utmost importance in evaluating splenic trauma and influences diagnostic capability more than for the other abdominal organs (see Chap. 3, "CT Examination Protocols in Abdominal Trauma"). X-ray of the thorax or the scout view obtained before CT scanning may evidence lower left rib fractures, medial displacement of gastric air, caudal displacement of the left colon flexure, and a high position of the left hemidiaphragm. These signs are suggestive of an enlarged spleen. A left pneumothorax or a left pleural effusion or lung contusion can also be noted. After IV injection of contrast medium, the spleen should not be evaluated during the early phase of arterial enhancement, when contrast medium pools between the white and red pulp. Scanning too early after contrast medium injection shows a heterogeneous mixing of contrast inside the spleen, which either completely obscures or at least does not reflect the true extent of contusion (Figs. 4.1, 4.5b). The diagnosis is easily missed when an injection-scan interval of 40 (20–50) s or less is applied, particularly in hypotensive patients (Berland and van Dyke 1985). The optimal injection-scan interval is 70 s, ranging from 60 to 90 s. An injection-scan interval longer than 100 s can also be responsible for false-negative diagnoses or of undergrading the severity of splenic damage (Ashlock et al. 1998b; Raptopoulos 1994). Hand injection and drip infusions of contrast medium should definitely be abandoned. Delayed scans are not useful overall and therefore are not obtained routinely in hepatic or splenic trauma. However, in rare instances, contrast extravasation is missed on early scanning and only recognized on delayed scans (Sivit

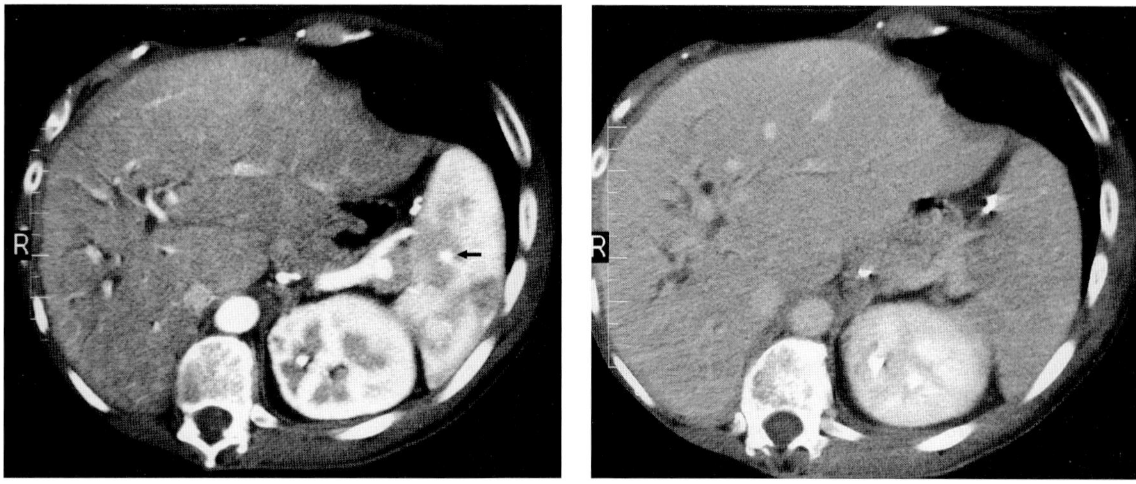

a b

Fig. 4.1a, b. A 52-year-old male admitted after abdominal contusion. **a** Early arterioportal phase of contrast enhancement shows on CT hypodense zones in the spleen and blushes of contrast (*arrow*), wrongly suggesting contusion and active bleeding. **b** Late scan shows no splenic injury. Notice moderate intrahepatic bile duct dilatation, not related to trauma

2000). Printing films with narrow window settings has no influence on lesion detection or injury grading and is no longer an issue, as the CT examinations are read on the console (Patten et al. 2000).

4.5.1.2
Positive Signs

In most cases, splenic injury is obvious on CT.

- The contused zones that have compromised vascularization show up as single or multiple hypodense, nonenhanced intrasplenic areas, with irregular limits, situated anywhere in the splenic tissue and most likely extending beneath the splenic capsule (Figs. 4.2, 4.8).
- A laceration of the spleen extends from one capsular surface to the opposite one; a small limited hypodense fracture line may be seen in low-grade trauma.
- The capsule may not be recognized as such, in contact with the contusion, but non-visibility of the capsular line does not necessarily indicate capsular disruption.

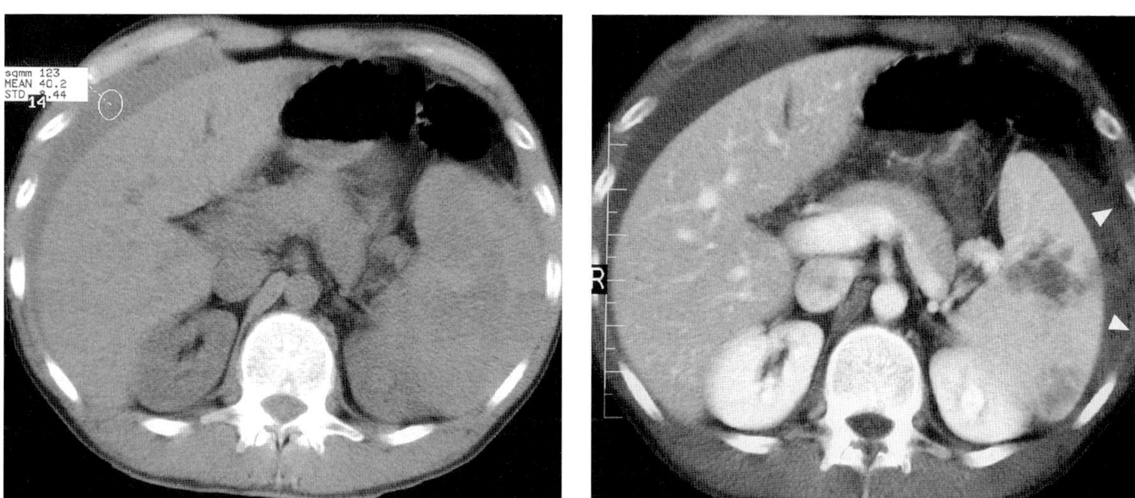

a b

Fig. 4.2a, b. A 35-year-old male admitted after a car accident. **a** CT prior to IV contrast injection shows an enlarged spleen, limited by high densities corresponding to a hematoma. Perihepatic hemoperitoneum at 40.2 HU. **b** After contrast injection, two hypodense areas of intrasplenic contusion are better seen than on nonenhanced scan. The splenic capsule (*arrowheads*) and subcapsular hematoma are more clearly delineated

- A subcapsular hematoma compresses the underlying splenic tissue. Its sharp limit, initially semilunar, may become convex toward the spleen when the hematoma has increased in size (Figs. 4.3, 4.25). Usually the hematoma extends over a large part or the entire external splenic surface and can surround the splenic tissue up to the hilum. Occasionally, it may be difficult to differentiate a subcapsular hematoma from a perisplenic effusion. A perisplenic collection does not exhibit a biconvex limit and does not exert compression on the splenic tissue. A subcapsular hematoma may show, prior to contrast injection, onion-skin-like layers of variable densities, which correspond to clots of different age (Fig. 4.4). The initial hyperdensity of splenic or subcapsular hematoma at the acute phase and its progressive change into hypodensities have been described since early CT reports and confirmed later (Wolverson et al. 1983; Boioli et al. 1994). The splenic pulp can also remain dense for a certain period of time due to retention of iodinated contrast medium, when blood spaces are compressed by a subcapsular or perisplenic hematoma (Fig. 4.5).
- A collected hematoma in the perisplenic space usually results from a splenic capsular tear. Subcapsular and perisplenic hematoma can coexist; neither is not enhanced. A hyperdense clot within a low-density perisplenic hemoperitoneum in contact with the spleen specifically suggests a splenic capsular tear (Federle et al. 1987). The splenic capsule is often identified with difficulties when subcapsular and perisplenic hemorrhage are present (Fig. 4.5b).

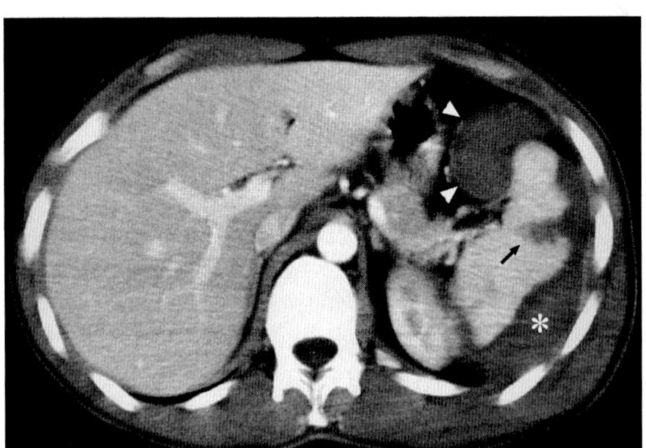

Fig. 4.3. CT obtained after blunt abdominal injury in a 29-year-old male. Compression of the splenic tissue by a large subcapsular hematoma (*asterisk*). A laceration of the spleen is seen at the lateral aspect (*arrow*). An associated localized hematoma, probably in a perisplenic location, is seen anterior to the spleen (*arrowheads*)

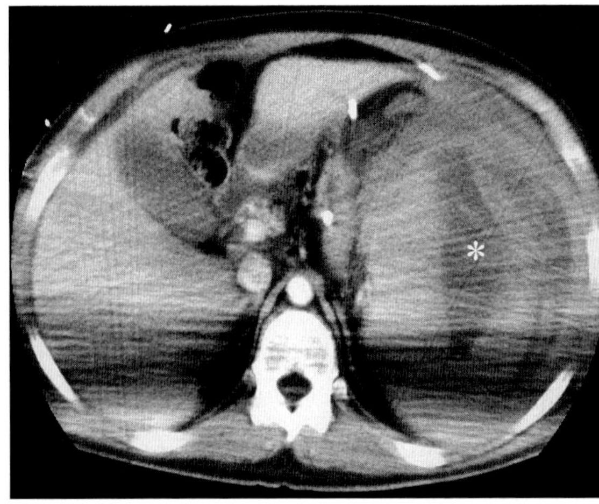

Fig. 4.4. A 45-year-old male, admitted after a car accident. Marked enlargement of the spleen on CT. Onion-skin densities corresponding to perisplenic and subcapsular hematoma. A hypodense intrasplenic contusion (*asterisk*) is also seen

- A large intrasplenic collected hematoma shows up as a round lesion, with clear margins and similar nonenhanced densities to a subcapsular hematoma. When multiple, hematomas should be differentiated from the mottled appearance of the normal spleen during the early phase of enhancement.
- Hemoperitoneum from splenic rupture initially accumulates at the convexity of the spleen. The spleen may be displaced caudally and medially. Usually the intact phrenicocolic ligament prevents direct overspilling of blood into the left paracolic gutter, but trauma can disrupt this anatomical barrier. Hemorrhage extends with increasing volume, preferentially cranially, in the left subphrenic and left subhepatic space. Spread to the right perihepatic spaces eventually occurs, either by crossing the midline beneath the diaphragm or by extension of blood from the left subhepatic space to Morison's pouch (Fig. 4.6). When hemoperitoneum is massive, it then fills the paracolic gutters, both subphrenic spaces and in the perivesical space. Fluid is found in less than 20% of patient in Morison's pouch and in less than 10% in the lesser sac. Fluid in the lesser sac is rather suggestive of gastric or pancreatic injury than splenic rupture. A collected hematoma can also be found in 10% in the left anterior pararenal space due to an associated retroperitoneal contusion (Balachandran et al. 1994).

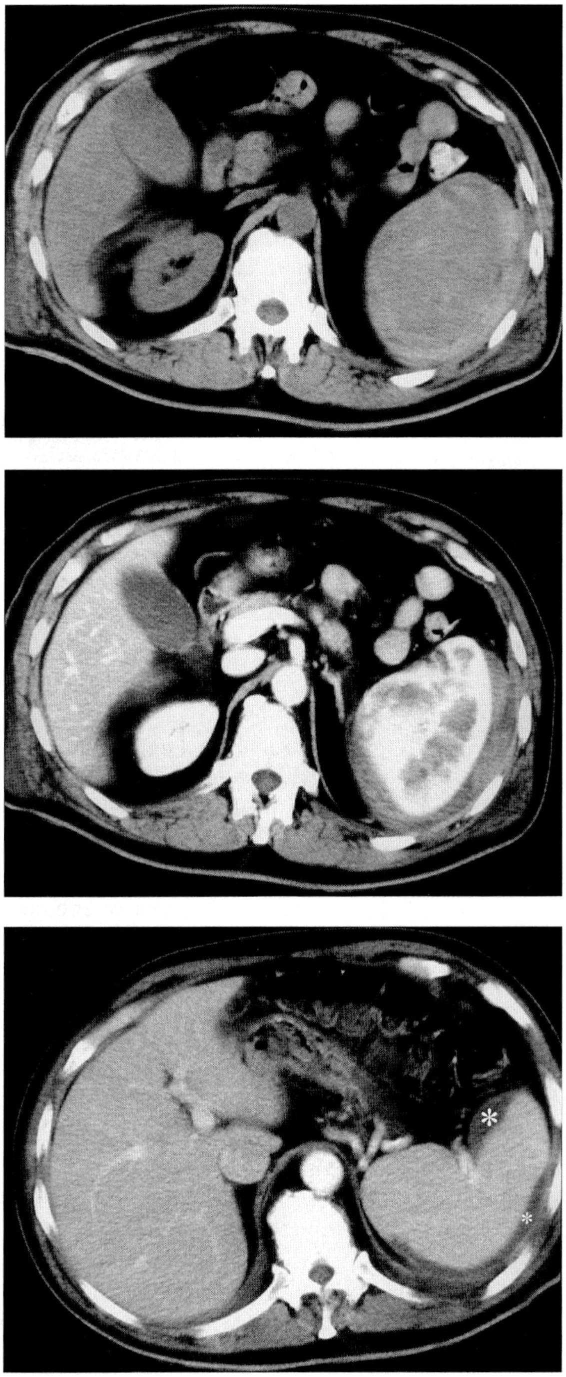

a b c

Fig. 4.5a–c. A 64-year-old male involved in a traffic accident. **a** On native scan, the spleen is enlarged, contains several hyperdense spots, and is surrounded by hyperdense layers corresponding to a fresh hematoma. **b** At the early phase after IV contrast injection, heterogeneous mixing of contrast in the white and red pulp mimics areas of splenic contusion. Despite contrast enhancement, it might be difficult to differentiate subcapsular from perisplenic hematoma. **c** Scan obtained 3 weeks later shows persistent minor subcapsular hematoma (*asterisks*) with fluid-like densities, whereas perisplenic hematoma has resorbed

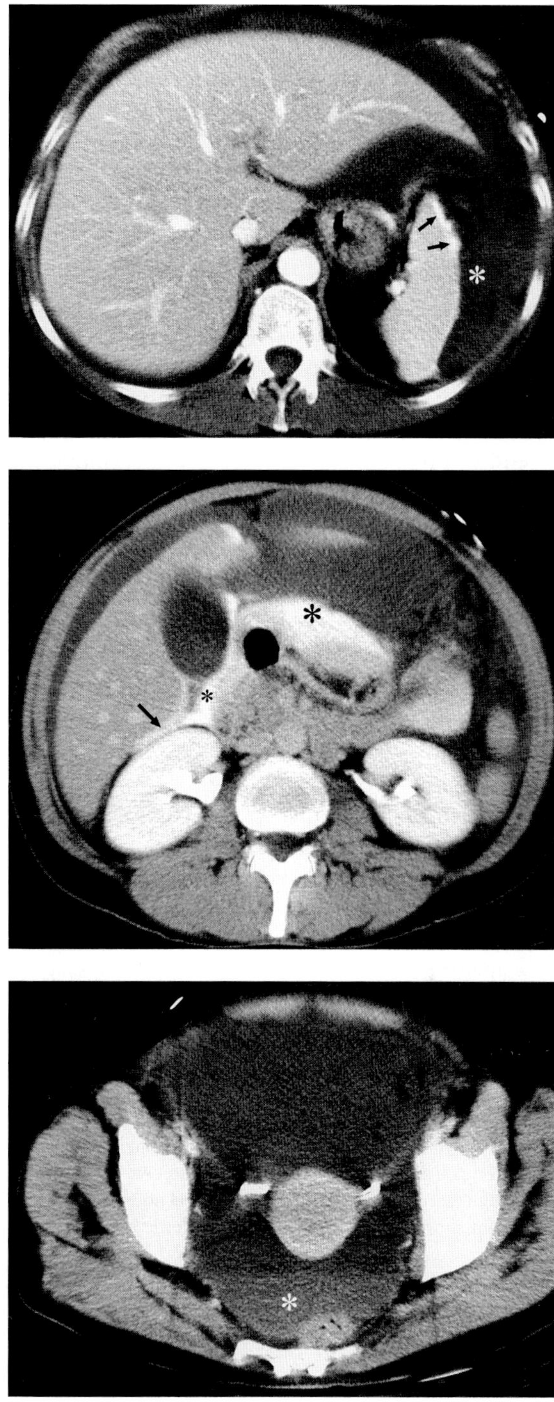

a b c

Fig. 4.6a–c. A 42-year-old female admitted after a traffic accident. **a** Flattening of the spleen by a subcapsular hematoma (*asterisk*). Subcapsular contrast medium deposit (*arrows*) in contact with the splenic tissue. Note absence of intrasplenic contusion and massive perisplenic hemoperitoneum. **b** Extravasated contrast medium accumulates in the left subhepatic space, crosses the midline (*asterisks*) and sedimentates in Morison's pouch (*arrow*). **c** Massive pelvic hemoperitoneum. Fresh blood has accumulated in the cul-de-sac (*asterisk*); peritoneal contrast has not yet reached the pelvis

With minimal hemoperitoneum, there is only fascial thickening, as the lateroconal fascia may be present (Wolfman et al. 1992). Cross-section imaging further demonstrated that a large splenic capsular rupture can be present without massive peritoneal bleeding (Fagelman et al. 1985). Conversely, in rare instances, splenic injury may remain undetected, and only the free intraperitoneal fluid is found (Eanniello et al. 1994).

- Active hemorrhage, seen as a hyperdense blush of contrast inside the spleen, as accumulated contrast medium under the capsule, layering of contrast in a hematoma, or lining the capsule and diluting progressively in the perisplenic or the upper abdominal peritoneal compartments is an unquestionable sign of active bleeding (Federle et al. 1998; Davis et al. 1998; Shammuganathan et al. 1993) (Figs. 4.7–4.10). It appears usually rapidly after the arterial phase of opacification. Massive and rapid contrast accumulation in the perisplenic space without continuity from an intrasplenic injury indicates rupture of a hilar vessel, either an artery or vein (Kluger et al. 1994a). Contrast extravasation is a good indicator for persistent bleeding and helps in identifying patients at high risk of failure of nonoperative treatment (Schurr et al. 1995). Rarely, extravasation appears only on delayed scans (Sivit 2000).

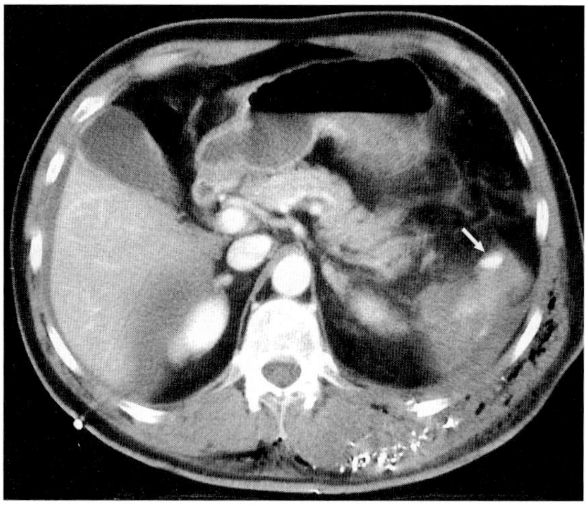

Fig. 4.7. A 59-year-old man admitted after a shotgun assault. Note radio-opaque pellets and gas bubbles in the left posterolateral subcutaneous tissue. Strong blush of contrast (*arrow*) at the anterior limit of the lower pole of the spleen. The spleen is nonenhanced, due to extensive contusion by energy accumulation from shotgun. Note moderate perisplenic hematoma

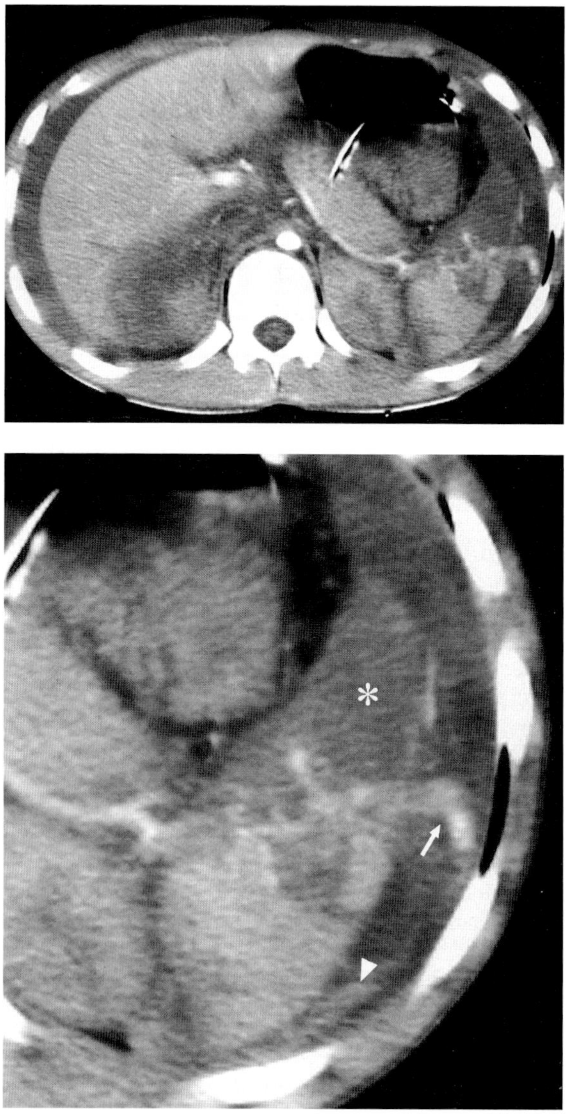

a

b

Fig. 4.8a, b. A 10-year-old boy hit by a truck. **a, b** Nonenhanced area of contusion (*asterisk*) in the anterior part of the spleen. Extravasation of contrast medium (*arrow*) through a capsular tear in the perisplenic space, where contrast sedimentates in a dependent position (*arrowhead*). Note perihepatic hemoperitoneum, showing lower densities than perisplenic blood clots. Severe vasoconstriction, caused by shock, of the abdominal aorta, splenic artery and renal arteries; the kidneys are only poorly enhanced

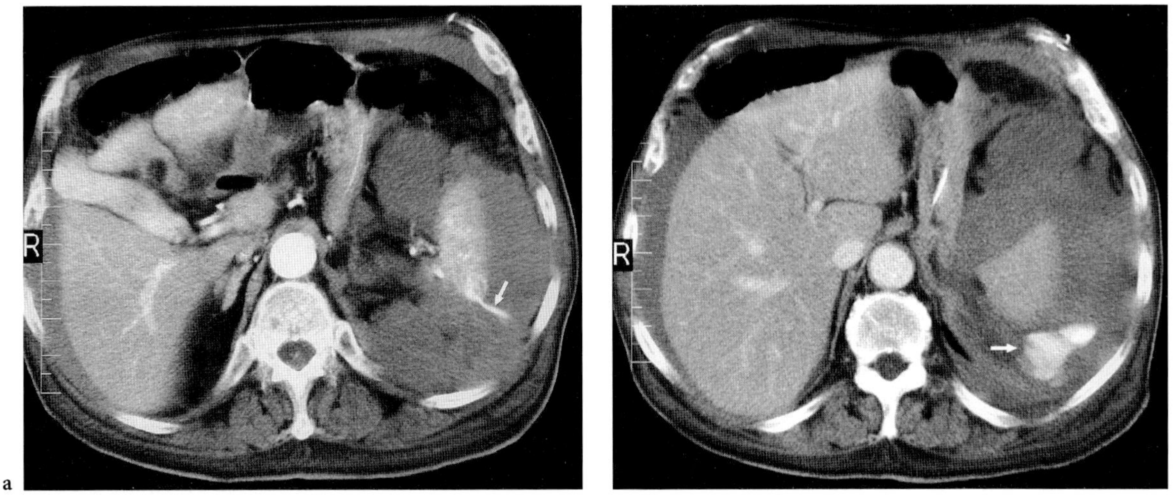

Fig. 4.9a, b. An 86-year-old male hit by a vehicle. CT at admission shows (a) massive hematoma surrounding the spleen and extravasation of contrast (*arrow*) (b) accumulating in a dependent position (*arrow*)

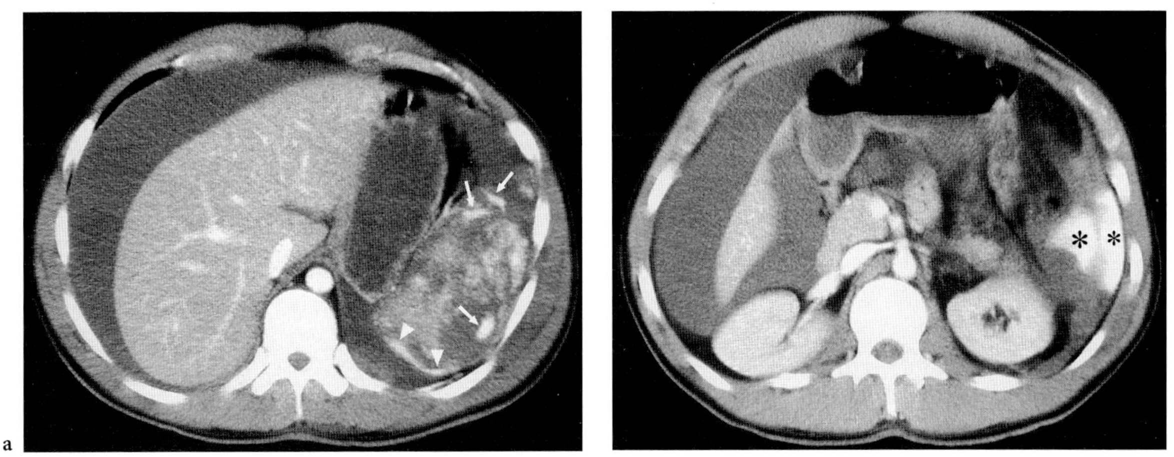

Fig. 4.10a, b. CT obtained after admission of a 37-year-old male following a car accident. a The spleen is enlarged. Diffuse areas of intrasplenic contusion and accumulation of contrast medium in the spleen (*arrows*) and in the dependent subcapsular space (*arrowhead*). b Extravasated contrast accumulates in the left paracolic gutter. Note also massive perihepatic hemoperitoneum and blood in the left anterior and posterior pararenal space

4.5.1.3 Pitfalls

Splenic Anomalies

Congenital and acquired abnormalities such as persistent splenic fissures, polysplenia, accessory spleen, wandering spleen and splenosis can be seen (Freeman et al. 1993; Kasales et al. 1994; Paterson et al. 1999).

Splenic Clefts

An insidious false-positive diagnosis of splenic rupture is congenital cleft or fissure (Figs. 4.11, 4.12). One or several clefts are normally present at the convexity of the spleen and represent embryological remnants. Splenic clefts divide the spleen according to its segmental arterial supply. They can extend from the capsule and progress deep down to the hilum, representing an intermediate state between polysplenia and a compact normal spleen. These local invaginations of

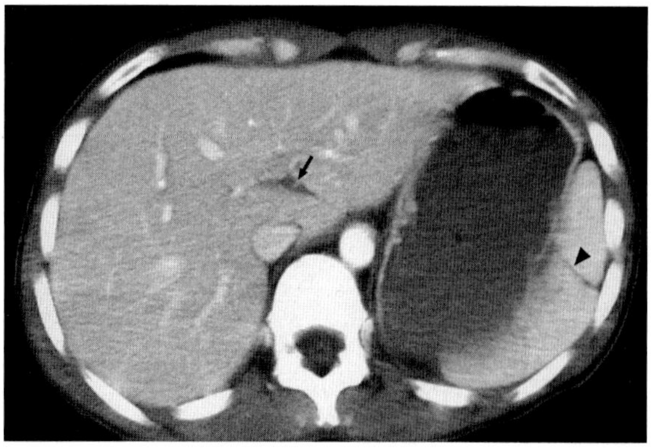

Fig. 4.11. CT in a 30-year-old male after a car accident. Small amount of blood in the fossa of the ligamentum teres of the liver (*arrow*), simulating a hepatic fracture. Normal splenic cleft (*arrowhead*), simulating a splenic fracture

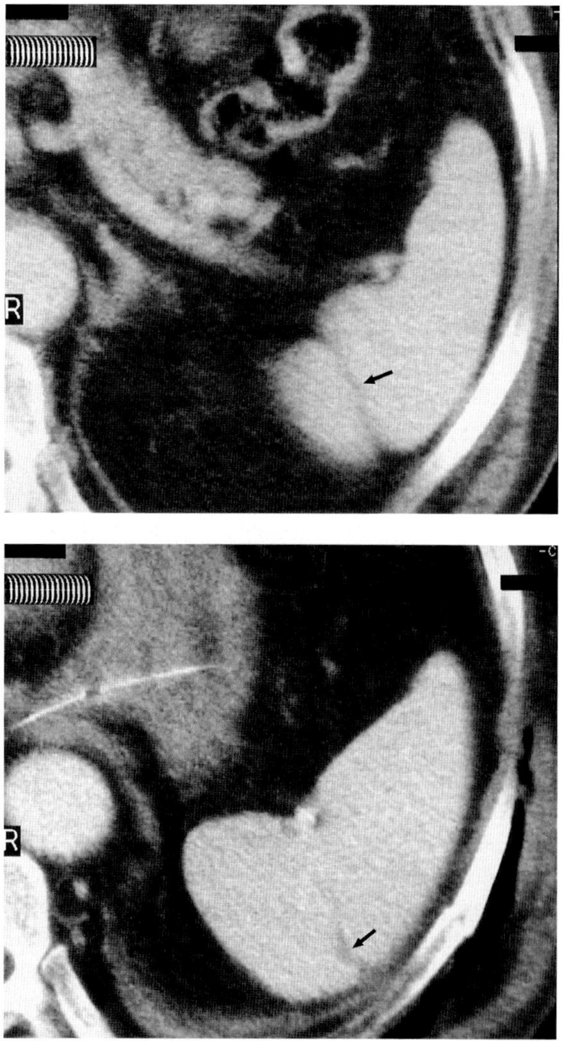

Fig. 4.12. **a** Splenic cleft (*arrow*) simulating on a more cranial slice, **b** a splenic fracture (*arrow*)

the splenic capsule show regular margins and become progressively thinner when progressing in depth. Splenic clefts are frequently seen on the lateral border, where they can be occasionally mistaken for a fracture, including on nuclear medicine studies (Hansen and Spiegelhoff 1981; Gay and Sistrom 1992). Usually they are easily recognized due to their characteristic regular cone shape. They can be particularly puzzling when a stab wound injury has occurred. A penetrating knife injury creates a larger splenic defect, with irregular margins and an adjacent subcapsular or perisplenic hematoma often present (Fig. 4.13).

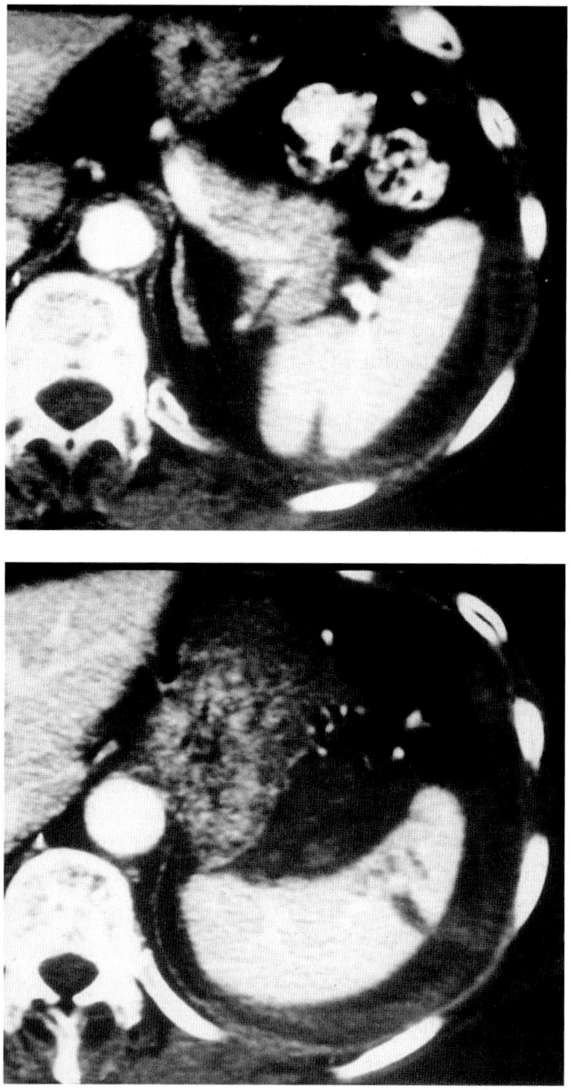

Fig. 4.13a, b. CT obtained in a 43-year-old male, who was stabbed in the back with a knife. **a** Perisplenic hematoma and a typical triangular-shaped splenic cleft in a posterior location. **b** More anteriorly, an ellipsoid hypodensity with more irregular margins is seen, corresponding to a splenic stab wound. The patient remained stable. Conservative treatment

Accessory Spleen

Accessory spleens are seen in 20%–33% of autopsies. They are usually located in the gastrosplenic ligament, anterior to the spleen or in the hilum in contact with the splenic vessels or close to the tail of the pancreas or in the greater omentum. They show a round shape and rarely exceed 2 cm in diameter. After splenectomy, splenic infarction or arterial embolization or when the spleen is diseased by an infiltrating process, an accessory spleen can enlarge, in some cases up to 6 cm. An accessory spleen is usually vascularized by a separate fine artery originating from the main splenic artery at the hilum (Fig. 4.14). On CT, an accessory spleen should not be mistaken for a nonopacified bowel loop.

Accessory spleens are small and therefore relatively protected in the abdomen and only rarely involved in blunt splenic trauma (Kumar 1962; Texeira and Hardin 1974; Richmond et al. 1992; Karam and Kozar 1998). Positive signs of injury are similar to those of the parent spleen. When perisplenic hematoma or effusion is seen and the parent spleen is normal, selective injury to an accessory spleen has to be considered. Injury to an accessory spleen can be managed following the same guidelines applicable to the parent spleen. Accessory spleens with normal histology also occasionally bleed spontaneously (Coote et al. 1999).

Polysplenia and Nodules of Splenosis

Congenital polysplenia simulates abdominal tumor. In case of trauma, it should not be mistaken for a shattered spleen. This rare abnormality consists of the non-union of multiple splenic units that develop on their own. They have regular limits and are homogeneously enhanced. Polysplenia is associated with many other congenital abnormalities and predominates in females (Derbekyan et al. 1999; Gayer et al. 1999).

Nodules of splenosis are splenic fragments that remain in the abdomen and grow on their own in situ after splenectomy and may also mimic a fragmented spleen, when multiple, of large size, and located in the splenic fossa.

Wandering Spleen

Wandering spleen is a rare congenital anomaly. It is explained by an incompetent splenorenal ligament, allowing the spleen to migrate caudally in the abdominal cavity. The spleen is found outside of its normal posterior subphrenic position, due to laxity or absence of gastrosplenic and splenorenal ligament. Usually the wandering spleen is located in an anterior abdominal position, against the abdominal wall and thus is more exposed to an abdominal impact (Horwitz and Black 1996). Torsion of a long pedicle of a wandering spleen following blunt trauma was described (Walcher et al. 1997).

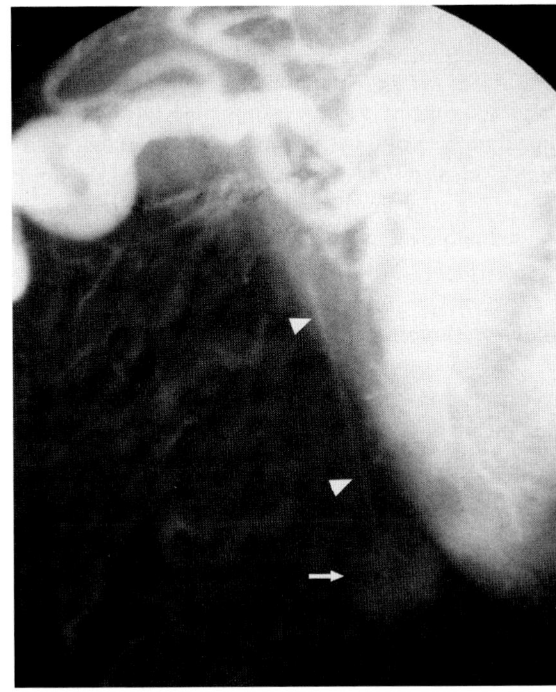

Fig. 4.14. Accessory spleens (*arrow*) are vascularized by a small artery (*arrowheads*) originating from the main splenic artery or a branch at the hilar division

Intrasplenic Lesions

A potentially false-positive diagnosis of active bleeding is a benign hypervascular splenic tumor or a pseudoaneurysm, which mimics hemorrhage. One or several intrasplenic aneurysms can be seen in patients with systemic arterial or portal hypertension and may simulate intrasplenic extravasation or posttraumatic pseudoaneurysm when located inside a contused zone. Conversely, an intrasplenic hemorrhagic blush should not be mistaken for an unexpected benign vascular tumor such as a hemangioma. A preexisting splenic infarct of any origin has an appearance similar to contusion, and may show an enhanced rim (Kluger et al. 1994b). Pathologies coexisting with injury are discussed in Chap. 13, "Blunt Abdominal Trauma in Patients with Preexisting Lesions."

At the chronic posttraumatic phase, differential diagnosis of splenic subcapsular hematoma may become problematic. Splenic cyst, hydatid disease, abscess, and intrasplenic pancreatic pseudocyst show a similar appearance on cross-section imaging. As it ages, chronic hematoma shows progressively decreased density values, responsible for a cyst-like appearance (Korobkin et al. 1978). Correct anatomical localization of a large splenic or perisplenic hematoma may be difficult on axial sections when the hematoma has replaced most of the normal spleen (Dondelinger and Fettes 1981).

Splenic Hypoperfusion Complex

In case of severe hypovolemic shock, the arteries contract due to output of vasoconstrictive agents. Spleen, kidney, pancreas and the gastrointestinal tract are often affected (Fig. 4.8)

The hypoperfusion complex may simulate disruption of the splenic artery by decreased enhancement or complete absence of splenic enhancement (Raptopoulos 1994; Ramsdell and Rao 1997). This syndrome occurs in 0.01%–2% of cases of major abdominal trauma in children with hypovolemic shock and may lead to unnecessary laparotomy. The CT appearance is particularly puzzling when no splenic enhancement at all is seen, whereas other solid organs are normally enhanced (Berland and van Dyke 1985) (Figs. 4.15, 4.16). The pancreas can be affected as an isolated organ in the same way as the spleen. When vasoconstriction resolves, progressive splenic enlargement may be seen on repeated CT examinations (Goodman and Aprahamian 1990). A sudden increase in intrasplenic blood inflow in an injured vasculature may be responsible for early rebleeding despite initial apparent hemostasis.

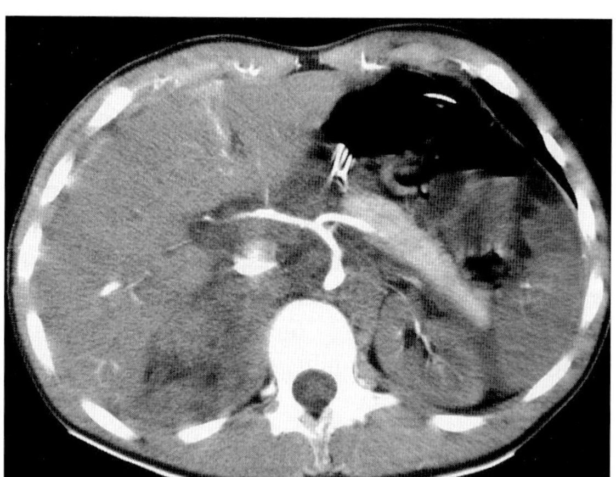

Fig. 4.15. A 44-year-old male ejected from his car after a collision. The patient was in shock at admission. Immediate CT shows no enhancement of the liver, spleen, and kidneys at the arterial phase, due to severe vasoconstriction, which also affects the aorta. Only the pancreas is normally enhanced. Massive retroperitoneal hematoma from right renal injury. Flattening of the IVC, surrounded by hematoma

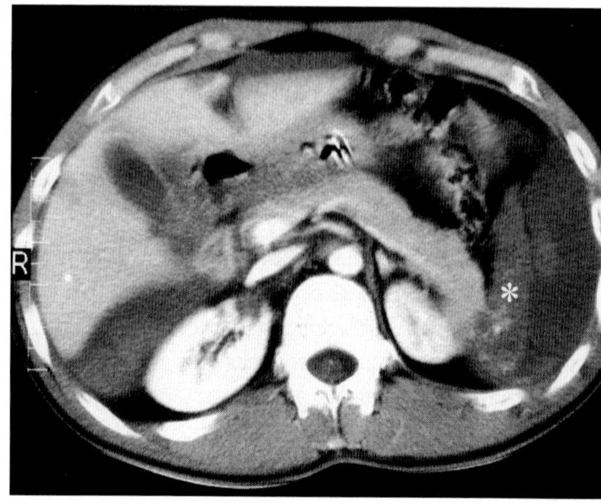

Fig. 4.16. A 32-year-old male admitted after blunt abdominal injury, involving deceleration forces. On contrast-enhanced CT, the spleen (*asterisk*) is nonenhanced due to arterial vasoconstriction and is displaced medially by massive perisplenic hemoperitoneum. Bleeding originated from mesenteric laceration

Other Pitfalls

Other pitfalls erroneously simulating splenic contusion include streak artifacts from gastric contrast and air, rib artifacts, beam hardening, and volume averaging artifacts. An elongated left lobe of the liver, which completely surrounds the splenic convexity, can mimic a perisplenic or subcapsular hematoma, using suboptimal CT technology (Cholankeril et al. 1984) (Fig. 4.17). Fluid in the posterior pleural sulcus can be mistaken for perisplenic hemorrhage. High densities in a rounded structure may correspond to hemorrhage in a preexisting splenic cyst.

4.5.1.4 Results

In early reports, CT was shown to carry a sensitivity and specificity of 95%–98% in the diagnosis of blunt splenic trauma, with the use of sequential scanning and long acquisition times (Wing et al. 1985; Jeffrey et al. 1981; Korobkin et al. 1978; Mall and Kaiser 1980; Sherck et al. 1984; Piekarski et al. 1980; Federle 1983, 1984; Federle et al. 1981). In the early literature, predominantly patients with an obvious clinical suspicion of splenic injury were scanned and CT was not evaluated as a systematic screening modality of trauma patients. However, the initial enthusiasm concerning selected patients with abdominal trauma was not denied by subsequent studies (Wing et al. 1985; Federle et al. 1987; Meredith and Trunkey 1988). The poor performance of CT when IV contrast was administered without a bolus injection was recognized early (Roberts 1996). CT had inferior results to radionuclide studies in such circumstances (Uthoff et al. 1983). Overall, CT was credited with an accuracy of 85% in detecting splenic injury and hemoperitoneum in the late 1980s (Shackford and Molin 1990). Today CT obtained with optimal technical parameters is able to evidence an intrasplenic contrast blush corresponding to acute pseudoaneurysm within the spleen in up to 8% of all patients with abdominal contusion, which eventually leads to arteriography and embolization in selected cases (Davis et al. 1998).

a

b

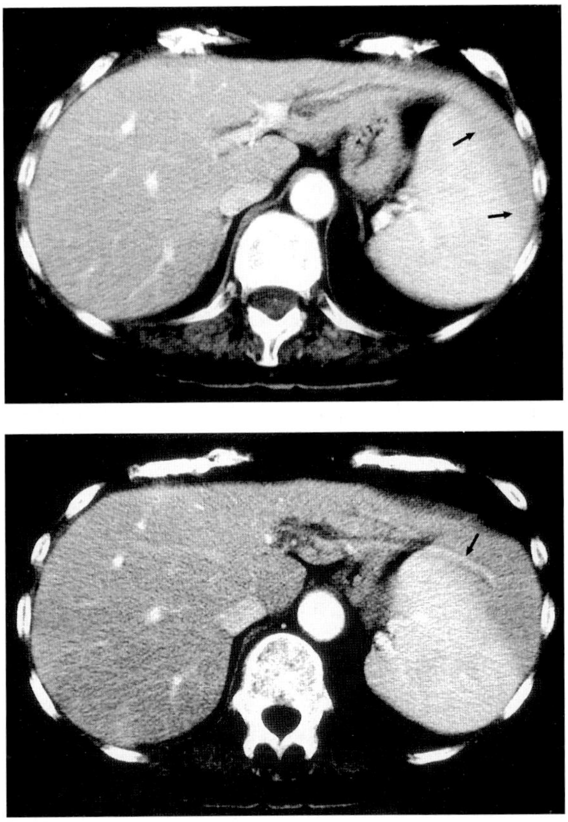

Fig. 4.17. **a** Elongated thin lateral segment of the left lobe of the liver, which might simulate a perisplenic hematoma (*arrows*). **b** A more cranial slice confirms continuity with the liver parenchyma and shows a portal branch (*arrow*) in the perisplenic liver segment

4.5.2 Ultrasound

Ultrasound (US) is less popular than CT in systematic screening of trauma patients. US may be used in patients to rule out an isolated splenic trauma after a minor trauma to the left upper quadrant, before discharge. High reliability in investigation of solid abdominal parenchyma, availability, short acquisition time and no ionizing radiation are well-known advantages of US, particularly in children. However, in large series of nonoperative management of splenic injury, US was used in only 4% of patients, whereas CT was used in 79%–87% and nuclear scan in 13%–21% in the USA and rarely in Europe (Cogbill et al. 1989; Koury et al. 1991).

4.5.2.1 Positive Signs

US signs of splenic injury include splenic enlargement, one or several zones of heterogeneous echogenicity, and intraparenchymal subcapsular or pericapsular fluid collection. Zones of contusion are delineated with an irregular contour, a round or wedged shape, and are generally hypo- or anechoic. Intrasplenic hyperechoic lines may be present in the acute posttraumatic phase. A double splenic contour suggests subcapsular hematoma. Initial collections of blood are hyperechoic and change rapidly within a few days into a hypo- or anechoic appearance (Fig. 4.18). US explores the capsule of the spleen with more confidence than CT and is able in some cases to demonstrate a localized interruption of the hyperechoic capsular line, even in the absence of parenchymal changes (Kuligowska et al. 1984). US is able to detect only minimal amounts of free abdominal fluid, but significant abdominal injuries can be present without hemoperitoneum (Chiu et al. 1997). Finally, a negative US examination does not eliminate splenic injury with absolute confidence (Krupnick et al. 1997).

4.5.2.2 Pitfalls

In about 12% of significant blunt splenic injury, no or minimal hemoperitoneum is seen on CT. Therefore US alone, relying only on the absence of hemoperitoneum as a screening method of trauma patients, is inadequate (Chiu et al. 1997; Ochsner et al. 2000).

US does not differentiate fresh clot from normal splenic tissue well (Benya and Bulas 1996). The

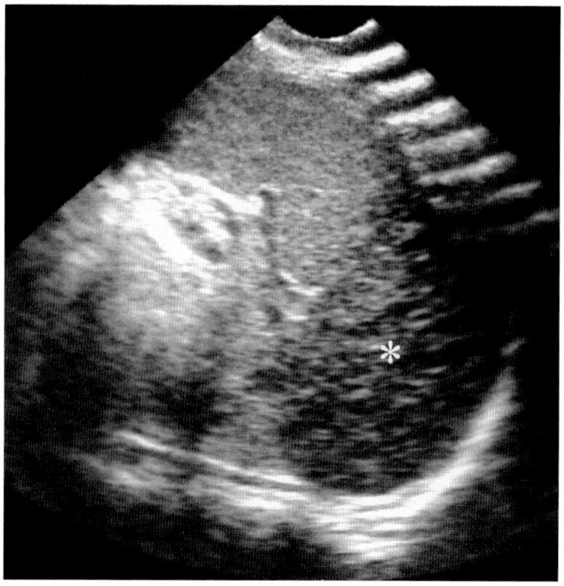

Fig. 4.18. A 16-year-old male admitted after a kick to the abdomen. Abdominal US shows a hypoechoic zone (*asterisk*) in the posterior part of the spleen, suggesting area of hemorrhage and contusion. No free intraperitoneal blood

elongated left lobe of the liver surrounding the spleen may simulate a perisplenic effusion on US, but is correctly identified on CT (Dunlop and Evans 1996). Splenic clefts are usually more evident in CT than on US. They are seen as a smooth disruption of the outline, and when combined with perisplenic fluid, may erroneously suggest rupture of the spleen (Mouaaouy et al. 1991; Benelli et al. 1992). US may be limited in the investigation of the upper pole of the spleen or of a horizontally oriented or a small sized spleen, or when the spleen is hidden cranially in the phrenic concavity. US examination is also limited by wound dressing, paralytic gastrointestinal ileus, tubes, and in the severely injured patient who is difficult to mobilize.

4.5.2.3
Results

US is sensitive in 86%–97% and specific in 71% in evidencing splenic contusion (Pignatelli et al. 1990; Becker et al. 1994). However, hemoperitoneum is shown accurately with US in 97% of patients, but the responsible splenic origin of bleeding is demonstrated in only 63%. Some reports underlined a high false-negative rate (up to 50%) of US compared to CT and difficulties in scanning with the probe when lower rib fractures were present and left upper abdominal quadrant pain limited the examination (Kaufman et al. 1984). US remains useful when CT is not available and in patients with benign trauma and localized pain in the left upper quadrant, without other posttraumatic abdominal findings (Asher et al. 1976). Repeated US examinations are more useful than repeated CT in evidencing splenic injury that was not visible at the initial examination (Siniluoto et al. 1992). US is also indicated as an alternative to CT during the follow-up observation period of conservative treatment. The examination can be easily repeated several times during the first 24–48 h after admission and later during the hospital stay, allowing for a closer imaging observation than CT, without the need for iodinated contrast medium injection and without radiation (Weill 1992). US is able to show the return to a normal echoic pattern of the contused zone and evidences a persistent echoic linear scar. Grade I splenic injuries require 7 weeks, grade II 9.5 weeks, and grade III 16 weeks for complete healing to be shown on US (Emery et al. 1999).

4.5.3
Magnetic Resonance Imaging

Magnetic Resonance Imaging (MRI) has obvious limitations in the investigation of acute trauma victims: equipment availability, patient transport, monitoring during the examination, and patient immobility are well-known limiting factors. Only limited experience is available in splenic trauma. MRI was credited with no significant advantage over CT in abdominal trauma in general. T1-weighted and gradient echo imaging were evaluated to be inferior to CT (McGehee et al. 1993). Multiplanar imaging is a definite but nonexclusive pictorial advantage of MRI. A pseudocapsule of the spleen is seen, produced by a chemical shift artifact between the spleen and surrounding fat, but recognition of this pseudocapsule is not absolutely necessary in evaluating splenic injury.

4.5.4
Arteriography

Splenic arteriography was decisive in the evaluation of splenic injury in the past, but became rapidly obsolete with the advent of CT and US. For many years arteriography was a reliable method to diagnose subcapsular hematoma, large intrasplenic contusion, posttraumatic vascular lesions, and contrast medium extravasation (Hebeler et al. 1982; Fisher et al. 1981; Haertel and Ryder 1979). Typical arteriographic findings include a parenchymal defect at the site of vascular interruption or contusion, intrasplenic blush of contrast medium, early venous return of an intrasplenic vein, displacement of intrasplenic arteries, enlargement of the spleen, detachment of the spleen from its contact with the diaphragm or the lateral abdominal wall, and spastic contraction of the splenic artery or branches (Berk and Wholey 1968; Love et al. 1968; Lundstrom 1970; Lepasoon and Olin 1971; Gold and Redman 1972). Causes of erroneous interpretation of splenic injury on angiography include the following: a false-positive diagnosis may be suggested by splenic fissure, a nonopacified polar artery, early venous return caused by massive injection of contrast medium, superposition of the gastric fundus, pancreatic tail, accessory spleen or left adrenal, and preexisting splenic infarct (Fig. 4.19). False-negative diagnoses are mainly due to minimal injury (Fig. 4.20). In a multicenter survey, arteriography is used today as a diagnostic modality in only 2% of patients treated by observation (Cogbill et al. 1989). Arteriography was re-introduced recently as a means of triage in groups with and without contrast extravasation: 50% of patients showing contrast extravasation were embolized, or otherwise would have been sent to surgery (Sclafani et al. 1991). However, contrast extravasation may be shown with more evidence on CT than on arteriography in some instances (Fig. 4.21). Contrast extravasation within the spleen does not necessarily mean that the bleeding will persist. A limited number of these patients could even be treated with bed rest alone, but close and strict clinical observation and imaging must be applied (Rees 1991). Transcatheter embolization of the splenic artery in patients with extravasation seen on angiography resulted in a successful outcome in 93% of the attempted cases (Sclafani et al. 1995).

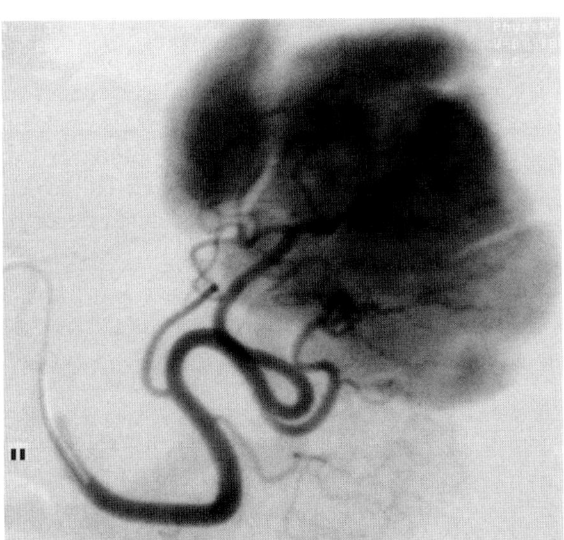

Fig. 4.19. Splenic arteriogram shows multiple splenic clefts or fissures at the splenic convexity, separating territories with different arterial supply. These fissures may simulate post-traumatic splenic fracture on cross-section imaging

4.6 Management

Management of splenic injury includes splenectomy, surgical or radiological spleen preserving techniques, and conservative treatment without any type of intervention.

4.6.1 Splenectomy

Splenectomy is the most efficient treatment of splenic injury. In almost all instances, penetrating splenic injury demands immediate surgical revision (Oreskovich and Carrico 1983). Splenectomy for acute splenic rupture, resulting from penetrating or blunt trauma, is advised in high-grade injury, shattered spleen, hilar disruption, avulsion of the vascular pedicle, multiple abdominal injuries requiring repair, massive blood loss, and wash-out coagulopathy (Wisner and Blaisdell 1992; Williams et al. 1997). Patients with a pathological splenomegaly, delayed splenic rupture, or spontaneous rupture with an unclear diagnosis most often undergo splenectomy. Elderly patients are also treated efficiently with splenectomy, as are trauma patients with head or spinal cord injuries precluding reliable physical examination. Splenectomy for trauma has an overall early mortality rate of 0%–5% or 12%–20%, including the most severe trauma cases and a morbidity rate of 13%–62% and a septic complication rate of 23% (Sekikawa and Shatney 1983; Hebeler et al. 1982; Steeke and Lim 1975). Splenectomy is the preferred surgical treatment in patients with HIV infections, even when minor-grade injury is present (Odom et al. 1991).

4.6.2 Overwhelming Postsplenectomy Infection

Overwhelming postsplenectomy infection (OPSI) was recognized in the early 1950s as a potentially late lethal complication from splenectomy in chil-

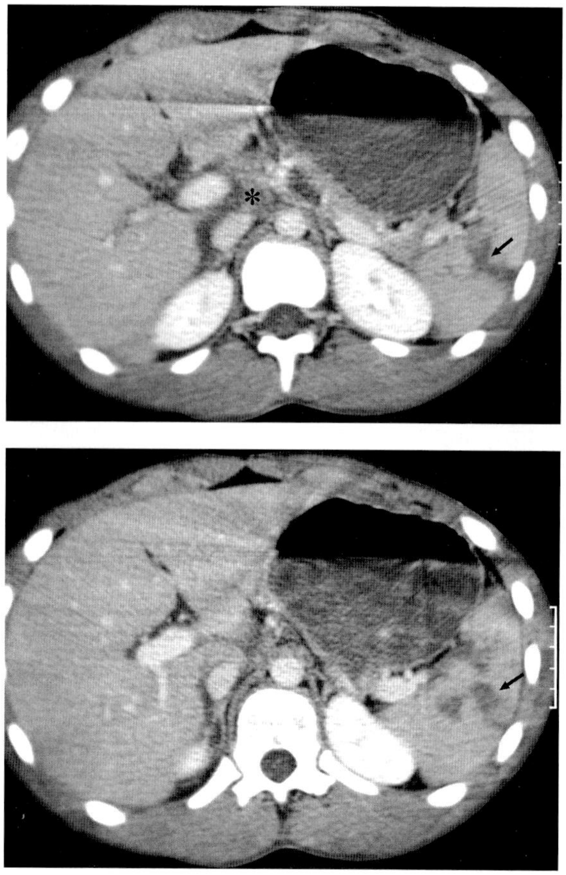

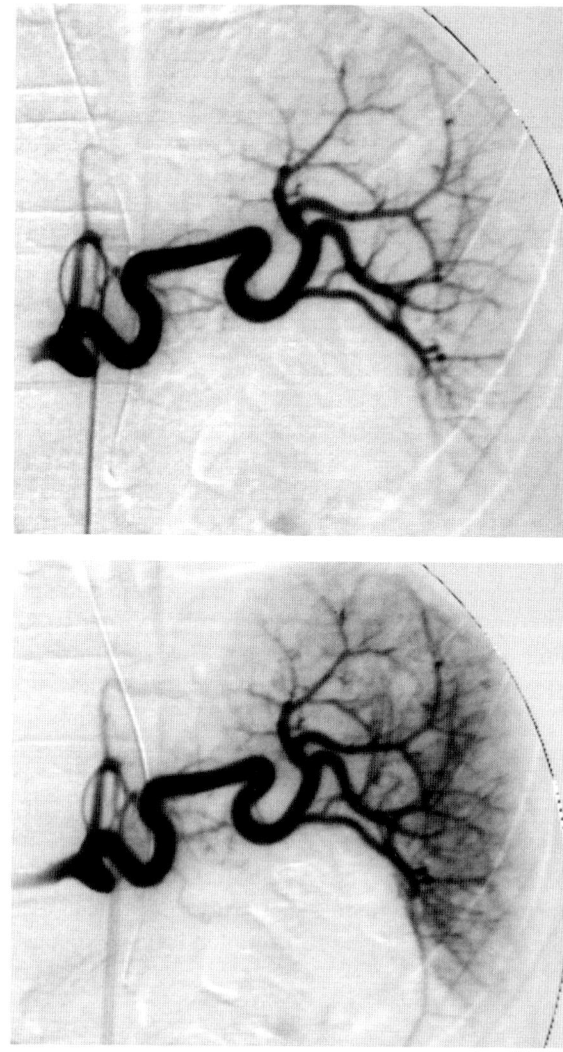

Fig. 4.20a–d. A 16-year-old male admitted after a traffic accident. **a, b** CT shows several hypodense areas of splenic contusion (*arrow*) and pericaval hematoma extending in the porta hepatis (*asterisk*) **c, d** Splenic arteriography shows moderate displacement of arterial branches in the upper pole. Hepatic arteriography had shown no vascular injury of hepatic vessels

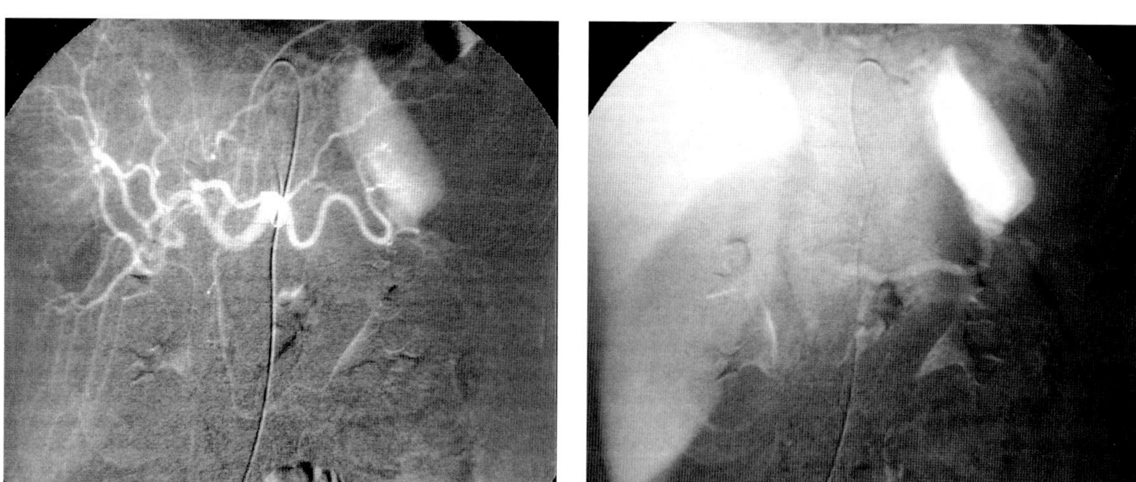

Fig. 4.21a, b. Same patient as in Fig. 4.6. **a, b** Celiac arteriography obtained immediately after CT shows compression and medial displacement of the spleen by a hematoma, but fails to demonstrate splenic contrast-medium extravasation, obvious on CT

dren, and challenged the rationale of systematic splenectomy (King and Shumacker 1952). This syndrome is characterized by fulminant pneumonia and meningitis, disseminated intravascular coagulation and rapid death (Grinblat and Gilboa 1975; Robinette and Fraumeni 1977). The mechanism of inadequate postsplenectomy immune function was described in subsequent reports. The principal immunological functions of the spleen concern clearance of antigens, bacteria and blood cells, by stimulation of phagocytosis and pinocytosis, production of IgM and opsonins (Constantopoulos et al. 1973; Claret et al. 1975; Dickerman 1976; Likhite 1976; Sullivan et al. 1978; Hosea et al. 1981; Downey et al. 1987; Traub et al. 1987). Splenectomy in children was shown to be followed in 4%–5% of patients by overwhelming postsplenectomy sepsis, with a mortality rate of 2%–3% (Singer 1973). Depending on the indication of splenectomy, mortality resulting from OPSI was 0.6% for splenectomy carried out for trauma, but 10% in hematological disorders. Subsequent observations have shown that complications from the postsplenectomy state occur in adults as well (King and Shumacker 1952; Singer 1973; Sekikawa and Shatney 1983). Early and late morbidity and mortality resulting from the asplenic state has been reported to be considerably more prevalent than in the population at large (Green et al. 1986; Pimpl et al. 1989; Sherman 1980; Di Cataldo et al. 1987; Singer 1973; Hebeler et al. 1982; Sekikawa and Shatney 1983). The risk of septicemia resulting from splenectomy done for trauma is estimated to be 140 times higher than in the general population (Green et al. 1986). In adults, incidence of OPSI is 0.3%–1% of splenectomies for trauma, with a mortality rate of 50%–80% (Singer 1973; Di Cataldo et al. 1987; Luna and Dellinger 1987). An incidence as high as 9% early serious infection with a mortality rate of 62% was reported during hospitalization for splenectomy done for multiorgan injury. Associated injuries to the pancreas, colon or central nervous system had a significantly increased risk of early sepsis, but only 2% of patients with isolated splenic injury had sepsis (Malangoni et al. 1984). Frequently found organisms are *Streptococcus pneumoniae*, *Neisseria meningitidis*, *Haemophilus influenzae*, *Escherichia coli*, *Staphylococcus aureus*, and *Pseudomonas*. Although the risk of dying from sepsis is relatively small (<1%), it is firmly established and can be prevented by spleen-preserving therapy. Immediate postsplenectomy administration of polyvalent pneumococcal vaccine is recommended (Caplan et al. 1983).

Furthermore, a survey of American veterans has shown a significant excess mortality not only from pneumonia, but also from ischemic heart disease following splenectomy. Myocardial ischemia could be related to thrombocytosis and hypercoagulability (Robinette and Fraumeni 1977).

4.6.3 Spleen-Preserving Techniques

4.6.3.1 Splenorrhaphy

Conservative management of splenic injury can be carried out with or without surgical revision in blunt trauma. The term "splenorrhaphy" designates all spleen-preserving interventions from topical packing, capping, wrapping, application or injection of glue or other local hemostatics (collagen fibrin) to splenic mesh wrapping (Ratner et al. 1977; Buntain and Lynn 1979; Strauch 1979; Weinstein et al. 1979). These alternative techniques, including partial splenectomy, have largely replaced total splenectomy whenever possible. Ligation of the splenic artery is another hemostatic spleen-preserving surgical technique (Andersson et al. 1985). Recently, high-intensity focused ultrasound (HIFU) was shown to induce hemostasis at adjustable depth in the spleen. HIFU could be used operatively and also in patients treated without surgery (Vaezy et al. 1999).

Today celioscopy, although not used as a routine procedure in trauma, may have a diagnostic role as an adjunct to CT in some patients, with incomplete or dubious findings or discrepant clinical and imaging findings. Celioscopy may also detect occult bowel injury or ongoing bleeding (Townsend et al. 1993). Direct observation, splenorrhaphy, and salvage of intraperitoneal blood with autotransfusion can be performed with celioscopy without the need for open surgery (Keramidas 1979; Sherman 1980; Traub and Perry 1982; Feliciano et al. 1985; Salvini 1993; Smith et al. 1993; Koehler et al. 1994; Poulin et al. 1995; Orcalli et al. 1998).

Splenorrhaphy is employed in 46%, splenectomy in 46%, and partial splenectomies based on vascular supply in 9% of cases in a recent analysis of 4076 patients (Christo and Didio 1997). Other reports confirmed that splenorrhaphy is applicable in 50%–70% of the patients with splenic hemorrhage and carries a limited risk of rebleeding when the spleen is fully mobilized and carefully inspected during repair (Feliciano et al. 1985, 1990; Ivatury et al. 1993). Intraoperative splenic injury is also preferentially treated by splenorrhaphy, as splenectomy performed for intraoperative rupture carries a higher mortality and morbidity rate than an elective procedure (Kremer et al. 1995). Splenorrhaphy has rare complications, but also has limitations and may fail in arresting splenic hemorrhage in up to 5%, necessitating conversion to splenectomy (Waninger et al. 1994). Experience with absorbable mesh wrapping is necessary to avoid rebleeding and other complications (Sondenaa et al. 1994).

In order to prevent OPSI after total splenectomy, surgeons have implanted small splenic fragments on the peritoneum between two layers of an omental pouch. These nodules of splenosis grow, increase in size, and are supposed to resume normal splenic function, as shown by IgM and tuftsin level as well as radioisotope and histological studies (Widman 1984; Tricario et al. 1993). However, heterotopic autotransplantation of the spleen does not show unequivocal results. Despite reimplantation of splenic fragments following splenectomy, cases of fatal postsplenectomy infection were described. In 1991, 18 such cases were reported in the literature (Michalski et al. 1991).

Overall, in longitudinal studies, no adverse outcome was noted during progressive change from splenectomy to splenorrhaphy and conservative nonoperative management (Morrell et al. 1995).

4.6.3.2
Hemostatic Arterial Embolization

Transcatheter hemostatic arterial embolization is a spleen-preserving hemostatic technique that can be carried out in selected patients as an alternative to surgical spleen-preserving operation (Chuang and Reuter 1975) (see also chapter 22 Arterial Lemostatic embolization in abdominal injuries). Indications are based on focal contrast-medium extravasation seen on CT. Helical CT correctly predicts extravasation seen on splenic arteriography and the need for hemostatic arterial embolization (Shanmuganathan et al. 2000). Angiography of the splenic artery confirms with confidence a pseudoaneurysm, an arteriovenous fistula, arterial thrombosis, disruption of an arterial branch, transcapsular stagnant or free diffusion of contrast medium (Fig. 4.22). Selective embolization by a femoral or sometimes axillary or brachial approach without need for subsequent splenic surgery is obtained in 93% of cases (Hagiwara et al. 1996) (see also Chap. 22,). In one study, in 8% of patients, an intrasplenic blush of contrast was seen on CT and confirmed to be a pseudoaneurysm on arteriography; 20 of 26 patients were successfully embolized, and 6 underwent splenectomy for technical failure of embolization (Davis et al. 1998). Hemostatic arterial embolization, being part of the initial management protocol and based on extravasation seen on CT or angiography, is successful in 87%–95% (Sclafani et al. 1991, 1995; Hagiwara et al. 1996). Patients with coagulation abnormalities such as intravascular coagulation can still be treated selectively with arterial embolization, but arteriography must document complete and permanent vascular occlusion at completion of the procedure (Ceelen et al. 1997). On postembolization examinations, CT shows splenic infarcts in two-thirds of patients after proximal embolization and in all cases after distal vaso-occlusion. Gas in the embolized area or in small arterial branches may be seen, particularly with Gelfoam embolization. Necrotic areas, liquefaction and air fluid level are suggestive of abscess formation (Killeen et al. 2001).

4.6.4
Nonoperative Conservative Treatment

Nonoperative management of splenic injury was implemented on a large clinical basis after recognition of septic complications caused by the asplenic state. Conservative treatment was first used in pediatric patients and subsequently in adults and was coincidental with the advent of reliable noninvasive splenic cross-section imaging techniques (Widman 1984; Cogbill et al. 1989; Longo et al. 1989; Pearl et al. 1989; Haller et al. 1994; Becker et al. 1994; Schweizer et al. 1992; Ashlock et al. 1998b; Garber et al. 1996; Mirvis et al. 1989; Godley et al. 1996; Barrett et al. 1983; Mucha 1986; Mucha et al. 1986; Resciniti et al. 1988; Zucker et al. 1984).

4.6.4.1
Inclusion Criteria

Selection criteria for nonoperative management are based on clinical findings and on results of CT imaging. Accepted inclusion criteria are:

- A hemodynamically stable patient with a systolic blood pressure more than 90 mmHg. Any patient, who remains hemodynamically stable after transient hypotension, can be managed nonoperatively, when no blush or contrast extravasation is seen on CT (irrespective of CT grading of splenic injury).
- No or a minimum of blood transfusion (less than 2 or 4 units).

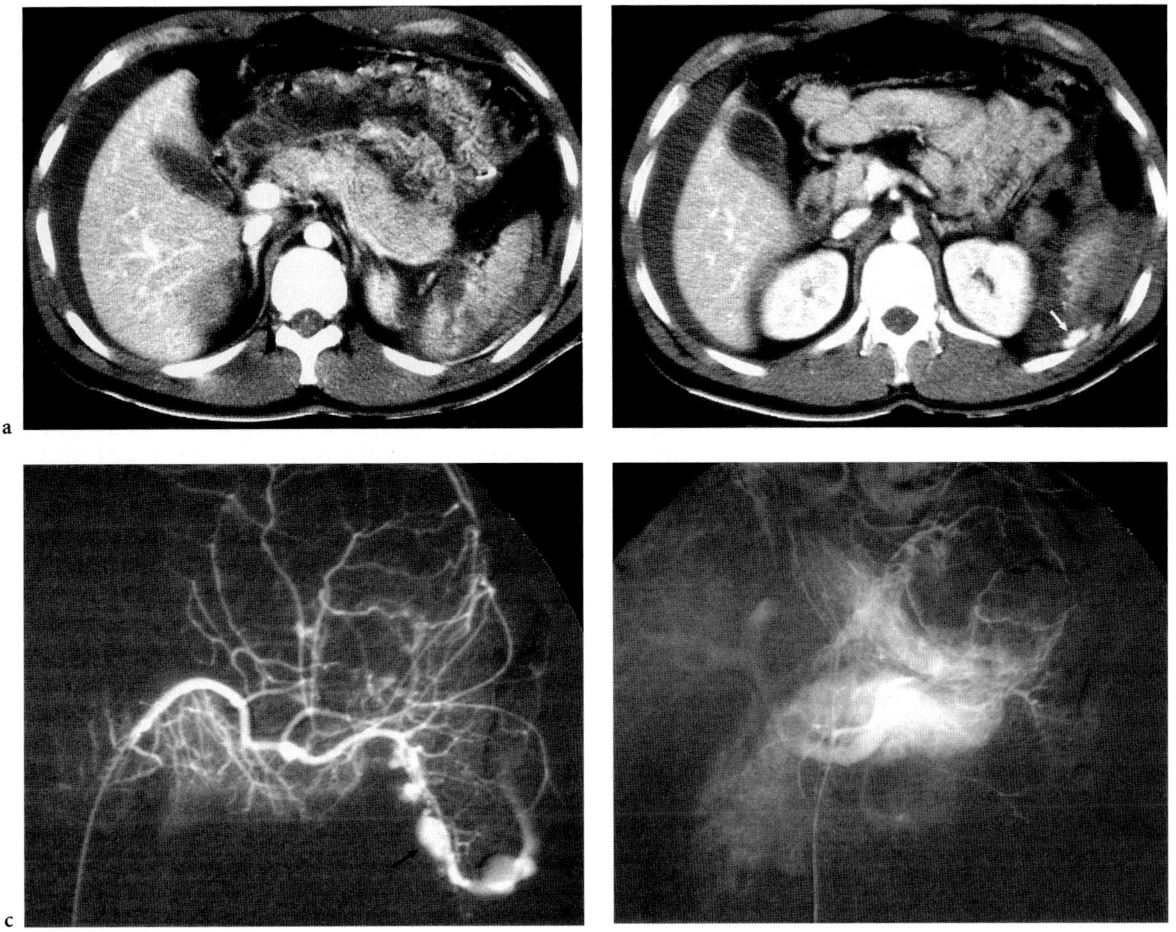

Fig. 4.22a–d. A 30-year-old male admitted after abdominal contusion. **a** Contrast-enhanced CT shows splenic contusion and moderate perisplenic hematoma. **b** Contrast medium has accumulated in the perisplenic space. **c** Splenic arteriography shows contrast extravasation (*arrow*) at the lower pole of the spleen and poor recognition of normal intrasplenic vasculature due to severe vasoconstriction. **d** Hemostatic embolization was obtained by injection of polyvinyl alcohol particles (500–700 μm)

- No peritoneal irritation.
- No free intraperitoneal air and no other documented or suspected abdominal injury needing surgical repair.
- Hematocrit stability should be obtained in 2 days.
- Low energy and localized traumatic impact.
- Opportunity for close observation and repeated imaging during hospital stay and after discharge must be given.
- Patient compliance is mandatory during conservative treatment and after discharge.
- Patients with associated head injury and neurological impairment can be safely included in a nonoperative management trial of blunt splenic injury in adults (Keller et al. 1996; Archer et al. 1996).
- Association of hepatic or renal injury that by itself does not require surgical hemostasis is not an exclusion criterion (Sartorelli et al. 2000).
- CT grading finally plays a relative role in the inclusion criteria of an individual patient. Patients with high-grade injury, but who remain hemodynamically stable, can be included in a conservative trial rather than systematically undergoing surgery. There is no consistent correlation between the splenic injury grade and success of conservative treatment. Statistically, minor injury and minimal hemoperitoneum has the tendency to do better than more severe cases, but experience shows that trivial splenic injury may suddenly bleed, whereas high grades may definitely do well without intervention (Fig. 4.23). A large nonperfused area in the spleen or a small localized intrasplenic blush in a stable patient is not a systematic indication for prompt intervention in our experience and other reports, but may require arteriography and embolization, as an alternative to urgent intervention

(Sclafani et al. 1991; Schurr et al. 1995; Gavant et al. 1997; Kos et al. 1999). Vascular injury at the splenic hilum or a severely shattered spleen are relative contraindications to expectant management.

- Patients without regular strenuous physical activity. Athletes or intense labor workers prone to trauma should be excluded from conservative management.
- Although age over 55 years was shown to carry a high failure rate of conservative treatment, more recent studies have shown that age over 55, abnormal Glasgow coma score, and transient hypotension are not determinant criteria of patient selection for a nonoperative trial (Falimirski and Provost 2000; Barone et al. 1999; Godley et al. 1996; Smith et al. 1996; Gaunt et al. 1999; Krause et al. 2000; Cocanour et al. 2000).
- In exceptional circumstances, neonates with splenic rupture can be included (Bickler et al. 2000).
- Although a diseased spleen or splenomegaly is a contraindication to conservative management, nonoperative management was successful in injured spleens with infectious mononucleosis with careful observation (Gauderer et al. 1989). Patients with multiple injuries of plain abdominal organs can be included in nonoperative management without increasing morbidity significantly (Sartorelli et al. 2000).

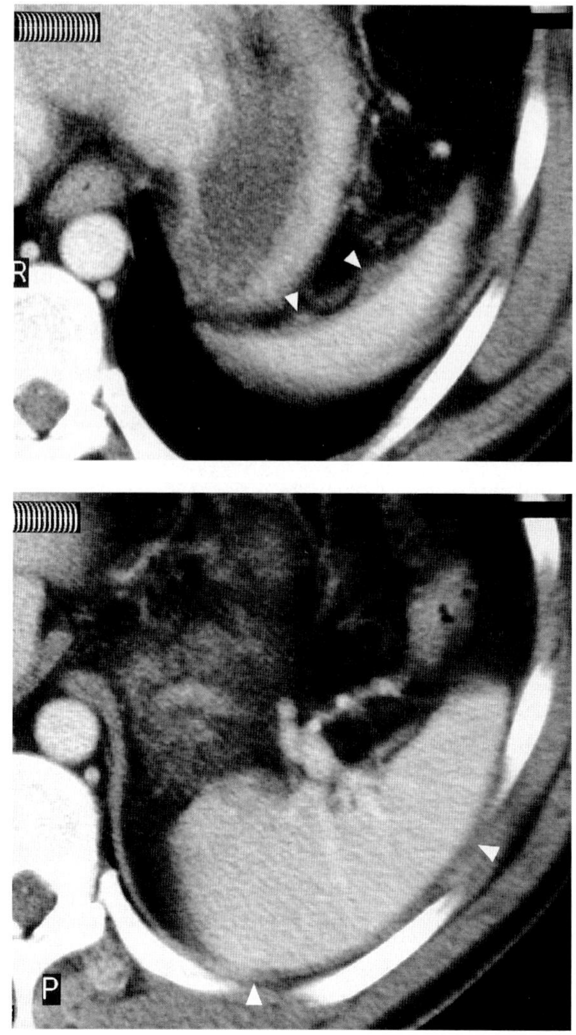

Fig. 4.23. a, b Teenager admitted after a motorcycle accident. CT at admission shows a minimal perisplenic effusion (*arrowheads*) without subcapsular or intrasplenic injury. Six hours later, the patient went in shock. Splenic laceration was found at laparotomy, treated by splenectomy

4.6.4.2
Results

Even before the advent of helical and multidetector CT technology, it was well established that a large number of blunt splenic injuries could be managed conservatively in children and adults. Figures of 87% of nonsurgical management are usually reported in large pediatric series. However, 23% of these patients required blood transfusions and splenectomy became necessary in 4% due to persistent bleeding or rebleeding. Stay in the intensive care unit is not necessarily required during observation of the most benign splenic injuries and hospital stay can be limited to 1 week in these cases. Reports that consider only grade I injury for conservative treatment showed an inclusion rate of only 12% (Olivero et al. 1994b). In adults, results tend to be similar to the pediatric experience: 87% of patients could be included in nonoperative management, but 13% required surgery for ongoing splenic hemorrhage. Overall, fewer blood transfusions were noted compared to the surgical group, no death and no missed abdominal injury was noted in the group of patients diagnosed with CT (Elmore et al. 1989). Some authors still oppose the pediatric age group to adults and claim an inclusion rate of children of 80% and only 25% or less in adults (Pachter et al. 1990; Cornwell 1993). It was shown that only 25% of adults with splenic injury could be included in a conservative treatment, when transfusion of four blood units was a criterion of exclusion (Koury et al. 1991; Umlas and Cronan 1991). An analysis of the literature showed that once an adult patient was given blood products, the advantages of nonoperative conservative management were lost, as the inherent risk of blood transfusions equaled that of postsplenectomy complications

(Beal and Spisso 1988; Luna and Dellinger 1987; Velanovich 1995).

Surveillance of a non-surgically treated patient consists of bed rest, daily physical examinations, serial hematocrit, nasogastric tube, and repeated imaging (Longo et al. 1989). Return to full activity is advised 3 months following trauma. Single-center experiences show that preservation of the spleen can be achieved in close to 100% of children and 90%–97% of adults (Villalba et al. 1990; Pearl et al. 1989; Berger and Kuhn 1981; Kaufman et al. 1984; Taylor et al. 1989; Brick et al. 1987; Davis et al. 1998; Buntain and Gould 1985; Smith et al. 1996; Guillon et al. 2000). In a large multicenter study, successful nonoperative management was 98% in children and 83% in adults ($p<0.05$) (Cogbill et al. 1989). However, in other large surveys, based on more than 2600 predominantly adult patients, the rate of nonoperative management was only 46% and splenectomy was performed in 43%. Operation was required later in 6% of adults and 0.4% of children. Reintervention for splenectomy was 3% in adults and 4% in children (Hunt et al. 1996). A review of the literature had shown that in those patients in whom conservative treatment has failed, the spleen could not be preserved in more than 75% of the cases (Nallathambi et al. 1988). Controversies remain, as in elderly patients, conservative management of splenic injury may fail more often than in the younger age group, probably due to changes that occur in the inner architecture of the spleen with age (Godley et al. 1996). Recent retrospective series still recognize a 30% failure rate of nonoperative management in adults, 86% of failures having a grade IV injury, whereas 87% with grade II or III in Buntain classification were successfully treated (Sanders and Civil 1999).

Serial CT examinations have shown that perisplenic fluid resolves completely in 1–4 weeks, and intrasplenic hematoma takes several months (Figs. 4.5, 4.24, 4.25). Complete return to normal appearance of the spleen may necessitate up to 4 months for low-grade injury and 1 year for multifocal and extended contusion (Schöpf et al. 1982; Benya and Bulas 1996; Roberts et al. 1993). In children, repeated CT examinations obtained during follow-up after nonoperative management showed that at 6 weeks 77% of grade I or II injures had completely resolved, but only 8% if trauma grading was III or IV. An average of 7 days of hospital stay in children was reported when conservative treatment was applied to single-organ splenic injury (Lynch et al. 1993). Complete healing, as demonstrated by CT, may require even much more time: 4 months for grade I and II injury, 6 months for grade III and up to 11 months for grade IV injury. Systematic follow-up CT examinations seem unnecessary and are not cost efficient in patients with clinically stable splenic injury (Lawson et al. 1995; Allins et al. 1996). Repeated CT findings affect conservative management only as an exception in children and adults, as sudden progression of the injury is rare, without clinical symptoms (Pranikoff et al. 1994; Benya et al. 1995; Lawson et al. 1995; Allins et al. 1996; Thaemert et al. 1997; Shafi et al. 1999). When worsening of splenic injury is noted, such as an increase in volume of hematoma, a vascular lesion, or an abdominal abscess, thorough reevaluation and treatment should not be delayed.

The quality-adjusted life expectancies (QALYs) in children were higher for observation than for splenorrhaphy or splenectomy (Velanovich and Tapper 1993). Patients should be followed clinically and with

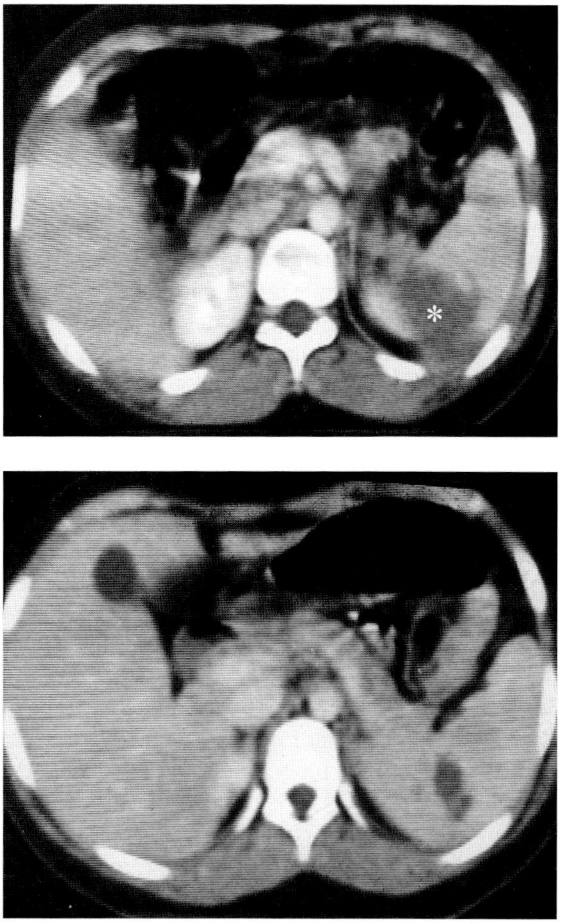

a

b

Fig. 4.24a, b. A 28-year-old male had a traffic accident. **a** CT at admission shows a large zone of contusion (*asterisk*) in the posterior part of the spleen, with possible rupture of the splenic capsule. Conservative management. **b** CT obtained 2 weeks following injury shows a small cyst-like residual intrasplenic lesion

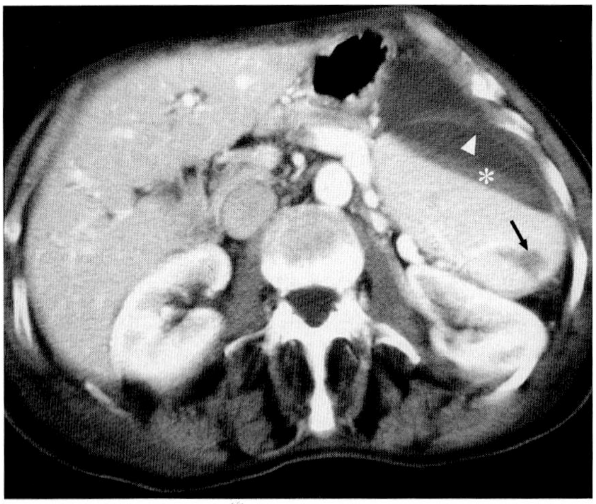

Fig. 4.25. A 57-year-old female had a car accident. CT at admission had evidenced intrasplenic contusion and subcapsular hematoma. On follow-up CT, small hypodense area of splenic contusion (*arrow*) and subcapsular hematoma, compressing the underlying splenic tissue. Fresh blood clots (*asterisk*) layer in a dependent location. The splenic capsule (*arrowhead*) is recognized by the subcapsular and perisplenic blood collection

cross-section imaging until scarring of the injured spleen is demonstrated. There is a good correlation between the rate of conservative nonoperative management and salvage rate of the spleen. In series containing a low nonoperative rate, definite preservation of the spleen is lower than in studies with a higher nonoperative rate (Williams et al. 1990). In patients with multiple blunt organ injuries, nonoperative treatment of splenic injury should be considered with caution, because of the risk of the higher failure rate in polytrauma patients (Rappaport et al. 1990).

4.6.5 Injury Grading Based on CT Findings

CT or US are unable alone to dictate the choice of management for splenic injury, but may contribute to the decision made on individual patient management (Conrad 1989; Lucas 1991; Wilson and Moorehead 1992; Raptopoulos 1994).

Many grading systems of splenic injury were described (see Chap. 27, "A Selection of Published Surgical and Radiological Classifications of Abdominal Injuries"). They contain four or five levels of severity (Shackford et al. 1981; Buntain et al. 1988; Resciniti et al. 1988; Mirvis et al. 1989; Scatamacchia et al. 1989; Mirvis and Shanmuganathan 1992; Schweizer et al. 1992; Becker et al. 1994; Moore et al. 1995). One classification also takes into account peritoneal effusion (Resciniti et al. 1988). Another grading considers devascularization and infarction (Ashlock et al. 1998b). The surgical classification given by Shackford considers splenorrhaphy as a treatment (Shackford et al. 1981). CT was shown to predict with accuracy the success of nonoperative conservative management, particularly in the papers in which the injury scaling system was described (Buntain et al. 1988; Resciniti et al. 1988; Cogbill et al. 1989) and in successfully selected patients (98% accuracy) for therapeutic laparotomy (86%) (Peitzman et al. 1986). However, many studies have shown that CT based on description of intrasplenic injury and grading systems is inaccurate in predicting patient selection for conservative management and in particular when none of the criteria considers intrasplenic blush of contrast material or contrast medium extravasation (Mirvis et al. 1989; Umlas and Cronan 1991; Smith et al. 1992; Becker et al. 1994; Kohn et al. 1994; Sutyak et al. 1995). Moreover, CT is inaccurate in predicting the blood transfusion frequency and volume needs in children included in nonoperative management (Ruess et al. 1995). When compared with surgical findings, two of the recently proposed CT grading systems were found to correlate only in 50% of the cases (Umlas and Cronan 1991). In another recent study, there was a clear correlation between the need for surgery and CT grading only when an optimal injection scan delay was considered, emphasizing the importance of CT technique (Ashlock et al. 1998b). Generally, most of grade IV and V splenic injuries using organ-injury scaling are treated by splenectomy, whereas lower grades are treated by splenorrhaphy or without surgery (Krahenbuhl and Berry 1994). Active hemorrhage, shown as contrast medium extravasation, is an absolute indication for treatment, either surgery or hemostatic arterial embolization, irrespective of the CT grading, and correlates best as a predictive criterion with success of conservative management (Federle et al. 1998). The ability of CT to show extravasation in the spleen was questioned, but actual CT technology has the potential to do as well as angiography (Sclafani 1994). Subcapsular hematoma observed on a single CT examination does not expose the patient to an increased risk of splenic rupture vs intraparenchymal injury and is not an isolated indicator of operative treatment (Black et al. 1992).

Success of conservative nonoperative management depends on clinical signs, young age, and Injury Severity Score rather than on injury grading by imaging (KOHN et al. 1994). The decision on whether surgical or conservative management should be adopted should not be based on CT imaging and CT grading alone, as it would lead to an overuse of splenectomy in high grades and an increased rate of delayed splenectomy in lower grades in symptomatic patients (BECKER et al. 1994). Although grading systems alone do not allow individual patient management, it is established that low-grade splenic injuries are not likely to be associated with other significant abdominal injury requiring surgical repair (FLAHERTY and JURKOVICH 1991).

4.7 Complications

Patients with surgical treatment who underwent either splenectomy or splenorrhaphy are usually not submitted to systematic imaging during follow-up, when clinical course is smooth.

CT and US should be used to monitor follow-up during conservative management of blunt splenic trauma. CT follow-up of splenic injury shows that all grades are able to return to an almost normal CT appearance when no intervention was performed. However, a late completely normal CT is noted in only 30%–44% of all patients and is more likely in moderate injury. Persistent cyst-like lesions, clefts, capsular retraction, and devascularized areas are seen more often in high-grade injury (PRANIKOFF et al. 1994; BLANE et al. 1999). Complications of splenic injury, which will be discussed below, are rebleeding, vascular lesions, hematoma, splenosis, and others.

4.7.1 Rebleeding

Before the era of CT examination of trauma patients, rebleeding or delayed rupture was highly overestimated and limited the acceptance of conservative therapy (MCINDOE 1932). Today, a 1% incidence of rebleeding requiring reoperation is anticipated after operative repair or partial splenectomy (BENJAMIN et al. 1976; OLSEN and POOLEY 1977; OLIVERO et al. 1994a). With nonoperative management, a rate of up to 6% of delayed bleeding occurring within the 1st week was reported (COCANOUR et al. 1998). Delayed splenic rupture does not necessarily occur only with major trauma treated conservatively without surgery. Minor injury, and particularly subcapsular, is more likely than central splenic hematoma to rupture with a delay (FARHAT et al. 1992; KLUGER et al. 1994a).

4.7.2 Posttraumatic Vascular Lesions

Pseudoaneurysm, arteriovenous fistula, or a combination of both may develop after organ-preserving management of posttraumatic splenic injury (Fig. 4.26). Their real frequency, which is unknown, may increase with generalized acceptance of conservative nonoperative management in which higher grades of splenic injury are included, and expose the patient to such complications (HIRAIDE et al. 1994; NOROTSKY et al. 1995; SUGG et al. 1995). Pseudoaneurysm, either single or multiple, is a well-known vascular complication following trauma and can occur in any incompletely sectioned artery. In the past, persistent intrasplenic pseudoaneurysm only rarely evolved to clinical significance, until occasional rupture had occurred, requiring emergency laparotomy and hemostatic splenectomy (MAHON and SUTTON 1985; HIRAIDE et al. 1994; SARIOGLU et al. 1996). Intense imaging at admission and during follow-up by CT, echo Doppler, or MRI will give a more precise indication on real frequency of splenic vascular lesions, but at present, only a few reports

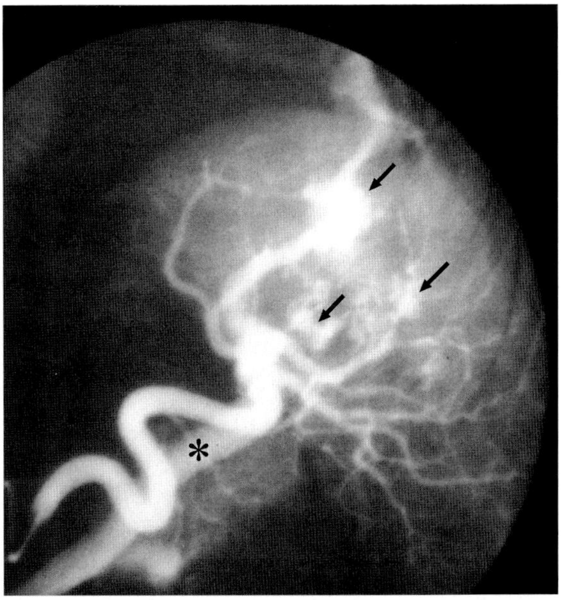

Fig. 4.26. Posttraumatic intrasplenic arteriovenous fistula with early venous return (*asterisk*) and several pseudoaneurysmal lesions (*arrows*). Treatment by selective arterial embolization

on imaging have been published (Davis et al. 1998; Nagar et al. 1997). Diagnosis can be established by CT with adequate contrast-medium enhancement, Doppler studies, or MRI, without the need of angiography. The fate of these lesions is still unknown and it is unclear if they might really favor delayed rupture of the spleen in all cases (Mahon and Sutton 1985). Delayed rupture of pseudoaneurysm is hypothesized to occur in 3%–46% of patients (Smith et al. 1989). Posttraumatic pseudoaneurysms and arteriovenous fistulas can also regress spontaneously and thrombose after several weeks or months, similarly to posttraumatic intrarenal or intrahepatic vascular lesions. The rate of spontaneous thrombosis is also unknown (Gow et al. 1996). Probably more systematic CT examinations with optimal technique of bolus injection would detect more of these lesions, allowing for preventive arterial embolization, before hemorrhagic complications arise (Norotsky et al. 1995). It is of major importance to note that almost 75% of false aneurysms of the spleen are detected only on follow-up CT examinations (Davis et al. 1998). Persistent arteriovenous fistulas probably have a lower risk of late bleeding than pseudoaneurysms, but may occasionally lead to high flow portal hypertension or acute myocardial ischemia (Sarioglu et al. 1996; Gunther et al. 1998). In practice, catheter arterial occlusion should be obtained only when the vascular lesion is persistent, increases in size, or is symptomatic (Henry et al. 1998; Nagar et al. 1997).

Selective arterial embolization of an intrasplenic pseudoaneurysm or arteriovenous fistula has only occasionally been reported (Chiarugi et al. 1995; Norotsky et al. 1995; James et al. 1996; Firstenberg et al. 1998; Patel et al. 1996; Davis et al. 1998; Salis et al. 1999). The presence of a splenic pseudoaneurysm during follow-up should be considered a predictor of failed nonoperative management, until more precise figures on their progression are available. Microcatheters and microcoils used as an occlusion agent provide a minimally invasive and effective treatment, preserving splenic tissue. Modern catheter and coil design makes it possible to reach any intrasplenic branch requiring embolization, even through a very tortuous splenic artery. In case of technical difficulties in microcatheterization, macrocoils can be placed in the proximal splenic artery at the splenic hilum. This technique can be valid in the acute phase after splenic trauma, but does not predict thrombosis of an intrasplenic pseudoaneurysm or arteriovenous fistula (Hagiwara et al. 1996).

Complications from selective intrasplenic embolization or proximal coil placement are infrequent. They include septicemia, splenic infarct, splenic abscess, rupture of the spleen, perisplenic or left pleural effusion, adynamic ileus, local pain, low grade fever, nausea, and vomiting.

4.7.3
Posttraumatic Hematoma or Abscess

An intrasplenic or subcapsular hematoma that is undrained may incompletely resolve and evolve into a chronic blood collection, also called chronic pseudocyst.

Posttraumatic splenic pseudocysts are frequently observed in some reports after nonoperative treatment and are almost absent in others depending on intensity of imaging during follow-up. Large subcapsular hematomas are prone to form such a persistent fluid collection, which contains brownish old blood (Figs. 4.27, 4.28). Isolated case reports advocate open or celioscopic decapsulation as treatment (van der Zee 1999). At surgery, a chronic hematoma may have an invasive, apparently neoplastic character (Lorimer 1964). Pathology shows a well-encapsulated mass, with a thick fibrous wall around the organized hematoma within or around the spleen, without epithelial cell lining. Pathology suggests that delayed rupture from an organized chronic hematoma is not more frequent than rupture of a pseudocyst of pancreatic origin, although it may occur several years after injury (Clark et al. 1975; Dondelinger and Fettes 1981). In some patients, it may not be possible to differentiate between a hemorrhagic pancreatic pseudocyst and a chronic hematoma. Chronic splenic hematomas may enlarge due to an osmotic pressure gradient more than 1 month after injury and become symptomatic and are known as chronic expanding hematoma (Grosdidier et al. 1974; Reid et al. 1980). Usual surgical treatment is conservative, with pseudocystectomy, which preserves the cyst wall and the spleen (Pachter et al. 1993). A conservative laparoscopic treatment of posttraumatic splenic cyst was advised in selected patients (Targarona et al. 1995). Splenectomy is the treatment of choice for cysts with unknown cause or uncertain diagnosis (Wolters et al. 1990). Surgery can be replaced by percutaneous aspiration or short-term catheter drainage with US or CT guidance (Gorg and Schwerk 1991) (Fig. 4.29). A chronic persistent intrasplenic hematoma may occasionally exhibit a calcified wall, which is indicative of its nature (Dreze 1993).

When a conservative management of chronic hematoma or pseudocyst is adopted, imaging should

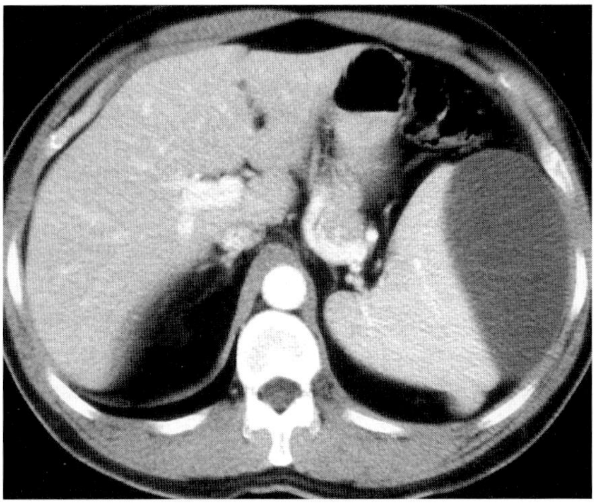

Fig. 4.27. A 45-year-old male, who had splenic contusion which was treated conservatively. CT obtained 3 weeks after injury shows a subcapsular splenic fluid collection, corresponding to a chronic hematoma. Note a thin, normal splenic capsule

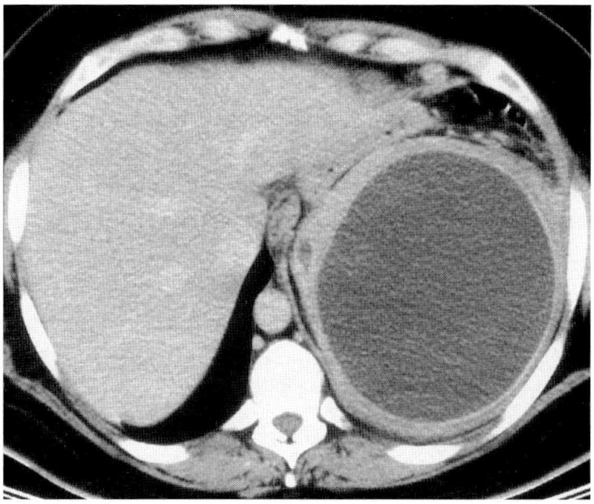

Fig. 4.28. A 54-year-old male who was managed conservatively for splenic contusion. CT obtained during follow-up showed a large fluid collection, limited by a thick wall that has almost completely replaced the normal splenic tissue. Old blood was aspirated form this chronic posttraumatic hematoma

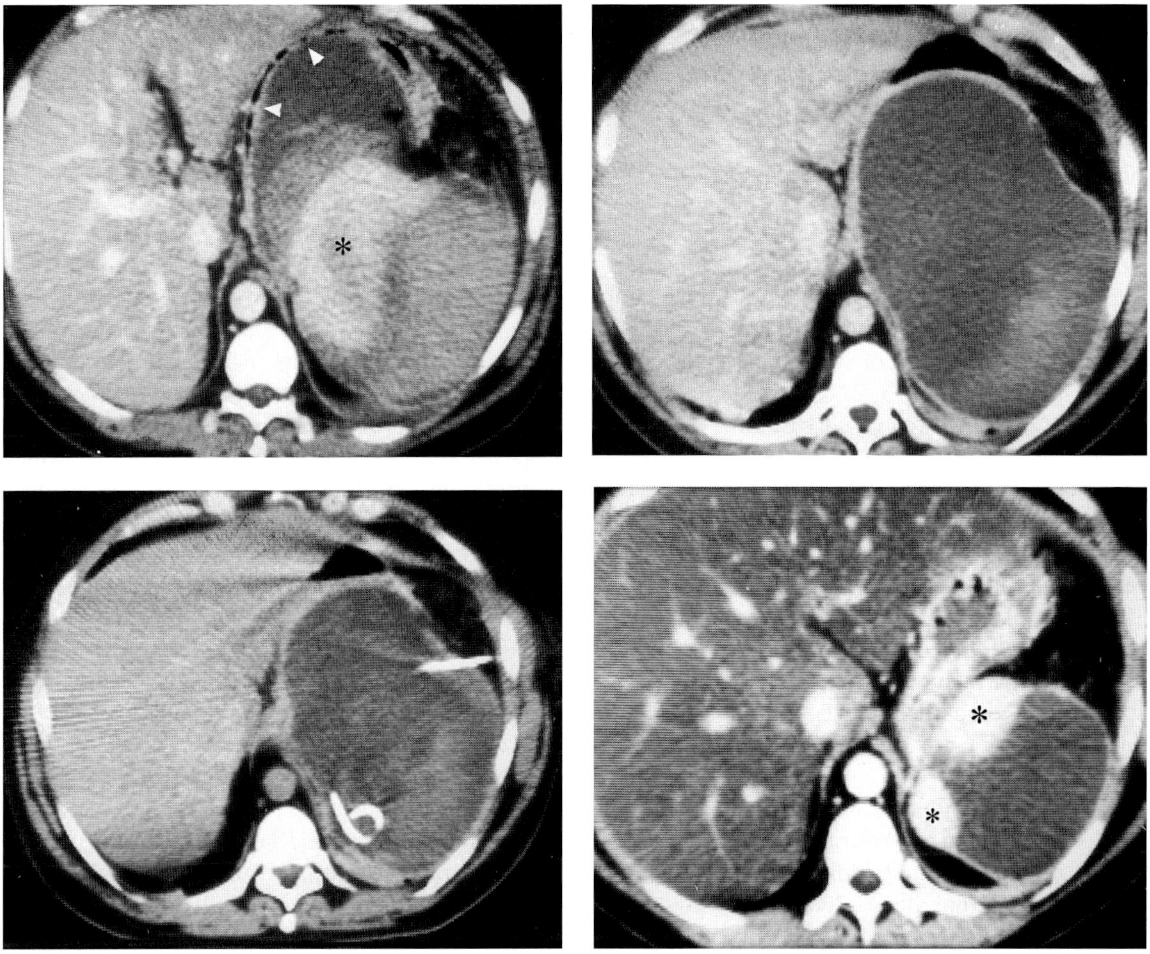

a b

c d

Fig. 4.29a–d. A 19-year-old male who had a car accident. A large subcapsular hematoma was present at admission. **a, b** Serial CT examinations showed progressive liquefaction of the dense hematic content (*arrowheads*). Normal splenic tissue (*asterisk*) and enlargement of the hematoma, compressing the stomach. **c** Serial percutaneous aspirations of chronic blood were performed with a 8-F catheter under CT guidance, until compression of the stomach was relieved (**d**) demonstrate regression and persistent healing after percutaneous aspiration or short-term catheter drainage (DONDELINGER and FETTES 1981). Posttraumatic splenic abscess that develops after spleen-preserving treatment can be drained by percutaneous catheter placement. Unilocular splenic abscesses have a better prognosis than multiloculated collections (SHAH et al. 1987).

4.7.4 Splenosis

4.7.4.1 Abdominal

Splenosis, as mentioned in "Polysplenia and Nodules of Splenosis," is an autonomous implantation and subsequent growth of fragments of splenic tissue that result from rupture of the splenic capsule. Nodules of splenosis are frequently found in the splenic space or on the peritoneal surface of any abdominal compartment, following posttraumatic splenic laceration and splenectomy, and also after conservative nonoperative treatment of splenic injury. Incidence following splenectomy for trauma is 26%–67% (LIVINGSTON et al. 1983; KIROFF et al. 1983; LUDTKE et al. 1989). Surgeons also deliberately implant small splenic fragments on the peritoneum during splenectomy to prevent OPSI (COONEY et al. 1979). Normal function of such implanted nodules of splenosis was proven by nuclear medicine studies, levels of IgM and tuftsin, and clearance of peripheral blood from Howell-Jolly bodies, red and white blood cell count, erythrocyte surface vacuoles, and complement and cutaneous skin testing with recall antigens. However, there is no irrefutable proof that reimplantation of splenic fragments provides an efficient resistance to infections after splenectomy (MOORE et al. 1983; LUDTKE et al. 1989). Nodules of splenosis can be isolated or be massively and widely spread in the abdomen, pelvis, thorax or limbs, as demonstrated by nuclear medicine studies (VENTO et al. 1999).

Usually these nodules of splenosis, in an abdominal or thoracic location, increase moderately in size and remain asymptomatic. Abdominal pain was reported for intra- or retroperitoneal locations of nodules of splenosis (SERVADIO et al. 1994). Others reported complications that include a mass effect, gastrointestinal bleeding, intestinal or urinary obstruction, splenic nodule infarction due to torsion, and spontaneous or posttraumatic bleeding (PRASAD and BECK 1968; BOCK et al. 1991; HEIDER et al. 1998; KATZ 1998; AL-AHMADI et al. 1998; SIKOV et al. 2000). Nodules of splenosis show as single or multiple round or oval masses that are enhanced after contrast administration, similar to the spleen (MENDELSON et al. 1982). Some abdominal nodules of splenosis could be mistaken for a malignant tumor of the liver, kidney, adrenal, appendix, pelvis and others, or for peritoneal metastases, hemangioma, mesothelioma, endometriosis, or an accessory spleen, and are erroneously investigated in depth or even operated upon (PRASAD and BECK 1968; WATSON et al. 1982; MBAKOP 1983; BOCK et al. 1991; YOSHIMITSU et al. 1993; SERVADIO et al. 1994; CHAGNAUD et al. 1998; HEIDER et al. 1998; KURTARAN et al. 1998; DEUTSCH et al. 1999; PIZARRO et al. 2000; STEIN et al. 2000). Among the late complications, intraperitoneal hemorrhage from a ruptured nodule of splenosis a few years to 22 years following initial splenic rupture was reported (CARREIRA et al. 1991; FEFERMAN and CRAMER 1991). Splenic tissue was demonstrated after splenectomy in the scrotum by nuclear medicine studies and was responsible for severe testicular pain. This finding should not be confused with a splenogonadal fusion, which is a rare congenital malformation resulting from fusion of splenic tissue with the left testicle, and rarely the ovary (CARRAGHER 1990; KOLESKI et al. 1999). Splenosis was also found after trauma treated with conservative treatment in the mesoappendix during appendectomy (AL-AHMADI et al. 1998). Intrahepatic splenosis probably results from portal seeding and may raise particular diagnostic problems by mimicking hepatic tumor such as adenoma, particularly when it occurs as an isolated finding or liver metastases in a patient with a primary malignancy (GRUEN and GOLLUB 1997; D'ANGELICA et al. 1998; FOROUDI et al. 1999). MRI shows hypointense signal on T1-weighted and hyperintense signal on T2-weighted images. After administration of SPIO, the lesions loose 50% of signal intensity but remain hyperintense compared to the hypointense normal liver (STORM et al. 1992; SERVADIO et al. 1994; DE VUYSERE et al. 2000).

4.7.4.2 Thoracic

After splenic rupture and left diaphragmatic laceration, fragments of spleen may migrate through a diaphragmatic tear and grow in the pleural or pericardial space, and mimic intrathoracic malignant pleural or pericardial tumor (OVNATANIAN 1966; KWAN et al. 1994). Tc 99m sulfur colloid liver–spleen nuclear medicine scans and clinical history are the clue to the correct diagnosis of intrathoracic splenosis, as for an abdominal location (MADJAR and WEISSBERG 1994; HARDIN and MORGAN 1994; KATRANCI et al. 1998). The combination of subcutaneous and thoracic nodules may be particularly suggestive of splenosis in a patient with a history of splenic injury (VELITCHKOV et al. 2000). Posttraumatic pseudoaneurysm of the thoracic aorta and thoracic splenosis can coexist and be incidentally discovered several decades after the injury (FIDVI et al. 1999). Scintigraphy has a high sensitivity in the detection of heterotopic splenosis, but serial nuclear medicine studies were not found helpful in children managed conservatively without taking into account clinical findings (BETHEL et al. 1992; GUNES et al. 1994). MRI appearance of splenosis is similar to that of normal splenic tissue (NORMAND et al. 1993). Fewer than 30 cases of thoracic splenosis were reported in 1999, with an interval between trauma and diagnosis of 3–42 years (BUCHINO and BUCHINO 1998; ROUCOS et al. 1990). Almost all were asymptomatic and were discovered on chest X-ray 9–32 years (mean, 16 years) after splenic injury. Occasionally, thoracic splenosis was demonstrated in association with symptoms of coronary heart disease (GAEDCKE et al. 1999). In 87% of the cases, a diagnostic thoracotomy was performed. However, the diagnosis should be established by imaging, including MRI, and careful patient history, as there is no reason to remove nodules of splenosis, unless they become symptomatic (BORDLEE et al. 1995). Fine-needle aspiration biopsy shows normal splenic tissue (RENNE et al. 1999).

4.7.4.3 Cerebral

Splenic tissue has also been found in remote sites such as the brain, probably as a result of hematogenous spread after posttraumatic fragmentation, and mimic brain tumor. Symptomatic cerebral splenosis was documented 15 years after posttraumatic splenectomy (RICKERT et al. 1998).

4.7.5 Other Complications

Postoperative complications following splenic intervention include wound infection, small bowel obstruction, abdominal abscess, pneumonia, pleural effusion or empyema, pancreatitis, urinary tract infection, bacteremia, and septicemia. Overall and late death and complication rates are similar in operative and nonoperative management of splenic trauma in children; conservative management does not worsen prognosis of splenic injury (SAUDEMONT et al. 1992). In rare cases, posttraumatic and apparently spontaneous rupture was reported as long as 2–5.5 years following trauma (DEVA and THOMPSON 1996; FERNANDES 1996). Compared to nonsplenectomized patients, postsplenectomy patients complain of an increased susceptibility to infections, accelerated exhaustion, and increased physical and mental weakness (KUNZ et al. 1990). When outcome of nonoperative management is considered, an increase in overall survival is noted compared to early laparotomy, but patients treated by observation alone carry a significantly increased risk of transfusion-related death (FELICIANO et al. 1992). Reinfusion of intraperitoneal blood using a cell saver obviates the risk of transfusion-related complications (WITTE et al. 1992).

Non-recognition of associated abdominal injuries requiring surgical repair is a permanent threat that is associated with nonoperative conservative treatment. However, the risk of missed abdominal injuries leading to late complications was minimal in children in a series studied retrospectively, with an 18% of associated abdominal injuries (MORSE and GARCIA 1994).

4.8 Conclusion

Special attention should be focused on the spleen on CT examinations obtained in trauma victims. Optimal contrast injection technique is mandatory for correct diagnosis of splenic injury. Intrasplenic blush of contrast extravasation should lead to angiographic evaluation and subsequent hemostatic embolization, preserving splenic tissue. A large number of patients who do not require surgical repair of associated abdominal lesions can be treated with nonoperative management of blunt splenic contusion. Contrary to the liver, some low-grade splenic injuries may suddenly profusely bleed, requiring urgent treatment. More intense imaging should be applied to demonstrate regression of injury and disclose vascular lesions, which can be treated by elective embolization.

References

Al-Ahmadi M, Brundage S, Brody F, Jacobs L, Sackier JM (1998) Splenosis of the meso-appendix: case report and review of the literature. J R Coll Surg Edinb 43:200–202

Allins A, Ho T, Nguyen TH, Cohen M, Waxman K, Hiatt JR (1996) Limited value of routine follow-up CT scans in non-

operative management of blunt liver and splenic injuries. Am Surg 62:883–886
Al-Obaidi SM (1989) Spontaneous rupture of the spleen due to metastatic carcinoma. Br J Clin Pract 43:385–386
Andersson R, Gustavsson T, Alwmark A (1985) Splenic artery ligation for traumatic rupture of the spleen. A case report. Acta Chir Scand 151:709–710
Archer LP, Rogers FB, Shackford SR (1996) Selective nonoperative management of liver and spleen injuries in neurologically impaired adult patient. Arch Surg 131:309–315
Asayama Y, Fukua T, Honda H et al (1998) Chronic expanding hematoma of the spleen by angiomyolipoma in a patient with tuberous sclerosis. Abdom Imaging 23:527–530
Asher WM, Parvins S, Virgilio RW et al (1976) Echographic evaluation of splenic injury after blunt trauma. Radiology 118:411–415
Ashlock SJ, Harris JH, Barron BJ (1998a) Traumatic rupture of an accessory spleen after prior splenectomy. Emerg Radiol 5:187–189
Ashlock SJ, Harris JH Jr, Kawashima A (1998b) Computed tomography of the spleen. Emerg Radiol 5:192–202
Asopa HS, Elhence IP (1965) Ruptured abscess of spleen. Indian J Med Sci 19:618–621
Autry JR, Weitzner S (1975) Hemangiosarcoma of spleen with spontaneous rupture. Cancer 35:534–539
Balachandran S, Leonard MH Jr, Kumar D, Goodman P (1994) Patterns of fluid accumulation in splenic trauma: demonstration by CT. Abdom Imaging 19:515–520
Baradaran S, Mischinger HJ, Bacher H, Werkgartner G, Karpf E, Linck FG (1995) Spontaneous splenic rupture during portal triad clamping. Langenbecks Arch Chir 380:266–268
Baumbach A, Brehm B, Sauer W, Doller G, Hoffmeister HM (1992) Spontaneous splenic rupture following acute Q fever. Am J Gastroenterol 87:1651–1653
Barone JE, Burn S, Svehlak SA et al (1999) Management of blunt splenic trauma in patient older than 55 years. Southern Connecticut Regional Trauma Quality Assurance Committee. J Trauma 46:87–90
Barrett J, Sheaff C, Abuabara S et al (1983) Splenic preservation in adults after blunt and penetrating trauma. Am J Surg 145: 313–317
Baudet R (1907) Ruptures de la rate. Med Prat 3:565–567
Beal SL, Spisso JM (1988) The risk of splenorrhaphy. Arch Surg 123:1158–1163
Becker MC, Brill R (1949) Hemorrhagic cyst of the spleen in a case of Gaucher's disease. Am J Surg 77:108–113
Becker CD, Spring P, Glättli A, Schweizer W (1994) Blunt splenic trauma in adults: can CT findings be used to determine the need for surgery. AJR 162:343–347
Benelli G, Bonardi R, Parziale M, Campari PF (1992) Role of echography in the differential diagnosis of accessory lobulations and small capsular traumatic fissures of the spleen. Radiol Med (Torino) 84:770–773
Benjamin CI, Engrav LH, Perry JF (1976) Delayed rupture or delayed diagnosis of rupture of the spleen. Surg Gynecol Obstet 142:171–172
Benya EC, Bulas DI (1996) Splenic injuries in children after blunt abdominal trauma. Semin Ultrasound CT MR 17:170–176
Benya EC, Bulas DI, Eichelberger MR, Sivit CJ (1995) Splenic injury from blunt abdominal trauma in children: follow-up evaluation with CT. Radiology 195:685–688
Berger PE, Kuhn JP (1981) CT of blunt abdominal trauma in childhood. AJR 136:105–110
Berk RN, Wholey MH (1968) Application of splenic arteriography in diagnosis of rupture of spleen. AJR 104:662–667
Berland LL, van Dyke JA (1985) Decreased splenic enhancement on CT in traumatized hypotensive patients. Radiology 156:469–471
Bernard SA, Jones BM, Scott WJ (1993) Intra-abdominal complications following prolonged cardiopulmonary resuscitation. Aust N Z J Surg 63:312–314
Bethel CA, Touloukian RJ, Seashore JH, Rosenfield NS (1992) Outcome of nonoperative management of splenic injury with nuclear scanning. Clinical significance of persistent abnormalities. Am J Dis Child 146:198–200
Bickler S, Ramachandran V, Gittes GK, Alonso M, Snyder CL (2000) Nonoperative management of newborn splenic injury. A case report. J Pediatr Surg 35:500–501
Black JJ, Sinow RM, Wilson SE et al (1992) Subcapsular hematoma as a predictor of delayed splenic rupture. Am Surg 58:732–735
Blane CE, Strouse PJ, Teitelbaum DH, Drongowski DH (1999) CT appearance of the spleen following conservative management of traumatic injury. Emerg Radiol 6:157–159
Blocker C, Brandon JC, Izenberg SD, Evankovich C, Teplick SK (1998) Posttraumatic enlargement of the spleen: a possible sign of delayed rupture. Emerg Radiol 5:263–265
Bock DB, King BF, Hezmall HP, Oesterling JE (1991) Splenosis presenting as a left renal mass indistinguishable from renal cell carcinoma. J Urol 146:152–154
Boioli F, Gattoni F, Tagliaferri B et al (1994) Blunt trauma of the spleen: the delayed rupture in computed tomography. Bildgebung 61:210–215
Bollinger JA, Fowler EF (1956) Traumatic rupture of the spleen with special reference to delayed splenic rupture. Am J Surg 91:561
Bonucci E, Piegaja (1964) Spontaneous rupture of the spleen during the course of occult Gaucher's disease. Arch It Anat Istol Pat 38:466–472
Bordlee RP, Eshaghi N, Oz O (1995) Thoracic splenosis: MR demonstration. J Thorac Imaging 10:146–149
Borgeat A, Tran-Thang C, Bachmann F (1989) Acute monoblastic leukemia complicated by fatal splenic rupture following initiation of chemotherapy. Schweiz Med Wochenschr 119: 227–229
Brick SM, Taylor GA, Ptter BM, Eichelberger MR (1987) Hepatic and splenic injury in children: role of CT in the decision for laparotomy. Radiology 165:643–646
Brissette M, Dhru RD (1992) Hodgkin's disease presenting as spontaneous splenic rupture. Arch Pathol Lab Med 116: 1077–1079
Broholm AL, Jans H (1995) Infectious mononucleosis and the risk of splenic rupture. Ugeskr Laeger 157:4579–4781
Buchino JJ, Buchino JJ (1998) Thoracic splenosis. South Med J 91:1054–1056
Buckman RF Jr, Piano G, Dunham CM, Soutter I, Ramzy A, Militello PR (1988) Major bowel and diaphragmatic injuries associated with blunt spleen or liver rupture. J Trauma 28:1317–1321
Bundy AL, Scott M, Druckman D, Siegal TL, Verdi TA (1985) Delayed and occult splenic rupture. Comput Radiol 9: 299–305
Buntain WL, Gould HR (1985) Splenic trauma in children and techniques of splenic salvage. World J Surg 9:398–409
Buntain WL, Lynn HB (1979) Splenorrhaphy: changing concepts for the injured spleen. Surgery 86:748–760

Buntain WL, Gould HR, Maull KI (1988) Predictability of splenic salvage by computed tomography. J Trauma 28: 24–34
Buzbee TM, Legha SS (1992) Spontaneous rupture of spleen in a patient with splenic metastasis of melanoma. A case report. Tumori 78:47–48
Cafferata EP, Mehta AC, Levine RA (1966) Gastric perforation caused by splenic sarcoma. Report of a case with associated hepatic schistosomiasis. Arch Intern Med 118:172–175
Caplan ES, Boltansky H, Snyder MJ et al (1983) Response of traumatized splenectomized patients to immediate vaccination with polyvalent pneumococcal vaccine. J Trauma 23:801–805
Carragher AM (1990) One hundred years of splenogonadal fusion. Urology 35:471–475
Carreira M, Conde R, Miranda C, Cerdeiras R, Curriaran MJ (1991) Posttraumatic hemoperitoneum: a rare complication of peritoneal splenosis. Rev Clin Esp 189:175–177
Caruso V, Hall WH (1984) Primary abdominal pregnancy in the spleen: a case report. Pathology 16:93–94
Ceelen W, de Waele J, Kunnen M, de Hemptinne B (1997) Non-operative management of a splenic laceration in a patient with the Proteus syndrome. J Accid Emerg Med 14: 111–113
Celebrezze JP Jr, Cottrell DJ, Williams GB (1998) Spontaneous splenic rupture due to isolated splenic peliosis. South Med J 91:763–764
Chadwick SJ, Huizinga WK, Backer LW (1985) Management of splenic trauma. The Durban experience. Br J Surg 72: 634–636
Chagnaud C, Champsaur P, di Costanzo V et al (1998) Peritoneal splenosis simulating a right retroperitoneal mass. J Radiol 79:1407–1409
Challis DE, Rew KJ, Steigrad SJ (1996) Choriocarcinoma complicated by splenic rupture: an unusual presentation. J Obstet Gynaecol Res 22:395–400
Chiarugi M, Goletti O, Pucciarelli M, Cioni R, Publisi A, Cavina E (1995) Post-traumatic intrasplenic pseudoaneurysm successfully managed by embolization. Injury 26:705–706
Chien RN, Liaw YF (1993) Pathological rupture of the spleen in hepatitis B virus-related cirrhosis. Am J Gastroenterol 88:1793–1795
Chiu WC, Cushing BM, Rodriguez A et al (1997) Abdominal injuries without hemoperitoneum: a potential limitation of focussed abdominal sonography for trauma (FAST). J Trauma 42:617–623
Cholankeril JV, Zamora BO, Ketyer S (1984) Left lobe of the liver draping around the spleen: a pitfall in computed tomography diagnosis of perisplenic hematoma. J Comput Tomogr 8:216–217
Christo MC, Didio LJ (1997) Anatomical and surgical aspects of splenic segmentectomies. Anat Anz 179:461–474
Chuang VP, Reuter SR (1975) Selective arterial embolization for the control of traumatic splenic bleeding. Invest Radiol 10:18–24
Claret I, Morales L, Mortner A (1975) Immunological studies in the postsplenectomy syndrome. J Pediatr Surg 10:59–64
Clark OH, Lim RC Jr, Margaretten W (1975) Spontaneous delayed splenic rupture: case report of five year interval between trauma and diagnosis. J Trauma 15:245–249
Clarnette TD, Beasley SW (1997) Handlebar injuries in children: patterns and prevention. Aust N Z J Surg 67:338–339
Cocanour CS, Moore FA, Ware DN et al (1998) Delayed complications of nonoperative management of blunt adult splenic trauma. Arch Surg 133:619–625
Cocanour CS, Moore FA, Ware DN, Marvin RG, Duke JH (2000) Age should not be a consideration for nonoperative management of blunt splenic injury. J Trauma 48:606–610
Cogbill TH, Moore EE, Jurkovich GJ et al (1989) Nonoperative management of blunt splenic trauma: a multi-center experience. J Trauma 29:1312–1317
Cohen SG, Pearlman CK (1967) Splenic rupture following foreign body perforation of the urinary bladder. Am Surg 33:830–834
Colarian J, Alousi M, Calzada R (1991) Splenic trauma during colonoscopy. Endoscopy 23:48–49
Cole WH, Walter L, Limarz LR (1949) Indications and result of splenectomy. Ann Surg 129:702
Conrad MR (1989) Blunt hepatic/splenic trauma in adults: CT based classification and correlation with prognosis and treatment. Radiology 173:285–286
Constantopoulos A, Najjar VA, Wish JB et al (1973) Defective phagocytosis due to Tuftsin deficiency in splenectomized subjects. Am J Dis Child 125:663–665
Cooney DR, Dearth JC, Swanson SE et al (1979) Relative merits of partial splenectomy, splenic implantation, and immunization in preventing post-splenectomy infection. Surgery 86:561–569
Cooray GH (1952) Spontaneous rupture of leukemic spleen. Br Med J 1:693–694
Coote JM, Eyers PS, Walker A, Wells IP (1999) Intra-abdominal bleeding caused by spontaneous rupture of an accessory spleen: the CT findings. Clin Radiol 54:689–691
Coughlin F, Aanning HL (1997) Delayed preservation of splenic trauma following colonoscopy. S D J Med 50:325–326
Cornwell EE III (1993) The role of nonoperative management of the injured spleen. J Nath Med Assoc 85:297–299
Cuckow P (1991) Spontaneous rupture: a new complication of splenosis. J R Coll Surg Edinb 36:186–187
D'Angelica M, Fong Y, Blumgart LH (1998) Isolated hepatic splenosis: first reported case. HPB Surg 11:39–42
Davis KA, Fabian TC, Croce MA et al (1998) Improved success in nonoperative management of blunt splenic injuries: embolization of splenic artery pseudoaneurysms. J Trauma 44:1008–1013
De Lajarte-Thirouard AS, Molina T, Audoin J et al (1999) Spleen localization of light chair deposition disease associated with sea blue histiocytosis revealed by spontaneous rupture. Virchows Arch 434:463–465
Delany HM, Janson RS (1981) Abdominal trauma: surgical and radiologic diagnosis. Springer, Berlin Heidelberg New York, pp 126–127
Derbekyan VA, Pham C, Emond C, Novales Diaz JA, Lisbona R (1999) Scintigraphic diagnosis of polysplenia in adult. Clin Nucl Med 24:161–163
Deutsch JC, Sandhu IS, Lawerence SP (1999) Splenosis presenting as an ulcerated gastric mass: endoscopic and endoscopic ultrasonographic imaging. J Clin Gastroenterol 28:266–267
Deva AK, Thompson JF (1996) Delayed rupture of the spleen 5 1/2 years after conservative management of traumatic spleen injury. Aust N Z J Surg 66:494–495
Devlin HB, Evans DS, Birkhead JS (1969) The incidence and morbidity of accidental injury to the spleen occurring during abdominal surgery. Br J Surg 56:446–448
De Vuysere S, van Steenbergen W, Aerts R, van Hauwaert H,

van Beckevoort D, van Hoe L (2000) Intrahepatic splenosis: imaging features. Abdom Imaging 25:187–189
De Waele JJ, Vermassen FEG (1999) Splenic herniation causing massive haemothorax after blunt trauma. J Accid Emerg Med 16:383–384
Di Cataldo A, Puelo S, Lidestri G et al (1987) Splenic trauma and overwhelming postsplenectomy infection. Br J Surg 74:343–345
Dickerman D (1976) Bacterial infection in the asplenic host: a review. J Trauma 16:662–668
Diebold J, Audouain J (1983) Peliosis of the spleen. Report of a case associated with chronic myelomonocytic leukemia presenting with spontaneous splenic rupture. Pathology 7: 197–204
Dobrow RB (1977) Spontaneous (pathologic) rupture of the spleen in previously undiagnosed Hodgkin's disease: report of a case with survival. Cancer 39:354–358
Dondelinger R, Fettes F (1981) Percutaneous aspiration of an occult splenic and perisplenic hematoma with computed tomography. Eur J Radiol 1:332–334
Douzdjian V, Broughan TA (1995) Spontaneous splenic rupture during total vascular occlusion of the liver. Br J Surg 82:406–407
Downey EC, Shackford SR, Fridlund PH et al (1987) Long-term depressed immune function in patients splenectomized for trauma. J Trauma 27:661–663
Drachenberg CB, Papadimitriou JC (1996) Splenic pathology in different forms of traumatic injury. Am J Clin Pathol 106:695
Drapanas T, Yates AJ, Brickman R, Wholey M (1969) The syndrome of occult rupture of the spleen. Arch Surg 99: 298–306
Drapiewski JF, Sternlieb SB, Jones R (1955) Primary amyloidosis with spontaneous rupture of the spleen and sudden death. Ann Intern Med 43:406–412
Dreze C (1993) Post-traumatic calcified hematoma of the spleen. Rev Med Liège 48:229–234
Druit T (1947) Spontaneous rupture of spleen after defecation. Lancet 2:652–653
Dunlop DG, Evans RM (1996) Congenital abnormality of the liver initially misdiagnosed as splenic haematoma. J R Soc Med 89:702–704
Eanniello VC, Gabram SG, Eusebio R, Jacobs LM (1994) Isolated free fluid on abdominal computerized tomographic scan: an indication for surgery in blunt trauma patients? Conn Med 58:707–710
Eklof B, Gjores JE, Lohi A, Norgren L, Stakiewicz W (1978) Spontaneous rupture of the liver and spleen during streptokinase treatment of deep venous thrombosis. Lakartidningen 75:777–778
Elmore JR, Clark DE, Isler RJ, Horner WR (1989) Selective nonoperative management of blunt splenic trauma in adults. Arch Surg 124:581–585
Emery KH (1997) Splenic emergencies. Radiol Clin North Am 35:831–843
Emery KH, Babcock DS, Borgman AS, Garci VF (1999) Splenic injury diagnosed with CT: US follow-up and healing rate in children and adolescents. Radiology 212:515–518
Espinal EA, Hoak T, Porter JA, Sleak FA (1997) Splenic rupture from colonoscopy. A report of two cases and review of the literature. Surg Endosc 11:71–73
Fabri PJ, Metz EM, Nick WV et al (1974) A quarter century with splenectomy: changing concepts. Arch Surg 180:569–575
Fagelman D, Hertz MA, Ross AS (1985) Delayed development of splenic subcapsular hematoma: CT evaluation. J Comput Assist Tomogr 9:815–816
Falimirski ME, Provost D (2000) Nonsurgical management of solid abdominal organ injury in patients over 55 years of age. Am Surg 66:631–635
Farhat GA, Abdu RA, Vanek VW (1992) Delayed splenic rupture: real or imaginary. Am Surg 58:340–345
Farhi DC, Ashfaq R (1996) Splenic pathology after traumatic injury. Am J Clin Pathol 105:474–478
Federle MP (1983) Computed tomography of blunt abdominal trauma. Radiol Clin North Am 21:461–475
Federle MP (1984) CT of upper abdominal trauma. Semin Roentgenol 19:269–280
Federle MP, Goldberg HI, Kaiser JA (1981) Evaluation of abdominal trauma by computed tomography. Radiology 136:637–644
Federle MP, Griffith B, Minagi H, Jeffrey RB (1987) Splenic trauma: evaluation with CT. Radiology 162:69–71
Federle MP, Courcoulas AP, Powell M, Ferris JV, Peitzman AB (1998) Blunt splenic injury in adults: clinical and CT criteria for management with emphasis on active extravasation. Radiology 206:137–142
Feferman I, Cramer J (1991) Splenosis: an unusual cause of intraabdominal hemorrhage. J Emerg Med 9:239–240
Feliciano DV, Bitondo CG, Mattox KL et al (1985) A four year experience with splenectomy versus splenorrhaphy. Ann Surg 201:568–575
Feliciano DV, Spjut-Patrinely V, Burch JM et al (1990) Splenorrhaphy. The alternative. Ann Surg 211:569–580
Feliciano PD, Mullins RJ, Trunkey DD, Crass RA, Beck JR, Helfand M (1992) A decision analysis of traumatic spleen injuries. J Trauma 33:340–347
Fernandes CM (1996) Splenic rupture manifesting two years after diagnosis of injury. Acad Emerg Med 3:946–947
Festa V, Falcetto G, Garrone C et al (1989) Spontaneous rupture of the spleen caused by primary amyloidosis. Description of a clinical case. Minerva Chir 44:1525–1528
Fidvi SA, Kroop SA, Klein SA (1999) Posttraumatic thoracic splenosis and chronic aortic pseudoaneurysm. J Thoracic Imaging 14:300–302
Firstenberg MS, Plaisier B, Newman JS, Malangoni MA (1998) Successful treatment of delayed splenic rupture with splenic artery embolization. Surgery 123:584–586
Fisher RP, Beverlin BC, Engrav LH (1978) Diagnostic peritoneal lavage: fourteen years and 2586 patients later. Am J Surg 136:701–704
Fisher RG, Foucar K, Estrada R, Ben-Menachem Y (1981) Splenic rupture in blunt trauma. Correlation of angiographic and pathologic records. Radiol Clin North Am 19:141–165
Flaherty L, Jurkovich GJ (1991) Minor splenic injuries: associated injuries and transfusion requirements. J Trauma 31: 1618–1621
Fletcher H, Frederick J, Barned H, Lizarraga V (1989) Spontaneous rupture of the spleen with splenic conservation. West Indian Med J 38:114–115
Flood MJ, Carpenter RA (1961) Spontaneous rupture of the spleen in acute myeloid leukemia. Br Med J 1:35–36
Foiada M, Muller W, Conti Rossini B, Pedrinis E (1993) Case report of spontaneous splenic rupture in splenoma. Helv Chir Acta 60:187–190
Foroudi F, Ahern V, Peduto A (1999) Splenosis mimicking metastases from breast carcinoma. Clin Oncol (R Coll Radiol) 11:190–192

Foster RP (1970) Delayed hemorrhage from the ruptured spleen. Br J Surg 57:189–192
Freeman JL, Jafri H, Roberts JL, Mezwa DG, Shirhoda A (1993) CT of congenital and acquired abnormalities of the spleen. Radiographics 13:597–610
Frizelle FA, Rietveld JA (1994) Spontaneous splenic rupture associated with Campylobacter jejuni infection. Br J Surg 81:718
Furman G, Morgenstern L (1993) Splenic injury and abscess complicating endoscopic retrograde cholangiopancreatography. Surg Endosc 7:343–344
Gaedcke G, Storz K, Braun S, Horny HP (1999) Thoracic splenosis with symptoms of coronary heart disease. Dtsch Med Wochenschr 20:958–961
Garber BG, Yelle JD, Smith RF, Lorimer JW, Garson C (1996) Management of splenic injuries in a Canadian trauma center. Can J Surg 39:474–480
Garre Sanchez MC, Garcia Munoz P, Torrella Cortes E, Alberca DE Las Parras F, Guillen Pardo B, Lopez Alanis A (1996) Splenic rupture in acute pancreatitis. Gastroenterol Hepatol 19:462–463
Gauderer MW, Stellato TA, Hutton MC (1989) Splenic injury: nonoperative management in three patients with infectious mononucleosis. J Pediatr Surg 24:118–120
Gaunt WT, McCarthy MC, Lambert CS et al (1999) Traditional criteria for observation of splenic trauma should be challenged. Am Surg 65:689–691
Gautier-Benoit C, Luez J, Cecile JP, Delepouille E, Pinchon-Marsy S (1973) Splenic rupture and chronic pancreatitis. Sem Hop 49:2693–2696
Gavant ML, Schurr M, Flick PA et al (1997) Predicting clinical outcome of nonsurgical management of blunt splenic injury: using CT to reveal abnormalities of splenic vasculature. AJR 168:207–212
Gay SB, Sistrom CL (1992) Computed tomographic evaluation of blunt abdominal trauma. Radiol Clin North Am 30:367–388
Gayer G, Apter S, Jonas T et al (1999) Polysplenia syndrome detected in adulthood: report of eight cases and review of the literature. Abdom Imaging 24:178–184
Gillet M, Randrianarivo P, Philippe E et al (1973) Hemangioendothelial sarcoma of the peritoneum revealed by an apparently spontaneous rupture of the spleen. Sem Hop 49:2159–2161
Godley CD, Warren RL, Sheridan RL, McCabe CJ (1996) Nonoperative management of blunt splenic injury in adults: age over 55 years as a powerful indicator of failure. J Am Coll Surg 183:133–139
Gold RE, Redman HC (1972) Splenic trauma: assessment of problems in diagnosis. AJR 116:413–418
Gorg C, Schwerk WB (1991) Sonographic investigation in the diagnosis of intrasplenic fluid collections. Bildgebung 58: 76–82
Goodman LR, Aprahamian C (1990) Changes in splenic size after abdominal trauma. Radiology 176:629–632
Gores PF, Simso LA (1989) Splenic injury during colonoscopy. Arch Surg 124:1342
Gorg C, Barth P, Weide R, Schwerk WB (1994) Spontaneous splenic rupture in acute amyloid leukemia: sonographic follow-up study. Bildgebung 61:37–39
Gow KW, Murphy JJ III, Blair GK, Stringer DA, Culhaim JA, Fraser GC (1996) Splanchnic artery pseudo-aneurysm secondary to blunt abdominal trauma in children. J Pediatr Surg 31:812–815
Green JB, Shackford SR, Sise MJ et al (1986) Late septic complications in adults following splenectomy for trauma: a prospective analysis of 144 patients. J Trauma 26:999–1004
Grinblat J, Gilboa Y (1975) Overwhelming pneumococcal sepsis 25 years after splenectomy. Am J Med Sci 270:523–524
Griswold RA, Collier HS (1961) Collective reviews: blunt abdominal trauma. Surg Gynecol Obstet 112:309–329
Grosdidier J, Boilear F, Richaume B (1974) Post-traumatic pseudocysts of the spleen (four observations). Sem Hop Paris 50:2556–2559
Gruen DR, Gollub MJ (1997) Intrahepatic splenosis mimicking hepatic adenoma. AJR 168:725–726
Guillon F, Borie F, Millat B (2000) Spleen trauma. J Chir (Paris) 137:205–213
Guleria S, Dorairajan LN, Sinha S, Khazanchi R, Bal S, Guleria R (1996) Spontaneous rupture of spleen in viral hepatitis A. Indian J Gastroenterol 15:30
Gunay K, Taviloglu K, Berber E, Ertekin C (1999) Traumatic rupture of hydatid cysts: a 12-year experience from an endemic region. J Trauma 46:164–167
Gunes I, Yilmazlar T, Sarikaya I, Akbunar T, Irgil C (1994) Scintigraphic detection of splenosis: superiority of tomographic spleen scintigraphy. Clin Radiol 49:115–117
Gunther K, Stangl R, Schweiger H, Rupprecht H (1998) Posttraumatic arteriovenous fistula between splenic artery and vein as a rare cause of acute myocardial ischemia. Chirurg 69:91–93
Habib E, Elhahad A, Slama JL (2000) Diagnosis and treatment of spleen rupture during pancreatitis. Gastroenterol Clin Biol 24:1229–1232
Haertel M, Ryder D (1979) Radiologic investigation of splenic trauma. Cardiovasc Radiol 2:27–33
Hagiwara A, Yukioka T, Ohta S, Nitatori T, Matsuda N, Shimazaki S (1996) Nonsurgical management of patients with blunt splenic injury: efficacy of transcatheter arterial embolization. Am J Roentgenol 167:159–166
Haj M, Zaina A, Wiess M et al (1999) Pathologic spontaneous rupture of the spleen as a presenting sign of splenic T-cell lymphoma – case report with review. Hepatogastroenterology 46:193–195
Haller JA, Papa P, Drugas C, Colombani P (1994) Nonoperative management of solid organ injuries in children: is it safe? Ann Surg 219:625–631
Hansen RM, Spiegelhoff DR (1981) Marked congenital fissure masquerading as splenic laceration: report of a case. J Nucl Med 22:151–152
Hardin VM, Morgan ME (1994) Thoracic splenosis. Clin Nucl Med 19:438–440
Heading RC, McClelland DB, Stuart AE, Hamilton T (1972) Ruptured angiomatous spleen presenting as a severe coagulation defect. Br J Surg 59:492–494
Heath B, Rogers A, Taylor A, Lavergne J (1994) Splenic rupture: an unusual complication of colonoscopy. Am J Gastroenterol 89:449–450
Hebeler RF, Ward RE, Miller PW, Ben-Menachem Y (1982) The management of splenic injury. J Trauma 22:492–495
Heider J, Winter P, Kreft B (1998) Symptomatic heterotopic splenic tissue in the adrenal gland area. Aktuel Radiol 8: 135–137
Henry C, Dettloff L, Mhiri R, Tournade A, Geiss S (1998) Post-traumatic intrasplenic arteriovenous fistula in a child. Spontaneous regression. J Radiol 79:271–273
Henry JJ (1978) Unusual presentation of splenic rupture. Soc Pediatr Urol Newslett 1:87

Hiraide A, Yamamoto H, Yahata K, Yoshioka T, Sugimoto T (1994) Delayed rupture of the spleen caused by an intrasplenic pseudoaneurysm following blunt trauma: case report. J Trauma 36:743–744
Hoagland RJ, Henson HM (1957) Splenic rupture in infectious mononucleosis. Ann Intern Med 46:1184–1191
Hopper KD, Chantelois AE (1989) The retrorenal spleen: implications for percutaneous left renal invasive procedures. Invest Radiol 24:592–595
Horie Y, Suou T, Hirayama C, Nagasako R (1982) Spontaneous rupture of the spleen secondary to metastatic hepatocellular carcinoma: a report of a case and review of the literature. Am J Gastroenterol 77:882–884
Horwitz JR, Black CT (1996) Traumatic rupture of a wandering spleen in a child: case report and literature review. J Trauma 41:348–350
Hosea SW, Brown EJ, Hamburger MI et al (1981) Opsonic requirements for intravascular clearance after splenectomy. N Engl J Med 304:245–250
Hunt JP, Lentz CW, Clairns BA et al (1996) Management and outcome of splenic injury: the results of a five-year statewide population-based study. Am Surg 62:911–917
Hurd WW, Katholi RE (1980) Acquired functional asplenia. Association with spontaneous rupture of the spleen and fatal spontaneous rupture of the liver in amyloidosis. Arch Intern Med 140:844–845
Huttunen R, Seppala A, Mokka R, Larmi TK (1975) Spontaneous rupture of the liver and the spleen: report of a successfully treated case with immunopathologic reaction. Surgery 77:722–725
Hynes HE, Silverstein MN, Fawcette KJ (1964) Spontaneous rupture of the spleen in acute leukemia. Cancer 17: 1356–1360
Ivatury RR, Simon RJ, Guignard J, Kazigo J, Gunduz Y, Stahl WM (1993) The spleen at risk after penetrating trauma. J Trauma 35:409–414
James CA, Emanuel PG, Vasquez D, Wagner CW, McFarland DR (1996) Embolization of splenic artery branch pseudoaneurysm after blunt abdominal trauma. J Trauma 40:835–837
Jeffrey HF (1991) An unusual case of tear of spleen. Can J Surg 34:315
Jeffrey RB, Laing FC, Federle MP (1981) Computed tomography of splenic trauma. Radiology 141:729–732
Johanet H, Melchior JC, Merrer J et al (1989) Hepatic and splenic contusion after external cardiac massage. A surgically treated case with favourable outcome. Ann Chir 43:760
Karam JA, Kozar RA (1998) Solitary blunt rupture of an accessory spleen. J Trauma 44:220–221
Kasales CJ, Patez S, Hopper KD et al (1994) Imaging variants of the liver, pancreas and spleen. Crit Rev Diagn Imaging 35:485–543
Katranci N, Parildar M, Goksel T, Savas R, Alper H (1998) Quiz case of the month. Posttraumatic intrathoracic splenosis. Eur Radiol 8:151–152
Katz DS, Moshiri M, Smith G, Meiner EM, Fruauff AA (1998) Spontaneous hemorrhage of abdominal splenosis. J Comput Assist Tomogr 22:725–727
Kaufman RA, Towbin R, Babcock DS et al (1984) Upper abdominal trauma in children: imaging evaluation. AJR 142:449–460
Keller MS, Sartorelli KH, Vane DW (1996) Associated head injury should not prevent nonoperative management of spleen or liver injury in children. J Trauma 41:471–475
Keramidas DC (1979) The ligation of the splenic artery in the treatment of traumatic rupture of the spleen. Surgery 85: 530–533
Killeen KL, Shanmuganathan K, Boydkranis R, Scalea TM, Mirvis SE (2001) CT findings after embolization for blunt splenic trauma. J Vasc Intervent Radiol 12:209–214
King H, Shumacker HB Jr (1952) Splenic studies 1: susceptibility to infection after splenectomy performed in infancy. Ann Surg 136:239–242
Kirks DR (1983) Radiological evaluation of visceral injuries in the battered child syndrome. Pediatr Ann 12:888–893
Kiroff GK, Mangos A, Cohen R, Chatterton BE, Jamieson GG (1983) Splenic regeneration following splenectomy for traumatic rupture. Aust N Z J Surg 53:431–434
Kluger Y, Paul DB, Raves JJ et al (1994a) Delayed rupture of the spleen: myths, facts, and their importance – case reports and a literature review. J Trauma 36:568–571
Kluger Y, Paul DB, Townsend RN, Diamond DL (1994b) Enhanced rim around infarcted, traumatized spleen on computed tomographic scans: case report. J Trauma 36: 436–437
Koehler RH, Smith RS, Fry WR (1994) Successful laparoscopic splenorrhaphy using absorbable mesh for grade III splenic injury: report of a case. Surg Laparosc Endosc 4:311–315
Kohn JS, Clark DE, Isler RJ, Pope CF (1994) Is computed tomographic grading of splenic injury useful in the nonsurgical management of blunt trauma? J Trauma 36:385–389
Kohr RM, Haendiges M, Taube RR (1993) Peliosis of the spleen: a rare cause of spontaneous splenic rupture with surgical implications. Am Surg 59:197–199
Koleski FC, Turk TM, Ouwenga M, Herrell SD, Borge MA, Albala DM (1999) Splenosis as a cause of testicular pain: laparoscopic management. J Endocrinol 13:373–375
Korobkin M, Moss AA, Callen PW, de Martini WJ, Kaiser JA (1978) Computed tomography of subcapsular splenic hematoma. Radiology 129:441–445
Kos X, Fanchamps JM, Trotteur G, Dondelinger RF (1999) Radiological damage control: evaluation of a combined CT and angiography suite with a pivoting table. Cardiovasc Intervent Radiol 22:124–129
Koumanidou C, Manopoulou E, Pantazis J et al (2000) Scrotal hematocele as an unusual presentation of blunt abdominal trauma in three male infants. J Clin Ultrasound 28: 190–193
Koury HI, Peschiera JL, Welling RE (1991) Non-operative management of blunt splenic trauma: a 10-year experience. Injury 22:349–352
Krahenbuhl L, Berry AR (1994) The management of splenic injuries in a District General Hospital. J R Coll Surg Edinb 39:249–252
Krause KR, Howells GA, Bair HA et al (2000) Nonoperative management of blunt splenic injury in adults 55 years and older: a twenty-year experience. Am Surg 66:636–640
Kremer B, Klomp HJ, Rothmund M et al (1995) Intraoperative splenic injury – organ preservation at any price? Langenbecks Arch Chir 380:125–129
Krupnick AS, Teitelbaum DH, Geiger JD et al (1997) Use of abdominal ultrasonography to assess pediatric splenic trauma. Potential pitfalls in the diagnosis. Ann Surg 225:408–414
Kubota K, Moteki M, Omine M, Tsuchiya J, Maekawa T (1974) Spontaneous splenic rupture related to anomalous loculation of the spleen in chronic myelogeneous leukemia. Rinsho Ketsueki 15:547–550

Kuligowska E, Mueller PR, Simeone JF, Fine C (1984) Ultrasound in upper abdominal trauma. Semin Roentgenol 19: 281–295

Kumar RA (1962) A case of traumatic rupture of an accessory spleen. Arch Dis Child 37:227

Kunz E, Buhler J, Gmohling M, Heinz C, Haubitz I, Klaue P (1990) Subjective sequelae of splenectomy. Langenbecks Arch Chir 375:214–219

Kurtaran A, Pangerl T, Scheuba C et al (1998) Visualization of intestinal splenosis by somatostatin receptor scintigraphy. Am J Gastroenterol 93:1375–1376

Kwan AJ, Drum DE, Ahn CS, Tow DE (1994) Intrathoracic splenosis mimicking metastatic lung cancer. Clin Nucl Med 19: 93–95

Lakhoo K, Bass DH, Cywes S (1991) Blunt splenic trauma in children. S Afr J Surg 29:108–109

Langevin J, Rothenbergher D, Goldbergs M (1984) Accidental splenic injury during surgical treatment of the colon and rectum. Surg Gynecol Obstet 159:139–144

Lannergren K, Tordai P, Linne T, Persson U (1990) Avoiding splenectomy in the treatment of children with splenic injury. Acta Chir Scand 156:359–365

Lansiaux S, Allaouchiche B, Gruner L, Barth X, Motin J (1998) Rupture of the intra-abdominal spleen as a cause of hemothorax. Ann Fr Anesth Reanim 17:58–60

Lawson DE, Jacobson JA, Spizarny KL, Pranikoff T (1995) Splenic trauma: value of follow-up CT. Radiology 194: 97–100

Lee RB, Bass SM, Morris JA Jr, McKenzie EJ (1990) Three or more rib fractures as an indicator for transfer to a level I trauma center: a population-based study. J Trauma 30:689–694

Lepasoon J, Olin T (1971) Angiographic diagnosis of splenic lesions following blunt abdominal trauma. Acta Radiol Diagn 11:257–273

Levy J (1994) Spontaneous rupture of the spleen in association with idiopathic thrombocytopenic purpura. Postgrad Med J 70:239

Lewis FW, Moloo N, Steigmann GV, Goff J (1991) Splenic injury complicating therapeutic upper gastrointestinal endoscopy and ERCP. Gastrointest Endosc 37:632–633

Likhite VV (1976) Immunological impairment and susceptibility to infection after splenectomy. JAMA 236:1376–1377

Lippstone MB, Sekula-Perlamna A, Tobin J, Callery RT (1998) Spontaneous splenic rupture and infectious mononucleosis in a forensic setting. Del Med J 70:433–437

Livingston CD, Sirinek KR, Levine BA, Aust JB (1982) Traumatic splenic injury: high incidence of associated injury. Arch Surg 117:670–674

Livingston CD, Levine BA, Lecklitner ML, Sirinek KR (1983) Incidence and function of residual splenic tissue following splenectomy for trauma in adults. Arch Surg 118:617–620

Longo WE, Baker CC, McMillen MA, Modlin IM, Degutis LC, Zucker KA (1989) Nonoperative management of adult splenic trauma. Criteria for successful outcome. Ann Surg 210:626–629

Longobardi Y, Lessin MS, Kleinman M, Wesselhoeft CW, Berns SD (2000) Unsuspected splenic rupture in a neonate. Pediatr Emerg Care 16:28–30

Lorimer WS Jr (1964) Occult rupture of the spleen. Arch Surg 89:434–440

Love L, Greenfield GB, Brown T, Moncada R, Freeark RJ, Baker TJ (1968) Arteriography of splenic trauma. Radiology 91: 96–102

Lowenfels AB (1966) Kehr's sign: a neglected aid in rupture of the spleen. N Engl J Med 274:1019

Lucas CE (1991) Splenic trauma: choice of management. Ann Surg 213:98–112

Ludtke FE, Mack SC, Schuff-Werner P, Voth E (1989) Splenic function after splenectomy for trauma. Role of autotransplantation and splenosis. Acta Chir Scan 155:533–539

Luna GK, Dellinger EP (1987) Non-operative observation therapy for splenic injuries: a safe therapeutic operation? Am J Surg 153:462–468

Lundström B (1970) Angiographic demonstration of rupture of the spleen. Acta Radiol (Diagn) 10:145–150

Lynch JH, Ford H, Gardner MJ, Weiner ES (1993) Is early discharge following isolated splenic injury in the hemodynamically stable child possible? J Pediatr Surg 28: 1403–1406

Madjar S, Weissberg D (1994) Thoracic splenosis. Thorax 49: 1020–1022

Mahon PA, Sutton JE (1985) Nonoperative management of adult splenic injury due to blunt trauma: a warning. Am J Surg 149:716–721

Malangoni MA, Dillon LD, Klamer TW, Condon RE (1984) Factory influencing the risk of early and late serious infection in adults after splenectomy for trauma. Surgery 96: 775–783

Mall JC, Kaiser JA (1980) CT diagnosis of the splenic laceration. AJR 131:265–269

Marin Leon I, Manzaneque Gonzalez L, Beiztegui Sillero A, Monteagudo Parreno A, Dastis Bendala C, Garcia Bragado F (1990) A traumatic rupture of the spleen. A proposal of new attitudes. A propos a case on brucellosis. Ann Med Intern 7:474–476

Martinazzi M, Lombardi C, Morosi G, Cavalleri M (1975) Splenohepatic hemangiosarcoma with laceration of the spleen. Tumori 61:575–580

Martinez Ruiz M, Boned J, Toral JR, Llobell G, Perablba JI (1990) Conservative treatment in spontaneous splenic rupture due to infectious mononucleosis. Ann Med Intern 7:578–580

Mbakop A (1983) Abdominal splenosis. Apropos of a case. Schweiz Med Wochenschr 113:191–193

McGehee M, Kier R, Cohn SM, McCarty SM (1993) Comparison of MRI with postcontrast CT for the evaluation of acute abdominal trauma. J Comput Assist Tomogr 17:410–413

McIndoe AH (1932) Delayed hemorrhage following traumatic rupture of the spleen. Br J Surg 20:249–268

Mendelson DS, Cohen BA, Armas PR (1982) CT appearance of splenosis. J Comput Assist Tomogr 6:1188–1190

Meredith JW, Trunkey DD (1988) CT scanning in acute abdominal injuries. Surg Clin North Am 68:255–268

Michalski S, Blankenhorn P, Lepsien G, Ludtke FE (1991) Fatal infection after splenectomy despite reimplantation of splenic tissue. Klin Wochenschr 69:375–378

Mirvis SE, Shanmuganathan K (1992) Abdominal computed tomography in blunt trauma. Seminars Radiol 27:150–183

Mirvis SE, Withley NO, Gens DR (1989) Blunt splenic trauma in adults: CT-based classification and correlation with prognosis and treatment. Radiology 171:33–39

Molina M, Ortega G, de Paco M, Buendia JL (1995) Spontaneous spleen rupture and liver cirrhosis. Med Clin (Barc) 104: 199

Moore EE, Cogbill TH, Jurkovich GJ, Shackford MD, Malangoni MA, Champion HR (1995) Organ injury scaling: spleen and liver (1994 revision). J Trauma 38:323–324

Moore GE, Stevens RE, Moore EE, Aragon GE (1983) Failure of splenic implants to protect against fatal postsplenectomy infection. Am J Surg 146:413–414

Morrell DG, Chang FC, Helmer SD (1995) Changing trends in the management of splenic injury. Am J Surg 170:686–689

Morris DH, Bullock FD (1919) The importance of the spleen in resistance to infection. Ann Surg 70:513–521

Morse MA, Garcia VF (1994) Selective nonoperative management of pediatric blunt splenic trauma: risk for missed associated injuries. J Pediatr Surg 29:23–27

Mouaaouy A, Zittel TT, Becker HD (1991) Blunt abdominal trauma: differential diagnosis of splenic lobulation and splenic rupture. Ultraschall Med 12:91–94

Mucha P (1986) Changing attitudes toward the management of blunt splenic trauma in adults. Mayo Clin Proc 61:472–477

Mucha P, Daly RC, Farnell MB (1986) Selective management of blunt splenic trauma. J Trauma 26:970–979

Nagar H, Kessler A, Weiss J (1997) Traumatic intraparenchymal splenic pseudoaneurysms in a child: nonoperative management. J Trauma 43:552–555

Nallathambi MN, Ivatury RP, Wapnir J, Rohman M, Stahl WM (1988) Nonoperative management versus early operation for blunt splenic trauma in adults. Surg Gynecol Obstet 166:252–258

Nieto Jimenez F, Tello Valero A, de Teresa Parreno L, Marzal Felici V, Grimalt Arrom M (1981) Spontaneous rupture of the spleen in a patient with diffuse histiocytic lymphoma, with reference to a case. Rev Clin Esp 162:221–224

Nincheri Kunz M, Evaristi L, Pera M, Veneroso A, Cozzani R, Caliendo L (1994) Splenic rupture in chronic pancreatitis. A clinical case. Observations. Minerva Chir 49:107–113

Nishida T, Ku Y, Saitoh Y (1995) Spontaneous splenic rupture during the course of a rubella infection: report of a case. Surg Today 25:83–85

Normand JP, Rioux M, Dumont M, Bouchard G, Letourneau L (1993) Thoracic splenosis after blunt trauma: frequency and imaging findings. AJR 161:739–741

Norotsky MC, Rogers FB, Shackford SR (1995) Delayed presentation of splenic artery pseudoaneurysms following blunt abdominal trauma: case reports. J Trauma 38:444–447

Ochsner MG, Knudson MM, Pachter HL et al (2000) Significance of minimal or no intraperitoneal fluid visible on CT scan associated with blunt liver and splenic injuries: a multicenter analysis. J Trauma 49:505–510

Odom JW, D'Amore TF, Meo MA, Lobbato V (1991) Splenectomy for minor splenic trauma in patients with HIV infections. Injury 22:85–88

Okazaki K, Moriyasu F, Shiomura T et al (1986) Spontaneous rupture of the spleen and liver in amyloidosis – a case report and review of the literature. Gastroenterol Jpn 21:518–524

Olivero G, Franchello A, Adduci A, Orlando E, Cotogni P (1994a) Lesions of the spleen caused by blunt trauma. Proposal of a classification based on CT and correlation with prognosis and treatment. Minerva Chir 49:751–757

Olivero G, Franchello A, Enrichens F, Orlando E, Adduci A, Cotogni P (1994b) Treatment of traumatic injuries of the spleen. Retrospective analysis of 164 cases. Minerva Chir 49:891–905

Olsen WR, Pooley TZ (1977) A second look at delayed splenic rupture. Arch Surg 112:422–425

Ong E, Gohmler U, Wurbs D (1991) Splenic injury as a complication of endoscopy: two case reports and a literature review. Endoscopy 23:302–304

Orcalli F, Elio A, Veronese E, Frigo F, Salvato S, Residori C (1998) Conservative laparoscopy in the treatment of post-traumatic splenic laceration using microfiber hemostatic collagen: three case histories. Surg Laparosc Endosc 8: 445–448

Oreskovich MR, Carrico CJ (1983) Stab wound in the anterior abdomen: analysis of a management plan using local wound exploration and quantitative peritoneal lavage. Ann Surg 194:262–269

Orloff MJ, Peskin GW (1958) Spontaneous rupture of the normal spleen: a surgical enigma. Surg Gynecol Obstet 106:1–11

Ovnatanian KI (1966) Splenosis of the pericardium. Vestn Khir Im II Grek 97:59–62

Paar WD, Look MP, Robertz Vaupel GM et al (1995) Non-operative management in a case of spontaneous splenic rupture in infectious mononucleosis. Z Gastroenterol 33:13–14

Pachter HL, Spencer FC, Hofstetter SR, Liang HG, Hoballah J, Coppa GF (1990) Experience with selective operative and nonoperative treatment of splenic injuries in 193 patients. Ann Surg 211:583–589

Pachter HL, Hofstetter SR, Elkowitz A, Harris L, Lian HG (1993) Traumatic cysts of the spleen – the role of cystectomy and splenic preservation: experience with seven consecutive patients. J Trauma 35:430–436

Papp JP, Penner JA (1971) Spontaneous splenic rupture in lymphoma: report of 3 cases. South Med J 64:631–632

Pappas D, Mirvis SE, Crepps JT (1987) Splenic trauma: false negative CT diagnosis in cases of delayed rupture. AJR 149: 727–728

Patel NY, Gogbill TH, Gundersen LH (1996) Angioembolization of multiple intrasplenic pseudoaneurysms as a result of blunt trauma. J Vasc Surg 24:299–301

Paterson A, Frush DP, Donnelly LF, Foss JN, O'Hara SM, Bisset GS III (1999) A pattern-oriented approach to splenic imaging in infants and children. Radiographics 19:1465–1485

Patrinou V, Skroubis G, Zolota V, Vagianos C (2000) Unusual presentation of pancreatic mucinous cystadenocarcinoma by spontaneous splenic rupture. Dig Surg 17:645–647

Patten RM, Gunberg SR, Brandenburger DK, Richardson ML (2000) CT detection of hepatic and splenic injuries: usefulness of liver window settings. AJR 175:1107–1110

Pearl RH, Wesson DE, Spence LJ et al (1989) Splenic injury: a 5-year update with improved results and changing criteria for conservative management. J Pediatr Surg 24:121–124

Peitzman AB, Makaroun MS, Slasky BS et al (1986) Prospective study of computed tomography in initial management of blunt abdominal trauma. Curr Prob Surg 26:585–592

Philipp H, Bohm N, Lesch R, Zimmermann WE, Heimbach W (1977) Acute hepatic-vein occlusive disease, associated with portal vein thrombosis, splenic rupture and hepatic failure. Med Welt 28:587–590

Piekarski J, Federle MP, Moss AA, London SS (1980) Computed tomography of the spleen. Radiology 135:683–689

Pignatelli V, Palumbo A, Savino A, Kiferle M (1990) Splenic echography in blunt abdominal trauma. Radiol Med (Torino) 80:661–664

Pimpl W, Dapunt O, Kaindl H et al (1989) Incidence of septic and thromboembolic related deaths after splenectomy in adults. Br J Surg 76:517–521

Pizzaro AR, Gallaspy JW, Herrera G, Gomila R (2000) Splenosis and the gynecologic patient: a case report and review of literature. J Louis State Med Soc 152:345–348

Poulin EC, Thibault C, Descoteaux JG, Cote G (1995) Partial laparoscopic splenectomy for trauma: technique and case report. Surg Laparosc Endosc 5:306–310
Powell DC, Bivins BA, Bell RM (1982) Diagnostic peritoneal lavage. Surg Gynecol Obstet 155:257–262
Pranikoff T, Hirschl RB, Schlesinger AE, Polley TZ, Coran AG (1994) Resolution of splenic injury after nonoperative management. J Pediatr Surg 29:1366–1369
Prasad C, Beck AR (1968) Splenosis and intestinal obstruction. J Mt Sinai Hosp N Y 35:534–540
Ramsdell MG, Rao PM (1997) Splenic nonenhancement at computed tomography: a sign of the hypoperfusion complex. Emerg Radiol 4:329–331
Rao PM, Novelline RA (1996) Computed tomographic diagnosis of splenic trauma presenting with Kehr's sign (referred left shoulder pain). Emerg Radiol 3:134–136
Rappaport W, McIntyre KE Jr, Carmona R (1990) The management of splenic trauma in the adult patient with blunt multiple injuries. Surg Gynecol Obstet 170:204–208
Raptopoulos V (1994) Abdominal trauma: emphasis on computed tomography. Radiol Clin North Am 32:969–987
Ratner MH, Garrow E, Valda V et al (1977) Surgical repair of the injured spleen. J Pediatr Surg 12:1019–1025
Rawsthorne GB, Cole TP, Kyle J (1970) Spontaneous rupture of the spleen in infections mononucleosis. Br J Surg 57: 396–398
Rees CR (1991) Blunt splenic trauma and the angiographer: will we go back to the future? Radiology 181:12–14
Rege JD, Kavischwar VS, Mopkar PS (1998) Peliosis of spleen presenting as splenic rupture with haemoperitoneum – a case report. Indian J Pathol Microbiol 41:465–467
Reid JD, Kommareddi S, Lankerani M, Park MC (1980) Chronic expanding hematomas. A clinicopathologic entity. JAMA 244:2241–2242
Resciniti A, Fink MP, Raptopoulos V, Davidoff A, Silva WE (1988) Nonoperative treatment of adult splenic trauma: development of a computed tomographic scoring system that detects appropriate candidates for expectant management. J Trauma 28:828–831
Renne G, Coci A, Biraghi T, Schmid C (1999) Fine needle aspiration of thoracic splenosis. A case report. Acta Cytol 43: 492–494
Rest G, Seid AS, Rogers O, Goldstein EJC (1985) Pathological rupture of the spleen due to Salmonella Dublin infection. J Trauma 25:366–367
Richmond R, Humphrey P, Nichols WK (1992) Isolated traumatic accessory splenic rupture: a case report and literature review. Mo Med 89:351–353
Rickert CH, Maasjosthusmann U, Probst-Cousin S, August C, Gullota F (1998) A unique case of cerebral spleen. Am J Pathol 22:894–896
Roback M, Battan KF, Koyle M, Meagher DP Jr (1996) Acute scrotal swelling after blunt thoracoabdominal trauma. J Trauma 40:155–156
Roberts JL (1996) CT of abdominal and pelvic trauma. Semin Ultrasound CT MR 17:142–169
Roberts JL, Dalen K, Bosanko CM, Jafir SZ (1993) CT in abdominal and pelvic trauma. Radiographics 13:735–752
Robinette CD, Fraumeni JF (1977) Splenectomy and subsequent mortality in veterans of the 1939–45 war. Lancet 2:127–129
Rogers JS Jr, Shah S (1980) Spontaneous splenic rupture in plasma cell leukemia. Cancer 46:212–214
Roucos S, Tabet G, Jebara VA, Ghossain MA, Baigini J, Saade B (1990) Thoracic splenosis. Case report and literature review. J Thoracic Cardiovasc Surg 99:361–363
Ruess L, Sivit CJ, Eichelberger MR, Taylor GA, Bond SJ (1995) Blunt hepatic and splenic trauma in children: correlation of a CT injury severity scale with clinical outcome. Pediatr Radiol 25:321–325
Saavedra RA (1965) Spontaneous rupture of the spleen with subacute bacterial endocarditis. Illinois Med J 127:279–281
Saladino R, Lund D, Fleisher G (1991) The spectrum of liver and spleen injuries in children: failure of the pediatric trauma score and clinical signs to predict isolated injuries. Ann Emerg Med 20:636–640
Salis A, Pais O, Vennos A, Scalea T (1999) Superselective embolization of a traumatic intrasplenic arteriovenous fistula. J Trauma 46:186–188
Salvini A (1993) The laparoscopic treatment of splenic rupture: a case report. Ann Ital Chir 64:225–228
Sandberg-Gertzen H, Ericzon BG, Blomberg B (1998) Primary amyloidosis with spontaneous splenic rupture, cholestasis, and liver failure treated with emergency liver transplantation. Am J Gastroenterol 93:2254–2256
Sanders MN, Civil I (1999) Adult splenic injuries: treatment patterns and predictive indicators. Aust N Z J Surg 69: 430–432
Sartorelli KH, Pilcher DB, Rogers FB (1995) Patterns of splenic injuries seen in skiers. Injury 26:43–46
Sartorelli KH, Frumiento C, Rogers FB, Osler TM (2000) Nonoperative management of hepatic splenic and renal injuries in adults with multiple injuries. J Trauma 49:56–61
Sarioglu A, Tanyel FC, Aryurek M, Balkanci F, Hicsonmez A (1996) Aneurysmatic arteriovenous fistula complicating splenic injury. Eur J Pediatr Surg 6:183–185
Saudemont A, Chambon JP, Wurtz A, Quandalle P (1992) Conservative treatment for trauma of the spleen in adults. Comparative study of 34 cases of conservative treatment and 61 cases of splenectomy. Ann Chir 46:324–329
Sayers RD, Bewes PC, Porter KM (1992) Emergency laparotomy for abdominal trauma. Injury 23:537–541
Scatamacchia SA, Raptopoulos V, Fink MP et al (1989) Splenic trauma in adults: impact of CT grading on management. Radiology 171:725–729
Schiodt I, Duun E, Fischer TK, Christiansen AP, Ralfkiaer E (2000) Fatal rupture of the spleen caused by infiltration of T-cell lymphoma. Ann Hematol 79:158–160
Schöpf R, Fretz C, Haertel M (1982) Computed tomography for injuries of the liver and spleen. Fortschr Rontgenstr 136: 681–684
Schultz DA, Froelich JW (1985) Delayed rupture of the spleen. A case report. Clin Nucl Med 10:642–645
Schurr MJ, Fabian TC, Gavant M et al (1995) Management of blunt splenic trauma: computed tomographic contrast blush predicts failure of nonoperative management. J Trauma 39:507–513
Schweizer W, Böhlen L, Dennison A, Blumgart LH (1992) Prospective study in adults of splenic preservation after traumatic rupture. Br J Surg 79:1330–1333
Sclafani SJA (1994) Editorial comment. J Trauma 36:390
Sclafani SJ, Weisberg A, Scalea TM, Philips TF, Duncan AO (1991) Blunt splenic injuries: nonsurgical treatment with CT, arteriography and transcatheter arterial embolization of the splenic artery. Radiology 181:189–196
Sclafani SJ, Shaftan GW, Scalea TM et al (1995) Nonoperative salvage of computed tomography – diagnosed splenic inju-

ries: utilization of angiography for triage and embolization for hemostasis. J Trauma 39:818–825
Sekikawa T, Shatney C (1983) Septic sequelae after splenectomy for trauma in adults. Am J Surg 145:667–673
Servadio Y, Leibovitch I, Apter S, Mor Y, Goldwasser B (1994) Symptomatic heterotopic splenic tissue in the left renal fossa. Eur Urol 25:174–176
Shackford SR, Molin M (1990) Management of splenic injuries. Surg Clin North Am 70:595–619
Shackford SR, Sise MJ, Virgilio RW, Peters RM (1981) Evaluation of splenorrhaphy: a grading system for splenic trauma. J Trauma 21:538–542
Shafi S, Gilbert JC, Irish MS, Glick PL, Caty MG, Azizkhan RG (1999) Follow-up imaging studies in children with splenic injuries. Clin Pediatr (Phila) 38:273–277
Shafiroff BB, Berkowitz D, Li JK, Fletcher P (1977) Splenic erosion and hemorrhage secondary to pancreatic pseudocyst. A review of the literature and additional case report. Am J Gastroenterol 68:145–153
Shafran N, Gewurtz G, Priel IE (1992) Splenic hemorrhage masquerading as myeloproliferative disease. Harefrah 122: 218–220
Shah HR, Cue JI, Boyd CM, Cone JB (1987) Solitary splenic abscess: a new complication of splenic salvage treated by percutaneous drainage. J Trauma 27:337–338
Shanmuganathan K, Mirvis SE, Sover ER (1993) Value of contrast-enhanced CT in detecting active hemorrhage in patient with blunt abdominal trauma or pelvic trauma. AJR 161:65–69
Shanmuganathan K, Mirvis SE, Boyd-Kranis R, Takada T, Scalea T (2000) Nonsurgical management of blunt splenic injury: use of CT criteria to select patients for splenic arteriography and potential endovascular therapy. Radiology 217:75–82
Sherck JP, McCort JJ, Oakes DD (1984) Computed tomography in thoraco-abdominal trauma. J Trauma 24:1015–1021
Sherman R (1980) perspectives in management of trauma to the spleen. J Trauma 20:1–13
Sherman HF (1989) The inguinal hernia: not always straightforward, not always a hernia. J Emerg Med 7:21–24
Shimono T, Yamaoka T, Nishimura K et al (1998) Peliosis of the spleen: splenic rupture with intraperitoneal hemorrhage. Abdom Imaging 23:201–202
Siegel JH, Dalal SA, Burgess AR, Young JW (1990) Pattern of organ injuries in pelvic fracture: impact force implications for survival and death in motor vehicle injuries. Accid Anal Prev 22:457–466
Sikov WM, Schiffman FJ, Weaver M, Dykman J, Shulman R, Torgan P (2000) Splenosis presenting as occult gastrointestinal bleeding. Am J Hematol 65:56–61
Singer DB (1973) Post splenectomy sepsis. Perspect Pediatr Pathol 1:285–311
Siniluoto TM, Paivansalo MJ, Lanning FP, Typpo AB, Lohela PK, Kotaniemi AE (1992) Ultrasonography in traumatic splenic rupture. Clin Radiol 46:391–396
Sivit CJ (2000) Detection of active intraabdominal hemorrhage after blunt trauma: value of delayed CT scanning. Pediatr Radiol 30:99–100
Skoog SJ, Belman AB (1986) The communicating hematocele: an unusual presentation for blunt splenic trauma. J Urol 136:1092
Slate RW, Getzen LC, Laning RC (1969) One hundred cases of traumatic rupture of the spleen. Arch Surg 99:498–500
Slater H (1973) Complications of splenectomy. Am Surgeon 39:221–223
Smith JA, Macleish DG, Collier NA (1989) Aneurysms of the visceral arteries. Aust N Z J Surg 59, 329–334
Smith JS, Wengrowitz MA, Delong BS (1992) Prospective validation of criteria, including age, for safe, nonsurgical management of the ruptured spleen. J Trauma 33:368–369
Smith JS Jr, Cooney RN, Mucha P Jr (1996) Nonoperative management of the ruptured spleen: a revalidation of criteria. Surgery 120:745–750
Smith RS, Meister RK, Tsoi EK, Bohman HR (1993) Laparoscopically guided blood salvage and autotransfusion in splenic trauma: a case report. J Trauma 34:313–314
Solomonov E, Hirsh M, Yahiya A, Krausz MM (2000) The effect of vigorous fluid resuscitation in uncontrolled hemorrhagic shock after massive splenic injury. Crit Care Med 28:749–754
Sondenaa K, Tasdemir I, Andersen E, Skadberg JE, Soreide JA (1994) Treatment of blunt injury of the spleen: is there a place for mesh wrapping. Eur J Surg 160:669–673
Spencer NJB, Arthur RJ, Stringer MD (1996) Ruptured splenic epidermoid cyst: case report and imaging appearances. Pediatr Radiol 26:871–873
Stallard N, Findlay G, Smithies M (1997) Splenic rupture following cardiopulmonary resuscitation. Resuscitation 35: 171–173
Steeke L, Lim RC Jr (1975) Advances in management of splenic injuries. Am J Surg 130:159–165
Stein S, Duarte PS, Alavi A, Zhuang H, Alavi JB (2000) Multiple intraabdominal soft-tissue masses in a man awaiting liver transplantation: a case study and discussion. Am J Clin Oncol 23:506–508
Stites TB, Ultmann JE (1996) Spontaneous rupture of the spleen in chronic lymphatic leukemia. Cancer 19:1578–1590
Stivelman RL, Glaubitz JP, Cramptom RS (1963) Laceration of the spleen due to non-penetrating trauma: one hundred cases. Am J Surg 106:888–891
Storm BL, Abbitt PL, Allen DA, Ros PR (1992) Splenosis: superparamagnetic iron oxide-enhanced MR imaging. AJR 159: 333–335
Stout C, Hampton JW, Anderson JD, Oruc N (1973) Fatal nontraumatic splenic rupture in hemophilia and the Kasabach-Merritt syndrome. South Med J 66:791–795
Strauch GO (1979) Preservation of splenic function in adults and children with injured spleens. Am J Surg 137:478–482
Su AS, Tran M-H, Larsen CR (1997) Spontaneous splenic rupture: report of five cases and a review of the literature. Emerg Radiol 4:415–418
Sugahara K, Togashi H, Aoki M et al (1999) Spontaneous splenic rupture in a patient with large hepatocellular carcinoma. Am J Gastroenterol 94:276–278
Sugg SL, Gerndt SJ, Hamilton BJ, Francis IR, Taheri PA, Rodriguez JL (1995) Pseudoaneurysms of the intraparenchymal splenic artery after blunt abdominal trauma: a complication of nonoperative therapy and its management. J Trauma 39:593–595
Sujka SK, Evans EJ, Nigam A (1986) Delayed rupture of the spleen presenting as a scrotal hematoma. J Trauma 26:85–86
Sullivan JL, Ochs HD, Schiffman G et al (1978) Immune response after splenectomy. Lancet 1:178–181
Sutyak JP, Chiu WC, D'Amelio LF, Amorosa JK, Hammond JS (1995) Computed tomography is inaccurate in estimating the severity of adult splenic injury. J Trauma 39:514–518

Tapp E (1969) Ruptured spleen associated with chicken-pox. Br Med J 1:617–618
Targarona EM, Martinez J, Ramos C, Becerra JA, Trias M (1995) Conservative laparoscopic treatment of a posttraumatic splenic cyst. Surg Endosc 9:71–72
Taxy JB (1978) Peliosis: a morphologic curiosity becomes an iatrogenic problem. Hum Pathol 9:331–340
Taylor GA, Rosenfield AT (1984) Limitations of computed tomography in the recognition of delayed splenic rupture. J Comput Assist Tomogr 8:1205–1207
Taylor GA, Guion CJ, Potter BM, Eichelberger MR (1989) CT of blunt abdominal trauma in children. AJR 153:555–559
Teniere P, Janer R, Michot F (1985) Les contusions de la rate. Rev Prat 35:19–26
Texeira MB, Hardin WJ (1974) Spontaneous rupture of accessory spleen. Am Surg 46:491–493
Thaemert BC, Cogbill TH, Lambert PJ (1997) Nonoperative management of splenic injury: are follow-up computed tomographic scans of any value. J Trauma 43:748–751
Thijs JC, Schneider AJ, van Kordelaar JM (1983) Spontaneous rupture of the spleen complicating portal hypertension. Intensive Care Med 9:299–300
Townsend MC, Flancbaum L, Choban PS, Cloutier CT (1993) Diagnostic laparoscopy as an adjunct to selective conservative management of solid organ injuries after blunt abdominal trauma. J Trauma 35:647–651
Traggis DG, Maunz DL, Baroudy R (1984) Splenic hemorrhage in a neonate of a mother on anticonvulsant therapy. J Pediatr Surg 19:598–599
Traub A, Perry JF (1981) Injuries associated with splenic trauma. J Trauma 21:840–847
Traub A, Perry JF Jr (1982) Splenic preservation following splenic trauma. J Trauma 22:496–501
Traub A, Giebink GS, Smith C et al (1987) Splenic reticuloendothelial function after splenectomy, spleen repair, and spleen transplantation. N Engl J Med 317:1559–1564
Tricario A, Sicoli F, Calise F, Iavazzo M, Salvatore M, Mans L (1993) Conservative treatment in splenic trauma. J R Coll Surg Edinb 38:145–148
Umlas SL, Cronan JJ (1991) Splenic trauma: can CT grading systems enable prediction of successful nonsurgical treatment? Radiology 178:481–487
Uthoff LB, Wyfells PL, Adams CS (1983) A prospective study comparing nuclear scintigraphy and computerized axial tomography in the initial evaluation of the trauma patient. Ann Surg 198:611–616
Vaezy S, Martin R, Keilman G et al (1999) Control of splenic bleeding by using high intensity ultrasound. J Trauma 47: 521–525
Van der Zee J (1999) Laparoscopic management of a large posttraumatic splenic cyst in a child. Surg Endosc 13:1241–1242
Vanhoenacker F, de Schepper A (2000) Spontaneous (nontraumatic) splenic rupture. In: De Schepper AM, Vanhoenacker F (eds) Medical imaging of the spleen. Springer, Berlin Heidelberg New York, p 153
Vas W, Friend WD (1981) Rupture of a normal spleen caused by vomiting following metrizamide myelogram. Diagn Imaging 50:309–312
Velanovich V (1995) Blunt splenic injury in adults: a decision analysis comparing options for treatment. Eur J Surg 161: 463–470
Velanovich V, Tapper D (1993) Decision analysis in children with blunt splenic trauma: the effects of observation, splenorrhaphy or splenectomy on quality-adjusted life expectancy. J Pediatr Surg 28:179–185
Velitchkov NG, Kjossev KT, Losanoff JE, Kavardjikova VA (2000) Subcutaneous splenosis: a clue to diagnosis of thoracic splenosis. J R Coll Surg Edinb 45:66
Vento JA, Peng F, Spencer RP, Ramsey WH (1999) Massive and widely distributed splenosis. Clin Nucl Med 24:845–846
Viamonte M, Wulkan M, Irani H (1992) Splenic trauma as a complication of colonoscopy. Surg Laparosc Endosc 2: 154–157
Viano DC, Andrzejak DV (1993) Biomechanics of abdominal injuries by armrest loading. J Trauma 34:105–115
Villalba MR, Howells GA, Lucas RJ et al (1990) Nonoperative management of the adult ruptured spleen. Arch Surg 125: 836–838
Vitello JM, Hartung R (1991) Splenic laceration secondary to closed chest massage: successful recognition and management – case report. J Trauma 31:426–428
Vizer G, Weiland O (1979) Spontaneous splenic rupture in influenza. Orv Hetil 120:1139–1140
Vock R (1992) Liver and splenic rupture as a complication of heart pressure massage. Beitr Gerichtl Med 50:193–203
Von der Walde J, Mashiah A, Berrebi A (1981) Spontaneous rupture of the spleen in hairy cell leukemia. Clin Oncol 7: 214–244
Walcher F, Schneider G, Marzi I, Kriener S, Kramann B, Mutschler W (1997) Torsion of a wandering spleen after blunt abdominal trauma. J Trauma 43:983–984
Waninger J, Haag K, Kohlberger E, Specht S (1994) Duplex ultrasound studies after organ saving intervention in traumatic splenic rupture. Zentralbl Chir 119:104–108
Watkins GI (1960) Blunt trauma to the abdomen. Arch Surg 80:187–191
Watson WJ, Sundwall DA, Benson WL (1982) Splenosis mimicking endometriosis. Obstet Gynecol 59:515–535
Weill F (1992) Grading of splenic trauma. Radiology 182:582
Weinstein ME, Govin GG, Rice CL et al (1979) Splenorrhaphy for splenic trauma. J Trauma 19:692–696
Welk E, Stein U, Bindewald H, Glogowski P (1991) Spontaneous splenic rupture in chronic pancreatitis. Dtsch Med Wochenschr 22:460–462
Wholey MH, Chamorro HA, Rao G, Chapman W (1978) Splenic infarction and spontaneous rupture of the spleen after therapeutic embolization. Cardiovasc Radiol 1:249–253
Widman WD (1984) Current concepts in the management of splenic trauma: a review. Mil Med 149:1–4
Wiig JN and the Splenic Injury Study Group (1987) Splenic injury: a prospective multicenter study on nonoperative and operative treatment. Br J Surg 74:310–313
Wiley AT, Teeter RR, Schnabel TG (1951) Rupture of the spleen in primary amyloidosis. Report of a case. Med Clin North Am 35:1841
Williams MD, Yong DH, Schiller WR (1990) Trend toward nonoperative management of splenic injuries. Am J Surg 160:588–592
Williams RA, Black JJ, Sinow RM, Wilson SE (1997) Computed tomography-assisted management of splenic trauma. Am J Surg 174:276–279
Wilson RH, Moorehead RJ (1992) Management of splenic trauma. Injury 23:5–9
Winde G, Sprakel B, Bosse A, Reers B, Wendt M (1991) Rupture of the spleen caused by primary angiosarcoma. Case report. Eur J Surg 157:215–217

Wing VW, Pederle MP, Morris JA, Jeffrey RB, Bluth R (1985) The clinical impact of CT for blunt abdominal trauma. AJR 145:1191–1194

Wisner DH, Blaisdell FW (1992) When to save the ruptured spleen. Surgery 111:121–122

Witte CL, Esser MJ, Rappaport WD (1992) Updating the management of salvageable splenic injury. Ann Surg 215: 261–265

Wolfman NT, Bechtold RE, Scharling ES, Meredith JH (1992) Blunt upper abdominal trauma: evaluation by CT. AJR 158: 493–501

Wolters U, Keller HW, Lorenz R, Pichlmaier H (1990) Splenic cysts: indications for surgery and surgical procedures. Langenbecks Arch Chir 375:231–234

Wolverson MK, Crepps LF, Sindaram M et al (1983) Hyperdensity of recent hemorrhage at body computed tomography: incidence and morphological variation. Radiology 148: 779–784

Wu WC, Katon RM (1993) Injury to the liver and spleen after diagnostic ERCP. Gastrointest Endosc 39:824–827

Yam LT, Crosby WH (1979) Spontaneous rupture of the spleen in leukemic reticuloendotheliosis. Am J Surg 137:270–273

Yoshimitsu K, Aibe H, Nobe T et al (1993) Intrahepatic splenosis mimicking a liver tumor. Abdom Imaging 18:156–158

Zabinski EJ, Harkins HN (1943) Delayed splenic rupture. A clinical syndrome. Arch Surg 46:186–189

Zingman BS, Viner BL (1993) Splenic complications in malaria: case report and review. Clin Infect Dis 16:223–232

Zucker K, Brows K, Rossman D et al (1984) Nonoperative management of splenic trauma. Arch Surg 119:400–404

5 Injuries of the Liver

R. F. Dondelinger, O. Cornet, J. H. Boverie

CONTENTS

R. F. Dondelinger, MD
Professor and Chairman, Department of Medical Imaging, University Hospital Sart Tilman, Domaine Universitaire du Sart Tilman B35, 4000 Liège, Belgium
O. Cornet, MD
Resident, Department of Medical Imaging, University Hospital Sart Tilman, Domaine du Sart Tilman B35, 4000 Liège, Belgium
J. H. Boverie, MD
Chef de Clinique, Department of Medical Imaging, University Hospital Sart Tilman, Domaine du Sart Tilman B35, 4000 Liège, Belgium

- Proper CT image acquisition and contrast enhancement technique is mandatory to disclose small-size posttraumatic intrahepatic vascular injuries.
- Retrohepatic hematoma and pericaval halo sign are suggestive of injury to the bare area of the liver. Potential laceration of the hepatic veins or the inferior vena cava, which may be responsible for catastrophic hemorrhage should be suspected.
- Conservative treatment of blunt liver injury should be based on a complete CT examination of the abdomen and thorax, in order to evidence those associated injuries that need surgical repair. An expectant nonoperative treatment option of liver injury should not be based exclusively on CT features or CT grading of liver contusion.
- Hemostatic arterial embolization should be performed in the hemodynamically stable patient in whom CT has evidenced contrast extravasation or an intrahepatic vascular lesion. Marginally stable patients with ongoing arterial bleeding can be included in centers with radiologists integrated into a trauma team and specialized in hemostatic embolization in acute trauma victims.

5.1 History

Liver injury has been known since ancient times. In Greek mythology, day per day, an eagle screwed out a fragment of Prometheus' liver , who was chained to a rock as a punishment for having robbed the Gods of fire and given it to mankind as a gift. This epos illustrates the capacity of the human liver to heal after injury and regenerate after resection. The rabbis of the Talmud theorized that a piece of liver the size of an olive was sufficient to sustain life. In the Old Testament, penetrating injury to the liver was considered lethal. Abner stabbed Asahel (Samuel 2:23) and was killed in turn by Asahel's brother Joab. Rashi (1040–1105 AD), a talmudic commentator, explained that both deaths were caused by liver injury (Westreich 1990). Hippocrates also recognized in his aphorisms that deep penetrating injury to the liver might be lethal. In more recent times, Berta in 1716 and Thompson at the battle of Waterloo in 1814 were credited with successful débridement of an injured liver, which was exteriorized through a penetrating battle wound. Further liver resections of tissue protruding through an open wound were reported by McPherson in 1846 and Massie in 1852. Other so-called hepatic resections of an injured liver, which were reported earlier, were probably all similar simple wound débridements of exteriorized liver fragments rather than real resections. The first reported laparotomy for hepatic contusion was performed by Willette in 1886. Von Burkhard successfully treated a traumatic liver laceration by tamponade in 1887 (Schwartz 1989, 1998).

At the turn of the nineteenth century, survival after attempts of surgical treatment of hepatic injury was 44%–69% (Tilton 1905; Edler 1986, 1987; Terrier and Auvray 1986). Pringle described intraoperative clamping of the portal triad for control of hepatic bleeding at the beginning of the twentieth century and already laid the basis of the later concept of surgical damage control (Pringle 1908). Although all patients died, the Pringle maneuver evolved as a valuable technique. Perihepatic surgical packing for treatment of liver injury was introduced by Halsted at the same time period and was also a kind of hepatic damage control (Halsted 1913). However, progress in resuscitation and in hepatic surgical techniques was an incentive for a more aggressive management of liver injury, based upon deep hepatotomies for effective vascular control, and lobectomies or more reduced resections, as an expeditious hemostatic treatment of the contused parenchyma. However, in the middle of the last century, mortality rates from liver injury were still similar to the figures recorded at the end of the nineteenth century (Kremer and Henne-Bruns 1993). The lack of improvement in survival was probably due to the high number of other significant associated injuries, or intractable hepatic hemorrhage and delayed complications leading to death of the trauma victim (Griswold and Collier 1961). Over the years, a better understanding of pathophysiology of polytrauma, a critical assessment of the complications resulting from aggressive liver surgery, more rapid patient rescue and transportation to the hospital, and more efficient organization of hospital emergency departments, combined with progress in resuscitation and anesthesia, brought a change in the surgical attitude, aiming at a more conservative treatment of the resuscitated victim (Frey et al. 1973).

The concept of damage control surgery revived perihepatic packing, with staged removal or brief hemostasis and rescheduled intervention for definitive repair, reducing mortality considerably (Feliciano 1981; Stone et al. 1983; Rotondo et al. 1993). Simultaneously, the advent of cross-section imaging confirmed the ground of the adopted surgical conservatism in abdominal parenchymal injury. The significant advantages of CT over radionuclide studies, diagnostic arteriography and peritoneal lavage, were rapidly recognized (Moon and Federle 1983). Selective arterial catheter embolization further contributed to nonaggressive management of liver hemorrhage (Jander et al. 1977; Rubin and Katzen 1977). Percutaneous drainage of abdominal fluid collections and nonoperative cannulation of the bile ducts and derived therapeutic procedures further contributed to the establishment of the currently prevailing intense diagnostic imaging, followed by conservatism in the management of pediatric and adult blunt hepatic injury.

5.2 Incidence

Hepatic injury represents 3%–11% of admissions in an urban city trauma center. These figures are stabilizing or even decreasing slightly in some areas due to a reduction in severe traffic accidents (Haney et al. 1982; Hanna et al. 1987; Cox et al. 1988; Strong 1999). Hepatic trauma comprises 5%–30% of all blunt abdominal injuries – some reports mention 45% – and probably is the most common finding at autopsy of trauma victims (McClelland and Shires 1965; McCort 1966; Dotzauer 1970; Hamelmann and Nitschke 1971; Peiper and Peitsch 1976; Reed et al. 1992). Frequency of liver injury was estimated to be higher in children than in adults before the era of cross-section imaging (Richardson et al. 1972). In the literature, the liver is said to be the second most frequently injured intraperitoneal organ, consistently surpassed by the spleen, even up to 50% in some series. But more recently, hepatic injury was found to occur with an equal or even a slightly higher frequency than splenic trauma. Systematic CT screening is capable of revealing subtle hepatic injury that otherwise might have gone unnoticed. Frequency of blunt hepatic contusion compared to penetrating injury varies according to the type of population, from 14%–96%. On the other hand, increasing civilian violence is responsible for the rising number of penetrating injuries in many urban areas. In the USA, penetrating injury accounted roughly for 80% –90% of hepatic trauma (Feliciano et al. 1986b; Hanna et al. 1987; Cogbill et al. 1988; Feliciano 1989; Wilson and Moorehead 1991). Blunt trauma largely predominates in Europe, and seems also to have increased to some degree in the USA over the last 25 years, compared to penetrating injury (Richardson et al. 1972, 2000; Lucas and Ledgerwood 2000).

5.3 Mechanism

5.3.1 Common

Livery injury resulting from blunt abdominal trauma is caused by a traffic accident in 66%–90% (Fekete et al. 1969; Hanna et al. 1985). The highest figures reported in a victim population include the driver, the passengers and the pedestrians involved together in the same accident. In children, similar figures are found; 54%–85% of blunt liver injuries are related to a traffic accident (Trauma Committee 1989; Cywes et al. 1991). Seatbelts certainly protect from a frontal impact during a car accident, but less from a lateral one. At high velocity deceleration, the liver may be crushed, fractured or avulsed due to the seatbelts, even when they are correctly placed or due to an improper use of shoulder harness or lap-type seatbelts or of an infant car seat (Junghanns 1978; Arajarvi et al. 1987; Contostavlos and Laposata 1992; Steinberg et al. 1996; Kloppel et al. 1997; Zuckerman et al. 1998). Other causes of blunt liver injury are falls, sport and work injuries and suicidal attempts. Sports injuries seem to occur with increasing frequency, compared to traffic accidents in recent literature. Bicycle handlebars, and in particular, the bar ends of bikes are responsible of hepatic injuries in children and adults similar to other organs like the pancreas and spleen (Clarnette and Beasley 1997; Nehoda and Hochleitner 1998; Spitz 1999). Finally liver injury, like other abdominal organs may be the result of a battered child (Heydenrich 1974; Sujka et al. 1988; Aoki et al. 1997; Cameron et al. 1997).

The large volume of the liver, the fragility of the liver parenchyma and the ease with which the hepatic attachments can rupture during an impact, explain the frequency of liver injury during abdominal contusion. The large right lobe of the liver, and particularly the lateral posterior sector is involved in 80% of the cases of blunt trauma, because of its location close to the ribs. Isolated injury to the left lobe or to the small left lateral segment is consequently rare.

Different mechanisms of blunt liver injury can act alone or in combination: a frontal or lateral high velocity impact with deceleration; or a direct blow to the right upper quadrant or the upper mid abdomen; or a crash of the liver over the spine or against the right rib cage; and finally a rupture of the liver capsule at the level of the attachments of the liver. As a consequence, the liver parenchyma ruptures, together with the liver capsule.

During a frontal impact consecutive to rapid deceleration, the heavier right lobe of the liver is projected anteriorly. Rupture tends to occur at the posterior aspect of the liver (bare area), where the right triangular ligament is attached to the liver capsule. The liver parenchyma ruptures in a direction parallel to the right hepatic vein towards the midline (Fig. 5.1). Such a parenchymal fracture may be further aggravated during surgical mobilization of the anterior part (segment V/VIII) of the right lobe, completing a partial disinsertion of the right hepatic vein and IVC intraoperatively, with the risk of exsanguination during surgery (Sherlock and Bismuth 1991). Orientation of the fracture line and depth depend on the orientation of large liver vessels and the direction and amount of energy of the impact.

Typical vertical contrecoup injury is caused by rapid deceleration after a fall, the victim landing on the feet or buttocks. Such a mechanism of injury is likely to produce retroperitoneal vascular laceration and in the liver a hepatic fracture in a sagittal

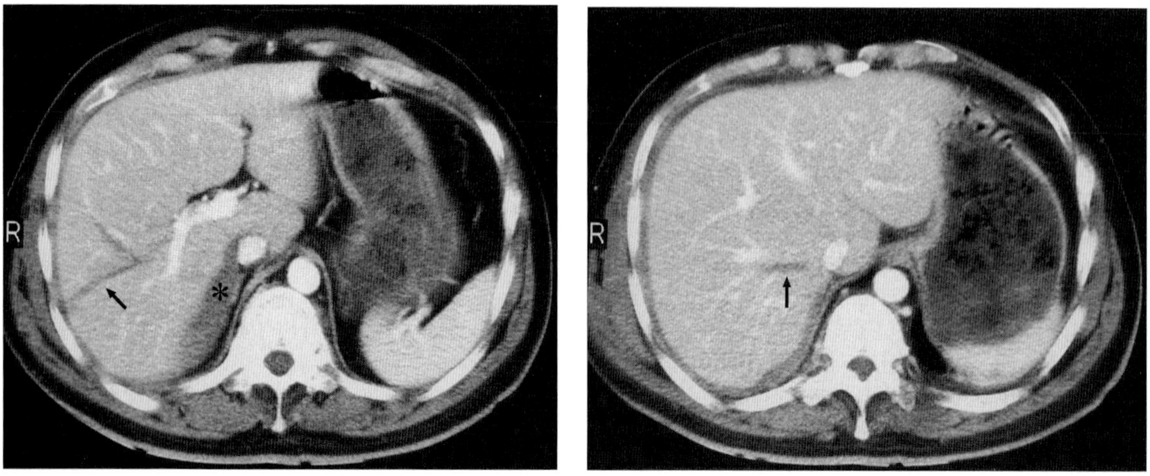

a b

Fig. 5.1a, b. A hypodense band (*arrow*) is seen in the right lobe of the liver, parallel to the course of the right hepatic vein. This type of parenchymal liver laceration is typical of a frontal impact consecutive to sudden deceleration. Notice a hypodense hematoma in contact with the inferior vena cava, adjacent to the bare area of the liver (*asterisk*)

plane or a separation of the parenchyma into fragments (Griswold and Collier 1961). During vertical deceleration, the left lobe is projected caudally and tends to create a short fracture line in contact with the ligamentum teres. Sagittal transection of the left lateral segment also typically results from improper placement of shoulder harness seatbelts (Contostavlos and Laposata 1992; Steinberg et al. 1996). A total avulsion of the left lateral segment may result from a malpositioned lap-type seatbelt (Radin 1992).

A crash of the liver against the rib or the spine or a direct blow creates a stellate burst or multiple fracture lines that radiate from the zone of impact and are most often located on the superior surface of the right lobe. The anterior or paramedian sector V/VIII of the right lobe and segment IV (left paramedian) and I (caudate lobe) of the left lobe are most often involved during this mechanism (Sherlock and Bismuth 1991). The left lobe is more frequently injured by a crash mechanism, as it has limited mobility in the upper abdomen compared to the right lobe, due to its fixation by the left triangular ligament and the falciform ligament and lies in close contact with the spine. Prolonged and severe compression of the liver results in ischemic necrosis, infarction and superinfection rather than in laceration (Jona and Goldstein 1977).

Knowledge of the trauma mechanism thus allows the medical team to anticipate expected pathological findings of a liver injury or it may give a clue to pathophysiology of the injuries seen on imaging. Hepatic hematoma results from injury to the superficial liver parenchyma, with an intact capsule. Blood collects preferentially in the subcapsular space and may spread over a great distance, particularly over the right lobe. Parenchymal fragility, such as steatosis or other diffuse infiltrating pathological processes, are promoting factors. Rupture of larger blood vessels, which are in a deeper location, result in a central hematoma, which may increase concentrically in volume or extend to the subcapsular space. The liver capsule, put under tension by an underlying hematoma, may rupture and result in severe hemorrhage, most easily at a distance of the fixation points of the liver (Roberts et al. 1993).

Hematomas represent around 40% and fractures around 60% of liver injuries. Hematomas and lacerations are associated together in only 7% of cases. Hematomas are seen in an equal proportion in a subcapsular, superficial and central location. Ruptured hematomas are found in a subcapsular, superficial, or central location, in 29%, 18%, and 11% respectively. Parenchymal fractures are hemorrhagic in 81%; about 20% are superficial and 40% extend into depth. One or two hepatic segments are involved in 33% and 50%, respectively, and three or four segments in 12% and 6%, respectively. Hemorrhage is related with a statistical significance to the extension of fracture in depth, length of fracture and the number of liver segments involved ($P<0.0003–0.00001$) (Letoublon and Castaing 1996).

Due to the great potential of the liver parenchyma to heal after injury, secondary delayed or occult bleeding is not a threat, conversely to the spleen (Wolfman et al. 1992).

5.3.2 Uncommon

5.3.2.1 External Cardiac Massage

Intensive external cardiac massage may be responsible for hepatic contusion in 3%–8.5% of the patients; the left lobe is particularly involved (LIGNITZ et al. 1977; DUMOULIN et al. 1981; ADLER et al. 1983; VOCK 1992; ZBAR 1993; DRUWE et al. 1996; FROMENT et al. 1998; ROSEN et al. 1999) (Fig. 5.2). In a review, an iatrogenic liver injury was found in about 3% of patients who died after cardiac massage and concomitant thrombolytic therapy, which may have precipitated hepatic hemorrhage. It is suggested in the literature that more than 10 min of cardiopulmonary resuscitation could be a contraindication to subsequent thrombolytic therapy for myocardial infarction, due to the risk of visceral hemorrhage (PEZZI et al. 1999). Heparin given in a trauma patient or in non-trauma conditions after cardiac massage may also precipitate hepatic hemorrhage. During external cardiac massage, the liver usually ruptures to the left of the falciform ligament. Rib fractures are associated in 73% of the cases, reflecting the intensity of resuscitation (ADAMS and SCHMITZ 1995). In the most dramatic cases, the left lobe may be completely separated, resulting in a posttraumatic left lobectomy. Simultaneous rupture of the liver and spleen was also reported after external cardiac massage (JOHANET et al. 1989). Curiously, one autopsy, which reported 140 unsuccessful resuscitations, which must have been intense, mentioned no liver injury, although splenic and even renal lacerations were observed (KLOSS et al. 1983).

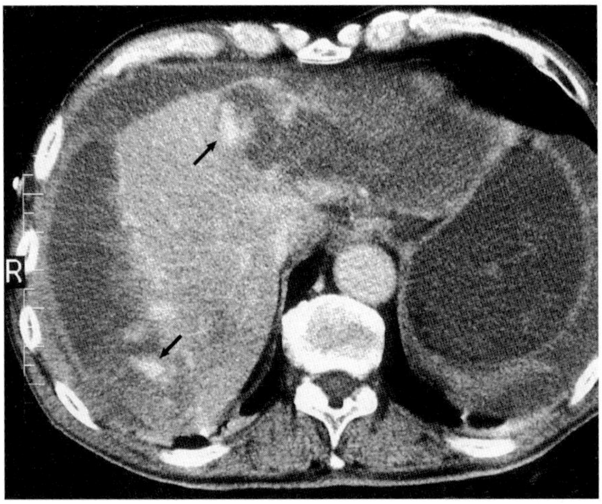

Fig. 5.2. This man collapsed after cardiac arrest. Vigorous external cardiac massage was undertaken for several minutes. The patient was resuscitated but became rapidly hypotensive again. CT at admission showed subcapsular hemorrhage in the right and left lobe of the liver, with blushes of extravasation of contrast medium (*arrows*) and supramesocolic hemoperitoneum. Conservative treatment was applied

5.3.2.2 Intraoperative Injury

Intraoperative liver injury may occur during open or laparoscopic surgery. Many causes are responsible for the injury: application of a surgical retractor, manual traction or mobilization of the liver. Perihepatic adhesions may become avulsed after pneumoperitoneum created for laparoscopy and bleed into the peritoneum. Liver injury caused by upper gastrointestinal surgery is usually located in the left lobe (HUNTER and REID 1983; FUSCO et al. 1994; ROGERS and MONAHAN 1996; YASSA and PETERS 1996; HASHIZUME and SUGIMACHI 1997; PASENAU et al. 2000). During mobilization of the right lobe of the liver in a trauma victim, a partial tear at the confluence of hepatic vein and IVC may become complete and result in profuse hemorrhage. In 4% of orthotopic liver transplantation, parenchymal liver injury may occur. In 50% of the organs, a grade IIb injury was present and was effectively treated by mesh wrapping, packing or other topical applications (SOLIMAN et al. 2000).

5.3.2.3 Nonoperative Iatrogenic Injury

Extracorporeal shock wave lithotripsy for renal or gallbladder stones is known to be responsible for renal or hepatic injury (MCGRATH et al. 1990; ROSSI and CATALANO 1992; MEYER and CASS 1995). Percutaneous transhepatic liver biopsy, puncture or catheterization of the intrahepatic bile ducts, portal vein, hepatic vein or hepatic artery, interstitial tumor therapy or percutaneous drainage procedures in the upper abdomen or even in the right hemithorax may result in hepatic hemorrhage (REICHERT et al. 1983; ORMANN et al. 1991; ZIRONI et al. 1999; AHMED et al. 2001). Transjugular intrahepatic portosystemic stent shunting (TIPS) may result in biliary or vascular injury, liver capsule perforation, intra- or retroperitoneal hemorrhage, hepatic infarction and bile leakage (HASKAL et al. 1993; PRAHLOW et al. 1997; SAWHNEY et al. 1997; OWEN and ROSE 2000). Even wedged hepatic vein phlebography done prior to TIPS for localizing the portal vein, may result in liver laceration and capsule perforation, when the catheter tip is

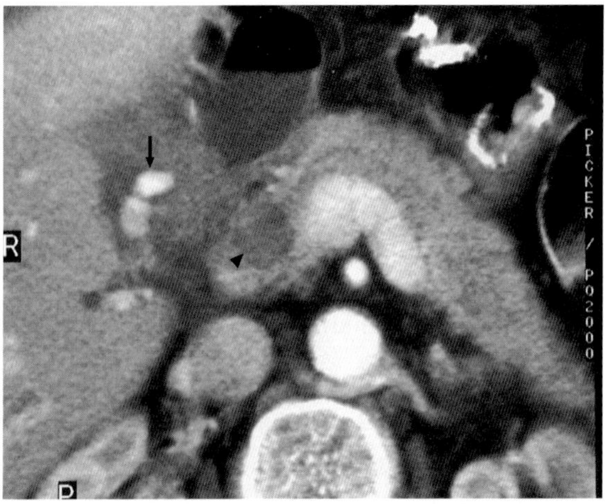

a

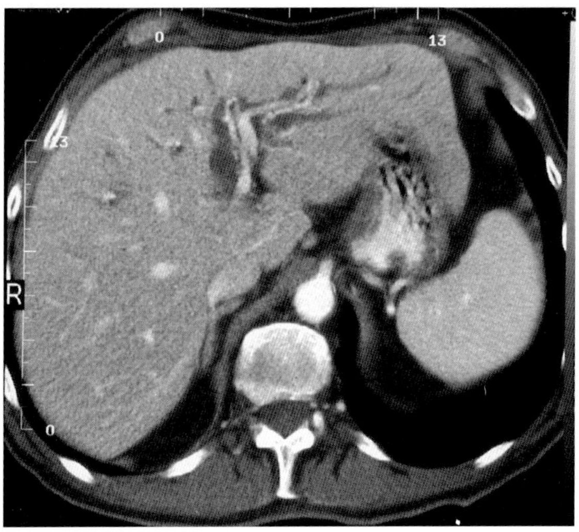

b

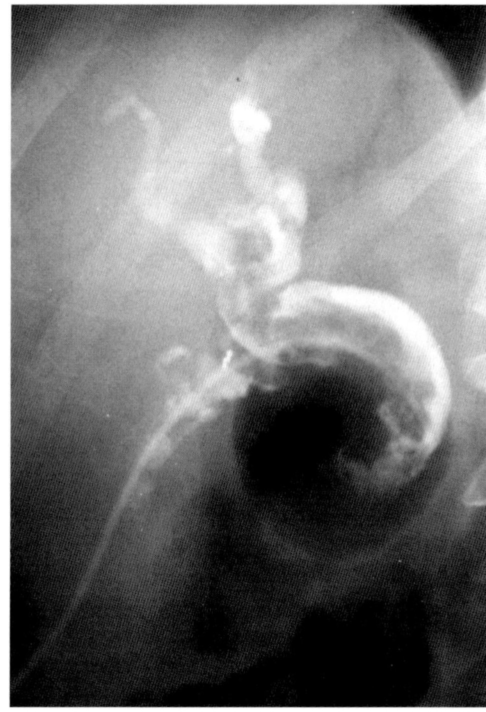

c

Fig. 5.3a–c. This patient showed upper gastrointestinal hemorrhage (hemobilia) after cholecystectomy. CT evidenced (**a**) a pseudoaneurysm located in the gallbladder fossa (*arrow*), a dilated choledochus filled with hyperdense material (*arrowhead*) and (**b**) dilatation of intrahepatic bile ducts predominating in the left lobe. (**c**) Opacification through a surgical biliary drain showed massive intraluminal defects within dilated intrahepatic and extrahepatic bile ducts, corresponding to duct obstruction with blood clots. The postoperative pseudoaneurysm was treated by selective arterial embolization

blocked in a peripheral hepatic vein branch directed towards the capsule, either injecting iodinated contrast medium or CO_2 (Semba et al. 1996). Finally, endoscopic retrograde cholangiography can be responsible for hepatic injury by perforation of the bile ducts by the guide wire or catheter (Wu and Katon 1993) (see also Chap. 6, "Injuries of the Bile Ducts").

5.3.2.4 Focal Hepatic Lesions

A great variety of intrahepatic focal lesions may rupture the liver capsule, either spontaneously or after a recognized or an unnoticed minimal trauma. Hypervascular lesions, large cystic lesions under tension and lesions that are in a subcapsular location are at particular risk.

Hepatocarcinoma may bleed spontaneously or rupture after a minor liver injury, or after arterial chemoembolization (Nagata et al. 1990; Schnarkowski et al. 1996; Rathod et al. 2000). The liver capsule may also rupture in case of malignant hepatic lymphoma, under aggressive chemotherapy (Tsutani et al. 1999). Other hepatic tumors such as hypervascular metastases from melanoma, another hypervascular primary or a vascular malformation may be the cause of intra- or extrahepatic hemorrhage. Prolonged use of contraceptive and hormonal therapy-induced adenoma is also a classic cause of spontaneous intra- and/or extrahepatic bleeding (Bottger et al. 1981). Spontaneous hemorrhage within a hepatic angiomyolipoma is less frequent and estimated to occur in up to 2% of cases (Manning et al. 1993; Nonomura et al. 1994). Hepatic cysts of any nature or abscesses are similarly exposed to rupture after trauma (Arcadio et al. 1968).

Finally, experimental work has shown that circulating cancer cells lodge in the liver within sites of injury, probably in relation with increased circulation around the trauma area (Agostino and Cliffton

1965). It is unknown if trauma to a malignant liver tumor accelerates systemic metastatic spread.

5.3.2.5
Non-posttraumatic Hepatic Hemorrhage

Spontaneous liver rupture has been described after coitus or vomiting (Horvath and Glasgow 1992; Davidson et al. 1993). Spontaneous liver laceration may also occur during labor or after cesarean section (Knoop et al. 1999). Pregnancy, toxemia of pregnancy, preeclampsia and hemolysis, elevated liver enzymes, and low platelet count (HELLP) syndrome may be responsible for nontraumatic liver rupture (Hibbard 1976; Sommer et al. 1979; Wagner et al. 1985; Risseeuw et al. 1999). The liver, due to its fragility caused by little stroma and thin capsule, may rupture in the neonate consecutive to birth injury, resulting in neonatal hemoperitoneum, in 0.13% of all newborns. The liver is five to six times more frequently involved than the spleen (Keuth et al. 1976; Menzel et al. 1977; Diez Pardo et al. 1979; Blocker and Ternberg 1986; Davies 1997).

Spontaneous rupture was also reported after thrombolytic therapy with streptokinase and in patients under coumarin anticoagulants. Ten cases of spontaneous liver rupture following lysis with streptokinase were described and four were lethal. Suggested favoring factors are a preexisting liver hemangioma, oral contraceptives, and hepatic steatosis (Ciorciaro et al. 1996; Hinterthaner et al. 1997). Some diffuse liver diseases such as amyloidosis can be responsible for spontaneous rupture of the liver and spleen (Okazaki et al. 1986).

5.3.3
Associated Injuries

Isolated liver injuries are seen in 10%–23% of cases of blunt hepatic trauma. As intense forces are involved in liver injury, a large number of associated abdominal injuries is expected. Recent studies have shown a high range of associated injuries in 41%–95% (Menegaux et al. 1993). Biliary, splenic, duodeno-pancreatic, bowel, right adrenal and right renal and transverse colon injuries are frequent observations. Midline organs such as the duodenum, pancreas and transverse colon are more likely to be injured together with the left lobe (Jeffrey and Olcott 1991). In some studies, 45% of victims also had an associated splenic injury (Roberts 1996). Conversely, when the spleen is primarily injured, an elongated left lobe of the liver covering the spleen is not necessarily damaged. Right pleural effusion, right lower rib fractures, hemothorax and pulmonary contusion are usual associated findings (McCort 1962, 1973; Kindling et al. 1969; Balasegaram 1976; Grasberger et al. 1985; Buckman et al. 1988). Associated rupture of the myocardium (right atrium) with tamponade is rare (Honda et al. 1996). IVC and portal vein lacerations are also seen infrequently in blunt liver injuries. Rupture of the right hemidiaphragm associated with liver injury raises special diagnostic problems, which are discussed in Chap. 9, "Injuries of the diaphragm".

5.4
Clinical Symptoms and Findings

5.4.1
General Symptoms and Clinical Signs

Clinical examination is not sufficiently reliable to establish the diagnosis of hepatic contusion and to evaluate its severity.

In the most severe injuries, during the initial phase of compensated hemorrhagic shock, clinical signs are subtle, until 40% of the blood volume is spoiled. Bradycardia can be puzzling, as it may be observed as a result of vagal stimulation. Due to its rich vascularization, the liver can bleed profusely and be responsible for rapidly progressive hypotension or shock. In the absence of rapid correction of blood volume, noncompensated hemorrhagic shock occurs, followed by metabolic acidosis, myocardial depression, diffuse intravascular coagulation and death. Multiple transfusions and hypothermia further contribute to metabolic acidosis, wash-out coagulopathy and other metabolic disorders.

In patients with less severe hepatic injury, abdominal pain, either diffuse or localized in the right upper quadrant is the most frequent complaint. Localizing abdominal symptoms are found in 27%, and nonspecific abdominal symptoms in 41%. Pain in the right shoulder (Kehr's sign) is indicative of phrenic, hepatic or biliary injury, and is specific if no trauma to the shoulder is evidenced. Singultus is rarely observed. A paralytic ileus can be present as a consequence of peritoneal irritation. In rare cases, patients may develop acute Budd-Chiari syndrome, due to compression, by a hematoma of the hepatic veins at the caval confluence (Izard et al. 1995).

It should be stressed that clinical symptoms can be absent in up to 19% of patients with documented liver injury (CORICA and POWERS 1975). In some cases, including the newborn, similarly to splenic injury, scrotal hematocele may be the only presentation of posttraumatic liver hemorrhage, due to a patent communication along the inguinal canal (HEYDENRICH et al. 1974; AMOURY et al. 1982).

Elevation of serum transaminase levels, in excess of 130 IU/l are an indicator of liver injury, even in the absence of clinical complaints (SAHDEV et al. 1991; COANT et al. 1992). In drug addicts, however, massive elevation of serum aminotransferases can be seen, even if only minimal liver contusion is present (LAM et al. 1999).

5.4.2 Hemobilia

Hemobilia is a sign of intrahepatic hemobiliary fistula and is estimated to develop in 2.5% of hepatic injuries (SCHORN and COLN 1977; CROCE et al. 1994). Possible causes are blunt or penetrating trauma, liver biopsy, surgery, and all types of simple or sophisticated transhepatic procedures, such as transhepatic cholangiography or biliary drainage, percutaneous bile duct stenting, local arterial chemoinfusion, TIPS, and percutaneous portal vein catheterization. Liver biopsy is the most frequent causal procedure, but hemobilia occurs only in 1–5 per 1,000 after needle puncture of the liver, although higher figures of 3%–7% were reported earlier (RAINES et al. 1979; ORMANN et al. 1991; JORNOD et al. 1999). Nontraumatic causes of hemobilia include inflammatory conditions, cholecystolithiasis, vascular disorders, tumor and coagulopathies. Major hemobilia was caused in more than 50% by trauma and in close to 20% by iatrogenic causes in 1980. Today, iatrogenic causes largely predominate and trauma accounts only for 5%–20% of hemobilia cases (SANDBLOM et al. 1984; YOSHIDA et al. 1987; GREEN et al. 2001).

Posttraumatic hemobilia is generally caused by an intrahepatic vascular lesion: a pseudoaneurysm or an arteriovenous fistula, which has eroded a bile duct wall. Therefore, hemobilia often coexists with biloma or a bile fistula. In some patients, persistent discrete extrahepatic hemorrhage is responsible for hemorrhagic ascites, which is diagnosed some time after the trauma. Persistent mixing of bile with a liver contusion prevents healing and explains recurrences of hemobilia. Significant bile duct obstruction caused by clot can occur, but is a rare event (Fig. 5.3). The bleeding is quite variable, either profuse, requiring urgent treatment, moderate or occult (SANDBLOM et al. 1984; SANDBLOM 1987). With the persistence of the lesion, which often remains unrecognized, hemobilia has the tendency to recur, sometimes for decades (SANDBLOM 1987). For hemobilia of posttraumatic and iatrogenic origin, the mean reported interval between injury and hemobilia is about 1 month, but a considerable time interval may separate injury from onset of symptoms (BISMUTH 1973). The classic clinical triad associates gastrointestinal hemorrhage, obstructive jaundice and biliary colic. The triad is incomplete in about 60%–70% of the cases (YOSHIDA et al. 1987). Hemobilia may be massive and patients present in shock (OKAZAKI et al. 1991).

The diagnosis of hemobilia is indirectly established by endoscopy. Endoscopic retrograde cholangiopancreatography (ERCP) confirms bleeding from the papilla only in a minority of the cases, but shows intraluminal choledochal defects, corresponding to clots, also occasionally seen in the pancreatic ducts, and evidences proximal biliary obstruction. ERCP does not show the intrahepatic bleeding site nor the nature of the vascular lesion responsible for hemobilia. Overall, ERCP is diagnostic in hemobilia in about one-third of cases and is able to rule out a gastroduodenal bleeding source. Bile duct dilatation often remains moderate, as clots are not totally obstructive. Endoscopic ultrasound (EUS) may be more contributive than ERCP because it more precisely shows mobile hyperechoic material without acoustic shadows in the gallbladder and the common bile duct, indicating endoluminal clot (CATTAN et al. 1999). Sphincterotomy as well as choledochal flushing removes clot from the bile ducts and exposes fragmented clot to the fibrinolytic activity of bile, accelerating regression of bile duct obstruction (CLANCY and WARREN 1997). Most often, clots dissolve spontaneously due to the intrinsic fibrinolytic properties of the bile.

US, CT and MRI can also suggest the diagnosis of hemobilia by showing echoic material in the bile ducts or hyperdense material and extra- and intrahepatic bile duct dilatation and sometimes the intrahepatic vascular lesion (SAX et al. 1988).

Blood pool scintigraphy may show accumulation at the site of an intrahepatic vascular lesion (NIELSEN et al. 1982), but arteriography is determinant, both for diagnosis and treatment. It locates the bleeding source in more than 90% of cases, evidencing either an underlying vascular lesion – a pseudoaneurysm or an arterioportal fistula – or shows, in a minority of cases, extravasation of contrast material into the bile ducts (VLAHOS et al. 1991). Arteriography is particularly useful for its therapeutic potential by allowing for selective hemostatic embolization (HEIMBACH et al. 1978; ROCHE et al. 1978a; CARR-LOCKE and WESTWOOD 1980; CURET et al. 1984; MCDOUGAL and MANDEL 1984; BRUNELLE et al. 1985; RICHARDSON et al. 1985; YOSHIDA et al. 1987; CZERNIAK et al. 1988; ROSCH et al. 1988; LEE and HIMAL 1992; SAVADER et al. 1992; TOMCZAK et al. 1997) (see also Chap. 23, "Imaging and Intervention of Posttraumatic Abdominal Complications"). A transient increase in liver enzymes may be noticed in nonselective hepatic embolization. In a review of 34 cases, two deaths were attributed to acute postembolization liver failure (VAUGHAN et al. 1984). In a review of 222 cases from the literature, 43% were managed conservatively and 36% by embolization. Surgery is indicated for repair of concomitant injuries or when embolization has failed. The overall mortality rate was 5% (GREEN et al. 2001).

Spontaneous definite resolution of hemobilia occurs only in a minority of patients without any kind of intervention. Bleeding may develop as a late recurrence even after several years (REUTER et al. 1980; CARR-LOCKE and WESTWOOD 1980; see also Chap. 6, "Injuries of the Bile Ducts").

5.4.3 Bilhemia

Bilhemia results from a posttraumatic communication established between a bile radicle and an intrahepatic vein (see also Chap. 6, "Injuries of the Bile Ducts") and is a rare event after blunt hepatobiliary injury, Fewer than 20 patients being reported. Due to low pressure in the hepatic venous system, bile drains into the vascular system. The jaundice caused by bilhemia cannot always be distinguished from jaundice caused by hemobilia (STRUYVEN et al. 1982). A patient may show a massive rise in direct bilirubin early after trauma and later in the course of follow-up of hemobilia, indicating that bilhemia and hemobilia may occur in the same patient.

Conversely to hemobilia, in bilhemia ERCP is able to show passage of bile in hepatic veins, and hepatic arteriography is usually nondiagnostic (STRUYVEN et al. 1982). Surgical treatment has shown that simple débridement and tamponade of the biliovenous fistula is therapeutic, avoiding hepatic resection (HABERLIK et al. 1992). Nonsurgical treatment of bilhemia can be obtained by endoscopic selective intrabiliary balloon placement to tamponade the leak with the liver for several days or sphincterotomy and bile duct stenting for decompression. If biliary obstruction is present, and responsible for elevated pressure in the bile ducts, balloon dilatation or stenting of a stricture should be obtained (STRUYVEN et al. 1982; VERHILLE and MUNOZ 1991; GABLE et al. 1997; SEARS et al. 1997).

Complete noninvasive therapy of the whole spectrum of bilhemia includes hemobilia and bile duct obstruction associates arterial embolization of the vascular lesion, endobiliary stenting for correction of bilhemia and bile duct obstruction, and percutaneous aspiration of an associated bile collection (EID et al. 1996).

5.4.4 Diagnostic Peritoneal Lavage

Diagnostic peritoneal lavage (DPL) confirms hemoperitoneum with a sensitivity over 95% and carries a false-positive or false-negative diagnosis in 1.5% (HANNA et al. 1987; HAWKINS et al. 1988; MEYER et al. 1989; REED et al. 1992; CROCE et al. 1995). Interpretation of peritoneal lavage is influenced by technique and the hemodynamic status of the patient. The severity of hemorrhage is imprecisely evaluated and no information is available on the source of bleeding. Undoubtedly, a positive peritoneal lavage is no longer a systematic indication for laparotomy and, if applied systematically, would lead to 30%–50% of unnecessary surgical interventions. In fact, about 80% of patients with blunt liver injury are hemodynamically stable and remain stable, without the need for urgent intervention despite hemoperitoneum being present (MALHOTRA et al. 2000). At present, DPL tends to be entirely replaced by imaging (DROST et al. 1991). A specific diagnosis of gastrointestinal or urinary bladder rupture or perforation of the bile ducts can, however, be reached by peritoneal lavage. This information is highly valuable if a stable patient should undergo other types of surgery than repair of hepatic injury.

5.5 Imaging

5.5.1 Ultrasound

5.5.1.1 Hemoperitoneum

Hemoperitoneum shows as a hypoechoic or anechoic pattern in the perihepatic spaces, which are investigated with high sensitivity by US. Mixed echoes or a hyperechoic dependent content corresponding to fresh clot may be seen in the perihepatic or pelvic compartments in the acute posttraumatic phase. Hemoperitoneum is best seen at the liver convexity, within the interlobar fissures, in Morrison's pouch, the paracolic gutters and pelvic perivesical spaces. Intestinal loops are separated by anechoic fluid, and seem to float in the fluid, when massive hemoperitoneum is present. Hemoperitoneum, ascites, bile effusion, intestinal fluid or intraperitoneal urine give similar US appearances. The amount of intraperitoneal hemorrhage can be approximately quantified on US appearance (McKenney et al. 1996). Significant injury to the bare area of the liver may be present without hemoperitoneum (Patten et al. 1993; Shuman 1997).

5.5.1.2 Hepatic Injuries

US findings can be described as follows:

- Small volumes of extravasated blood (0.5–2 ml) give intrahepatic linear echoic foci, as shown experimentally (Van Sonnenberg et al. 1983).
- Acute intrahepatic hematoma shows as a hyperechoic rounded image with sharp demarcation (Fig. 5.4); when in a subcapsular location, the shape is lenticular and the normal hepatic parenchyma is displaced centrally with scalloping limits. When noncoagulated blood and clot coexist, fresh clot is recognized as more hyperechoic and gravity-dependent signals. As for splenic injury, a perihepatic hematoma may be difficult to separate from a subcapsular blood collection. With ongoing spontaneous clot lysis, hematomas progressively change into an anechoic pattern. Brisk intrahepatic hemorrhage may also show as anechoic in the acute phase, compared with normal liver parenchyma (Fig. 5.5).
- Hepatic contusion is defined as an area of abnormal vascularization and edema, but with only little collected hemorrhage; it shows as a hypoechoic area (Fig. 5.6). This aspect is not as much emphasized in the literature as hyperechoic hemorrhagic contusion or hematoma. Differential diagnosis between a collected hematoma and hepatic contusion remains equivocal. When geographical hypoechoic areas are seen, they predominantly correspond to a mild or moderate contusion, Mirvis grade II or III (Ohta et al. 1998). Power Doppler could be helpful to demonstrate contused areas, which do not show any signal of perfusion.
- Parenchymal tears or fractures show as bands, lines or stellate hyperechoic strands, which may coalesce.

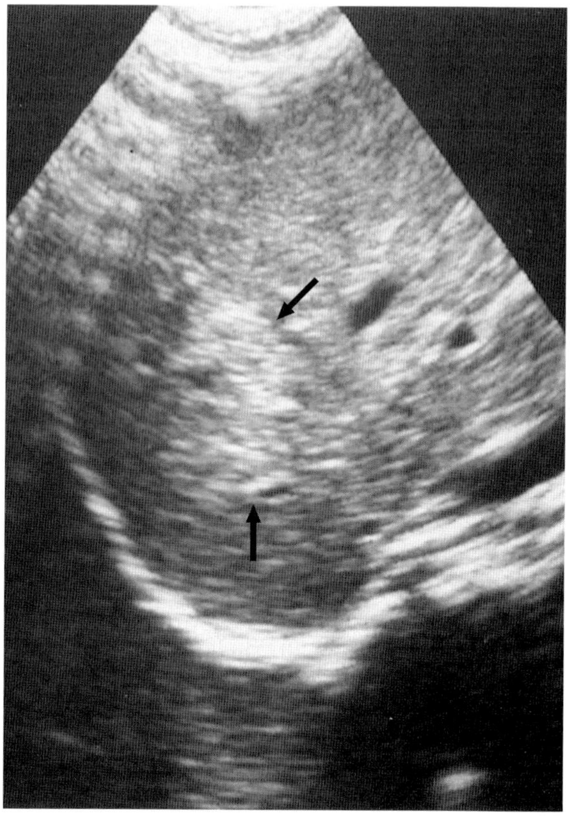

Fig. 5.4. A 6-year-old boy was admitted after having been involved in a traffic accident. Moderate abdominal pain in the right upper quadrant. Ultrasound shows a focal hyperechoic area (*arrows*) located in the right lobe of the liver, without intraperitoneal fluid, typical of a fresh intrahepatic hematoma. Conservative management was applied

- US could be more efficient than CT sections, which are limited to the axial plane, to evidence a hepatic hernia through a right diaphragmatic tear (see Chap. 9, "Injuries of the diaphragm").

5.5.1.3 Results

US evidences an intraperitoneal effusion with high confidence even if of small amount: sensitivities of 82%–88% and specificities of 94%–100% are reported (Kimura and Otsuka 1991; Jehle et al. 1993; Lucciarini et al. 1993; Goletti et al. 1994; Rozycki et al. 1995; McKenney et al. 1996; McKenney 1999). Isoechoic intraperitoneal hemorrhage adjacent to the liver may not be recognized in some cases. Changes in the liver texture, even discrete ones, are revealed in more than 90% of hepatic injury. The examination at the bedside can be accomplished in 1 min (Jehle et al. 1993). Quantification of hemoperitoneum using a

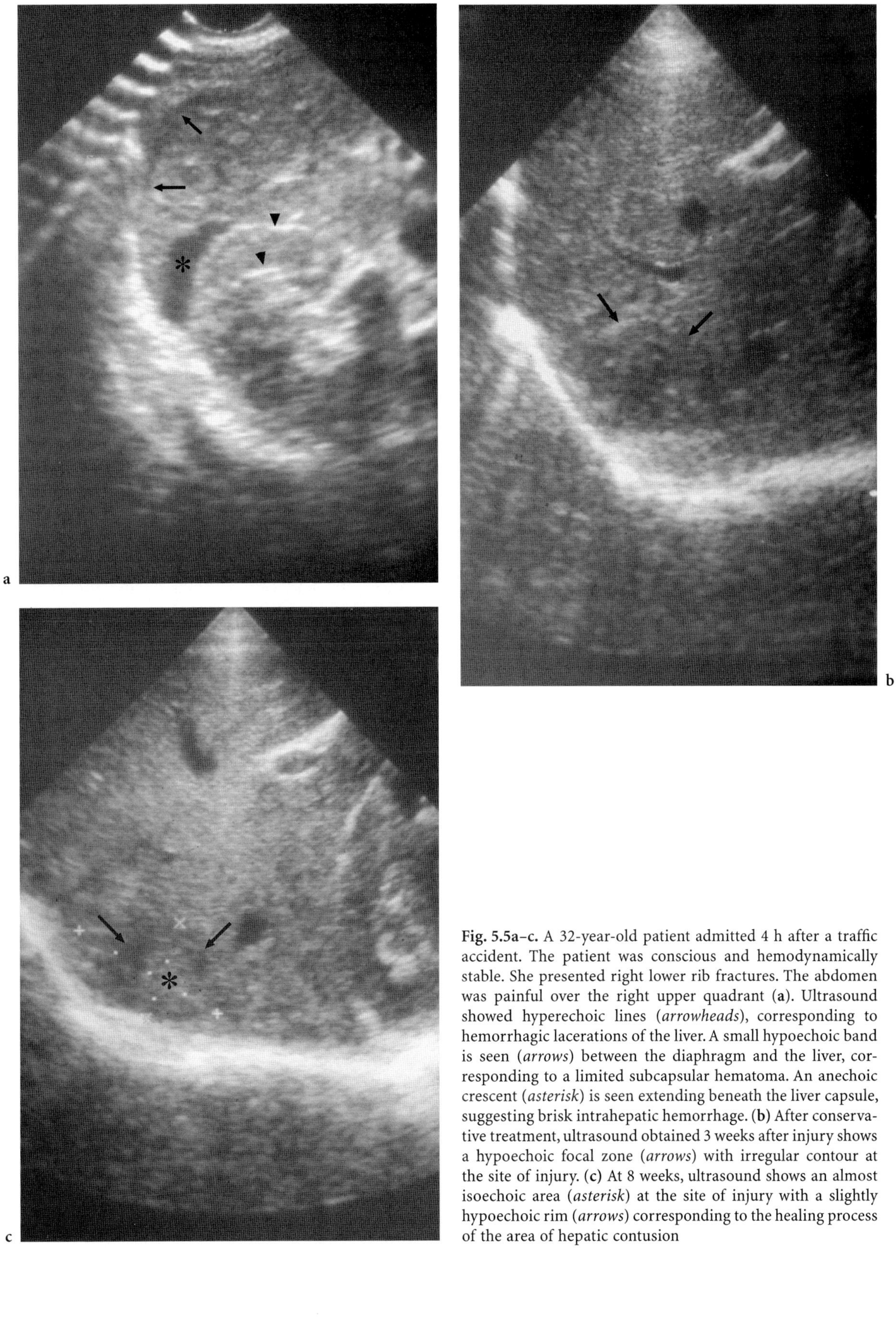

Fig. 5.5a–c. A 32-year-old patient admitted 4 h after a traffic accident. The patient was conscious and hemodynamically stable. She presented right lower rib fractures. The abdomen was painful over the right upper quadrant (**a**). Ultrasound showed hyperechoic lines (*arrowheads*), corresponding to hemorrhagic lacerations of the liver. A small hypoechoic band is seen (*arrows*) between the diaphragm and the liver, corresponding to a limited subcapsular hematoma. An anechoic crescent (*asterisk*) is seen extending beneath the liver capsule, suggesting brisk intrahepatic hemorrhage. (**b**) After conservative treatment, ultrasound obtained 3 weeks after injury shows a hypoechoic focal zone (*arrows*) with irregular contour at the site of injury. (**c**) At 8 weeks, ultrasound shows an almost isoechoic area (*asterisk*) at the site of injury with a slightly hypoechoic rim (*arrows*) corresponding to the healing process of the area of hepatic contusion

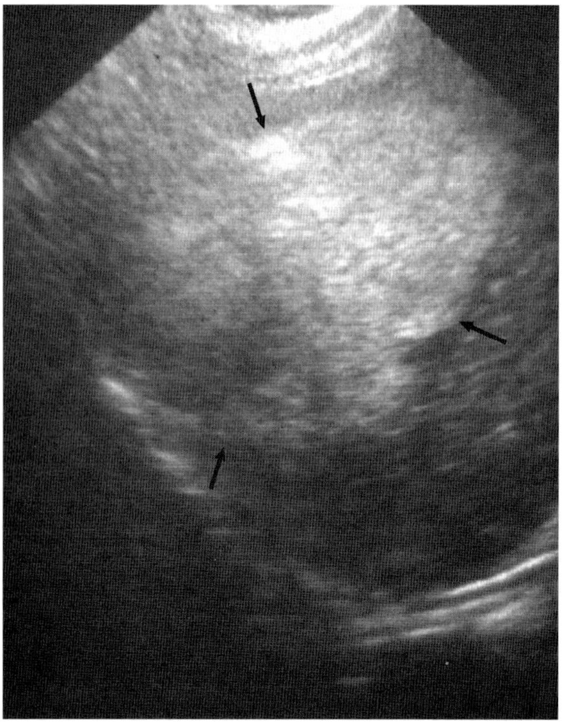

Fig. 5.6. This patient, aged 69 years, was admitted for acute abdominal pain, 24 h after a fall. She was hemodynamically stable. Abdominal ultrasound showed a focal heterogeneous and hyperechoic area in the right lobe (*arrows*), suggesting an area of contusion and hemorrhage

scoring system can suggest the potential risk of failure of conservative treatment of parenchymal injury (see Chap. 27, "A Selection of Published Surgical and Radiological Classifications of Abdominal Injuries"): a score equal or less than 2 was correlated with successful conservative management in 90%, whereas a score higher than 2 required laparotomy in 75% of cases, but these correlations have little practical value in patient management (McKenney et al. 1996; McKenney 1999). The major drawback of US is the limited information gained on the bare area and the perfusion of the liver. No reliable information is given on the digestive tract, thorax and bone. However, US is helpful in single trauma of moderate severity in a hemodynamically stable patient and in patients with minimal trauma, to exclude abdominal injury before the patient's discharge. On the other end of the spectrum of severity, US quickly answers the question if a hemorrhagic pericardial and/or hemoperitoneum or both are present to decide if a damage control laparotomy or thoracotomy should be done. US should in any case be supplemented in pediatric victims by CT, when no definite source of a visualized hemoperitoneum is evidenced (Akgur et al. 1997). Other limitations of US are patient obesity, subcutaneous emphysema, massive pneumoperitoneum and wound dressing.

5.5.2 Computed Tomography

5.5.2.1 Technique

With the use of slow scanners, a precontrast CT examination was obtained, which was only occasionally useful in detecting moderately hyperdense collected hematomas (Fig. 5.7). Minimal contusion was sometimes difficult to see on postcontrast scans alone that were obtained at the phase of equilibrium of parenchymal enhancement. A large contusion or hematoma was usually not overlooked in the absence of a precontrast scan. Actually, with rapid scanners with helical single-slice or multislice capability, precontrast scans are no longer routinely obtained. Scanning direction is craniocaudal during arterial enhancement, and caudocranial during the portal phase. A third scanning at the phase of equilibrium may be helpful for optimal delineation of contused areas or hematomas. Usually, the liver is scanned during a complete abdominal survey, including the entire thorax. Three-dimensional display of the liver gives a more detailed spatial display of injuries and normal intrahepatic structures, although all the

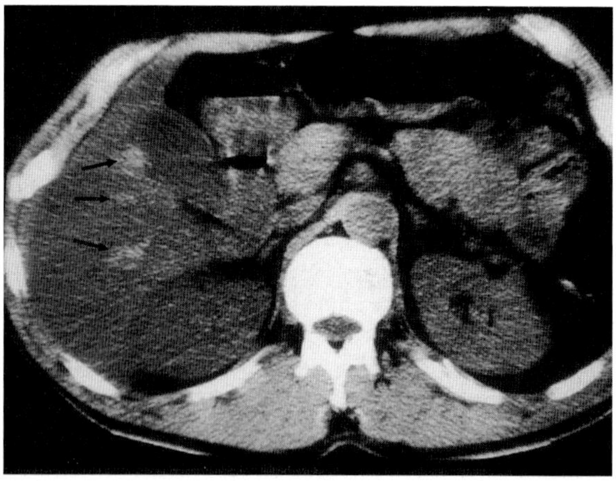

Fig. 5.7. Precontrast scan at admission, after a moderate abdominal impact, shows small hyperdense foci (*arrows*) in the right lobe of the liver, corresponding to minimal areas of intraparenchymal hemorrhage, which were no longer visible on postcontrast scan

information necessary for treatment was contained in the native axial slices (GOODMAN et al. 1995). Lesions located at the liver dome, diaphragmatic rupture and liver herniation in the thorax benefit from the images displayed in a frontal or sagittal plane. Printing of CT images at different window settings, using an additional narrow windowing, did not influence results of film reading of liver injury using conventional abdominal window settings and is no longer an issue of debate, as examinations are exclusively read on the console (PATTEN et al. 2000).

5.5.2.2 Positive Signs

Positive CT signs of hepatic injury are:

- A hypodense area with irregular margins in the liver parenchyma, or a stellate configuration: these features correspond to a hepatic contusion. Hypodensity can be subtle and visible only after IV contrast injection (Fig. 5.8). An area of contusion infiltrates the parenchyma and does not displace major intrahepatic vascular structures.
- A collected hematoma, either in an intraparenchymal or a subcapsular location, results from intraparenchymal hemorrhage. Fresh collected blood is spontaneously hyperdense vs normal liver on nonenhanced scans (Fig. 5.9). An intraparenchymal hematoma shows as a round area with regular limits and displaces or compresses intrahepatic vascular structures. A subcapsular hematoma has a lenticular shape and compresses the underlying parenchyma, with a scalloping limit (Figs. 5.10, 5.11). The involved lobe may show increased contrast staining between the hematoma and the liver capsule, due to reduced flow in the compressed sinusoids.
- Hypo- and hyperdense parenchymal areas may coexist, associating contusion and hemorrhage.
- Tears or laceration of the liver parenchyma present as thick, linear hypodensities similar to contusion, which may be parallel, resembling bear claws (Fig. 5.12). These lines often extend parallel to the plane of a large hepatic vein. Extent in depth is variable; lines may remain short and superficial, or extend deep to the liver hilum or may join the confluence of the hepatic veins and IVC. It can be difficult to distinguish between contusion and fracture or laceration in all cases. Rupture of the liver capsule may also be difficult to diagnose in a closed abdomen, when no separation of the capsular limit and of the parenchyma is seen.
- A hepatic fracture is recognized with confidence when a thick hypodense irregular line extends

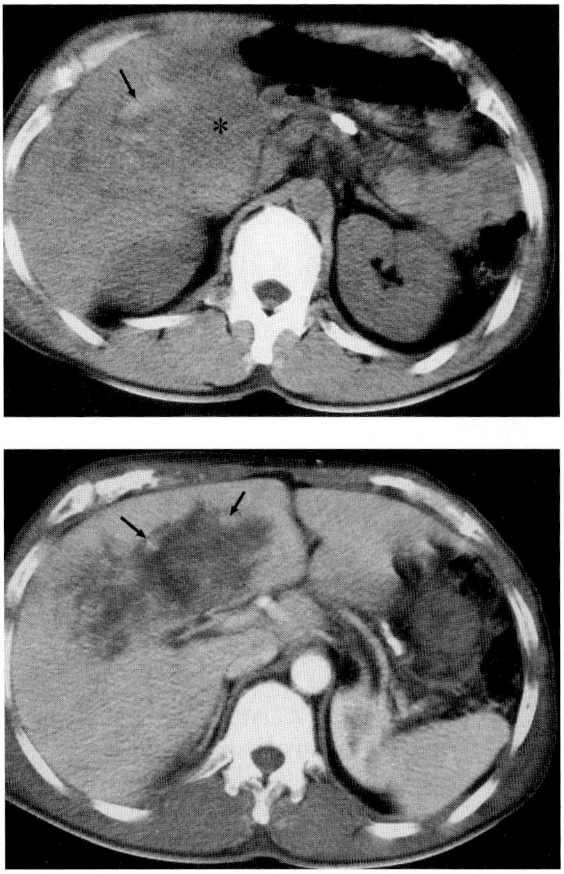

Fig. 5.8a, b. (**a**) On a precontrast scan, a focal hyperdense area (*arrows*) is faintly visible in the central zone of the liver, associated with a slightly hypodense surrounding area (*asterisk*). (**b**) On postcontrast scan, an extensive hypodense hepatic contusion with irregular margins and slight blushes of contrast (*arrows*) is better visible than on nonenhanced scan

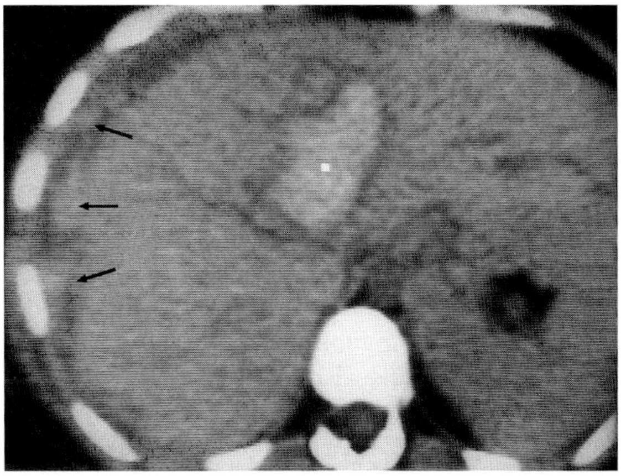

Fig 5.9. Nonenhanced CT of the abdomen shows a hyperdense collection of fresh blood (caliper) (63.4 HU), within the central region of the liver, corresponding to acute collected hemorrhage. Fresh blood clots (arrows) are seen in the perihepatic hemoperitoneum

from one liver surface to another, or from the liver surface to the hilum or to the IVC, and the liver capsule is clearly interrupted (Fig. 5.13).

- Liver contusion to the bare area is associated with hemoperitoneum in 20% of cases only. However, retroperitoneal hematoma may be seen in 88%, and (peri)-adrenal hematoma in 48% (Patten et al. 1993). An extraperitoneal hematoma can occur as an isolated finding, and is located in contact with the bare area, at the posterior aspect of the liver, or in the periadrenal or perirenal space (Fig. 5.14). When no liver injury is seen, an IVC laceration, a duodenopancreatic injury or a right phrenic rupture should be sought first.
- Effusion of blood around the IVC is shown as a hypodense pericaval halo sign; frequently a retroperitoneal hematoma in the right adrenal space is associated (Stalker et al. 1986; Radin 1992; Patten et al. 1993) (Figs. 5.15–5.17). This perivenous caval tracking may be considered as an equivalent of periportal tracking. Curiously, a halo sign is not found around the hepatic veins, probably due to the lobular structure of the liver, favoring accumulation of blood in the portal triad spaces and not in the centrilobular area.
- Periportal tracking is often seen at the acute posttraumatic phase and may regress within 1 day (Koslin et al. 1987; Macrander et al. 1989; Patrick et al. 1992; Wolfman et al. 1992; Lawson et al. 1993; Shanmuganathan et al. 1993). A hypodense periportal ring is seen on axial cuts or a hypodense lining parallel to the portal vein on tangential sections (Fig. 5.18). A classification of four grades was described (Vade et al. 1994; see Chap. 27, "A Selection of Published Surgical and Radiological Classifications of Abdominal Injuries"). The mechanism of periportal tracking is not univocal: elevated venous pressure, dilated lymphatics by lymphedema and hemorrhage probably play a simultaneous role when periportal tracking is diffuse. The sign seems to predominate in the right lobe of the liver, but can be confined to a particular area of the liver. Periportal tracking can be found as an isolated finding following moderate abdominal contusion (see also Chap. 6, "Injuries of the Bile Ducts").
- Rarely, air bubbles or tubular or branching air may be seen within a large area of contusion in the acute posttraumatic phase. When seen several days later, gas is likely, but not necessarily caused by hepatic necrosis or infection (Abramson et al. 1989). If air is seen in a portal branch in normal liver outside an area of contusion, preferentially in the left lobe, gastrointestinal or colon rupture should be suspected (Ho and Hu 1995) (Fig. 5.19).
- Nonenhancement of the liver, including on delayed scanning, may be due to complete interruption of flow in the hepatic artery and portal vein (Gay and Sistrom 1992; Hatten and Hamrick-Turner 1996). Arterial, portal, or arterial and portal devascularization, may lead to hepatic infarction and later to secondary posttraumatic intrahepatic abscess formation (Eng et al. 1981). Patients with major injury to the portal triad are usually in shock and operated upon without imaging, but patients with partial tears or vascular occlusion may undergo imaging. Isolated rupture of the hepatic artery is confirmed when no enhancement is visible at the arterial phase (Fig. 5.20). Severe arterial vasoconstriction can also occur, as it is occasionally seen in the pancreas and spleen (hypoperfusion complex) and may simulate hepatic artery disruption.
- Occasionally, thrombus of a large intrahepatic portal branch may be seen as an intraluminal hypodensity, within an area of contusion (Fig. 5.21).
- Compression or thrombosis of a major hepatic vein, usually the right, or the IVC may lead to a classic staining of contrast medium at the periphery of the liver parenchyma, mimicking Budd-Chiari Syndrome.
- Contrast extravasation staining within the liver parenchyma or diffusing through the liver capsule and diluting in the hemoperitoneum in the perihepatic spaces is an unequivocal sign of active bleeding or free intraperitoneal hemorrhage originating from the liver (Toombs et al. 1982; Meyer et al. 1985; Whitten et al. 1990; Fig. 5.22). Intrahepatic extravasation shows characteristic attenuation values of 80–130 HU, usually surrounded by a hematoma with lower densities. Densities of extravasated contrast are similar to those measured in large opacified vessels. Clotted blood, in the absence of extravasation, has density values around 60 HU and unclotted free intraperitoneal blood that is not mixed with contrast, 35–45 HU (Orwig and Federle 1989; Jeffrey et al. 1991; Radin 1992; Figs. 5.9, 5.11).
- Perihepatic or inframesocolic hemoperitoneum. Hemoperitoneum shows as a hypodense perihepatic fluid collection, which does not enhance after IV contrast injection, unless free intraperitoneal contrast extravasation is present. Average densities are around 45 HU and exceed

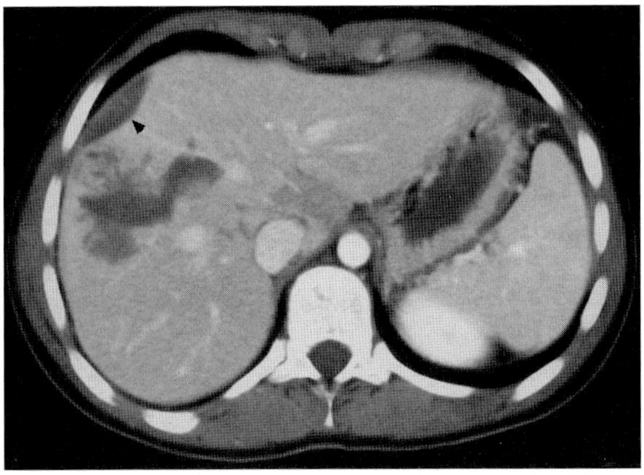

Fig. 5.10. Postcontrast scan shows an irregular hypodense area of contusion in the right lobe of the liver, without displacement of major intrahepatic vessels, and a small lenticular shaped, hypodense subcapsular hematoma (*arrowhead*)

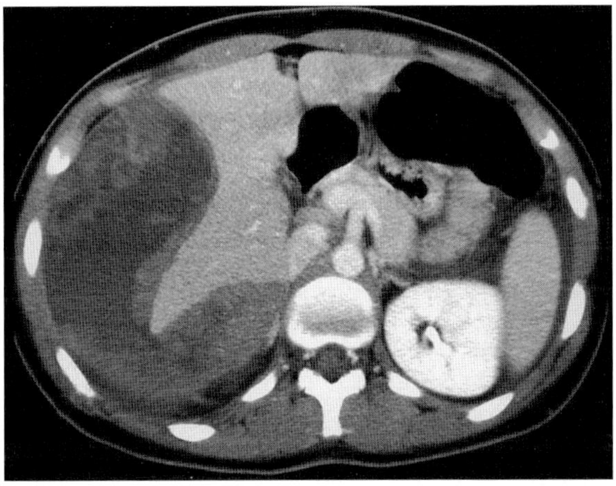

Fig. 5.11. Massive subcapsular hematoma of the liver is shown on a postcontrast scan, with a scalloping limit of the underlying parenchyma. Mixed densities correspond to fresh clots and fluid content within the hematoma

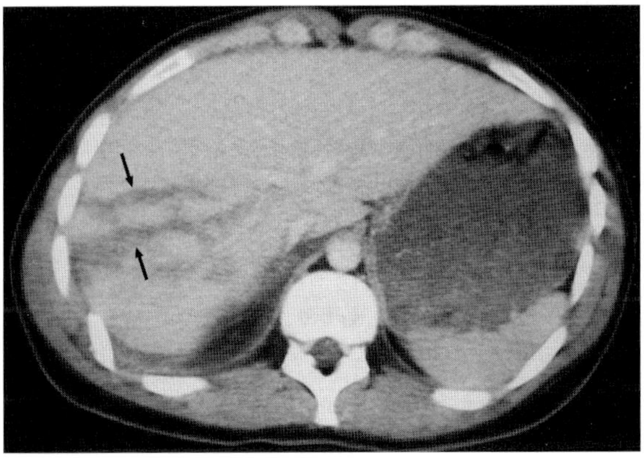

Fig. 5.12. Postcontrast scan shows thick irregular hypodensities (*arrows*) resembling bear claws, corresponding to post-traumatic lacerations of the right lobe of the liver

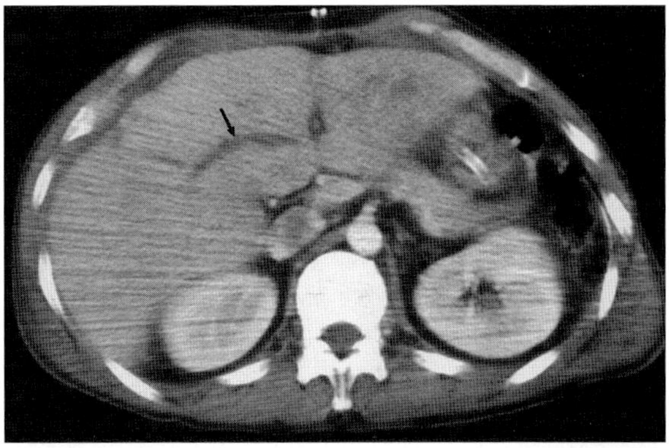

a

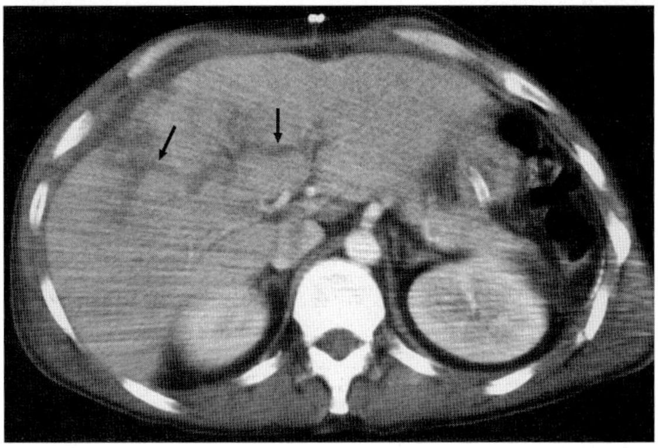

b

Fig. 5.13a, b. On postcontrast scan, an irregular hypodense band (*arrows*) is seen, extending from the right anterolateral surface of the liver to the ligamentum teres. Interruption of the liver capsule may be difficult to see on the closed abdomen, as in this case

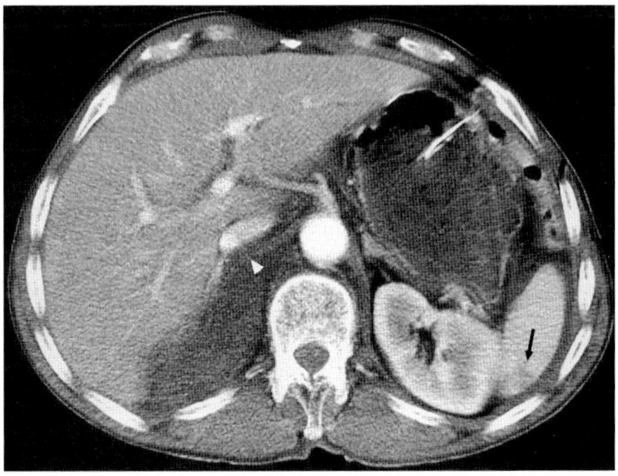

Fig. 5.14. On postcontrast scan, an extensive hematoma is visible at the bare area of the liver, with indistinct margins of the right crus of the diaphragm (*arrowhead*). The inferior vena cava and right adrenal gland are moderately displaced anteriorly. Note a small area of contusion in the lower pole of the spleen (*arrow*). When retroperitoneal hematoma is present at the bare area, injury at the hepatic vein-caval confluence should be suspected first. Rupture of the right hemidiaphragm and other sources of retroperitoneal bleeding should be ruled out

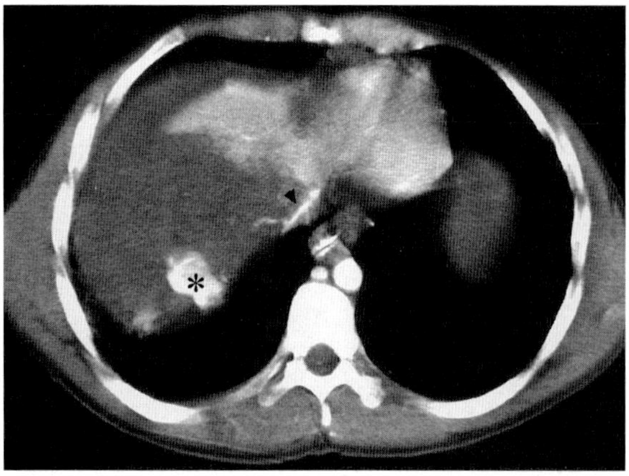

Fig. 5.15. On postcontrast CT, an extensive contusion and laceration of the right lobe of the liver is seen with massive extravasation of contrast material (*asterisk*). The inferior vena cava is flattened and shows irregular margins (*arrowhead*). At laparotomy, a laceration of the retrohepatic caval wall was confirmed

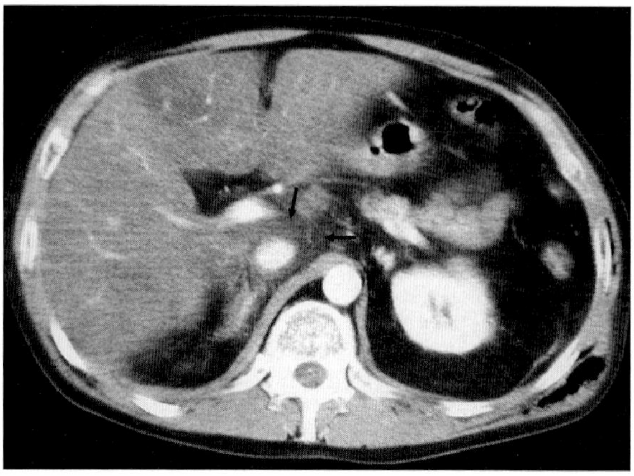

Fig. 5.17. A pericaval (*arrows*) and a right periadrenal hematoma is seen, without signs of caval laceration. No intervention was performed

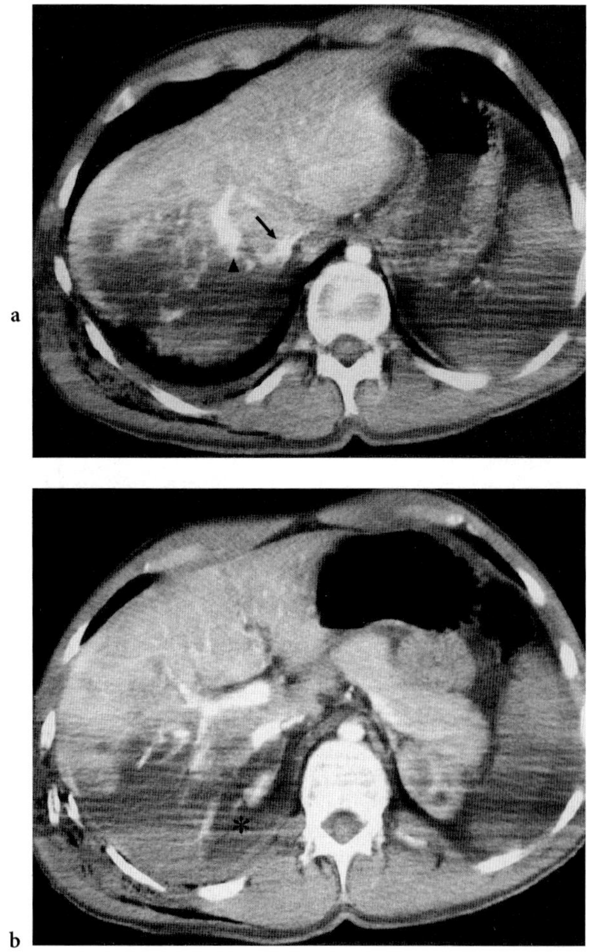

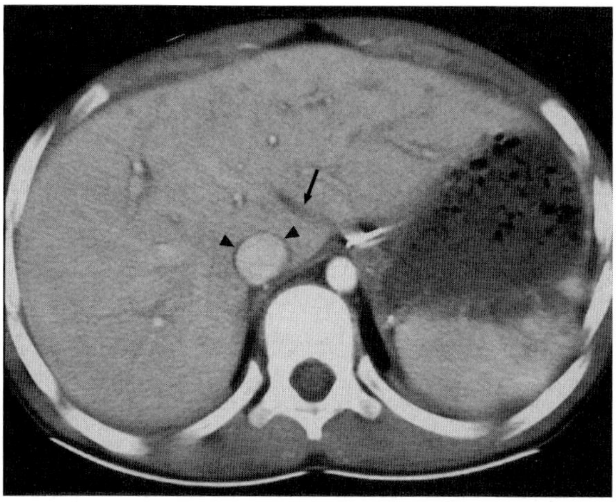

△
Fig. 5.18. Hypodense rings or lines are seen around the intrahepatic portal vein branches, and much less around the hepatic veins. A hypodense pericaval halo is also seen (*arrowheads*). Periportal tracking corresponds to minor hepatic contusion (see text). The ligamentum teres (*arrow*) should not be confused with a hepatic fracture. Note a minor splenic contusion

◁ Fig. 5.16a, b. On postcontrast scan, an extensive contusion of the right lobe of the liver is seen (**a**). The inferior vena cava shows irregular contour (*arrow*). The right hepatic vein is displaced anteriorly and partially obstructed (*arrowhead*). At a more caudal level (**b**), a retrohepatic hematoma (*asterisk*) is seen involving the adrenal space. The patient remained stable. No laparotomy was performed

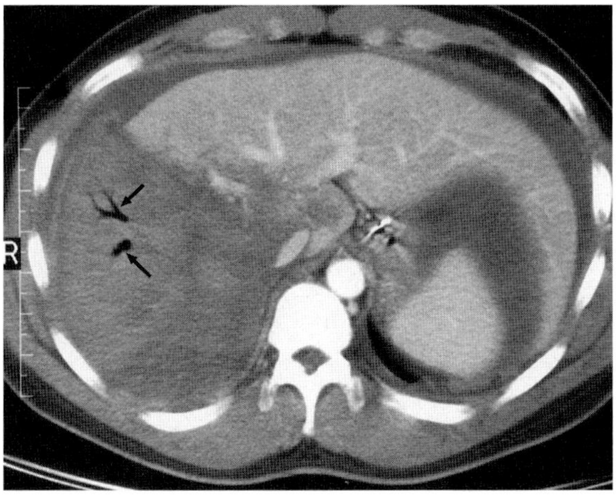

Fig. 5.19. A large hemorrhagic contusion with mixed densities is seen in the right lobe of the liver. The liver capsule is interrupted. Gas has accumulated in peripheral portal vein branches (*arrows*), in the area of contusion. Massive hemoperitoneum

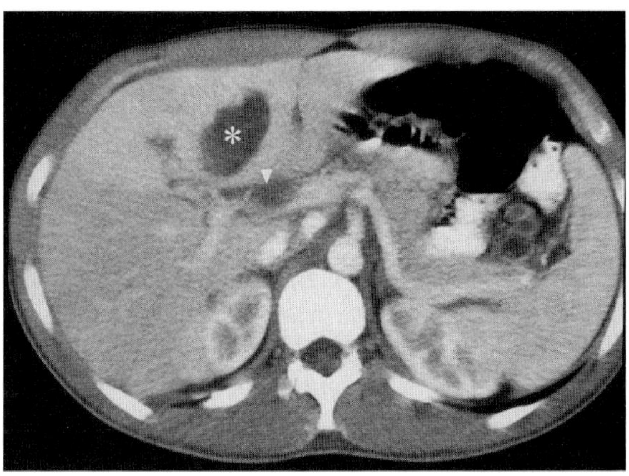

Fig. 5.20. A collected hematoma is noted in the left lobe of the liver (*asterisk*) and in the porta hepatis (*arrowhead*). The right lobe of the liver shows decreased enhancement at the arterial phase of opacification due to impairment of arterial flow to the right liver, probably by injury to the right hepatic artery. Right portal vein branches are normally enhanced

30 HU in all emergency cases. Fresh clots show as hyperdense zones and predominate at the site of hemorrhage: such differences in densities may be clearly visible when comparing the perihepatic and the perisplenic compartment. They are useful to predict what organ is actively bleeding, when splenic and hepatic injuries coexist (Federle and Jeffrey 1983; Levine et al. 1995). Hemoperitoneum is most frequently shown in the dependent perihepatic compartments, the right paracolic gutter and the perivesical space.

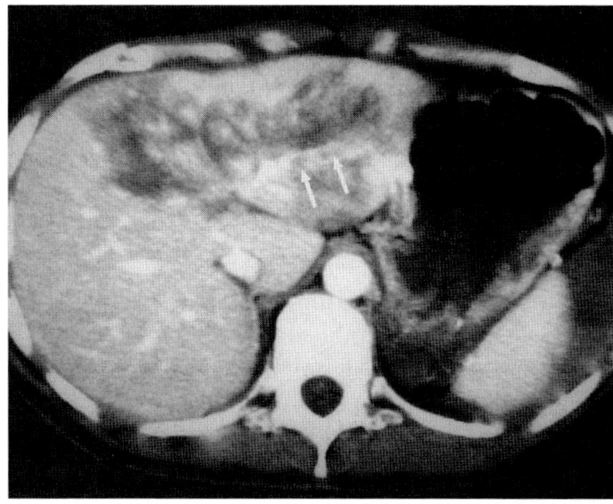

Fig. 5.21. On contrast-enhanced CT, extensive areas of contusion are seen in the left lobe of the liver, and a perisplenic hemoperitoneum is evidenced. Intraluminal thrombus (*arrows*) is seen in the left intrahepatic portal vein branch

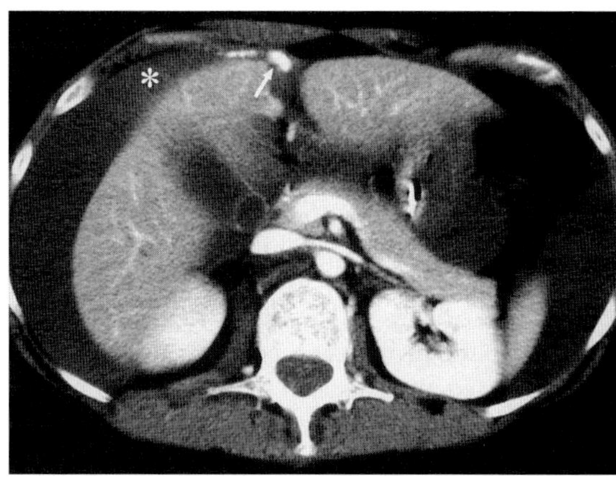

Fig. 5.22. Contrast-enhanced CT shows no intrahepatic parenchymal injury. Extravasation of contrast medium is seen at the arterial phase originating from the ligamentum teres (*arrow*), and diluting progressively in the anterior perihepatic peritoneal space (*asterisk*). Massive supramesocolic hemoperitoneum distends the abdominal cavity

- Occasionally, bowel loops can herniate through a defect of the liver capsule and simulate cavitating liver injury with air.

5.5.2.3 Pitfalls

With the advent of multislice scanners, most of the pitfalls that occurred in the past are overcome by the actual rapid scanning and optimal image quality, including multiplanar viewing.

Some potential pitfalls are listed below:

- A hyperdense hematoma could theoretically escape CT examination, which is obtained only after minimal IV contrast enhancement, when densities of the hematoma and enhanced liver parenchyma become similar, but generally a hypodense delineating ring is seen.
- Scanning too early without imaging at the portal phase or at the equilibrium phase may obscure discrete areas of hepatic contusion, particularly when no precontrast scan was obtained.
- Deep fissures filled with fat may simulate an intrahepatic linear laceration (Fig. 5.18).
- Absence of perihepatic hemoperitoneum is not an indicator of absence of liver injury: 11% of liver injuries and 12% of splenic injuries show no or only minimal hemoperitoneum on CT at admission (Ochsner et al. 2000).
- Ascites showing low water-like densities, caused by an acute Budd-Chiari syndrome, should not be confused with posttraumatic hemoperitoneum, bile ascites, intraperitoneal intestinal fluid or urine (Markert et al. 1997).
- On delayed scans, triangular or wedge-shaped, or more diffuse hypodensities may become apparent only on follow-up CT examinations obtained several days or weeks after admission. These changes can be caused by hepatic necrosis induced by hepatotoxic drugs (acetaminophen) given during hospitalization (Anderson et al. 1997).
- Unsuspected intrahepatic neoplasias with puzzling density, when of hypervascular nature, may be occasional pitfalls, and should not be confused with a posttraumatic vascular lesion or contrast extravasation (Cook et al. 1986).
- Preexisting liver cirrhosis may be responsible of deformed liver contour, lobar or segmental hypertrophies and atrophies, mosaic perfusion, portal vein thrombosis, focal areas of steatosis, which might complicate the diagnosis of liver contusion (Fig. 5.23).
- Streak artifacts could simulate a hepatic fracture on slow scanners in the past . They could also hide thrombus or intraluminal fat in the retrohepatic IVC, precisely at the diaphragmatic junction (Sheafor et al. 1998).

5.5.2.4 Classification

Early surgical classifications, based on lesion morphology, distinguished between linear contusion, burst or stellate fracture, and subcapsular or central hematoma (Fekete and Guillet 1969). Other classifications adapted to blunt hepatic trauma considered four grades: grades I and II include simple laceration with a benign prognosis. Stage III includes more complex injuries such as a central hepatic hematoma, stellate fractures and long linear fractures. Stage IV includes laceration of several segments and injury of the portal vein or hepatic vein (Guiset et al. 1980). The classification given by Moore et al. and its revision is the most widely used and considers an additional stage V for venous injury and a stage VI corresponding to hepatic avulsion, incompatible with survival (Moore 1984; Moore et al. 1989). Other classifications combine the surgical description of injury and clinical findings (Calne et al. 1979). A radiological classification, based on CT findings and derived from the surgical classification by Moore, is given by Mirvis and is largely used in the radiological literature (Mirvis et al. 1989). Many similar classifications of blunt hepatic injuries are available in the literature (see Chap. 27, "A Selection of Published Surgical and Radiological Classifications of Abdominal Injuries"). Intraoperative findings correlated well with CT description of injury, particularly in the papers in which the classification was described. Other studies, however, found a poor correlation between CT grading and surgery, but CT technique is a crucial factor in establishing such comparisons within a single study and also when comparing studies from different centers (Croce et al. 1991).

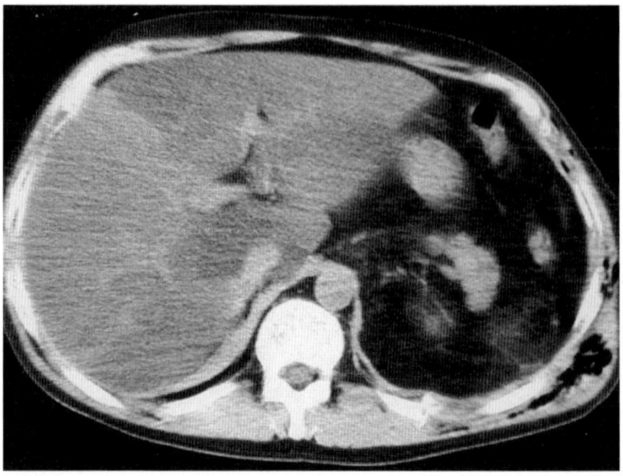

Fig. 5.23. CT was obtained at admission after a left lateral thoracoabdominal impact. Heterogeneous enhancement of the liver is seen, with hypodense areas located in the left lobe and in the caudate lobe, corresponding to diffuse steatosis, in a patient with liver cirrhosis. No posttraumatic liver injury was seen

5.5.2.5 Results

CT is the most sensitive test for the detection of hepatic contusion. The early literature and the more recent publications agree that overall diagnostic sensitivity of CT is about 93% and specificity reaches 98%. In the subgroup of patients with grade II or III injury, sensitivity was 100% and specificity 94% (McCort 1987; Watanabe et al. 1990; Raptopoulos 1994). However, CT was found only 65% sensitive and 85% specific in the detection of specific hepatic vascular injury in a comparison with arteriography (Poletti et al. 2000). When aiming at a detailed description of liver lesions, contusion, tear, fracture, and hematoma can be distinguished with more or less ease on CT, although, as for the spleen, it may be difficult to see a rupture of the capsule or a clear separation of liver fragments when the liver is maintained compressed in the closed abdomen.

The significance of periportal tracking needs comment. Periportal tracking may be present in 22%–62% of cases (Koslin et al. 1987; Macrander et al. 1989; Patrick et al. 1992; Wolfman et al. 1992; Lawson et al. 1993; Shanmuganathan et al. 1993). In patients with minor hepatic trauma, i.e., 60% of all patients with periportal tracking, it may be the only positive finding of an impact on the liver, without contusion or hematoma being present (Patrick et al. 1992). Progress to more severe injury was never seen on follow-up scans. Patients with circumferential periportal tracking without liver injury had significantly elevated liver enzymes, as compared with lower grades or noncircumferential periportal tracking (Vade et al. 1994). In one study, patients with periportal tracking had a higher number of extrahepatic associated injuries and more complications irrespective of operative or nonoperative treatment. When portal tracking is seen in a focal area of the liver, other signs of injury should be thoroughly sought (Yokota and Sugimoto 1994).

5.5.3 Arteriography

Before the advent of cross-sectional imaging, hepatic arteriography was used as the only imaging technique that was able to show posttraumatic vascular changes (Boijsen et al. 1966; Schorn and Coln 1977). Arteriography in trauma has almost no false-positive results and 1%–2% false-negative diagnoses of active hemorrhage (Ben-Menachem 1981; Gilliland et al. 1982; Sclafani et al. 1986). However, arteriography is much less useful to evidence areas of contusion, tears, fractures, small hematomas or hepatic vein or IVC injury. Angiographic signs of liver injury include spots or blush of contrast extravasation, which accumulates inside the liver or outside the liver capsule, vascular displacement, or compression, pseudoaneurysm or arteriovenous, arterioportal or arteriobiliary fistulae, and arterial, portal or hepatic vein thrombus. An avascular zone with marked displacement of vessels and surrounding dense parenchymal staining caused by compression usually corresponds to hematoma or biloma (Figs. 5.26b; 5.27a; 5.31b, c; 5.32b; 5.34b). Hepatic vein injury is demonstrated by angiography only in exceptional circumstances (Sclafani et al. 1983). Arteriography obtained in the first days after injury has shown arterial hypervascularization and amputation of the portal flow in the contused areas. Arterioportal flow may also be seen in the absence of a gross posttraumatic arterioportal fistula. These phenomena are transient and not related to severity of the injury (L'Hermine et al. 1978).

Hepatic arterial anatomy and variants must be kept in mind to obtain a complete arteriographic work-up. As a reminder, the right hepatic artery or the right lateral hepatic artery, or the celiac artery may originate from the superior mesenteric artery; the left hepatic artery or the branches of the left lateral sector may originate from the left gastric artery. Vascular anatomy and variants of the liver should be known in order to diagnose any parenchymal filling defect correctly, caused by a nonopacified aberrant hepatic artery (Konstam et al. 1979).

5.5.4 Magnetic Resonance Imaging

Magnetic resonance imaging (MRI) has no role in the assessment of acute hepatic injury, even though an examination could be concluded in a short time (Yamamoto and Pu 1992). MRI may be indicated in the subacute, delayed posttraumatic or convalescent phase, to confirm presence and extent of contusion, location and nature of a posttraumatic collection – hematoma or biloma – to demonstrate biliary obstruction, a vascular lesion or liver infarction and for follow-up of these lesions (Takakuwa et al. 1993; Balci et al. 1999; Hamil et al. 2000). Hepatic laceration at the acute stage is slightly hypointense on T1-weighted images and hyperintense on T2-weighted images and proton density sequences. Within

1 month, the laceration becomes hyperintense on all sequences (YAMAMOTO and PU 1992). In case reports, results of T2-weighted imaging and CT were judged of equal value and T1-weighted and gradient recalled sequences inferior to CT (MCGEHEE et al. 1993). Contrast-enhanced MR offers a better delineation of liver injury than nonenhanced MR (TERK and ROZENBERG 1998). MR has the potential to confirm blood in the gallbladder in the investigation of hemobilia, and also to evidence occasionally active bleeding from a liver laceration (YAMAMOTO et al. 1994).

5.6 Management

5.6.1 Surgical

5.6.1.1 Prognosis

Mortality of blunt liver injury depends on type and severity of hepatic injury, number and type of associated injuries and type of treatment. Overall mortality of hepatic injury caused by blunt contusion is 10%–64%, with a mean around 30% in the past and 10% in more recent reports. Among nonsurvivors from hepatic contusion after a car accident, 82% were drivers and 18% passengers. Among survivors, 68% were drivers, 32% were passengers and 7% were ejected from the car (FREY et al. 1973). Mortality resulting from penetrating trauma is about 10%–17%, and injury caused by a stab wound is responsible for the lowest mortality rates, of 0.6–5%, and gunshots for about 12% (MORTON et al. 1972; TRUNKEY et al. 1974; DEFORE et al. 1976; LEVIN et al. 1978; CARMONA et al. 1982; OLSEN 1982; ANDERSON and BALLINGER 1985; FELICIANO et al. 1986a,b; WALT 1986; HANNA et al. 1987; COGBILL et al. 1988; COX et al. 1988; BEAL 1990; MAIONE et al. 1994; MARR et al. 2000).

The cause of death, directly related to liver injury, is uncontrolled hemorrhage in 75%–82% (LEVIN et al. 1978; ELERDING et al. 1979; FELICIANO et al. 1986a,b; COX et al. 1988; BEAL 1990). Aggressive resuscitation was able to limit early mortality of liver injury to less than 4% in the most optimistic reports. Intraoperative and perioperative mortality is actually around 2%–8% and the mortality rate directly related to hepatic injury is 5%–8% (MALHOTRA et al. 2000). Generally, the majority of liver injuries, around 70%–80%, are grade I–III. However, in those series where 40% of patients had severe injury (grade IV–V) and five or more associated lesions, overall mortality was 41%–73% and liver-related mortality 36% after surgical treatment (REIFFERSCHELD 1958; DEFORE et al. 1976; TRUNKEY et al. 1974; SAYERS et al. 1992; MAIONE et al. 1994). Outcome is also related to management options. The mortality rate for patients with blunt liver injury that was treated conservatively is around 13%, and patients who required surgery had the highest mortality rate, around 36% or more (MAIONE et al. 1994; BRAMHALL and BUCKELS 2000). Mortality is also related to the type of surgical treatment. When only sutures or drainage is required in low-grade liver injury, mortality is 5%, whereas hepatic resection, required in more extended injuries, carried a mortality of up to 52% (LEVIN et al. 1978). The number of peri- and postoperative transfusions is also correlated to the mortality rate caused by hepatic contusion (SCOTT et al. 1988). The figures for direct liver-related mortality tend to be similar, between blunt or penetrating injury, but postoperative complications are more frequent after surgical repair of penetrating trauma (MARR et al. 2000). In recent surgical experience with high-grade liver injuries (grades IV and V) that were managed with surgical, angiographic and endoscopic biliary approaches, overall mortality was 14% and hepatic mortality 9% (8% for grade IV and 22% for grade V; ASENSIO et al. 2000).

Severity of associated injuries and delayed posttraumatic multiorgan failure are responsible for an additional mortality rate of 11%–23% in liver trauma. Roughly half of all lethal outcomes are caused by associated injuries. Extra-abdominal-associated lesions that significantly increase mortality rates are trauma to the brain or the thorax and delayed septic complications (RIVKIND et al. 1989). Imaging should recognize the liver injury, but also signs of liver cirrhosis, as mortality in the cirrhotic patient is increased by a factor of five in trauma patients and the hospital stay of injured cirrhotic patients is lengthened by 36% (GOMEZ et al. 1994).

Surgical and CT-based classifications of liver injury reflect the severity of lesions and contribute to optimal therapeutic management (MOORE et al. 1994). Grades I, II and III, which are the most frequent, show a mortality rate ranging from 0% to 14%, grade IV a mortality rate from 7% to 56%, and grade V a mortality rate from 33% to 100%. The lowest figures correspond to single liver injury, the highest figures to multiple associated injuries. In grade V, 55% are intraoperative death, and 28% are caused by intractable hemorrhage, whereas intraoperative death accounts only for 17% and 20% in grades I and II, respectively (Letoublon and Castaing 1996). Many prognostic factors predicting early death in liver injury have been analyzed in retrospective and prospective studies: shock, number of blood units given, Glasgow coma score, associated injuries, postoperative blood urea nitrogen, preoperative alanine and aspartate aminotransferase, base excess, and platelet count. The three last factors were recognized as most prognostic for hemorrhagic death (Chen et al. 1995; Sim et al. 1995; Nishida et al. 1996).

5.6.1.2 Hemostasis

The objective of treatment is to stop bleeding originating from the liver. The following surgical treatment modalities are applied: simple peripheral hemostatic sutures, closure of fracture by large sutures, the Pringle maneuver, vascular tourniquets or ligatures, glue, perihepatic mesh, hepatorrhaphy, perihepatic packing, hepatostomy (in gunshots), atypical liver resection, and regular lobectomies or segmentectomies.

Major hepatic hemorrhage is caused by a transcapsular hepatic fracture and arterial bleeding, portal vein, hepatic vein or venocaval rupture or disinsertion, which might lead to death in tabula, during excessive liver mobilization (Klein et al. 1994; Jurkovich et al. 1995). Damage control or abbreviated surgery is a deliberately incomplete operation to avoid irreversible complications of hypothermia, acidosis and washout coagulopathy. The intervention takes a few minutes and is limited to control of hemorrhage and repair of gastrointestinal or other hollow viscus rupture. Reoperation is scheduled 2–24 h later in the resuscitated and stabilized patients who have survived. Damage control surgery may be required in up to 18% of patients with the most severe blunt liver injury. In a series of 200 patients treated, 50% survived damage-control surgery, and 67% of survivors stayed alive (Stone et al. 1983; Burch et al. 1992). Survival of damage-control laparotomy is significantly higher than after a conventional laparotomy in the most severe patient group. Indications for abbreviated damage control surgery are estimated hemorrhage of 4–5 l, control body temperature inferior to 34°C, and pH less than 7.25 (Carrillo et al. 1993). Clamping of the thoracic aorta in hemostasis of blunt abdominal contusion is an extreme operation and carries a mortality of 88%–100% (Harnar et al. 1981; Flynn et al. 1982). Perihepatic packing, (followed by wrapping) (Cirocchi et al. 1999) is a life-saving maneuver, similar to a damage-control intervention, and may allow patient transfer to a trauma center after resuscitation (Calne et al. 1979; Feliciano 1981; Pachter et al. 1983; Carmona et al. 1984; Baracco-Gandolfo et al. 1986; Feliciano et al. 1986a,b; Ivatury et al. 1986; Sherlock and Bismuth 1991; Fig. 5.24).

In complex hepatic injury and irreversible hepatic failure, orthotopic liver transplantation was considered in the subacute posttraumatic phase (Esquivel et al. 1987; Ringe et al. 1988, 1991; Oldhafer et al. 1993; Demirbas et al. 1997; Ginzburg et al. 1998). On the other hand, livers with low-grade injury, considered marginal organs, were successfully transplanted (Broering et al. 1999; Avolio et al. 2000). Injured liver transplantation has no effect on patient survival when high-risk candidates are avoided. Therefore, in view of liver transplantation from a trauma victim, careful imaging of the liver is necessary, even in patients with apparently low-grade liver injury, but other associated lethal injuries.

Hepatic Veins and Inferior Vena Cava

Hepatic veins or IVC hemorrhage is profuse and has no tendency to stop, as veins do not contract to stop extravasation. Disinsertion of a main hepatic vein at the venocaval confluence or rupture of the retrohepatic IVC after blunt trauma is often lethal (grade V injury), whereas injury to the suprarenal and

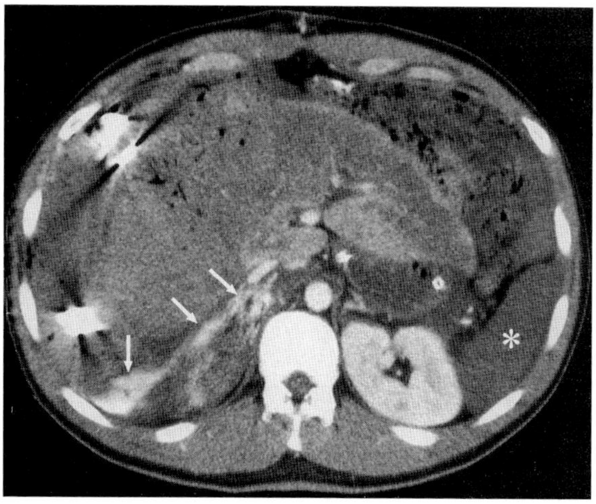

Fig. 5.24. Contrast-enhanced CT obtained after emergent laparotomy for massive hepatic posttraumatic laceration. Note the faint enhancement of the liver parenchyma, absence of splenic enhancement (*asterisk*) caused by severe vasoconstriction, and massive contrast extravasation (*arrows*) originating from the bare area of the liver around the inferior vena cava. The liver is compressed by operative perihepatic packing. Multiple air bubbles are seen within the packing material, and within the liver parenchyma at the site of laceration

infrarenal IVC has a somewhat better prognosis. An overall mortality rate of 33%–85% was reported, and a rate of close to 100% when complete transection of the IVC has occurred in the supradiaphragmatic IVC (ALLEN and BLASIDELL 1972; TURPIN et al. 1977; HALPERN and ALDRETE 1979; BYRNE et al. 1980; KASHUK et al. 1982; MILIKAN et al. 1983; BURCH et al. 1988; WIENCEK and WILSON 1988; COIMBRA et al. 1993, 1994a,b; LEPPANIEMI et al. 1994; CARILLO et al. 1997; CHEN et al. 2000).

Hepatic veins are involved in about 13% of liver injuries (SHANMUGANATHAN and MIRVIS 1995). Injury to the right hepatic vein is the most frequent (6%), followed by the IVC and median hepatic vein (2.5%), and left hepatic vein (1%). Venous injury is significantly more frequent with liver laceration than with isolated intrahepatic hematoma (LETOUBLON and CASTAING 1996). Imaging plays a limited role in evidencing venous laceration, as the majority of patients are hemodynamically unstable and are immediately directed to the operating room. Venous injury must be suspected when an area of contusion or a hematoma is located at the junction of the hepatic vein confluence, or when a retrohepatic hematoma is seen around the IVC (Figs. 5.16, 5.24). Surgical treatment includes primary venorraphy with atriocaval shunt, venovenous bypass, a nonshunting caval isolation approach, perihepatic packing, or ligation without resection (ALLEN and BLASIDELL 1972; DEPINTO et al. 1976; MCMASTER 1976; PILCHER et al. 1977; WALT 1978; KUDSK et al. 1982; BROTMAN et al. 1984; MOORE 1984; PACHTER et al. 1986; COGBILL et al. 1988; KRIGE et al. 1992; YOKOTA et al. 1993; BAUMGARTNER et al. 1995; TAGA et al. 1997; THOMFORD et al. 1998; CHEN et al. 2000). An intraoperatively localized tear in a hepatic vein or IVC can be treated by emergent endoluminal intracaval placement of a covered metal stent, without a direct surgical approach (BURCH 1997).

Portal Vein

Portal vein injury is caused by blunt trauma in 5%–10% of cases. Injury to the extrahepatic segment of portal vein branches seems more frequent than portal vein trunk injury during blunt trauma (Fig. 5.25). The right portal vein branch is more frequently involved than the left and association with hepatic laceration is almost the rule (BUSUTTIL et al. 1980; SHELDON et al. 1985; LETOUBLON and CASTAING 1996). Patients with injury to the porta hepatis require urgent intervention. Mortality, caused by exsanguination, is 41%–80% (MATTOX et al. 1975; BOSTWICK and STONE 1975; BUSUTTIL et al. 1980; COLLINS et al. 1988; JURKOVICH et al. 1995). Portal vein injury is controlled by a Pringle maneuver, and repaired by primary lateral venorraphy, vein patch interposition, splenic-mesenteric bypass, or end-to-end suture or ligation of the portal vein as a last resort and followed by a second-look operation in survivors. Associated injuries to the IVC, aorta, liver, pancreas, or bile ducts are common in these severe injury grades (MATTOX et al. 1975). Concomitant bile duct transection is treated by biliary-enteric bypass or more conservatively if tangential rupture is present (FISH 1966; BUSUTIL et al. 1980). Severe rupture of the pancreas may also be associated with portal vein rupture (HENNE-BRUNS and KREMER 1992). In rare instances, the portal vein or a branch may undergo occult self-tamponaded rupture and occasionally obstructive jaundice can be caused by a hematoma in the porta hepatis resulting from partial portal vein (left branch) laceration (LAU and DIAMOND 1997).

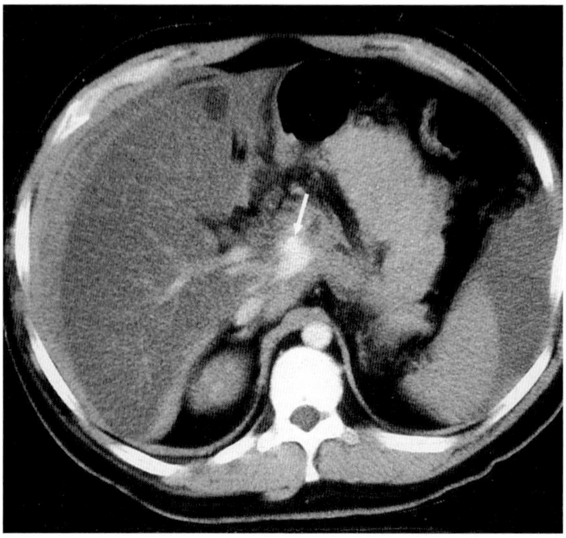

Fig. 5.25. Rupture of the portal vein trunk. Massive extravasation of contrast medium (*arrow*) has accumulated in contact with the extrahepatic portal vein trunk. Faint opacification of the intrahepatic portal vein branches. Massive perihepatic and perisplenic hemoperitoneum

Hepatic Artery

It has been shown that the liver parenchyma usually tolerates proximal ligation of the common hepatic artery or proximal arterial embolization well. Hepatic infarction is rarely observed, provided the liver has not suffered from anoxia, hepatocyte function is intact, the portal vein is patent and arterial collateral circulation is able to develop immediately, particularly through the peribiliary arterial plexus (Burton-Opitz 1910; Bengmark and Rosengren 1970; Lewis et al. 1974; Mays 1974; Jander et al. 1977; Fuller and Anderson 1978; Walt 1978; Flint and Polk 1979; Feliciano and Pachter 1989).

Ligation of one or both lobar hepatic arteries can be done, usually without complications. Arterial ligation aims at rapid hemostasis in so-called explosion injury of the liver, without long-term complications (Musiani et al. 1993). The literature reports arterial ligation to be applied in around 10% of severe injuries, with a 70%–80% successful control of hemorrhage. However, liver necrosis following hepatic artery ligation or arterial embolization was reported in a few cases, despite patency of the portal vein (Lucas and Ledgerwood 1978; Flint and Polk 1979). Cholecystectomy can be performed prophylactically after hepatic artery ligation to prevent ischemic gallbladder wall necrosis.

5.6.2 Conservative

5.6.2.1 Surgical

Surgical treatment of blunt hepatic injury is predominantly conservative. Lobar resections were replaced by tamponade packing and peripheral sutures or hepatorrhaphy, use of topical hemostatic agent or simple peritoneal drainage (Witte and Zukoski 1983; Cox 1984; Moore et al. 1985; Baracco-Gandolfo et al. 1986; Giuliano et al. 1987; Shah et al. 1993; Fang et al. 2000). Minor surgery without deep hepatotomy and without resection can be applied in 60%–90% of hepatic contusions, resulting in an overall mortality of 10%–14% and only 5% or less when the liver is the only organ injured (McInnis et al. 1977; Walt 1980; Pachter et al. 1983; Hanna et al. 1987). Patients with the most severe injuries – predominantly grade III to V– and with a 95% rate of associated injuries, however, have a 34% perioperative mortality with conservative surgery (Menegaux et al. 1993). Resorbable mesh or pads of polyglycolic acid can be placed around the liver, but indication in liver contusion is not well established. Due to the great variety of patients selection for perihepatic packing, results vary greatly, with mortality between 0% and 58%. Patients who have an additional extrahepatic bleeding site have the highest mortality, varying from 45% to 58% (Feliciano et al. 1986a; Cogbill et al. 1988; Cue et al. 1990; Sharp and Locicero 1992; Morris and Crane 1993). Smaller series show more optimistic results depending on patient selection.

Pregnant women should be treated conservatively, but surgical exploration is mandatory when fetal monitoring is not reassuring (Icely and Chez 1999).

The use of controlled surgical biliary drainage in major liver injury was largely debated in the literature (Merendino et al. 1963; Longmire and Cleveland 1972; Lucas and Ledgerwood 1973; Pickleman and Block 1973; Mays 1974). Increased morbidity, resulting from bile decompression and the inability to prevent other injury-related complications, led to the nonacceptance of T-tube, or systematic, cholecystostomy.

5.6.2.2 Arterial Embolization

Hepatic artery embolization was shown to be a valuable adjunct in the management of severe hepatic hemorrhage (Allison et al. 1985; see also Chap. 22, "Aterial hemostatic embolization in abdominal injuries"). Embolization on an emergency basis and as a primary hemostatic treatment, including patients with hemoperitoneum, has been reported in small series of patients (Jander et al. 1977; Rubin and Katzen 1977; Hashimoto et al. 1990; Dondelinger and Kurdziel 1991; Kos et al. 1999; Yitzhak et al. 2001; Figs. 5.26, 5.27). However, even in marginally stable or unstable patients with complex liver injury, emergency arterial liver embolization can be performed in specialized departments. Other reports illustrated the value of arterial embolization for ongoing or recurrent hemorrhage, despite initial laparotomy and reintervention (Bass and Crosier 1977; Wagner et al. 1985; De Toma et al. 1994; Yitzhak et al. 2001).

In one recent study, arterial embolization was shown to be 100% effective for treating extravasation of contrast medium in the liver, following blunt hepatic injury, in a cohort of hemodynamically stabilized patients, with 52% grades III and IV injury (Hagiwara et al. 1997). In another study, 16 of 30 markedly unstable patients with blunt liver injury underwent arterial hemostatic embolization. Patients were stabilized after embolization and no major complication was observed (Murakami et al. 1993). In another study of 24 patients with posttraumatic vascular lesions, transcatheter occlusion was successful in 88% (Schwartz et al. 1993). Patients with grades IV and V hepatic injury, who remained hemodynamically stable only with continued resuscitation, could undergo hepatic arteriography and embolization, bridging the therapeutic option of nonoperative

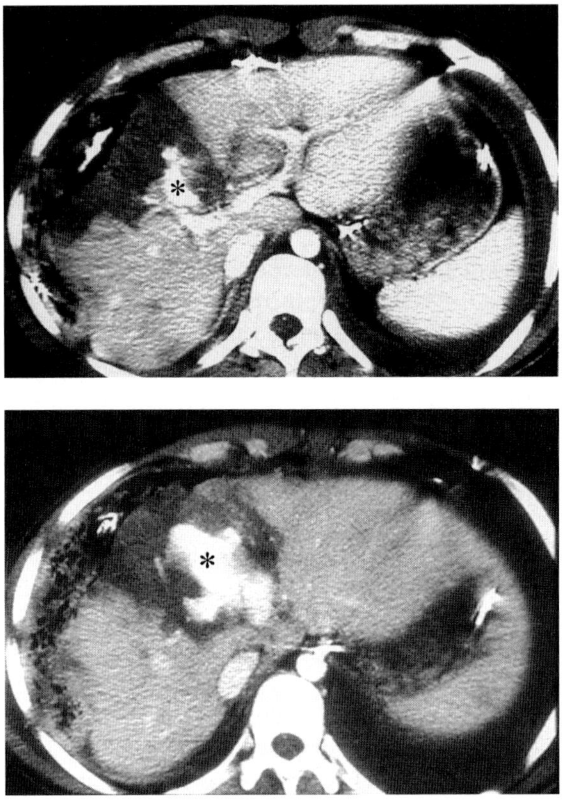

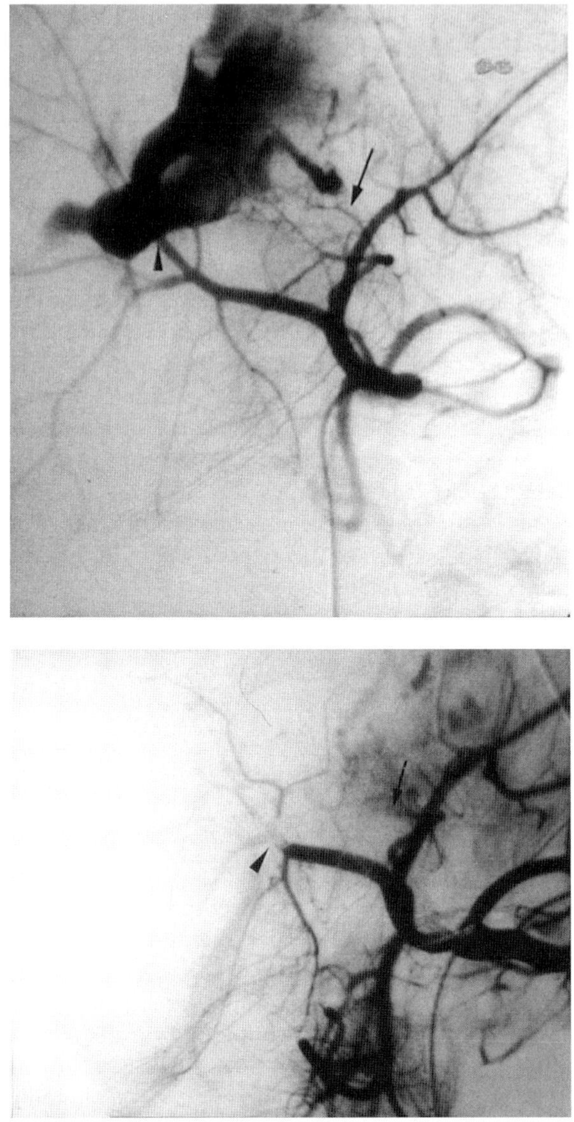

Fig. 5.26a–d. This patient had a crash laparotomy at another hospital, where he was admitted after a car accident. (**a,b**) CT obtained after transfer of the patient shows perihepatic packing and massive extravasation of contrast medium (*asterisk*) within the zone of extensive hepatic contusion. (**c**) Immediate hepatic arteriography confirmed massive extravasation originating from right (*arrowhead*) and left (*arrow*) intrahepatic arterial branches. (**d**) Embolization was obtained by selective occlusion of left hepatic arterial branches (*arrow*) and a more proximal embolization of the right hepatic artery (*arrowhead*) with gel foam pledgets. The patient survived and required an additional embolization 24 h later for contrast oozing from arterial branches in the left lobe

intervention and surgery. Treatment was effective in 10 of 11 patients (Ciraulo et al. 1998).

Indications for angiography and embolization are evidence of continuous hemorrhage or patients who remain borderline after resuscitation and in whom contrast medium extravasation, intraparenchymal blush, or contrast staining is seen on CT (Sherman 1996; Gorich et al. 1999; Harper and Maull 2000). Such management requires optimal organization and skills in the radiology department (Sugimoto et al. 1994). Arterial embolization is said to be contributive to the overall better outcome of liver injuries, which is explained by a relative decrease in major liver injuries and improved surgical results for major injury (Richardson et al. 2000). Patients with early ongoing bleeding after primary surgical hemostasis and patients who are referred after a crash laparotomy should also undergo arteriography and when necessary possible embolization avoiding reoperation (De Toma et al. 1994). Patients who rebleed after an initially successful embolization should be treated again angiographically.

Complications of arterial hepatic embolization mainly include rebleeding due to incomplete vaso-occlusion or coagulopathy and later hepatic infarction or abscess, bile duct necrosis, biloma, and pseudoaneurysm.

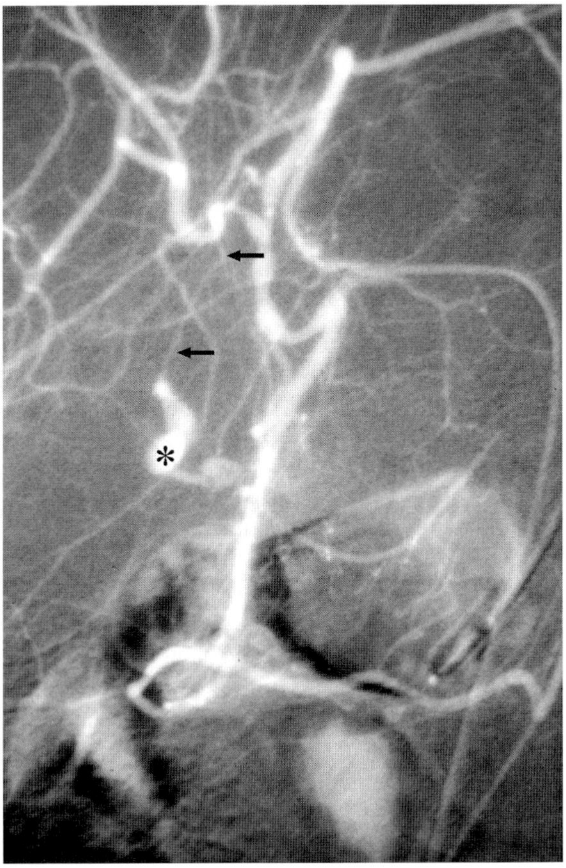

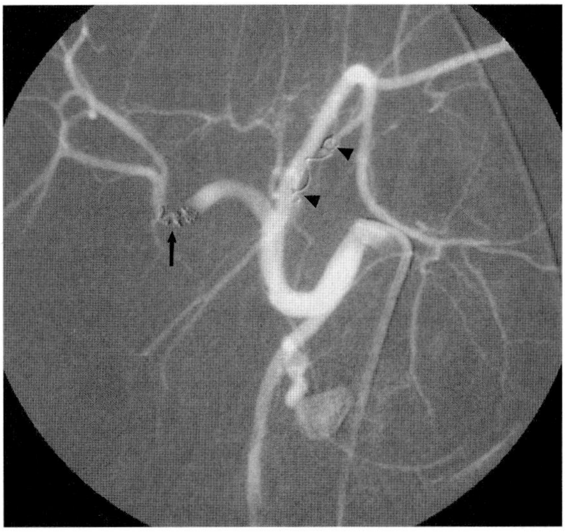

Fig. 5.27a, b. Same patient than in Fig. 5.22. (**a**) Hepatic arteriography confirms extravasation (*asterisk*) of contrast medium shown on CT at admission in Fig. 5.22.. The bleeding (*asterisk*) originates from a branch of the middle hepatic artery (*arrows*). (**b**) Hemostasis was obtained by selective placement of two microcoils in the artery of the quadrate segment (segment IV) (*arrowheads*). Additional coils (*arrow*) were placed in the proximal right hepatic artery to decrease flow and prevent rebleeding from intrahepatic revascularization of the left lobe. Conservative treatment was successful after embolization

5.6.2.3
Expectant Nonsurgical

Inclusion Criteria

One of the major rationales in favor of nonsurgical management is the observation that 50%–80% of all hepatic injuries have stopped bleeding at time of operation (Meredith et al. 1994). In fact, conservative treatment of blunt liver contusion was already suggested by Pringle (1908).

Conservative therapy of blunt liver injuries was advocated in the early 1980s in the pediatric age group based on clinical criteria and CT findings (Karp et al. 1983; Brick et al. 1987). Nonoperative treatment was extended to the stable adult population (Geis et al. 1981; Moon and Federle 1983; Meyer et al. 1985; Foley et al. 1987; Farnell et al. 1988; Mirvis et al. 1989; Knudson et al. 1990; Federico et al. 1990; Hiatt et al. 1990; Croce et al. 1991, 1995; Dondelinger and Kurdziel 1991; Sherman et al. 1994; Pachter and Hofstetter 1995; Boone et al. 1995; Goff and Gilbert 1995; Becker et al. 1996; Bond et al. 1996; Pachter et al. 1996; Brasel et al. 1997). Meredith concluded in his paper advocating conservative treatment and mobilization of the traumatized patient: "if the Oldsmobile striking the patient did not stimulate sufficient hemorrhage to warrant surgery, then it is unlikely that walking to the bathroom will" (Meredith et al. 1994).

Inclusion criteria are:

- Hemodynamically stable, or rapidly and definitely stabilized patient after admission, with a minimum of blood transfusions required
- Absence of peritoneal irritation
- Absence of pneumoperitoneum
- Absence of contrast extravasation
- Absence of extrahepatic abdominal surgery requiring surgical repair
- Surgical and radiological facility for rapid hepatic intervention or hemostatic arterial embolization

Patients should not be selected for conservative treatment on the basis of lesion grading only, as grade III and IV contusions may entirely regress without complications and moderate injury may occasionally bleed severely (Mirvis et al. 1989; Schweizer et al. 1993; Fig. 5.28). However, the risk of delayed bleeding or rebleeding is much less in hepatic than in splenic injury. Hypoechoic geographical areas of contusion on US in the majority of cases indicate a Mirvis grade II or III injury, which usually do not require surgical intervention (Ohta et al. 1998). Injury to the bare area of the liver, with retroperitoneal hematoma and with or without hemoperitoneum is also an indication for nonoperative management in the stable patient (Patten et al. 1993). The presence of periportal tracking is irrelevant to the decision of conservative management. The age limit of 55 years, which has been debated in the literature, is not a criterion of exclusion from expectant nonsurgical management of liver injury (Falimirski and Provost 2000). Furthermore – at least in children

a

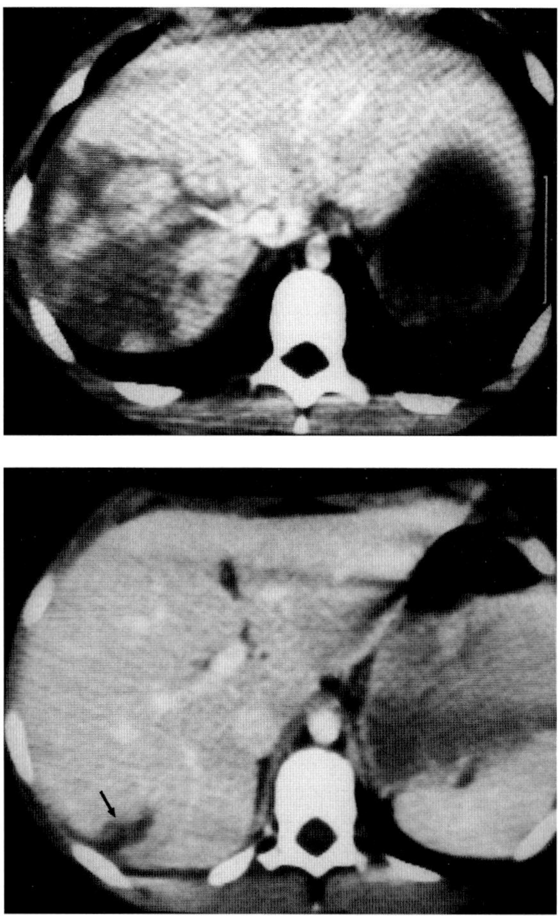

b

Fig. 5.28a, b. Conservative treatment of hepatic contusion grade III in a child. **(a)** CT at admission shows a hypodense area of contusion in the right lobe of the liver, without contrast medium extravasation and without significant perihepatic hemoperitoneum. **(b)** CT obtained 10 days after trauma shows a significant regression of the area of hepatic contusion. A small hypodense area is visible at the limit between segment VII and VIII (*arrow*)

– it was shown that associated head injury should not rule out nonoperative management of hepatic trauma. In groups stratified for type of injury and severity, abdominal and neurological morbidity was improved with nonoperative abdominal treatment (Keller et al. 1996).

The early literature reported that limited hemoperitoneum, smaller than an estimated volume of 0.2 l, did not require urgent intervention (Meyer et al. 1985). Our experience has shown that liver injury without hemoperitoneum seen on CT obtained at admission is benign, without risk of delayed bleeding. Furthermore, the velocity of resorption of hemoperitoneum within 1 week estimated on imaging should not be a criterion to guide conservative treatment, as hemoperitoneum usually increases in volume in the pelvic compartments and decreases in the perihepatic spaces during the first days following trauma (Foley et al. 1987).

Posttraumatic hepatic hematomas were a great concern in the past and were included in injury grading systems (Lambeth and Rubin 1979; Cheatham et al. 1980). The presence of a large hematoma that is not expanding should not contraindicate expectant conservative treatment. Associated injuries of other solid abdominal organs also do not contraindicate nonoperative management (Sartorelli et al. 2000). Diagnostic laparoscopy was advocated as an adjunct for patient selection for conservative management, but its use has not spread (Townsend et al. 1993). It may be useful to evacuate massive hemoperitoneum, to detect occult gastrointestinal injury and reveal ongoing hepatic hemorrhage.

A minority of penetrating liver injuries (about 5%) in children and adults can also be treated conservatively: injuries caused by low-velocity stab wounds, without cavitation effect, show a similar behavior to blunt injuries, and some victims of a low-grade and isolated liver injury caused by gunshot, who are hemodynamically stable, can also be selected for nonsurgical management (Fig. 5.29). However, there is a risk of peritonitis, abdominal compartment syndrome or biloma (Demetriades et al. 1999). In these cases, imaging has to eliminate the possibility of any intrahepatic or extrahepatic injury that requires repair (Talbert et al. 1980; Moore et al. 1980; Demetriades et al. 1986, 1991; Renz and Feliciano 1994; Dicker et al. 1996; Renz et al. 1996; Pal and Khan 2000).

Results

Imaging obtained during follow-up in conservative treatment of liver injury showed that most lesions

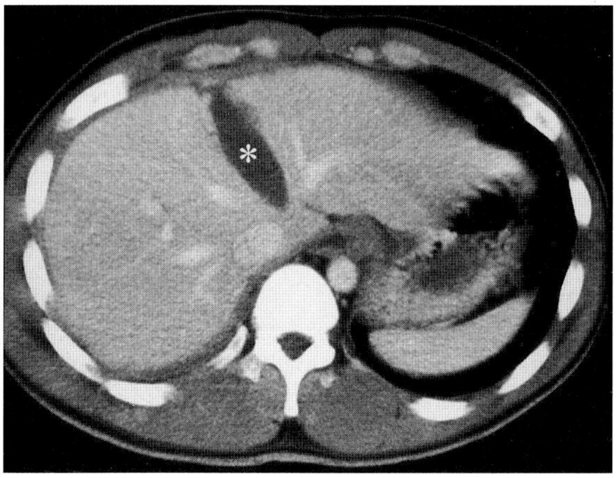

Fig. 5.29. CT obtained in a patient after a stab wound in the epigastrium. A typical ellipsoid hypodense area (*asterisk*) with distinct margins is seen in the liver, without contrast medium extravasation or injury to the inferior vena cava or hepatic veins. Minimal perihepatic hemoperitoneum is noted. Conservative management without surgical exploration was applied successfully

regress spontaneously without causing symptoms. Currently, 80%–86% of all blunt liver injuries in adults and more than 90% in children are treated nonoperatively, although other reports still indicate a lower percentage of about 56%, according to variable patient populations and differences in severity of injury and associated injuries (CROCE et al. 1991, 1995; CARLES et al. 1994; MEREDITH et al. 1994; SHERMAN et al. 1994; BOONE et al. 1995; GOFF and GILBERT 1995; BOND et al. 1996; PACHTER et al. 1996; BRUNERO et al. 1996; LUCAS and LEDGERWOOD 2000; MALHOTRA et al. 2000; RICHARDSON et al. 2000). Nonoperative treatment significantly decreases the rate of nontherapeutic laparotomy. The number of transfusions is usually decreased with conservative treatment, but might be higher in some cases and surgery, if necessary, might become delayed (BRASEL et al. 1997; FANG et al. 2000). In fact, nonoperative management fails in 0%–19% of the cases according to patient selection. Liver related failures are present in half of cases and are associated with high-grade injury and large hemoperitoneum (CARLES et al. 1994; CHEN et al. 1998; MALHOTRA et al. 2000). In series with predominantly grade II and III injury, success of nonoperative management is as high as 98% (CUFF et al. 2000). Hospital stays of 2–7 days (mean 3) were reported in patients with conservatively treated grade III hepatic injury to the bare area and retroperitoneal hematoma (PATTEN et al. 1993). In a prospective comparative trial with laparotomy, patients were included on the basis of hemodynamic stability. There was no death, no delayed laparotomy and no complication in the group with conservative management (SHERMAN et al. 1994). Patients who fail conservative nonsurgical treatment or hemostatic arterial embolization can still benefit from laparoscopy and topical fibrin glue application to avoid a nontherapeutic laparotomy (CHEN et al. 1998; FEMI-PEARSE et al. 1998). In patients with low-grade penetrating injury, conservative management is successful in 70% of included patients (DEMETRIADES et al. 1999).

5.6.3 Follow-up

Follow-up imaging studies are necessary both after surgical intervention and conservative treatment of liver injury (SCHÖPF et al. 1982; Fig. 5.28). Recent studies suggest that no clinically useful information is gained from systematic follow-up examinations for patients included in a nonoperative trial, without a clinical change (CIRAULO et al. 1996). Information affecting management was obtained in 9% of cases, but the CT examination was prompted by clinical findings (CUFF et al. 2000; Fig. 5.30). It was found that patients who fail conservative nonsurgical management have accelerated heart rate, abdominal pain, skin color changes, or fever ; they require blood transfusions, and serial hemoglobin test and CT scans are usually ordered in emergency situations. Subtle clinical findings and nursing observations should be analyzed carefully as a clue to early diagnosis of failed expectant management of blunt liver injury (SHREVE 1999). Severity of the hepatic lesions, associated injuries, and clinical status should be considered together to initiate posttraumatic follow-up imaging. After surgical repair, CT best shows the result of omental packing by typical heterogeneous filling of the parenchymal laceration and showing fat densities. Patients who underwent hemostatic arterial embolization at admission should also undergo repeat CT imaging during a minimum of 3 weeks, as the risk for pseudoaneurysm and recurrent bleeding caused by delayed rupture may occur despite arterial embolization (HAGIWARA et al. 1997).

Generally, US and CT allow an adequate follow-up of liver injury. The role of radionuclide studies is discussed in the following chapter on bile duct injuries. On US, hyperechoic hemorrhage changes into hypoechoic areas, which returns to a normal hepatic echoic pattern within several weeks, due to

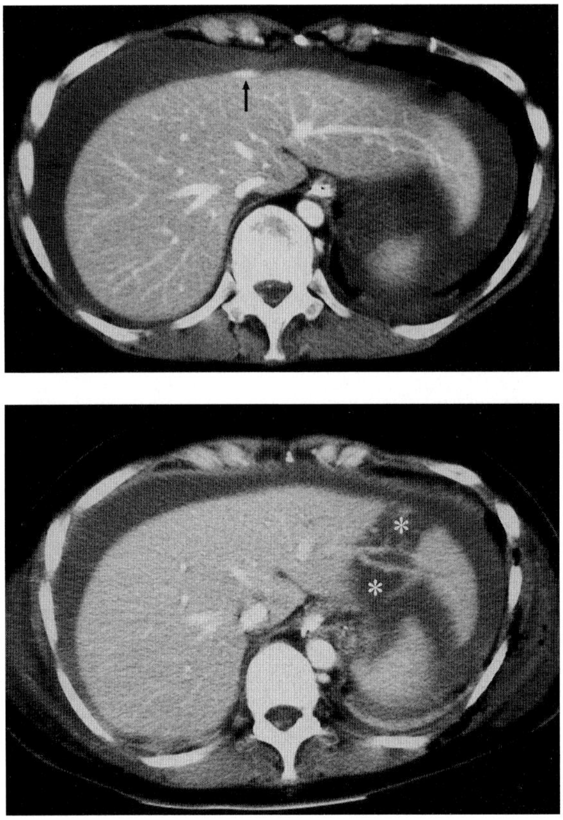

Fig. 5.30a, b. Same patient than in Fig. 5.22. and 5.27. (**a**) CT at admission shows extravasation (*arrow*) of contrast medium at the anterior liver surface, without area of contusion seen in the left lobe of the liver. Massive perihepatic and perisplenic hemoperitoneum is seen. (**b**) CT obtained 4 days later shows complete fracture (*asterisks*) of the left lateral segment of the liver. The free end of the left lobe is retained only by the intrahepatic portal vein branches. A left lateral segmentectomy was obtained

resorption of blood, edema and granulation tissue formation (Van Sonnenberg et al. 1983). Central hematomas show a similar pattern of regression. On CT, hematomas change into a hypodense content and progressive enlargement at the phase of liquefaction, followed by slow regression of the diameter. A small cyst-like lesion may persist for several months or indefinitely. Patients with central or subcapsular hematoma should be controlled at least for 1 month, and patients who receive anticoagulation should be observed particularly closely. Patients with blood loss, peritoneal irritation and sudden increase of volume of the hematoma or intrahematoma hemorrhage or rupture, as observed on imaging, should receive prompt treatment (Geis et al. 1981). Hepatic contusion regresses more rapidly than hematomas, in approximately 2 weeks and may leave a localized capsular retraction and scar calcification, or a decrease in the volume of a sector or lobe due to vascular compromise.

In conclusion, systematic follow-up studies at regular intervals are not obtained routinely if the clinical course is smooth, although total regression of lesions should be documented when conservative, nonsurgical treatment has been applied. This might also be important for medicolegal reasons. In case of a suspected complication, imaging should not be delayed (Meredith et al. 1994). Patients with grade IV or V injury usually need closer clinical follow-up and more imaging than patients with lower grades, as complications requiring treatment are more frequent (Pachter et al. 1996). CT evidence of healing may take 1–6 months. Complete healing of the most severe liver injuries on CT may take 12–15 months, even in children (Bulas et al. 1993).

5.7 Posttraumatic Complications

5.7.1 Vascular

The liver is a vascular sponge composed of an arterial and a venous portal inflow system and a large venous draining system. All intrahepatic vascular components can become involved in posttraumatic vascular lesions.

5.7.1.1 Delayed Hemorrhage

Ongoing internal hemorrhage or oozing of blood through a surgical drain may be seen after an initial laparotomy in a small number of cases. These patients are either operated on again or investigated with arteriography and subsequent embolization. Patients who underwent a crash laparotomy and are transferred to a referral center should systematically undergo angiography before reoperation if the hemodynamic status allows such testing (Clark et al. 1994). Delayed hemorrhage in patients with conservative management can occur within days or a week and is scantly reported (Lambeth and Rubin 1979; Fig. 5.31). The literature suggests that nonsurgical expectant or angiographic management of delayed hemorrhage in these patients is safe (Gates 1994). However, in patients with the

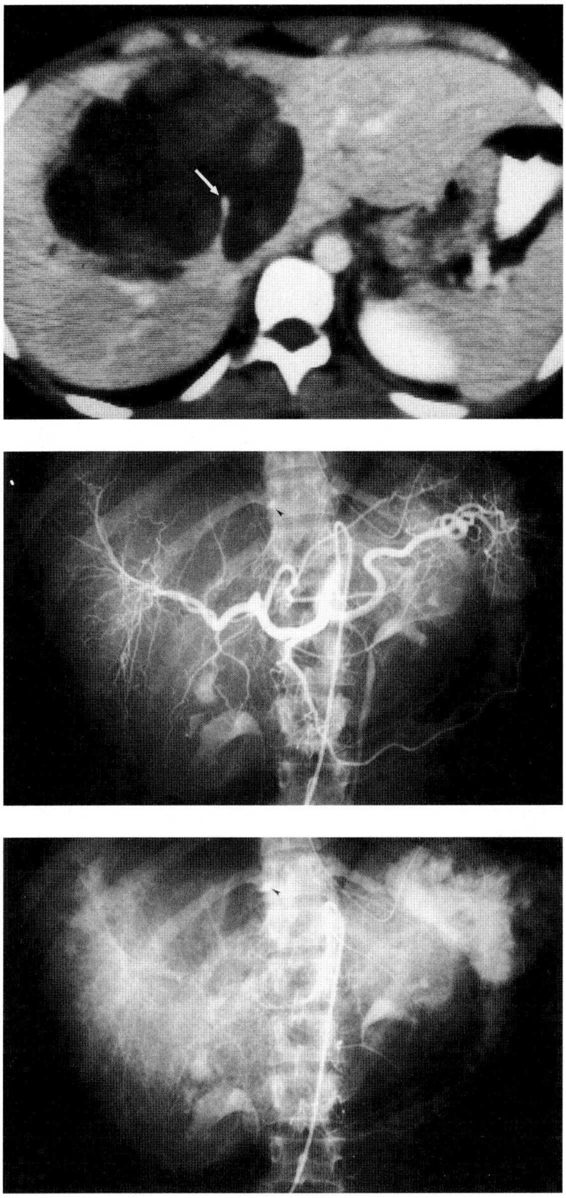

a b c

Fig. 5.31a–c. (**a**) CT obtained 24 h after admission for blunt hepatic contusion shows an expanding intrahepatic hematoma with mixed densities and suspicion of a focal contrast medium extravasation (*arrow*) within the hematoma. (**b,c**) Hepatic arteriography confirms contrast extravasation (*arrowhead*) originating from a small intrahepatic arterial branch within the left lobe. Note a large avascular zone and displacement of intrahepatic arterial branches by the hematoma

most severe grades of liver injury, postoperative lethal complications are caused in 50% by delayed hemorrhage (Aldrete et al. 1979; Brotman et al. 1984). Expanding hematomas should be managed without delay, either surgically or in selected cases, by arterial embolization.

5.7.1.2 Pseudoaneurysm

Posttraumatic hepatic pseudoaneurysm occasionally occurs in adults and children. Estimated frequency is 2%–3% and predominates in patients with grade IV injury (Schweizer et al. 1993; Croce et al. 1994). Pseudoaneurysm was described in a few children with blunt trauma and one child after penetrating injury (McGillibray and Valentine 1989; Schwartz et al. 1993; Basile et al. 1999; Sidhu et al. 1999). A pseudoaneurysm forms at the site of arterial injury and results from a self-limited blood cavity, surrounded by liver parenchyma, contained by a pseudo-wall and still connected to a ruptured vessel. Pseudoaneurysms may arise from a lobar or segmental intrahepatic artery or from an extrahepatic artery (Reber et al. 1998). They predominate in the right lobe (Mathisen et al. 1982; Basile et al. 1999). Persistent bilomas or bile fistulae are probably responsible for some of these pseudoaneurysms, due to the erosive potential of bile on the vascular wall (Hagiwara et al. 1993; Croce et al. 1994; Steiner et al. 1994). Posttraumatic stenosis of the bile ducts may also be associated with pseudoaneurysm, emphasizing the correlation between biliary and arterial injury in liver trauma (Halme et al. 1994).

US color Doppler, CT and MR should be able to disclose all significant pseudoaneurysms, unless they are of small size, with a diameter of less than 1 cm (Mallek et al. 1990). Noninvasive imaging is indicated first when unexplained sepsis, or gastrointestinal hemorrhage occurs in the posttraumatic phase. However, in comparison with angiography, CT may miss one-third of all angiographically confirmed pseudoaneurysms, and US half to two-thirds of all vascular lesions occurring after liver transplantation (Tobben et al. 1988; Zajko et al. 1989). The fate of these posttraumatic hepatic pseudoaneurysms is not well known. The smaller ones may thrombose spontaneously, others may remain patent, persist, or enlarge rapidly (Mallek et al. 1990). Enlargement up to 9 cm in diameter in 10 years was reported (Mathisen et al. 1982). Pseudoaneurysms may become complicated when they rupture into the biliary system and are responsible for hemobilia. They may also be at the origin of recurrent septic complications or rupture secondarily inside the liver parenchyma, erode in a vein or perforate through the liver capsule in the upper gastrointestinal tract (Kestenberg and Mittal 1992).

Accepted treatment of hepatic pseudoaneurysm is selective angiographic coil embolization, including extraparenchymal pseudoaneurysm located on the proper hepatic artery. Gelfoam pledgets were the usual embolization agent for many years. Now, placement of coils in the parent artery at the site of the pseudoaneurysm or using the sandwich embolization technique for larger vessels, by placing coils proximal and distal to the pseudoaneurysm, preventing recanalization of its lumen, is the standard technique (Heimbach et al. 1978; Roche et al. 1978a,b; Mathisen et al. 1982; Vadon et al. 1984; Lee and Himal 1992; Lerut et al. 1992; Hagiwara et al. 1993; Schwartz et al. 1993; Knowdley et al. 1994; Steiner et al. 1994; Gow et al. 1996; Sidhu et al. 1999; Inoguchi et al. 2001). Some pseudoaneurysms located in the periphery of the liver parenchyma and that are difficult to reach because of the small size of arteries, spasm, thrombosis or previous embolization or ligation can be treated by intrasaccular embolization, using a direct percutaneous transhepatic needle placement in the aneurysmal sack with cross-sectional imaging guidance (Lukancic et al. 1991; Merhav et al. 1993).

Embolization techniques are 90% effective in elective interventions to treat hemobilia by occlusion of a pseudoaneurysm or an arteriovenous fistula (Schwartz et al. 1993; Hidalgo et al. 1995). Recurrence of a vascular lesion after correct vaso-occlusion is rare. Fatal hemorrhage from a hepatic pseudoaneurysm from liver biopsy, despite repeat embolization and surgery was reported (Ahmed et al. 2001). Each coil should be tightly packed individually without residual coil elongation and all coils should be tightly packed together without interstices, to avoid late recanalization and coil migration (Garby et al. 1997). Complete and persistent vaso-occlusion of the parent vessel, proximal and distal to the pseudoaneurysm, allowing no revascularization by backflow should be documented angiographically before catheter withdrawal.

Surgery should be avoided, as attempts at débridement of a large vascular cavity in the liver may fail before vascular control is gained and lead to massive bleeding (Croce et al. 1994). However, direct ligation is applied in some patients with severe hemorrhage, requiring immediate surgical control (Gow et al. 1996).

5.7.1.3
Arterioportal and Arteriovenous Fistula

Arterioportal or arteriovenous fistula results from arterial rupture into an adjacent portal vein or a hepatic vein. This type of posttraumatic vascular injury is said to occur in 5%–20% of percutaneous transhepatic procedures. In fact, after blunt hepatic injury, arteriovenous fistula is seen with a frequency equal to pseudoaneurysm during conservative management (Schweizer et al. 1993). Arterioportal, arteriovenous (hepatic vein), or complex arterioportovenous fistula or portovenous communications can be seen. Small and peripherally located arterioportal fistulae and those with small flow pure venous shunts can close spontaneously, because of the low-pressure system, while fistulae with a high-pressure gradient involving the artery usually grow and enlarge to a certain point. Some may remain quiescent for long periods of time, up to 36 years (Balci et al. 1999). Arteriovenous fistulae usually also show a component of pseudoaneurysm, or may coexist with a separate pseudoaneurysm (Lerut et al. 1992; Galeon et al. 1997).

Intra- or extrahepatic rupture of an arterioportal or arteriovenous fistula can occur and various other complications can be seen. Rupture into the bile ducts with hemobilia is an infrequent event (Dunlop et al. 1977). Large arteriovenous fistulae can lead to overload of the right heart and a large hepatic arterioportal fistula can lead to dynamic portal hypertension with esogastric varices, variceal bleeding ascites or mesenteric ischemia, which in turn develop symptoms sometimes more than 20 years after trauma (Harada et al. 1975; Missavage et al. 1984; Chavan et al. 1993; Oishi et al. 1993; Kayser et al. 1996; Kirchgatterer et al. 1998; Wolf et al. 1998; English et al. 2001). Hepatic infarct or abscess, as may be seen with diffuse arteriohepatic vein shunting in hepatic vascular malformations, is uncommon following trauma. In this case, the diagnosis of an arterioportal fistula can be established with gadolinium-enhanced 3D MRA (Balci et al. 1999).

CT detects large pseudoaneurysms rather easily, but associated arteriovenous fistulae may not be seen (Galeon et al. 1997). A typical sign of an arterioportal shunt on CT is a wedge-shaped transient parenchymal enhancement seen at the portal phase (Lee et al. 1997). An arterioportal fistula detectable by CT can suggest the need for intervention, particularly when centrally located (Tanaka et al. 1991). Nuclear medicine is rarely used in Europe to confirm the diagnosis of a posttraumatic vascular fistula. Simultaneous appearance of the radionuclide in the liver and down the aorta suggests the diagnosis (Sziklas and Spencer 1975). Large or complicated vascular fistulae, like pseudoaneurysms, are best treated by selective coil embolization, avoiding parenchymal resection or laparotomy for simple ligation (Lerut et al. 1992; Chavan et al. 1993; Galeon et al. 1997; Tomczak et al. 1997; Kirchgatterer et al. 1998; Balci et al. 1999; English et al. 2001; Fig. 5.32).

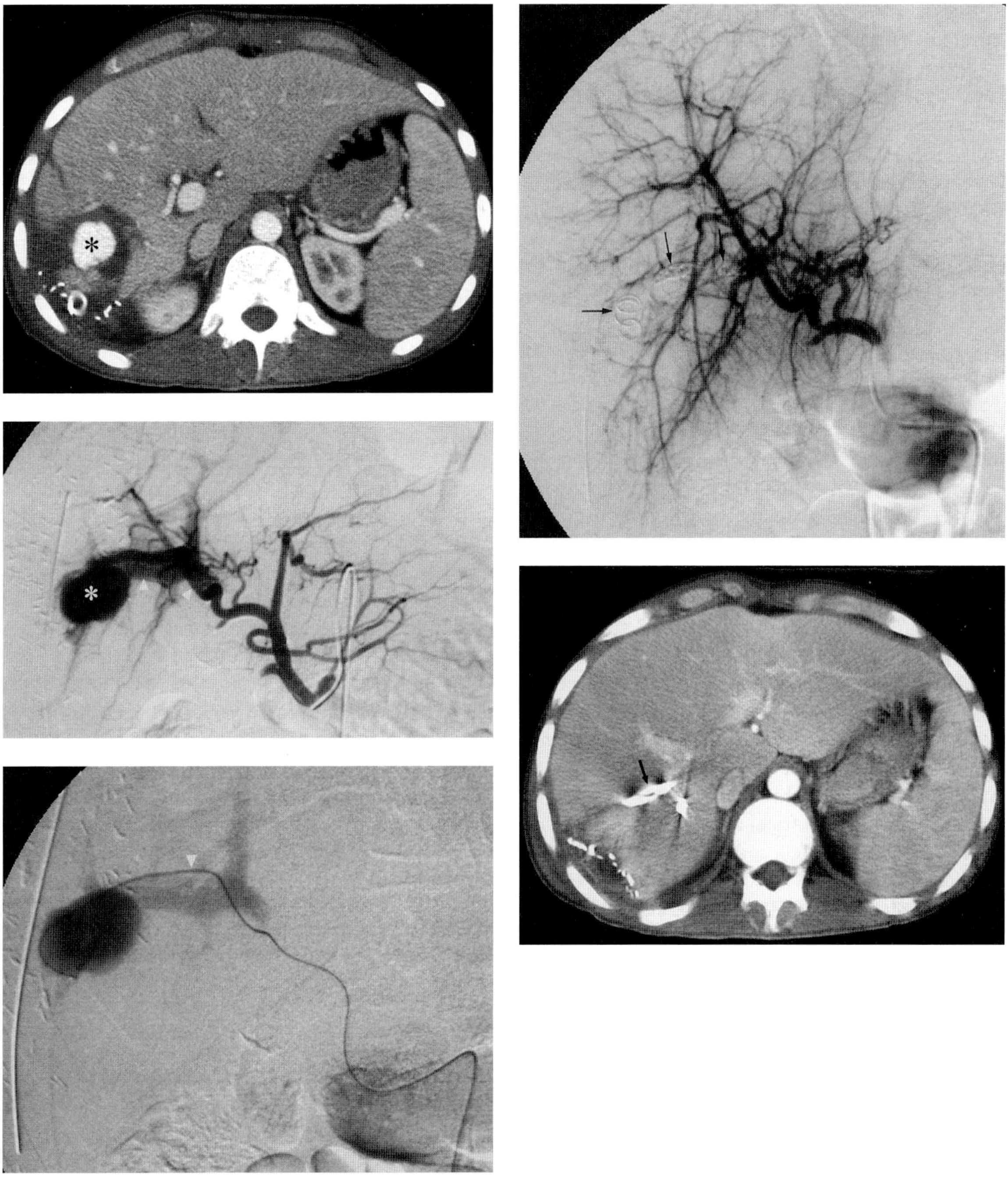

a b c d e

Fig. 5.32a–e. This patient, admitted after a traffic accident, had immediate surgery for repair of a liver laceration. Peripheral sutures and a surgical drain were placed. Continuous blood oozing through the surgical drain was observed after surgery. (**a**) CT showed a pseudoaneurysm (*asterisk*), 2 cm in diameter, within the area of contusion in the right lobe of the liver. (**b**) Hepatic arteriography confirms a pseudoaneurysm (*asterisk*) and arterioportal fistula. Note the opacified right hepatic portal vein (*arrowheads*). (**c**) Selective catheterization of the feeding artery of the pseudoaneurysm with a microcatheter (*arrowhead*). (**d**) Embolization was obtained by placement of microcoils within the feeding artery (*arrows*). One coil protruded in the pseudoaneurysmal sac. Postembolization hepatic arteriography shows minimal intrahepatic vascular amputation. (**e**) CT obtained 2 weeks after embolization shows no enhancement at the location of the embolized pseudoaneurysm. Note coils (*arrow*) within intrahepatic arterial branches. Clinical course was uneventful

5.7.1.4
Thromboembolism

Local posttraumatic thrombosis, either partial or complete, of hepatic veins, the portal vein or branches, or IVC can occur and is sometimes detected several days or months after conservative or surgical treatment. Postinjury hypercoagulable and hypofibrinolytic state favors venous thrombosis and pulmonary embolism (KIMOTO et al. 1998). An intraparenchymal or subcapsular hematoma or biloma may be responsible in the acute or late posttraumatic phase of compression of hepatic veins or IVC and responsible for acute Budd-Chiari syndrome, with or without venous thrombosis, associating hepatomegaly and ascites. Percutaneous or surgical drainage of the hepatic collection relieves the syndrome, but can also initiate clot migration (IZARD et al. 1995; MARKERT et al. 1997). Fatal pulmonary embolism was reported (NICOLOFF et al. 1964; FRANK et al. 1994). Thrombolytic therapy, balloon angioplasty or endoluminal stenting can be indicated in selected cases of posttraumatic thrombosis of the IVC and hepatic veins (FRANK et al. 1994; PATEL et al. 1996).

A concomitant posttraumatic arteriovenous fistula may favor large clot migration, for instance during reintervention, and lead to lethal pulmonary embolism (HUGUET et al. 1975). Recognition of thrombosis of the hepatic vein or IVC is therefore of utmost importance, particularly when reintervention is scheduled.

Foreign bodies such as shot-gun pellets or bullets may migrate from the portal vein to the liver, or from the liver into the IVC and to the pulmonary circulation, or from the heart to the hepatic vein (WALLACE and SLOVIS 1987; EZBERCI and KARGI 1999). Fragments of liver tissue may become detached by contusion and migrate to a large hepatic vein and to the pulmonary arteries, responsible for pulmonary embolism. Some embolisms are composed of macroscopic tissue fragments; in other cases, only microscopic investigation of the lung at autopsy showed multiple foci of hepatic tissue embolized to the pulmonary arteries (MOAR 1984; GREENBERG 1986; VOITK and MUNKITTRICK 1986; WALZ and WALZ 1992; YATES et al. 1996; MICHALODIMITRAKIS and TSATSAKIS 1998). In some cases, macroscopic liver fragments were driven directly through a laceration of the IVC wall and obstructed the caval lumen, then extended to the right atrium or embolized to the lung (VOITK and MUNKITTRICK 1986; TAKATSU et al. 1988). Not only liver fragments, but also perihepatic fat can enter the IVC through a caval wall tear. CT shows typical fat intraluminal densities. MRI shows low-signal T1 and high-signal T2 filling defect corresponding to subcutaneous fat (SHEAFOR et al. 1998).

Pulmonary bile emboli can occur when severe bile duct obstruction communicates through a posttraumatic intrahepatic biliary-venous fistula (BALOGH 1984).

5.7.2
Nonvascular

5.7.2.1
Abdominal Compartment Syndrome

Damage-control laparotomy, with temporary perihepatic packing, associated with visceral edema due to shock and reperfusion might be responsible for an abdominal compartment syndrome with an intra-abdominal pressure less than 15 or 20 mmHg, resulting in impaired cardiopulmonary and renal function (MELDRUM et al. 1995, 1997). Compression of the IVC by a subcapsular hematoma can lead to a pseudo-Budd-Chiari syndrome; as discussed in the preceding section. In other cases, a subcapsular hematoma may compress the portal vein and induce portal hypertension with reversal of portal flow, deteriorating liver function, and ascites (SOMMER et al. 1979; PETRI et al. 1993; PRETRE et al. 1993; PEARL and TRUNKEY 1999). Surgical or percutaneous catheter drainage of the compressing fluid collection should be applied urgently.

5.7.2.2
Chronic Hematoma

Posttraumatic hematomas need surgical or conservative treatment, depending on their progression. When the patient remains stable, and the hematoma is not expanding and induces no further complication by compression due to large volume, expectant therapy is indicated (BRUNERO et al. 1996). Most hematomas will resorb, but some may persist, evolving into so-called chronic hematoma (Fig. 5.33). When blood clots have completely resorbed, a chronic hematoma may not be distinguished from a biloma or any other cyst or pseudocyst or a cystic tumor. Such so-called posttraumatic cysts are rare in adults and even more so in children, an incidence of 0.5% being reported. There seems to be no relation between the severity of injury and the occurrence of chronic hematoma (SUGIMOTO et al. 1982; CHUANG and HUANG 1996). These chronic hematic cysts have an inflammatory or fibrous pseudocapsule, and can undergo compli-

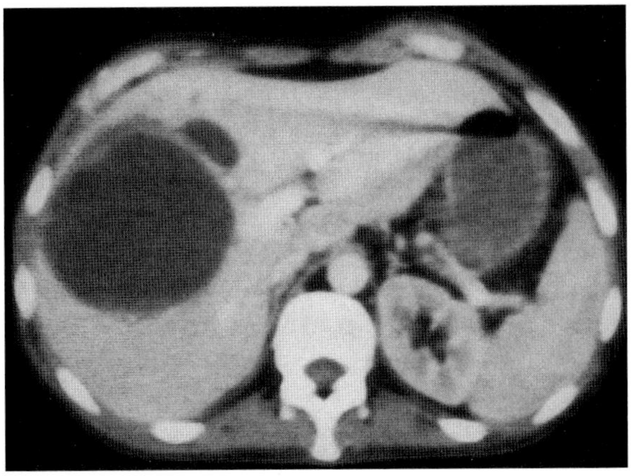

Fig. 5.33. Abdominal CT obtained 1 month after blunt hepatic contusion. CT at admission had shown a hyperdense intrahepatic hematoma similar to that shown in Fig. 5.9., that is actually replaced by a large hypodense fluid collection. Persistent chronic hematomas may show homogeneous fluid-like densities, which cannot be distinguished from a biloma. Percutaneous aspiration was successful

cations such as hemorrhage, rupture, transformation into abscess, hemobilia, bile duct obstruction, peritonitis, compression of adjacent structures and others. Patients usually tolerate uncomplicated posttraumatic cysts well unless they increase considerably in size. Before the era of intense imaging, some cysts persisted for years undetected before symptoms developed (Henson et al. 1957; Jones and Harley 1970; Chuang and Huang 1996). Usual clinical symptoms are abdominal discomfort or pain, cholangitis, obstructive jaundice, sepsis, or shock caused by massive hemorrhage inside the hematic cavity (Chuang and Huang 1996). In uncomplicated chronic hematoma, US shows relatively anechoic fluid collections and CT fluid-like densities. The cyst is unilocular without tissue component. Nonregressive fluid collections should be aspirated systematically to avoid abscess formation. Rarely, large chronic posttraumatic cysts regress spontaneously, as was reported in a 30-cm giant cyst (Sugimoto et al. 1982; Eber et al. 1995).

5.7.2.3
Hepatic Necrosis

Severe and extensive hepatic necrosis can occur following a burst or a crush injury with arterial occlusion or combined arterial and portal occlusion. Thrombosis of an intrahepatic portal branch is not enough to induce necrosis. CT shows a nonenhanced lobe or a well-demarcated segmental hypodense area without enhancement. Later gas bubbles or intravascular branching gas patterns develop within the infarcted parenchyma. Arterial hemostatic embolization can further contribute to parenchymal necrosis (Fig. 5.34). MRI shows low intensity on T1- and T2-weighted images, without enhancement. When unrecognized, abscess formation, sepsis, and multi-organ failure are dreadful complications of hepatic tissue necrosis. The radiologist should be aware of complete nonenhancement of a liver lobe, indicating liver resection in selected patients to shortcut escalating complications (Hatten et al. 1996).

5.7.2.4
Abscess

Prophylactic surgical drainage of severe liver injuries is rarely used, postoperative fluid collections are frequent and those in which infection is suspected can be aspirated or drained percutaneously with imaging control (Reed et al. 1992). Posttraumatic liver abscess is twice as common as persistent biloma and three times more frequent than chronic hematoma (Olsen 1982). So-called secondary pyogenic abscess may form on the floor of an ischemic contusion, leading to parenchymal necrosis, particularly after conservative treatment without débridement. A persistent biloma, hematoma, or mixed fluid collection may become infected at any time. In patients treated with systematic laparotomy for blunt liver injury, and particularly after major trauma, a 7% abscess rate is found (Shah et al. 1993). In patients treated conservatively, the risk of developing liver abscess should not be underestimated; an incidence of 1.4% is reported (Eng et al. 1981; Carles et al. 1994). Massive, nonselective arterial embolization has to be avoided, to minimize necrosis and superinfection of hepatic tissue. Posttraumatic liver abscesses can be treated with imaging-guided percutaneous aspiration or drainage techniques, but have a higher failure rate than abscesses that develop in normal liver parenchyma, as is the case with a bile fistula, and vascular lesions can coexist. Posttraumatic liver abscess may develop several months or 1–2 years after trauma (Dondelinger et al. 1990; Haight et al. 1994).

5.7.2.5
Biloma

Biloma or bile fistula may develop after any type of intervention or expectant nonsurgical treatment (Sharudin and Noori 1997). After systematic sur-

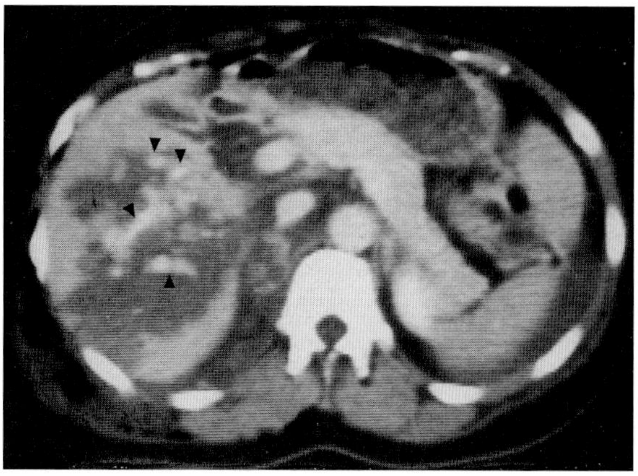
a

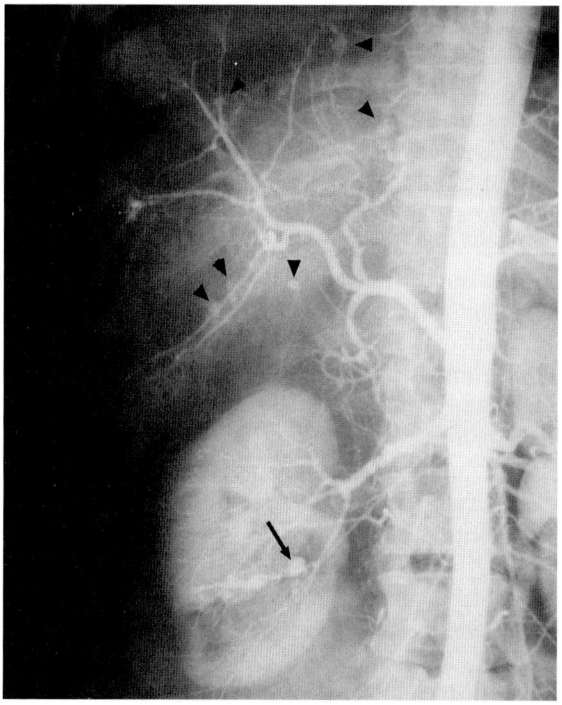
b

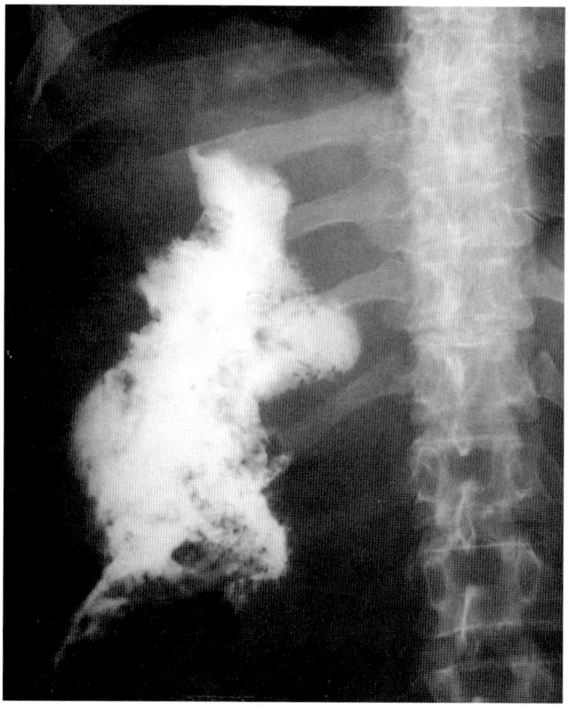
c

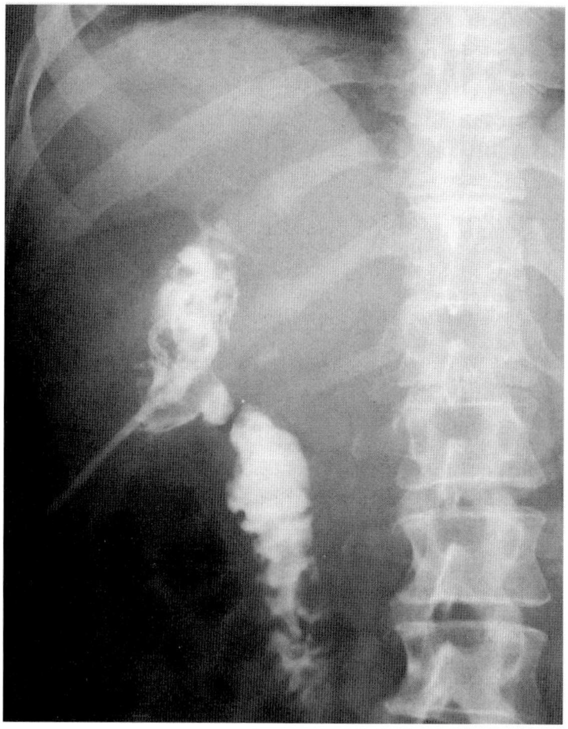
d

Fig. 5.34a–d. (**a**) CT of this unstable patient at admission shows extensive areas of contusion within the right lobe of the liver and areas of contrast extravasation (*arrowheads*). Note perihepatic and perisplenic hemoperitoneum, and right adrenal hematoma. Extensive right renal contusion was present (not shown). (**b**) Abdominal aortogram obtained immediately after CT confirms vasoconstriction and multiple foci of intrahepatic contrast extravasation (*arrowheads*) and shows a right intrarenal pseudoaneurysm (*arrow*). After extensive intrahepatic arterial embolization, the patient developed right liver lobe necrosis, managed by percutaneous large-bore catheter drainage. (**c**) Contrast opacification of the necrotic cavity through the drainage catheter showed no biliary or extrahepatic fistula. (**d**) After 3 weeks of external catheter drainage, opacification through the catheter showed an extrahepatic fistula between the necrotic cavity and the duodenum, which subsequently closed after prolonged drainage gery, a 3% rate of prolonged bile leak has been noted (SHAH et al. 1993). Following conservative treatment with restrictive patient inclusion, 11.5% of patients develop biloma and 8% a free peritoneal bile leak (BYNOE et al. 1992). Biliary cysts may develop secondary to hepatic infarction, consecutive to arterial trauma or arterial hemostatic embolization. This complication is discussed in detail in the following chapter on bile injury.

5.7.2.6
Posthepatectomy Biliary Stricture

A biliary stricture may occur in the intra- or extrahepatic biliary tract, several months or more than 1 year following hepatectomy for traumatic rupture, without evidence of a bile duct injury at the time of trauma. Proposed mechanisms are anatomical distortion of the bile duct wall secondary to hepatic resection and subsequent regeneration, followed by inflammation and fibrosis. Repeated percutaneous transhepatic balloon dilatation of this type of benign bile duct stricture was proven successful in 50% only of patients (LITTLE et al. 1986).

5.7.2.7
Fatty Replacement

Fatty replacement was described following liver trauma, exhibiting decreased or negative absorption values on CT on the contused area (PARDES et al. 1982).

5.7.2.8
Other

Hepatic US examination may be abnormal in 22% of the cases in the posttraumatic phase, showing capsular retraction, calcifications, or segmental bile duct obstruction. Cholelithiasis may develop over the long term following hemobilia in children and adults (OLSEN 1982; FARRON et al. 1996). Coagulopathy may be seen in 5% of cases (SHAH et al. 1993). Ectopic nodules of hepatic tissue, not connected to the liver, may grow, independently, as in splenosis, following blunt liver trauma (LASSER and WILSON 1975).

5.8
Conclusion

Evaluation of blunt hepatic injury raises more concern than injury to other solid abdominal organs, because of the complex vascularization of the liver, the presence of the biliary system and the high frequency of hepatic involvement during abdominal contusion. Hepatic contusion presents with equal or greater frequency to splenic trauma. Location of impact forces determines the type of injury and orientation of hepatic fracture lines. The CT examination technique is of paramount importance for evaluation of vascular intrahepatic injury.

US and CT show with similar ease areas of contusion, hematomas, and perihepatic peritoneal effusion, but both modalities have a certain number, although limited, of pitfalls. Disruption of the liver capsule may be difficult to evidence, particularly on CT in the closed abdomen. The decision to initiate a conservative treatment of blunt hepatic injury is based on the observation that the vast majority of minor or moderate liver injury is nonhemorrhagic at the time of operation. Imaging findings and injury classification are helpful in when deciding on the type of management, but are not absolute criteria.

Hemostatic arterial embolization is an adjunct therapy in the frame of conservative management of hepatic contusion. Indications of arteriography and subsequent embolization are based on contrast extravasation or blush on CT in most cases. During follow-up of conservative management, cross-sectional imaging is mandatory, when clinical progression deviates from its smooth course. Planned interventional procedures are required with increasing frequency for treatment of posttraumatic intrahepatic vascular injuries that are diagnosed on delayed CT examinations or aspiration and drainage of intrahepatic or perihepatic fluid collections.

References

Abramson SJ, Berdon WE, Kaufman RA, Ruzal-Shapiro C (1989) Hepatic parenchyma and subcapsular gas after hepatic laceration caused by blunt abdominal trauma. AJR 153:1031–1032
Adams HA, Schmitz CS (1995) Intra-abdominal bleeding after myocardial infarction with cardiopulmonary resuscitation and thrombolytic therapy (abstract). Anaesthesist 44: 585–589
Adler SN, Klein RA, Pellecchia C, Lyon DT (1983) Massive hepatic hemorrhage associated with cardiopulmonary resuscitation. Arch Intern Med 143:813–814
Agostino D, Cliffton EF (1965) Organ localization and the effect of trauma on the fate of circulating cancer cells. Cancer Res 25:1728–1732
Ahmed A, Samuels SL, Keefe EB, Cheung RC (2001) Delayed fatal hemorrhage from pseudoaneurysm of the hepatic

artery after percutaneous liver biopsy. Am J Gastroenterol 96:233–237
Akgur FM, Aktug T, Olguner M, Kovanlikaya A, Hakguder G (1997) Prospective study investigating routine usage of ultrasonography as the initial diagnostic modality for the evaluation of children sustaining blunt abdominal trauma. J Trauma 42:626–628
Aldrete JS, Halpern NB, Ward S, Wright JO (1979) Factors determining the mortality and morbidity in hepatic injuries. Ann Surg 189:466–501
Allen RE Jr, Blasidell FW (1972) Injuries to the inferior vena cava. Surg Clin North Am 52:699–710
Allison DJ, Jordon H, Hennessy O (1985) Therapeutic embolization of the hepatic artery : a review of 75 procedures. Lancet 1:595
Amoury RA, Barth GW, Hall RT, Rhodes PG, Holder TM, Ashcraft KW (1982) Scrotal ecchymosis: sign of intraperitoneal hemorrhage in the newborn. South Med J 75: 1471–1475
Anderson CB, Ballinger WF (1985) Abdominal injuries. In: Zuidema GD, Rutherford RB, Ballinger WF (eds) The management of trauma, 4th edn. Saunders, Philadelphia
Anderson B, Cluroe A, Duncan D (1997) Hepatic necrosis masquerading as trauma. Pediatr Radiol 27:82–83
Aoki Y, Nata M, Hashiyada M, Sagisaka K (1997) Laceration of the liver with delayed massive intra-abdominal hemorrhage: a case report of child abuse. Nippon Hoigaku Zasshi 51:44–47
Arajarvi E, Sanavirta S, Tolonen J (1987) Abdominal injuries sustained in severe traffic accidents by seatbelt wearers. J Trauma 27:393–397
Arcadio F, Requin JL, Neidhart JH et al (1968) Medico-legal notes concerning the post-traumatic hydatid cyst of the liver. Soc Med Légale 4:386–388
Asensio JA, Demetriades D, Chahwan S et al (2000) Approach to the management of complex hepatic injuries. J Trauma 48:66–69
Avolio AW, Agnes S, Chirico ASA, Cillo U, Frongillo F, Castagneto M (2000) Successful transplantation of an injured liver. Transplant Proc 32:131–133
Balasegaram M (1976) The surgical management of hepatic trauma. J Trauma 16:141–148
Balci NC, Semelka RC, Sandhu JS (1999) Intrahepatic arterioportal fistula: gadolinium-enhanced 3D magnetic resonance angiography findings and angiographic embolization with steel coils. Magn Reson Imaging 17:475–478
Balogh K (1984) Pulmonary bile emboli. Sequelae of iatrogenic trauma. Arch Pathol Lab Med 108:814–816
Baracco-Gandolfo V, Vidarte O, Baracco-Miller V, Del-Castillo M (1986) Prolonged closed liver packing in severe hepatic trauma: experience with 36 patients. J Trauma 26:754–756
Basile KE, Sivit CJ, Sachs PB, Stallion A (1999) Hepatic artery pseudoaneurysm: a rare complication of blunt abdominal trauma in children. Pediatr Radiol 29:306–308
Bass EM, Crosier JH (1977) Percutaneous control of post-traumatic hepatic hemorrhage by gelfoam embolization. J Trauma 17:61–63
Baumgartner F, Scudamore C, Nair C, Karusseit O, Hemming A (1995) Venovenous bypass for major hepatic and caval trauma. J Trauma 39:671–673
Beal SL (1990) Fatal hepatic hemorrhage: an unsolved problem in the management of complex liver injuries. J Trauma 30: 163–169
Becker CD, Gal I, Baer HU, Vock P (1996) Blunt hepatic trauma in adults: correlation of CT injury grading with outcome. Radiology 201:215–220
Ben-Menachem Y (1981) Logic and logistics of radiography, angiography and angiographic intervention in massive blunt trauma. Radiol Clin North Am 19:9–15
Bengmark S, Rosengren K (1970) Angiographic study of collateral circulation after ligation of the hepatic artery in man. Am J Surg 119:620–625
Bismuth H (1973) Hemobilia. N Engl J Med 288:617–619
Blocker SH, Ternberg JL (1986) Traumatic liver laceration in the newborn: repair with fibrin glue. J Pediatr Surg 21:369–371
Boijsen E, Judkins MP, Simay A (1966) Angiographic diagnosis of hepatic rupture. Radiology 86:66–72
Bond SJ, Eichelberger MR, Gotschall CS, Sivit CJ, Randolph JG (1996) Nonoperative management of blunt hepatic and splenic injuries in children. Ann Surg 223:286–289
Boone DC, Federle M, Billiar TR, Udekwu AO, Pietzman AB (1995) Evolution of management of major hepatic trauma: identification of patterns of injury. J Trauma 36:529–536
Bostwick J III, Stone HH (1975) Trauma to the portal venous system. South Med J 68:1369–1372
Bottger G, Schiebold KD, Uhlmann B, Rockel A (1981) Liver rupture after prolonged use of contraceptive. Z Gesamte Inn Med 36:226–267
Bramhall SR, Buckels JA (2000) Management of liver trauma. Br J Surg 87:519–520
Brasel KJ, Delisle CM, Olson CJ, Borgstrom DC (1997) Trends in the management of hepatic injury. Am J Surg 174:674–677
Brick SH, Taylor GA, Potter BM, Eichelberger MR (1987) Hepatic and splenic injury in children: role of CT in the decision for laparotomy. Radiology 165:643–646
Broering DC, Gundlach M, Bockhorn M, Malago M, Rogiers X (1999) Transplantation of traumatized livers: is it safe? Transplant Proc 31:540
Brotman S, Oliver G, Oster-Granite ML, Cowley RA (1984) The treatment of 179 blunt trauma-induced liver injuries in a statewide trauma center. Am Surg 50:603–608
Brunelle F, Maurage C, Lacombe A, Chaumont P (1985) Emergency embolization in posttraumatic hemobilia in a child. J Pediatr Surg 20:172–174
Brunero M, Balossini F, Falzoni PU, Sorrentino G, Zilioli M, La Capria A (1996) Conservative treatment of post-traumatic hepatic hematoma. Minerva Pediatr 48:387–391
Buckman RF, Piano GP, Dunham M, Soutter I, Ramzy A, Militello PR (1988) Major bowel and diaphragmatic injuries associated with blunt spleen or liver rupture. J Trauma 28:1317–1321
Bulas DI, Eichelberger MR, Sivit CJ et al (1993) Hepatic injury from blunt trauma in children: follow-up evaluation with CT. AJR 160:347–351
Burch JM (1997) New concepts in trauma. Am J Surg 173:44–46
Burch JM, Feliciano D, Mattox KL, Edelman M (1988) Injuries of the inferior vena cava. Am J Surg 156:548–552
Burch JM, Ortiz VB, Richardson RJ, Martin RR, Mattox KL, Jordan GL Jr (1992) Abbreviated laparotomy and planned reoperation for critically injured patients. Ann Surg 215: 476–484
Burton-Opitz R (1910) The vascularity of the liver. I. The flow of blood in the hepatic artery. Q J Exp Physiol 3:20
Busuttil RW, Kitahama A, Cerise E, McFadden M, Lo R, Longmire WP Jr (1980) Management of blunt and penetrating injuries to the porta hepatis. Ann Surg 191:641–648

Bynoe RP, Bell RM, Miles WS, Close TP, Ross MA, Fine JG (1992) Complications of nonoperative management of blunt hepatic injuries. J Trauma 32:308–314, discussion 314–315
Byrne DE, Pass HI, Crawford FA Jr (1980) Traumatic vena caval injuries. Am J Surg 140:600–602
Calne RY, McMastar P, Pentlow BD (1979) The treatment of major liver trauma by primary packing with transfer of the patient for definitive treatment. Br J Surg 66:338–339
Cameron CM, Lazoritz S, Calhoun AD (1997) Blunt abdominal injury: simultaneously occurring liver and pancreatic injury in child abuse. Pediatr Emerg Care 13:334–336
Carles J, Dubuisson V, Douws C, Chahine Z, Gernier N, Videau J (1994) Conservative treatment of hepatic injuries. Management and course. Chirurgie 120:444–450
Carmona RH, Lim RC Jr, Clark GC (1982) Morbidity and mortality in hepatic trauma. A 5-year study. Am J Surg 144: 88–94
Carmona RH, Peck DZ, Lim RC (1984) The role of packing and planned reoperation in severe hepatic trauma. J Trauma 24: 779–782
Carrillo C, Fogler RJ, Shaftan GW (1993) Delayed gastrointestinal reconstruction following massive abdominal trauma. J Trauma 34:233–235
Carrillo EH, Spain DA, Miller FB, Richardson JD (1997) Intrahepatic vascular clamping in complex hepatic vein injuries. J Trauma 43:131–133
Carr-Locke DL, Westwood CA (1980) Endoscopy and endoscopic retrograde cholangiopancreatography finding in traumatic liver injury and hemobilia. Am J Gastroenterol 73:162–164
Cattan P, Cuillerier E, Cellier C et al (1999) Hemobilia caused by a pseudoaneurysm of the hepatic artery diagnosed by EUS. Gastrointest Endosc 49:252–255
Chavan A, Harms J, Pichlmayr R, Galanski M (1993) Transcatheter coil occlusion of an intrahepatic arterioportal fistula in a transplanted liver. Bildgebung 60:215–218
Cheatham JE Jr, Smith EI, Tunell WP et al (1980) Nonoperative management of subcapsular hematomas of the liver. Am J Surg 140:852–857
Chen RJ, Fang JF, Lin BC, Wang YD, Chen MF (1995) Factors that influence the operative mortality after blunt hepatic injuries. Eur J Surg 161:811–817
Chen RJ, Fang JF, Lin BC et al (1998) Selective application of laparoscopy and fibrin glue in the failure of nonoperative management of blunt hepatic trauma. J Trauma 44: 691–695
Chen RJ, Fang JF, Lin BC, Hsu YP, Kao JL, Chen MF (2000) Factors determining operative mortality of grade V blunt hepatic trauma. J Trauma 49:886–889
Chuang JH, Huang SC (1996) Posttraumatic hepatic cyst – an unusual sequela of liver injury in the era of imaging. J Pediatr Surg 31:272–274
Ciorciaro C, Hartmann K, Stoller R, Kuhn M (1996) Liver injury by coumarin anticoagulants: experience of the IKS (Intercanton Monitoring Station) and the SANZ. Schweiz Med Wochenschr 126:2109–2113
Ciraulo DL, Nikkanen HE, Palter M et al (1996) Clinical analysis of the utility of repeat computed tomographic scan before discharge in blunt hepatic injury. J Trauma 41:821–824
Ciraulo DL, Luk S, Palter M et al (1998) Selective hepatic arterial embolization of grade IV and V blunt hepatic injuries: an extension of resuscitation in the nonoperative management of traumatic hepatic injuries. J Trauma 45:353–358
Cirocchi R, Contine A, Mazieri M et al (1999) Perihepatic packing combined with wrappings in the treatment of major bilobar hepatic trauma. Chir Ital 51:259–264
Clancy TE, Warren RL (1997) Endoscopic treatment of biliary colic resulting from hemobilia after nonoperative management of blunt hepatic injury: case report and review of the literature. J Trauma 43:527–529
Clark DE, Cobean RA, Radke FR, Abourjaily GS, Curci MR (1994) Management of major hepatic trauma involving interhospital transfer. Am Surg 60:881–885
Clarnette TD, Beasley SW (1997) Handlebar injuries in children: patterns and prevention. Aust N Z J Surg 67:338–339
Coant PN, Kornberg AE, Brody AS, Edwards-Holmes K (1992) Markers for occult liver injury of physical abuse in children. Pediatrics 89:274–278
Cogbill TH, Moore EE, Jurkovich GJ, Feliciano DV, Morris JA, Mucha P (1988) Severe hepatic trauma: a multi-center experience with 1335 liver injuries. J Trauma 28:1433–1438
Coimbra R, Santos PE, Caffaro RA, Rasslan S, Rahal F (1993) Inferior vena cava trauma: analysis of 36 cases. Rev Assoc Med Bras 39:229–233
Coimbra R, Prado PA, Araujo LH (1994a) Factors related to mortality. Int Surg 79:138–143
Coimbra R, Prado PA, Araujo LH, Candelaria PA, Caffaro RA, Rasslan S (1994b) Factors related to mortality in inferior vena cava injuries. A 5-year experience. Int Surg 79:138–141
Collins PS, Golocovsky M, Salander JM et al (1988) Intraabdominal vascular injury secondary to penetrating trauma. J Trauma 28:S165–S170
Contostavlos DL, Laposata EA (1992) Sagittal liver transection – an injury from improperly worn shoulder harness seatbelts: a report of two cases. J Trauma 33:637–640
Cook DE, Walsh JW, Withley VC, Brewer WH (1986) Upper abdominal trauma: pitfalls in CT diagnosis. Radiology 159: 65–69
Corica A, Powers SR Jr (1975) Blunt liver trauma: an analysis of 75 treated patients. J Trauma 15:751–756
Cox EF (1984) Blunt abdominal trauma. A 5-year analysis of 870 patients requiring coeliotomy. Ann Surg 199:467–474
Cox EF, Flancbaum L, Dauterive AH, Paulson RL (1988) Blunt trauma to the liver. Analysis of management and mortality in 323 consecutive patients. Ann Surg 207:126–134
Croce MA, Fabian TC, Kudsk KA et al (1991) AAST organ injury scale: correlation of CT-graded liver injuries and operative findings. J Trauma 31:806–812
Croce MA, Fabian TC, Spiers JC, Kudsk KA (1994) Traumatic hepatic artery pseudoaneurysm with hemobilia. Am J Surg 168:235–238
Croce MA, Fabian TC, Menke PG et al (1995) Nonoperative management of blunt hepatic trauma is the treatment of choice for hemodynamically stable patients: results of a prospective trial. Ann Surg 221:744–755
Cue JI, Cryer HG, Miller FB, Richardson JD, Polk HC Jr (1990) Packing and planned reexploration for hepatic and retroperitoneal hemorrhage: critical refinements of a useful technique. J Trauma 30:1007–1011
Cuff RF, Cogbill TH, Lambert PJ (2000) Nonoperative management of blunt liver trauma: the value of follow-up abdominal computed tomography scans. Am Surg 66:332–336
Curet P, Baumer R, Roche A, Grellet J, Mercadier M (1984) Hepatic hemobilia of traumatic or iatrogenic origin: recent advances in diagnosis and therapy, review of the literature from 1976 to 1981. World J Surg 8:2–8

Cywes S, Bass DH, Rode H, Millar JW (1991) Blunt liver trauma in children. Injury 22:310–315

Czerniak A, Thompson JN, Hemingway AP et al (1988) Hemobilia. A disease in evolution. Arch Surg 123:718–721

Davidson PG, Ozuner G, Silich RJ (1993) Hemoperitoneum as a result of coital injury to the liver. A case report. J Reprod Med 38:472–474

Davies MR (1997) Iatrogenic hepatic rupture in the newborn and its management by pack tamponade. J Pediatr Surg 32: 1414–1419

Defore WW Jr, Mattox KL, Jordan GL Jr, Beall AC Jr (1976) Management of 1590 consecutive cases of liver trauma. Arch Surg 111:493–497

Demetriades D, Rabinowitz B, Sofianos C (1986) Non-operative management of penetrating liver injuries: a prospective study. Br J Surg 73:736–737

Demetriades D, Charambides D, Lakhoo M et al (1991) Gunshot wounds of the abdomen: role of selective conservative management. Br J Surg 78:220–224

Demetriades D, Gomez H, Chahwan S et al (1999) Gunshot injuries to the liver: the role of selective nonoperative management. J Am Coll Surg 188:343–348

Demirbas A, Fragulidis GP, Karatzas T (1997) Role of liver transplantation in the management of liver trauma. Transplant Proc 29:2848

Depinto DJ, Mucha SJ, Powers PC (1976) Major hepatic vein ligation necessitated by blunt abdominal trauma. Ann Surg 183:243–246

De Toma G, Mingoli A, Modini C, Cavallaro A, Stipa S (1994) The value of angiography and selective hepatic artery embolization for continuous bleeding after surgery in liver trauma: case reports. J Trauma 37:508–511

Dicker RA, Sartorelli KH, McBrids WJ, Vane DW (1996) Penetrating hepatic trauma in children: operating room or not. J Pediatr Surg 31:1189–1191

Diez Pardo JA, Tovar JA, Herrero E, Lassaletta L, Vellibre D (1979) Neonatal laceration of liver and spleen. An Esp Pediatr 12:159–162

Dondelinger RF, Kurdziel JC (1991) A plea for conservative nonoperative management of hepatic contusion. Ann Chir 45:863–876

Dondelinger RF, Kurdziel JC, Gathy C (1990) Percutaneous treatment of pyogenic liver abscess: a critical analysis of results. Cardiovasc Intervent Radiol 13:174–182

Dotzauer G (1970) Organ injuries caused by blunt abdominal trauma (Hefte zur Unfallheilkunde 107). Springer, Berlin Heidelberg New York, pp 63–81

Drost TF, Rosemurgy AS, Kearney RE, Roberts P (1991) Diagnostic peritoneal lavage. Limited indications due to evolving concepts in trauma care. Am Surg 57:126–128

Druwe PM, Cools FJ, De Raedt HJ, Bossaert LL (1996) Liver rupture after cardiopulmonary resuscitation in a patient receiving thrombolytic therapy. Resuscitation 32:213–216

Dumoulin P, Hannoun L, Menu P et al (1981) Rupture of the liver secondary to external cardiac massage in a patient with coronary disease: recovery after partial hepatectomy and aortocoronary by-pass. Ann Med Interne (Paris) 132:261–264

Dunlop W, Lindsay R, Morrish HF, Preshaw RM (1977) Hemobilia associated with a traumatic arteriovenous fistula. Can J Surg 20:441–443

Eber B, Schafhalter-Zoppoth I, Schumacher M, Krejs GJ (1995) Giant cyst of the liver with complete resolution following blunt trauma to the abdomen. Z Gastroenterol 33:709–710

Edler L (1986) Die traumatische Verletzungen der parenchymatösen Unterleibsorganen (Leber, Milz, Pancreas, Nieren). Arch Klin Chir 34:343

Edler L (1987) Die traumatische Verletzungen der parenchymatösen Unterleibsorganen (Leber, Milz, Pancreas, Nieren). Arch Klin Chir 34:373, 378

Eid A, Almogy G, Pikarsky AJ, Binenbaum Y, Shiloni E, Rivkind A (1996) Conservative treatment of a traumatic tear of the left hepatic duct: case report. J Trauma 41:912–913

Elerding SC, Aragon GE, Moore EE (1979) Fatal hepatic hemorrhage after trauma. Am J Surg 138:883–888

Eng RH, Tecson-Tumang F, Corrado ML (1981) Blunt trauma and liver abscess. Am J Gastroenterol 76:252–255

English WP, Johnson MB, Borman KR, Turner WW Jr (2001) Mesenteric ischemia: an unusual presentation of traumatic intrahepatic arterioportal fistula. Am Surg 67:865–867

Esquivel CO, Bernardos A, Makowka L, Iwatsuki S, Gordon RD, Starzl TE (1987) Liver replacement after massive hepatic trauma. J Trauma 27:800–803

Ezberci F, Kargi H (1999) Surgical management of a pulmonary artery missile embolism after an air rifle wound to the liver. South Med J 92:1207–1209

Falimirski ME, Provost D (2000) Nonsurgical management of solid abdominal organ injury in patients over 55 years of age. Am Surg 66:631–635

Fang JG, Chen RJ, Lin BC, Hsu YB, Kao JL, Chen MF (2000) Blunt hepatic injury: minimal intervention is the policy of treatment. J Trauma 49:722–728

Farnell MB, Spencer MP, Thompson E et al (1988) Nonoperative management of blunt hepatic trauma in adults. Surgery 104:748–756

Farron F, Gudinchet F, Genton N (1996) Hepatic trauma in children: long term follow-up. Eur J Pediatr Surg 6:347–349

Federico JA, Horner WR, Clark DE, Isler RJ (1990) Blunt hepatic trauma. Arch Surg 125:905–909

Federle MP, Jeffrey RB (1983) Hemoperitoneum studied by computed tomography. Radiology 143:187–192

Fekete F, Guillet R (1969) Les traumatismes du foie. Rapport au 71è Congrès Français de Chirurgie, Paris, pp 213–382

Fekete F, Guillet R, Giuli R, Goyer B (1969) Considérations thérapeutiques sur les traumatismes du foie. A propos de 1062 observations. Ann Chir 23:1207–1216

Feliciano DV (1981) Intra-abdominal packing for control of hepatic hemorrhage: a reappraisal. J Trauma 21:285–290

Feliciano DV (1989) Surgery for liver trauma. Surg Clin North Am 69:273–284

Feliciano D, Pachter H (1989) Hepatic trauma revisited. Curr Probl Surg 26:453–524

Feliciano DV, Mattox KL, Burch JM, Bitondo CG, Jordan GJ (1986a) Packing for control of hepatic hemorrhage. J Trauma 26:738–743

Feliciano DV, Mattox KL, Jordan GL Jr, Burch JM, Bitando CG, Cruse PA (1986b) Management of 1000 consecutive cases of hepatic trauma (1979–1984). Ann Surg 204:438–445

Femi-Pearse J, Mahmoud A, Kolachalam RB (1998) Laparoscopic control of bleeding liver laceration. Surg Endosc 12: 1171–1172

Fish JC (1966) Reconstruction of the portal vein. Case reports and literature review. Am Surg 32:472–478

Flint LM, Polk HC (1979) Selective hepatic artery ligation: limitations and failures. J Trauma 19:319–323

Flynn TC, Ward RE, Miller PW (1982) Emergency department thoracotomy. Ann Emerg Med 11:413–416

Foley WD, Cates JD, Kellman GM et al (1987) Treatment of blunt hepatic injuries: role of CT. Radiology 164:635–638
Frank MS, Stern EJ, Foy HM (1994) Occult complication of nonoperative treatment of blunt liver injury: detection by CT. AJR 163:333–334
Frey CF, Trollope M, Harpster W, Snyder R (1973) A fifteen-year experience with automotive hepatic trauma. J Trauma 13: 1039–1049
Froment P, Savioz D, Roberson M, Morel P (1998) Hepatic lesions after effective external cardiac massage – an iatrogenic complication not to be overlooked. Swiss Surg 5:225–227
Fuller JW, Anderson PH (1978) Operative management of combined injuries to the portal vein and hepatic artery. South Med J 71:423–424
Fusco MA, Scott TE, Paluzzi MW (1994) Traction injury to the liver during laparoscopic cholecystectomy. Surg Laparosc Endosc 4:454–456
Gable DR, Allen JW, Harrell DJ, Carillo EH (1997) Endoscopic treatment of posttraumatic «bilhemia» case report. J Trauma 43:534–536
Galeon M, Goffette P, van Beers BE, Pringot J (1997) Posttraumatic intrahepatic pseudoaneurysm: diagnosis with helical CT angiography and management with embolization. J Belge Radiol 80:287–288
Garby KB, King TS, Tsai FY (1997) Recurrence of pseudoaneurysm after successful embolization. J Endovasc Surg 4: 385–388
Gates JD (1994) Delayed hemorrhage with free rupture complicating the nonsurgical management of blunt hepatic trauma: a case report and review of the literature. J Trauma 36:572–575
Gay SB, Sistrom CL (1992) Computed tomographic evaluation of blunt abdominal trauma. Radiol Clin North Am 30: 367–388
Geis WP, Schulz KA, Giacchino JL, Freeark RJ (1981) The fate of unruptured intrahepatic hematomas. Surgery 90:689–697
Gilliland MG, Ward RE, Flynn TC, Miller PW, Ben-Menachem Y, Duke JH Jr (1982) Peritoneal lavage and angiography in the management of patients with pelvic fractures. Am J Surg 144:744–747
Ginzburg E, Shatz D, Lynn M et al (1998) The role of liver transplantation in the subacute trauma patient. Am Surg 64:363–364
Giuliano F, Haas O, Rat P, Barry P, Favre JP (1987) Injuries to the liver. Study of fifty-four cases. J Chir (Paris) 124:103–107
Goff CD, Gilbert CM (1995) Nonoperative management of blunt hepatic trauma. Am Surg 61:66–68
Goletti O, Ghiselli G, Lippolis PR, Chiarugi M, Braccini G, Macaluso C, Cavina E (1994) The role of ultrasonography in blunt abdominal trauma: results in 250 consecutive cases. J Trauma 36:178–181
Gomez GA, Jacobson LE, Asensio JA, Nauta RJ (1994) Pre-existing liver disease in the trauma patient. Crit Care Clin 10: 555–566
Goodman DA, Ararwal N, Tiruchelvam V et al (1995) CT reconstruction in the surgical management of hepatic injuries. Ann R Coll Surg Engl 77:7–11
Gorich J, Rilinger N, Brado M et al (1999) Non-operative management of arterial liver hemorrhages. Eur Radiol 9:85–88
Gow KW, Murphy JJ III, Blair GK, Stringer DA, Culham JA, Fraser GC (1996) Splanchnic artery pseudo-aneurysms secondary to blunt abdominal trauma in children. J Pediatr Surg 31:812–815
Grasberger RC, Scott CM, McCormick JR, Birkett DH, Hirsch EF (1985) Pericardial complications in hepatic trauma. J Trauma 25:322–325
Green MH, Dvell RM, Johnson CD, Jamieson NV (2001) Haemobilia. Br J Surg 88:773–786
Greenberg MJ (1986) Pulmonary artery embolism with liver tissue. Ann Emerg Med 184:1119–1120
Griswold, Collier (1961) Collective review : blunt abdominal trauma. Surg Gynecol Obstet 112:309–329
Guiset J, Combemale B, Lagache G (1980) Contusions du foie ; proposition d'une classification. Nouv Presse Méd 9: 189–190
Haberlik A, Cendron M, Sauer H (1992) Biliovenous fistula in children after blunt liver trauma: proposal for a simple surgical treatment. J Pediatr Surg 27:1203–1206
Hagiwara A, Yukioka T, Shimazaki S, Megawa T, Matuda H (1993) Delayed hemorrhage following catheter arterial embolization for blunt hepatic injury. Cardiovasc Intervent Radiol 16:380–383
Hagiwara A, Yukioka T, Ohta S et al (1997) Nonsurgical management of patients with blunt hepatic injury: efficacy of transcatheter arterial embolization. AJR 169:1151–1156
Haight DO, Toney JF, Greene JN, Sandin RL, Vincent AL (1994) Liver abscess following blunt trauma: a case report and review of the literature. South Med J 87:811–813
Halme L, Orko R, Tieral E, Hockerstedt K (1994) Late biliary stenosis after conservative management of traumatic liver rupture: case report. J Trauma 36:740–742
Halpern NB, Aldrete JS (1979) Factors influencing mortality and morbidity from injuries, the abdominal aorta and inferior vena cava. Am J Surg 137:384–388
Halsted WS (1913) The employment of fine silk in preference to catgut and advantage of transfixing tissues and vessels in controlling hemorrhage: also an account of the introduction of gloves, gutta-percha tissue and silver fail. JAM 60: 1119–1126
Hamelmann H, Nitschke J (1971) Intraperitoneal hemorrhage in blunt abdominal trauma. Chirurg 42:433–438
Hamil J, Civil ID, McCall JL (2000) Traumatic liver necrosis diagnosed by magnetic resonance imaging. Aust N Z J Surg 70:379–381
Haney PJ, Whitley NO, Brotman S, Cunat JS, Whitley J (1982) Liver injury and complications in the postoperative trauma patient: CT evaluation. AJR 139:271–275
Hanna SS, Maheshwari Y, Harrison AW, Taylor GA, Miller HAB, Maggisano R (1985) Blunt liver trauma at the Sunnybrook regional trauma unit. Can J Surg 28:220–223
Hanna SS, Gorman PR, Harrison AW, Taylor G, Miller HA, Pagliarello G (1987) Blunt liver trauma at Sunnybrook Medical Center. J Trauma 27:965–969
Harada N, Ito T, Taura S, Tsuchiya R, Koga Y (1975) Portal hypertension due to hepatic artery-portal vein arteriovenous fistula – a case report. Jpn J Surg 5:145–152
Harnar TJ, Oreskovich MR, Copass MK, Heimbach DM, Herman CM, Carrico CJ (1981) Role of emergency thoracotomy in the resuscitation of moribund trauma victims: 100 consecutive cases. Am J Surg 142:96–99
Harper HC III, Maull KI (2000) Transcatheter arterial embolization in blunt hepatic trauma. South Med J 93:663–665
Hashimoto S, Ido K, Hiramatsu K et al (1990) Expanding role of emergency embolization in the management of severe blunt hepatic trauma. Cardiovasc Intervent Radiol 13: 193–197

Hashizume M, Sugimachi K (1997) Needle and trocar injury during laparoscopic surgery in Japan. Surg Endosc 11: 1198–1201
Haskal ZJ, Pentecost MJ, Rubin RA (1993) Hepatic arterial injury after transjugular intrahepatic portosystemic shunt placement: report of two cases. Radiology 188:85–88
Hatten M, Hamrick-Turner JE (1996) Segmental hepatic necrosis after blunt abdominal trauma: CT findings. AJR 167:769–770
Hawkins ML, Scofield WM, Carraway RP, Laws HL (1988) Diagnostic peritoneal lavage in blunt trauma. South Med J 81:293–296
Heimbach DM, Ferguson GS, Harley JD (1978) Treatment and traumatic hemobilia with angiographic embolization. J Trauma 18:221–224
Henne-Bruns D, Kremer B (1992) Injuries of the portal vein and vena cava in severe blunt abdominal trauma. Zentralbl Chir 117:343–347
Henson SW Jr, Gray HK, Dockerty MB (1957) Benign tumors of the liver. V Traumatic cysts. Surg Gynaecol Obstet 104: 302–306
Heydenrich JJ (1974) Haemoperitoneum and associated torsion of the testicle in the newborn. S Afr Med J 48:2221
Hiatt JR, Harrier HD, Koenig BV, Randon KJ (1990) Nonoperative management of major blunt liver injury with hemoperitoneum. Arch Surg 125:101–103
Hibbard L (1976) Spontaneous rupture of the liver in pregnancy: a report of eight cases. Am J Obstet Gynecol 126: 334–338
Hidalgo F, Narvaez J, Rene M, Dominguez J, Sancho C, Montanya X (1995) Treatment of hemobilia with selective hepatic artery embolization. J Vasc Interv Radiol 6:793–798
Hinterthaner M, Kaminski M, Hirner A, Fischer HP (1997) Spontaneous rupture of the liver following lysis with streptokinase. Zentralbl Chir 122:49–51
Ho MC, Hu RH (1995) Hepatic portal vein gas following blunt colon injury: report of a case. J Formos Med Assoc 94: 578–580
Honda K, Koishizawa T, Nonaka K et al (1996) A case report of surgical management of blunt ruptured right atrium with blunt ruptured liver. Kyobu Geka 49:471–474
Horvath KA, Glasgow AH (1992) Massive intra-abdominal hemorrhage from a hepatic laceration caused by vomiting. Arch Surg 127:1361
Huguet C, Callot D, Charles JF, Coloigner M, Marre P, Tiengou L (1975) Pulmonary embolism, an unrecognized risk of posttraumatic arterio-venous fistulae of the hepatic veins. J Chir (Paris) 110:341–348
Hunter V, Reid MH (1983) Computed tomography of liver trauma due to surgical retraction. J Comput Tomogr 7: 381–383
Icely S, Chez RA (1999) Traumatic liver rupture in pregnancy. Am J Obstet Gynecol 180:1030–1031
Inoguchi H, Mii S, Sakata H, Orita H, Yamashita S (2001) Intrahepatic pseudoaneurysm after surgical hemostasis for a delayed hemorrhage due to blunt liver injury: report of a case. Surg Today 31:367–370
Ivatury RR, Nallathambi M, Gunduz Y, Constable R, Rohman M, Stahl WM (1986) Liver packing for uncontrolled hemorrhage: a reappraisal. J Trauma 26:744–749
Izard G, Houri R, Randrianasolo S, Gailleton R (1995) Acute Budd-Chiari syndrome of traumatic origin. Presse Med 24: 1209–1210
Jander HP, Laws HL, Kogutt MS, Mihas AA (1977) Emergency embolization in blunt hepatic trauma. AJR 129:249–252
Jeffrey RB Jr, Olcott EW (1991) Imaging of blunt hepatic trauma. Radiol Clin North Am 29:1299–1310
Jeffrey RB Jr, Cardoza JD, Olcott EW (1991) Detection of active intra-abdominal arterial hemorrhage: value of dynamic contrast-enhanced CT. AJR 156:725–729
Jehle D, Guarino J, Karamanoukian H (1993) Emergency department ultrasound in the evaluation of blunt abdominal trauma. Am J Emerg Med 11:342–346
Johanet H, Melchior JC, Merrer J, Rabault N, Oberlin P, Etienne JC, Fingerhut A (1989) Hepatic and splenic contusion after external cardiac massage. A surgically treated case with favourable outcome. Ann Chir 43:760
Jona JZ, Goldstein IR (1977) Compression hepatic necrosis in a child. J Trauma 17:402–404
Jones HV, Harley HR (1970) Traumatic cyst of the liver. Br J Surg 57:449–464
Jornod P, Wiesel PH, Pescature P, Gonvers JJ (1999) Hemobilia, a rare cause of acute pancreatitis after percutaneous liver biopsy: diagnosis and treatment by endoscopic retrograde cholangiopancreatography. Am J Gastroenterol 94: 3051–3054
Junghanns K (1978) Seatbelt-related abdominal injuries. Langenbecks Arch Chir 347:373–376
Jurkovich GJ, Hoyt DB, Moore FA et al (1995) Portal triad injuries. J Trauma 39:426–434
Karp MP, Cooney DR, Pros GA, Newman BM, Jewett TC (1983) Nonoperative management of pediatric hepatic trauma. J Pediatr Surg 18:512–518
Kashuk JL, Moore EE, Milikan JS, Moore JB (1982) Major abdominal vascular trauma: a unified approach. J Trauma 22:672–679
Kayser S, Marincek B, Schlumpf R, Fried M, Wirth HP (1996) Rapidly progressive portal hypertension 23 years posttraumatic arterioportal fistula of the liver. Am J Gastroenterol 91:1442–1446
Keller MS, Sartorelli KH, Vane DW (1996) Associated head injury should not prevent nonoperative management of spleen or liver injury in children. J Trauma 41:471–475
Kestenberg W, Mittal VK (1992) Post-traumatic pseudoaneurysm of the left hepatic artery initially appearing as upper gastrointestinal hemorrhage secondary to hepatic artery-duodenal fistula. A case study. Am Surg 58:451–454
Keuth U, Althaus W, Feldmann EM (1976) X-ray diagnosis of hepatic rupture in a newborn. Monatschr Kinderheilkd 124:138–140
Kimoto T, Kohno H, Uchida M et al (1998) Inferior vena caval thrombosis after traumatic liver injury. HPB Surg 11: 111–116
Kimura A, Otsuka T (1991) Emergency center ultrasonography in the evaluation of hemoperitoneum: a prospective study. J Trauma 31:20–23
Kindling PH, Wilson RF, Watt AJ (1969) Hepatic trauma with particular reference to blunt injury. J Trauma 9:17–26
Kirchgatterer A, Baldinger C, Kenglinger F et al (1998) Portal hypertension due to traumatic hepatic arterioportal fistula: report of successful embolization. Eur J Gastroenterol Hepatol 10:1057–1059
Klein SR, Baumgartner FJ, Bongard FS (1994) Contemporary management strategy for major inferior vena caval injuries. J Trauma 37:35–41
Kloppel R, Brock D, Kosling S, Benneg J, Hormann D (1997)

Spiral computerized tomography diagnosis of abdominal seat belt injuries in children. Aktuel Radiol 7:19–22
Kloss T, Puschkel K, Wishhusen F, Welk I, Roewer N, Jungck E (1983) Resuscitation injuries. Anaesth Intensivther Notfallmed 18:199–203
Knoop M, Neumann U, Neuhaus P (1999) Bilobar liver hematoma and spontaneous rupture after cesarean section. Chirurg 70:214–216
Knowdley D, Aggarwal A, Sachs P (1994) Delayed hemorrhage after percutaneous liver biopsy: role of therapeutic angiography. J Clin Gastroenterol 19:50–53
Knudson MM, Lim RC, Oakes DD, Jeffrey RB Jr (1990) Nonoperative management of blunt liver injuries in adults: the need for continued surveillance. J Trauma 30:1494–1500
Konstam MA, Novelline RA, Athanasoulis C (1979) Aberrant hepatic artery: a potential cause for error in the angiographic diagnosis of traumatic liver hematoma. Gastrointest Radiol 30:43–45
Koslin DB, Stanley RJ, Berland LL, Shin MS, Dalton SC (1987) Hepatic perivascular lymphoedema: CT appearance. AJR 150:111–113
Kos X, Fanchamps JM, Trotteur G, Dondelinger RF (1999) Radiologic damage control: evaluation of a combined CT and angiography suite with a pivoting table. Cardiovasc Intervent Radiol 22:124–129
Kremer B, Henne-Bruns D (1993) Evaluation of different techniques in liver rupture. Chirurg 64:852–859
Krige JE, Bornman PC, Terblanche J (1992) Therapeutic perihepatic packing in complex liver trauma. Br J Surg 79: 43–46
Kudsk KA, Sheldon JF, Lim RC Jr (1982) Atrial-caval shunting (ACS) after trauma. J Trauma 22:81–85
Lam EC, Janzen RM, Meloche RM, Trepanier PJ, Yoshida EM (1999) Acute pseudohepatitis in a chronic substance abuse secondary to occult seat belt injury. Can J Gastroenterol 13: 155–158
Lambeth W, Rubin BE (1979) Nonoperative management of intrahepatic hemorrhage and hematoma following blunt trauma. Surg Gynecol Obstet 148:507–511
Lasser A, Wilson GL (1975) Ectopic liver tissue mass in the thoracic cavity. Cancer 36:1823–1826
Lau LL, Diamond T (1997) Delayed presentation of porta hepatis injury following blunt abdominal trauma. HPB Surg 10: 249–252
Lawson TL, Thorsen MK, Erickson SJ, Perret RS, Quiroz FA, Foley WD (1993) Periportal halo: a CT sign of liver disease. Abdom Imaging 18:42–46
Lee M, Himal HS (1992) Hemobilia – successful treatment by angiographic embolization. Surg Endosc 6:75–77
Lee SJ, Lim JH, Lee HJ, Lim HK, Choo SW, Choo IW (1997) Transient subsegmental hepatic parenchymal enhancement on dynamic CT: a sign of postbiopsy arterioportal shunt. J Comput Assist Tomogr 21:355–360
Leppaniemi AK, Savolainem HO, Salo JA (1994) Traumatic inferior vena caval injuries. Scand J Thorac Cardiovasc Surg 28:103–108
Lerut J, Vauthey N, Triller J, Gertsch P, Schweizer W (1992) Intrahepatic arterioportal fistula following conservative treatment of a traumatic liver rupture: case report. J Trauma 33:760–764
Letoublon C, Castaing D (1996) Blunt injuries of the liver. Arnette Blackwell, Paris
Levin A, Gover P, Nance FC (1978) Surgical restraint in the management of hepatic injury: a review of Charity Hospital experience. J Trauma 18:399–404
Levine CD, Patel VS, Wachsberg RH et al (1995) CT in patients with blunt abdominal trauma: clinical significance of intraperitoneal fluid detected on a scan with otherwise normal findings. AJR 164:1381–1385
Lewis FR, Lim RC Jr, Blaisdell FW (1974) Hepatic artery ligation: adjunct in the management of massive hemorrhage from the liver. J Trauma 14:743–755
L'Hermine C, Grand M, Remond A, van Kemmel M, Quandalle P (1978) Inversion of intrahepatic portal flow in contusions of the liver: a new concept of traumatic arterioportal fistulas. J Radiol Electrol Nucl Med 58:609–619
Lignitz E, Gillner E, May D (1977) Complications of resuscitative measures with special regard to liver damage. Prakt Anaesth 12:523–526
Little JM, Wong KP, Simmons K (1986) Percutaneous dilatation in the management of bile duct strictures. Aust N Z J Surg 56:697–700
Longmire WP Jr, Cleveland RJ (1972) Surgical anatomy and blunt trauma of the liver. Surg Clin North Am 52:687–692
Lucas CE, Ledgerwood AM (1973) Controlled biliary drainage for large injuries of the liver. Surg Gynecol Obstet 137: 585–589
Lucas CE, Ledgerwood AM (1978) Liver necrosis following hepatic artery transection due to trauma. Arch Surg 113: 1107
Lucas CE, Ledgerwood AM (2000) Changing times and treatment of liver injury. Am Surg 66:337–341
Lucciarini P, Ofner D, Weber F, Lungenschmid D (1993) Ultrasonography in the initial evaluation and follow-up of blunt abdominal injury. Surgery 114:506–512
Lukancic SP, Nemcek AA Jr, Vogelzang RL (1991) Posttraumatic intrahepatic arterial pseudoaneurysm: treatment with direct percutaneous puncture. J Vasc Interv Radiol 2:335–337
Macrander SJ, Lawson TL, Foley WD, Dodds WJ, Erickson SJ, Quiroz FA (1989) Periportal tracking in hepatic trauma: CT features. J Comput Assist Tomogr 13:952–957
Maione G, Tommasini Degna C, Baticci F, Gerosa E, Grassi G, Forti D (1994) Contusion of the liver. Importance of associated lesions in polytraumatized patients. J Chir 131: 194–200
Malhotra AK, Fabian TC, Croce MA, Gavin TJ, Kudsk KA, Minard G, Pritchard FE (2000) Blunt hepatic injury: a paradigm shift from operative to nonoperative management in the 1990s. Ann Surg 231:804–813
Mallek R, Mostbeck G, Gebauer A et al (1990) Posttraumatic pseudoaneurysm of the hepatic artery. Radiology 30:484–486
Manning MM, Murray KD, Townsend MC (1993) The laparoscopic diagnosis and treatment of cavernous hemangioma hemorrhage following blunt trauma. J Laparoendosc Surg 3:399–403
Markert DJ, Shanmuganathan K, Mirvis SE, Nakajima Y, Hayakawa M (1997) Budd-Chiari syndrome resulting from intrahepatic IVC compression secondary to blunt hepatic trauma. Clin Radiol 52:384–387
Marr JD, Krige JE, Terblanche J (2000) Analysis of 153 gun shot wounds of the liver. Br J Surg 87:1030–1034
Mathisen DJ, Athanasoulis CA, Malt RA (1982) Preservation of arterial flow to the liver: goal in treatment of extrahepatic and post-traumatic intrahepatic aneurysms of the hepatic artery. Ann Surg 196:400–411

Mattox KL, Espada R, Beall AR (1975) Traumatic injury to the portal vein. Ann Surg 181:519–522
Mays E (1974) Demonstration of collateral arterial flow after interruption of hepatic arteries in man. N Engl J Med 290: 993–995
McClelland RN, Shires GT (1965) Management of liver traumas in 259 consecutive patients. Ann Surg 161:248–253
McCort JJ (1962) Rupture or laceration of liver by non-penetrating trauma. Radiology 78:49–57
McCort JJ (1966) Radiographic examination in blunt abdominal trauma. Saunders, Philadelphia
McCort JJ (1973) Abdominal trauma. In: Margulis AR, Burhenne HJ (eds) Alimentary tract roentgenology, vol I. Mosby, St Louis, pp 228–270
McCort JJ (1987) Caring for the major trauma victim: the role for radiology. Radiology 163:1–9
McDougal EG, Mandel SR (1984) Traumatic hemobilia. Successful nonoperative treatment in two cases. Am Surg 50: 169–172
McGehee M, Kier R, Cohn SM, McCarthy SM (1993) Comparison of MRI with post contrast CT for the evaluation of acute abdominal trauma. J Comput Assist Tomogr 17:410–413
McGillibray D, Valentine R (1989) Nonoperative management of blunt pediatric liver injury – late complications: case report. J Trauma 29:251–254
McGrath FP, Lee SH, Gibney RG, Burhenne HD (1990) Hepatic subcapsular hematoma: an unusual complication of biliary lithotripsy. AJR 154:1015–1016
McInnis WD, Richardson JD, Aust JB (1977) Hepatic trauma: pitfalls in management. Arch Surg 112:157–161
McKenney MG, Martin L, Lentz K et al (1996) 1000 consecutive ultrasounds for blunt abdominal trauma. J Trauma 40: 607–612
McKenney KL (1999) Ultrasound of blunt abdominal trauma. Radiol Clin North Am 37:879–893
McMaster P (1976) Hepatic trauma involving the hepatic veins and vena cava. Injury 7:299–305
Meldrum DR, Moore FA, Moore EE, Haenel JB, Cosgriff N, Burch JM (1995) Jack A. Barney Resident Research Award. Cardiopulmonary hazards of perihepatic packing for major liver injuries. Am J Surg 170:537–540
Meldrum DR, Moore FA, Moore EE, Franciose RJ, Sauaia A, Burch JM (1997) Prospective characterization and selective management of the abdominal compartment syndrome. Am J Surg 174:667–672
Menegaux F, Langlois P, Chigot JP (1993) Severe blunt trauma of the liver: study of mortality factors. J Trauma 35: 865–869
Menzel K, Niedner W, Topke B (1977) Hemoperitoneum in the newborn infant. Zentralbl Gynakol 99:240–244
Meredith JW, Young JS, Bowling J, Roboussin D (1994) Nonoperative management of blunt hepatic trauma: the exception or the rule. J Trauma 36:529–535
Merendino KA, Dillard DH, Gammock DE (1963) The concept of surgical biliary decompression in the management of liver trauma. Surg Gynecol Obstet 117:285–290
Merhav H, Zajko A, Dodd G et al (1993) Percutaneous transhepatic embolization of an intrahepatic pseudoaneurysm following liver biopsy in a liver transplant patient. Transplant Int 6:239–241
Meyer AA, Crass RA, Lim RC et al (1985) Selective nonoperative management of blunt liver injury using computed tomography. Arch Surg 120:550–554
Meyer DM, Thal ER, Weigelt JA, Redman HC (1989) Evaluation of computed tomography and diagnostic peritoneal lavage in blunt abdominal trauma. J Trauma 29:1168–1171
Meyer JJ, Cass AS (1995) Subcapsular hematoma of the liver after renal extracorporeal shock wave lithotripsy. J Urol 154:516–517
Michalodimitrakis M, Tsatsakis A (1998) Massive pulmonary embolism by liver tissue. Med Sci Law 38:85–87
Milikan JS, Moore EE, Cogbill TH, Hashuk JL (1983) Inferior vena cava injuries: a continuing challenge. J Trauma 23: 207–212
Mirvis SE, Whitley NO, Vainwright JR, Gens DR (1989) Blunt hepatic trauma in adults: CT-based classification and correlation with prognosis and treatment. Radiology 171:27–32
Missavage AE, Hones AM, Walt AJ, Hans B, Jacobs LA (1984) Traumatic hepatic arteriovenous fistula causing portal hypertension and variceal bleeding. J Trauma 24:355–358
Moar JJ (1984) Pulmonary embolism due to hepatic tissue – a forensic vital sign? A case report. S Afr Med J 66:669–670
Moon KL, Federle MP (1983) Computed tomography in hepatic trauma. AJR 141:309–314
Moore JB, Moore EE, Thompson JS (1980) Abdominal injuries associated with penetrating trauma in the lower chest. Am J Surg 140:724–730
Moore EE (1984) Critical decisions in the management of hepatic trauma. Am J Surg 148:712–716
Moore FA, Moore EE, Seagraves A (1985) Nonresectional management of major hepatic trauma. An evolving concept. Am J Surg 150:725–729
Moore EE, Shackford SR, Pachter HL et al (1989) Organ injury scaling: spleen, liver, and kidney. J Trauma 29:1664–1666
Moore EE, Cogbill TH, Jurkovich GJ, Shackford MD, Malangoni MA, Champion HR (1994) Organ injury scaling: spleen and liver (1994 revision). J Trauma 38:323–324
Morris DL, Crane M (1993) 911 access and trauma deaths: a complex association. Ann Emerg Med 22:1777–1779
Morton JR, Roys GD, Bicker DL (1972) The treatment of liver injuries. Surg Gynecol Obstet 134:298–303
Murakami R, Tajima H, Kumazaki T (1993) Transcatheter hepatic arterial embolization for the treatment of blunt hepatic injury. Nippon Igaku Hoshasen Gakkai Zasshi 53: 395–402
Musiani R, Bartoli R, Barlettani P (1993) Ligation of the hilar arteries in hemorrhages due to traumatic rupture of the liver. Minerva Chir 48:317–323
Nagata Y, Kohno T, Saga K et al (1990) CT manifestations of a ruptured hepatic tumor after transcatheter arterial embolization. Comput Med Imaging Graph 72:497–499
Nehoda H, Hochleitner BW (1998) Subcapsular liver hematomas caused by bar ends in mountain bike crashes. Lancet 351:342
Nicoloff DM, Fortuny IE, de Wall RA (1964) Acute Budd Chiari syndrome secondary to intrahepatic hematoma following blunt abdominal trauma: treatment by open intracardiac surgery. J Thoracic Cardiovasc Surg 163:333–334
Nielsen SL, Mygind T, Miskowiak J (1982) Blood pool scintigraphy and arterial embolization in traumatic hemobilia. Eur J Nucl Med 7:389–390
Nishida T, Fujita N, Nakao K (1996) A multivariate analysis of the prognosis factors in severe liver trauma. Surg Today 26: 389–394
Nonomura A, Mizukami Y, Kadoya M (1994) Angiomyolipoma of the liver: a collective review. J Gastroenterol 29:95–105

Ochsner MG, Knudson MM, Pachter HL et al (2000) Significance of minimal or no intraperitoneal fluid visible on CT scan associated with blunt liver and splenic injuries: a multicenter analysis. J Trauma 49:505–510
Ohta S, Hagiwara A, Yukioka T et al (1998) Hypoechoic appearance of hepatic parenchyma on ultrasound examination of patients with blunt hepatic injury. J Trauma 44:135–138
Oishi AJ, Nagorney DM, Cherry KJ (1993) Portal hypertension, variceal bleeding and high output cardiac failure secondary to an intrahepatic arterioportal fistula. HPB Surg 7:53–59
Okazaki K, Moriyasu F, Shiomura T et al (1986) Spontaneous rupture of the spleen and liver in amyloidosis – a case report and review of the literature. Gastroenterol Jpn 21: 518–524
Okazaki M, Ono H, Higashihara H et al (1991) Angiographic management of massive hemobilia due to iatrogenic trauma. Gastrointest Radiol 16:205–209
Oldhafer KH, Ringer B, Pichlmayr R (1993) Therapy of severe liver trauma – is there an indication for liver transplantation. Unfallchirurg 96:497–498
Olsen WR (1982) Late complications of central liver injuries. Surgery 92:733–743
Ormann W, Starck E, Pausch J (1991) Arterial embolization of an arteriovenous fistula with hemobilia after fluid liver puncture. Z Gastroenterol 29:153–155
Orwig D, Federle MP (1989) Localized clotted blood as evidence of visceral trauma on CT: the sentinel clot sign. AJR 153:747–749
Owen RJ, Rose JD (2000) Endovascular treatment of a portal vein tear during TIPSS. Cardiovasc Intervent Radiol 23: 230–232
Pachter HL, Hofstetter SR (1995) The current status of nonoperative management of adult blunt hepatic injuries. Am J Surg 169:442–453
Pachter HL, Spencer FC, Hofstetter SR, Coppa GF (1983) Experience with the finger fracture technique to achieve intrahepatic hemostasis in 75 patients with severe injuries of the liver. Ann Surg 197:771–778
Pachter HL, Spencer FC, Hofstetter SR, Liang HC, Coppa GF (1986) The management of juxtahepatic venous injuries without an atriocaval shunt: preliminary clinical observations. Surgery 99:569–575
Pachter HL, Knudson MM, Esrig B et al (1996) Status of nonoperative management of blunt hepatic injuries in 1995: a multicenter experience with 404 patients. J Trauma 40:31–38
Pal KM, Khan A (2000) Nonoperative management of penetrating liver trauma. Injury 31:199–201
Pardes JG, Haaga JR, Borkowski G (1982) Focal hepatic fatty metamorphosis secondary to trauma. J Comput Assist Tomogr 6:769–771
Pasenau J, Mamazza J, Schlachta CM, Seshadri PA, Poulin EC (2000) Liver hematoma after laparoscopic Nissen fundoplication: a case report and review of retraction injuries. Surg Laparosc Endosc Percutan Tech 10:178–181
Patel NH, Bradshaw B, Meissner MH, Towsend MF (1996) Posttraumatic Budd-Chiari syndrome treated with thrombolytic therapy and angioplasty. J Trauma 40:294–298
Patrick LE, Ball TI, Atkinson GO, Winn KJ (1992) Pediatric blunt abdominal trauma: periportal tracking with CT. Radiology 183:689–691
Patten RM, Spear RP, Vincent LM, Hesla RB, Jurkovich GJ (1993) Traumatic laceration of the liver limited to the bare area: CT findings in 25 patients. AJR 160:1019–1022
Patten RM, Gunberg SR, Brandenburger DK, Richardson ML (2000) CT detection of hepatic and splenic injuries: usefulness of liver window settings. AJR 175:1107–1110
Pearl L, Trunkey DD (1999) compartment syndrome of the liver. J Trauma 47:769–798
Peiper HJ, Peitsch W (1976) Blunt upper abdominal injury. Unfallheilkunde 79:341–346
Petri A, Sandor L, Adam E, Bozo A (1993) Acute venous liver circulatory disorder caused by blunt abdominal trauma: is it a compartment syndrome? Unfallchirug 96:625–627
Pezzi A, Pasetti G, Lombardi F, Fiorentini C, Iapichino G (1999) Liver rupture after cardiopulmonary resuscitation (CPR) and thrombolysis. Intensive Care Med 25:1032
Pickleman J, Block GE (1973) Adjuncts to the operative management of penetrating liver injuries. Arch Surg 106: 402–406
Pilcher DB, Harmann PK, Moore EE (1977) Retrohepatic vena cava balloon shunt introduced via the sapheno-femoral junction. J Trauma 17:837–841
Poletti PA, Mirvis SE, Shanmuganathan K, Killeen KL, Coldwell D (2000) CT criteria for management of blunt liver trauma: correlation with angiographic and surgical findings. Radiology 216:418–427
Prahlow JA, O'Bryant TJ, Barnard JJ (1997) Cardiac perforation due to Wallstent embolization: a fatal complication of the transjugular intrahepatic portosystemic shunt procedure. Radiology 205:170–172
Pretre R, Mentha G, Robert J, Schneider PA, Rohner A (1993) Acute segmental arterioportal shunt with reversal of portal blood flow after atypical resection for hepatic injury. Eur J Surg 159:313–315
Pringle JH (1908) Notes on the arrest of hepatic hemorrhage due to trauma. Ann Surg 48:541–549
Radin DR (1992) Liver trauma and transsection in the inferior vena cava. Sentinel contrast sign and perivenous tracking. Acta Radiol 33:255–257
Raines DR, van Heertum RL, Johnson LF (1979) Intrahepatic hematoma: a complication of percutaneous liver biopsy. Gastroenterology 76:284–289
Raptopoulos V (1994) Abdominal trauma: emphasis on computed tomography. Radiol Clin North Am 32:969–987
Rathod K, Sheth R, Shah P, Rege S (2000) Active contrast extravasation in spontaneous rupture of hepatocellular carcinoma: a rare CT finding. J Postgrad Med 46:35–36
Reber PU, Baer HU, Patel AG, Wildi S, Triller J, Buchler MR (1998) Superselective microcoil embolization: treatment of choice in high-risk patients with extrahepatic pseudoaneurysm of the hepatic arteries. J Am Coll Surg 186: 325–330
Reed RL, Merrel C, Meyers WC, Fischer RP (1992) Continuing evolution in the approach to severe liver trauma. Ann Surg 216:524–538
Reichert CM, Weisenthal LM, Klein HG (1983) Delayed hemorrhage after percutaneous liver biopsy. J Clin Gastroenterol 5:263–266
Reifferscheid M (1958) Clinics of hepatic injuries. Langenbecks Arch Clin Chir 288:361–367
Renz BM, Feliciano DV (1994) Gunshot wounds to the right thoracoabdomen: a prospective study of nonoperative management. J Trauma 37:737–744
Renz BM, Bott J, Feliciano DV (1996) Failure of nonoperative treatment of a gunshot wound to the liver predicted by computed tomography. J Trauma 40:191–193

Reuter G, Heller K, Munster W (1980) Traumatic haemobilia in childhood. Zentralbl Chir 105:1148–1153
Richardson A, Simmons K, Gutmann J, Little JM (1985) Hepatic hemobilia: nonoperative management in eight cases. Aust N Z J Surg 55:447–451
Richardson JD, Belin RP, Griffen WO Jr (1972) Blunt abdominal trauma in children. Ann Surg 176:213–216
Richardson DJ, Franklin GA, Lukan JK et al (2000) Evolution in the management of hepatic trauma: a 25-year perspective. Ann Surg 232:324–330
Ringe B, Pinchlmayr R, Lübbe N, Bornscheuer A, Kuse E (1988) Total hepatectomy as temporary approach to acute or primary graft failure. Transplant Proc 20:552–555
Ringe B, Pinchlmayr R, Ziegler H (1991) Management of severe hepatic trauma by two-stage total hepatectomy and subsequent liver transplantation. Surgery 109:792–796
Risseeuw JJ, de Vries JE, van Eyck J, Rabin B (1999) Liver rupture postpartum associated with preeclampsia and HELLP syndrome. J Matern Fetal Med 8:32–35
Rivkind AI, Siegel JH, Dunham M (1989) Patterns of organ injury in blunt hepatic trauma and their significance for management and outcome. J Trauma 29:1398–1415
Roberts JL (1996) CT of abdominal and pelvic trauma. Semin Ultrasound CT MR 17:142–169
Roberts JL, Dalen K, Bosanko CM, Jafir SZ (1993) CT in abdominal and pelvic trauma. Radiographics 13:735–752
Roche A, Doyon D, Harry G, Benozio M (1978a) Therapeutic arterial embolization in hemobilia. A propos of 3 cases. J Radiol Electrol Med Nucl 59:191–196
Roche A, Doyon D, Harry G, Weingarten A, Edouard A (1978b) Hepatic arterial embolization: 35 cases. Nouv Presse Med 7:633–637
Rogers RG, Monahan EG (1996) Postoperative hemorrhage due to avulsion of perihepatic adhesions after pneumoperitoneum. J Am Assoc Gynecol Laparosc 3:631–633
Rosch J, Putnam JS, Keller FS (1988) Diagnosis and management of hemobilia. Semin Intervent Radiol 5:49–60
Rosen J, Tuchek JM, Hartmann JR (1999) Liver laceration in the hemodynamically unstable post-cardiac massage patient: early recognition and management – case report. J Trauma 47:408–409
Rossi G, Catalano O (1992) A rare complication of renal and biliary lithotripsy: subcapsular hematoma of the liver. Radiol Med 83:646–647
Rotondo MF, Schwab CW, McGonigal MD et al (1993) "Damage control": an approach for improved survival in exsanguinating penetrating abdominal injury. J Trauma 35:375–382
Rozycki GS, Ochsner MG, Schmidt JA et al (1995) A prospective study of surgeon-performed ultrasound as the primary adjuvant modality for injured patients assessment. J Trauma 39:492–500
Rubin BE, Katzen BT (1977) Selective hepatic artery embolization to control massive hepatic hemorrhage after trauma. AJR 129:253–256
Sahdev P, Garramone RR, Schwartz RJ, Steelman SR, Jacobs LM (1991) Evaluation of liver function tests in screening for intra-abdominal injuries. Ann Emerg Med 20:838–841
Sandblom P (1987) Hemobilia. In: Way LW, Pellegrin CA (eds) Surgery for the gallbladder and bile ducts. Saunders, Philadelphia, pp 643–654
Sandblom P, Saegesser F, Mirkovitch V (1984) Hepatic hemobilia: hemorrhage from the intrahepatic biliary tract, a review. World J Surg 8:41–50
Sartorelli KH, Frumiento C, Rogers FB, Osler TM (2000) Nonoperative management of hepatic, splenic, and renal injuries in adults with multiple injuries. J Trauma 49:56–61
Savader SJ, Trerotola SO, Merine DS, Venbrux AC, Osterman FA (1992) Hemobilia after percutaneous transhepatic biliary drainage: treatment with transcatheter embolotherapy. J Vasc Intervent Radiol 3:345–352
Sawhney R, Wall SD, Yee J, Haynard I (1997) Hepatic infarction: unusual complication of a transjugular intrahepatic portosystemic shunt. J Vasc Interv Radiol 8:129–132
Sax SL, Athey PA, Lamki N (1988) Sonographic findings in traumatic hemobilia: report of two cases and review of the literature. J Clin Ultrasound 16:29–34
Sayers RD, Bewes PC, Porter KM (1992) Emergency laparotomy for abdominal trauma. Injury 23:537–541
Schnarkowski P, Klüppelberg U, Lienemann A, Reiser MF (1996) Rupture of a liver cell carcinoma after chemoembolization. Fortschr Röntgenstr 164:341–343
Schöpf F, Fretz CH, Haertel M (1982) Computed tomography for injuries of the liver and spleen. Fortschr Rontgenstr 136:681–684
Schorn L, Coln D (1977) Hepatic arteriographic changes after trauma. Am J Surg 134:754–757
Schwartz SI (1989) Surgery of the liver. Historical background. In: McDermott Jr (ed) Surgery of the liver. Blackwell Scientific, Boston, pp 3–12
Schwartz SI (1998) The James Ewing Lecture: one life, many livers. Am Surg Oncol 5:573–579
Schwartz RA, Teitelbaum GP, Katz MD, Pentecost MJ (1993) Effectiveness of transcatheter embolization in the control of hepatic vascular injuries. J Vasc Interv Radiol 4:359–365
Schweizer W, Becker C, Tanner S, Schaeppi B, Huber A, Blumgart LH (1993) The significance of computed tomography for conservative treatment of liver trauma. Helv Chir Acta 59:717–724
Sclafani SJ, Gordon DH, Mitchell W (1983) Laceration of the inferior vena cava of angiographic demonstration. Cardiovasc Intervent Radiol 6:164–166
Sclafani SJ, Cooper R, Shaftlan GW, Goldstein AS, Glanz S, Gordon DH (1986) Arterial trauma: diagnostic and therapeutic angiography. Radiology 161:165–172
Scott CM, Grasberger RC, Heeran TF, Williams LF, Hirsch EF (1988) Intra-abdominal sepsis after hepatic trauma. Am J Surg 155:284–288
Sears RJ, Ishitani MB, Bickston SJ (1997) Endoscopic diagnosis and therapy of a case of bilhemia after percutaneous liver biopsy. Gastrointest Endosc 46:276–279
Semba CP, Saperstein L, Nyman U, Dake MD (1996) Hepatic laceration from wedged venography performed before transjugular intrahepatic portosystemic shunt placement. J Vasc Interv Radiol 7:143–146
Shah PA, Kulkarni SS, Joshi N, Lakshmy MV, Dewoolkar VV (1993) Hepatic trauma: experience of 110 cases. Injury 24: 303–305
Shahrudin MD, Noori SM (1997) Biloma and biliary fistula associate with hepatorraphy for liver injury. Hepatogastroenterology 44:519–521
Shanmuganathan K, Mirvis SE (1995) CT evaluation of the liver with acute blunt trauma. Crit Rev Diagn Imaging 36: 73–113
Shanmuganathan K, Mirvis SE, Amoroso M (1993) Periportal low density on CT in patients with blunt trauma: association with elevated venous pressure. AJR 160:279–283

Sharp KW, Locicero RJ (1992) Abdominal packing for surgically uncontrollable hemorrhage. Ann Surg 215:467–475
Sheafor DH, Foti TM, Vaslef S, Nelson RC (1998) Fat in the inferior vena cava associated with caval injury. AJR 171:181–182
Sheldon GF, Lim RC, Yee ES et al (1985) Management of injuries to the porta hepatis. Ann Surg 202:539–545
Sherlock DJ, Bismuth H (1991) Secondary surgery for liver trauma. Br J Surg 78:1313–1317
Sherman HF (1996) Letter to the editor. J Trauma 40:171
Sherman HF, Savage BA, Jones LM et al (1994) Nonoperative management of blunt hepatic injuries: safe at any grade? J Trauma 37:616–621
Shreve WS (1999) Nursing assessment in adult trauma patients with nonoperative management of spleen and liver lacerations. J Trauma Nurs 6:37–41
Shuman WP (1997) CT of blunt abdominal trauma in adults. Radiology 205:297–306
Sidhu MK, Shaw DWW, Daly CP, Waldhausen JH, Coldwell D (1999) Post-traumatic hepatic pseudoaneurysm in children. Pediatr Radiol 29:46–52
Sim PH, Razack AH, Jalleh RP (1995) A preliminary study of possible prognostic factors of traumatic liver injury seen at University Hospital 1984–1991. Med J Malaysia 50:346–352
Soliman T, Langer F, Puhalla H et al (2000) Parenchymal liver injury in orthotopic liver transplantation. Transplantation 9:2079–2084
Sommer DG, Greenway GD, Bookstein JJ, Orloff MJ (1979) Hepatic rupture with toxemia of pregnancy: angiographic diagnosis. AJR 132:455–456
Spitz DJ (1999) Unrecognized fatal liver injury caused by a bicycle handlebar. Am J Emerg Med 17:244
Stalker HP, Kaufman RA, Towbin R (1986) Patterns of liver injury in childhood: CT analysis. AJR 147:1199–1205
Steinberg ML, Birnbaum BA, Jacobs JE, Schwab CW (1996) Shoulder harness seatbelt injury: CT appearance of hepatic avulsion with active arterial hemorrhage. J Comput Assist Tomogr 20:938–939
Steiner Z, Brown RA, Jamieson DH, Millar AJ, Cywes S (1994) Management of hemobilia and persistent biliary fistula after blunt liver trauma. J Pediatr Surg 29:1575–1577
Stone HH, Strom PR, Mullins RJ (1983) Management of the major coagulopathy with reset during laparotomy. Ann Surg 197:532–535
Strong RW (1999) The management of blunt liver injuries. Aust N Z J Surg 69:609–616
Struyven J, Cremer M, Pirson P, Jeanty P, Jeanmart J (1982) Posttraumatic bilhemia: diagnosis and catheter therapy. AJR 138:746–747
Sugimoto T, Yoshioko T, Sawada Y, Sugimoto H, Maemura K (1982) Posttraumatic cyst of the liver found on CT – a new concept. J Trauma 22:797–800
Sugimoto K, Horiike S, Hirata M, Ohwada T, Maekawa K (1994) The role of angiography in the assessment of blunt liver injury. Injury 25:283–287
Sujka SK, Jewett TC Jr, Karp MP (1988) Acute scrotal swelling as the first evidence of intraabdominal trauma in a battered child. J Pediatr Surg 23:380
Sziklas JJ, Spencer RP (1975) Hepatic artery-portal vein fistula detected on hepatic flow study: case report. J Nucl Med 16: 910–911
Taga S, Ezaki T, Yano K et al (1997) Hepatic venous injury: a case report of atriocaval shunt by a centrifuged pump. Hepatogastroenterology 44:1219–1221
Takakuwa T, Yokota J, Sugimoto T (1993) Liver infarction produced by dual vessels occlusion due to trauma and TAE: long follow-up using CT, US and MRI. Med J Osaka Univ 41/42:23–27
Takatsu A, Shigeta A, Abe M, Kitune K, Kawai T (1988) Embolism of massive hepatic tissue in inferior vena cava and right atrium after closed liver injury. Am J Forensic Med Pathol 9:233–235
Talbert J, Gruenberg JC, Sy G, Brown RS (1980) Peritoneal lavage in penetrating thoracic trauma. J Trauma 20:979–981
Tanaka H, Iwai A, Sugimoto H, Yoshioka T, Sugimoto T (1991) Intrahepatic arterioportal fistula after blunt hepatic trauma: case reports. J Trauma 31:143–146
Terk MR, Rozenberg D (1998) Gadolinium-enhanced MR imaging of traumatic hepatic injury. AJR 171:665–669
Terrier F, Auvray M (1986) Les traumatismes du foie et des voies biliaires. Rev Chir 16:717–721
Tilton BT (1905) Some considerations regarding wounds of the liver. Ann Surg 41:20
Thomford NR, Papouras WC, Durzinsky DS (1998) Active venovenous bypass of the retrohepatic vena cava utilizing two atrial cannullae. Am Surg 64:791–794
Tobben P, Zajko A, Sumkin J et al (1988) Pseudoaneurysms complicating organ transplantation: roles of CT, duplex sonography, and angiography. Radiology 169:65–70
Tomczak R, Helmberger T, Gorich J et al (1997) Abdominal arteriovenous and arterioportal fistulas: etiology, diagnosis, therapeutic possibilities. Z Gastroenterol 35:555–562
Toombs BD, Sandler CM, Rauschkolb EN, Strax R, Harle TS (1982) Assessment of hepatic injuries with computed tomography. J Comput Assist Tomogr 6:72–75
Townsend MC, Flancbaum L, Choban PS, Cloutier CT (1993) Diagnostic laparoscopy as an adjunct to selective conservative management of solid organ injuries after blunt abdominal trauma. J Trauma 35:647–651
Trauma Committee (1989) C.A.P.S. Canadian Association of Pediatric Surgeons: liver trauma study. J Pediatr Surg 24: 1035–1040
Trunkey DD, Shires GT, McClelland R (1974) Management of liver trauma in 811 consecutive patients. Ann Surg 179: 722–726
Tsutani H, Inai K, Kishi S, Morinaga K, Naiki H, Ueda T (1999) Hepatic tumor rupture following effectual treatment with irinotecan in a patient with highly refractory malignant lymphoma. Int J Hematol 70:178–180
Turpin I, State D, Schwartz A (1977) Injuries to the inferior vena cava and their management. Am J Surg 134:25–32
Vade A, Demos TC, Salvino C, Korach JL (1994) Periportal tracking in pediatric blunt abdominal trauma. Correlation with liver enzymes and liver injury. Clin Imaging 18:189–194
Vadon G, Karacsony S, Englоner L (1984) Transcatheter embolization for the control of posttraumatic hemobilia. Eur J Radiol 4:190–192
Van Sonnenberg E, Simeone JF, Mueller PR, Wittenberg J, Hall DA, Ferrucci JT (1983) Sonographic appearance of hematoma in the liver, spleen, and kidney: a clinical, pathologic and animal study. Radiology 147:507–510
Vaughan R, Rosch J, Keller FS, Antonovic R (1984) Treatment of hemobilia by transcatheter vascular occlusion. Eur J Radiol 4:183–189
Verhille MS, Munoz SJ (1991) Acute biliary-vascular fistula following needle aspiration of the liver. Gastroenterology 101:1731–1733

Vlahos L, Kalovidouris A, Gouliamos A, Kailidou E (1991) Posttraumatic hemobilia. Eur J Radiol 13:199–202

Vock R (1992) Liver and splenic ruptures as a complication of heart pressure massage. Beitr Gerichtl Med 50:193–203

Voitk AJ, Munkittrick RC (1986) A fatal pulmonary embolus composed of gross liver tissue. Can J Surg 29:218–219

Wagner WH, Lundell CJ, Donovan AJ (1985) Percutaneous angiographic embolization for hepatic arterial hemorrhage. Arch Surg 120:1241–1249

Wallace KL, Slovis CM (1987) Hepatic vein bullet embolus as a complication of left ventricular gunshot injury. Ann Emerg Med 16:102–104

Walt AJ (1978) The mythology of hepatic trauma – or Babel revisited. Am J Surg 135:12–18

Walt AJ (1980) Hepatic injuries. A 1980 overview. S Afr Med J 57:658–661

Walt AJ (1986) Liver injuries. In: Bengmark S, Blumgart LH (eds) Liver surgery. Churchill Livingstone, London, p 130

Walz MV, Walz MK (1992) Pulmonary embolism caused by liver tissue. Aktuel Traumatol 22:102–103

Watanabe S, Ishi T, Kamachi M, Takahashi T (1990) Computed tomography and non-operative treatment for blunt abdominal trauma. Jpn J Surg 20:56–63

Westreich M (1990) Liver disease in the Talmud. J Clin Gastroenterol 12:57–62

Whitten C, Grimes C, Isler R, Curch M, Diggins A (1990) CT of actively haemorrhaging liver laceration in a 9-year-old child. Pediatr Radiol 25:1162–1165

Wiencek RG Jr, Wilson RF (1988) Inferior vena cava injuries: the challenge continues. Am Surg 54:423–428

Wilson RH, Moorehead RJ (1991) Hepatic trauma and its management. Injury 22:439–445

Witte CL, Zukoski CF (1983) A rational approach to serious blunt hepatic injury. Am Surg 49:446–453

Wolf S, Berger H, Jauch KW (1998) Arterioportal fistula with portal hypertension after liver trauma and resection: case report and review of the literature. Hepatogastroenterology 45:821–826

Wolfman NT, Bechthold RE, Scharling ES, Meredith JH (1992) Blunt upper abdominal trauma: evaluation by CT. AJR 158: 493–501

Wu WC, Katon RM (1993) Injury to the liver and spleen after diagnostic ERCP. Gastrointest Endosc 39:824–827

Yamamoto F, Pu Y (1992) MR imaging of hepatic laceration. AJR 158:1170

Yamamoto F, Pu Y, Mori A, Shilpakar SK, Rikitake K, Yamamoto H (1994) A case report of MR imaging of traumatic hemobilia. J Gastroenterol 29:511–513

Yassa NA, Peters JH (1996) CT of focal injury due to surgical retractor. AJR 166:599–602

Yates TE, Riddick L, Carter RD, Izenberg S (1996) Portal vein embolization following shotgun-pellet injuries to the abdomen. Am J Forensic Med Pathol 17:151–154

Yitzhak A, Shaked G, Lupu L, Mizrahi S, Kluger Y (2001) Selective embolization of hepatic arteries an additional precaution to control hemorrhage in the management of severe liver trauma. Harefuah 140:193–196

Yokota J, Mizobata Y, Mitani K, Matsuoka T, Sugimoto T (1993) The surgical management of blunt liver trauma. Nippon Geka Gakkai Zasshi 94:604–610

Yokota J, Sugimoto T (1994) Clinical significance of periportal tracking on computed tomographic scan in patients with blunt liver trauma. Am J Surg 168:247–250

Yoshida J, Donajue PE, Nyhus LM (1987) Hemobilia: review of recent experience with a worldwide problem. Am J Gastroenterol 82:448–453

Zajko A, Tobben P, Esquivel C et al (1989) Pseudoaneurysm following orthotopic liver transplantation: clinical and radiologic manifestations. Transplant Proc 21:2457–2459

Zbar RIS (1993) Liver laceration after cardiopulmonary resuscitation: a case report. Heart Lung 22:463–465

Zironi G, Piscaglia F, Gaiana S, Masi L, Bolondi L (1999) Intrahepatic artery pseudoaneurysm: a possible complication of blind thoracocentesis. J Clin Ultrasound 27:151–155

Zuckerman GB, Lucas MJ, Holmes NJ, Underberg-Davis SJ (1998) Hepatic and oral trauma in an infant related to improper use of an infant car seat. J Trauma 45:838–840

6 Injuries of the Bile Ducts

R. F. Dondelinger, O. Cornet, J. H. Boverie

CONTENTS

- Intraluminal clot, a thickened gallbladder wall or other wall anomalies and pericholecystic fluid are the most frequent findings of blunt gallbladder injury on CT.
- Indirect signs of extrahepatic bile duct injury are hematoma in the porta hepatis, hemoperitoneum and liver contusion in adjacent segments (segment IV).
- Cholescintigraphy and endoscopic cholangiography should be used liberally in posttraumatic patients with suspicion of a bile duct fistula in the early posttraumatic phase or a delayed stenosis.

6.1 History

Posttraumatic rupture of the gallbladder was first documented on a pathological specimen at the end of the fourteenth century (Griswold and Collier 1961; Alawneh 1981). The first description of a clinical case of blunt injury to the gallbladder was given in 1691 (Lewerenz 1903). At least five more cases of injury to the extrahepatic bile ducts were described in the eighteenth century and about 19 additional cases were reported in the nineteenth century; all patients had died from the injury (Wainwright 1799; Drysdale 1861; Uhde 1880; Kernes 1892; Kehr 1892; Battle 1894; Whipple 1898; Porter 1898; Spencer 1898; Garrett 1900; Lewerenz 1903; Alawneh

R. F. Dondelinger, MD
Professor and Chairman, Department of Medical Imaging, University Hospital Sart Tilman, Domaine Universitaire du Sart Tilman B35, 4000 Liège, Belgium
O. Cornet, MD
Resident, Department of Medical Imaging, University Hospital Sart Tilman, Domaine du Sart Tilman B35, 4000 Liège, Belgium
J. H. Boverie, MD
Chef de Clinique, Department of Medical Imaging, University Hospital Sart Tilman, Domaine du Sart Tilman B35, 4000 Liège, Belgium

1981; Delany and Jason 1981). Fizeau gave the first detailed description of posttraumatic rupture of the choledochus responsible for bile ascites (Fizeau 1806). Quincke described in 1871 the classic triad of hemobilia, and Dixon is credited with the first cholecystectomy performed for posttraumatic gallbladder rupture (Dixon 1887). Kehr operated on the first patient with penetrating injury to the gallbladder, performing a cholecystostomy (Kehr 1892). Battle gave the initial description of complete transection of the common bile duct by blunt injury in a child in 1894 (Battle 1894). In a review of the literature, Zollinger reported 74 patients with extrahepatic bile duct injuries collected since 1890 (Zollinger et al. 1972). About 500 cases of injuries to the extrahepatic bile ducts were published until 1981 in the world literature; 300 of these were reported after the end of World War II (Alawneh 1981). At the same time, 101 cases of gallbladder injuries secondary to blunt trauma were collected in the English literature (Soderstrom et al. 1981).

This chapter is focused on noniatrogenic injuries of the bile ducts. Injury following open or celioscopic cholecystectomy or instrumental endoluminal intervention in the ductal system will only be mentioned.

6.2 Incidence

Noniatrogenic injury of the bile ducts is rare compared to injury to the liver, spleen or pancreas. Incidence of extrahepatic bile ducts injury varies from 1%–5%, as confirmed during laparotomy indicated for trauma. Young male adults with a median age of 25–30 years are predominantly affected, due to the predominance of penetrating injury. Indeed, the vast majority of reported injuries to the extrahepatic bile ducts result from penetrating trauma, accounting for 75%–90%. Blunt trauma is consequently uncommon, about 300 cases being reported at present, and roughly one-third in the pediatric age group, where blunt trauma predominates (Hall et al. 1956; Hopson et al. 1966; Tonnesen 1970; Zollinger et al. 1972; Busuttil et al. 1980; Spigos et al. 1981; Soderstrom et al. 1981; Kitahama et al. 1982; Khodadadi et al. 1983; Posner and Moore 1985; Michelassi and Ranson 1985; Ivatury et al. 1985; Sheldon et al. 1985; Bourque et al. 1989; Bade et al. 1989; McNabney et al. 1990; Feliciano 1994; Bar-Maor and Shoshany 1994; Sharma 1995; Letoublon and Castaing 1966).

The gallbladder is involved in 2%–8% of all abdominal injuries and the common bile duct in 0.5%. The gallbladder is involved in 70%–85% of all extrahepatic bile duct injuries, and the common bile duct in 15%–30% (Penn 1962; Diethrich et al. 1966; Haynes et al. 1969; Estrada and Sutherland 1969; Soderstrom et al. 1981; Hockerstedt et al. 1982; Cox 1984; Scaglione et al. 1998; Shanmuganathan and Mirvis 1998). In a recent multicenter review, 35 patients with blunt injury to the extrahepatic bile ducts were recorded in a cumulated 60-year experience, accounting for less than 0.03% of admissions (Jurkovich et al. 1995).

Injury to the bile ducts occurs most commonly in association with other abdominal injuries. Isolated gallbladder injury occurs only in 3% of all bile duct injuries, but minimal intraluminal bleeding in the gallbladder is probably more frequent than assumed in the past (Wright 1976; Soderstrom et al. 1981; Soyer et al. 1981; Thibodeau and Illescas 1988). Isolated injury to the extrahepatic bile ducts is even more rare; approximately 40 cases have been reported in the literature (Kitahama et al. 1982; Ivatury et al. 1985; Kernohan and Humphreys 1985; Michelassi and Ranson 1985; Bade et al. 1989; Monk et al. 1991; Eid et al. 1996; Krishna et al. 1992; Sharma et al. 1997; Simstein 2000). In children, less than 20 cases of isolated and complete transection of the common bile duct were reported following blunt trauma, in the English-language literature (Fletcher et al. 1961; Shorthouse et al. 1978; Janss and Freimark 1979; Carmichael 1980; Bourque et al. 1989; Dawson and Jurkovich 1991; Chung et al. 1993; Miyakawa et al. 1996; Krishnamurthy et al. 1997; Arkovitz et al. 1999). Blunt injury to both hepatic ducts, either at the confluence or in their intrahepatic portion was reported in less than 30 patients (Zollinger et al. 1972; Charters and Bardin 1978; Philippe et al. 1982; Michelassi and Ranson 1985; Bade et al. 1989; Muin et al. 1992; Krishna et al. 1992; Bin Yahib et al. 1999). Blunt rupture of the common bile duct in its intrapancreatic course is extremely rare (Chow et al. 1996; Soffer et al. 1996; Depolo et al. 1999). Combined posttraumatic transection of the common bile duct, duodenum, pancreatic duct, or papilla of Vater has been reported in a few publications (Fish and Johnson 1965; Parkinson and Wisniewski 1978; Kawarada et al. 1984; Ito et al. 1993; McLindon et al. 1998). Twelve cases of combined rupture of the common duct and ampulla of Vater due to blunt injury were collected in 1973 (Balsano and Reynolds 1973).

6.3 Classification

6.3.1 Gallbladder Injuries

Blunt trauma to the gallbladder can be classified in mural contusion, which is the most benign form of injury, perforation, partial or complete avulsion and intraluminal hemorrhage (SMITH and HASTINGS 1954; SODERSTROM et al. 1981; POSNER and MOORE 1985; THIBODEAU and ILLESCAS 1988). The Organ Injury Scaling (OIS) Committee of the American Association for the Surgery of Trauma (AAST) has formulated a combined injury scale for gallbladder and bile duct trauma (MOORE et al. 1995) (see also Chap. 27, "A Selection of Published Surgical and Radiological Classifications of Abdominal Injuries"). Gallbladder wall rupture or perforation is more frequent than avulsion, which refers to partial or complete detachment of the gallbladder from the cystic duct, the cystic artery, and the liver surface, and was termed posttraumatic cholecystectomy (BROWN 1932; BOSWORTH 1948; KAEHR et al. 1984; XEROPOTAMOS et al. 1992). A completely avulsed gallbladder can subsequently be dislodged to remote anatomical compartments, such as the pelvis (ALI 1975). Posttraumatic acute cholecystitis is a particular condition, in which no significant injury of the gallbladder wall is detected. Cholecystitis is explained by blockage of the cystic duct by blood clots, irritating the gallbladder mucosa, but acute acalculous cholecystitis can be confusing, as it may also arise early in the posttraumatic period in the absence of intraluminal hemorrhage. Acute inflammation can evolve into gangrenous cholecystitis after traumatic hemobilia (IRENEUS 1942; SANDBLOM 1948; EPSTEIN and LIPSHUTZ 1952; HOFFMAN 1956; PENN 1962; SOLHEIM 1972; DELAITRE et al. 1976; DUPRIEST et al. 1979; SODERSTROM et al. 1981; SPIGOS et al. 1981; KAEHR et al. 1984; KRAMER et al. 1985; OLDHAM et al. 1986; DE LUNA et al. 1996).

6.3.2 Ductal Injuries

Injuries to the common bile duct are classified in partial or tangential tear and complete ductal transection. There is no radiological classification of noniatrogenic bile duct injury available. Trerotola divided complications from iatrogenic injury into minor and major. Minor complications included bile leakage and biloma, responding to percutaneous management or simple surgical repair. The term "biloma" was coined to describe an encapsulated bile collection of traumatic origin (GOULD and PATEL 1979). Major complications included common hepatic duct injuries or strictures, requiring surgical repair (TREROTOLA et al. 1992). In practice, classifications used in iatrogenic bile duct injury can also be applied to noniatrogenic injury (STRASBERG et al. 1995). The Bismuth classification, which is basically used in tumor obstruction at the liver hilum, is accurate for localization of postoperative bile duct stenoses demonstrated on cholangiography (BISMUTH 1982; BLUMGART et al. 1984; CHARTRAND-LEFÈBVRE et al. 1994). This classification is particularly valuable when percutaneous transhepatic cholangiography is used.

6.4 Mechanism

Several mechanisms of blunt trauma to the bile ducts may be hypothesized and are discussed below (LEWIS 1938; FLETCHER et al. 1961; FISH and JOHNSON 1965; ZOLLINGER et al. 1972; KITAHAMA et al. 1982; GATELY and THOMAS 1985). Frequently found causes of blunt injury are traffic accidents (65%), followed by occupational and sports injuries (10%), falls (7%), blows during physical fighting (8%) and unknown causes (10%) (MICHELASSI and RANSON 1985).

6.4.1 Gallbladder

The gallbladder is only relatively protected by the liver from a direct abdominal impact. Many predisposing factors for gallbladder injury can be listed: its superficial abdominal location, increased mobility of the gallbladder attached by a long meso, the thin normal gallbladder wall, and congenital abnormalities such as an adjacent, mobile accessory lobe of the liver that may undergo torsion, implicating torsion of the meso of the gallbladder (KOPLEWITZ et al. 1999). A midline position of the gallbladder may facilitate injury by compression against the spine. A distended gallbladder after fasting is at increased risk and alcohol ingestion further contributes to the increase in pressure in the ductal lumen, due to increased tone of the sphincter of Oddi and stimulation of secretion and gastrin secretin, which accelerate production and flow of bile (SMITH and SODERBERG 1964;

Pirola and Davis 1968). Preexisting obstruction of the common bile duct or cystic duct by cholelithiasis may also lead to gallbladder rupture during minimal or (pseudo)spontaneous rupture due to elevated pressure (Wiener et al. 1982; McLindon et al. 1998). Conversely, a chronic cholecystitis, by its thick wall, is better protected from rupture than a normal or an acutely inflamed gallbladder (Foley et al. 1987).

The wall of the gallbladder is commonly ruptured at the fundus and in some cases, the gallbladder is completely disrupted from the main bile duct, at the junction of the cystic duct with the common bile duct. Avulsion of the gallbladder is usually secondary to a high-speed impact during blunt trauma and can be associated with massive hemorrhage from the cystic artery. Posttraumatic torsion of the gallbladder or cystic duct is another rare mechanism of trauma and may lead to ischemic gallbladder wall necrosis, which is complicated by rupture several days or weeks following trauma (Coulter 1948; Fielding and Strachan 1975; Salman et al. 1996). Minor trauma is frequently seen on CT and is responsible for gallbladder wall contusion, intraluminal hematoma, or hematocele or pericholecystic fluid (Saad et al. 1979). A distended gallbladder may rupture together with the distended urinary bladder, resulting in urobilohemoperitoneum (Blumgart 1969). A limited tear in the gallbladder wall may be responsible for a slow increase of bile extravasation, accumulating first in the gallbladder fossa, before extending to other peritoneal compartments (Coulter 1948; Brickley et al. 1960; Fielding and Strachan 1975).

In iatrogenic injury, the gallbladder can be perforated during percutaneous liver biopsy, transhepatic or subhepatic catheter drainage procedures, percutaneous transhepatic cholangiography (PTC) and endoscopic retrograde cholangiography (ERCP), percutaneous transhepatic portal vein catheterization, transjugular intrahepatic portosystemic shunt (TIPS), hepatic tumor ablation, and other upper abdominal procedures, including complete gallbladder wall disruption during percutaneous gallbladder drainage or other instrumental procedures carried out in the gallbladder (Smadja et al. 1993; Dennison et al. 1990). A traumatic perforation of the gallbladder or of the adjacent liver may be responsible for hemobilia, caused by gallbladder wall or liver hemorrhage extending directly into the gallbladder lumen (Saad et al. 1979). Occult gallbladder perforation was described as a complication of extracorporeal shock wave gallstone lithotripsy (Janowitz et al. 1992). Transcatheter arterial hepatic embolization or chemoembolization may result in toxic and ischemic gallbladder wall necrosis and subsequent perforation (Sata et al. 1986).

6.4.2
Extrahepatic Bile Ducts

6.4.2.1
Common

The extrahepatic common bile duct is better protected than the gallbladder by its small caliber, deep abdominal location, the thoracic rib cage, the liver, epiploon, and intestine, and therefore is less frequently involved during blunt abdominal trauma. Iatrogenic cause, during elective cholecystectomy, is mainly responsible for tangential injury to the bile duct, and rarely of complete transection (Neeman et al. 1988). Most injuries of the choledochal wall created by guidewire perforation, catheters, or other small-caliber devices are without consequence, provided a drainage catheter is left in place in the bile ducts. Extracorporeal shock wave lithotripsy of gallbladder or kidney stones may create common bile duct injury (Hung et al. 2000).

During noniatrogenic penetrating trauma, the common bile duct may be transected or ruptured at any level (Burt and Nelson 1981). However, during blunt injury, maximum shear stress force leading to disruption is exerted at the fixed superior limit of the pancreas, which is the most frequently involved (40%), and is most commonly consecutive to high-speed deceleration or squeezing the liver against the ribs and displacement in a cranial direction (Fish and Johnson 1965; Shorthouse et al. 1978). The next most frequent location of extrahepatic bile duct injury is the bifurcation of the common bile duct (30%) and the origin of the left hepatic duct. The left hepatic duct is more sensitive to laceration, due to its frequently longer extracapsular course than the right duct (Vanneuville et al. 1977; Busuttil et al. 1980; Michelassi and Ranson 1985; Parks and Diamond 1995; Bin Yahib et al. 1999). A sudden displacement of the liver in a cranial direction is likely to produce a rupture at the hilar bifurcation (Elmslie and White 1966). Rupture of the retropancreatic segment occurs in less than 10% of cases and rupture at the site of the cystic duct occurs in 5%–20% (Kitahama et al. 1982; Posner and Moore 1985; Soderstrom et al. 1981; Busuttil et al. 1980; Bourque et al. 1989; Rydell 1970; Michelassi and Ranson 1985; Bade et al. 1989; Dawson et al. 1991; Parks and Diamond 1995).

A livery injury extending into the porta hepatis is very much prone to injury of the extrahepatic bile ducts (Moulton et al. 1993). The choledochus may also rupture, when compressed against the upper lumbar spine during a crush–compression injury (Lewis 1938; Lee and Wherry 1961). It was anticipated that disruption of the small blood vessels of the peribiliary plexus may be responsible for biliary duct ischemia leading to delayed necrosis, even when no complete transection was initially present. However, ischemic necrosis after trauma is not likely to occur when normal anatomy is preserved, due to the rich peribiliary ductal network and the collateral arterial plexus present at the liver hilum (Gately and Thomas 1985; Vellar 1999).

Probably there is no unique, unequivocal mechanism to explain blunt rupture of the extrahepatic bile ducts. A compression–crush injury of the upper abdomen, implicating a crush of the common bile duct over the spine, a sudden increase in ductal pressure, due to gallbladder compression with concomitant "duct blow-out," shear forces displacing the two upper thirds of the choledochus away from the intrapancreatic segment are some of the potential mechanisms of injury which may act together (Mason et al. 1954; Fletcher et al. 1961; Fish and Johnson 1965; Maier et al. 1968; Rydell 1970). A short cystic duct and a distended gallbladder may not only favor gallbladder rupture, but also the blow-out mechanism of the choledochus, by rapid increase in ductal pressure during sudden gallbladder compression. Complete laceration of the bile duct is more likely to occur distally than at the level of the cystic duct (Michelassi and Ranson 1985). Associated tears of the hepatic artery, the gastroduodenal artery, or the portal vein are rare. These structures can escape compression or elongation forces, as they are more elastic and less fixed than the bile duct in the porta hepatis (Mason et al. 1954; Fletcher et al. 1961; Rydell 1970; Leber and Hume 1971; Carabalona et al. 1973; Forster et al. 1977; Shorthouse et al. 1978; Kitahama et al. 1982; Theunis et al. 1989; Bunt et al. 1990; Zbar 1993; Kruuna et al. 1994).

A biliary leak, when persistent through a traumatic tear, extends into the peritoneal cavity, or retroperitoneal space, or thorax. Most leaks originate from the common bile duct, but they may also extend from a small intrahepatic bile radicle. Bile leaks through the tear and generally fills the adjacent intraperitoneal compartments, or occasionally the retroperitoneal space, until pressure is equalized between the bile duct lumen and the biloma. Some bile collections may simulate a posttraumatic pancreatic pseudocyst (Bourque et al. 1989; Colovic and Perisic-Savic 1991).

Bile induces peritoneal irritation, possible sepsis and on rare occasions, evolves into a biliary cutaneous fistula (Brase et al. 1976; Goldin et al. 1990; Steiner et al. 1994). A bile fistula may also extend to the thorax, establishing a communication with the pleural cavity or the bronchi (Oparah and Mandal 1978; Straaten and Engel 1978; Franklin and Mathai 1980; Haddad et al. 1986; Rothberg et al. 1994). Even when complete transection of the common bile duct is present, bile duct dilatation above the site of rupture occurs neither immediately, nor constantly.

Bile extravasation, hemorrhage, and inflammation at the site of bile duct laceration may result in delayed bile duct stricture and obstruction (Skow and Longmire 1974; Busuttil et al. 1980). A posttraumatic stenosis may occur in the late posttraumatic phase, at the same site than the initial bile duct laceration, and in some cases as a consequence of hepatectomy for traumatic hepatic rupture (Kasai et al. 1993). Stenosis in the intrapancreatic portion of the common bile duct does not necessarily result from ductal transection, but can be secondary to posttraumatic pancreatitis, evolving into chronic inflammatory foci, which compress the distal bile duct (Yoon et al. 1998).

6.4.2.2
Uncommon

Seatbelts may be responsible of gallbladder injury, or transection of the common bile duct and the pelviureteral junction (Wright 1976; Spitz and Van Blerk 1971). Bicycle handlebar injury is a classic mechanism of pancreatic injury in children and a rare cause of extrahepatic bile duct injury (Rohatgi and Gupta 1987).

Other rare mechanisms of injury are briefly mentioned. Idiopathic spontaneous perforation in the newborn, probably related to birth trauma, has been reported (Marshall et al. 1984; Topuzlu et al. 1994). In adults, spontaneous perforation of the left hepatic duct and perforation after a session of bodybuilding exercise have been described (Muller et al. 1993; Wang et al. 1995). Chronic choledocholithiasis may ulcerate the common bile duct wall at the prepapillary level and facilitate perforation, which can occur spontaneously or after minor trauma (Huljic and Knaepler 1982). Any severe inflammatory reaction in the common bile duct wall may cause spontaneous nontraumatic perforation (Golematis et al. 1978). Other uncommon causes of bile duct perforation are surgical, endoscopic, or percutaneous intrabiliary or intraparenchymal hepatic instrumentation (SCHRIEFERS 1968). Percutaneous ethanol injection in hepatocarcinoma or in a cystic cavity can occasionally result in inadvertent leakage of alcohol in the bile duct wall and either result in ductal atrophy or in obstruction above an ethanol-induced bile duct stenosis (KODA et al. 1992). A choledochal cyst may rupture spontaneously, due to obstruction of the lumen by protein plugs, or rupture like the gallbladder, when involved in blunt injury, resulting in hemoperitoneum and bile peritonitis (BATTERSBY 1978; ANDO et al. 1995).

6.4.3
Intrahepatic Bile Ducts

Intrahepatic bile ducts can rupture concomitantly to a hepatic parenchymal laceration. Hepatic lacerations that are located or extend around the porta hepatis should be particularly suspected (SEWELL 1966; CHARTERS and BARDIN 1978; VERRAN and SCHROEDER 1988).

Rupture of the segmental or smaller intrahepatic bile ducts is not routinely searched for after trauma and minor injuries remain frequently undetected (MOSER et al. 1995; FROMENT et al. 1998). Rarely, an intrahepatic bile duct cyst may rupture after blunt abdominal trauma (SANDOR et al. 1991). Rupture of small intrahepatic bile ducts is responsible for a biloma or bilohematoma which accumulates inside the liver parenchyma, in a subcapsular location, or around the liver through a capsular rupture, but is only rarely responsible for massive or persistent choleperitoneum or bile peritonitis (LEHTO and VILKKI 1985; SOULIER and VALAYER 1987) (Fig. 6.1). Transcapsular fistulae can communicate with the peritoneal cavity, the kidney or the retroperitoneal space, the colon, the inferior vena cava, pleura, bronchi, or establish an intrahepatic-cutaneous fistula (SAFRANY et al. 1978; SAMHOURI et al. 1980; IVATURY et al. 1984; THORSEN et al. 1984; RYU et al. 1998; SHEIK-GAFOOR et al. 1998). Blunt hepatic injury carries a rate of biloma formation of 6%–8% (SUGIMOTO et al. 1993; HOWDIESHELL et al. 1995; DE BACKER et al. 1998).

Trauma to the intrahepatic bile ducts does not result only in innocuous biloma, but may be followed by a large number of other potentially significant complications: hemorrhage, abscess, bilhemia, bile embolization, hemobilia, bile duct necrosis, cholangitis and bile duct stricture. It has been suggested that mixing of extravasated bile into an intrahepatic

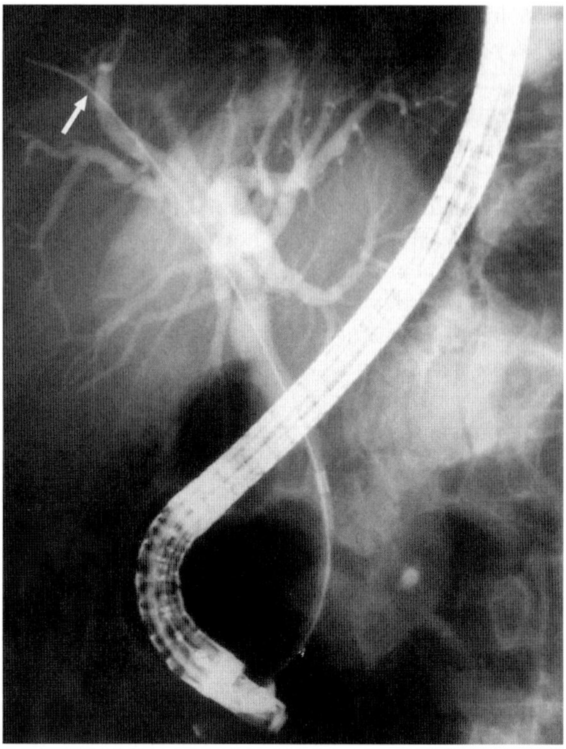

a

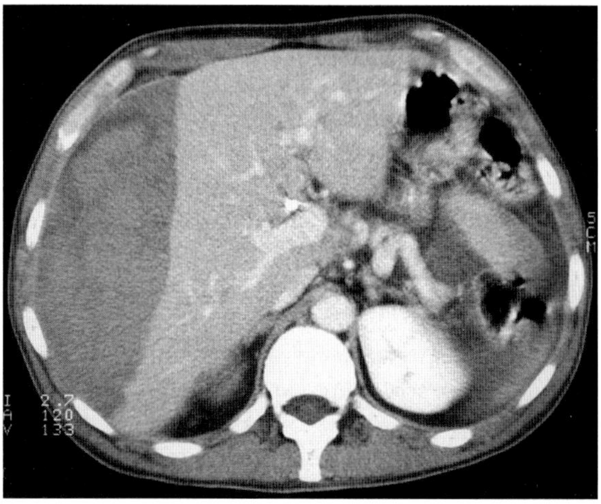

b

Fig. 6.1a, b. A 41-year-old male underwent endoscopic retrograde cholangiography, sphincterectomy, mechanical stone extraction and temporary plastic stent placement for treatment of choledocholithiasis causing obstructive jaundice. **a** During placement of a 10F plastic stent in the choledochus, the guidewire was pushed far into the intrahepatic bile ducts and perforated a segmental bile duct of the right lobe (*arrow*). **b** The next day, the patient complained of persistent abdominal pain in the right upper quadrant. CT obtained 2 days after ERCP showed a massive subcapsular bilohematoma with mixed densities in the right lobe of the liver, resulting from perforation with the guidewire. Conservative treatment was given hematoma produces hepatic tissue necrosis and favors the accumulation of bile, and subsequently irritation of the arterial wall and pseudoaneurysm formation, which is prone to hemobilia, requiring arterial embolization, which may also result in return in formation of a biloma (SUGIMOTO et al. 1993; HAGIWARA et al. 1997; CIRAULO et al. 1998) (Fig. 6.2). Pulmonary or systemic, intracerebral bile emboli can occur after percutaneous biliary drainage and also after penetrating or blunt injury with a bile-hepatic vein communication, and occasionally be lethal (BALOGH 1984; HABERLIK et al. 1992) (see also Chap. 19).

Iatrogenic causes of intrahepatic biliary-arteriovenous fistula or extrahepatic fistulizations mainly include hepatic surgery, percutaneous transhepatic cholangiography that is not followed by drainage, blind and forceful intrabiliary instrumentation, including the use of balloon-tipped Fogarty catheters, biliary spoon or forceps, Bakes dilators, percutaneous liver biopsy or biliary drainage, tumor embolization, percutaneous tumor ablation, forceful injection of contrast medium in the bile ducts during cholangiography, TIPS, portal vein catheterization, and others (KOCH and GORDER 1969; HENZEL et al. 1971; VAN WAY and SAWYERS 1973; GOLDMAN et al. 1976; FRAHM and FREESE 1980; RUBIO et al. 1986; SCHUSTER et al. 1990; VERHILL and MUNOZ 1991; PAYMANI et al. 1993).

6.4.4 Associated Injuries

Isolated traumatic injury to the extrahepatic bile ducts is rare. In most published series, which con-

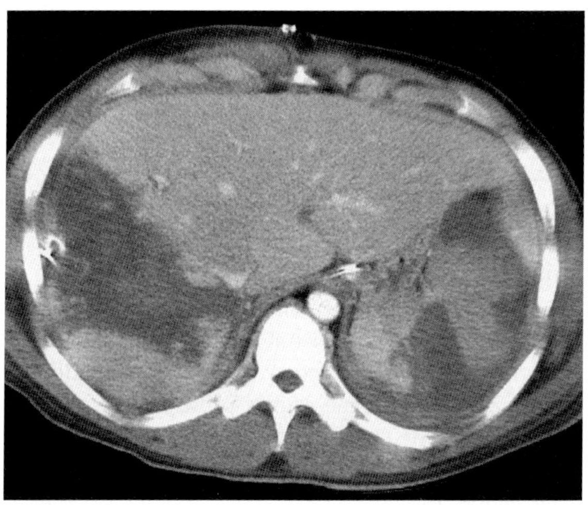
a

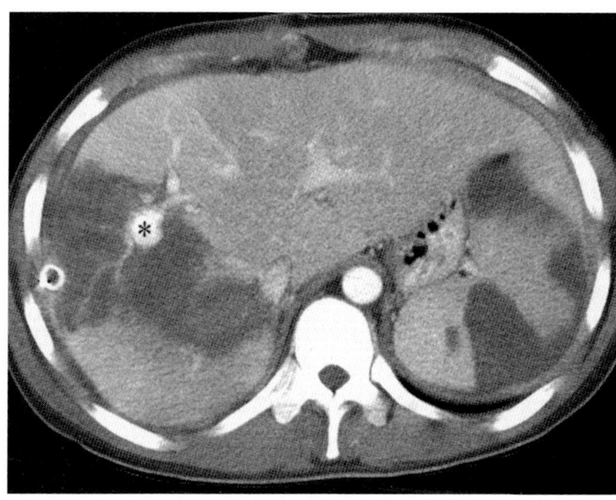
b

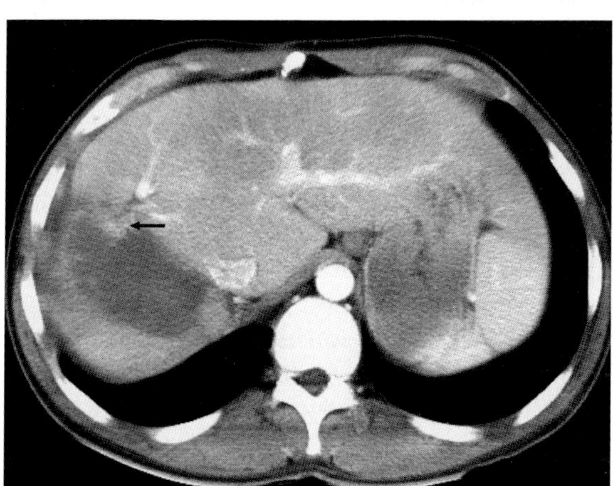
c

Fig. 6.2a–c. A 24-year-old alcoholic male was involved in a motorcycle accident. Imaging at admission to another hospital showed hemoperitoneum, splenic rupture and contusion of the liver and right kidney. The patient was transferred for arterial splenic embolization after transfusion of eight blood units. Three days later, the patient was operated on for abdominal revision, evacuation of a massive hemoperitoneum, and cholecystectomy was performed. No hepatic or splenic hemorrhage or bile fistula was seen intraoperatively. **a** CT obtained 5 days after surgery showed extensive areas of contusion in the right lobe of the liver. Notice also splenic infarcts resulting from hemostatic splenic embolization. Bile oozed through a surgical drain that was placed in contact with the liver with a daily output of 600 ml. **b** CT obtained 2 weeks later showed an arterial pseudoaneurysm in the right lobe of the liver (*asterisk*), 2 cm in diameter, located within the area of hepatic contusion. This pseudoaneurysm, which was not seen at admission, was probably caused by erosion of the arterial wall by the fistulized bile. No hemobilia occurred and no specific treatment was given. **c** On CT obtained 2 months later, the intrahepatic pseudoaneurysm had thrombosed spontaneously and only a slight blush (*arrow*) was seen. The external bile fistula through the surgical catheter had closed spontaneously tain a majority of penetrating injuries, 92%–100% of patients had other associated abdominal injuries, with a mean of 2–2.5 injuries per patient. Gallbladder injury is five times more often associated with other lesions than ductal injury (SODERSTROM et al. 1981; KITAHAMA et al. 1982; POSNER and MOORE 1985; IVATURY et al. 1985; BADE et al. 1989; ERB et al. 1994; PARKS and DIAMOND 1995; ZANTUT et al. 1995; SHANMUGANATHAN and MIRVIS 1995; SHARMA 1995). The liver is injured together with the bile ducts in about 80%–90% of cases: liver laceration, contusion or hematoma in the quadrate lobe are common observations (FLETCHER 1972). Other neighboring organs that can be implicated are small bowel and mesentery, duodeno-pancreas, colon, stomach, spleen, right kidney or ureter, right adrenal gland, right lower rib fractures, lung and pleura. Rare associations are injury to the heart, inferior vena cava, portal vein and diaphragm, and urinary bladder.

6.5 Clinical Symptoms and Findings

Little is published in the radiological literature on the diagnosis of noniatrogenic bile duct injury, as preoperative diagnosis is notoriously problematic with noninvasive cross-section imaging, and patients are often operated on without imaging for repair of other associated abdominal injuries. Prior to the systematic use of CT, none of the injuries of the gallbladder was diagnosed preoperatively (SODERSTROM et al. 1981). Clinical presentation can be subdivided into early, delayed, and late.

6.5.1 Presentation at Admission

At admission, patients may be divided into two categories (MICHELASSI and RANSON 1985); patients in the first group present with an acute abdomen and are in shock. Urgent laparotomy is performed and bile duct injury is primarily recognized and repaired or a life-saving operation is performed and the porta hepatis region is adequately drained and operative revision is rescheduled in survivors. In the second group of patients with apparently benign abdominal trauma, in whom surgery was not obtained, bile duct injury is not initially recognized until delayed or late clinical symptoms develop.

There are no specific acute clinical symptoms that are suggestive of injury to the bile ducts. In a series of 31 patients, the diagnosis of injury to the gallbladder was not suspected clinically in any patient before surgery (SODERSTROM et al. 1981). Symptoms and clinical signs may be discrete or absent at admission and develop only days or weeks after trauma, following a "period of illusion" or a "two-phase illness" (SCHECHTER 1969; FLETCHER 1972; SHORTHOUSE et al. 1978; HULJIC and KNAEPLER 1982). When rupture of the gallbladder has occurred with massive free flow of concentrated or infected bile in the peritoneal cavity, peritoneal irritation can be present already at admission, leading to immediate surgery, but this is far from being the rule. In many cases, extravasation of sterile bile is reabsorbed by the peritoneal serosa and gives only progressive and mild clinical signs of bile peritonitis. Fifty percent of patients with peritoneal bile effusion have no localizing abdominal symptoms (ELLIS and CRONIN 1960; FISH and JOHNSON 1965; BUSUTTIL et al. 1980; FELICIANO 1994). Similarly, even complete transection of the common bile duct may not necessarily induce bile peritonitis in the early posttraumatic phase.

When the patient is either in shock or shows signs of an acute abdomen at admission or when imaging demonstrates abdominal injuries that lead to immediate laparotomy, the diagnosis of injury to the bile ducts should be established intraoperatively, during meticulous revision of the porta hepatis. Avulsion of the cystic artery may lead to significant peritoneal hemorrhage and is promptly recognized intraoperatively (JEFFREY et al. 1986). Hematoma or blood oozing at the porta hepatis should always raise the suspicion of a bile duct injury (IVATURY et al. 1985; DAWSON et al. 1991). A bile leak is present at operation in 23% of the cases of bile duct injury, but in practice, significant bile duct injury may not be noticed during initial laparotomy done for repair of associated abdominal injuries in about 3%–20% of cases, and in up to 84% of cases, hepatic duct lesions may escape diagnosis with an average delay of 3 weeks (HAYNES et al. 1969; ZOLLINGER et al. 1972; KITAHAMA et al. 1982; JONES and THOMAS 1985; MICHELASSI and RANSON 1985; IVATURY et al. 1985; THOMSON and BADE 1989; BIN YAHIB et al. 1999).

Overall, clinical symptoms, laboratory tests and physical examination are poor predictors of a posttraumatic biliary leak, except when bilhemia is present in 1% of the cases (CROCE et al. 1995). Signs of bilhemia are jaundice that becomes profound in the early posttraumatic phase and a rapid increase of direct and total serum bilirubin up to extreme values

(61 mg/dl) and an increase in bile acids in the serum (BLUM et al. 1987; BLUM et al. 1993; VISNER et al. 1994; GLASER et al. 1994; GABLE et al. 1997). A biliovenous pressure gradient of 15–20 cm H_2O is necessary to maintain passage of bile into the venous circulation. Liver enzymes are only moderately elevated and patients have no pain, unless choledochal obstruction by clot has occurred.

Hemobilia is not discussed in detail here, as it was discussed with liver injury in Chap. 5.

6.5.2 Delayed Presentation

Delayed presentation is more common in ductal injury than in gallbladder rupture. In blunt trauma, frequently, only partial rupture of the extrahepatic bile ducts has occurred, which accounts for the fact that more than 50% of patients present with delayed symptoms days or weeks after the trauma, particularly when no emergency laparotomy was required at admission for treatment of associated injuries (MOYLE and KARL 1969; TONNESEN 1970; ZOLLINGER et al. 1972; ABOU-MOURAD and ROGERS 1980; MICHELASSI and RANSON 1985).

Bile leakage in conjunction with blunt hepatic injury occurs in 0.5%–21% (HOLLANDS and LITTLE 1991; SUGIMOTO et al. 1993; CROCE et al. 1995; PACHTER et al. 1996). Many leaks are transient and biliary fistulae persist in 4% of cases (MCGILLIVRAY and VALENTINE 1989; BYNOE et al. 1992). In about 0.6% of cases, a biliary fistula or biloma may also develop after liver resection or hepatorrhaphy for liver injury (MICHEL et al. 1992; SHAHRUDIN and NOORI 1997). In other patients, bile peritonitis progressively develops during the follow-up of expectant nonsurgical management of liver injury after a delay of several weeks (HARTMAN and GREANEY 1964; BARKER and FROMM 1987). In the literature, the diagnosis of a bile leak is established 4–13 days after the onset of symptoms and even after more than 1 month, when hepatorrhaphy was performed at admission. Patients in whom diagnosis is delayed for several weeks or 1 month have a higher mortality rate than patients with an early diagnosis (CARMICHAEL 1980). Therefore, rapid and aggressive imaging of the biliary system is mandatory when the suspicion of posttraumatic bile duct rupture is raised.

Most common delayed clinical symptoms of bile duct injury are nonlocalized abdominal pain, right shoulder pain (Kehr's sign), bile straining from a surgical drain, jaundice, acholic stool, abdominal distension or tenderness, fever and leukocytosis, or persistent ileus. However, jaundice is not a pathognomonic sign, as it may be caused by many other conditions after abdominal trauma: multiple blood transfusions, liver failure, hematoma, abscess, intrahepatic bile-vein fistula, iatrogenic surgical injury, cholecystitis, and general anesthesia. Other nonspecific symptoms of a bile fistula are loss of appetite, nausea, vomiting and anorexia, and loss of weight. In some patients, a painless progressive distension of the abdomen is seen, caused by massive biliary ascites or a giant biloma without other clinical signs of bile peritonitis (HAYNES et al. 1969; MCFADDEN et al. 1980; SPIGOS et al. 1981; ACKERMAN et al. 1985; PANDIT et al. 2000). Peritoneal tap confirms biliary ascites or biloma with great certainty (FLETCHER 1972; ACKERMAN et al. 1985; ROHATGI and GUPTA 1987). Finally, a biliobronchial fistula can be diagnosed on the observation of bilioptysis (HADDAD et al. 1986).

In rare circumstances, a hematoma of the porta hepatis, caused by portal vein laceration, can be responsible for biliary obstruction by external compression in the early posttraumatic phase (LAU and DIAMOND 1997). Some patients may develop hemobilia from a hematocele in the gallbladder lumen and cholecystitis, by the irritation from intraluminal blood (GLASER et al. 1994; HANAZAKI et al. 1995).

6.5.3 Late Presentation

In patients in whom nonoperative management of liver injury was adopted and who show a mild clinical course, the diagnosis of isolated injury to the bile ducts may be missed (FLETCHER et al. 1961; SHORTHOUSE et al. 1978; BUSUTTIL et al. 1980; SHERMAN et al. 1992; HALME et al. 1994). Some of these patients may develop obstructive jaundice several weeks or months after blunt abdominal trauma, caused by a posttraumatic bile duct stricture (HORIGUCHI et al. 1998). Clinical symptoms of posttraumatic bile duct stricture associate abdominal pain in the right upper quadrant, jaundice, and cholangitis (SKOW and LONGMIRE 1974; SHERMAN et al. 1992; YOON et al. 1998). Patients who were operated for a bile duct rupture or hepatic parenchymal rupture by hepatectomy may also develop a late postoperative bile duct stenosis (KASAI et al. 1993). A rate of 55% of strictures was noted for end-to-end repair, compared to a 16% stricture rate for biliary-enteric anastomosis (IVATURY et al. 1985). Anecdotally, biliary obstruction may result from an intraductal bullet or shrapnel migration after penetrating liver injury 2–64 years earlier or migration of a fragment of liver parenchyma into the common bile duct (Möller and Schroeder 1985; Lifshits et al. 1989; Mitchell et al. 1991; Rescorla et al. 1996). Late bile duct obstruction, caused by a posttraumatic pancreatic granuloma, has also been reported (Douglas and Luck 1974). Finally, cholelithiasis secondary to hemobilia has been documented in children (Farron et al. 1996). In severe liver injury, late bile duct stenosis can be revealed in the late phase together with other vascular lesions (pseudoaneurysm) (Halme et al. 1994).

6.6 Imaging

6.6.1 Nuclear Medicine

Nuclear medicine studies with iminodiacetic acid derivatives (technetium 99m-dimethyl iminodiacetic acid: HIDA, EHIDA, DISIDA, PIPIDA) evaluate if hepatocytes can synthesize and excrete bile. Nuclear medicine studies are not routine in the acute posttraumatic phase in Europe, but are obtained later, when a biliary leak or biliary obstruction is suspected (Reichelt 1978; Weissmann et al. 1979; Christensen et al. 1981; Sty et al. 1982; Powers and Melton 1982; Zeman et al. 1984; Lineaweaver et al. 1985; Gartman et al. 1985; Savitch et al. 1986; Salam et al. 1987; Itoh et al. 1987). Bile scintigraphy traces the flow of bile in the abdomen or thorax, but lacks anatomical precision in location of a fistula and in the distinction between partial or complete bile duct disruption (Haddad et al. 1986). Bile extravasation through a tear is documented by extrahepatic bile accumulation or excretion into surgical catheters without emptying of the scintigraphic agent into the digestive tract lumen. Delayed scanning, 4 h after injection should always be obtained to confirm extraluminal accumulation of bile. Cholescintigraphy easily differentiates a bile collection from other nonbiliary collections, such as an hematoma, seroma or ascites, seen on US or CT (Fig. 6.3). Intrahepatic bilhemia can also be diagnosed by hepatobiliary scintigraphy. A biliovenous fistula is suggested by persistent blood pool activity of the tracer, bile duct visualization without tracer pooling, and nonvisualization of the opacified bowel (Francois et al. 1994). A nuclear medicine scan can be falsely negative, as extravasated bile may simulate opacified bowel loops (Meyers 1994). Scintigraphy is also able to detect gallbladder rupture, although nonfilling of the gallbladder is not specific for gallbladder injury or cholecystitis and findings should be correlated with cross-section imaging (Zeman et al. 1984). Traumatic pancreatitis, (acalculous) cholecystitis, or hyperalimentation are among other causes of a negative gallbladder cholescintigram. Cholescintigraphy is 83%–87% accurate for predicting the presence of a bile leak after laparoscopic cholecystectomy (Brugge et al. 1994). In one study, hepatobiliary scintigraphy performed within 1 week of abdominal trauma showed a biloma in 20% and bile leakage in 16% (Coletti et al. 1987). Another study reported 33% of bile duct leakage in blunt and penetrating injury (Zeman et al. 1984). After surgical repair of ductal rupture, cholescintigraphy is also indicated to demonstrate ductal integrity (Wig et al. 1988). In case of bile duct obstruction, cholescintigraphy shows retained intrahepatic activity and no passage of the isotope into the gastrointestinal tract. When clinical symptoms suggestive of bile duct rupture are present, an apparently normal scan requires endoscopic retrograde cholangiopancreatography (ERCP).

Tc-99m sulfur colloid scans seem to offer no significant advantage over cholescintigraphy in the detection of hepatic parenchymal injury (Zeman et al. 1984).

6.6.2 Computed Tomography

6.6.2.1 Technique

At admission, helical single-slice or multislice abdominal CT is obtained with routine protocols for polytrauma patients concerning IV injection of contrast medium and scanning parameters.

Helical CT cholangiography was described as a reliable method of detection and localization of a bile leakage when large ducts are affected (Dinkel et al. 1999; Borocco et al. 1996). The method is reliable, but necessitates a slow IV infusion of iodinated bile-specific contrast medium, which is known to carry potential adverse reactions; it acts in competition with the metabolism of bilirubin and is therefore not applicable in biliary obstruction. Good contrast is obtained in the bile ducts when serum bilirubin level is less than 2 mg/dl, but uncertain opacification for levels over 5 mg/dl (Stockberger et al. 1996). Case reports have confirmed that correct location of a posttraumatic bile leak could be demonstrated by cholangio-spiral CT (Wicky et al. 1999) (Fig. 6.4). At present, CT cholan-

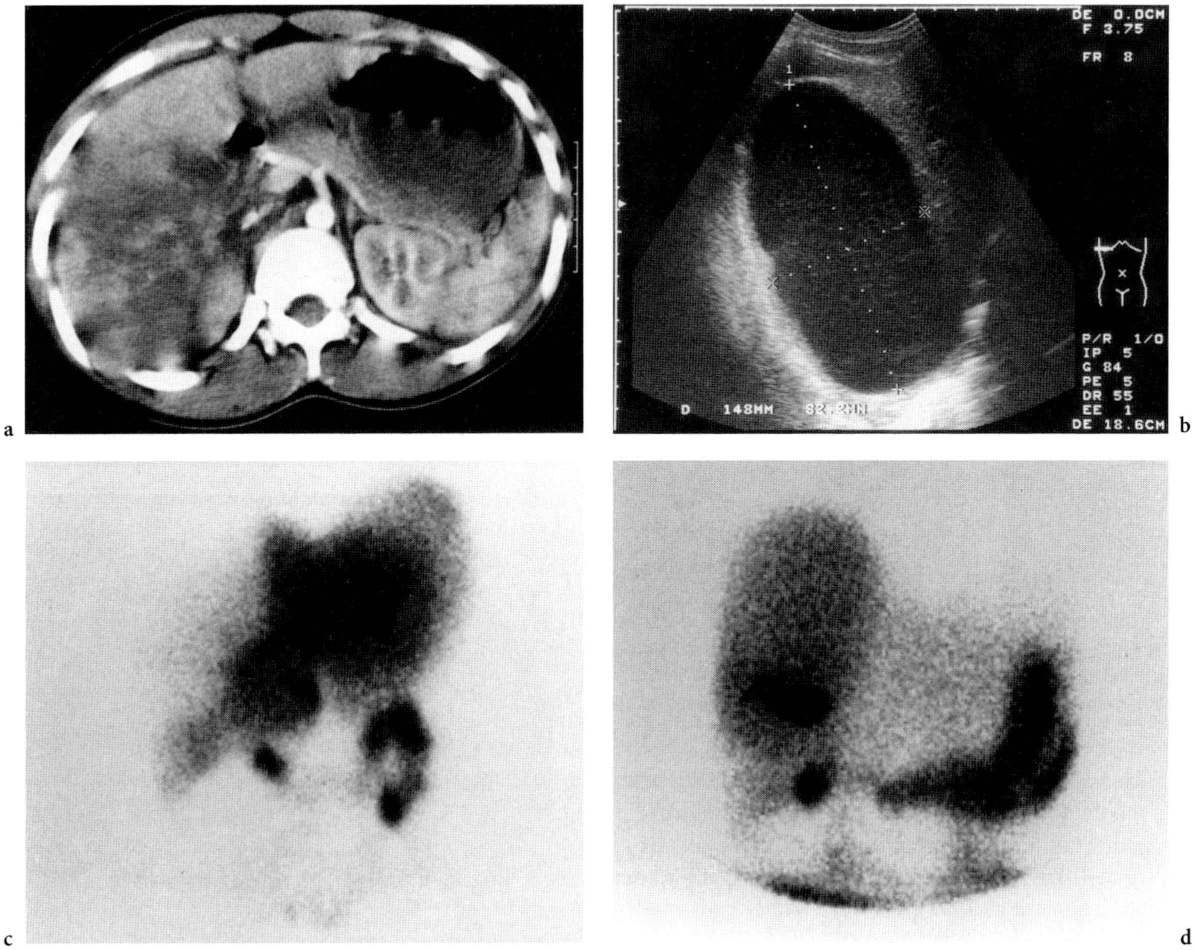

Fig. 6.3a–d. A 15-year-old girl was admitted after a motor vehicle accident. **a** Spiral CT of the abdomen shows hepatic contusion of segment V and VI, extending to the area of inferior vena cava, which is surrounded by a hematoma. **b** US obtained 3 days later demonstrated a hypoechoic fluid collection, with distinct margins, located lateral to the right lobe of the liver and compatible with a biloma. **c** Iminodiacetic acid (IDA) bile scintigraphy (early phase at 5 min) shows normal activity of the left lobe of the liver. A lateral mass effect with no activity compresses the right lobe. **d** At the late phase (30 min after injection), enhancement disappeared in the normal liver; the gallbladder is filled and the lateral mass effect shows relatively homogeneous activity corresponding to a biloma, which is progressively filled with the radionuclide (from Wicky et al. 1999, with permission)

giography is largely replaced by magnetic resonance cholangiopancreatography (MRCP).

6.6.2.2 Gallbladder Injury

CT signs of gallbladder injury are occasionally described in isolated reports or in series containing a limited number of patients (Daneman et al. 1983; Gottesman et al. 1984; Jeffrey et al. 1986; Ball et al. 1988; Erb et al. 1994; Scaglione et al. 1998). Many CT signs are not specific of gallbladder rupture.

CT at admission may show:

- A hyperdense intraluminal clot in the gallbladder lumen and in some cases in the common bile duct, which may be dilated by the hematoma. Fresh clot is best seen with narrow window settings on the nonenhanced scan; when present as an isolated finding, it indicates minimal contusion. A blood-bile level can be seen (Figs. 6.5, 6.15a). Other causes of high intraluminal densities are retained contrast from a previous contrast medium injection or milk of calcium bile.
- Pericholecystic fluid is almost always present when significant injury to the gallbladder has occurred, but a hematoma in the porta hepatis may extend from liver injury, without injury to the bile ducts (Fig. 6.6). Fluid-like densities indicate extravasation of bile, but are not specific. Ascites, diluted blood, or lymphoedema exhibit similar

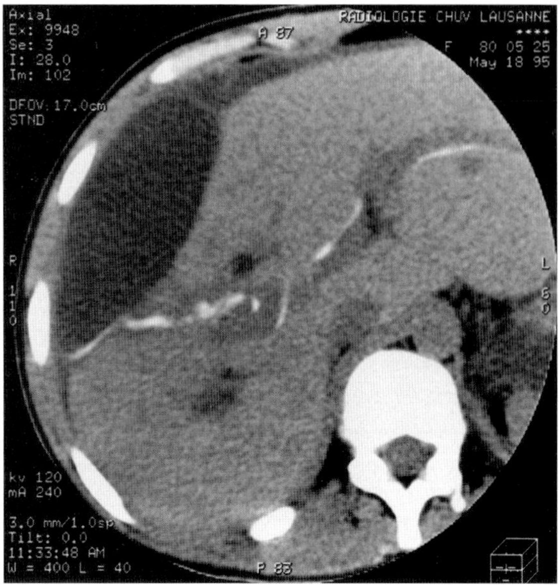

Fig. 6.4. Same patient as Fig. 6.3. Spiral CT obtained after intravenous injection of 20 ml of iodoxamic acid shows extravasation of opaque bile from the right hepatic duct into the biloma

density values. High fluid densities indicate pericholecystic hemorrhage or a bilohematoma. A small amount of pericholecystic fluid results from a self-sealed microperforation of the gallbladder wall (Erb et al. 1994) (Fig. 6.7).

- A mass effect by the pericholecystic fluid collection may be seen on the duodenum adjacent to the gallbladder (Berland et al. 1980; Daneman et al. 1983; Yoon et al. 1998; Erb et al. 1994).
- When the gallbladder has ruptured, it is partially or completely collapsed.
- An ill-defined and thickened contour of the gallbladder indicates mural hematoma of the gallbladder wall (normal <3 mm) and may be present in case of wall contusion or partial gallbladder avulsion.
- The dissected gallbladder wall may show as an intraluminal double contour.
- When extensive gallbladder wall rupture has occurred, gallstones may be found outside the gallbladder lumen, which is collapsed (Wolfson et al. 1984).
- An incompletely avulsed gallbladder is usually displaced towards the midline.
- The gallbladder may be completely avulsed and found in a remote peritoneal compartment, such as the pelvis (Vajdic et al. 1979; Ball et al. 1988).
- The injured gallbladder wall or mucosa is usually enhanced by IV contrast. An enhanced gallblad-

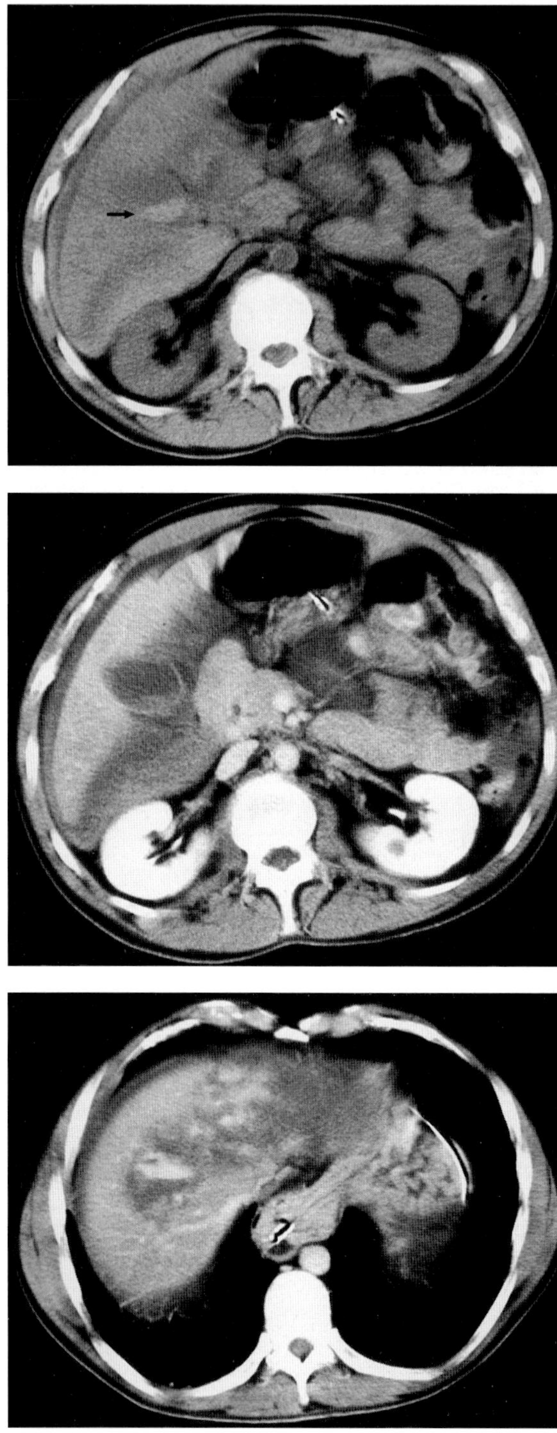

a

b

c

Fig. 6.5a–c. A 47-year-old male was involved in a traffic accident. **a, b** CT at admission without contrast injection (**a**) showed hemoperitoneum in Morrison's pouch and similar high densities in the gallbladder lumen (*arrow*). Fresh clot is better seen without contrast and narrow window settings than after intravenous contrast injection (**b**). **c** Diffuse areas of contusion are seen predominantly in the left lobe of the liver, with multiple intrahepatic blushes of contrast extravasation. No arteriography was performed

a

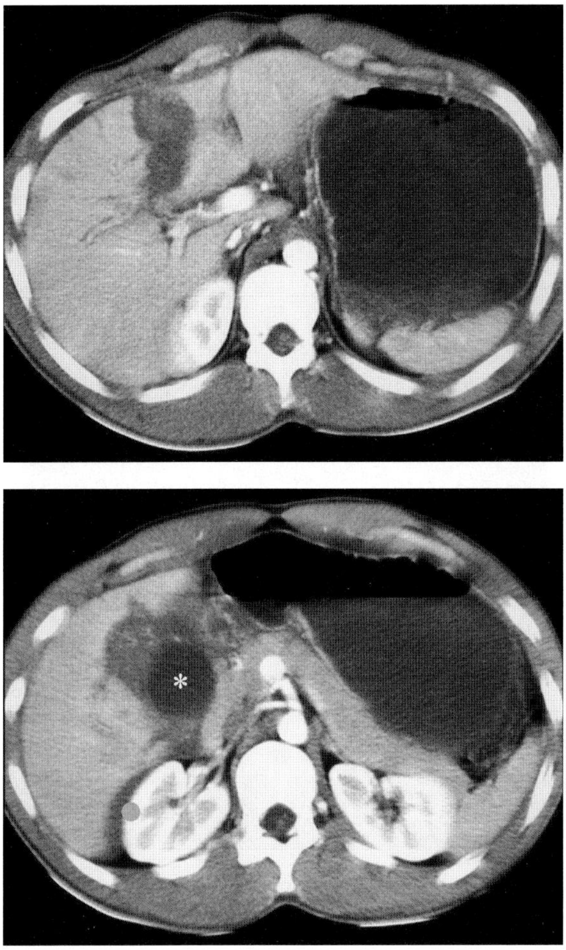

b

Fig. 6.6a, b. A 27-year-old male was involved in a traffic accident. **a** CT at admission showed a hepatic hematoma located in segment IV. **b** The hematoma extended in the porta hepatis and surrounded the gallbladder (*asterisk*), which contained water density bile. No bile injury was noted during follow-up, after conservative treatment

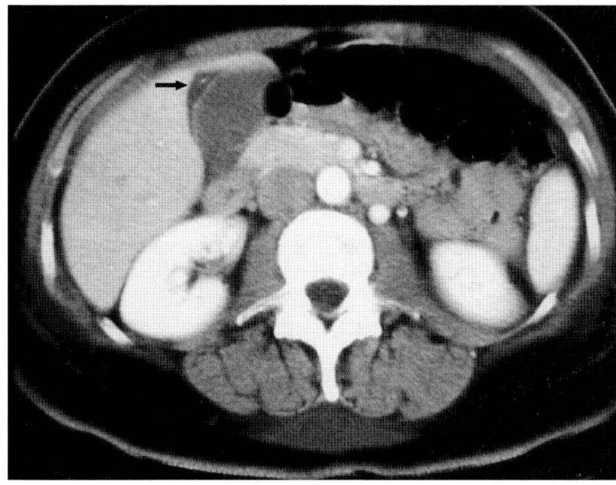

Fig. 6.7. A 45-year-old female underwent CT at admission for moderate blunt abdominal trauma. A minimal low-density pericholecystic fluid collection (*arrow*) is noted and probably corresponds to a minimal bile extravasation. No other significant upper abdominal injury is noted

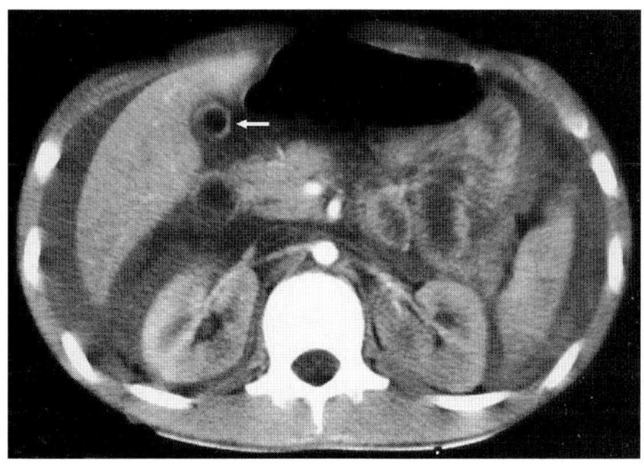

Fig. 6.8. A 10-year-old child was involved in a traffic accident. CT obtained after resuscitation showed diffuse arterial vasoconstriction due to shock, massive hemoperitoneum and retroperitoneal hematoma. The wall of a non-distended gallbladder (*arrow*) is moderately thickened. Enhancement of the gallbladder wall is caused by low arterial flow in the cystic artery, related to shock

der wall suggests that the cystic artery is patent (Fig. 6.8).

- A free mucosal flap that is enhanced after IV contrast medium injection may project into the gallbladder lumen.
- An air–fluid level in the gallbladder or in the main bile duct can be seen, caused by an internal fistula with the stomach or duodenum. This sign usually appears in delayed complications (Hoff et al. 1998).
- Massive upper abdominal or subhepatic hemoperitoneum may be present after rupture of the cystic artery (Jeffrey et al. 1986).
- A heterogeneous avascular liver mass and a thickened wall gallbladder with a transverse orientation of its long axis may be seen in case of combined torsion of an accessory liver lobe and the gallbladder meso (Koplewitz et al. 1999).
- On delayed CT studies, stigmata of chronic cholecystitis with a thickened wall and persistent retracted clot simulating an intraluminal soft tissue mass may be seen (Hanazaki et al. 1995).
- Focal intrahepatic periportal tracking in hepatic parenchyma adjacent to the gallbladder should draw the attention to possible gallbladder or bile duct injury.

6.6.2.3
Extrahepatic Ductal Injury

Direct signs of common bile duct rupture are rarely observed on CT. Suggestive, but nonspecific signs are:

- Thickening of the common bile duct wall by hematoma
- High-density content in the choledochal lumen (Fig. 6.15a)
- Contusion of the pancreatic head or posttraumatic pancreatitis and intrapancreatic common bile duct indistinctly seen
- Fluid in the porta hepatis and extending in the perihepatic peritoneal spaces or in the lesser sac
- Focal liver laceration in the quadrate lobe (segment IV) or a major hepatic fracture extending through the porta hepatis (Moulton et al. 1993; Eid et al. 1996)
- Biliary ascites (proven by percutaneous fluid aspiration)
- Occasionally a retroperitoneal or peripancreatic biloma; the latter can be mistaken for a posttraumatic pancreatic pseudocyst (Cope 1925; Kalderon and Sobel 1965; Bourque et al. 1989)

In the late phase, when biliary obstruction has occurred due to a posttraumatic bile duct stenosis, CT shows intra- and extrahepatic bile duct dilatation and an abrupt narrowing of the common bile duct, mimicking malignancy. Generally, other signs of injury, which were obvious on the initial CT examination, have resolved at this time (Yoon et al. 1998). Knowledge of previous abdominal contusion is essential for the interpretation of images of posttraumatic bile duct obstruction without other evident cause of a tumor or lithiasis.

6.6.2.4
Intrahepatic Bile Duct Injury

Rupture of intrahepatic bile ducts results in intraparenchymal or subcapsular bilohematoma with mixed densities, evolving into a collection with nonspecific fluid densities. Segmental bile duct dilatation may be seen, caused by bile duct laceration and obstruction. Posttraumatic periportal tracking, caused by lymphoedema, should not be mistaken for diffuse intrahepatic bile duct dilatation (Koslin et al. 1988) (Fig. 6.9).

6.6.2.5
Results

No combination of CT findings is specific for a particular type of gallbladder injury or able to predict surgical treatment (Scaglione et al. 1998). Percutaneous US- or CT-guided needle aspiration of an intrahepatic or perihepatic fluid collection is highly accurate in confirming extravasation of bile. Diagnosis of injury to the extrahepatic ductal system is difficult. A normal CT does not exclude isolated injury to the extrahepatic bile ducts, but absence of pericholecystic fluid reasonably excludes significant gallbladder wall rupture (Erb et al. 1994).

There is no series available in the literature assessing the diagnostic accuracy of CT in extrahepatic bile duct injury.

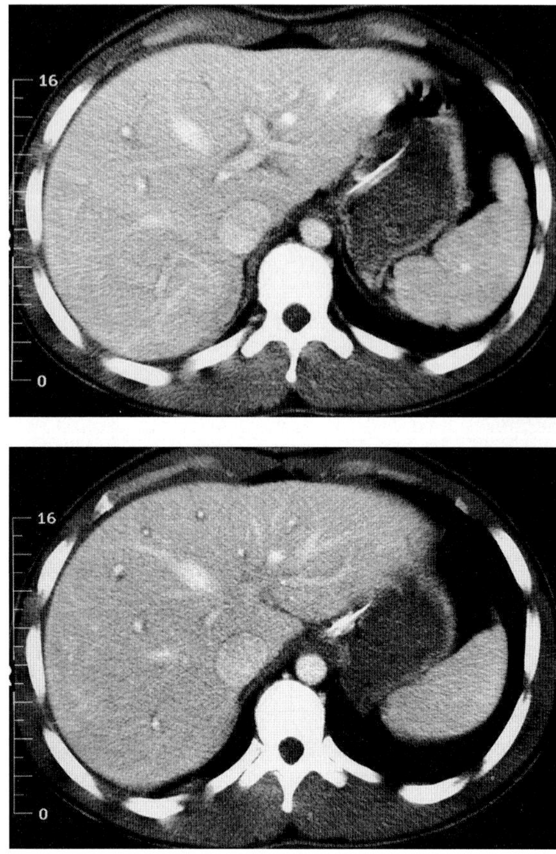

Fig. 6.9. a, b Diffuse periportal tracking is seen, as collar-shaped low densities around the intrahepatic portal vein sections in a patient with abdominal contusion on CT. Periportal tracking is an unspecific sign of hepatic contusion and should not be confused with intrahepatic bile duct dilatation

6.6.3
Ultrasound

Ultrasound (US) reproduces similar findings to CT and is also more efficient in the diagnosis of gallbladder injury than common bile duct injury. US signs are not well correlated with the pathological findings at cholecystectomy (SCAGLIONE et al. 1998). Intraluminal blood clot and pericholecystic fluid seen on US are not specific for gallbladder or choledochal injury. Fresh intraluminal blood shows as nonshadowing mobile echoic material or mass, which must be distinguished from sludge or pus in the gallbladder lumen. Clotted blood shows an echo pattern, which may simulate a soft tissue mass. Other US appearances are scattered or evenly distributed intraluminal echoes (ALANEN and KORMAND 1985; KAUZLARIC and BARMIER 1985; LAFFEY et al. 1988; SAX et al. 1988; NISHIWAKI et al. 1999). Serial US examinations show progressive liquefaction of an intraluminal gallbladder hematoma and rapid resolution of pericholecystic fluid. The gallbladder remains distended when no rupture has occurred. Small lacerations of the gallbladder wall, which are not shown by CT, can be detected by US by focal hypoechoic mural thickening (SATA et al. 1986). If the gallbladder is not found in its usual position, it may have become completely avulsed or partial inversion of the liver with a suprahepatic gallbladder should be considered (LEEKAM et al. 1987).

US is not efficient in the diagnosis of injury to the bile duct in the porta hepatis. In case of bile leakage, US evidences a free peritoneal effusion or collected bile in the porta hepatis or in the perihepatic spaces, or moderate dilatation of intra- or extrahepatic bile ducts (GOULD and PATEL 1979). Bilomas are circumscribed, echo-free with an excellent posterior shadowing, but can show debris or septations and are readily distinguished from hematomas, which show as a focal echoic mass (ESENSTEN et al. 1983) (Figs. 6.3b, 6.10). Both types of fluid collections are rapidly surrounded by a pseudocapsule, generated by an inflammatory reaction, which is absent in the acute phase. Dilatation of intrahepatic bile ducts, which is easily shown by US, can occur when obstruction is due to stenosis. In case of a bile leak, no or moderate bile duct dilation is seen (SPIGOS et al. 1981; THIBODEAU and ILLESCAS 1988).

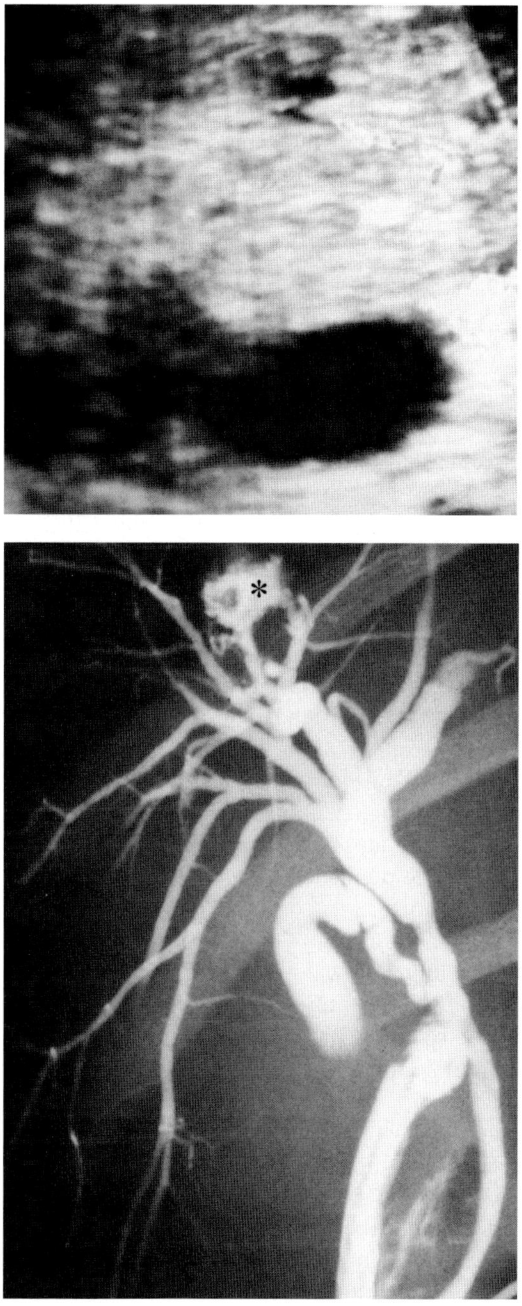
a
b

Fig. 6.10a, b. A 17-year-old male had sustained blunt abdominal trauma. The patient was admitted with delay for abdominal pain, fever, and jaundice. No investigation had been obtained at time of injury. **a** Compound-mode US showed an anechoic fluid collection in the right lobe of the liver. **b** PTC confirmed an intrahepatic bile duct fistula, opacifying an intrahepatic biloma (*asterisk*)

6.6.4 Cholangiography

6.6.4.1 Intraoperative

Intraoperative cholangiography, performed during urgent laparotomy or cholecystectomy, is able to detect a leak of the intra- or extrahepatic bile ducts, allowing for appropriate surgical treatment. Integrity of the bile ducts should be confirmed intraoperatively, particularly when extensive hematoma is present in the porta hepatis, or after surgical repair of a bile duct laceration or emergency liver resection. Manual compression of the distal common bile duct is necessary to increase the pressure upstream and produce contrast extravasation through a small proximal tear. Intraoperative cholangiography reduces the need for reoperation following inadequate surgical bile duct exploration (Mason et al. 1954; Graff 1963; Spencer et al. 1963; Steichen and Sheiner 1966; Richter 1969; Fletcher 1972; Sandblom 1973; Atik 1976; Huguet and Bloch 1977; McFadden et al. 1980; Kitahama et al. 1982; Michelassi and Ranson 1985; Feliciano et al. 1985; Muin et al. 1992; Froment et al. 1998).

6.6.4.2
Endoscopic Retrograde

Endoscopic retrograde cholangiography (ERC) is indicated in only 0.05% of all abdominal trauma patients (Harrell et al. 1998). ERC is useful in the subacute and delayed posttraumatic period to document bile duct laceration and bile extravasation, and in the delayed or late phase to evaluate posttraumatic bile duct stenosis (Tanaka et al. 1977; Safrany et al. 1978; Jones and Thomas 1985). In 3%–20%, a bile duct tear with a biliary fistula may not be recognized immediately at laparotomy; the mean time lapse between injury and ERC was 22 days in the published series, and in some cases several months, or up to 1 year, due to nonspecific clinical symptoms and a low index of suspicion of bile duct injury (Harrell et al. 1998). Therefore nuclear medicine studies and ERC should be liberally used in trauma patients with a suspicion of bile duct injury. Patients with high-grade liver injury or fracture of segment IV who are considered for conservative management should be investigated by ERC, if a suspicion of bile duct rupture is raised (Sugimoto et al. 1993). Trauma patients undergoing ERC should be hemodynamically stable; gastroduodenal perforation is a contraindication. The procedure is technically successful in 76%–95% and fails in case of preexisting enteric anastomosis or for other technical reasons. A morbidity rate of 5% is reported (Buckley and Connon 1990).

ERC has been recognized as the modality of choice to confirm the presence of injury to the extrahepatic bile ducts (Barclay and Crampton 1987; Sugimoto et al. 1993; Scioscia et al. 1994; Gerndt et al. 1995; Harrell et al. 1998). In case of partial tear of the main bile duct with a bile fistula, ERC shows the location and size of the leakage precisely and may also establish the diagnosis of gallbladder rupture, although its role is limited in practice to injury of the extra- or intrahepatic ducts (Boll and Belber 1978; Mitre and Brodmerkel 1979).

Bile duct fistulae of blunt posttraumatic origin are rare compared to iatrogenic causes such as laparoscopic, open cholecystectomy, or interventional hepatobiliary procedures and therefore little specific information is available in the literature on ERC in noniatrogenic trauma, but the basic abnormal imaging findings are similar (Burt and Nelson 1981; Michelassi and Ranson 1985; McLindon et al. 1998). In case of complete rupture of the main bile duct, no information can be obtained on the proximal bile ducts by ERC, and even in some cases of incomplete bile duct transection, contrast medium may not progress to the proximal part of the injured bile duct and catheterization may fail (Jones and Thomas 1985). In these cases, percutaneous transhepatic cholangiography is indicated in addition to ERC to depict exact location and extent of ductal rupture (Arkovitz et al. 1999).

ERC is also useful to evidence bile leakage from intrahepatic bile duct rupture and is suggested by some on a routine basis in high-grade liver injury. Intrahepatic bile leak can result from penetrating or blunt trauma and result in bilhemia from direct bile drainage into a hepatic vein , in an intrahepatic bile collection, or in a transcapsular fistula. Peripheral intrahepatic bile radicle tear remains a more difficult diagnosis than laceration of a major duct close to the hilar bifurcation and is frequently overlooked (Moser et al. 1995). A rate of up to 21% of injury to intrahepatic bile ducts was found and 84% of patients developed a biloma. However, the impact of these injuries on conservative management of liver injury is modest and not well defined (Sugimoto et al. 1993; De Backer et al. 1998).

In the late posttraumatic phase, ERC shows, in case of biliary obstruction, a stenosis or a complete stop. Abrupt narrowing of the common bile duct, most frequently seen at the superior limit of the pancreas, may mimic infiltrating malignancy. In other cases, progressive tapering of the intrapancreatic portion of the common bile duct can be seen, but can be caused by a posttraumatic focus of pancreatitis compressing the bile duct. The extra- and intrahepatic bile ducts are moderately or severely dilated depending on the degree of stenosis.

6.6.4.3
Percutaneous Transhepatic

Percutaneous transhepatic cholangiography (PTC) is not used as a primary diagnostic modality in the acute posttraumatic phase to evidence bile duct injury, as ERC is usually obtained first. PTC is indicated when ERC has failed or has evidenced a complete stop of the main bile duct, or when the endoscopist was unable to catheterize the papilla or the common bile duct above a fistula or an obstruction. Its definite place is a complement in mapping the injured bile ducts and a means of conservative management of bile duct injury. PTC is the first step to give a map of the intra- and extrahepatic bile ducts serving for subsequent percutaneous catheter-mediated interventions. The main goals of percutaneous opacification are (Dawson and Mueller 1994):

- Bile duct decompression in critically ill patients
- Location of bile duct leakage or stricture, evaluation of extent, and recognition of anatomical variants of the bile ducts (Figs. 6.11, 6.12)
- Planning of optimal percutaneous transhepatic approach for either unilobar or bilobar biliary drainage
- Plastic stent placement or balloon angioplasty for treatment of leakage/stricture

When a biliary fistula is present, intrahepatic bile ducts are usually not dilated or moderately dilated. PTC and catheter insertion are, however, still successful in 90% of patients and the total complication

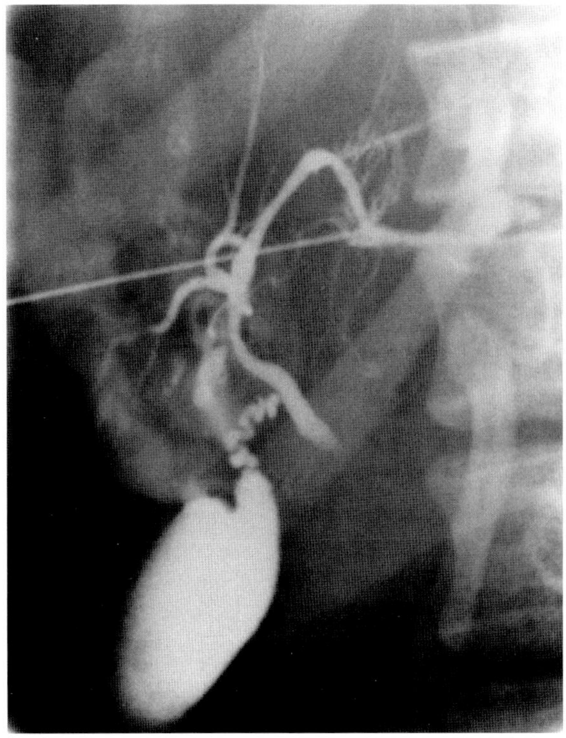

Fig. 6.11. Same patient as Fig. 6.3. Percutaneous transhepatic cholangiography: the left intrahepatic duct, the common bile duct and the gallbladder are normal. A contrast leak is evidenced, which fills the biloma located lateral to the right lobe of the liver

a 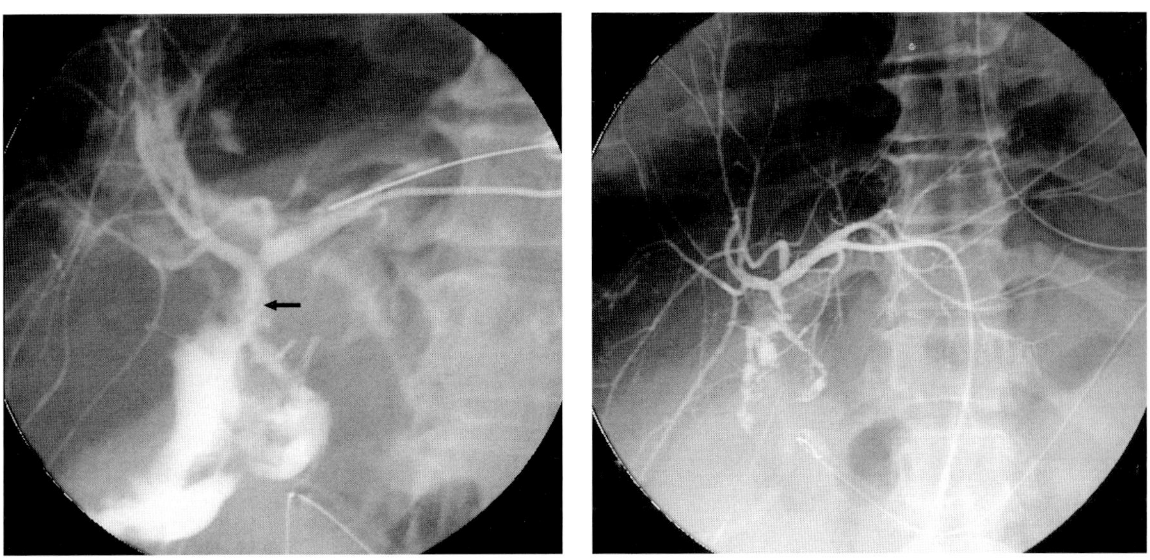 b

Fig. 6.12a, b. Celioscopic cholecystectomy in an 89-year-old female was followed by a bile fistula. A subhepatic drain was placed surgically, which exteriorized a massive bile fistula. **a** PTC showed moderately dilated intrahepatic bile ducts and extravasation of bile from the proximal part of the choledochus (*arrow*). **b** A 7F pigtail catheter was placed by a percutaneous transhepatic puncture and located at the hilar bifurcation for bile diversion from the origin of the fistula, before choledochojejunostomy was performed rate is 9% (Funaki et al. 1999). Occasionally, PTC, like ERC, evidences rupture of the gallbladder (Frank et al. 1976).

6.6.5 Magnetic Resonance Cholangiography

Magnetic resonance cholangiography (MRC) has been advocated as a noninvasive imaging modality of the biliary system. Imaging techniques include gradient echo sequences, rapid acquisition with relaxation enhancement (RARE), fast spin echo sequences, and half Fourier acquisition single short turbo spin echo (HASTE), 3D reverse flash imaging with steady-state precession (FISP) with breath holds, single-shot acquisitions at a single breath hold, and others.

Specific application of MRC in acute trauma patients is rarely reported in the literature. However, MRC has the potential to depict with precision the bile ducts and evaluate bile duct obstruction, as shown in other conditions than acute trauma (Wallner et al. 1991; Lauenberger et al. 1995; Lee et al. 1997; Mehta et al. 1997; Irie et al. 1998; Fulcher et al. 1998; Yeh et al. 1999). MRC has the advantage of evidencing the entire biliary system above or below a complete obstruction and also the pancreatic ducts. During the same examination, other fluid collections are depicted. MRI differentiates a biloma from a subacute hematoma: a biloma is heterogeneous and intense on T1-weighted images and homogeneously hyperintense on T2-weighted images, whereas a hematoma is hyperintense on T1- and T2-weighted images (Shigemura et al. 1995).

6.6.6 Diagnostic Peritoneal Lavage

Abdominal paracentesis has been advocated as a valuable diagnostic test of injury to the extrahepatic bile ducts (Rohatgi and Gupta 1987). Diagnostic peritoneal lavage (DPL) at admission is not of great help to document bile in the peritoneal fluid, as it may not yet have spread in the peritoneal cavity. No obvious bile was seen in the lavage fluid in 90% of patients, who were operated on for gallbladder injury (Soderstrom et al. 1981). When lavage fluid contains bile, it may not originate from the extrahepatic bile ducts, but from a ruptured liver or gastroduodenal tract. The bile may also form a biloma in the retroperitoneal space, escaping recognition by DPL. An elevated amylase level in the lavage fluid should not be misleading for pancreatic injury, as pancreatic juice may reflux in the ruptured bile ducts; many other different conditions are responsible for elevated amylase in the peritoneal fluid (see Chap. 7, "Injuries of the Pancreas"). In case of bile duct injury, however, DPL is often positive for hemoperitoneum, because of the high incidence of associated abdominal injuries or the hemorrhaging gallbladder wall.

6.6.7 Arteriography

In the acute posttraumatic period, hepatic arteriography might be able to demonstrate an occluded cystic artery or an abnormal gallbladder wall at the capillary phase or contrast extravasation, but angiography is not used routinely. Occasionally, following penetrating injury, angiography may be helpful to establish the diagnosis of arterial or portal trauma associated with bile duct laceration (Kruuna et al. 1994). Arteriography is more useful later, in the diagnostic work-up of hemobilia and treatment of pseudoaneurysm or arterioportal fistula (Okazaki et al. 1991; Vlahos et al. 1991; Hagiwara et al. 1997) (Fig. 6.13).

6.7 Management

6.7.1 Surgical

6.7.1.1 Damage Control Laparotomy

In the patient in shock, requiring immediate surgical control with minimal or without preoperative imaging, the diagnosis of laceration of the extrahepatic bile ducts may be established or suspected, or overlooked, the attention being focused on other life-threatening injuries. A life-saving operation may be deliberately terminated by simple external drainage and a second elective operation is scheduled for bile duct repair (McFadden et al. 1980). All hematomas in the porta hepatis should be completely explored to detect extrahepatic bile duct injury (Ivatury et al. 1985). The most critical patients are those with injury to the portal triad which is mainly caused by penetrating injury. Overall mortality in these complex injuries is 51%–80% and intraoperative death

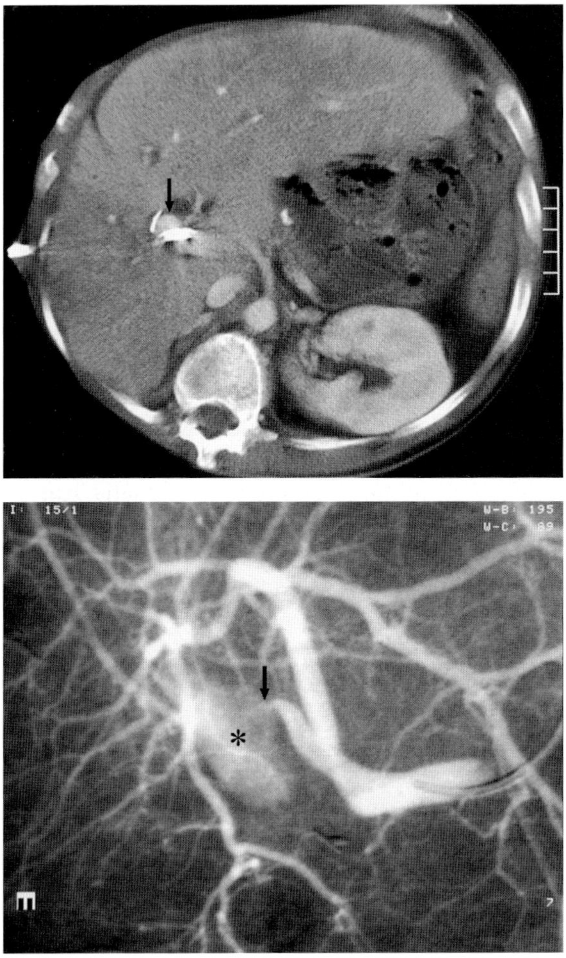

a

b

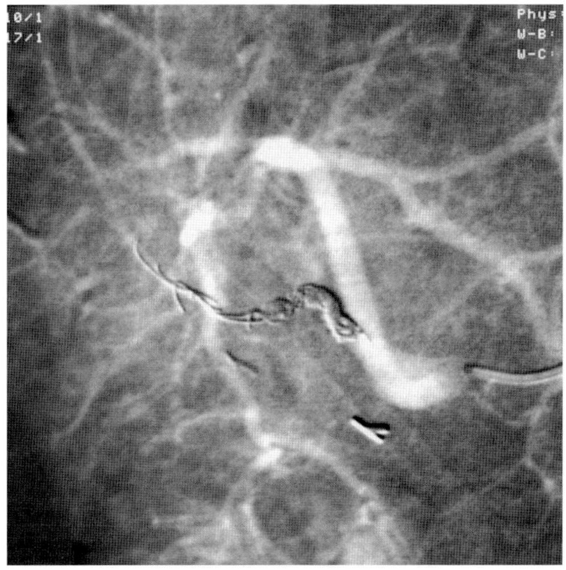

c

Fig. 6.13a–c. A 37-year-old male underwent percutaneous transhepatic mechanical extraction of a choledochal stone, because total gastrectomy prevented an endoscopic approach. The patient presented with persistent hemobilia after the percutaneous procedure. **a** CT showed an intrahepatic vascular lesion (*arrow*) in contact with the percutaneous transhepatic drainage catheter. **b** Hepatic arteriography obtained 2 days later showed an almost complete interruption of the right hepatic artery (*arrow*) and opacification of a pseudoaneurysm (*asterisk*), which had considerably enlarged in size compared to the previous CT examination. **c** Treatment was obtained by vaso-occlusive placement of coils in the ruptured right hepatic artery, distal, and proximal to the vascular tear, to avoid rebleeding by backflow

is mainly caused by exsanguination (Busuttil et al. 1980; Jurkovich et al. 1995).

6.7.1.2 Gallbladder Injury

Gallbladder injury is recognized intraoperatively. In case of gallbladder laceration or avulsion, a cholecystectomy and intraoperative cholangiography is performed (Parks and Diamond 1995). In case of minimal contusion of the gallbladder wall, expectant treatment can be advocated, followed by percutaneous imaging-guided aspiration of a pericholecystic biloma. In one report, four of seven patients (43%) with blunt gallbladder injury (three had partial avulsion, one had contusion) had no cholecystectomy (Posner and Moore 1985). Cholecystostomy or suture of the gallbladder (cholecystorrhaphy) wall are rarely performed, because of the risk of secondary perforation and the potential of late gallstone formation due to impaired gallbladder function. Post-traumatic cholecystitis due to cystic duct obstruction by blood clots responds to temporary percutaneous cholecystostomy and flushing of the gallbladder with heparinized saline through the drainage catheter (Rathnaraj et al. 1994). In selected cases of isolated penetrating injury of the gallbladder, laparoscopic cholecystectomy was performed (Velez et al. 1999).

6.7.1.3 Ductal Injury

Early Intervention

In a review of the literature based on a limited number of publications with small numbers of patients, reported operative therapy was variable, including drainage, primary suture repair, stenting, choledochoduodenostomy, end-to-end anastomosis with mucosa-to-mucosa reconstruction after obtaining adequate width of the main bile duct, cholecystojejunostomy and choledochojejunostomy, and hepatic and/or pancreatic/

duodenal injury repair. Parameters guiding surgical treatment are the hemodynamic and metabolic status of the patient, type of associated injuries, and extent of injury to the bile ducts, the liver and duodeno-pancreas (MICHELASSI and RANSON 1985).

In patients with portal triad injury (resulting mainly from penetrating trauma), survival after biliary enteric anastomosis was 89% and 50% after primary repair (JURKOVICH et al. 1995). In blunt trauma of the extrahepatic bile ducts without portal vein injury, laparotomy was obtained within 24 h only in 32% of cases, due to difficulties in establishing a correct diagnosis (MICHELASSI and RANSON 1995). Reported mortality of blunt injury to the bile ducts was about 20%, but in some reports it was significantly higher than that of penetrating injury (50% vs 8.3%) (IVATURY et al. 1985; JURKOVICH et al. 1995; ZANTUT et al. 1995). A simple external drainage operation without reintervention was associated with a 100% mortality rate and is not recommended (BOURQUE et al. 1989). Simple drainage is carried out only in unstable patients and requires reintervention, with a higher risk of sepsis and bile fistula formation. Hepatic resection or right or left hepatic duct ligation may be required in extensive proximal duct injury. Simple ligation can be performed irrespective of their size without significant complications (HADJIS and BLUMGART 1988; HOWDIESHELL et al. 1990). Distal composite biliary and duodeno-pancreatic injury may be treated by primary repair or by a Whipple procedure (LEE et al. 1976; BUSUTTIL et al. 1980; KITAHAMA et al. 1982; FELICIANO 1994).

At the other end of the spectrum, a limited or partial ductal tear, which is less than 50% of the ductal circumference without defect, is repaired by suture with or without T-tube placement. In this setting, late bile duct stricture is infrequent (FELICIANO et al. 1985; SHELDON et al. 1985; PARKS and DIAMOND 1995). Surgical stenting without suture repair or defect plasty was applied in exceptional cases and seemed to give adequate healing of the rupture, thus validating the principles of simple endoscopic or percutaneous bile duct stenting (SAKAMOTO et al. 1997). Complete laceration or transection is treated by end-to-end anastomosis or biliary enteric anastomosis. The latter operation was shown to carry significantly fewer postoperative strictures (4% vs 55%), less cholangitis, and less late liver cirrhosis (CARMICHAEL 1980; IVATURY et al. 1985). In children, complete laceration or avulsion of the main bile duct is also treated by a biliary enteric anastomosis (MOULTON et al. 1993; ARKOVITZ et al. 1999). Reoperation for biliary fistula should be avoided, as it carries a mortality of 5%–8%. Actually, a Roux-en-Y biliary enteric anastomosis was shown to give optimal long term results, when complete bile duct transection with loss of ductal tissue had occurred at the liver hilum (LONGMIRE 1966; WARREN and HARDY 1967; BUSUTTIL et al. 1980; MCFADDEN et al. 1980; KITAHAMA et al. 1982; POSNER and MOORE 1985; MICHELASSI and RANSON 1985; BADE et al. 1989; FELICIANO 1994; KOZAREK 1994; PARKS and DIAMOND 1995). In some cases with complex hepatobiliary injury, a partial hepatectomy is carried out in addition to biliary surgery.

Surgical repair of an intrahepatic leak is more difficult than repair of the extrahepatic duct and carries a higher complication rate. However, operation for an intrahepatic bile duct leak by reconstruction or hepatic segmental resection is rarely required (ROCHE et al. 1993). A limited traumatic tear of a lobar duct can be treated conservatively with adequate drainage (SEWELL 1966; CHARTERS and BARDIN 1978; VERRAN and SCHROEDER 1988; EID et al. 1996; VERRAN 1997).

Late Surgery

Late posttraumatic bile duct stenosis is treated by Roux-en-Y hepaticojejunostomy. A recent study has shown that in postoperative stenosis, surgical reconstruction with a Roux-en-Y hepaticojejunostomy preceded by preoperative cholangiography is associated with a successful outcome in up to 98% of patients, without the need for a biliary stent after a mean follow-up close to 5 years (LILLEMOE et al. 2000). In a comparative study, surgery had an actuarial success rate of 89% and balloon dilatation of 55% at 72 months of follow-up (PITT et al. 1989). Repeated interventions may become necessary over the years, in up to 10%–30% and even 55% according to duration of follow-up, due to recurrent bile duct stenosis at the site of anastomosis (IVATURY et al. 1985). In general, surgical repair of benign bile duct stenosis has a 70%–90% long-term success rate, but lesions at the hepatic duct confluence are the most difficult to treat (HAFF et al. 1969; PELLEGRINI et al. 1984; SABER and EL-MANIALOW 1984; PITT et al. 1989; JARNAGIN and BLUMGART 1999). Biliary cirrhosis and portal hypertension are potential late complications.

6.7.1.4
Results

Missed bile duct injuries have a 75% severe complication rate (JURKOVICH et al. 1995). Mortality of reintervention for persistent biliary fistula is 5%–8%. Mortality during hospital stay after blunt injury to the bile ducts is 13% and mortality from concomitant injury 10%. Overall mortality of patients with extrahepatic bile duct injury is 24% and greater in blunt than in penetrating trauma (Kitahama et al. 1982; Michelassi and Ranson 1985; Zantut et al. 1995).

6.7.2 Endoscopic

6.7.2.1 Fistulae

Management of bile duct fistulae that are recognized or persist after initial management of the trauma patient may be controversial. The basic principle of endoscopic or percutaneous treatment is localization of the biliary leak, decompression, and diversion of bile flow (Horattas et al. 1994). Posttraumatic bile leakage trough a partial tear of the common bile duct can be treated by endoscopic sphincterotomy, a nasobiliary catheter or placement of a 10F plastic stent bridging the gap (Burmeister et al. 1985; Smith et al. 1986; Sauerbruch et al. 1986; Deviere et al. 1987; Leung et al. 1988; Barthel et al. 1989; Goldin et al. 1990; Durham et al. 1992; Kozarek et al. 1994; Pachter et al. 1996; Sharma et al. 1997; Sugiyama et al. 2000) (Fig. 6.14). Sphincterotomy lowers the bile-duodenum pressure gradient and the peak sphincter pressure, thus increasing flow of bile directly to the duodenum. Sphincterotomy was advocated as a treatment of bile duct fistula, but when performed alone without stenting it is not efficient in all cases, as the fistula may persist in up to 24% (Del Olmo et al. 1988; Ponchon et al. 1989; Liguory et al. 1991; Scioscia et al. 1994). Nasobiliary drainage was recognized as an adequate treatment of bile leak (Burmeister et al. 1985; Deviere et al. 1987; Leung et al. 1988; Barthel et al. 1989). When a nasobiliary drainage was established, suction can be applied for 24–48 h. As an alternative to a protruding catheter, endoscopic stenting of a biliary fistula can be performed. A plastic F10 stent is left in place during several months for appropriate calibration of the bile duct lumen at the site of injury and healing (Smith et al. 1986; Hartle et al. 1993; Horattas et al. 1994; Jenkins and Ponsky 1995; Eid et al. 1996; Hoff et al. 1998; De Backer et al. 1998; Harrell et al. 1998; McLindon et al. 1998; Griffen et al. 2000). On an experimental basis, it has also been shown that biliary stenting is more effective than sphincterotomy in the resolution of biliary leaks (Marks et al. 1998). Stent placement may fail when complete separation of both ends of the ruptured bile duct is present.

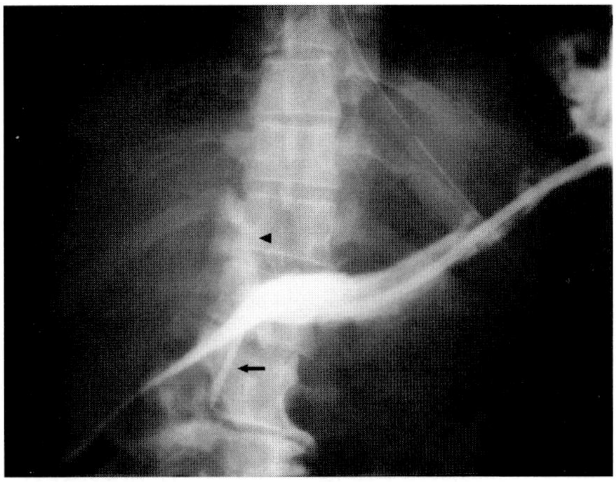

a

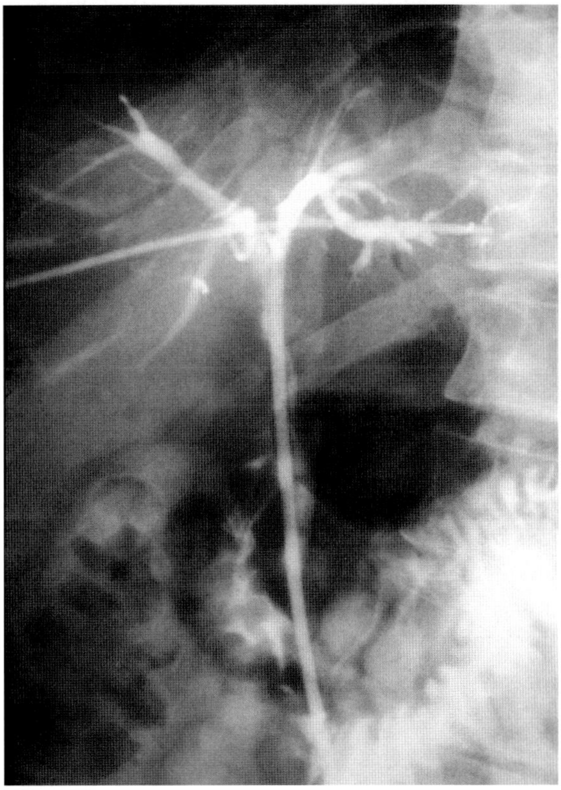

b

Fig. 6.14a, b. A middle-aged man was admitted in shock after a traffic accident. Laparotomy showed injuries to the liver and spleen. An intrasplenic arteriovenous fistula was embolized angiographically. During the hospital stay, the patient presented with an upper abdominal abscess, which was treated surgically and by additional percutaneous catheter drainage. **a** Opacification through the left subhepatic drainage catheter showed a fistula with the choledochus at the level of the superior pancreatic limit. The distal choledochus is normal (*arrow*) and contrast spreads in the porta hepatis (*arrowheads*). **b** The choledochal rupture had been missed intraoperatively and was treated by endoscopic insertion of a 10F plastic stent, which remained in place for 6 months. PTC was necessary to display the proximal bile ducts and guide stent placement. Opacification of the bile ducts through a 5F percutaneous transhepatic catheter shows normal function of the biliary stent

"Peripheral" leaks originating from a small intrahepatic bile radicle may also give profuse bile extravasation in some cases, when intraductal pressure remains elevated. Intrahepatic biliary leakage, either with biloma formation or a bile–hepatic vein communication resulting from blunt liver trauma can be treated nonoperatively with a plastic stent, sealing the bilio-venous communication or by inflating a balloon in the bile ducts at the level of the bilio-venous communication, expecting to seal the fistula by tamponade (Struyven et al. 1982; Poli et al. 1995; Gable et al. 1997; Harrell et al. 1998). When associated with a large necrotic cavity, a hepatic lobectomy may be associated (Glaser et al. 1994). Intrahepatic bile duct rupture resulting in biloma may occasionally, if persistent, give raise to an arterial pseudoaneurysm, by corrosive erosion, and if ruptured, delayed bleeding (Hagiwara et al. 1993). Bile peritonitis resulting from a biliary leak can also be treated by a minimally invasive approach, associating celioscopic peritoneal irrigation and drainage and endoscopic bile duct stenting (Griffen et al. 2000).

ERC is actually recognized as a valuable method for diagnosis and management of biliary fistulae in a subgroup of patients requiring no immediate abdominal surgery, but in whom a high index of suspicion of biliary fistulae is raised (Harrell et al. 1998). In large series of postoperative bile leaks, endoscopic drainage was feasible in 89% and successful in 90% in treated patients (80% on an intention-to-treat basis) (Davids et al. 1992). A few cases of nonoperative management of biliary tract fistula after blunt abdominal trauma were reported in children, in whom a nasobiliary drain was placed to treat the fistula (Poli et al. 1995).

6.7.2.2 Stenosis

Endoscopic placement of stents is also regarded today as a first option for benign posttraumatic stenosis occurring during follow-up, as an alternative to surgery (Ott et al. 1992; Dumonceau et al. 1998). An F10–F12 plastic stent is placed over the site of stenosis and exchanged on a regular basis, every 4–6 months to avoid stent clogging, or earlier if cholangitis or jaundice develop, caused by stent obstruction. Balloon dilatation of the stricture can be performed in addition during stent exchange. Mean duration of stenting was about 8 months. Endoscopic stenting carried a late recurrence rate of stenosis of 19% after a mean follow-up of 44 months (Dumonceau et al. 1998). During endoscopic management of bile duct stricture, sphincterotomy is helpful for multiple manipulations (Kozarek et al. 1994). Recent experience has shown that calibration with a stent or catheter should be prolonged for 12 months to optimize results.

Posttraumatic hemobilia is occasionally responsible for intermittent biliary obstruction, which may occur several days or weeks following injury, and is caused by residual intraductal clots that have not dissolved spontaneously. Endoscopic sphincterotomy and ductal lavage is the treatment of choice (Clancy and Warren 1997).

6.7.2.3 Results

Results of endoscopic management of posttraumatic noniatrogenic bile duct stenosis cannot be definitely assessed, as experience is too limited. As a comparison, endoscopic treatment of iatrogenic postoperative stenosis shows a successful balloon dilatation and successful stent insertion in 86%–88%. Efficient treatment of biliary obstruction, and in some patients of concomitant bile leakage, was obtained in 75%–83% after a follow-up period of 2–6.5 years. In the remaining patients, symptoms of cholangitis and biliary obstruction recurred, due to stricture formation (Huibregtse et al. 1986; Berkelhammer et al. 1989; Geenen et al. 1989; Davids et al. 1992, 1993; Walden et al. 1993; Kozarek et al. 1994). Stents may migrate in 2%–5% and clog in 30% within 3 months of insertion, requiring repeated interventions (Speer et al. 1988; Gilbert et al. 1991). In a comparative study with surgery, comorbidity and mortality rates were similar in both groups (Davids et al. 1993).

6.7.3 Percutaneous Transhepatic

Percutaneous transhepatic biliary drainage can be considered in particular situations, when endoscopic catheterization has failed due to complete disruption of bile ducts (Scioscia et al. 1994). Similarly, late obstruction of the bile ducts caused by a tight stenosis may not be successfully managed by an endoscopic access and requires a percutaneous transhepatic approach.

6.7.3.1 Fistulae and Bilomas

Percutaneous treatment of a posttraumatic bile leak has been reported in a few patients (Kaufman et al.

1985; GOLDIN et al. 1990; LIGUORY et al. 1991; BLUM et al. 1993; SCIOSCIA et al. 1994; SHAHRUDIN and NOORI 1997). Even when intrahepatic bile ducts are only minimally dilated, PTC may still be successful, but percutaneous placement of a biliary catheter or stent requires at least mild intrahepatic bile duct dilatation (SMITH et al. 1986; VACCARO et al. 1991; HARRIS et al. 1993; ERNST et al. 1999; FUNAKI et al. 1999) (Fig. 6.12). A rendezvous procedure using a combined percutaneous transhepatic and peroral approach can be carried out, which minimizes the hepatic trauma by limiting the size of the transhepatic catheter to F5 (MONTESANO et al. 1999). However, a combined procedure is cumbersome and has no real advantage over an exclusive percutaneous procedure with puncture of an intrahepatic bile duct in the periphery of the liver. The catheter or a plastic stent should be left in place until complete resolution of the bile fistula has occurred. Other means of closure of a fistula are local tetracycline instillation and fibrin glue injection through a drainage catheter, but any additional local inflammatory reaction in the wall of the bile ducts may end up in late bile duct stricture (DINKEL et al. 1999).

An intra- or extrahepatic biloma should be treated by US- or CT-guided percutaneous catheter drainage, when its size is larger than 3 cm or when symptomatic, to avoid secondary transformation in an abscess or compression of the bile ducts or the upper gastrointestinal tract (SCLAFANI et al. 1984; BYNOE et al. 1992; MOOSA et al. 1992; HORATTAS et al. 1994; PACHTER and HOFSTETTER 1995; PONSKY 1996; SHAHRUDIN and NOORI 1997) (Fig. 6.15). Pure bilomas without hemorrhagic content require only small-bore catheters that are well tolerated by the patient (VAZQUEZ et al. 1985). Contrast injection in the biloma following aspiration of its content, may confirm a biliary fistula, by showing the communication with the bile ducts. When a stent has been placed in the injured bile duct, effectiveness of the stenting procedure can be monitored by measuring the decreasing daily output trough the drainage catheter of a concomitant biloma. Treatment limited to catheter drainage of the cavity alone without sphincterotomy or stenting may be effective in some patients with a small bile duct tear (GARCIA URGUELLES et al. 1996).

In one series, biliary leaks treated by percutaneous transhepatic catheter drainage, healed in 81% after about 2.5 months of drainage after a mean follow-up period of 38 months (ERNST et al. 1999). In another report of biliary complications following hepatorrhaphy for liver injury, bile fistula or biloma healed after a mean of 6 weeks after percutaneous catheter drainage (SHAHRUDIN and NOORI 1997). Embolization of a fistulous tract with Gelfoam and coils has been described, but this technique cannot replace catheter drainage of the bile collection, and bile flow diversion from the fistulous site by a stent (HUNT et al. 1997; OLIVA et al. 1997; RYU et al. 1998). Coils can migrate through the fistulous tract and be expelled at a cutaneous orifice.

Pleurobiliary and bronchobiliary fistulae are more complex to treat than a short fistulous tract. Clinical symptoms include fever, cough, chest and right upper quadrant pain, and bilioptysis. A bile empyema develops frequently. In addition to bile diversion with biliary drainage or temporary stenting, pleural and abdominal drainage of bile collections is required. As a preventive treatment, posttraumatic diaphragmatic tears should be diagnosed and closed early to avoid chronic fistulization (OPARAH and MANDAL 1978). Occasionally, a foreign body such as a bullet, lodged in an intrahepatic abscess cavity, requires percutaneous transhepatic extraction (CHACKO et al. 1996).

6.7.3.2
Stenosis

PTC is more frequently used to investigate biliary duct obstruction than a biliary fistula (BURT and NELSON 1981). PTC seems particularly indicated when a stenosis has formed after laceration at the common bile duct bifurcation or when a complete stop is seen on ERCP at any level. There are no large series of patients available with specifically noniatrogenic posttraumatic bile duct stenosis, treated by percutaneous balloon dilatation or catheter calibration, but percutaneous transhepatic balloon dilatation has been largely reported in the treatment of benign bile duct strictures of other causes. A posttraumatic bile duct stenosis is ischemic in nature and therefore prone to fail with balloon dilatation. It was shown that primary strictures following laparoscopic cholecystectomy responded poorly to percutaneous management. In contrast, strictures resulting from primary repair had a better response rate (TREROTOLA et al. 1992). At the present time, we apply balloon dilatation only once, followed by a 1 year of catheter drainage, which calibrates the stenosis with one or two F14 catheters for strictures involving both lobar ducts.

An overall success rate of percutaneous dilatation of 55%–85% was obtained after a follow-up of 24–59 months (GALLACHER et al. 1985; VOGEL et al. 1985; MUELLER et al. 1986; WILLIAMS et al. 1987; MOORE et al. 1987; PITT et al. 1989; CITRON and

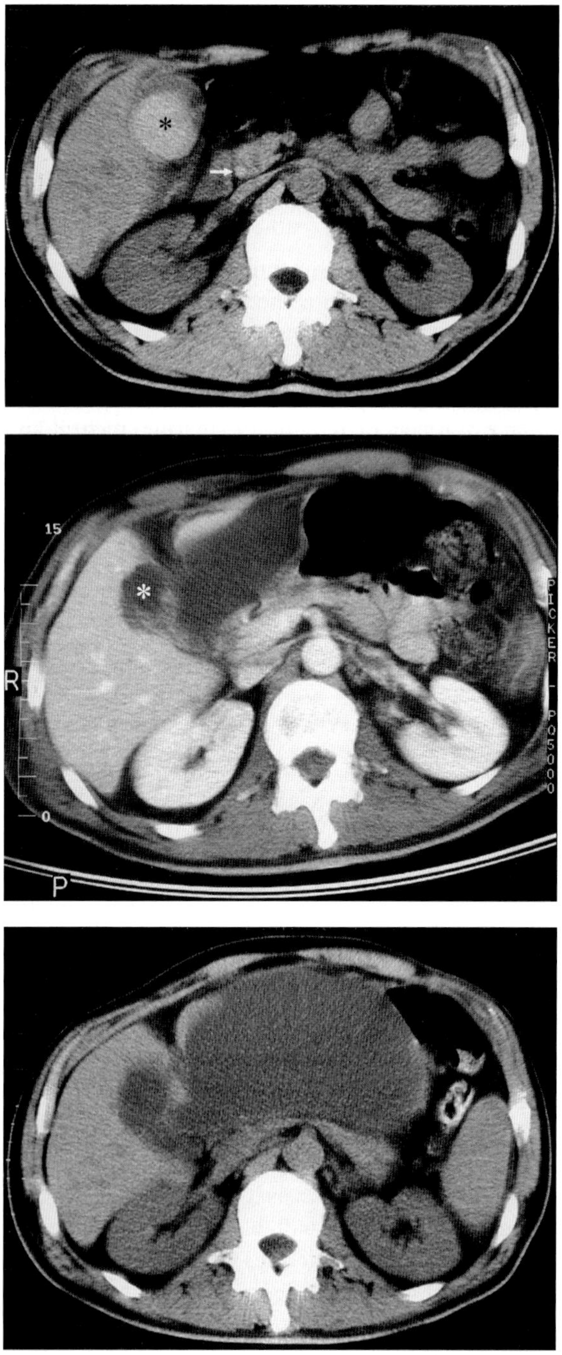

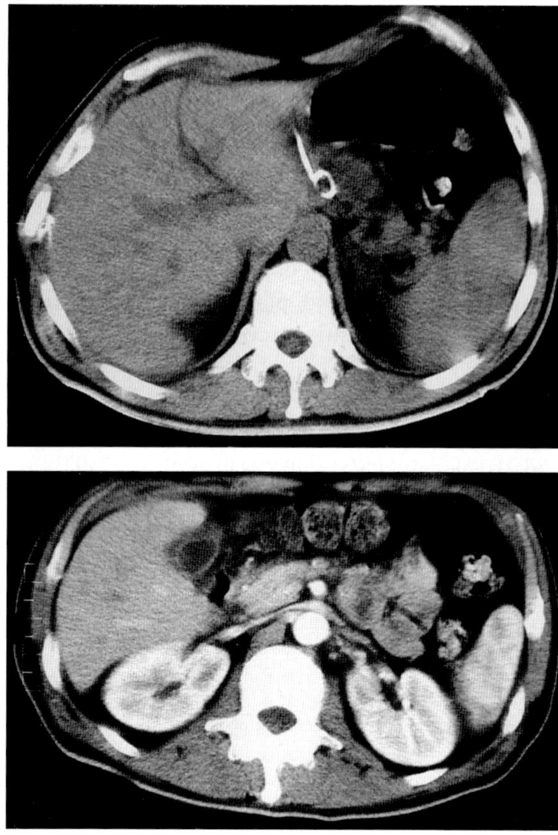

Fig. 6.15a–e. A 41-year-old male was admitted following blunt trauma from a car accident. **a** CT at admission without contrast showed high density, fresh clot in the gallbladder lumen (*asterisk*) and in the intrapancreatic choledochus (*arrow*). An area of moderate liver contusion was seen in segment IV (not shown). Conservative treatment was given. **b** CT performed 16 days after admission showed a nondistended gallbladder (*asterisk*) and a fluid collection in the left subhepatic space. Needle aspiration showed a bilohematoma. Note residual dependent clot in the gallbladder lumen. **c** During the following days, the patient became febrile and complained of upper abdominal discomfort. CT performed 6 days after percutaneous aspiration showed a large fluid collection, extending from the gallbladder fossa to the left subhepatic space. **d** Percutaneous drainage was applied with a 5F pigtail catheter: 1600 ml of bile was evacuated, resulting probably from a microperforation of the gallbladder. **e** CT obtained 3 days later showed a small residual fluid collection around the gallbladder. No further treatment was given

Martin 1991). A restenosis rate of 22%–34% was reported, which is better than surgical results (Way et al. 1981; Blumgart et al. 1984). Complications are noted in up to 29% and include cholangitis, pancreatitis, fever, general sepsis, and hemobilia (Williams et al. 1987).

Placement of metal stents should be considered only as a last resort in the treatment of benign bile duct obstruction. Regardless of the type of stent used, only 50% of patients remained symptom free after 18 months of follow-up (Rossi et al. 1990).

6.7.4 Conservative Nonoperative

Nonoperative management of bile duct injuries can be followed in patients with a limited contusion of the gallbladder. Some patients fall necessarily into this category, when a minimal gallbladder or bile duct perforation has occurred, but was not recognized at time of injury and remained occult during follow-up. When expectant therapy is deliberately applied, repeated CT or US examinations are necessary to confirm resolution of an intraluminal gallbladder clot, return to normal aspect of a thickened gallbladder wall, and resolution of a pericholecystic fluid collection. In blunt injury, nonoperative treatment was followed in the past in only 3% of cases (Michelassi and Ranson 1985).

Intrahepatic bilomas may require up to 3–4 months for complete absorption, whereas hepatic contusions regress in 4–6 weeks (Sugimoto et al. 1993). An intra- or extrahepatic biloma can be aspirated or drained without surgery (Howdieshell et al. 1995; De Backer et al. 1998). Some intrahepatic bile-vein communications of limited size may heal spontaneously, when no biliary obstruction is present.

It should be noticed that among 100 patients reported with blunt injury to the extrahepatic bile ducts, none was treated nonoperatively for associated hepatic injury (Michelassi and Ranson 1985; Mangiante et al. 1987). On the other hand, in nonoperative management of blunt liver injury in children, a biliary leak requiring delayed treatment was noticed in 3% (Moulton et al. 1993).

Spontaneous closure of major or peripheral bile duct leaks has occasionally been reported in patients with liver injury. Patients had either bile peritonitis or bile discharge through a surgical drain. Mean duration for closure of the fistula was 33 days. Although there was no mortality, a median of four complications occurred, reflecting severity of associated liver injury (Hollands and Little 1991).

6.8 Conclusion

As most significant injuries to the bile ducts are caused by penetrating injury, detailed preoperative imaging is often not obtained. US or CT are able to establish the diagnosis of injury to the gallbladder, but injury to the extrahepatic bile ducts is a difficult diagnosis. Nuclear medicine studies and ERC are more powerful diagnostic modalities than cross-section imaging. A high index of suspicion is necessary to establish the diagnosis early, before complications occur. Endoscopic or percutaneous temporary stenting has a definite role in the treatment of posttraumatic biliary fistulae or late stricture. Intrahepatic or perihepatic bilomas should be liberally aspirated or drained with cross-section imaging guidance for diagnosis and treatment, to avoid chronic fistulization, bile duct obstruction, abscess, and hemorrhage.

References

Abou-Mourad NN, Rogers LS (1980) Extrahepatic biliary steering wheel trauma simulating pancreatic carcinoma – a dilemma in management. J Trauma 20:180–182

Ackerman NB, Sillin LF, Suresh K (1985) Consequences of intraperitoneal bile: bile ascites versus bile peritonitis. Am J Surg 149:244–246

Alanen A, Kormand M (1985) Correlation of the echogenecity and structure of clotted blood. J Ultrasound Med 4:421–425

Alawneh I (1981) Historische Bemerkungen über Gallenwegtrauma. Aktuel Traumatol 11:231–233

Ali M (1975) Avulsion of the gallbladder in blunt abdominal trauma. Injury 6:334

Ando H, Ito T, Watanabe Y, Seo T, Kanebo K, Nagaya M (1995) Spontaneous perforation of choledochal cyst. J Am Coll Surg 181:125–128

Arkovitz MS, Liang H, Pachter HL, Alexander P, Newman RM, Gittes GK (1999) Complete biliary avulsion from blunt compression injury. J Pediatr Surg 34:1559–1562

Atik M (1976) Operative cholangiography and special technical consideration in the management of severe injury of the liver. Surg Gynecol Obstet 143:741–748

Bade PG, Thomson SR, Hirschberg A, Robbs JV (1989) Surgical options in traumatic injury to the extrahepatic biliary tract. Br J Surg 76:256–258

Ball DS, Friedman AC, Radecki PD, Caroilne DF (1988) Avulsed gallbladder: CT appearance. J Comput Assist Tomogr 12: 538–539

Balogh K (1984) Pulmonary bile emboli. Sequelae of iatrogenic trauma. Arch Pathol Lab Med 108:814–816

Balsano N, Reynolds B (1973) Rupture of the common duct and ampulla of Vater due to blunt trauma. Ann Surg 178: 200–203

Barclay GR, Crampton JR (1987) ERCP in late post-traumatic biliary fistula. Postgrad Med J 63:147–149

Barker SL, Fromm D (1987) Bile peritonitis following expectant management of liver fracture. N Y State J Med 87:565–567

Bar-Maor JA, Shoshany G (1994) Traumatic rupture of the choledochus treated temporarily by Roux-en-Y entero-hepato-duodenal ligamentostomy. J Pediatr Surg 29:1578–1579

Barthel JS, Sastri SV, Landsbaum C (1989) Closure of cystic duct stump leak by nasobiliary tube drainage. J Clin Gastroenterol 11:574–577

Battersby C (1978) Ruptured choledochal cyst: recognition and management. Aust N Z J Surg 48:515–517

Battle WH (1894) Traumatic rupture of the common bile duct. Transact Clin Soc 27:144–148

Berkelhammer C, Kortan P, Haber GB (1989) Endoscopic biliary prostheses as treatment for benign postoperative bile duct strictures. Gastrointest Endosc 35:95–101

Berland LL, Doust BD, Foley WD (1980) Acute hemorrhage into the gallbladder diagnosed by computed tomography and ultrasonography. J Comput Assist Tomogr 4:260–262

Bin Yahib S, Al Rabeeah A, Al Sammarrai A (1999) An unusual bile duct injury in a child after blunt abdominal trauma. J Pediatr Surg 34:1161–1163
Bismuth H (1982) Postoperative strictures of the bile duct. In: Blumgart LH (ed) The biliary tract. Churchill Livingstone, Edinburgh, pp 209–218
Blum M, Fiedler C, Winde G, Pircher W, von Bassewitz B (1987) Bilhemia – a review of diagnosis and therapy. Chirurg 58: 482–486
Blum U, Buitrago-Tellez C, El Seif M, Wimmer B (1993) Posttraumatic bilhemia: conservative management by percutaneous drainage. Cardiovasc Intervent Radiol 16:55–57
Blumgart LH (1969) Rupture of gallbladder associated with intraperitoneal rupture of urinary bladder. Br J Surg 56:76–77
Blumgart LH, Kelly CJ, Benjamin IS (1984) Benign bile duct stricture following cholecystectomy: critical factors in management. Br J Surg 71:836–843
Boll K, Belber JP (1978) Diagnosis of gangrene and perforation of the gallbladder by endoscopic retrograde cholangiography. Ann Surg 191:641–648
Borocco A, Bosson N, Leroux C, Ducou-Le-Pointe H, Montagne JP (1996) Cholangioscanner en mode spiralé et reconstructions tridimensionnelles de l'arbre biliaire chez l'enfant. J Radiol 77:663–666
Bosworth BM (1948) Perforation of the small intestine from non-penetrating abdominal trauma. Am J Surg 76:472–479
Bourque MD, Spigland N, Bensoussan AL, Garel L, Blanchard H (1989) Isolated complete transection of common bile duct due to trauma in a child, and review of the literature. J Pediatr Surg 24:1068–1070
Brase A, Neuhaus P, Nvic M (1976) External biliary fistula following severe rupture of the liver. Röntgenblätter 29: 529–532
Brown HP Jr (1932) Traumatic cholecystectomy. Ann Surg 95: 952–953
Brugge WR, Rosenberg DJ, Alavi A (1994) Diagnosis of postoperative bile leaks. Am J Gastroenterol 89:2178–2183
Buckley A, Connon JJ (1990) The role of ERCP in children and adolescents. Gastrointest Endosc 36:369–372
Bunt TJ, Weimar R, Malone JM (1990) Porta hepatitis disruption from blunt trauma. Am Surg 56:695–696
Burmeister W, Koppen MO, Wurbs D (1985) Treatment of a biliocutaneous fistula by endoscopic insertion of a nasobiliary tube. Gastrointest Endosc 31:279–281
Burt TB, Nelson JA (1981) Extrahepatic biliary duct trauma – a spectrum of injuries. West J Med 134:283–289
Busuttil RW, Kitahama A, Cerise E, McFadden M, Lo R, Longmire WP Jr (1980) Management of blunt and penetrating injuries to the porta hepatis. Ann Surg 191:641–648
Bynoe RP, Bell RM, Miles WS et al (1992) Complications of nonoperative management of blunt hepatic injury. J Trauma 32:308–315
Carabalona P, Vernhet J, Bonnel F (1973) Associated rupture of the liver, both hepatic arteries, the portal vein and the common bile duct following abdominal contusion. Chirurgie 98:764–767
Carmichael DH (1980) Avulsion of the common bile duct by blunt trauma. South Med J 73:166–168
Chacko KN, Jesudason SRB, Ninan S (1996) Percutaneous removal of a bullet from the liver. Br J Surg 83:180
Charters AC, Bardin J (1978) Intrahepatic bile duct rupture following blunt abdominal trauma. Arch Surg 113:873–876
Chartrand-Lefèbvre C, Dufresne MP, Lafortune M, Lapointe R, Dagenais M, Roy A (1994) Iatrogenic injury to the bile duct: a working classification for radiologists. Radiology 193:523–526
Chow LW, Gertsch P, Cheung KL, Leung SY (1996) Intrapancreatic avulsion of common bile duct after blunt abdominal trauma. Eur J Surg 162:519–521
Christensen PB, Joergensen EO, Schoubye J et al (1981) Scintigraphy with 99m-Tc-HIDA (2–6 diethyl acetanildeiminodiacetic acid) as a diagnostic test in traumatic lesions of the liver and biliary tract. Gastrointest Radiol 6:43–46
Chung YC, Lee PH, Huang MT, Chang CN (1993) Complete transection of common bile duct due to blunt abdominal trauma: a case report and literature review. J Formos Med Assoc 92:78–81
Ciraulo DL, Luk S, Palter M et al (1998) Selective hepatic arterial embolization of grade IV and V blunt hepatic injuries: an extension of resuscitation in the nonoperative management of traumatic hepatic injuries. J Trauma 45:353–359
Citron SJ, Martin LG (1991) Benign biliary strictures: treatment with percutaneous cholangioplasty. Radiology 178:339–341
Clancy T, Warren RL (1997) Endoscopic treatment of biliary colic resulting from hemobilia after nonoperative management of blunt hepatic injury: case report and review of the literature. J Trauma 43:527–529
Coletti PM, Barakos JM, Ralls RE et al (1987) Hepatobiliary scintigraphy and scintiangiography in abdominal trauma. Clin Nucl Med 12:901–905
Colovic R, Perisic-Savic M (1991) Retroperitoneal biloma secondary to operative common bile duct injury. HPB Surg 3:193–197
Cope Z (1925) Extravasation of bile. Br J Surg 13:120
Coulter DF (1948) Traumatic delayed rupture of the gallbladder in a child aged 9. Br Med J i:198
Cox EF (1984) Blunt abdominal trauma, a 5-year analysis of 870 patients requiring celiotomy. Ann Surg 199:467–474
Croce MA, Fabian TC, Menke PG et al (1995) Nonoperative management of blunt hepatic trauma is the treatment of choice for hemodynamically stable patients: result of a prospective trial. Ann Surg 221:744–755
Daneman A, Matzinger MA, Martin DJ (1983) Posttraumatic hemorrhage into the gallbladder. J Comput Tomogr 7: 59–61
Davids PHP, Rauws EAJ, Coene PP et al (1992) Endoscopic stenting for post-operative biliary strictures. Gastrointest Endosc 38:12–18
Davids PHP, Tanka AKF, Rauws EAJ et al (1993) Benign biliary strictures. Surgery or endoscopy? Ann Surg 217:237–243
Dawson DL, Jurkovich GJ (1991) Hepatic duct disruption from blunt abdominal trauma: case report and literature review. J Trauma 31:698–702
Dawson SL, Mueller PR (1994) Interventional radiology in the management of bile duct injuries. Surg Clin North Am 74: 865–874
Dawson DL, Johansen KH, Jurkovich GJ (1991) Injuries to the portal triad. Am J Surg 161:545–551
De Backer A, Fierens H, de Schepper A, Pelckmans P, Jorens PG, Vaneerdeweg W (1998) Diagnosis and nonsurgical management of bile leak complicated by biloma after blunt liver injury: report of two cases. Eur Radiol 8:1619–1622
Delaitre B, Meradji B, Mentouri B, Lemaigre G (1976) Gangrenous cholecystitis during traumatic hemobilia. Nouv Presse Med 5:2169

Delany HM, Jason RS (1981) Abdominal trauma: surgical and radiologic diagnosis. Springer, Berlin Heidelberg New York, p 153
Del Olmo L, Merona E, Moreira VF et al (1988) Successful treatment of postoperative external biliary fistulas by endoscopic sphincterotomy. Gastrointest Endosc 34:307–309
De Luna Vargas MA, Gonzalez-Ojeda A, Cardenas-Chavez O et al (1996) Acute acalculous cholecystitis in patients with severe trauma. Rev Gastroenterol Med 61:348–355
Dennison KG, Khoury D, Heironiums JD (1990) Gallbladder perforation during liver biopsy diagnosed using hepatobiliary scintigraphy: a case report. J Clin Nucl Med 15:95–96
Depolo A, Rahelic V, Uravic M (1999) Intra-pancreatic rupture of the bile duct. Hepatogastroenterology 46:2616–2620
Deviere J, van Gansbeke D, Ansay J, de Toeuf J, Cremer M (1987) Endoscopic management of a posttraumatic biliary fistula. Endoscopy 19:136–139
Diethrich EB, Beall AC Jr, Jordan GL Jr, de Backey ME (1966) Traumatic injuries to the extrahepatic biliary tract. Am J Surg 112:756–759
Dinkel HP, Moll R, Gassel HJ et al (1999) Helical CT cholangiography for the detection and localization of bile duct leakage. AJR 173:613–617
Dixon A (1887) A case of rupture of gallbladder "cholecystectomy" subsequent obstruction of common bile duct by overlooked impacted calculous death. Ann Surg 5: 321–325
Douglas JN, Luck RJ (1974) Late obstructive jaundice due to traumatic pancreatic granuloma. Injury 6:60–62
Drysdale TM (1861) Case of rupture of the common duct of the liver. Formation of a cyst containing bile. Death occurring on the fifty-third day. Autopsy. Am J Med Sci 12:399–404
Dumonceau JM, Deviere J, Delhaye M et al (1998) Plastic and metal stents for postoperative benign bile duct strictures: the best and the worst. Gastrointest Endosc 47:8–17
Dupriest RW Jr, Khaneja SC, Cowley RA (1979) Acute cholecystitis complicating trauma. Ann Surg 189:84–89
Durham RM, Buckley J, Keegan M, Fravell S et al (1992) Management of blunt hepatic injuries. Am J Surg 164: 477–481
Eid A, Almogy G, Pikasky AJ, Binenbaum Y, Shiloni E, Rivkind A (1996) Conservative treatment of a traumatic tear of the left hepatic duct: case report. J Trauma 41:912–913
Ellis H, Cronin K (1960) Bile peritonitis. Br J Surg 48: 166–171
Elmslie R, White TT (1966) An investigation into trypsin in the pancreaticobiliary tree. Br J Surg 53:586–593
Epstein HJ, Lipshutz B (1952) Hemobilia, cholecystitis and gastrointestinal bleeding with rupture of the liver. JAMA 149:1132–1133
Erb RE, Mirvis SE, Shanmuganathan K (1994) Gallbladder injury secondary to blunt trauma: CT findings. J Trauma 18:778–784
Ernst O, Sergent G, Mizrahi D, Delemazure O, L'Hermine C (1999) Biliary leaks: treatment by means of percutaneous transhepatic biliary drainage. Radiology 21:345–348
Esensten M, Ralls PW, Colletti P, Halls J (1983) Posttraumatic intrahepatic biloma: sonographic diagnosis. AJR 140: 303–305
Estrada RL, Sutherland NG (1969) Subparietal or non-penetrating traumatic rupture of the biliary tree. Br J Surg 56:85–91
Farron F, Gudinchet F, Genton N (1996) Hepatic trauma in children: long-term follow-up. Eur J Pediatr Surg 6: 347–349
Feliciano DV (1994) Biliary injuries as a result of blunt and penetrating trauma. Surg Clin North Am 74:897–907
Feliciano DV, Bitondo CG, Burch JM, Mattox KL, Beall AC Jr, Jordan GL Jr (1985) Management of traumatic injuries to the extrahepatic biliary ducts. Am J Surg 150:705–709
Fielding JWL, Strachan CJL (1975) Jaundice as a sign of delayed gallbladder perforation following blunt abdominal trauma. Injury 7:66–67
Fish JC, Johnson GL (1965) Rupture of the duodenum following blunt trauma: report of a case with avulsion of papilla of Vater. Ann Surg 162:917–919
Fizeau M (1806) Observation sur une rupture du conduit cholédoque, avec épanchement de bile dans le ventre; suivie d'autres observations analogues, puisées dans les auteurs, et de réflexions sur la couleur jaune des ictériques. J Med Chir Pharma Col 12:171–184
Fletcher WS (1972) Nonpenetrating trauma to the gallbladder and extrahepatic bile ducts. Surg Clin North Am 52: 711–717
Fletcher WS, Mahnke EE, Dunphy JE (1961) Complete division of the common bile duct due to blunt trauma. J Trauma 1: 87–95
Foley DW, Cates JD, Kellman GM et al (1987) Treatment of blunt hepatic injuries: role of CT. Radiology 164:635–638
Forster E, Wyart A, Peter C, Mariano A, Kassen S (1977) Rupture of the choledochus and the gastroduodenal artery, portal lesion and laceration of the liver caused by a closed injury. Chirurgie 103:714–716
Frahm W, Freese P (1980) Injury of the right hepatic duct following percutaneous transhepatic cholangiography. Zentralbl Chir 105:611–613
Francois D, Warland S, van Nieuwenhuize JP, de Ville de Goyet J, Pauwels S (1994) Hepatobiliary scintigraphy in a patient with bilhemia. Eur J Nucl Med 21:1020–1023
Frank DJ, Pereiras R, Souza-Lima MS et al (1976) Traumatic rupture of the gallbladder with massive biliary ascites. JAMA 240:252–253
Franklin DC, Mathai J (1980) Biliary pleural fistula: a complication of hepatic trauma. J Trauma 20:256–258
Froment P, Pelloni A, Rouijel J, Gertsch P (1998) Closed injuries of the intrahepatic bile ducts – clinical presentation, diagnosis and treatment. Swiss Surg 5:228–231
Fulcher AS, Turner MA, Capps GW, Zfass AM, Baker KM (1998) Half-Fourier RARE MR cholangiopancreatography: experience in 300 subjects. Radiology 207:21–32
Funaki B, Zaleski GX, Straus CA et al (1999) Percutaneous biliary drainage in patients with nondilated intrahepatic bile ducts. AJR 173:1541–1544
Gable DR, Allen JW, Harrell DJ, Carillo EH (1997) Endoscopic treatment of posttraumatic "bilhemia": case report. J Trauma 43:534–536
Gallacher DJ, Kadir S, Kaufman SL et al (1985) Nonoperative management of benign postoperative biliary strictures. Radiology 156:625–629
Garcia Urguelles X, Uroz Tristan J, Avila Suarez R, Alonso Jimenez L (1996) Intrahepatic biloma. Conservative management with external drainage. CIR Pediatr 9:85–87
Garrett RW (1900) Traumatic rupture of the bile duct. Ann Surg 31:227
Gartman DM, Zeman RK, Cahow CE, Baker CC (1985) The

value of hepatobiliary scanning in complex liver trauma. J Trauma 25:887–891

Gately JF, Thomas EJ (1985) Post-traumatic ischemic necrosis of the common bile duct. Can J Surg 28:32–33

Geenen DJ, Geenen JE, Hogan WJ et al (1989) Endoscopic therapy for benign bile duct strictures. Gastrointest Endosc 35:367–371

Gerndt SJ, Seidel SP, Taheri PA, Rodriguez JL (1995) Biliary tract injury following blunt abdominal trauma: case reports. J Trauma 39:612–615

Gilbert D, Dimarino AJ Jr, Jensen DM et al (1991) Status evaluation of biliary stents. Position paper by American Society of Gastroenterologists, Technology Assessment Committee, December

Glaser K, Wetscher G, Pointner R et al (1994) Traumatic bilhemia. Surgery 116:24–27

Goldin E, Katz E, Wengrower D et al (1990) Treatment of fistulas of the biliary tract by endoscopic insertion of endoprostheses. Surg Gynecol Obstet 170:418–423

Goldman SM, Diamond A, Salik JO (1976) Intrahepatic rupture secondary to duct exploration demonstration by cholangiography. Radiology 118:13–17

Golematis B, Bramis J, Antonopoulos K, Charitopoulos N, Melissas J, Papalabros E (1978) Spontaneous (nontraumatic) perforation of the common bile duct: report of three cases. Am Surg 44:734–741

Gottesman L, Marks RA, Khoury PT, Moallem AG, Wichern WA (1984) Diagnosis of isolated perforation of the gallbladder following blunt trauma using sonography and CT scan. J Trauma 24:280–281

Gould L, Patel A (1979) Ultrasound detection of extrahepatic encapsulated bile: "biloma". AJR 132:1014–1015

Graff RJ (1963) Considerations in the treatment of traumatic hemobilia. Am J Surg 105:662

Griffen M, Ochoa J, Boulanger BR (2000) A minimally invasive approach to bile peritonitis after blunt liver injury. Am Surg 66:309–312

Griswold RA, Collier HS (1961) Collective review: blunt abdominal trauma. Surg Gynecol Obstet 112:309–329

Haberlik A, Cendron M, Sauer H (1992) Biliovenous fistula in children after blunt liver trauma: proposal for a simple surgical treatment. J Pediatr Surg 27:1203–1206

Haddad M, Aoun N, Rizk G (1986) Demonstration of a traumatic bronchobiliary fistula by cholescintigraphy with 99m technetium-EHIDA. J Radiol 67:345–347

Hadjis NS, Blumgart LH (1988) Injury to segmental bile ducts. A reappraisal. Arch Surg 123:351–353

Haff RC, Butcher HR Jr, Ballinger WF Jr (1969) Biliary tract operations: a review of 1000 patients. Arch Surg 98: 428–434

Hagiwara A, Yukiota T, Shimazaki S, Megawa T, Matuda H (1993) Delayed hemorrhage following transcatheter arterial embolization for blunt hepatic injury. Cardiovasc Interv Radiol 16:380–383

Hagiwara A, Yukiota T, Ohta S et al (1997) Nonsurgical management of patients with blunt hepatic injury: efficacy of transcatheter arterial embolization. AJR 169:1151–1156

Hall ER, Howard JM, Jordan GL, Mikesky WE (1956) Traumatic injuries of the gallbladder. Ann Surg 72:520–524

Halme L, Orko R, Tierala E, Hockerstedt K (1994) Late biliary stenosis after conservative management of traumatic liver rupture: case report. J Trauma 36:740–742

Hanazaki K, Machida E, Sodeyama H et al (1995) Chronic cholecystitis following hemobilia due to traumatic intrahepatic injury. Surg Endosc 9:1004–1007

Harrell DJ, Vitale GC, Larson GM (1998) Selective role for endoscopic retrograde cholangiopancreatography in abdominal trauma. Surg Endosc 12:400–404

Harris VJ, Kopecky KK, Harman JT, Crist DW (1993) Percutaneous transhepatic drainage of the nondilated biliary system. J Vasc Intervent Radiol 4:591–595

Hartle RJ, McGarrity TJ, Conter RL (1993) Treatment of a giant biloma and bile leak by ERCP stent placement. Am J Gastroenterol 88:2117–2118

Hartman SW, Greaney EM Jr (1964) Traumatic injuries to the biliary system in children. Am J Surg 108:150–153

Haynes CD, Given KS, Stone HH et al (1969) Nonsurgical trauma to the extrahepatic bile ducts. South Med J 62:1323–1326

Henzel JH, Belssing WD, Deweese MS (1971) Intrahepatic biliary disruption. Report of two cases occurring during use of balloon-tipped biliary catheters. Arch Surg 102:218–220

Hockerstedt K, Airo I, Karaharju AE, Sundin A (1982) Abdominal trauma and laparotomy in 158 patients, a comparative study of penetrating and blunt injury. Acta Chir Scand 148:9–14

Hoff WS, Ginsberg GG, Grossman MD, Reilly PM, Kauder DR, Schwab CW (1998) Traumatic choledochogastric fistula: endoscopic evaluation and treatment with biliary stent. J Trauma 45:1094–1096

Hoffman E (1956) Acute gangrenous cholecystitis secondary to trauma. Am J Surg 91:288–289

Hollands MJ, Little JM (1991) Post-traumatic bile fistulae. J Trauma 31:117–120

Hopson WB, Sherman RT, Sanders JW (1966) Stab wounds of the abdomen: 5-year review of 297 cases. Am Surg 32: 213–218

Horattas MC, Lewis RD, Fenton AH, Awender HM (1994) Modern concepts in nonsurgical management of traumatic biliary fistulas. J Trauma 36:186–189

Horiguchi J, Ohwada S, Tanahashi Y et al (1998) Traumatic biliary stricture successfully treated by percutaneous transhepatic bile duct dilatation; a case report. Hepatogastroenterology 45:2038–2041

Howdieshell TR, Hawkins ML, Osler TM, Demarest GB (1990) Management of blunt hepatic duct transection by ligation. South Med J 83:579–583

Howdieshell TR, Purvis J, Bates WB, Teeslink CR (1995) Biloma and biliary fistula following hepatorrhaphy for liver trauma: incidence, natural history and management. Am Surg 61: 165–168

Huguet C, Bloch P (1977) Peroperative cholangiography in liver trauma. J Chir (Paris) 114:351–360

Huibregtse RM, Kanton RM, Tytgat GNJ (1986) Endoscopic treatment of postoperative biliary strictures. Endoscopy 18:133–137

Huljic P, Knaepler H (1982) Stumpfes Bauchtrauma und Choledochusruptur bei Choledochuskonkrementen – Fragen des Zusammenhangs. Chirurg 53:137–139

Hung SY, Chen HM, Jan YY, Chen MF (2000) Common bile duct and pancreatic injury after extracorporeal shock wave lithotripsy for renal stone. Hepatogastroenterology 47:1162–1163

Hunt JA, Gallagher PJ, Heintze SW, Waugh R, Shiel BG (1997) Percutaneous microcoil embolization of intraperitoneal intrahepatic and extrahepatic biliary fistulas. Aust N Z J Surg 67:424–427

Ireneus C Jr (1942) Traumatic hemorrhagic cholecystitis with hematemesis and shock as the presenting symptoms. Am J Surg 56:655–658

Irie H, Honda H, Taijma T et al (1998) Optimal MR cholangi opancreaticographic sequence and its clinical application. Radiology 206:379–387

Ito T, Yamamoto M, Machida H, Hashiguichi Y, Yatsuda N, Yasuda M (1993) Complete avulsion of the papilla of Vater and gastroduodenal artery due to blunt abdominal trauma: report of a case. Surg Today 23:172–175

Itoh H, Shimono R, Hamamoto K (1987) Liver trauma with bile leakage by hepatobiliary scintigraphy. Clin Nucl Med 12:72–73

Ivatury RR, O'Shea J, Rohman M (1984) Posttraumatic thoracobiliary fistula. J Trauma 24:438–442

Ivatury RR, Rohman M, Nallathambi M et al (1985) The morbidity of injuries of the extrahepatic biliary system. J Trauma 25:967–973

Janowitz P, Janowitz A, Schumacher KA, Wechsler JG, Ditschuneit H (1992) Occult gallbladder perforation: an unusual complication of gallstone lithotripsy. Hepatogastroenterology 39:43–46

Janss G, Freimark L (1979) Isolated transection of the common duct. JACEP 8:161–163

Jarnagin WR, Blumgart LH (1999) Operative repair of bile duct injuries involving the hepatic duct confluence. Arch Surg 134:769–775

Jeffrey RB, Federle MP, Laing FC, Wing VW (1986) Computed tomography of blunt trauma to the gallbladder. J Comput Assist Tomogr 10:756–758

Jenkins MA, Ponsky JL (1995) Endoscopic retrograde cholangiopancreatography and endobiliary stenting in the treatment of biliary injury resulting from liver trauma. Surg Laparosc Endosc 5:118–120

Jones KB, Thomas E (1985) Traumatic rupture of the hepatic duct demonstrated by endoscopic retrograde cholangiography. J Trauma 25:448–449

Jurkovich GJ, Hoyt DB, Moore FA et al (1995) Portal triad injuries. J Trauma 39:426–434

Kaehr D, Jones LM, Miller SF, Finley RK (1984) Traumatic cholecystectomy. J Trauma 24:544–545

Kalderon AE, Sobel HJ (1965) Retroperitoneal rupture of the common bile duct. Arch Surg 90:188

Kasai T, Nakatani T, Hirosawa K, Kobayashi K (1993) Benign stricture of the extrahepatic bile duct following hepatectomy for traumatic hepatic rupture. Intensive Care Med 19:472–477

Kaufman SL, Kadir S, Mitchell SE et al (1985) Percutaneous transhepatic biliary drainage for bile leaks and fistulas. AJR 144:1055–1058

Kauzlaric D, Barmier E (1985) Sonography of intraluminal gallbladder hematoma. J Clin Ultrasound 13:291–294

Kawarada Y, Tani K, Yoshimine S, Mizumoto R (1984) Blunt injury of duodenum with avulsion of papilla of Vater – report of a case. Jpn J Surg 14:499–504

Kehr H (1892) Über einen durch ideale Cholezystostomie geheilten Fall von Schussverletzungen der Gallenblase. Zentralbl Chir 19:645–647

Kernes z (1892) A case of lesion of the gall-ducts. Ann Surg 16:393

Kernohan RM, Humphreys WG (1985) Closed abdominal trauma in a child causing avulsion of the common bile duct and gastric stasis. Injury 16:235–237

Khodadadi J, Mihich M, Finally R, Milleritzky M (1983) Avulsion of common bile duct after blunt abdominal injury: a review of the literature. Injury 14:447–450

Kitahama A, Elliott LF, Overby JL, Webb WR (1982) The extrahepatic biliary tract injury: perspective in diagnosis and treatment. Ann Surg 196:536–540

Koch RL, Gorder JL (1969) Bile-blood fistula: a complication of percutaneous transhepatic cholangiography. Radiology 93:67–68

Koda M, Okamoto K, Miyoshi Y, Kawasaki H (1992) Hepatic vascular and bile duct injury after ethanol injection therapy for hepatocellular carcinoma. Gastrointest Radiol 17:167–169

Koplewitz BZ, Manson DE, Ein SH (1999) Posttraumatic torsion of accessory lobe of the liver and the gallbladder. Pediatr Radiol 29:799–802

Koslin DB, Stanley RJ, Berland LL, Shin MS, Dalton SC (1988) Hepatic perivascular lymphoedema: CT appearance. AJR 150:111–113

Kozarek RA (1994) Endoscopic techniques in management of biliary tract injuries. Surg Clin North Am 74:883–893

Kozarek RA, Ball TJ, Patterson DJ et al (1994) Endoscopic treatment of biliary injury in the era of laparoscopic cholecystectomy. Gastrointest Endosc 40:10–16

Kramer W, Veihelmann D, Neugebauer W (1985) Acute post-traumatic cholecystitis. Caused by or following polytrauma? Aktuel Traumatol 15:73–75

Krishna A, Kaul PB, Murali MV et al (1992) Isolated extrahepatic bile duct injury: diagnosis and surgical management. Pediatr Surg Int 7:143–145

Krishnamurthy B, Jagdish S, Pai D, Babu P (1997) Transection of common bile duct following blunt injury to abdomen. Indian J Gastroenterol 16:109–110

Kruuna OJ, Haapiainen RK, Kivilaadso EO (1994) Penetrating liver laceration with complete transgression of hilar structures presenting with minimal clinical signs. Ann Chir Gynaecol 83:73–75

Laffey PA, Brandon JC, Teplick SK, Haskin PH, Pavlides CA (1988) Ultrasound of hemobilia: a clinical and experimental study. J Clin Ultrasound 16:167–170

Lau LL, Diamond T (1997) Delayed presentation of porta hepatis injury following blunt abdominal trauma. HPB Surg 10:249–252

Lauenberger J, Bücheri M, Schneider B, Blum U, Hennig J, Langer M (1995) Breath-hold projection magnetic resonance-cholangiopancreaticography (MRCP): a new method for the examination of the bile and pancreatic ducts. Magn Reson Med 33:18–23

Leber RE, Hume HA (1971) Blunt rupture of the hepatic artery: a report of two unusual cases. J Trauma 11:625–628

Lee JG, Wherry DC (1961) Traumatic rupture of the extrahepatic biliary ducts from external trauma. J Trauma 1:105

Lee D, Zacher J, Vogel TT (1976) Primary repair in transection of duodenum with avulsion of the common duct. Arch Surg 111:592–593

Lee MG, Lee HJ, Kim MH, Kang EM, Kim YH, Lee SG, Kim PN, Ha HK, Auh YH (1997) Extrahepatic biliary diseases: 3DMR cholangiopancreaticography compared with endoscopic retrograde cholangiopancreaticography. Radiology 202: 663–669

Leekam RN, Ilves R, Shankar L (1987) Inversion of gallbladder secondary to traumatic herniation of liver: CT findings. J Comput Assist Tomogr 11:163–164

Lehto M, Vilkki P (1985) Intraperitoneal hepatic bile duct fistulae following blunt abdominal contusion. Ann Chir Gynaecol 74:296–298

Letoublon C, Castaing D (1996) Blunt injuries of the liver. Blackwell, Paris

Leung JWC, Chung SCS, Sung JY, Metreweli C (1988) Endoscopic management of postoperative biliary fistula. Surg Endosc 2:190–193

Lewerenz z (1903) Über die subkutanen Verletzungen der Gallenwege traumatischen Ursprungs nebst einem kasuistischen Beitrag. Langenbecks Arch Klin Chir 71: 111–146

Lewis KM (1938) Traumatic rupture of the bile ducts. Ann Surg 108:237–242

Lifshits IZ, Semin MD, Usenko AI, Zamskova MV (1989) Migration of a fragment of liver parenchyma into the common bile duct. Vrach Delo 1:87–88

Liguory C, Vitale GC, Lefebre JF et al (1991) Endoscopic treatment of postoperative biliary fistulae. Surgery 110: 779–784

Lillemoe KD, Melton GB, Cameron JL et al (2000) Postoperative bile duct strictures: management and outcome in the 1990. Ann Surg 232:430–441

Lineaweaver W, Robertson J, Rumley T (1985) PIPIDA scan diagnosis of traumatic rupture of the gallbladder. Injury 16:238–240

Longmire W Jr (1966) Early management of injury to the extrahepatic biliary duct. JAMA 195:623

Maier WP, Lightfoot WP, Rosemond GP (1968) Extrahepatic biliary ductal injury in closed trauma. Am J Surg 116: 103–108

Mangiante EC, Brown L, Fabian TC (1987) Isolated blunt disruption of the common bile duct. J Tenn Med Assoc 80: 484–484

Marks JM, Ponsky JL, Shililngstad RB, Singh J (1998) Biliary stenting is more effective than sphincterotomy in the resolution of biliary leaks. Surg Endosc 12:327–330

Marshall DG, Brabyn DG, Vezina WC (1984) Spontaneous perforation of the common bile duct in infancy detected by 99mTc HIDA scanning. Can J Surg 27:590–591

Mason LB, Sidbury JB, Guiarg S (1954) Rupture of the extrahepatic bile ducts from nonpenetrating trauma. Ann Surg 140:234–241

McFadden PM, Tanner G, Kitihama A (1980) Traumatic hepatic duct injury. Am J Surg 139:268–271

McGillivray DC, Valentine RJ (1989) Nonoperative management of blunt pediatric liver injury – late complications: case report. J Trauma 29:251–254

McLindon JP, England RE, Martin DF (1998) Causes, clinical features and non-operative management of bile leaks. Eur Radiol 8:1602–1607

McNabney WK, Rudek R, Pemberton LB (1990) The significance of gallbladder trauma. J Emerg Med 3:277–280

Mehta SN, Reinhold C, Barkun AN (1997) Magnetic resonance cholangiopancreatography. Gastrointest Endosc Clin North Am 7:247–270

Meyers WC (1994) Commentary. Interventional radiology in the management of bile duct injuries. Surg Clin North Am 74:875–877

Michel P, Passicos J, Pagliano G (1992) External biliary fistula after right lateral sectorial hepatectomy for liver injury. Recovered by cholecysto-fistulous anastomosis. Ann Chir 46:940–943

Michelassi F, Ranson JHC (1985) Bile duct disruption by blunt trauma. J Trauma 25:454–457

Mitchell R, Kerr R, Barton J, Schmidt A (1991) Biliary obstruction secondary to a shrapnel. Am J Gastroenterol 86:153–154

Mitre RJ, Brodmerkel GJ Jr (1979) Traumatic rupture of the gallbladder: preoperative diagnosis by endoscopic retrograde cholangiopancreatography (ERCP). Gastrointest Endosc 25:74–75

Miyakawa S, Mizuno K, Horiguchi A, Hayakawa M, Ischimara S, Miura K (1996) Complete transection of the left hepatic duct due to blunt abdominal trauma. Hepatogastroenterology 43:1395–1398

Moller R, Schroeder U (1985) [Obstructive jaundice 64 years after a grenade splinter injury of the liver.] Chirurg 56: 532–534

Monk JS, Church JS, Agarawal N (1991) Repair of a traumatic noncircumferential hepatic bile duct using a vein patch: case report. J Trauma 31:1555–1557

Montesano G, Bezzi G, Turano R, Gallinaro L, Forte A, Bezzi MC (1999) Lesions of the main bile duct: combined percutaneous endoscopic treatment. Ann Ital Chir 70: 421–424

Moore AV, Illescas FF, Mills SR et al (1987) Percutaneous dilation of benign biliary strictures. Radiology 156:625–629

Moore EE, Jurkovich GJ, Knudson MM et al (1995) Organ injury scaling VI: extrahepatic biliary, esophagus, stomach, vulva, vagina, uterus (nonpregnant), uterus (pregnant), fallopian tube, and ovary. J Trauma 39:1069–1070

Moosa AR, Easter DW, van Sonnenberg E et al (1992) Laparoscopic injuries to the bile duct: a cause of concern. Ann Surg 215:203–208

Moser JM, Schweizer W, Czermiak A, Baer HU (1995) Segmental bile duct injury after blunt abdominal trauma: a difficult diagnosis. Hepatogastroenterology 42:103–105

Moulton SL, Downey EC, Anderson DS, Lynch FP (1993) Blunt bile duct injuries in children. J Pediatr Surg 28:795–797

Moyle WD, Karl RC (1969) Rupture of the extrahepatic biliary ducts by external blunt trauma. J Trauma 9:623–628

Mueller PR, van Sonnenberg E, Ferrucci JT Jr et al (1986) Biliary stricture dilatation: multicenter review of clinical management in 73 patients. Radiology 160:17–22

Muin A, Leong YP, Tay SK (1992) Laceration of the common hepatic duct bifurcation by blunt abdominal trauma. Injury 23:422–423

Muller MF, Krestin GP, Weder W, Munch R, Wegmann A (1993) Spontaneous rupture of the left hepatic duct. Dtsch Med Wochenschr 118:377–380

Neeman A, Koren A, Reiss R, Kadish U (1988) Complete transection of the common bile duct diagnosed by endoscopic retrograde cholangiography. Gastrointest Radiol 13:167–168

Nishiwaki M, Ashida H, Nishimura T et al (1999) Posttraumatic intra-gallbladder hemorrhage in a patient with liver cirrhosis. J Gastroenterol 34:282–285

Okazaki M, Ono H, Higashi Hara H et al (1991) Angiographic management of massive hemobilia due to iatrogenic trauma. Gastrointest Radiol 16:204–205

Oldham KT, Guice KS, Ryckman F et al (1986) Blunt liver injury in childhood, evolution of therapy and current perspective. Surgery 100:542–549

Oliva VL, Nicolet V, Soulez G et al (1997) Bilomas developing after laparoscopic biliary surgery: percutaneous management

with embolization of biliary leaks. J Vasc Intervent Radiol 8:469–472
Oparah SS, Mandal AK (1978) Traumatic thoracobiliary (pleurobiliary and bronchobiliary) fistulas: clinical and review study. J Trauma 18:539–544
Ott DJ, Gilliam JH, Zagoria RJ, Young GP (1992) Intervention endoscopy of the biliary and pancreatic duct: current indications and methods. AJR 158:243–250
Pachter HL, Hofstetter SR (1995) The current status of nonoperative management of adult blunt hepatic injuries. Am J Surg 169:442–453
Pachter HL, Knudson MM, Esrig B, Ross S, Hoydt D, Cogbill T (1996) Status of nonoperative management of blunt hepatic injuries in 1995: a multicenter experience with 404 patients. J Trauma 40:31–38
Pandit SK, Budhiraja S, Rattan KN (2000) Posttraumatic bile ascites. Indian J Pediatr 67:72–73
Parkinson SW, Wisniewiski ZS (1978) Avulsion of the ampulla of Vater: an isolated injury following blunt abdominal trauma. Aust N Z J Surg 48:562–564
Parks RW, Diamond T (1995) Non-surgical trauma to the extrahepatic biliary tract. Br J Surg 82:1303–1310
Paymani M, Zajko AB, Campbell WL (1993) Bile leakage as a complication of liver biopsy in liver transplants. Abd Imaging 18:258–260
Pellegrini CA, Thomas MJ, Way LW (1984) Recurrent biliary stricture: patterns of recurrence and outcome of surgical therapy. Am J Surg 147:175–180
Penn I (1962) Injuries of the gallbladder. Br J Surg 49:636–641
Philippe JM, Tenière P, Testart J, Menard A, Bridoux J, Boutry P (1982) Rupture of the biliary tract in the liver hilum region following closed abdominal injuries. General review about 2 cases. J Chir (Paris) 1119:177–182
Pirola RC, Davis AE (1968) Effects of ethyl alcohol on sphincteric resistance at the choledochoduodenal junction in man. Gut 9:557–560
Pitt HA, Kaufman SL, Coleman J et al (1989) Benign postoperative biliary strictures. Operate or dilate. Ann Surg 210:417–427
Poli ML, Lefèbvre F, Ludot H, Bouche-Pillon MA, Daoud S, Tiefin G (1995) Nonoperative management of biliary tract fistulas after blunt abdominal trauma in a child. J Pediatr Surg 30:1719–1721
Ponchon T, Galez JF, Valette PJ et al (1989) Endoscopic treatment of biliary tract fistulas. Gastrointest Endosc 35:490–498
Ponsky JL (1996) Endoscopic approaches to common bile duct injuries. Surg Clin North Am 76:505–513
Porter MF (1898) Injuries of the gall ducts. Am J Obstet Dis Women 38:693–695
Posner MC, Moore EE (1985) Extrahepatic biliary tract injury: operative management plan. J Trauma 25:833–837
Powers TA, Melton RE (1982) Diagnosis of gallbladder perforation by Tc-99m disofenin cholescintigraphy. Clin Nucl Med 7:701–702
Rathnaraj S, Aggarwal S, Satija V, Verghese M (1994) Clot cholecystitis. Indian J Gastroenterol 13:69
Reichelt HG (1978) Hepatobiliary sequential scintigraphy. Chirurg 49:167–171
Rescorla FJ, Schlatter M, Hawes RH, Grosfeld JL (1996) Delayed presentation of a penetrating biliary tract injury in a child. J Trauma 40:157–158
Richter J (1969) Zur traumatischen Hemobilie. Zentralbl Chir 94:464–470
Roche B, Mentha G, Bugmann P, La Scala G, Le Coultre C (1993) Intrahepatic biliary lesions following blunt liver trauma in children – is nonpenetrative management or conservative operative treatment always safe? Eur J Pediatr Surg 3: 209–212
Rohatgi M, Gupta DK (1987) Isolated complete transection of common bile duct following blunt bicycle handlebar injury. J Pediatr Surg 22:1029–1030
Rossi P, Bezzi M, Salvatori F et al (1990) Recurrent benign biliary strictures: management with self-expanding metal stents. Radiology 175:661–665
Rothberg ML, Klingman RR, Peetz D, Ferraris VA, Berry WR (1994) Traumatic thoracobiliary fistula. Ann Thorac Surg 57:472–475
Rubio PA, Farrell EM, Berkman NL, Coan J (1986) Extravasation of contrast material due to rupture of intrahepatic duct: eight additional cases. South Med J 79:1165–1167
Rydell WB Jr (1970) Complete transection of the common bile duct due to blunt abdominal trauma. Arch Surg 100: 724–728
Ryu R, Novak Z, Coldwell D (1998) Percutaneous embolization of a posttraumatic nephrobiliary fistula. J Trauma 44: 389–391
Saad SA, Rush BF Jr, Devanesan JD, Lazaro EJ (1979) Traumatic hematocele of the gallbladder with hemobilia. J Trauma 19: 67–69
Saber K, El-Manialow M (1984) Repair of bile duct injuries. World J Surg 8:82–89
Safrany L, van Husen N, Kautz G, Wittrin G, Clemens M, Weitemeyer R (1978) Endoscopic retrograde cholangiography (ERC) in surgical emergencies. Ann Surg 187:20–23
Sakamoto Y, Tanaka N, Furuya T et al (1997) A simple stenting method for management of hepatic ductal injury secondary to blunt abdominal trauma: two case reports. J Trauma 42: 1165–1168
Salam M, Glowniak JV, Vetto RM, Jarboe JE, Haines JE, Krishnamurthy GT (1987) Detection of bile leakage from traumatic right hepatic duct laceration with technectium-99m DISIDA cholescintigraphy. Clin Nucl Med 12:589–591
Salman AB, Yildirgan MI, Celebi F (1996) Posttraumatic gallbladder torsion in a child. J Pediatr Surg 31:1586
Samhouri F, Gruenberg JC, Brown RS (1980) Intrahepatic-cutaneous biliary fistulas secondary to trauma. Henry Ford Hosp Med J 28:63–66
Sandblom P (1948) Hemorrhage into the biliary tract following trauma – traumatic hemobilia. Surgery 24:571–586
Sandblom P (1973) Hemobilia. Surg Clin North Am 53: 1191–1201
Sandor L, Bali I, Bozo A, Farkas G (1991) Ruptured retroperitoneal bile duct cyst. An extremely rare injury after blunt abdominal trauma. Unfallchirurg 94:360–362
Sata T, Higashi Y, Ono Y (1986) Sonography of gallbladder perforation: a complication of transcatheter hepatic arterial embolization. J Ultrasound Med 5:715–718
Sauerbruch T, Weinzierl M, Holl J et al (1986) Treatment of postoperative bile fistulas by internal endoscopic biliary drainage. Gastroenterology 90:1998–2003
Savitch I, Esser JD, Springolo E, Kew MC (1986) Demonstration of posttraumatic bile leak using technetium-99m DISIDA. Clin Nucl Med 11:873–874
Sax SL, Athey PA, Lamki N, Cadavid GA (1988) Sonographic findings in traumatic hemobilia: report of two cases and review of the literature. J Clin Ultrasound 16:29–34

Scaglione M, Rossi G, Pinto F et al (1998) Gallbladder blunt trauma: comparison between radiologic and anatomo-surgical findings. Radiol Med (Torino) 96:592–595
Schechter DS (1969) Solitary wounding of the gallbladder from blunt abdominal trauma. N Y State J Med 69:2895–2901
Schriefers KH (1968) The problem of bile duct injuries in stomach resection. Langenbecks Arch Chir 322:203–204
Schuster JA, Gutierrez OH, Azodo MV (1990) Erosion of portal vein catheter into the biliary system. Gastrointest Radiol 15:47–48
Scioscia PJ, Dillon PW, Cilley RE, Hoover WC, Krummel TM (1994) Endoscopic sphincterotomy in the management of posttraumatic biliary fistulae. J Pediatr Surg 29:3–6
Sclafani SJA, Shaftan GW, McAuley J, Nayaranaswamay T et al (1984) Interventional radiology in the management of hepatic trauma. J Trauma 24:256–262
Sewell JH (1966) Avulsion of the left hepatic duct. Ann Surg 165:628–631
Shahrudin MD, Noori SM (1997) Biloma and biliary fistula associated with hepatorrhaphy for liver injury. Hepatogastroenterology 44:519–521
Shanmuganathan K, Mirvis SE (1995) CT evaluation of the liver with acute blunt trauma. Crit Rev Diagn Imaging 36: 73–113
Shanmuganathan K, Mirvis SE (1998) CT scan evaluation of blunt hepatic trauma. Radiol Clin North Am 36:399–411
Sharma O (1995) Blunt gallbladder injuries: presentation of twenty-two cases with review of the literature. J Trauma 39:576–580
Sharma BC, Maini A, Saraswat VA (1997) Endoscopic management of perforation of right hepatic duct following non-surgical abdominal trauma. HPB Surg 10:245–247
Sheik-Gafoor MH, Singh B, Moodley J (1998) Traumatic thoracobiliary fistula: report of a case successfully managed conservatively, with an overview of current diagnostic and therapeutic options. J Trauma 45:819–821
Sheldon GF, Lim RC, Yee ES et al (1985) Management of injuries to the porta hepatis. Ann Surg 202:539–545
Sherman HF, Hilger JS, Jones LM, McAuley CE, Barrette RR (1992) Delayed diagnosis of extrahepatic biliary injury. Eur J Surg 158:575–578
Shigemura T, Yamamoto F, Shilpakar SK, Kojima T, Yamamoto S, Pu Y (1995) MRI differential diagnosis of intrahepatic biloma from subacute hematoma. Abdom Imaging 20: 211–213
Shorthouse AJ, Singh MP, Treasure T, Franklin RH (1978) Isolated complete transection of the common bile duct by blunt abdominal trauma. Br J Surg 65:543–545
Simstein NL (2000) Isolated blunt trauma to the hepatic duct. Int Surg 85:55–56
Skow JR, Longmire WP (1974) Common duct stricture secondary to blunt abdominal trauma. Am Surg 40: 576–587
Smadja C, Ratziu V, Poynard T, Chaput JC, Franco D (1993) Laparoscopic treatment without cholecystectomy for gallbladder perforation after biopsy. J Hepatol 18:381
Smith AC, Schapiro RH, Kelsey PB et al (1986) Successful treatment of nonhealing biliary-cutaneous fistulas with biliary stents. Gastroenterology 90:764–769
Smith EH, Soderberg CH Jr (1964) Traumatic rupture of the gallbladder. Rhode Island Med J 47:29–30
Smith SW, Hastings TN (1954) Traumatic rupture of the gallbladder. Ann Surg 139:517–520
Soderstrom CA, Maekawa K, Dupriest RW Jr, Cowley RA (1981) Gallbladder injuries resulting from blunt abdominal trauma: an experience and review. Ann Surg 193:60–66
Soffer D, Pamoukian VN, Minski Z, Aladgem D, Kluger Y (1996) Traumatic transection of the intrapancreatic common bile duct due to blunt injury: a case report and literature review. Injury 27:672–674
Solheim K (1972) Blunt gallbladder injury. Injury 3:246–248
Soulier Y, Valayer J (1987) Choleperitoneum due to rupture of the intrahepatic bile duct caused by a closed injury of the abdomen. A propos of 2 pediatric cases. Chir Pediatr 28: 322–324
Soyer MT, Mirelman D, Campbell ES (1981) Isolated gallbladder rupture secondary to blunt trauma. Ala J Med Sci 18:100
Speer AG, Cotton PB, Rode J (1988) Biliary stent blockage with bacterial biofilm. Ann Intern Med 108:546–553
Spencer W (1898) A case of rupture of the common bile-duct. Lancet 37:100
Spencer FC, Menguy R, Eiseman B (1963) Operative cholangiography in the management of traumatic hemobilia. Surgery 54:376–377
Spigos DG, Tan WS, Larson G (1981) Diagnosis of traumatic rupture of the gallbladder. Am J Surg 141:731–735
Spitz L, van Blerk PJ (1971) Transection of the common bile duct and pelvi-ureteric junction due to seat belt. J Trauma 11:266–269
Steichen FM, Sheiner NM (1966) Traumatic intrahepatic hemobilia. Arch Surg 92:838–847
Steiner Z, Brown RA, Jamieson DH, Millar AJ, Cywes S (1994) Management of hemobilia and persistent biliary fistula after blunt liver trauma. J Pediatr Surg 29:1575–1577
Stockberger SM, Sherman S, Kopecky KK (1996) Helical CT cholangiography. Abdom Imaging 21:98–104
Straaten HG, Engel C (1978) The traumatic broncho-biliary fistula. Zentralbl Chir 103:815–817
Strasberg SM, Hert M, Soper NJ (1995) An analysis of the problem of biliary injury during laparoscopic cholecystectomy. J Am Coll Surg 180:101–125
Struyven J, Cremer M, Pirson P, Jeanty P, Jeanmart J (1982) Posttraumatic bilhemia: diagnosis and catheter therapy. AJR 138:746–747
Sty JR, Starshak RJ, Hubbard AM (1982) Radionuclide hepatobiliary imaging in the detection of traumatic biliary tract disease in children. Pediatr Radiol 12:115–118
Sugimoto K, Asari Y, Sakaguchi T, Owada T, Maekawa K (1993) Endoscopic retrograde cholangiography in the nonsurgical management of blunt liver injury. J Trauma 35:192–199
Sugiyama M, Atomi Y, Matsuoka T, Yamaguhi Y (2000) Endoscopic biliary stenting for treatment of persistent biliary fistula after blunt hepatic injury. Gastrointest Endosc 51:42–44
Tanaka M, Uchiyama M, Umezaki T et al (1977) A new diagnostic aid in traumatic hemobilia. Endoscopy 9:54–57
Theunis P, Coenen L, Brouwer J (1989) Traumatic injuries to the porta hepatis: case report and review of the literature. Injury 20:152–156
Thibodeau M, Illescas FF (1988) Sonographic diagnosis of isolated gallbladder trauma. J Can Assoc Radiol 39:280–281
Thomson SR, Bade PG (1989) Penetrating bile duct trauma. Injury 20:215–216
Thorsen WB Jr, Lynd CW, Bhyun DS (1984) Traumatic external biliary fistula. Pa Med 87:48–49

Tonnesen P (1970) Rupture of extrahepatic biliary ducts from blunt external trauma. Dan Med Bull 17:238–245
Topuzlu Tekant G, Yigit U, Bulut M (1994) Is birth trauma responsible for idiopathic perforation of the biliary tract in infancy? Turk J Pediatr 36:263–266
Trerotola SO, Savader SJ, Lund GB et al (1992) Biliary tract complications following laparoscopic cholecystectomy: imaging and intervention. Radiology 184:195–200
Uhde (1880) Zerreissung eines Gallenganges mit glücklichem Ausgang. Arch Klin Chir 25:485
Vaccaro JP, Dorfman GS, Lambiase RE (1991) Treatment of biliary leaks and fistulae by simultaneous percutaneous drainage and diversion. Cardiovasc Intervent Radiol 14: 109–115
Vajdic J, Mirkovic M, Patrnogic D, Danicici B, Preradov S (1979) Injuries of the extrahepatic biliary tract. Acta Chir Jugosl 26:281–283
Vanneuville G, Chipponi J, Floucaud D, Aussilhou A, Fermaud H, Veyret E (1977) Traumatic rupture of the left hepatic duct. A propos of a case. Med Chir Dig 6:95–98
Van Way CW III, Sawyers JL (1973) Damage to the intrahepatic biliary system from the use of the balloon tipped catheter. Am J Surg 125:343–344
Vazquez JL, Thorsen MK, Dodds WJ et al (1985) Evaluation and treatment of intraabdominal bilomas. AJR 144:933–938
Velez SE, Llaryora RG, Lerda FA (1999) Laparoscopic cholecystectomy in penetrating trauma. J Laparoendosc Adv Surg Tech 9:291–293
Vellar ID (1999) The blood supply of the biliary ductal system and its relevance to vasculobiliary injuries following cholecystectomy. Aust N Z J Surg 69:816–820
Verhill MS, Munoz ST (1991) Acute biliary vascular fistula following needle aspiration of the lesion. Gastroenterology 101:1731–1733
Verran DJ (1997) Conservative treatment of a traumatic tear of the left hepatic duct: case report. J Trauma 43:728–729
Verran D, Schroeder D (1988) Management of intrahepatic bile duct injuries: presentation of two cases. Aust N Z J Surg 58: 674–678
Visner SL, Helling TS, Watkins M (1994) Early profound jaundice following blunt hepatic trauma: resolution after lobectomy – case report. J Trauma 36:576–579
Vlahos L, Kalovidouris A, Gouliamos A, Kailidou E (1991) Post-traumatic hemobilia. Eur J Radiol 13:199–202
Vogel SB, Howard RJ, Caridi J (1985) Evaluation of percutaneous transhepatic balloon dilatation of benign biliary strictures in high-risk patients. Am J Surg 149:73–79
Wainwright T (1799) Letter. Med Phys J 362–364
Walden D, Raijman L, Fuchs E et al (1993) Long term follow-up of endoscopic stenting (ES) for benign postoperative bile duct strictures (BPBDS) (abstract). Gastrointest Endosc 39:335
Wallner BK, Schumacher KA, Weidenmaier W, Friedrich JM (1991) Dilated biliary tract: evaluation with MR cholangiography with a T2-weighted contrast-enhanced fast sequence. Radiology 181:805–808
Wang CH, Lin RC, Mo LR, Yau MP, Tsai CC (1995) Spontaneous perforation of the left hepatic duct – a case report. Hepatogastroenterology 42:77–79
Warren KW, Hardy KJ (1967) The damaged bile duct. Surg Clin North Am 47:1077–1094
Way LW, Bernhoft RA, Thomas MJ (1981) Biliary stricture. Surg Clin North Am 61:963–972
Weissmann HS, Chun KJ, Frank M, Koenigsberg M, Milstein DM, Freeman LM (1979) Demonstration of traumatic bile leakage with cholescintigraphy and ultrasonography. AJR 133:843–847
Whipple C (1898) A case report of traumatic rupture of the liver: formation of cystic swelling containing bile-stained fluid. Lancet 1:719
Wicky S, Gudinchet F, Barghouth G, Shnyder P (1999) Three-dimensional cholangio-spiral CT demonstration of a posttraumatic bile leak in a child. Eur Radiol 9:99–102
Wiener I, Watson LC, Wolma FJ (1982) Perforation of the gallbladder due to blunt abdominal trauma. Arch Surg 117: 805–807
Wig J, Romslo I, Thoresen JE, Myrvold H (1988) Cholescintigraphy in the diagnosis and follow-up of hepatobiliary injury. Clin Nucl Med 13:751–755
Williams HJ, Bender CE, May GR (1987) Benign postoperative biliary strictures: dilation with fluoroscopic guidance. Radiology 163:629–634
Wolfson RH, Moore EE, Murr PC (1984) Free intraperitoneal cholelithiasis: a sign of traumatic perforation of the gallbladder. J Emerg Med 1:223–225
Wright JE (1976) Gallbladder rupture, an isolated seat belt injury. Med J Aust 1:785–786
Xeropotamos N, Baltoyannis G, Nastos D, Giannoukas A, Cassioumis A (1992) Traumatic cholecystectomy. Eur J Surg 158:249–250
Yeh TS, Jan YY, Tseng JH, Hwang TL, Jeng LB, Chen MF (1999) Value of magnetic resonance cholangiopancreatography in demonstrating major bile duct injuries following laparoscopic cholecystectomy. Br J Surg 86:181–184
Yoon KH, Ha HK, Kim MH et al (1998) Biliary stricture caused by blunt abdominal trauma: clinical and radiologic features in five patients. Radiology 207:737–741
Zantut LF, Machado MA, Volpe P, Poggetti RS, Birolini D (1995) Traumatic injuries of the gallbladder and the extrahepatic biliary tract: analysis of 45 cases. Rev Assoc Med Bres 41: 53–59
Zbar RIS (1993) Liver laceration after cardiopulmonary resuscitation: a case report. Heart Lung 22:463
Zeman RK, Lee CH, Stahl R et al (1984) Strategy for the use of biliary scintigraphy in non-iatrogenic biliary trauma. Radiology 151:771–777
Zollinger RM Jr, Keller RT, Hubay CA (1972) Traumatic rupture of the right and left hepatic ducts. J Trauma 12:563–569

7 Injuries of the Pancreas

R. F. Dondelinger, O. Cornet, J. H. Boverie

CONTENTS

- A high clinical index of suspicion is required to recognize pancreatic injury on CT examination at admission.
- In doubtful cases, or when serial serum amylase levels increase, CT examination should be repeated.
- Rupture of the pancreatic duct is best evidenced by endoscopic retrograde pancreatography.
- Multislice CT or MRI might increase the potential of demonstrating pancreatic ductal injury.

7.1 History

Injury to the pancreas did not attract much attention in the past before the advent of modern abdominal surgery. A first necropsy report of posttraumatic laceration of the pancreas was given in the Lancet in 1827 (Travers 1827). Carré is credited with the first reported suture of a ruptured pancreas (Delany and Jason 1981).

7.2 Incidence

In children and in adults, major pancreatic injury is rare, compared to other solid abdominal organs. In the USA, most pancreatic injuries result from penetrating trauma, but a relative increase of blunt trauma has been noticed recently. Roughly, about one-third of pancreatic injuries are caused by blunt contusion in large American surgical series published during the last decade (Glancy 1989; Linker and DeLuca 1989; Akhrass et al. 1996, 1997). In European countries, blunt contusion largely predominates in children and in adults (Wilkinson 1989). In adults, pancreatic trauma is diagnosed in about 3% of surgical interventions indicated for abdominal injuries. Incidence of pancreatic contusion is estimated at 0.4 per 100,000

R. F. Dondelinger, MD
Professor and Chairman, Department of Medical Imaging, University Hospital Sart Tilman, Domaine Universitaire du Sart Tilman B35, 4000 Liège, Belgium
O. Cornet, MD
Resident, Department of Medical Imaging, University Hospital Sart Tilman, Domaine du Sart Tilman B35, 4000 Liège, Belgium
J. H. Boverie, MD
Chef de Clinique, Department of Medical Imaging, University Hospital Sart Tilman, Domaine du Sart Tilman B35, 4000 Liège, Belgium

population and 0.2%–14% of abdominal injury. In fact, only about 100 cases of major posttraumatic pancreatic transection, diagnosed at surgery or autopsy, were reported in the medical literature in 1987 (VAN STEENBERGEN et al. 1987). Predominantly males less than 40 years old are involved. In children, the pancreas is the fourth most commonly injured abdominal organ, and is found in 7%–15% of laparotomies done for blunt abdominal trauma (NILSSON et al. 1986; ALANEN et al. 2000; McGAHREN et al. 1995). Penetrating injury is obviously rare in the pediatric age group. In children, up to 80% of pancreatic injuries occur in boys, related to playing or sports injuries (GROSFELD and COONEY 1975; HEITSCH et al. 1976; LABORDE et al. 1982; JEFFREY et al. 1983; COOK et al. 1986; NILSSON et al. 1986; GLANCY 1989; CHAPMAN and MORRIS 1989; HORST and BIVINS 1989; DODDS et al. 1990; WILSON and MOOREHEAD 1991; SUKUL et al. 1992; RAPTOPOULOS 1994; PATTON and FABIAN 1996; AKHRASS et al. 1996, 1997; TIMBERLAKE 1997; LUDWIG et al. 1998; FIRSTENBERG et al. 1999; JOBST et al. 1999).

As penetrating wounds are surgically explored shortly after admission and preoperative diagnosis of blunt pancreatic injury is frequently missed, the radiological diagnosis of pancreatic trauma is only rarely reported in detail in the literature (Fig. 7.1). Even in blunt trauma, despite systematic imaging of the traumatized patient with CT, the majority of pancreatic contusion is still diagnosed at time of operation, done for repair of associated abdominal injuries, or with delay, when no immediate surgery was indicated (BALTHAZAR et al. 1985; CHAPMAN and MORRIS 1989; HORST and BIVINS 1989; GLANCY 1989; AKHRASS et al. 1997). In large surgical reports, radiological contribution is hardly mentioned or remains limited. Consequently there are only few radiological studies available and each report refers to a small number of patients, imaged each year in an urban general hospital in Europe (BAKER et al. 1982; JEFFREY et al. 1983; COOK et al. 1986; VAN STEENBERGEN et al. 1987; DODDS et al. 1990; CRAIG et al. 1995; AKHRASS et al. 1996, 1997; PROCACCI et al. 1997; MIELE et al. 1998; BIGATTINI et al. 1999).

In a recent surgical review, the contribution of CT to the diagnosis of pancreatic trauma, either benign or severe, was still called "anecdotal" (BRADLEY et al. 1998).

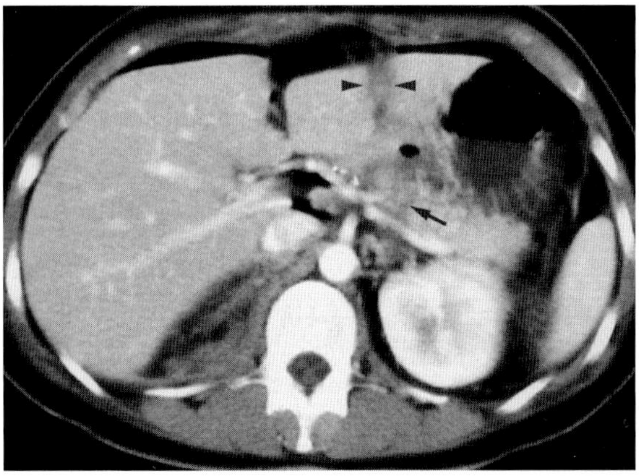

Fig. 7.1. A 32-year-old female was admitted after a suicide attempt by gunshot in the abdomen. She was surgically explored immediately after admission: hepatic and gastric wounds were sutured. Hemostasis of a pancreatic transsection of the body was achieved and drainage catheters were placed. Postoperative abdominal CT, which was obtained 1 week later, showed an irregular hypodense area of the body of the pancreas (*arrow*) and a sagittal hypodense hepatic tract (*arrowheads*) created by the bullet traversing the left lobe of the liver. Persistent postoperative pneumoperitoneum

7.3 Mechanism

Although the pancreas is apparently protected from contusion by its deep location in the abdominal cavity and by the surrounding retroperitoneal fat and surrounding viscera, its relation to the lumbar spine explains the possible mechanism of injury. It is known that a fracture of the upper lumbar spine increases the likelihood of pancreatic damage. Classically, pancreatic contusion results from a direct impact, frequently with the handlebar of a bicycle or motorcycle or the steering wheel of a car, or from a blow to the abdomen or a fall. In some series, 40%–80% of blunt pancreatic injuries were caused by an impact of the steering wheel of a car or bicycle handlebar (FRASER 1969; ANDERSON et al. 1974; HAGER and MENARDI 1982; SPARNON and FORD 1986; BASS et al. 1988; LOVELL et al. 1992; ROBERTS 1996; SMITH et al. 1996; ARKOVITZ et al. 1997; CLARNETTE and BEASLEY 1997; JOBST et al. 1999; KOESTNER and HOAK 1999; HOLLAND et al. 1999; BERLETTI et al. 2000; GRAHAM et al. 2000). The use of seatbelts was particularly incriminated in the mechanism of duodenopancreatic trauma, but remains controversial (BUXTON 1969; FREEMAN 1985; BARKIN et al. 1988; CRAIG et al. 1995). Bicycle or scooter handlebars or ski poles are responsible for a particular "almost penetrating" injury, without an external wound, but which can injure a deeply located organ such as the pancreas. Probably, the absence of peripancreatic fat in young individuals makes the pancreas more vulnerable to blunt injury.

Rather than the classic sharp blow to the upper abdomen, the trauma victim may have experienced only a light blow, but injury may occur during acute flexion of the trunk during sport injuries in boxing, football or baseball games, or the injury is produced by a sustained and severe flexion of the trunk. Pancreatic damage caused by constant pounding motion of long distance and marathon running were shown to be responsible for anecdotal "posttraumatic" acute pancreatitis (Campero and Campbell 1974; Wohlwend and Hirata 1975; Speakman and Reece-Smith 1983; Harrison et al. 1985; Nielsen and Jensen 1986; Holmich et al. 1988; Ficarra 1996).

Child abuse must also be mentioned as a cause of major pancreatic trauma or posttraumatic pancreatitis, and should be suspected in children without a clear history of accident or with a fraudulent description of trauma by adults (Touloukian 1968; O'Neill et al. 1973; Pena and Medovy 1973; Kirks 1983; Gonzalez et al. 1987; Tolia et al. 1990; Hilfer and Holgersen 1995; Cameron et al. 1997; Van Winckel et al. 1997; De Roux and Prendergast 1998).

The effect of sudden bending or compression of the flexible pancreas over the lumbar spine is either a superficial or a deep and complete transverse pancreatic fracture, which is classically located at the isthmus, to the left of the superior mesenteric vessels (Holmes 1973; Rommens et al. 1989). However, in practice, all portions of the pancreas can be involved, including the uncinate process or the distal "intraperitoneal" portion of the tail (Craig et al. 1995; Bigattini et al. 1999). The pancreatic ducts are at permanent risk of being partially or completely ruptured during pancreatic injury. Occasionally, selective rupture of the main pancreatic duct, without laceration of the pancreatic parenchyma, was reported at laparotomy (Van Hee et al. 1993). Due to its deep location, isolated blunt and penetrating injury of the pancreas is rare (Fischer et al. 1996). When pancreatic injury is obvious, other traumatic lesions, either intraperitoneal or retroperitoneal, should always be searched for (Cleveland and Waddell 1963; Guerriero et al. 1973; Jeffrey et al. 1983). The adjacent duodenum is the most likely organ to be injured together with the pancreas (Anderson et al. 1973). Overall, figures of 50%–98% of associated abdominal injuries are reported with an average of 2.5–3.5 associated injuries per patient (Northrup and Simmons 1972; Heyse-Moore 1976; Graham et al. 1978; Laborde et al. 1982; Balasegaram 1979; Stone et al. 1981; Federle et al. 1982; Friend et al. 1985; Rubio and Dichoso 1987; Glancy 1989; Wilson and Moorehead 1991; Machado et al. 1994; Timberlake 1997; Carboni et al. 1999).

Injuries to the spleen, liver, diaphragm, large vessels, kidney, intestine, and colorectum, particularly after penetrating injury, are the most frequent (Anderson et al. 1973; Dodds et al. 1990; Cogbill et al. 1991; Johanet et al. 1991; Machado et al. 1994; Rosen and McAninch 1994; Smith et al. 1996). Associations of hepatic and right kidney contusion or splenic and left kidney injury suggest a line of compression force that might also have involved the pancreas, which lies between these organs (Dodds et al. 1990). Furthermore, when pancreatic injury occurs in combination with any other solid abdominal organ injury, a rate of hollow viscus injury up to 33% can be expected (Nance et al. 1997). In the most severe blunt trauma, resulting in duodenal rupture, avulsion of the pancreatic duct, the ampulla of Vater, the common bile duct and gastroduodenal artery may occur in various combinations (Fish and Johnson 1965; Balsano and Reynolds 1973; Lee et al. 1976; Metzger and Jenny 1980; Schimpl et al. 1992; Ito et al. 1993; Cox and Eastman 1994). Despite their frequent occurrence, associated abdominal injuries do not seem to influence operation on the pancreas, particularly in children (Keller et al. 1997).

Other anecdotal mechanisms of pancreatic injury are mentioned below. Like for the liver and the spleen, the pancreas may be injured by repeated compression forces caused during cardiac resuscitation (Waldman et al. 1984). Iatrogenic causes of pancreatic trauma include percutaneous pancreatic biopsy, catheter drainage of pancreatic pseudocyst or abscess, endoscopic sphincterotomy, and cholangiopancreatography, arterial embolization procedures of peripancreatic vessels, extracorporeal shock wave lithotripsy of intraductal stones, and various upper abdominal surgical interventions, particularly splenectomy, during which the tail of the pancreas may be injured (Maingot 1970, 1978; Vora and Wakamatsu 1980; Florence et al. 1981; Winter et al. 1982; Balthazar et al. 1985; Sisley et al. 1987; Mullen et al. 1991; Khan et al. 1993; Ochiai et al. 1997; Hung et al. 2000).

7.4 Clinical Diagnosis

7.4.1 Symptoms and Findings

The diagnosis of blunt pancreatic injury is notoriously difficult, because the retroperitoneal location of the pancreas delays the clinical symptoms and physical findings (Smith et al. 1996). The typical, but nonspecific clinical triad of pancreatic trauma is: upper abdominal pain or tenderness, elevated serum amylase level, and elevated leukocyte count. Severe acute posttraumatic pancreatitis or pancreatic hemorrhage may occasionally give a dramatic picture of an acute abdomen with shock, intense and diffuse abdominal pain, and vomiting. In general, however, at admission, only mild or moderate upper abdominal pain is present. Rebound tenderness and adynamic ileus develop progressively. Trivial symptoms and physical findings at admission or decreasing in severity during the first hours following trauma may give a false sense of security (Lucas 1977; Linos et al. 1983). Particularly in children, who suffered from sports or playing trauma, the interval from trauma to diagnosis can be delayed to several days (Shilyansky et al. 1998). In rare cases, a lumbar skin discoloration (Turner's sing) can be noticed after a couple of days and is caused by posterior diffusion of catabolic enzyme secretions by the pancreas (Ficarra 1996). Some patients, who remained asymptomatic for weeks to months, despite pancreatic duct transection being present, have been reported (Anderson et al. 1974; Berni et al. 1982; Smego et al. 1985). In a few cases, nonspecific chronic abdominal pain was the main symptom of remote blunt pancreatic injury (Gholson et al. 1994) and in other cases, obstructive jaundice, occurring several weeks after abdominal injury, revealed isolated contusion of the head of the pancreas (Emmick and Petersen 1996).

7.4.2 Serum Amylase

Serum isoamylase levels and urine amylase or lipase levels are not good predictors of the presence or the severity of pancreatic injury, nor of the need for exploratory laparotomy. Figures of 18%–78% elevated serum amylase levels, up to 40% of false negative, and up to 90% of false positive results were reported in pancreatic injury (White and Benfield 1972; Donovan et al. 1972; Olsen 1973; Moretz et al. 1975; Graham et al. 1978; Stone et al. 1981; Berni et al. 1982; Cogbill et al. 1982; Farkouh et al. 1982; Bouwman et al. 1984; Greenlee et al. 1984; Kudsk et al. 1986; Wilson and Moorehead 1991; Roberts et al. 1993; Craig et al. 1995; Yagi et al. 1997; Jobst et al. 1999).

This is not surprising, as amylase levels at admission were shown to be normal in acute nontraumatic pancreatitis in 19%–32% of the cases (Spechler et al. 1983; Clavien et al. 1989). Serum amylase is not diagnostic for pancreatic injury, within the first 3 h of trauma, irrespective of the type of injury and can remain within normal limits during the first 24 h or several days of trauma, particularly in adults, sometimes even despite complete pancreatic transection being present (Dickerman and Dunn 1981; Jeffrey et al. 1983; Meredith and Trunkey 1988; Wilson and Moorehead 1991; Takishima et al. 1997; Arkowitz et al. 1997).

Further confusion is added to the difficulty of diagnosis, as many other trauma-related conditions can be responsible for elevated serum amylase such as recent alcohol intake, cerebral bleeding, thermal burns, mesenteric infarction, salivary gland trauma, rupture of the gastrointestinal tract, and endoscopic retrograde pancreatography (ERP) (Bouwman et al. 1983; Cook et al. 1986; Vitale et al. 1987; Chapman and Morris 1989; Justice et al. 1994; Pezzilli et al. 1997). The proposed mechanisms to explain elevated serum amylase in intracranial bleeding include vagal stimulation, release of cholecystokinin from the brain, and disturbance of central control of pancreatic enzyme secretion (Justice et al. 1994). Furthermore, serial amylase levels, which are important to suggest the presence of pancreatic injury, do not correlate well with severity of pancreatic injury, nor with the need for intervention (Firstenberg et al. 1999; Jobst et al. 1999). Fractionated amylase, with measurement of elevated salivary isoamylase and serum lipase levels, is useful to rule out pancreatic injury in case of combined facial and abdominal trauma (Burkhardt et al. 1967; Goyne and Alexander 1980; Greenlee et al. 1984; Jobst et al. 1999). In patients without pancreatic injury, salivary type amylase level may be elevated in 94%, due to the permeability of its cell membrane (Takamashi et al. 1980).

In practice, correlation between pancreatic injury and serum amylase level is somewhat better in children than in adults (Takishima et al. 1996a). Serum amylase greater than 200 UI/l and serum lipase greater than 1800 UI/l are useful clinical markers for major pancreatic duct injury, when combined with positive clinical and imaging findings (Nadler et al. 1999). Rising levels of serum amylase and clinical deterioration are the best indices of suspicion of significant pancreatic trauma and should lead to repeated abdominal imaging if initial US or CT were negative or questionable (Lucas 1977; Cogbill et al. 1982).

7.5 Imaging

The surgical adage "the pancreas is not your friend" can be extended to radiologists, as diagnosis of pancreatic trauma remains problematic despite significant progress made in cross-section imaging (Jurkovich and Carrico 1990).

7.5.1 Computed Tomography

7.5.1.1 Technique

CT is the most effective and efficient imaging modality for diagnosing pancreatic injury, provided a high index of suspicion is raised and proper examination technique is used (Strax et al. 1980; Federle et al. 1981; Jeffrey et al. 1983; Meredith and Trunkey 1988; Dodds et al. 1990; Mirvis and Shanmuganathan 1992; Nelson et al. 1994; Fischer et al. 1996; Lane et al. 1996; Coppola et al. 1997; Giovnie et al. 1997; Shuman 1997; Procacci et al. 1997; Wong et al. 1997; Miele et al. 1998; Bigattini et al. 1999).

Intravenous bolus injection of contrast medium is always mandatory. Thin collimation and overlapped reconstructions are the rule and can be obtained in a second intent, after a rush screening examination of the entire abdomen and the thorax has been obtained. Oral contrast is not part of a systematic CT examination protocol of polytrauma patients at admission in most European centers. It may improve sensitivity for pancreatic and duodenal injury, but was not found superior to CT examinations without gastrointestinal enhancement and did not contribute to patient selection for operative treatment (Tsang et al. 1997; Ryan et al. 2000).

7.5.1.2 Positive Signs of Injury

Irrespective of single or multislice CT technique, the basic positive CT signs of pancreatic injury include the following:

- A hypodense zone within the pancreatic gland with unsharp demarcation on CT obtained rapidly after trauma (Figs. 7.1, 7.2a); limits of contusion become better defined after 24–48 h (Fig. 7.2b).

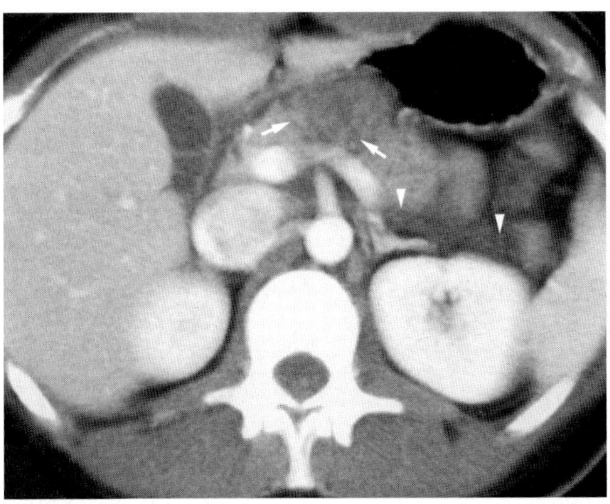
a

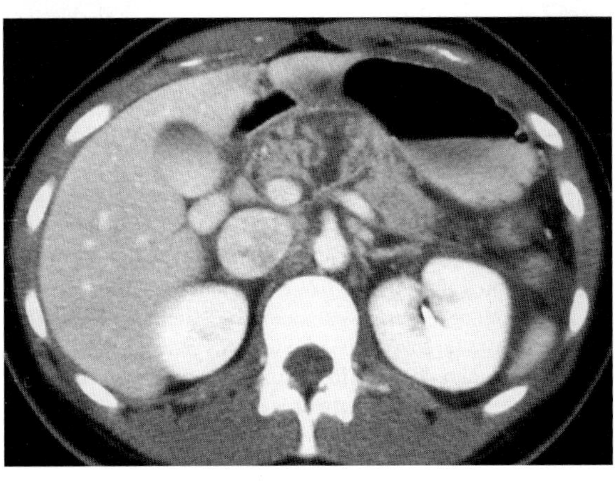
b

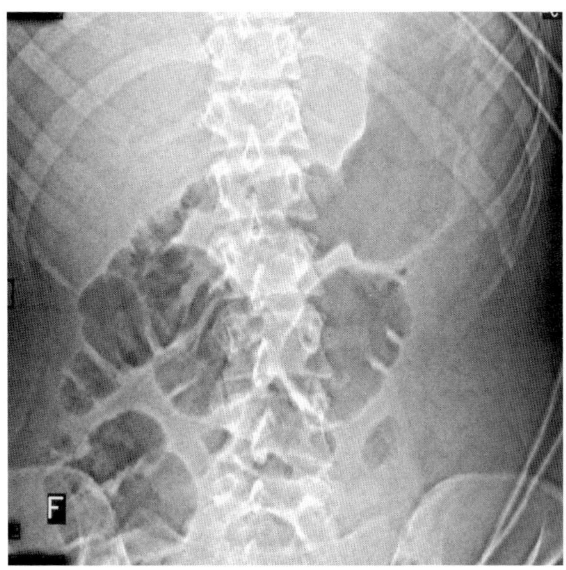
c

Fig. 7.2a–c. An 18-year-old female had sustained a frontal impact from the steering wheel of a go-cart. She was admitted 5 hours following the accident. Serum amylase at admission was 375 UI/l. **a** CT at admission showed a focal hypodense enlargement of the body of the pancreas (*arrows*) and a peripancreatic effusion in the left anterior pararenal space (*arrowheads*). Conservative nonoperative treatment was given for 3 days. **b** CT, repeated 2 days after admission, showed the hypodense area of pancreatic contusion more clearly. **c** The CT scout view showed nonspecific passive dilatation of the stomach and duodenum and cut-off of the distal transverse colon. A pancreatic gastric derivation was performed 3 days after admission

- A distinct partial or complete sagittal fracture line, showing most often as a cleft, a complete transsection, or a stellate fragmentation separating two segments of normally enhanced pancreas (TOOMBS et al. 1981; BAKER et al. 1982; HERMAN and SIEGEL 1991) (Figs. 7.3a, 7.4a, 7.5a, 7.6a).
- Focal or diffuse pancreatic enlargement.
- Edema in the peripancreatic fat planes.
- A fluid collection in contact with the contused pancreatic zone (Fig. 7.7 and 7.3a) or in the peripancreatic space, that can extend along the same anatomical pathways as acute pancreatitis. Classic spread involves the left or right anterior pararenal space (Figs. 7.2a and 7.7), the perirenal space (Fig. 7.8b), the splenic hilum (Fig. 7.5b), the transverse mesocolon (Fig. 7.3c), the lesser sac, the paracolic gutters, the posterior pararenal space, and pelvis. Fluid around the superior mesenteric vessels (Fig. 7.3b) or portal vein is particularly suggestive of pancreatic or duodenal injury (BLEICHNER et al. 1998).
- Intraperitoneal effusion or chylous ascites (HILFER and HOLGERSEN 1995).
- A collected hematoma with mixed or hypodense densities in or around the pancreas, displacing peripancreatic abdominal structures or fluid separating pancreas and duodenum (Fig. 7.6c).
- Duodenal involvement may show as a dilatation by air of the duodenal lumen, fluid around the duodenal loop, or local or circumferential thickening of the duodenal wall by a mural hematoma (Figs. 7.8a, 7.3c). In case of duodenal rupture, retroperitoneal gas bubbles or intraperitoneal air, extravasation of orally given gastroduodenal contrast material or intraportal gas can be seen. The avulsed duodenal

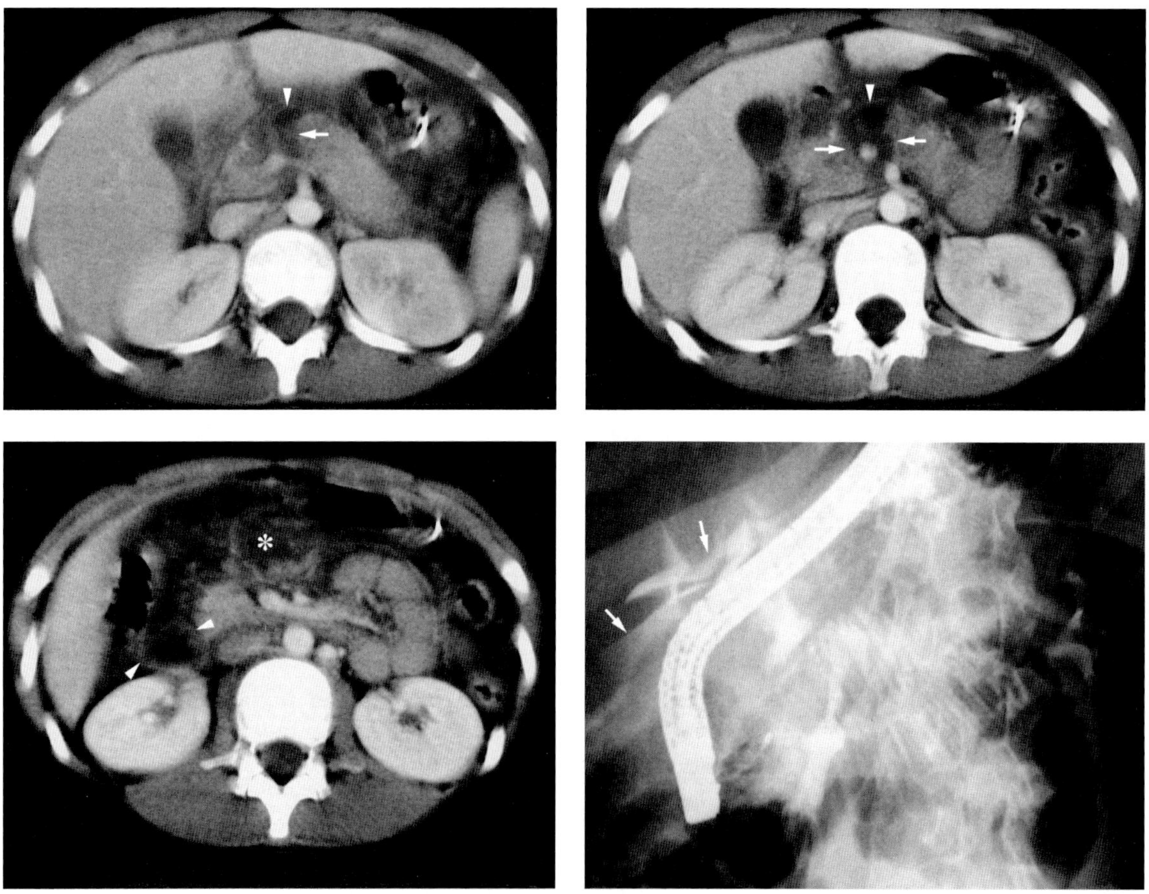

a b c d

Fig. 7.3a–d. A 9-year-old girl had an epigastric impact of the handlebar during a fall from a bicycle. She was admitted to another hospital where the diagnosis of posttraumatic pancreatitis was established. Serum amylase level at admission was 325 UI/l and 1765 UI/l on the next day. The patient was transferred 2 days after the accident. **a, b** CT at admission showed a hypodense, thick, transverse fracture (*arrow*) of the isthmus of the pancreas (**a**), with ill-defined margins and a small adjacent fluid collection (*arrowhead*) (**b**). The superior mesenteric vessels are surrounded by hematoma. **c** Extensive edema in the transverse mesocolon (*asterisk*) and circumferential thickening of the duodenal wall superior to 3 mm (*arrowheads*) was seen. CT also showed hepatic grade II contusion and peritoneal effusion. **d** Late film of ERCP, which was obtained 1 day after admission, showed intraperitoneal extravasation of contrast medium (*arrow*), confirming pancreatic duct rupture. The patient was operated on: the head of the pancreas was sutured and the distal part of the transected pancreas was anastomosed with the stomach loop, consequent to a fracture of the uncinate process is seen to be displaced laterally (FISHER et al. 1996).

- Subtle signs, which reflect minor pancreatic injury are: failure to recognize a portion of the pancreas (Fig. 7.9), blurring of the contour of the pancreatic gland or peripancreatic vessels, and discrete thickening of the anterior pararenal fascia, as seen in acute pancreatitis (JEFFREY et al. 1983; DODDS et al. 1990; HERMAN and SIEGEL 1991).
- Unspecific signs – pneumoperitoneum, sentinel loop, paralytic ileus, transverse colon cut-off injury – should indicate the search for other associated abdominal injuries (COPPOLA et al. 1997) (Fig. 7.2c).

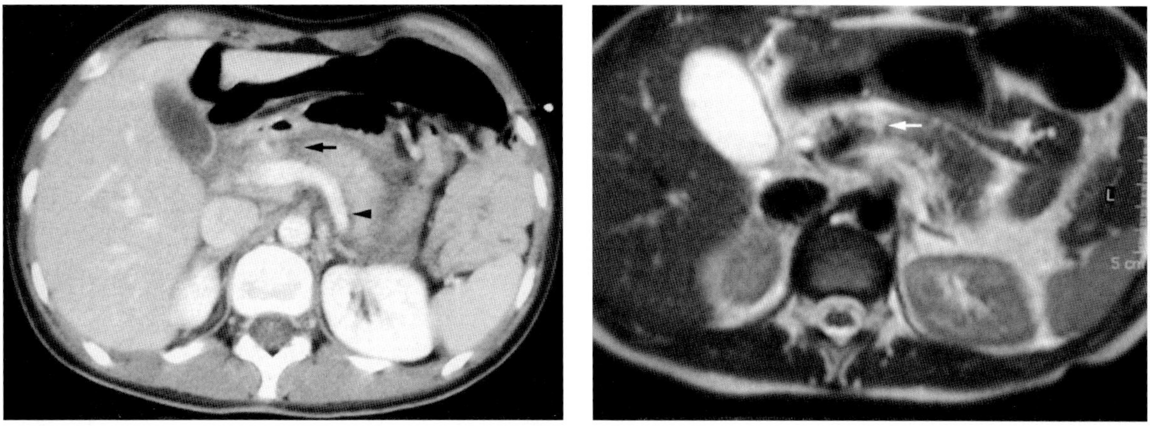

a b

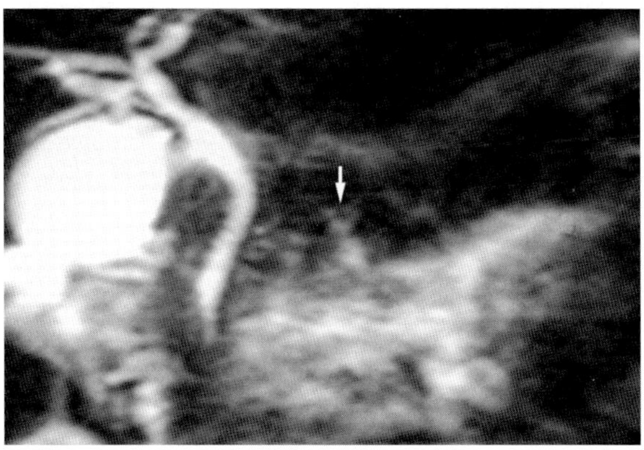

c

Fig. 7.4a–c. A 26-year-old female, who was involved in a car accident, experienced a frontal impact by the steering-wheel. Serum amylase at admission was 1408 UI/l. **a** CT showed a hypodense cleft with irregular margins (*arrow*), located at the isthmus and perpendicular to the long axis of the pancreas. Blurring of the peripancreatic fat and of the space between the splenic vein and pancreas (*arrowhead*). **b** MRI showed the pancreatic fracture (*arrow*) and the peripancreatic fluid as a hyperintense signal on T2-weighted images. **c** Magnetic resonance cholangiopancreatography (MRCP) demonstrated the interruption of the main pancreatic duct (*arrow*) at the level of the pancreatic contusion. The patient underwent surgery: the proximal pancreas was sutured and a distal pancreatic gastrostomy was performed. (From CROMBE et al. 2001, with permission)

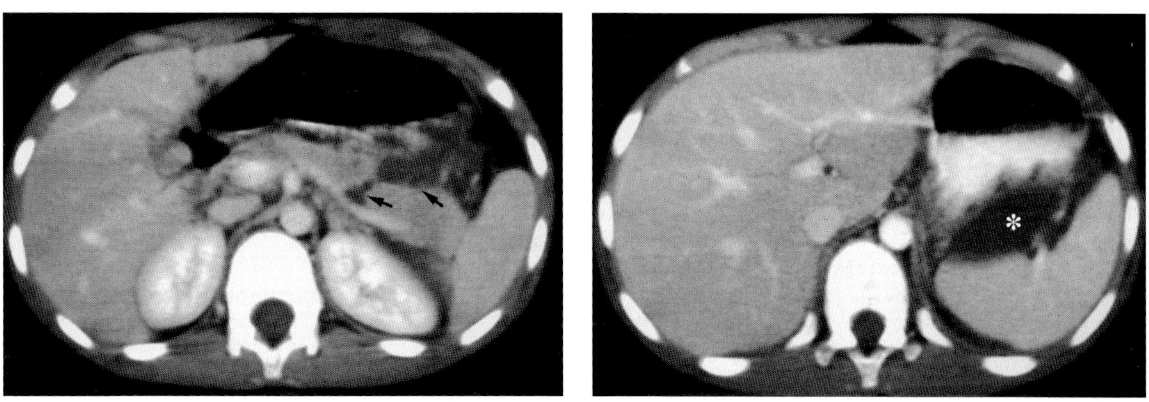

a b

Fig. 7.5a, b. A 10-year-old girl had a bicycle accident with an upper abdominal impact of the handlebar. An initial CT obtained immediately after admission to another hospital was read normal. A second CT performed 3 days later was read as positive for pancreatic injury. The patient was transferred for further management. The initial serum amylase level was 1110 UI/l. Three days later, the amylase level had decreased to 272 UI/l. **a** CT showed complete transection (*arrows*) of the tail of the pancreas, with clear margins, indicating that organization of the pancreatic injury had occurred. **b** A homogeneous water density fluid collection (*asterisk*), corresponding to a posttraumatic pancreatic pseudocyst, is located at the hilum of the spleen, compressing the posterior aspect of the stomach. A distal caudal pancreatectomy was performed the day of admission

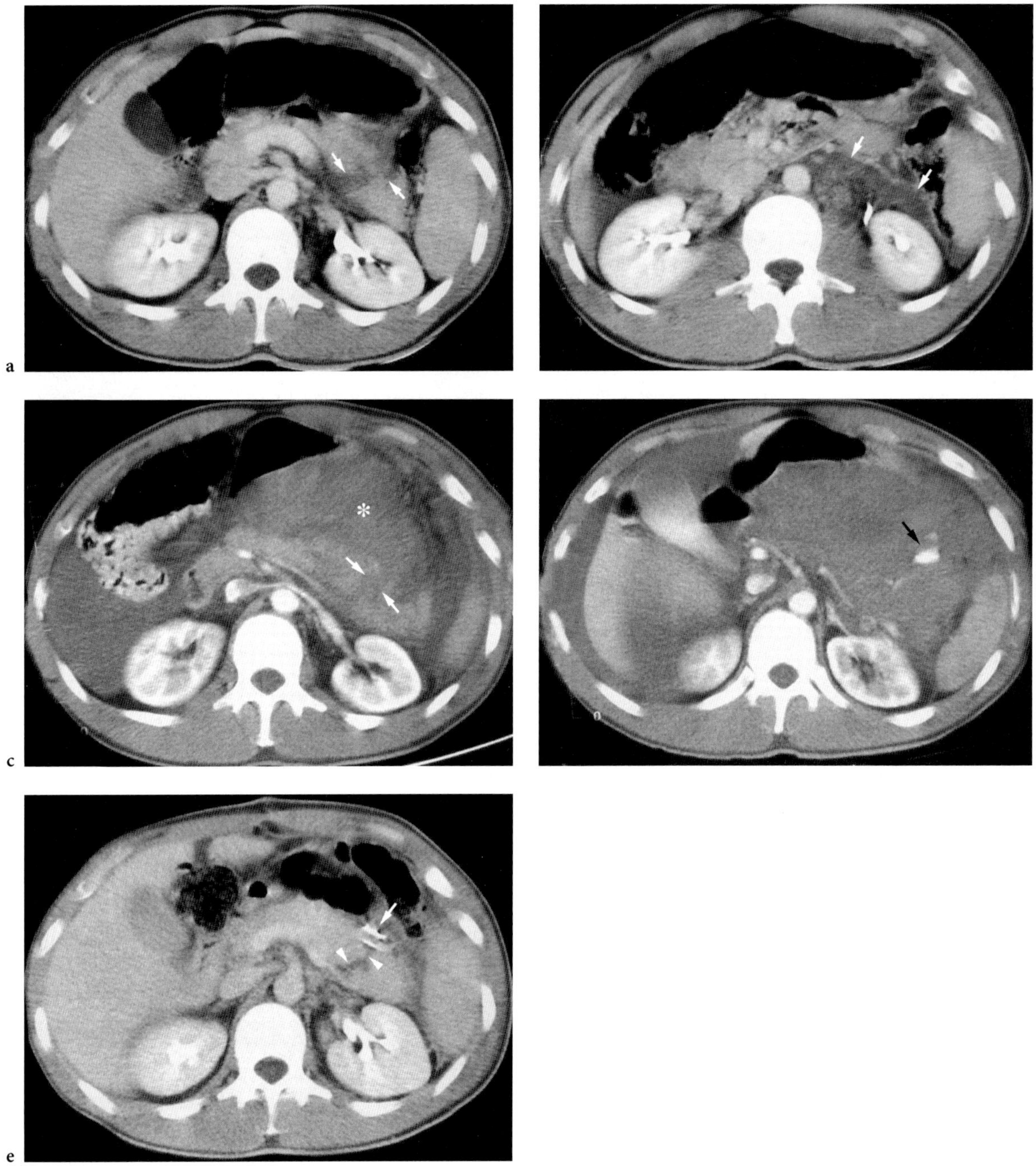

Fig. 7.6a–e. A 26-year-old male was involved in a car accident as a driver. He was in hemodynamic shock at admission. The amylase level was 75 UI/l. CT was obtained within 1 hour of the accident. **a** Hypodense, thick transverse fracture (*arrows*) of the tail of the pancreas. **b** Extensive retroperitoneal fluid in the left anterior pararenal and left perirenal space (*arrows*). **c** Forty hours after admission the patient presented with an acute abdomen. Repeated CT showed a large hematoma (*asterisk*) adjacent to the pancreatic tail and massive hemoperitoneum, particularly in the right paracolic gutter. The pancreatic fracture (*arrows*) is still visible in a faintly enhanced pancreas, due to diffuse hypoperfusion caused by vasoconstriction. Note the contracted splenic and left renal vein. d Extravasation of contrast (*arrow*) is seen at the arterial phase of enhancement inside the hematoma. The patient was treated surgically. A prepancreatic sump drain was placed. **e** CT obtained 3 days after surgery showed a persistent thin, transverse fracture line at the tail of the pancreas (*arrowheads*). Prepancreatic sump drain (*arrow*)

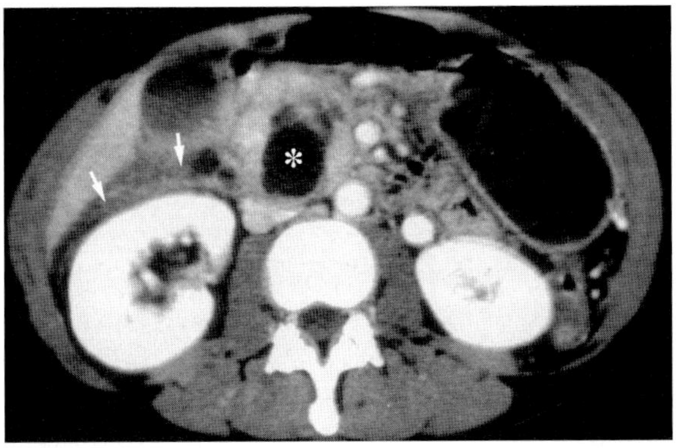

Fig. 7.7. A 47-year-old female was involved as a driver in a car accident. She was admitted for fracture of the left tibia and complained of abdominal pain. Diffuse abdominal tenderness was present at examination. Serum amylase at admission was 1.125 UI/l. Abdominal CT showed a 4-cm fluid collection (*asterisk*) in the head of the pancreas and fluid in the right anterior pararenal space (*arrows*). The patient was operated on and a sump drain was placed

a 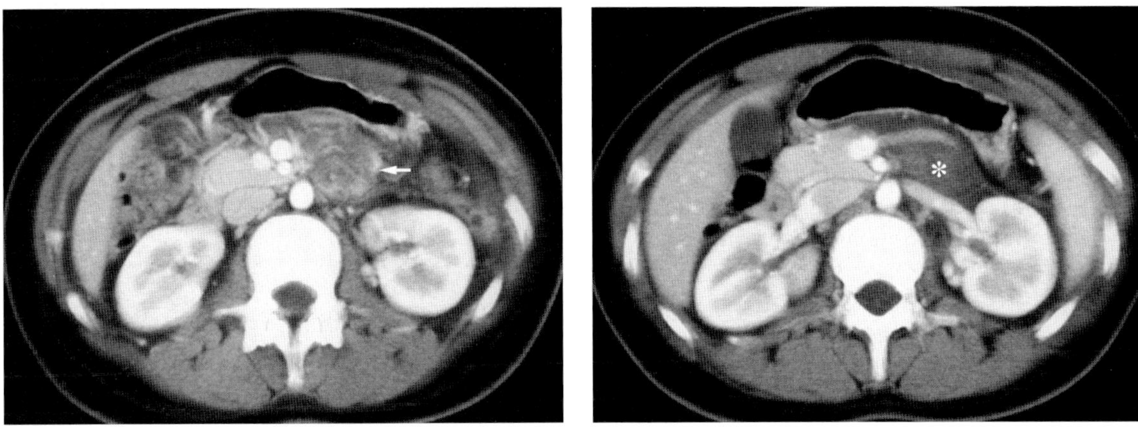 b

Fig. 7.8a, b. A 13-year-old girl was admitted after a fall from a horse. **a, b** She complained of abdominal pain. Serum amylase at admission was 141 UI/l. Similar levels were noted in the following days (112–139 UI/l). **a** CT at admission showed replacement of the horizontal duodenum by a hypodense fluid collection with indistinct limits (*arrows*), situated to the left of the superior mesenteric vessels, which are slightly displaced to the right. **b** A large peripancreatic fluid collection was seen (*asterisk*), demarcated by the left renal vein and surrounding the splenic vein. No pancreatic injury and no extraluminal gas was observed. The diagnosis of injury to the horizontal duodenum was formulated and confirmed at surgery

a 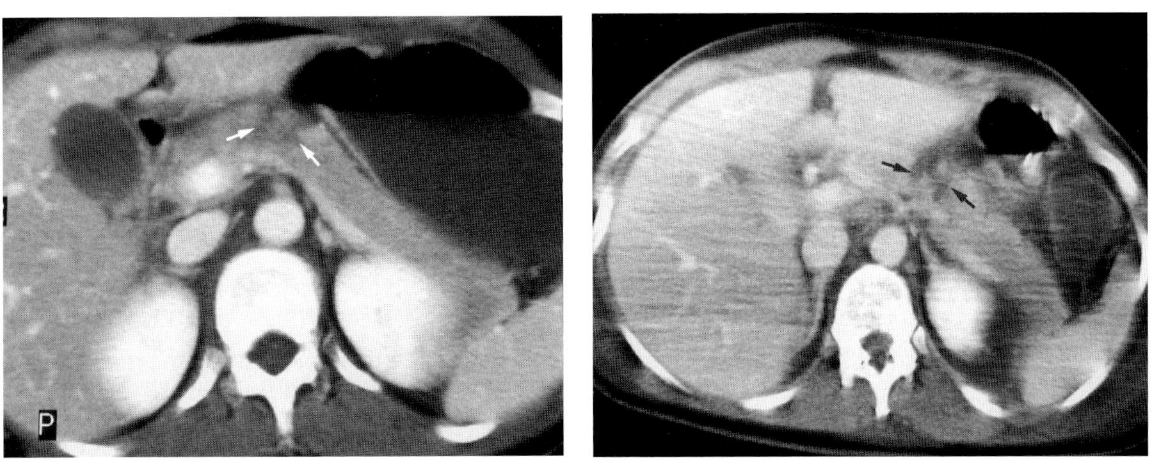 b

Fig. 7.9a, b. A 28-year-old female was transferred from another hospital after having been involved, as a driver, in a car accident. CT at admission showed hepatic and pancreatic injury. **a, b** A subtle hypodense area (*arrows*) is seen at the isthmus of the pancreas on initial CT (**a**) and was better demonstrated on CT 3 days later (*arrows*) (**b**) with no increase in retroperitoneal fluid. Limited pancreatic injury should not be mistaken for streak artifacts by the stomach. Conservative nonoperative treatment was applied

7.5.1.3 Pitfalls

False-Negative Diagnosis

False-negative CT findings were caused in the past by inadequate examination technique, such as sequential scanning with separate slices or a 10-mm slice thickness. Perception errors are responsible for misdiagnosis in many cases. Posttraumatic changes that are not clearly demarcated in the pancreas immediately following trauma and an initially absent or limited peripancreatic effusion further complicate CT diagnosis. Pancreatic contusion can also be missed, when it is associated with other major abdominal lesions or when acute contrast extravasation is seen in another abdominal organ, which focuses the attention (Akhrass et al. 1996; Bigattini et al. 1999). A hematoma adjacent to the pancreas may obscure a pancreatic fracture. Complete pancreatic transection may not be seen or be difficult to distinguish from simple contusion due to close appositions of the fracture margins in the closed abdomen (Jeffrey et al. 1983; Procacci et al. 1997). Moreover, complete posttraumatic necrosis of the pancreatic head was reported despite normal anatomy on CT at admission, using single-slice technology (Doctor et al. 1995).

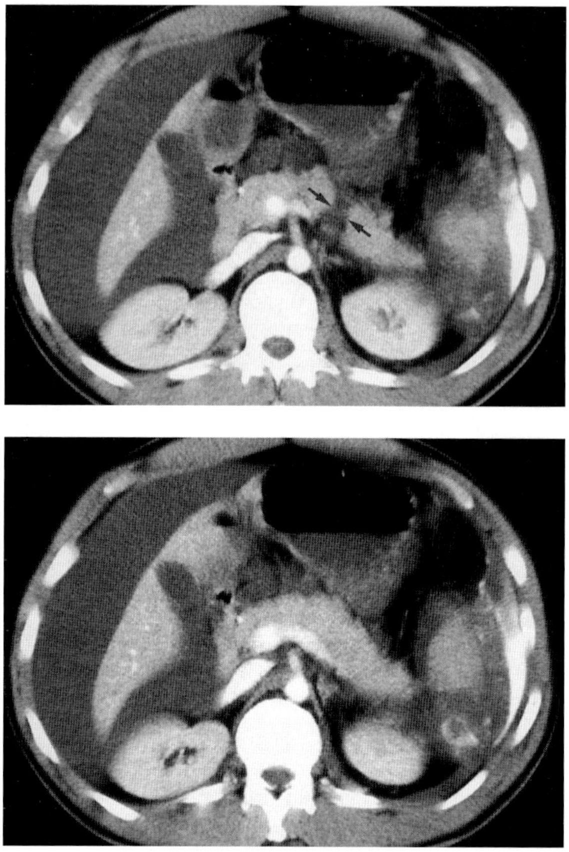

Fig. 7.10a, b. A 30-year-old male had a motorcycle accident. At admission, the serum amylase level was 52 UI/l and remained normal in the following days. **a, b** CT at admission showed a shattered spleen with contrast extravasation and massive hemoperitoneum. A partial thickness transection of the tail of the pancreas (*arrows*) is wrongly suggested, but caused by partial volume artifact (**a**). Adjacent slices show normal pancreas (**b**). Laparotomy confirmed splenic laceration, intra- and retroperitoneal hematoma and normal pancreas

False-Positive Diagnosis

The pancreas was known to be a large provider of false-positive diagnoses in blunt abdominal trauma. A false-positive rate of 9% was reported in early publications (Jeffrey et al. 1983; Cook et al. 1986). Most of these sources of error in film reading can be avoided:

- Streak artifacts from gastroduodenal contrast or from a nasogastric tube can simulate a pancreatic fracture.
- Unopacified bowel loops can mimic peripancreatic hematoma.
- Peripancreatic effusion, fluid in the lesser sac, or a hematoma originating from a surrounding contused organ can be erroneously attributed to pancreatic injury (Cook 1986).
- Loculations of the pancreatic contour created by penetrating fat lobules or partial volume that is caused by the variable orientation of the gland in the axial plane can simulate a pancreatic fracture, particularly at the level of the isthmus or in other segments (Fig. 7.10).
- Fluid separating the splenic vein from the pancreas can suggest a pancreatic injury (Fig. 7.4a), but the fluid can also originate from the left anterior pararenal space (Lane et al. 1994; Sivit and Eichelberger 1995). Vigorous fluid perfusion, for example, given during resuscitation, is sometimes responsible for obliteration of retroperitoneal fat planes, simulating peripancreatic hemorrhage or effusion on CT (Chamrova et al. 1994). A more reliable indicator of pancreatic injury is isolated fluid in the lesser sac (Sivit et al. 1992).
- Finally, the uninjured pancreas can remain totally unenhanced, simulating major peripancreatic vascular rupture. Nonenhancement can be caused by generalized vasoconstriction, major hypoperfusion, particularly in children with trauma to the central nervous system, acidemia, or profuse bleeding from any source, including pancreatic injury (Taylor et al. 1987) (Fig. 7.6c).

7.5.1.4
Classification

Several surgical classifications of pancreatic damage are available. The classification given by Lucas is widespread and considers parenchymal and ductal transection (LUCAS 1977). Four degrees are defined:

1. Superficial contusion or limited hematoma with intact duct
2. Deep laceration, transection, or hematoma with possible duct injury
3. Severe transection with crash injury to the pancreatic head
4. Variable degree of pancreatic injury with associated duodenal trauma

Two other generally accepted classifications, the classic grading given by Moore and the classification by Jurkovich and Carrico, consider five levels of severity of parenchymal and ductal damage (MOORE et al. 1990; JURKOVICH and CARRICO 1990). Surgical classifications of pancreatic injury are not directly applicable CT or US, as pancreatic ductal rupture remains generally undetected without the use of endoscopic retrograde pancreatography (ERP) (TAKISHIMA et al. 2000). The authors of a radiological classification of blunt pancreatic trauma attempted to correlate CT findings with ductal injury in a limited series of patients:

Grade A Pancreatitis and/or superficial laceration at any site
Grade BI Deep laceration at distal pancreas
Grade BII Transection at distal pancreas
Grade CI Deep laceration at proximal pancreas
Grade CII Transection at proximal pancreas (WONG et al. 1997)

No ductal rupture was seen in grade A and no main pancreatic duct was intact in grades BII and CII. The diagnosis of pancreatic duct injury is not only problematic with cross-section imaging, but can also remain unrecognized during celiotomy or laparotomy in up to 8% of cases, with potentially disastrous consequences (LUCAS 1977).

7.5.1.5
Results

Published Reports

CT obtained at admission is much less effective in evidencing injury to the pancreas than to other solid abdominal organs. Using the single-slice technique, a normal CT examination cannot rule out pancreatic contusion or ductal injury (JEFFREY et al. 1983; PEITZMAN et al. 1986; DODDS et al. 1990; PEVEC et al. 1991; AKHRASS et al. 1996, 1997).

Many radiological reports have emphasized the difficulties in diagnosing pancreatic trauma with CT (STRAX et al. 1980; JEFFREY et al. 1983; FEDERLE 1983; COOK et al. 1986; RESCORLA et al. 1995; BRADLEY et al. 1998). CT performed shortly after admission or within 12 h of trauma, is read as normal in about 40%–70% of cases, despite significant pancreatic injury having been proven present by subsequent surgery or repeated imaging. Sensitivity of CT is between 33% and 85%, depending on CT technique, experience of the radiologist with pancreatic trauma, and index of clinical suspicion (PATTZMAN et al. 1986; BARKIN et al. 1988; SIVIT et al. 1992; NELSON et al. 1994; SMITH et al. 1996; AKHRASS et al. 1996; ARKOVITZ et al. 1997; JOBST et al. 1999; BIGATTINI et al. 1999; EL-BOGHDADLY et al. 2000). Sensitivity of 0% in the detection of pancreatic injury was reported (UDEKWU et al. 1996). In one surgical report, CT was said to be no better than flipping a coin in diagnosing injury to the main pancreatic duct and therefore should not be used to guide therapy (BRADLEY et al. 1998). When clinical suspicion is high, despite a normal examination obtained within a few hours of admission, CT should be repeated, with thin reconstructions 12 or 24 h later. CT should also be repeated in all cases, when the serum amylase level has increased or when clinical symptoms or abdominal clinical findings persist or increase (MEREDITH and TRUNKEY 1988; HORST and BIVINS 1989). A 100% sensitivity can be reached in a selected patient group, with a high index of suspicion and when CT examination is repeated (LANE et al. 1994; EL-BOGHDADLY et al. 2000). Hepatic, splenic, left renal, gastrointestinal, and mesenteric injury associated with massive hemoperitoneum or hematoma in the upper abdomen should not obscure pancreatic injury. In a recent surgical series, the main reasons for the delay in diagnosis of pancreatic trauma were missed injury at initial operation, failure to exclude blunt pancreatic trauma before nonsurgical treatment, delay in presentation and underestimation of severity of injury on CT, and missed duodenal rupture (LEPPANIEMI and HAAPIAINEN 1999). The possibility of a pancreatic injury should always be considered in children with bicycle falls, when the mechanism of injury was a direct frontal upper abdominal impact, and in child abuse. In children, diagnostic sensitivity is 85% at admission and 90% on delayed examination. This score is higher than in adults, although some publications claim that CT is also relatively insensitive for diagnosing pancreatic fracture in children, due to the absence of peripancreatic fat planes (Feliciano et al. 1987; Nelson et al. 1994; Arkowitz et al. 1997).

Personal Series

In a personal series, 10 patients, 5 male and 5 female, aged 10–47 years (mean, 22.3) were investigated at admission within 2 and 6 h of blunt abdominal trauma. In one patient, time from injury to CT was unknown. Six patients were involved in a car accident, three had a bicycle accident and one had been kicked by a horse. Serum amylase level at admission varied from 28 to 1225 UI/l (normal, 30–110) with a median level of 255 UI/l. Four patients had a normal serum amylase at admission. All patients complained of abdominal pain, two were in hemodynamic shock, one of them was comatose. The diagnosis of pancreatic injury was missed on initial CT in 6 of 10 patients. Reviewing the films, pancreatic contusion was confirmed in two cases that were initially missed. CT was repeated in four patients, at 15 and 39 h, 2 days, and 3 days, respectively, and confirmed pancreatic injury in all cases. ERP was obtained in two patients with a positive CT and confirmed main pancreatic duct rupture. Other abdominal injuries that were evidenced on CT at admission were duodenal contusion or rupture in two cases, rupture, hepatic contusion in two cases, splenic contusion in two cases, retroperitoneal hemorrhage in one case, and left renal contusion in another patient. All patients were operated: a caudal pancreatectomy was performed in three. One patient had pancreatic injury grade I, six had grade II, one grade III and two grade IV. One patient died from associated brain damage. A pancreatic fistula was observed in one case and treated by percutaneous catheterization (Bigattini et al. 1999).

7.5.2 Ultrasound

Ultrasound (US) was largely replaced by CT in the systematic screening of adult trauma patients. US may be helpful in addition to a doubtful CT in patients with minimal intraabdominal fat planes and in children with a suspicion of trauma that might be limited to the pancreas, but generally US is considered less reliable than CT in adults and in children, particularly in the assessment of the severity of injury (Jeffrey et al. 1986; Gorenstein et al. 1987; Van Steenbergen et al. 1987; Bass et al. 1988; Lane et al. 1996; Bang and Bentzon 1997; Giovine et al. 1997; Shuman 1997; Yoshii et al. 1998).

Focal or diffuse pancreatic gland enlargement can be seen, with areas of intrapancreatic hypoechogenicity or band-like structures. Frequently, peripancreatic fluid, similar to the findings in acute pancreatitis, is observed (Kuligowska et al. 1984). Pancreatic fractures can be exquisitely shown by US in some cases, but can also remain undetected in others, similarly to CT (Bozymski et al. 1981). The pancreatic duct is correctly investigated only in exceptional cases with US. It is generally agreed that the sensitivity of US is less for pancreatic injury than for other plain abdominal organs. A sensitivity of 71% was reported for the pancreas, whereas for injuries to the liver, spleen, and kidney a detection rate higher than 90% was found (Yoshii et al. 1998). When a conservative treatment of pancreatic injury was adopted in children, US is particularly useful during follow-up to depict biliary dilatation or a peripancreatic fluid collection or pseudocyst (Garel et al. 1983). The usefulness of the combination of US and ERP for effective patient management was stressed (Vallon et al. 1979; Gothi et al. 1993; Gothi 1998).

Endoscopic US (EUS) has been advocated in the diagnosis of blunt pancreatic trauma, but is too invasive for systematic use (Sugiyama et al. 1996). EUS is able to show hypoechoic areas at the site of injury, a complete transection, or hypoechoic peripancreatic fluid. No consistent data on EUS in pancreatic trauma are available: it is reported to be at least as sensitive as CT. Similarly to EUS, intraoperative US has not gained large popularity in the assessment of pancreatic injury.

7.5.3 Endoscopic Retrograde Pancreatography

Endoscopic retrograde pancreatography (ERP) is performed in 0.05% of all admitted trauma patients (Harrell et al. 1998). Preoperative or intraoperative ERP is claimed to be the gold standard for the diagnosis of pancreatic ductal injury in adults and is credited with the highest sensitivity and specificity in evidencing rupture of the main pancreatic duct compared to other imaging tests (Barkin et al. 1988; Whittwell et al. 1989; Hayward et al. 1989; Clements and Reisser 1996; Coppola et al. 1997). Positive signs of ductal injury include interruption of the main duct, showing a complete stop, local extravasation of contrast, remote diffusion, or filling

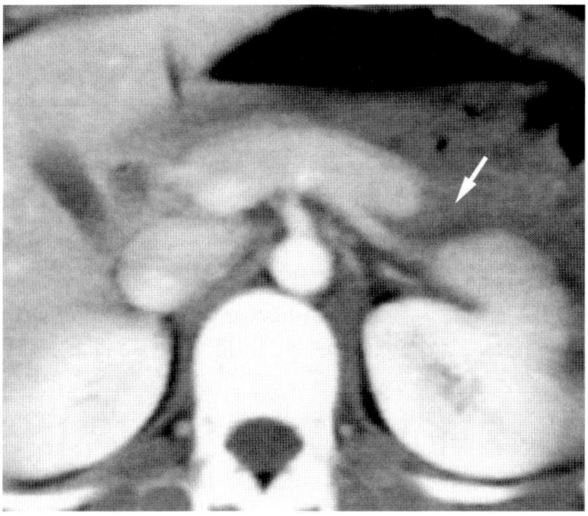

a

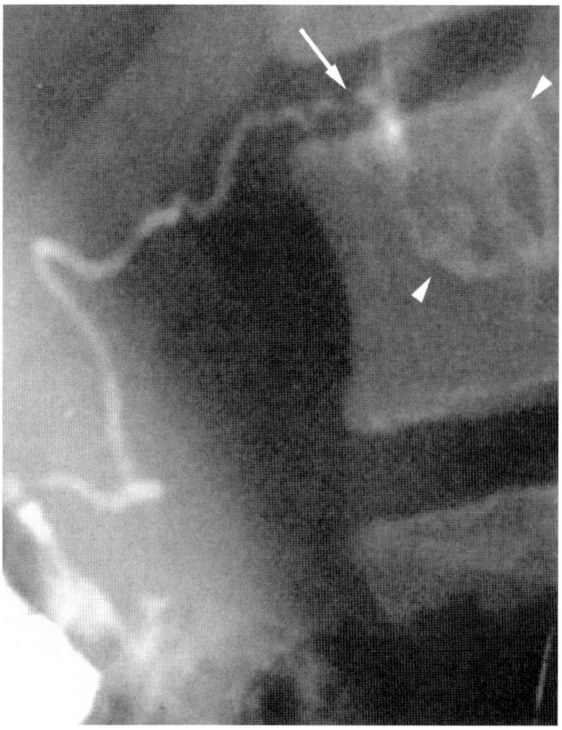

b

Fig. 7.11a, b. A 17-year-old male was kicked by a horse in the upper abdomen. Serum amylase at admission, 4 hours after trauma was at 45 UI/l. **a** CT showed complete transection of the tail of the pancreas (*arrow*). **b** ERP showed disruption of the main pancreatic duct in its distal segment (*arrow*) and extravasation of contrast medium (*arrowheads*). The patient was operated on: a caudal pancreatectomy was performed and a sump drain was placed

of a cavity (Figs. 7.11b, 7.3d). However, cannulation of the pancreatic duct may fail in 4%–10%, and a complication rate of 3%–5% is expected (Eimiller 1992; Takehara 1998; Nirula et al. 1999). Systematic use of ERP is questioned, because of the relatively invasive nature of the procedure in the acute post-traumatic phase and the relatively low frequency of ductal rupture, which occurs in about 15% of cases, and less often in contusion than in penetrating injury (Gougeon et al. 1976; Ham and Yeo 1976; Lucas 1977; Belhohlavek et al. 1978; Graham et al. 1978; Taxier et al. 1980; Bozymski et al. 1981; Berni et al. 1982; Jones 1985; Hall et al. 1986; Laraja et al. 1986; Feliciano et al. 1987; Keeling et al. 1987; Barkin et al. 1988; Sugawa and Lucas 1988; Whittwell et al. 1989; Stone et al. 1990; Blind et al. 1994, 1996; Doctor et al. 1995; Rescorla et al. 1995; Clements and Reisser 1996; Hirata et al. 1997).

In practice, ERP is rarely performed in the acute setting (Hayward et al. 1989). In an unstable patient, intraoperative ERP can be obtained during urgent laparotomy, but usually ERP is performed with some delay or in the early convalescent phase, when a peripancreatic or retroperitoneal fluid collection develops, persists or increases, when conservative management has failed and the clinical condition deteriorates, or when imaging gives equivocal results on pancreatic and ductal integrity (Barkin et al. 1988; Doctor et al. 1995).

Recognition of ductal rupture is a determining factor for proper management and to avoid prolonged morbidity and delayed complications (Taxier et al. 1980; Berni et al. 1982; Smego et al. 1985; Whittwell et al. 1989). In case of penetrating trauma, transection of the pancreatic duct and the common bile duct can be documented by the combined opacification of the pancreatic ducts and the bile ducts (McLindon et al. 1998). In a multi-institutional review, injury to the main pancreatic duct was the principal cause of post-traumatic pancreas-specific morbidity. As diagnostic delay of ductal rupture leads to an increased complication rate, the selection of the type of management should rather be based on pancreatic duct integrity established by ERP than on cross-section imaging alone (Bradley et al. 1998). Repeated CT after emergency ERP was claimed to enhance diagnostic sensitivity (Takishima et al. 1996b).

Finally, ERP has its own potential pitfalls. Rarely, a major pancreatic fracture or duodenal avulsion can be present without any abnormality seen on ERP, when the fracture line does not involve the main pancreatic duct (Fischer et al. 1996). Acquired or nontraumatic congenital anomalies such as pancreas divisum, choledochal cyst, and anomalous pancreatobiliary junction have to be correctly recognized and not be confused with posttraumatic changes (SUGIYAMA et al. 1998; PORTIS et al. 1994).

At present, the tendency is to adhere to CT investigation at admission, to repeat a negative or doubtful CT in patients with suspicion of pancreatic trauma, and to obtain ERP in selected cases, when clinical and laboratory findings and/or a peripancreatic fluid collection suggest pancreatic duct transection.

7.5.4 Angiography

In practice, pancreatic arteriography provides no significant contribution to the diagnosis of posttraumatic pancreatic injury. Celiomesenteric arteriography may confirm contrast medium extravasation from an intra- or peripancreatic artery, may occasionally show passage of contrast in the pancreatic duct or other signs of arterial trauma such as arterial occlusion, arteriovenous shunt, vessel irregularities, false aneurysm, arterial stretching or displacement, an intraparenchymal avascular zone at the parenchymal phase, and finally displacement, compression, or thrombosis of the splenic vein or other peripancreatic veins. Angiographic signs of pancreatic injury are nonspecific and may remain subtle despite significant pancreatic injury being shown on CT (CHVOJKA 1970; HAERTEL and FUCHS 1974; SOROUDI and BOOKSTEIN 1975).

7.5.5 Magnetic Resonance Imaging

Magnetic resonance imaging (MRI) so far has little role to play in the assessment of the acute abdominal trauma victim. MRI and magnetic resonance cholangiopancreatography (MRCP) can be indicated in the postoperative, subacute, convalescent, or chronic phase to confirm disruption of the main pancreatic duct or of a side branch that may escape ERP, to show a pseudocyst or a ductal stricture with duct obstruction. Sensitivities for pancreatic duct dilatation of 87%–100% and a specificity of 81% were reported (MAMMONE et al. 1998; TAKEHARA 1998; NIRULA et al. 1999; FULCHER and TURNER 1999a, b; FULCHER et al. 2000; SOTO et al. 2001). On T2-weighted sequences, pancreatic rupture appears as a hyperintense signal and rupture of the pancreatic duct can be evidenced on MRCP (CROMBE et al. 2001) (Fig. 7.4b, c). The widespread availability of noninvasive imaging of the pancreatic ducts by MRCP – and multislice CT – will be a major advance in the management of pancreatic injury.

7.5.6 Diagnostic Peritoneal Lavage

There is agreement that diagnostic peritoneal lavage (DPL) is not a reliable indicator of blunt pancreatic trauma; neither is the lavage fluid amylase level (JEFFREY et al. 1983; FREEMAN 1985; COOK et al. 1986; WALKER 1986; MEREDITH and TRUNKEY 1988; GLANCY 1989; LINKER and DELUCA 1989; CHAPMAN and MORRIS 1989; WISLON and MOOREHEAD 1991; CRAIG et al. 1995).

False-positive results are common. Only a minority of patients with elevated lavage fluid amylase have proven pancreatic injury. Amylase is not specific for pancreatic injury and may also be elevated in injury to the gastrointestinal tract (JEFFREY et al. 1983; COOK et al. 1986; LINKER and DELUCA 1989). False-negative results are also observed. A complete pancreatic transection, caused by injury confined to the retroperitoneal space, can be accompanied by normal lavage amylase. However, patients with persistent ascites in the posttraumatic period and constantly elevated amylase and protein levels in the ascites fluid should undergo intense pancreatic imaging to confirm a pancreatic duct fistula.

7.6 Management

7.6.1 Surgical

Pancreatic injuries have a low priority versus hemorrhage from solid viscera and rupture of the gastrointestinal tract (JONES et al. 1991).

Surgery is formally indicated in all penetrating pancreatic injuries and generally in pancreatic duct rupture, duodenal rupture, persistent hemorrhage, free abdominal air, and other associated injuries that require repair, and finally in any equivocal situation requiring surgery for diagnosis. Management of blunt pancreatic trauma has evolved over the years, but is still controversial. The principal question is whether there is a rupture of the main pancreatic duct. Surgical exploration is reliable in evaluating pancreatic duct rupture (SMEGO et al. 1985). Systematic early surgical intervention also shortcuts escalation into delayed mortality and morbidity, as a delay in diagnosis of ductal rupture beyond 24 h was shown to worsen the outcome significantly (Lucas 1977; Jones et al. 1990; Bradley et al. 1998; Meier et al. 2001). Arrest of hemorrhage, débridement, and active drainage are basic principles of surgical treatment. In penetrating injury, complete disruption of the pancreas can be treated with primary repair of the pancreatic duct, when possible (Martin et al. 1968; Raymond and Dane 1987; Hashimoto et al. 1998). In case of combined pancreatic and duodenal injury, surgical intervention is always mandatory. In the most severe forms of injury with duodenopancreatic devascularization and lesions that preclude conservatism, cephalic pancreaticoduodenectomy is required (Foley et al. 1969; Anderson et al. 1973; Cogbill et al. 1982; Oreskovich and Carrico 1984). In case of pancreatic duct transection, an efficient treatment is spleen-preserving, caudal pancreatectomy or, when the duct lesion is located to the right of the mesenteric vessels, a Whipple procedure. Duct ligation was proposed as an alternative to pancreatojejunostomy during a Whipple procedure in the unstable patient (Strauch 1972; Yellin et al. 1972; Babb and Harmon 1976; Robey et al. 1982; Fitzgibbons et al. 1982; Dawson and Scott-Conner 1986; Henriques et al. 1986; Cremer and Becker 1987; Carr et al. 1989; Pachter et al. 1989; Stone et al. 1990; Gentilello et al. 1991; Schein et al. 1991; Sukul et al. 1992; Delcore et al. 1994; Sheridan and Mitchell 1994; McGahren et al. 1995; Jobst et al. 1999; Kurisu et al. 1999; Thomson and Ghimenton 2000).

As indicated above, urgent laparotomy reduces septic complications and the number of posttraumatic pancreatic pseudocysts, filled by persistent ductal leakage. Conservative surgery, which consists of drainage without resection, does not necessarily decrease late complications and may even increase their rate and carry more death than resection (Anane-Sefah et al. 1975; Wisner et al. 1990; Akhrass et al. 1996). In minor pancreatic injury in children, the advantage of surgical drainage versus nondrainage is still being debated (Jobst et al. 1999). As the majority of pancreatic injuries are grade I to II, in these minor injuries, passive closed drainage is usually applied, and in more advanced injury – grade III – débridement and evacuation of hematoma. Active sump drainage and catheter jejunostomy for early parenteral feeding is performed in the majority of these patients.

Overall, surgical exploration is mandatory in about one-third of the patients, mainly because of the frequently associated injuries (Akhrass et al. 1997). Two-thirds of patients with blunt pancreatic trauma were shown to have trivial injury at operation and radical pancreatic resection is only rarely required.

7.6.2
Conservative Nonoperative

When minor pancreatic injury can be ascertained by imaging, some advocate conservative nonoperative management, guided by clinical, laboratory, and imaging findings, but accepting the risk of a missed ductal rupture. Main pancreatic duct disruption treated with total parenteral nutrition was sporadically reported (Shirai et al. 1995). Conservative management intends to reduce the number of unnecessary laparotomies in benign and single-organ contusion, but on the other hand, isolated pancreatic damage rarely occurs and the potential complications resulting from unrecognized pancreatic duct rupture and an associated duodenal or intestinal perforation or other significant injuries are a permanent threat with potentially severe consequences (Hilfer and Holgersen 1995; Fischer et al. 1996; Keller et al. 1997; Timberlake 1997; Bigattini et al. 1999; Nance et al. 2000). When conservative management is adopted, ERP is mandatory to confirm main pancreatic duct integrity, particularly when the patient had abdominal pain and elevated serum amylase at admission (Chandler and Waxman 1996; Harrell et al. 1998).

Another drawback of conservative, nonsurgical treatment is possible delayed hemorrhage. Unrecognized pancreatic hemorrhage is uncommon, but can be life-threatening, with an early mortality rate from exsanguination of 20%–50%. Furthermore, posttraumatic hemorrhage can also originate from an unrecognized extrapancreatic abdominal bleeding source. Contrast-enhanced CT images have to be scrutinized with utmost attention, in order to correctly localize a bleeding source in the pancreatic area (Stone et al. 1981; Freeman 1985; Cook et al. 1996) (Fig. 7.6d).

In the pediatric age group, isolated and benign pancreatic contusions (grade I or II) without major ductal rupture are more frequent than in adults and therefore more often allow for a conservative nonsurgical management, which is actually adopted in 50%–90% of cases (Gorenstein et al. 1987; Keller et al. 1997; Shilyansky et al. 1998; Jobst et al. 1999). Successful attempts at conservative treatment in children with combined injury of the liver or spleen or complete transection of the pancreas and duodenum were occasionally reported (Ohno et al. 1995;

Arkowitz and Garcia 1996; Keller et al. 1997; Yagi et al. 1997).

Recently, early endoscopic placement of a stent in the disrupted pancreatic duct after sphincterotomy was reported (Bendahan et al. 1995; Canty and Weinman 2001). Stenting of the pancreatic duct was followed by a rapid clinical improvement and the stent was removed within 12 days of placement.

7.6.3 Prognosis

Despite the diagnostic difficulties and frequent delays, the percentage of patients who die primarily from pancreatic trauma is actually low, from 0%–10%. In several large studies, more than 90% of direct admissions with pancreatic injury survived (Anderson et al. 1974; Grosfeld and Cooney 1975; Kudsk et al. 1986; Timberlake 1997; Graham et al. 2000). In other large series of pediatric pancreatic trauma, no deaths were directly attributable to isolated pancreatic injury.

The reported overall mortality rates following blunt pancreatic injury average 10%–30%, although higher rates of up to 50% were reported. Isolated pancreatic injury carries an overall lower death rate of 3%–10% and injury to the head of the pancreas or combined pancreatic and duodenal injury a death rate of 20%–30%, but death may be caused by other extrapancreatic injuries (Bach and Frey 1971; Olsen 1973; Heitsch et al. 1976; Graham et al. 1978, 1979; Balasegaram 1979; Stone et al. 1981; Cogbill et al. 1982; Laborde et al. 1982; Sims et al. 1984; Jones 1985; Smego et al. 1985; Peitzman et al. 1986; Chapman and Morris 1989; Keller et al. 1997; Gothi 1998; Carboni et al. 1999). Death is more common in the presence of duct injury and duct injury is more often associated with bowel injury, reflecting severity of trauma (Heitsch et al. 1976). The death rate is also correlated with the type of surgery: mortality is higher with a drainage procedure than with resection (Anane-Sefah et al. 1975). Associated abdominal or extraabdominal injuries, profound hemorrhagic shock, suppurative pancreatitis, and posttraumatic respiratory insufficiency are among the most frequent overall causes of fatalities (Stone et al. 1981).

Penetrating pancreatic injury carries an overall mortality rate of 23%–66%, mainly due to severe vascular and other associated injuries (Young et al. 1998; Firstenberg et al. 1999). In a review of the literature of patients with predominantly penetrating injury (73%), the highest mortality rates were found in patients who underwent total pancreatectomy, duct reanastomosis, and those who had no surgical treatment (Glancy 1989). There seems to be no significant difference in mortality between isolated blunt and penetrating pancreatic injury (Karl and Chandler 1977; Jones 1978).

7.7 Complications

7.7.1 Frequency and Prevention

Early or delayed posttraumatic complications include pseudocyst, internal and external pancreatic fistulas, hemorrhage, acute pancreatitis, anastomotic breakdown, pancreatic ascites, sepsis and abscess formation, multiorgan failure, peripheral fat necrosis, and thromboembolic complications (Toftdahl et al. 1984; Adams 1993; Tyburski et al. 2001). Gram-negative sepsis is one of the most frequent causes of death and sepsis is correlated with duct rupture and bowel perforation (Heitsch et al. 1976). As interruption of pancreatic duct integrity accounts for half of all complications, persistent elevated amylase should always prompt intensive pancreatic imaging (Roberts 1975; Heitsch et al. 1976).

Late complications may occur several months or even years after trauma and include chronic pancreatitis, pancreatic duct stricture, bile duct obstruction, diabetes, and exocrine pancreatic insufficiency. The latter complication is rare, even after extensive pancreatic resection (Douglas and Luck 1974; Rubio and Dichoso 1987; Bradley 1991; Wilson and Moorehead 1991).

Overall estimated frequency of complications is 20%–70% with an additional mortality rate of 10%–20% (Bach and Frey 1971; Anane-Sefah et al. 1975; Campbell and Kennedy 1980; Cogbill et al. 1982; Laborde et al. 1982; Moore and Moore 1984; Sims et al. 1984; Smego et al. 1985; Rubio and Dichoso 1987; Leppaniemi et al. 1988; Carr et al. 1989; Wilson and Moorehead 1991; Moncure and Goins 1993; Riedl et al. 1994; Madiba and Mokoena 1995; Emmick and Pertersen 1996; Lane et al. 1996; Akhrass et al. 1997; Carboni et al. 1999; Thanh et al. 1999).

Complications are best avoided by prompt recognition of pancreatic injury and rapid and proper initial therapy.

7.7.2 Pancreatic Pseudocyst and Abscess

Necrotic pseudocyst formation is a common complication of pancreatic injury and is observed more frequently in children than in adults (Fig. 7.7, 7.5b). Overall, pseudocysts have been noted in up to 60% or 80% of children with blunt pancreatic trauma. (GROSFELD and COONEY 1975; PEDINIELLI et al. 1979; POKORNY et al. 1980; SIVIT et al. 1992; MCGAHREN et al. 1995; ARKOWITZ et al. 1997; GRAHAM et al. 2000).

Postoperative pancreatitis is observed in 3%–10% after pancreatic resection and usually has a smooth course; the feared hemorrhagic pancreatitis is rare (SPITZ 1965; GRAHAM et al. 1978; JONES 1985; COGBILL et al. 1991). Serial CT or US examinations are best suited to following regression of peripancreatic fluid collections. In fact, in adults, pancreatic trauma is the third cause of pseudocyst formation, following alcohol abuse and biliary calculi, and accounts for 3% or 8% of all pseudocysts for operative and nonoperative causes, respectively (MAULE and REBER 1993). With early surgical revision, the number of posttraumatic pseudocysts was reduced, whereas with conservative treatment, 40% of children who have sustained pancreatic trauma develop pseudocysts (BURNWEIT et al. 1990; WILSON and MORREHEAD 1991). Posttraumatic pseudocysts are often a self-limiting process and show a tendency of spontaneous resolution similar to pseudocysts of nontraumatic origin (BASS et al. 1988). Pseudocysts detected in pancreatic laceration and main pancreatic duct injury, and with a diameter of less than 10 cm, usually spontaneously regressed (KOUCHI et al. 1999).

Persistent or enlarging pseudocysts or those that become symptomatic should be treated. Pseudocysts may become complicated even weeks, months or more than a decade after trauma, by hemorrhage, superinfection, abscess, rupture, fistulization, or bowel obstruction or compression of other adjacent structures (NAGY 1990; YOSHII et al. 1998; LUCAYA et al. 1998). Patients with symptomatic pseudocysts may be seriously ill and sometimes require a prolonged hospital stay of several months (DAHMAN and STEPHENS 1981). A pseudocyst can rupture into adjacent bowel or solid viscera, mainly the liver, spleen, or left kidney, or the pseudocyst may extend through the diaphragm into the pleura, mediastinum, or pericardium (HARDIKAR et al. 1986; WHITMAN et al. 1988; OKUDA et al. 1991).

When a pseudocyst shows a fluid-like echo-free content, it can be successfully drained externally by percutaneous catheter placement or internally in the upper gastrointestinal tract with US or endoscopic control (BASS et al. 1988). When the pseudocyst is communicating with an unobstructed pancreatic duct, it usually heals with prolonged drainage (FUNNELL et al. 1994; SHILYANSKY et al. 1998; HOLLAND et al. 1999; JOBST et al. 1999). Rarely, healing of complete disruption of the main pancreatic duct was reported following simple percutaneous catheter drainage of a communicating pseudocyst (OHNO et al. 1995). Needle aspiration alone of a pseudocyst without placing a catheter is usually ineffective in about two-thirds of patients, as fluid regularly reaccumulates within the pseudocyst (SHILYANSKY et al. 1998). Absence of pancreatic duct disruption should be checked by ERP, before percutaneous pseudocyst drainage is considered, but ductal catheterization and contrast injection itself can carry a risk of pseudocyst infection or hemorrhage: the place of ERP is therefore not clearly defined, but early drainage prevents secondary complications of the pseudocyst (JAFFE et al. 1989).

In anecdotal cases, a cystic pancreatic tumor diagnosed shortly after trauma was mistaken for a posttraumatic pseudocyst (PERSSON et al. 1986; HANSSON et al. 1999). When reading ERP or magnetic resonance pancreatography (MRP) in trauma patients, the possibility of a congenital underlying pancreatobiliary anomaly should be recognized, although the practical implication is low (SUGIYAMA et al. 1998).

Posttraumatic pancreatic abscesses develop in 8%–25% and are most frequent after penetrating injury, incomplete débridement and drainage, or when other abdominal injuries including bowel rupture are associated (WYNN et al. 1985; FELICIANO et al. 1987; BOFFARD and BROOKS 2000). The rate of abdominal abscesses following pancreatic and duodenal injuries may amount to 61% and predominate in patients who required relaparotomy (COGBILL et al. 1991; MONCURE and GOINS 1993). Drainage of a pancreatic abscess can be performed either by an exclusive percutaneous catheter drainage or by a synchronous anterior celiotomy and posterior drainage or by intraoperative endoscopic transpancreatic drainage (BERNE et al. 1981; KOPELMAN et al. 1998).

A biloma in contact with the pancreas, resulting from laceration of the common bile duct at the level of the superior margin of the pancreas, may mimic a pancreatic pseudocyst. When a fluid collection extends in the porta hepatis, an associated bile duct rupture should be suspected (BOURQUE et al. 1989).

Finally, a pancreatic sequestrum, that was not evacuated surgically, may be responsible for abdominal pain developing or persisting months or years after trauma (KUDSK et al. 1986).

7.7.3 Pancreatic Fistulas

Posttraumatic pancreatic fistulas are common and were called rather a desired result than a complication after ductal rupture. Incidence varies from 7%–35% and was highest when the diagnosis was delayed or after injury of the pancreatic head; 26% occur after a combined pancreatic and duodenal injury and 14% after a partial pancreatic resection (Graham et al. 1978; Balasegaram 1979; Stone et al. 1981; Fitzgibbons et al. 1982; Cogbill et al. 1982, 1991; Moore and Moore 1984; Jones 1985; Moncure and Goins 1993; Madiba and Mokoena 1995; Akhrass et al. 1997).

Pancreatic fistulas preferentially develop after drainage procedures and may lengthen considerably the duration of hospital stay (Lucas 1977). With conservative medical treatment, 70% of a low-output pancreatic fistula closes within 2 weeks, when no obstruction to flow is present (Feliciano et al. 1987). Some pancreatic fistulas are complex, also involving the gastrointestinal tract. They most likely occur in connection with posttraumatic abscess formation, and are of increased output (Lal et al. 1978) (Fig. 7.12). Other fistulas develop after external drainage of a pseudocyst (Pokorny et al. 1980; Farrell et al. 1996). Low-output fistulas may occasionally close spontaneously. In case of nonresponse of a high-output fistula after a trial with octreotide or somatostatin treatment, percutaneous catheter drainage can be applied before more radical surgery is considered (Cabay et al. 1998). Depending on the localization of the ductal fistula and therapeutic response to medical treatment and catheter drainage, distal pancreatic resection, pancreaticojejunostomy of the injured segment or cephalic pancreaticoduodenectomy are required (Klar et al. 1999). Sinograms and ERP can be both diagnostic and therapeutic, by insertion of a percutaneous drainage catheter or a plastic stent, which bridges the gap in a ruptured main pancreatic duct, similarly to the accepted surgical technique (Fabre et al. 1995; McGahren et al. 1995; Huckfeldt et al. 1996; Thanh et al. 1999; Canty and Weinman 2001). The procedure can also be performed percutaneously in selected patients when the endoscopic route is impossible or has failed (Dondelinger and Kurdziel 1991) (Fig. 7.12). In this respect, routine intraoperative ERP in case of proximal duct laceration was shown to reduce postoperative morbidity from 55% to 15% (Berni et al. 1982).

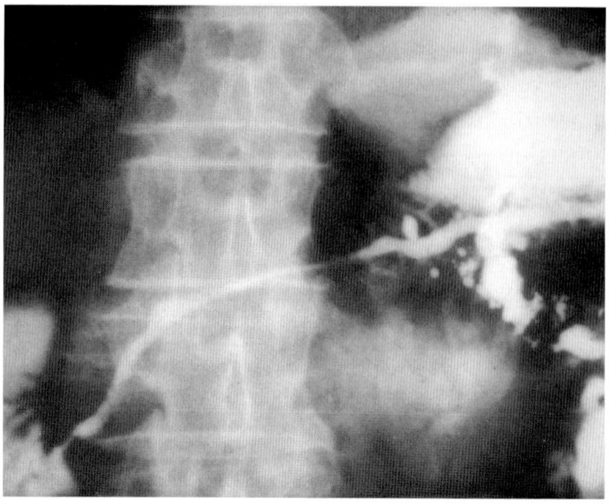
a

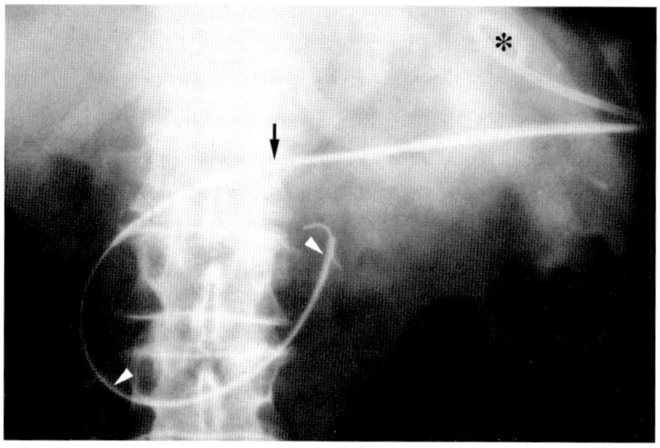
b

Fig. 7.12a, b. An 81-year-old male was involved in a traffic accident. A splenectomy was carried out for splenic rupture and pancreatic contusion was diagnosed at laparotomy. A pancreatic duct laceration was confirmed at postoperative ERP and treated with a 7F plastic stent. Thereafter, the patient developed a left subphrenic abscess. **a** Percutaneous catheter drainage of the subphrenic abscess was performed. Contrast abscessogram showed a communication of the abscess cavity with the pancreatic duct, stomach, and left colon. **b** The pancreatic duct was separately catheterized by a percutaneous left lateral approach. The 7F plastic stent (*arrowheads*) was pushed over the wire in the duodenum. The transpapillary drainage catheter (*arrow*) was exchanged for two metal Strecker stents (4 cm, 4 mm) placed in a posttraumatic narrowing of the pancreatic duct, which had formed at the site of disruption. Note the pigtail drainage catheter in place in the left subphrenic abscess (*asterisk*). The subphrenic abscess regressed and the pancreatic fistula closed. The patient died several months later from pneumonia. (From Dondelinger and Kurdziel 1991, with permission)

7.7.4 Hemorrhage

Some pancreatic trauma victims present at admission with shock or with the full range of symptoms of acute hemorrhagic pancreatitis, which is immediately diagnostic (Spitz 1965). Immediate or delayed hemorrhage can also develop some time after admission or a quiescent pseudoaneurysm may form, which is at risk of delayed rupture and bleeding at any time, either in the peritoneal cavity or the retroperitoneal space, the gastrointestinal tract or inside a posttraumatic pseudocyst (Fig. 7.6d). Perioperative hemorrhage from an associated injury may be responsible for a mortality rate of 9% (Fitzgibbons et al. 1982). Figures of 5%–10% of significant postoperative secondary hemorrhage were reported, often in connection with abdominal sepsis and abscess formation (Campbell and Kennedy 1980; Cogbill et al. 1982; Moore and Moore 1984; Mansour et al. 1989).

Patients present either with intraabdominal bleeding or upper gastrointestinal hemorrhage, when blood is removed through the pancreatic duct (hemosuccus pancreaticus). Upper gastrointestinal tract endoscopy may confirm the origin of bleeding through the papilla. About 2% of all hemobilia are in fact of pancreatic origin (Sandblom 1972). Intracystic hemorrhage and sepsis are also classic complications of pseudocysts, which can occasionally be fatal (Cogbill 1968; Greenstein et al. 1971; Lewis et al. 1993). Emergent angiography and selective arterial embolization is the treatment of choice for a pancreatic posttraumatic pseudoaneurysm, arteriovenous fistula, or active bleeding of a pancreatic or peripancreatic artery and should immediately follow the recognition of any intra- or peripancreatic contrast extravasation or a pancreatic blush seen on CT (Kadell et al. 1967; Brintnall et al. 1974; Freeman et al. 1985; Baker et al. 1987; Shah et al. 1988).

7.8 Conclusion

A direct frontal mid to upper abdominal impact and a bicycle fall on the handlebar in a child are classic mechanisms of blunt pancreatic injury. Clinical symptoms are not specific. The serum amylase level is frequently normal during the first 3 h and peritoneal lavage fluid amylase is not a reliable diagnostic test. CT is the most powerful imaging technique to evidence pancreatic injury and associated lesions, but remains normal or doubtful at admission in about 40% of adults. Neither CT nor US are able to visualize pancreatic duct rupture. As ERP cannot be performed in all trauma patients, only patients with minor or moderate pancreatic injury can be enrolled in a conservative management without surgical revision. The role of multislice CT at admission and MRP has to be investigated in the future, with the hope of increasing diagnostic efficiency in the demonstration of pancreatic duct rupture. Early recognition of pancreatic injury and efficient proper management reduce the number of delayed posttraumatic complications.

References

Adams DB (1993) Peripheral fat necrosis after penetrating pancreatic trauma: a case report. Am Surg 59:769–771

Akhrass R, Kim K, Brandt CP (1996) Computed tomography: an unreliable indicator of pancreatic trauma. Am Surg 62: 647–651

Akhrass R, Yaffe MB, Brandt CP, Reigle M, Fallow WF Jr, Mallangoni MA (1997) Pancreatic trauma: a ten-year multi-institutional experience. Am Surg 63:598–604

Alanen M, Pajulo O, Reunanen M (2000) Pancreatic injuries in children. Ann Chir Gynaecol 89:277–280

Anane-Sefah J, Norton LW, Eiseman B (1975) Operative choice and technique following pancreatic injury. Arch Surg 110: 161–166

Anderson CB, Weisz D, Rodger MR, Tucker GL (1973) Combined pancreaticoduodenal trauma. Am J Surg 125:530–534

Anderson CB, Connors JP, Mejia DC et al (1974) Drainage methods in the treatment of pancreatic injuries. Surg Gynecol Obstet 138:587–590

Arkowitz MS, Garcia VF (1996) Spontaneous recanalization of the pancreatic duct: case report and review. J Trauma 40: 1014–1016

Arkowitz MS, Johnson N, Garcia VF (1997) Pancreatic trauma in children: mechanism of injury. J Trauma 42:49–53

Babb J, Harmon H (1976) Diagnosis and management of pancreatic trauma. Am Surg 42:390–394

Bach RD, Frey CF (1971) Diagnosis and treatment of pancreatic trauma. Am J Surg 121:20–29

Baker KS, Tisnado J, Cho S-R, Beachley MC (1987) Splanchnic artery aneurysms and pseudoaneurysms: transcatheter embolization. Radiology 163: 135–139

Baker LP, Wagner EJ, Brotman S, Whitley NO (1982) Transection of the pancreas. J Comput Assist Tomogr 6:411–412

Balasegaram M (1979) Surgical management of pancreatic trauma. Curr Probl Surg 16:1–59

Balsano NA, Reynolds BM (1973) Rupture of the common duct and ampulla of Vater due to blunt trauma. Ann Surg 178: 200–203

Balthazar EJ, Megibow A, Rothberg M, Lefleur RS (1985) CT evaluation of pancreatic injury following splenectomy. Gastrointest Radiol 10:139–144

Bang N, Bentzon N (1997) Pancreatic fracture diagnosed by ultrasound. Ugeskrift for Laeger 159:7989–4990

Barkin JS, Ferstenberg RM, Panullo W, Manten HD, Davis RC Jr (1988) Endoscopic retrograde cholangiopancreatography in pancreatic trauma. Gastrointest Endosc 34:102–105

Bass J, Di Lorenzo M, Desjardins JG, Grignon A, Ouimet A (1988) Blunt pancreatic injuries in children: the role of percutaneous external drainage in the treatment of pancreatic pseudocysts. J Pediatr Surg 23:721–724

Belohlavek D, Merkle P, Probst M (1978) Identification of traumatic rupture of the pancreatic duct by endoscopic retrograde pancreatography. Gastrointest Endosc 24: 255–256

Bendahan J, Van Rewsburg CJ, Van Vuren B, Muller R (1995) Endoscopic intrapancreatic stent for traumatic duct injury. Injury 8:553–554

Berletti R, Cavagna E, Carubia G, Schiavon F, Tedeschi U (2000) An isolated complete fracture of the pancreas due to skiing trauma. Integrated imaging in a case. Radiol Med (Torino) 100:81–84

Berne TV, Donovan AJ (1981) Synchronous anterior coeliotomy and posterior drainage of pancreatic abscess. Arch Surg 116:527–533

Berni GA, Bandyk DF, Oreskovich MR, Carrico CJ (1982) Role of intra-operative pancreatography in patients with injury to the pancreas. Am J Surg 143:602–605

Bigattini D, Boverie JH, Dondelinger RF (1999) CT of blunt trauma of the pancreas in adults. Eur Radiol 9:244–249

Bleichner JP, Guillou YM, Martin L, Sequin P, Malledant Y (1998) Pancreatitis after blunt injuries to the abdomen. Ann Fr Anesth Reanim 17:250–253

Blind PJ, Mellbring G; Hjertkvist M, Sandzen B (1994) Diagnosis of traumatic pancreatic duct rupture by on-table endoscopic retrograde pancreatography. Pancreas 9:387–389

Blind PJ, Norrgard O, Oberg A (1996) Intraoperative endoscopic retrograde pancreatography reveals traumatic pancreatic duct rupture. Lakartidningen 93:3473–3474

Boffard KD, Brooks AJ (2000) Pancreatic trauma – injuries to the pancreas and pancreatic duct. Eur J Surg 166:4–12

Bourque MD, Spigland N, Bensoussan AL, Garel L, Blanchard H (1989) Isolated complete transection of the common bile duct due to blunt trauma in a child, and review of the literature. J Pediatr Surg 24:1068–1070

Bouwman DL, Altshuler J, Weaver DW (1983) Hyperamylasemia: a result of intracranial bleeding. Surgery 94:318–323

Bouwman DL, Weaver DW, Walt AJ (1984) Serum amylase and its isoenzymes: a clarification of their implications in trauma. J Trauma 24:573–578

Bozymski EM, Orlando RC, Holt JW III (1981) Traumatic disruption of the pancreatic duct demonstrated by endoscopic retrograde pancreatography. J Trauma 21:244–245

Bradley EL III (1991) Chronic obstructive pancreatitis as a delayed complication of pancreatic trauma. HPB Surg 5: 49–59; discussion 59–60

Bradley EL III, Young PR Jr, Chang MC et al (1998) Diagnosis and initial management of blunt pancreatic trauma: guidelines from a multi-institutional review. Ann Surg 227: 861–869

Brintnall BB, Laidlaw WW, Papp JP (1974) Hemobilia: pancreatic pseudocyst hemorrhage demonstrated by endoscopy and arteriography. Dig Dis 19:186–188

Burkhardt G, Gabsch HC, Lantsch H (1967) Serum lipase determination within the scope of pancreas diagnosis. Z Gesamte Inn Med 22:112–117

Burnweit C, Wesson D, Stringer D, Filler R (1990) Percutaneous drainage of traumatic pancreatic pseudocysts in children. J Trauma 30:1273–1277

Buxton B (1969) Rupture of the duodenum produced by a safety belt. Aust N Z J Surg 38:315–320

Cabay JE, Boverie JH, Dondelinger RF (1998) Percutaneous catheter drainage of external fistulas of the pancreatic duct. Eur Radiol 8:445–448

Cameron CM, Lazoritz S, Calhoun AD (1997) Blunt abdominal injury: simultaneously occurring liver and pancreatic injury in child abuse. Pediatr Emerg Care 13:334–336

Campbell R, Kennedy T (1980) The management of pancreatic and pancreaticoduodenal injuries. Br J Surg 67:845–850

Campero AA, Campbell GD (1974) Intra-pancreatic pseudocyst following a rugby injury. N Z Med J 79:1068–1071

Canty TG Sr, Weinman D (2001) Treatment of pancreatic duct disruption in children by an endoscopically placed stent. J Pediatr Surg 36:345–348

Carboni GL, Rothlin MA, Trentz O (1999) Management of pancreatic injuries. Unfallchirurg 102:298–304

Carr ND, Caims SJ, Lees WR, Russell RC (1989) Late complications of pancreatic trauma. Br J Surg 76:1244–1246

Chamrova Z, Shanmuganathan K, Mirvis SE, Erb RE (1994) Retroperitoneal fluid resulting from rapid intravascular resuscitation in trauma: CT mimic of retroperitoneal injury. Emerg Radiol 1:85–88

Chandler C, Waxman K (1996) Demonstration of pancreatic ductal integrity by endoscopic retrograde pancreatography allows conservative surgical management. J Trauma 40:466–468

Chapman WC, Morris JA Jr (1989) Diagnosis and management of blunt pancreatic injury. J Tenn Med Assoc 82:84–85

Chvojka J (1970) Ein Beitrag der gezielten Angiographie zur Diagnostik der Pankreasverletzungen. ROFO 113:336–339

Clarnette TD, Beasley SW (1997) Handlebar injuries in children: patterns and prevention. Aust N Z J Surg 67:338–339

Clavien PA, Robert J, Meyer P et al (1989) Acute pancreatitis and normo-amylasemia. Ann Surg 210:614–620

Clements RH, Reisser JR (1996) Urgent endoscopic retrograde pancreatography in the stable trauma patient. Am Surg 62: 446–448

Cleveland HC, Waddell WR (1963) Retroperitoneal rupture of the duodenum due to non-penetrating – penetrating trauma. Surg Clin North Am 43:413–423

Cogbill CL (1968) Hemorrhage in pancreatic pseudocysts: review of literature and report of two cases. Ann Surg 167:112–115

Cogbill TH, Moore EM, Kashuk JL (1982) Changing trends in the management of pancreatic trauma. Arch Surg 117: 722–728

Cogbill TH, Moore EE, Morris JA et al (1991) Distal pancreatectomy for trauma: a multicenter experience. J Trauma 31:1600–1606

Cook DE, Walsh JM, Vick CW, Brewer WH (1986) Upper abdominal trauma: pitfalls in CT diagnosis. Radiology 159: 65–69

Coppola V, Vallone G, Verrengia D et al (1997) Pancreatic fractures: the role of CT and the indications for endoscopic retrograde pancreatography. Radiol Med (Torino) 94:335–340

Cox MR, Eastman MC (1994) Traumatic duodenal rupture and avulsion of the ampulla of Vater. HPB Surg 7: 225–229

Craig MH, Talton DS, Hauser CJ, Poole GV (1995) Pancreatic injuries from blunt trauma. Am Surg 61:125–128

Cremer H, Becker JH (1987) A spleen-preserving procedure in traumatic transection of the pancreas. A case report and evaluation of experimental data. S Afr J Surg 25:76–77

Crombe D, Ghijseling L, Van Campenhoudt M, Landen S, Pringot J (2001) Pancreatic duct rupture in a 26-year-old patient. J Belge Radiol 84:125

Dahman B, Stephens CA (1981) Pseudocysts of the pancreas after blunt abdominal trauma in children. J Pediatr Surg 16:17–21

Dawson DL, Scott-Conner CE (1986) Distal pancreatectomy with splenic preservation: the anatomic basis for a meticulous operation. J Trauma 26:1142–1145
De Roux SJ, Prendergast NC (1998) Laceration of the hepatoduodenal ligament, pancreas and duodenum in a child due to blunt impact. J Forensic Sci 43:222–224
Delany HM, Jason RS (1981) Abdominal trauma: surgical and radiological diagnosis. Springer, New York
Delcore R, Stauffer JS, Thomas JH, Pierce GE (1994) The role of pancreatogastrostomy following pancreatoduodenectomy for trauma. J Trauma 37:395–400
Dickerman RM, Dunn EL (1981) Splenic, pancreatic and hepatic injuries. Surg Clin North Am 61:3–16
Doctor N, Dodley JS, Davidson BR (1995) Assessment of pancreatic duct damage following trauma: is endoscopic retrograde cholangiopancreatography the gold standard. Postgrad Med J 71:116–117
Dodds WJ, Taylor AJ, Erickson SJ, Lawson TL (1990) Traumatic fracture of the pancreas: CT characteristics. J Comput Assist Tomogr 14:375–378
Dondelinger RF, Kurdziel JC (1991) Percutaneous placement of expandable metal stents in the main pancreatic duct. Seminars Intervent Radiol 8:316–320
Donovan AJ, Turrill F, Berne CJ (1972) Injuries of the pancreas from blunt trauma. Surg Clin North Am 52:649–665
Douglas JN, Luck RJ (1974) Late obstructive jaundice due to traumatic pancreatic granuloma. Injury 6:60–62
Eimiller A (1992) Complications in endoscopy (review) Endoscopy 24:176–184
El-Boghdadly S, Al-Yousef Z, Al Bedah K (2000) Pancreatic injury: an audit and a practical approach. Ann R Coll Surg Engl 82:258–262
Emmick RH, Petersen SR (1996) Evaluation of pancreatic injury after blunt abdominal trauma. Ann Emerg Med 27:658–661
Fabre JM, Bauret P, Prudhomme M et al (1995) Posttraumatic pancreatic fistula cured by endoprosthesis in the pancreatic duct. Am J Gastroenterol 90:804–806
Farkouh E, Wassef R, Henri A, Allard M (1982) Importance of the serum amylase level in patients with blunt abdominal trauma. Can J Surg 25:626–628
Farrell RJ, Krige JE, Bornman PC, Knottenbelt JD, Terblanche J (1996) Operative strategies in pancreatic trauma. Br J Surg 83:934–937
Federle MP (1983) Computed tomography of blunt abdominal trauma. Radiol Clin North Am 21:461–475
Federle MP, Goldberg HI, Kaiser JA, Moss AA, Jeffrey RB Jr, Mall JC (1981) Evaluation of abdominal trauma by computed tomography. Radiology 138:637–644
Federle MP, Crass RA, Jeffrey RB, Trunkey DD (1982) Computed tomography in blunt abdominal trauma. Arch Surg 117:645–650
Feliciano DV, Matin TD, Cruse PA, et al (1987) Management of combined pancreatoduodenal injuries. Ann Surg 205:673–679
Ficarra BJ (1996) Diseases and injuries in athletes. A review. J Med 27:241–275
Firstenberg MS, Volsko TA, Sivit C, Stallion A, Dudgeon DL, Grisoni ER (1999) Selective management of pediatric pancreatic injuries. J Pediatr Surg 34:1142–1147
Fischer JH, Carpenter KD, O'Keefe GE (1996) CT diagnosis of an isolated blunt pancreatic injury. AJR 167:1152
Fish JC, Johnson GL (1965) Rupture of duodenum following blunt trauma: report of a case with avulsion of papilla of Vater. Ann Surg 162:917–920
Fitzgibbons TS, Yellin AE, Maruyama MM, Donovan AJ (1982) Management of the transsected pancreas following distal pancreatectomy. Surg Gynecol Obstet 154:225–231
Florence MG, Hart MJ, White TT (1981) Ampullary disconnection during the course of biliary and duodenal surgery. Am J Surg 142:100–105
Foley WJ, Gaines RD, Fry WJ (1969) Pancreaticoduodenectomy for severe trauma to the head of the pancreas and the associated structures: report of three cases. Ann Surg 170:759–765
Fraser GC (1969) "Handlebar" injury of the pancreas. Report of a case complicated by pseudocyst formation with spontaneous internal rupture. J Pediatr Surg 4:216–219
Freeman CP (1985) Isolated pancreatic damage following seat belt injury. Injury 16:478–480
Freeman MP, Tisnado J, Cho SR (1985) Transcatheter embolization of the dorsal pancreatic artery to control massive postoperative bleeding. Am J Gastroenterol 80:185–187
Friend PJ, Jamieson NV, McFarlane R (1985) Blunt pancreatic injury: two case reports and a review of the literature. Injury 16:391–392
Fulcher AS, Turner MA (1999a) Magnetic resonance pancreatography. Crit Reviews Diagn Imaging 40:285–322
Fulcher AS, Turner MA (1999b) MR pancreatography: a useful tool for evaluating pancreatic disorders. Radiographics 19: 5–24
Fulcher AS, Turner MA, Yelon JA et al (2000) Magnetic resonance cholangiopancreatography (MRCP) in the assessment of pancreatic duct trauma and its sequelae: preliminary findings. J Trauma 48:1001–1007
Funnell IC, Bornman PC, Krige JE, Beningfield SJ, Terblanche J (1994) Endoscopic drainage of traumatic pancreatic pseudocyst. Br J Surg 81:879–881
Garel L, Brunelle F, Lallemand D et al (1983) Pseudocysts of the pancreas in children: which cases require surgery ? Pediatr Surg 13:120–124
Gentilello LM, Cortes V, Buechter KJ, Gomez GA, Castro M, Zeppa R (1991) Whipple procedure for trauma: is duct ligation a safe alternative to pancreaticojejunostomy? J Trauma 31:661–667
Gholson CF, Sittig K, Favrot D, McDonald JC (1994) Chronic abdominal pain as the initial manifestation of pancreatic injury due to remote blunt trauma of the abdomen. South Med J 87:902–904
Giovine S, Romano L, Rossi G, Ragozino A (1997) Computed tomography in the diagnosis of posttraumatic pancreatic lesions. Radiol Med 94:341–345
Glancy KE (1989) Review of pancreatic trauma. West J Med 151:45–51
Gonzalez R, Heiss WH, Rauh W (1987) Blunt abdominal trauma caused by child abuse. Monatsschr Kinderheilkd 135:692–695
Gorenstein A, O'Halpin D, Wesson DE, Daneman A, Filler RM (1987) Blunt injury to the pancreas in children: selective management based on ultrasound. J Pediatr Surg 22: 1110–1116
Gothi R (1998) US of pancreas in blunt abdominal trauma. Radiology 209:283
Gothi R, Bose NC, Kumar N (1993) Case report: ultrasound demonstration of traumatic fracture of the pancreas with pancreatic duct disruption. Clin Radiol 47:434–435
Gougeon FW, Legros G, Archambault A, Bessette G, Bastien E (1976) Pancreatic trauma: a new diagnostic approach. Am J Surg 132:400–402

Goyne WB, Alexander JM (1980) Use of fractionated amylase to distinguish between pancreatic and parotid injury: report of cases. J Oral Surg 38:522–524

Graham CA, O'Toole SJ, Watson AJ, Munro FD, Haddock G (2000) Pancreatic trauma in Scottish children. J R Coll Surg Edinb 45:223–226

Graham JM, Mattox KL, Jordon GL (1978) Traumatic injuries of the pancreas. Am J Surg 136:744–748

Graham JM, Mattox KL, Vauchan GD III, Jordan GL Jr (1979) Combined pancreatoduodenal injuries. J Trauma 19:340–346

Greenlee T, Murphy K, Ram MD (1984) Amylase isoenzymes in the evaluation of trauma patients. Am Surg 50:637–640

Greenstein A, Demaio EF, Nabseth DC (1971) Acute hemorrhage associated with pancreatic pseudocyst. Surgery 69: 56–62

Grosfeld JL, Cooney DR (1975) Pancreatic and gastrointestinal trauma in children. Pediatr Clin North Am 22:365–377

Guerriero WG, Carlton CE Jr, Jordan GL Jr (1973) Management of combined injury to the pancreas and upper urinary tract. J Urol 110:622–624

Haertel M, Fuchs WA (1974) Angiography in pancreatic trauma. Br J Radiol 47:641–645

Hager J, Menardi G (1982) Blunt abdominal injuries in children following winter sports accidents. ZFA (Stuttgart) 58: 1757–1760

Hall RI, Lavelle MI, Venables CW (1986) Use of ERCP to identify the site of traumatic injuries of the main pancreatic duct in children. Br J Surg 73:411–412

Ham JM, Yeo BW (1976) Operative pancreatography. Aust N Z J Surg 46:387–390

Hansson B, Hubens G, Hagendorens M, Deprettere A, Colpaert C, Eyskens E (1999) Frantz's tumour of the pancreas presenting as a post-traumatic pancreatic pseudocyst. Acta Chir Belg 99:82–84

Hardikar JV, Mistry RC, Patel CV (1986) Hydropneumopericardium due to ruptured traumatic pseudocyst of pancreas (a case report). J Postgrad Med 32:241–242

Harrell DJ, Vitale GC, Larson GM (1998) Selective role for endoscopic retrograde cholangiopancreatography in abdominal trauma. Surg Endosc 12:400–404

Harrison JD, Branicki FJ, Makin GS (1985) Pancreatic injury in association football. Injury 16:232

Hashimoto T, Otobe Y, Matsuo Y et al (1998) Successful primary repair of complete pancreatic disruption caused by blunt abdominal trauma: a report of two cases. Surgery 123:702–705

Hayward SR, Lucas CE, Sugawa C, Ledgerwood AM (1989) Emergent endoscopic retrograde cholangiopancreatography: a highly specific test for acute pancreatic trauma. Arch Surg 124:745–746

Heitsch RC, Knutson CO, Fulton RL, Jones CE (1976) Delineation of critical factors in the treatment of pancreatic trauma. Surgery 80:523–529

Henriques HF, Soderstrom CA, Crittenden MD, Gens DR (1986) Distal pancreatectomy with splenic preservation: a blunt trauma patient report. Md Med J 35:285–287

Herman TE, Siegel MJ (1991) CT of the pancreas in children. AJR 157:375–379

Heyse-Moore GH (1976) Blunt pancreatic and pancreaticoduodenal trauma. Br J Surg 63:226–228

Hilfer CL, Holgersen LO (1995) Massive chylous ascites and transected pancreas secondary to child abuse: successful nonsurgical management. Pediatr Radiol 25:117–119

Hirata K, Ohta R, Tsurudome Y et al (1997) Traumatic pancreatic duct rupture in a child diagnosed by endoscopic retrograde pancreatography. Eur J Pediatr Surg 7:48–49

Holland AJ, Davey RB, Sparnon AL, Chapman M, Lequesne GW (1999) Traumatic pancreatitis: long-term review of initial non-operative management in children. J Paediatr Child Health 35:78–81

Holmes G (1973) Flexion injuries of the pancreas. N Z Med J 79:302–303

Holmich P, Darre E, Jahnsen F et al (1988) The elite marathon runner: problems during and after competition. Br J Sports Med 22:19–21

Horst HM, Bivins BA (1989) Pancreatic transection. A concept of evolving injury. Arch Surg 124:1093–1095

Huckfeldt R, Agee C, Nicholds WK, Barthel J (1996) Nonoperative treatment of traumatic pancreatic duct disruption using an endoscopically placed stent. J Trauma 41:143–144

Hung SY, Chen HM, Jan YY, Chen MF et al (2000) Common bile duct and pancreatic injury after extracorporeal shock wave lithotripsy for renal stone. Hepatogastroenterology 47: 1162–1163

Ito T, Yamamoto M, MachidA H, Hashiguchi Y, Yatsuda N, Yasuda M (1993) Complete avulsion of the papilla of Vater and gastroduodenal artery due to blunt abdominal trauma: report of a case. Surg Today 23:172–175

Jaffe RB, Arata JA, Matlak ME (1989) Percutaneous drainage of traumatic pancreatic pseudocysts in children. AJR 152: 591–595

Jeffrey RB Jr, Federle MP, Crass RA (1983) Computed tomography of pancreatic trauma. Radiology 147:491–494

Jeffrey RB, Laing FC, Wing VW (1986) Ultrasound in acute pancreatic trauma. Gastrointest Radiol 11:44–46

Jobst MA, Ganty TG Sr, Lynch FP (1999) Management of pancreatic injury in pediatric blunt abdominal trauma. J Pediatric Surg 34:818–823

Johanet H, Fasano JJ, Marmuse JP et al (1991) Traumatismes du pancréas: urgence diagnostique et thérapeutique. Chirurgie 128:337–342

Jones RC (1978) Management of pancreatic trauma. Ann Surg 187:555–564

Jones RC (1985) Management of pancreatic trauma. Am J Surg 150:698–704

Jones WG, Finkelstein J, Barie PS (1990) Managing pancreatic trauma. Infect Surg 9:29–35

Jones WG II, Reilly DM, Baries PS (1991) Pancreatic injuries. Diagnosis, treatment. AORN J 53:917–918, 920–921, 924–933

Jurkovich GJ, Carrico CJ (1990) Pancreatic trauma. Surg Clin North Am 70:575–593

Justice AD, Dibenedetto RJ, Stanford E (1994) Significance of elevated pancreatic enzymes in intracranial bleeding. South Med J 87:889–893

Kadell BM, Riley JM (1967) Major arterial involvement by pancreatic pseudocysts. AJR 99:632–636

Karl HW, Chandler JG (1977) Mortality and morbidity of pancreatic injury. Am J Surg 134:549–554

Keeling P, Calthorpe D, Lane B, Collins PG (1987) Blunt injury of the neck of the pancreas: a report of nine patients. Injury 18:93–95

Keller MS, Stafford PW, Vane DW (1997) Conservative management of pancreatic trauma in children. J Trauma 42: 1097–1100

Khan KN, Nakata K, Shima H et al (1993) Pancreatic tissue

damage by transcatheter arterial embolization for hepatoma. Dig Dis Sci 38:65–70
Kirks DR (1983) Radiological evaluation of visceral injuries in the battered child syndrome. Pediatr Ann 12:888–893
Klar E, Angelescu M, Richter G, Herfarth C (1999) Current management of hepatic, biliary and pancreatic trauma. Chirurg 70:1255–1268
Koestner AJ, Hoak S (1999) A 6-year-old with a pancreatic injury from bicycle handlebars. J Emerg Nurs 25:84–87
Kopelman D, Suissa A, Klein Y, Hashmonai M (1998) Pancreatic duct injury: intraoperative endoscopic transpancreatic drainage of parapancreatic abscess. J Trauma 44:555–557
Kouchi K, Tanae M, Yoshida H et al (1999) Nonoperative management of blunt pancreatic injury in childhood. J Pediatr Surg 34:1736–1739
Kudsk KA, Temizer D, Ellison EC, Cloutier CT, Buckley DC, Carey LC (1986) Post-traumatic pancreatic sequestrum: recognition and treatment. J Trauma 26:320–324
Kuligowska E, Mueller PR, Simeone JF, Fine C (1984) Ultrasound in upper abdominal trauma. Seminars Roentgenol 19:281–295
Kurisu A, Kobayashi H, Kawashima K (1999) Pancreaticogastrostomy after pancreaticoduodenectomy: a rational approach to severe combined pancreaticoduodenal injury. J Trauma 46:970–972
Laborde Y, Champetier J, Letoublon C et al (1982) Pancreatic injuries. Report on 42 cases. J Chir (Paris) 119:47–54
Lal SK, Gross E, Holbrook IB, Irving MM (1978) Metabolic problems in the management of a traumatic pancreatic fistula. Injury 9:323–326
Lane MJ, Mindelzun ER, Sandu JS, McCormick VD, Jeffrey RB (1994) CT diagnosis of blunt pancreatic trauma: importance of detecting fluid between the pancreas and the splenic vein. AJR 163:833–835
Lane MJ, Mindelzun RE, Jeffrey RB (1996) Diagnosis of pancreatic injury after blunt abdominal trauma. Semin Ultrasound CT MR 17:177–182
Laraja RD, Lobbato VJ, Cassaro S, Reddy SS (1986) Intraoperative endoscopic retrograde cholangiopancreatography (ERCP) in penetrating trauma of the pancreas. J Trauma 26:1146–1147
Lee D, Zacher J, Vogel TT (1976) Primary repair in transsection of duodenum with avulsion of the common duct. Arch Surg 111:592–593
Leppaniemi AK, Haapiainen RK (1999) Risk factors of delayed diagnosis of pancreatic trauma. Eur J Surgery 165:1134–1137
Leppaniemi AK, Haapiainen RK, Kiviluoto T, Lempinen M (1988) Pancreatic trauma: acute and late manifestations. Br J Surg 75:165–167
Lewis G, Krige JE, Bornman PC, Terblanche J (1993) Traumatic pancreatic pseudocysts. Br J Surg 80:89–93
Linker CS, Deluca SA (1989) Traumatic pancreatic transection. Am Fam Physician 40:127–128
Linos DA, King RM, Much P, Farnell MB (1983) Blunt pancreatic trauma. Minn Med 66:153–160
Lovell ME, Brett M, Enion DS (1992) Mountain bike injury to the abdomen, transection of the pancreas and small bowel evisceration. Injury 23:499–500
Lucas CE (1977) Diagnosis and treatment of pancreatic and duodenal injury. Surg Clinics North Am 57:49–64
Lucaya J, Vazquez E, Caballero F, Chait PG, Daneman A, Wesson D (1998) Non-operative management of traumatic pancreatic pseudocysts associated with pancreatic duct laceration in children. Pediatr Radiol 28:5–8
Ludwig K, Petermann J, Lorenz D (1998) Diagnosis and therapy of traumatic injury of the pancreas. Zentralblatt Chir 123:245–250
Machado MA, Volpe P, Souza AL Jr, Poggetti RS, Branco PD, Birolini D (1994) Traumatic injuries of the pancreas: report of 65 cases. Rev Hosp Clin Fac Med Sao Paulo 49:238–242
Madiba TE, Mokoena TR (1995) Favourable prognosis after surgical drainage of gunshot stab or blunt trauma of the pancreas. Br J Surgery 82:1236–1239
Maingot R (1970) Operative injuries to the duct of Santorini. Br J Clin Pract 24:1–2
Maingot R (1978) Injuries to the pancreas and its ducts during upper abdominal operations. Br J Clin Pract 32:37–43
Mammone JF, Siegelman ES, Outwater EK (1998) Magnetic resonance imaging of the pancreas and biliary tree. Sem Ultrasound CT MR 19:35–52
Mansour MA, Moore JB, Moore EE, Moore FA (1989) Conservative management of combined pancreatoduodenal injuries. Am J Surg 158:531–535
Martin LW, Henderson BM, Welsh N (1968) Disruption of the head of the pancreas caused by blunt trauma in children: a report of two cases treated with primary repair of the pancreatic duct. Surgery. 63:697–700
Maule WF, Reber HA (1993) Diagnosis and management of pancreatic pseudocysts, pancreatic ascites and pancreatic fistulas. In: Go VLW et al (eds) The pancreas. Raven Press, New York, pp 741–750
McGahren ED, Magnuson D, Schaller RT, Tapper D (1995) Management of transected pancreas in children. Aust N Z J Surgery 65:242–246
McLindon JP, England RE, Martin DF (1998) Causes, clinical features and non-operative management of bile leaks. Eur Radiol 8:1602–1607
Meier DE, Coln CD, Hicks BA, Guzzetta PC (2001) Early operation in children with pancreas transection. J Pediatr Surg 36: 341–344
Meredith JW, Trunkey DD (1988) CT scanning in acute abdominal injuries. Surg Clin North Am 68:255–268
Metzger U, Jenny M (1980) Traumatic duodeno-pancreatic dehiscence with avulsion of Vater's ampulla. Helv Chir Acta 46:815–817
Miele V, Patti G, Galluzzo M, Bibbolino C, Adami L (1998) Isolated pancreatic rupture caused by abdominal blunt trauma in a child. Study with spiral computerized tomography. Radiol Med (Torino) 96:256–258
Mirvis SE, Shanmuganathan K (1992) Abdominal computed tomography in blunt trauma. Semin Roentgenol 27:150–183
Moncure M, Goins WA (1993) Challenges in the management of pancreatic and duodenal injuries. J Nat Med Assoc 85: 767–772
Moore EE, Cogbill TH, Malangoni MA et al (1990) Organ injury scaling, II: pancreas, duodenum, small bowel, colon, and rectum. J Trauma 30:1427–1429
Moore JB, Moore EE (1984) Changing trends in the management of combined pancreatoduodenal injuries. World J Surg 8:791–797
Moretz JA III, Campbell DP, Parker DE, Williams GR (1975) Significance of serum amylase level in evaluation of pancreatic trauma. Am J Surg 130:739–741
Mullen KD, Hoofnagle JH, Jones EA (1991) Shock wave-induced pancreatic trauma. Am J Gastroenterol 86:630–632
Nadler EP, Gardner M, Schall LC, Lynch JM, Ford HR (1999) Management of blunt pancreatic injury in children. J Trauma 44:1098–1103

Nagy D (1990) A rare case of pancreatic cyst. Acta Morphol Hung 38:225–228
Nance ML, Peden GW, Shapiro MB, Kauder DR, Rotondo MF, Schwab CW (1997) Solid viscus injury in blunt abdominal trauma. J Trauma 43:618–622
Nance ML, Keller MS, Stafford PW (2000) Predicting hollow visceral injury in the pediatric blunt trauma patients with solid visceral injury. J Pediatr Surg 35:1300–1303
Nelson MG, Jones DR, Vasilakis A, Timberlake GA (1994) Computed tomographic diagnosis of acute blunt pancreatic transection. W V Med J 90:274–278
Nielsen TH, Jensen LS (1986) Pancreatic transection during karate training. Br J Sports Med 20:82–83
Nilsson E, Norrby S, Skullman S, Sjodahl R (1986) Pancreatic trauma in a defined population. Acta Chir Scand 152:647–651
Nirula R, Velmahos GC, Demetriades D (1999) Magnetic resonance cholangiopancreatography in pancreatic trauma: a new diagnostic modality? J Trauma 47:585–587
Northrup WF III, Simmons RL (1972) Pancreatic trauma: a review. Surgery 71:27–43
O'Neill JA Jr, Meacham WF, Griffin JP, Sawyers JL (1973) Patterns of injury in the battered child syndrome. J Trauma 13: 332–339
Ochiai H, Nakamura S, Suzuki S, Baba S (1997) Pancreatic damage resulting from temporary portal triad interruption during partial hepatectomy: protective effect of a prostaglandin I2 analogue. J Surg Res 73:129–136
Ohno Y, Ohgami H, Nagasaki A, Hirose R (1995) Complete disruption of the main pancreatic duct: a case successfully managed by percutaneous drainage. J Pediatr Surg 30:1741–1742
Okuda K, Sugita S, Tsukada E, Sakuma Y, Ohkubo K (1991) Pancreatic pseudocyst in the left hepatic lobe: a report of two cases. Hepatology 13:359–363
Olsen WR (1973) The serum amylase in abdominal blunt trauma. Trauma 13:200–204
Oreskovich MR, Carrico CJ (1984) Pancreaticoduodenectomy for trauma: a viable option? Am J Surg 147:618–623
Pachter HL, Hofstetter SR, Liang HG, Hoballah J (1989) Traumatic injuries to the pancreas: the role of distal pancreatectomy with splenic preservation. J Trauma 29:1352–1355
Patton J, Fabian T (1996) Complex pancreatic injuries. Surg Clin North Am 76:783–795
Pattzman AB, Makaraoun MS, Slasky BS, Ritter P (1986) Prospective study of CT in initial management of blunt abdominal trauma. J Trauma 26:585–592
Pedinielli L, Marinetti C, Felix M (1979) Acute pancreatitis and posttraumatic pseudocysts of the pancreas. Report of 12 cases. J Chir (Paris) 116:97–105
Peitzman AB, Makaroun MS, Slasky BS, Ritter P (1986) Prospective study of computed tomography in initial management of blunt abdominal trauma. J Trauma 26:585–592
Pena SD, Medovy H (1973) Child abuse and traumatic pseudocyst of the pancreas. J Pediatr 83:1026–1028
Persson M, Bisgaard C, Nielsen BB, Christiansen T, Kroustrup JP (1986) Solid and papillary epithelial neoplasm of the pancreas presenting as a traumatic cyst. Case report. Acta Chir Scand 152:223–226
Pevec WC, Peitzman AB, Udekwu AO, McCoy B, Straub W (1991) Computed tomography in the evaluation of blunt abdominal trauma. Surg Gynecol Obstet 173:262–267
Pezzilli R, Billi P, Barakat B et al (1997) Serum pancreatic enzymes in patients with coma due to head injury or acute stroke. Int J Clin Lab Res 27:244–246
Pokorny WJ, Raffensperger JG, Harberg FJ (1980) Pancreatic pseudocysts in children. Surg Gynecol Obstet 151:182–184
Portis M, Meyers P, McDonald JC, Gholson CF (1994) Traumatic pancreatitis in a patient with pancreas divisum: clinical and radiographic features. Abdom Imaging 19: 162–164
Procacci C, Graziani R, Bicego E et al (1997) Blunt pancreatic trauma. Role of CT. Acta Radiol 38:543–549
Raptopoulos V (1994) Abdominal trauma: emphasis on computed tomography. Radiol Clin North Am 32:969–987
Raymond SP, Dane TE (1987) A case of primary repair of pancreatic transection. Injury 1987 18:354–355
Rescorla FJ, Plumley DA, Sherman S, Scherer LR III, West KW, Grosfeld JL (1995) The efficacy of early ERCP in pediatric pancreatic trauma. J Pediatr Surg 30:336–340
Riedl S, Buhr HJ, Herfarth C (1994) Effect of diagnostic imaging techniques on choice of therapy and prognosis of traumatic pancreas and duodenal injuries. Largenbecks Arch Chir 379:38–43
Roberts JC (1975) Traumatic pancreatitis and pleural effusion. Aust N Z J Surg 45:90–93
Roberts JL (1996) CT of abdominal and pelvic trauma. Semin Ultrasound CT MR 17:142–169
Roberts JL, Dalen K, Bosanko CM, Jafir SZ (1993) CT in abdominal and pelvic trauma. Radiographics 13:735–752
Robey E, Mullen JT, Schwab CW (1982) Blunt transection of the pancreas treated by distal pancreatectomy, splenic salvage and hyperalimentation. Four cases and review of the literature. Ann Surg 196:695–699
Rommens P, Christiaens R, Mulier K, Broos PL (1989) Flexion-distraction injuries of the thoracolumbar spine with complete pancreatic rupture. Description of a case. Unfallchirurg 92:26–28
Rosen MA, McAninch JW (1994) Management of combined renal and pancreatic trauma. J Urol 152:22–25
Rubio PA, Dichoso C (1987) Traumatic transection of the pancreas with subsequent chronic pancreatitis. South Med J 80:272–273
Ryan SP, Gaisie G, Kraus RA (2000) CT scanning of children with blunt abdominal trauma – is oral contrast useful? Emerg Radiol 7:712–717
Sandblom P (1972) 100 years of surgery, development and outlook of clinical research. Chirurg 43:206–216
Schein M, Freinkel W, D'Egidio A (1991) Splenic conservation in distal pancreatic injury: stay away from the hilum! J Trauma 31:431
Schimpl G, Sauer H, Schober PH, Weber G (1992) Rupture of the duodenum with avulsion of the papilla of Vater due to blunt trauma in a child, and review of the literature. Eur J Pediatr Surg 2:291–294
Shah PA, Nagral SS, Bhansali S et al (1988) Control of secondary haemorrhage from a pancreatic abscess by embolization. J Postgrad Med 34:119–121
Sheridan RL, Mitchell J (1994) Blunt pancreatic transection: management by distal pancreatectomy with splenic salvage. Injury 25:677–678
Shilyansky J, Sena KL, Kreller M et al (1998) Nonoperative management of pancreatic injuries in children. J Pediatr Surg 33:343–349
Shirai Y, Tsukada K, Yamadera Y et al (1995) Blunt pancreatic trauma with main pancreatic duct disruption managed successfully with total parenteral nutrition: report of a case. Surg Today 25:76–78

Shuman WP (1997) CT of blunt abdominal trauma in adult. Radiology 205:297–306
Sims EH, Mandal AK, Schlater T, Fleming AW, Lou MA (1984) Factors affecting outcome in pancreatic trauma. J Trauma 24:125–128
Sisley JF, Bowden TA, Mansberger AR Jr (1987) Pancreatic duct disruption and duodenal hematoma associated with endoscopic retrograde cholangiopancreatography. South Med J 80:1441–1443
Sivit CJ, Eichelberger MR (1995) CT diagnosis of pancreatic injury in children: significance of fluid separating the splenic vein and the pancreas. AJR 165:921–924
Sivit CJ, Eichelberger MR, Taylor GA, Bulas DI, Gotschall CS, Kushner DC (1992) Blunt pancreatic trauma in children: CT diagnosis. AJR 158:1097–1100
Smego DR, Richardson JD, Flint LM (1985) Determinants of outcome in pancreatic trauma. J Trauma 25:771–776
Smith DR, Stanley RJ, Rue LW (1996) Delayed diagnosis of pancreatic transection after blunt abdominal trauma. J Trauma 40:1009–1013
Soroudi M, Bookstein JJ (1975) Angiography in acute pancreatic transsection. Radiology 115:309–311
Soto JA, Alvarez O, Munera F, Yepes NL, Sepulveda ME, Perez JM (2001) Traumatic disruption of the pancreatic duct: diagnosis with MR pancreatography. AJR 176:175–178
Sparnon AL, Ford WD (1986) Bicycle handlebar injuries in children. J Pediatr Surg 21:118–119
Speakman M, Reece-Smith H (1983) Gastric and pancreatic rupture due to a sports injury. Br J Surg 70:190
Spechler SJ, Dalton JW, Robbins AH et al (1983) Prevalence of normal serum amylase levels in patients with acute alcoholic pancreatitis. Dig Dis Sci 28:865–869
Spitz WU (1965) Hemorrhagic pancreatitis following a kick in the abdomen. Report of a case. J Forensic Med 12:105–107
Stone A, Sugawa C, Lucas C, Hayward S, Nakamura R (1990) The role of endoscopic retrograde pancreatography (ERP) in blunt abdominal trauma. Am Surg 56:715–720
Stone HH, Fabian TC, Satiani B, Turkleson ML (1981) Experiences in the management of pancreatic trauma. J Trauma 21:257–262
Strauch GO (1972) The use of pancreatogastrostomy after blunt traumatic pancreatic transection: a complete and efficient operation. Ann Surg 176:16–18
Strax R, Sandler CM, Toombs BD (1980) CT demonstration of pancreatic transsection: case report and comparison with other diagnostic modalities in the evaluation of blunt pancreatic trauma. J Comput Tomogr 4:319–322
Sugawa C, Lucas CE (1988) The case for preoperative and intraoperative ERCP in pancreatic trauma. Gastrointest Endosc 34:145–147
Sugiyama M, Atomi Y, Kuroda A, Muto T, Wada N (1996) Endoscopic ultrasonography for diagnosing blunt pancreatic trauma. Gastrointest Endosc 44:723–725
Sugiyama M, Atomi Y, Naka S, Nagashima Y, Kozawa K, Wada N (1998) Pancreatic trauma in patients with pancreatobiliary anomaly. Hepatogastroenterology 45:1141–1144
Sukul K, Lont HE, Johannes EJ (1992) Management of pancreatic injuries. Hepatogastroenterology 39:447–450
Takamashi M, Maemura K, Sawada Y, Yoshioka T, Sugimoto T (1980) Hyperamylasemia in critically injured patients. J Trauma 20:951–955
Takehara Y (1998) Can MRCP replace ERCP? J Magnet Reson Imaging 8:517–534
Takishima T, Sugimoto K, Asari Y et al (1996a) Characteristics of pancreatic injury in children: a comparison with such injury in adults. J Pediatr Surg 31:896–900
Takishima T, Horiike S, Sugimoto K et al (1996b) Role of repeat computed tomography after emergency endoscopic retrograde pancreatography in the diagnosis of traumatic injury to pancreatic ducts. J Trauma 40:253–257
Takishima T, Sugimoto K, Hirata M, Asari Y, Ohwada T, Kakita A (1997) Serum amylase level on admission in the diagnosis of blunt injury to the pancreas: its significance and limitations. Annals Surg 226:70–76
Takishima T, Hirata M, Kataoka Y et al (2000) Pancreatographic classification of pancreatic ductal injuries caused by blunt injury to the pancreas. J Trauma 48:745–751
Taxier M, Sivak MV Jr, Coopeman AM, Sullivan BH Jr (1980) Endoscopic retrograde pancreatography in the evaluation of trauma to the pancreas. Surg Gynecol Obstet 150:65–68
Taylor GA, Fallat ME, Eichelberger MR (1987) Hypovolemic shock in children: abdominal CT manifestations. Radiology 164:479–481
Thanh LN, Duchmann JC, Latrive JP, That BT, Huguier M (1999) Conservation of the left pancreas in rupture of the pancreatic isthmus. A propos of 3 cases. Chirurgie 124: 165–170
Thomson SR, Ghimenton F (2000) Pancreaticogastrostomy for trauma: an alternative to distal pancreatectomy. Injury 31: 394–395
Timberlake GA (1997) Blunt pancreatic trauma: experience at a rural referral center. Am Surg 63:252–286
Toftdahl D, Rasmussen A, Jespersen J (1984) Acute pancreatitis with thromboembolic complications. Physiopathological aspects. Ugeskr Laeger 146:2093–2095
Tolia V, Patel AS, Amundson GM (1990) Pancreatic fracture secondary to child abuse: the role of computed tomography in its diagnosis. Clin Pediatr (Phila) 29:667–668
Toombs BD, Lester RG, Ben-MEnachem Y, Sandler CM (1981) Computed tomography in blunt trauma. Radiol Clin North Am 19:17–35
Touloukian RJ (1968) Abdominal visceral injuries in battered children. Pediatrics 42:642–646
Travers B (1827) Rupture of the pancreas. Lancet 12:384
Tsang BD, Panacek EA, Brant WE, Wisner DH (1997) Effect of oral contrast administration for abdominal computed tomography in evaluation of acute blunt trauma. Ann Emerg Med 30:7–13
Tyburski JG, Dente CJ, Wilson RF, Shanti C, Steffes CP, Carlin A (2001) Infectious complications following duodenal and/or pancreatic trauma. Am Surg 67:227–230
Udekwu PO, Gurkin B, Oller DW (1996) The use of computed tomography in blunt abdominal injuries. Am Surg 62: 56–59
Vallon AG, Lees WR, Cotton PB (1979) Grey-scale ultrasonography and endoscopic pancreatography after pancreatic trauma. Br J Surg 66:169–172
Van Hee R, Van Genderen B, Van Hee W, Hubens A, Creve U (1993) Selective rupture of the Wirsung duct: a rare form of pancreatic trauma. Acta Chir Belg 93:46–48
Van Steenbergen W, Samain H, Pouillon M et al (1987) Transection of the pancreas demonstrated by ultrasound and computed tomography. Gastrointest Radiol 12:128–130
Van Winckel M, Robberecht E, Afschrift M, Smets A, Wood BP (1997) Radiological case of the month. Battered child syndrome. Arch Pediatr Adolesc Med 151:621–622

Vitale GC, Larson GM, Davidson PR, Bouwman DL, Weaver DW (1987) Analysis of hyperamylasemia in patients with severe head injury. J Surg Res 43:226–233

Vora NM, Wakamatsu T (1980) Delayed massive bleeding from gastroduodenal artery due to transduodenal needle biopsy of pancreas. Del Med J 52:323–326

Waldman PJ, Walters BL, Grunau CF (1984) Pancreatic injury associated with interposed abdominal compressions in pediatric cardiopulmonary resuscitation. Am J Emerg Med 2:510–512

Walker ML (1986) Management of pancreatic trauma: concepts and controversy. J Nat Med Assoc 78:1177–1183

White PH, Benfield JR (1972) Amylase in management of pancreatic trauma. Arch Surg 105:158–163

Whitman GJ, Pearce WH, Moore EE, Barton B (1988) Free intraperitoneal rupture of a pancreatic pseudocyst: a presentation of acute abdominal trauma. J Trauma 28: 555–556

Whittwell AE, Gomez GA, Byers P, Kreis DJ Jr, Manten H, Casillas VJ (1989) Blunt pancreatic trauma: prospective evaluation of early endoscopic retrograde cholangiopancreatography. South Med J 82:586–591

Wilkinson AE (1989) Injuries of the pancreas. S Afr Surg 27: 67–68

Wilson RH, Moorehead RJ (1991) Current management of trauma to the pancreas. Br J Surg 78:1196–1202

Winter J, Ulatowski L, Hoffmann E (1982) The disinsertion of Vater's papilla in stomach resection. Causes, diagnosis and therapy. Chirurg 53:574–580

Wisner DL, Wold RL, Frey CF (1990) Diagnosis and treatment of pancreatic injuries: an analysis of management principles. Arch Surg 125:1109–1113

Wohlwend D, Hirata I Jr (1975) Pancreatic injury in intercollegiate football. J Am Coll Health Assoc 23:223–224

Wong Y-C, Wang LJ, Lin BC, Chen CJ, Lim KE, Chen RJ (1997) CT grading of blunt pancreatic injuries: prediction of ductal disruption and surgical correlation. J Comput Assist Tomogr 21:246–250

Wynn M, Hill DM, Miller DR et al (1985) Management of pancreatic and duodenal trauma. Am J Surg 150:327–332

Yagi M, Mishina T, Fujishima T, Date K, Saito H, Suzuki N (1997) Successful treatment of blunt trauma involving complete laceration of the pancreas and duodenum in a 7-year-old child: report of a case. Surg Today 27:84–87

Yellin AE, Vecchione TR, Donovan AJ (1972) Distal pancreatectomy for pancreatic trauma. Am J Surg 124:135–142

Yoshii H, Sato M, Yamamoto S et al (1998) Usefulness and limitations of ultrasonography in the initial evaluation of blunt abdominal trauma. J Trauma Inj, Infect Crit Care 45:45–51

Young PR Jr, Meredith JW, Baker CC, Thomason MH, Chang MC (1998) Pancreatic injuries resulting from penetrating trauma: a multi-institution review. Am Surg 64:838–843

8 Injuries of the Gastrointestinal Tract

G. Ponghis, M. Lewin, J. H. Boverie, R. F. Dondelinger

CONTENTS

G. Ponghis, MD
Resident, Department of Medical Imaging, University Hospital Sart Tilman, Domaine du Sart Tilman B35, 4000 Liège, Belgium
M. Lewin
Department of Medical Imaging, University Hospital Sart Tilman, Domaine du Sart Tilman B35, 4000 Liège, Belgium
J. H. Boverie, MD
Chef de Clinique, Department of Medical Imaging, University Hospital Sart Tilman, Domaine du Sart Tilman B35, 4000 Liège, Belgium
R. F. Dondelinger, MD
Professor and Chairman, Department of Medical Imaging, University Hospital Sart Tilman, Domaine Universitaire du Sart Tilman B35, 4000 Liège, Belgium

- Absence of pneumoperitoneum or retropneumoperitoneum on CT at admission should not be used as the sole negative predictor of bowel wall perforation.
- A large amount of peritoneal fluid, that is not explained by hemorrhage of a parenchymal organ, or a central mesenteric distribution on CT is a strong indicator of bowel wall injury.
- When bowel wall hematoma is evidenced, perforation should be ruled out by intense imaging, as conservative nonoperative management can be applied in many cases of isolated hematoma, in particular in a duodenal location.
- Serial clinical and CT examinations should be obtained in case of high suspicion of bowel perforation to reach a timely diagnosis and avoid complications of delayed treatment.
- Peroral administration of contrast material is not indicated on a routine basis to evidence gastrointestinal tract injury with CT.

8.1 History

Aristotle was aware of the possible rupture of the small intestine after nonpenetrating trauma to the abdominal wall. Sacherus is credited for the first successful repair of ruptured intestine in 1720 and Rambdohr anastomosed a transected segment of intestine in 1730. Precise description of posttraumatic injuries of the gastrointestinal (GI) tract and of pathophysiological mechanisms of small bowel and mesentery injuries were given during the 19th century. In the USA, the first case of ruptured intestine was published in 1837. Sperling and Rigler are believed to have published the first case of radiographically demonstrated duodenal perforation in 1937 (Mc Laughlan 1839; Sperling and Rigler 1937; Griswold and Collier 1961).

In the 20th century, before the era of cross-section imaging, radiological evidence of trauma to the GI tract was limited to plain films of the thorax and abdomen and luminal contrast studies. Useful radiographic signs in the acute posttraumatic phase are few and centered on pneumoperitoneum, indicating bowel perforation. Arteriography was advocated in the 1960s of last century for screening of patients with abdominal trauma, but did not greatly contribute to the specific diagnosis of GI tract wall injuries (Freeark et al. 1968a, 1968b, 1969; Osborn et al. 1973). The introduction of diagnostic peritoneal lavage (DPL) was a major innovation in trauma management. Since the first description by Root et al., repeated analyses of results have documented excellent sensitivity, and variable specificity for GI tract perforation (Root et al. 1965; Feliciano 1991a). Today, systematic cross-section imaging in trauma patients depicts directly the presence and extent of GI tract injury, including refined posttraumatic changes such as small mural or mesenteric hematoma and minute pneumoperitoneum, and consequently has largely replaced DPL in most cases of blunt abdominal trauma. There has also been an interest in the use of US (ultrasound) for evaluating patients with blunt abdominal trauma for more than 20 years. With improved technology and clinical experience, this interest has increased in recent years, more in children than in adults, but without replacing CT as the primary screening modality.

8.2 Incidence

GI tract injuries occur roughly in 5%–25% of trauma victims. Frequency varies according to the mechanism of trauma and the considered segment of the GI tract. In adults, penetrating trauma predominates, but blunt trauma is steadily increasing since several decades, due to strong forces exerted during violent traffic collisions on the GI tract, which exhibits considerable mobility (Griswold and Collier 1961; Ting and Reuter 1973; Westcott and Smith 1975; Williams and Sargeant 1963). In the pediatric age group, penetrating trauma is rare for obvious reasons (Grosfeld et al. 1989). In blunt abdominal trauma, due to its length and location, small bowel injury is the most frequent, followed by colorectal, duodenal, and gastric involvement (Shuck and Lowe 1978; Davis et al. 1976; Hunt et al. 1980; Cox 1984; Dauterive et al. 1985; Talton et al. 1995). Overall, hollow viscus injury shows a strong preponderance for the duodenum in children and for the small bowel and colon in adults (Allen et al. 1998).

- Oesophageal perforation occurs almost exclusively with penetrating injury. Closed injury is rare, and predominates in the upper third (Dupont Le Priol et al. 1992). Isolated mural hematoma of the esophagus after blunt trauma is extremely rare (De Vries et al. 1991; Perniceni and Gayet 1995).
- Perforation of the stomach occurs mainly after penetrating trauma to the upper abdomen (Wilkinson 1989; Allen et al. 1998). In blunt trauma, gastric rupture is seen in 0.9%–1.7%, and more frequently in children than in adults (Yajko et al. 1975). A common finding in patients with this injury is a distended stomach after eating. Total gastric transsection is rare (Leddy and Frew 1977). Usually, partial rupture is observed: the anterior wall of the stomach is the most common site, followed by the greater curvature, the lesser curvature, and the posterior wall in order of decreasing frequency. Occasionally, ischemic necrosis of a portion of the gastric wall may result from mesenteric avulsion (Garfinkle and Matolo 1976).
- Trauma of the duodenum occurs in 1%–12% of all intra-abdominal injuries (Feliciano 1989; Carillo et al. 1996; Ballard et al. 1997). The majority of cases are caused by abdominal penetration (Morton and Jordan 1968; Asensio et al. 1993; Tyburski et al. 2001). Duodenum and pancreas are often involved together in major trauma. In almost 50% of the cases of rupture or duodenal wall hematoma, the second segment of the duodenum is involved, followed by the other portions (Nelson 1966; Morton and Jordan 1968; Ting and Reuter 1973; Love 1975; Lucas and Ledgerwood 1975; Margolis et al. 1976; Flint et al. 1980; Thoms and Ricketts 1988; Contostavlos et al. 1996; Ballard et al. 1997). Of all bowel segments, the duodenum is the most frequent site of posttraumatic hematoma without perforation and is most commonly injured in children, accounting in this group for 2%–3% of blunt abdominal injuries (Jewett et al. 1988; Nghiem et al. 1993; Strouse et al. 1999).
- Small bowel and mesentery are also most commonly injured as a result of penetrating trauma, like the other GI tract segments, but 5%–15% of these injuries are secondary to blunt trauma, and small bowel represents the third or fourth most commonly injured abdominal organ. Isolated GI tract injury is a rare finding and occurs in only 1%–2% of the cases (Feliciano 1991a; Chiang 1993; Metzger et al. 1995; Nghiem et al. 1995;

FRICK et al. 1999; BROWSTEIN et al. 2000). The jejunum is generally more frequently injured than the ileum (JACOBSON and CARTER 1951; TING and REUTER 1973; FISCHER et al. 1988; FRICK et al. 1999). Perforations are most common at the upper and lower ends of the small bowel near a point of fixation, such as the ligament of Treitz and ileocaecal valve and jejunal perforations raise usually more diagnostic problems than the ileum (DAUTERIVE et al. 1985; GRASSI et al. 1998). One third of mesenteric injuries involving mesenteric arteries and/or veins result in a devascularized bowel segment, which requires resection and is most common in the distal ileum (DAUTERIVE et al. 1985; WISNER et al. 1990; FRICK et al. 1999).

- Trauma to the colon is less common than to the small bowel. However, increasing frequency accounts for 3%–5% of all blunt abdominal injuries (MCKENZIE and BELL 1972; HAYES et al. 1991; BROWN et al. 1992; WISNER and BLAISDELL 1992; SCHUMPELICK et al. 1999; YIN et al. 2000). The transverse colon (40%) and sigmoid are the most common sites of blunt injury, followed by the ascending colon (16%), caecum (12%), and descending colon (8%) (HOWELL et al. 1976). Injury of the anteriorly located transverse colon often involves intramural hematomas or serosal tear without fecal spillage. The most serious injuries, including avulsion of the meso, full thickness laceration, transection, and devascularization of a segment of the colon are most often seen in the ascending colon (DAUTERIVE et al. 1985; NGHIEM et al. 1993).

8.3 Mechanism

8.3.1 Common

The mechanism of perforation and rupture caused by penetrating stab and gunshot guns of the GI tract wall wound is obvious.

During blunt trauma, four possible and still valid mechanisms were postulated: a crushing force applied to the bowel against the spine, shearing forces to the bowel and mesentery along the lines of attachment during deceleration, and bursting forces occurring secondary to increased intraluminal pressure and perforation by sharp objects or bone fragments (MACKERSIE et al. 1989).

- The horizontal segment of the duodenum and the pancreas cross the vertebral column and are easily compressed against the spine by a direct blow, but small bowel segments can be affected as well (NGHIEM et al. 1993; CARILLO et al. 1996). Anecdotally, a bowel segment can be entrapped and incarcerated between two fractured vertebral bodies (ELDRIDGE et al. 1993).
- Lesions created by shearing forces can occur at any site of the bowel, but preferentially near fixed points. They consist of a tear in the serosa-muscularis propria portion of the bowel, with varying degrees of avulsion of that layer from the intact mucosa-sub mucosa layer ending in either partial or complete rupture (DAUTERIVE et al. 1985; CONTOSTAVLOS et al. 1996). Multiple transverse split-thickness laceration are distinctive seatbelt lacerations, where the muscular layer ruptures, when intestinal loops are compressed against the abdominal restraint, while the inner layers resist (LEGIER 1992). Peritoneal adhesions favor the occurrence of traumatic intestinal injuries by increasing shearing forces (WEISS and DREILING 1968). Shearing forces are also responsible for avulsion of large arteries and veins, leading to ischemic necrosis of the GI tract.
- Bursting forces resulting in „blow-out" are preferentially seen in the pharynx and the upper portion of the oesophagus and in the duodenum, but any bowel segment dilated with air can be involved. Duodenal „blow-out" is explained by simultaneous contraction of the pylorus and distal duodenum (COCKE and MEYER 1964). „Blow-out" rupture of the small bowel occurs most frequently on the antimesenteric border (NGHIEM et al. 1993; HAGIWARA et al. 1995). Experimental studies on dogs showed that shearing forces between 2 opposite surfaces resulted in intestinal injury and were unrelated to intraluminal pressure (WILLIAMS and SARGENT 1963). Presence of fluid or gas within the bowel seemed to provide some protection against intestinal injury (FRICK et al. 1999).
- Displaced fractured bone fragments in the pelvis may perforate the rectal wall during blunt trauma (CERISE and SCULLY 1970; SHUCK and LOWE 1978; STRATE and GRIECO 1983; DAUTERIVE et al. 1985).

The bowel injuries resulting from these mechanisms can be divided into major and less critical injuries. Major injuries are large perforation or rupture of the bowel wall, and interruption of arterial and venous flow leading to bowel ischemia and necrosis. Significant bowel injuries are found in about 5%

of blunt abdominal trauma (Nghiem et al. 1995). Minor injuries include hematoma of the bowel wall or limited blood collected in the adjacent mesentery (Mirvis et al. 1992; Nghiem et al. 1993).

Motor vehicle collisions, being probably the most common cause of blunt trauma in general, are also the most common cause of blunt bowel injury (Frick et al. 1999; Hugues et al. 2002). The proper use of seat belts has resulted on one hand in lower injury severity and fatality rates, on the other hand lap belt use only and also nonproper seat belt use have resulted in an increased rate of duodenal or intestinal injuries in adults and children, due to sudden deceleration, involving in various combinations the above-described mechanisms. In children, „almost penetrating injury" from the handlebars of a bicycle is an additional classical mechanism of GI tract injury (Arajarvi et al. 1987; Appleby and Nagy 1989; Absun et al. 1990; Newman et al. 1990; Anderson et al. 1991; Rutledge et al. 1991; Sivit et al. 1991; Kloppel et al. 1997; Browstein et al. 2000). In the „jumper syndrome," after a fall from a height, hollow viscus perforation accounts for 50% of the abdominal injuries (Scalea et al. 1986).

8.3.2 Uncommon

In Europe, penetrating trauma by gunshots and stab wounds is less frequent than in the USA (Chihombori et al. 1991; Udobi et al. 2001).

Iatrogenic injuries of the GI tract are multiple and diverse and may be responsible of a great variety of injuries at various sites. GI tract wall hematoma or perforation can occur during any endoscopic procedure, using rigid or flexible instruments for diagnostic or therapeutic purposes. Classical causes are deep mural biopsy, laser ablation of mucosal lesions, polypectomy, bouginage, and luminal stenting, endoscopic retrograde cholangiography, sphincterotomy, local mural injection of vasoconstrictive drugs or sclerosing agents, endoscopic gastrostomy or any other type of endoscopic intervention, and including placement of nasojejunal feeding tubes and transrectal prostate biopsy. In particular, many case reports describe oesophageal perforation during cardiac echography (Meyers and Ghahremani 1975; Siegle et al. 1976; Nelson et al. 1982; Fernandez et al. 1988; Bogan and Conces 1989; Diner 1988; Kuhlman et al. 1989; Zinelis et al. 1989; Cotton et al. 1991; Hulyalkar and Ayd 1993; Polhamus et al. 1993; Latham and Hodgins 1995; Guzman et al. 1998; Kos et al. 1998; St Pierre et al. 1998; Hernandez et al. 1999; Kihara et al. 1999; Kinoshita et al. 1999; Kallmeyer et al. 2000; Maatman et al. 2002).

GI tract necrosis and perforation can also be consecutive to arterial embolism or thrombosis in the coeliomesenteric circulation, either during diagnostic catheterization or therapeutic vaso-occlusion or due to reflux of toxic drugs during chemoembolization in the liver.

Diagnostic radiographic examinations may also result in GI tract injuries: perforation during enteroclysis, transanal colostomy, or enterostomy opacifications, often combined with inflation of intraluminal balloons in an inappropriate location, such as colostomy or enterostomy, responsible for either barium peritonitis or barium intravasation in the portal system up to the intrahepatic branches (Goff et al. 1982; Ott et al. 1985; Diner 1988; Walker et al. 1989; Williams and Harned 1991).

Besides iatrogenic injury, the GI tract wall can be perforated by a great variety of sharp objects, animal or fish bone, toothpick or needle, predominantly in the stomach, or in the small intestine. Transmural rectal perforation can be caused by insertion of foreign bodies for erotic purposes (Grass et al. 1981; Gonzalez et al. 1988; Cranston et al. 1993; Rioux and Langis 1994; Chan et al. 1999; Porcu et al. 1999; Cheung et al. 2000; Zingg et al. 2000; Kerschner et al. 2001; Lam et al. 2001; Toyonaga et al. 2001). Accidental acid ingestion, especially by children, is another uncommon cause of injuries to the esophagus and stomach, which can result in perforation (Mitani et al. 1996; Millar at al. 2001; Bernhardt et al. 2002). Electrocution may result in mural necrosis, predominantly in the colon, or intestine (Williams and Karl 1981).

Finally, seromuscular rupture of the intestine may be observed in the acute or chronic form in battered children (Kirks 1983; Gonzalez et al. 1987; Shah et al. 1997). In particular, in the chronic form, reparative processes and cicatrisation tend to obscure its true nature and may result in the failure to recognize its traumatic origin. In one case, a volvulus with strangulation of a loop of the transverse colon that had become herniated through a defect in the transverse mesocolon led to lethal peritonitis as a late complication (Contostavlos et al. 1996).

8.3.3 Associated Injuries

GI tact injuries consecutive to penetrating or blunt abdominal trauma are rarely isolated. In blunt trauma, patients have additional injuries in 30%–75%, and associated injuries to abdominal organs in more than 50%, most frequently to the liver, followed by the spleen and pancreas (Pokorny et al. 1986; Grosfeld et al. 1975, 1989; Wisner et al. 1990; Hayes et al. 1991; Ballard et al. 1997; Nance et al. 1997; Frick et al. 1999). Adults with blunt liver or spleen injury have an about 4%–11% risk for hollow viscus injury. In the pediatric age group, solid organ injury, except the pancreas, is less often associated with hollow viscus injury than in adults (Nance et al. 2000). Pancreatic injuries in particular are useful indicators for searching for associated hollow viscus injury. Injury to the pancreas is associated with hollow viscus injury in 30% of children and 50% of adults, and duodenal injury is associated with trauma to other organs in 30%–87% including the common bile duct (Snyder et al. 1980; Adkins and Keyser 1985; Buckman et al. 1988; Asensio et al. 1993). Trauma to the left side of the body is present in many patients with gastric perforation and the most common associated injury is rupture of the spleen (Nghiem et al. 1993). Lumbar vertebral fractures, and in particular the Chance type fracture, proved also to be a useful marker for hollow viscus injury, involving the small bowel, particularly in children (36% vs. 16% in adults) (Kloppel et al. 1997; Allen et al. 1998; Rabinovici et al. 1999).

8.4 Clinical Symptoms and Findings

8.4.1 Symptoms and Signs

The prompt identification of significant blunt hollow viscus injury remains a diagnostic challenge for all age groups, as it may remain occult or give only minimal symptoms at presentation, which is responsible for diagnostic delay of several days and sometimes more than a week (Chiang 1993; Allen et al. 1998). A combination of clinical suspicion, and proper and serial physical examination and imaging is required for a timely diagnosis, and rapid surgical repair (Rouse et al. 1984; Sherck and Oakes 1990; Albanese et al. 1996; Frick et al. 1999). Abdominal pain and signs of peritoneal irritation develop slowly in small bowel perforation, because the jejunal bowel contents usually have neutral pH, low bacterial count, and are not enzymatically active (Nghiem et al. 1993). Retroperitoneal perforation, in particular of the duodenum or rectum, is even more treacherous, and often not immediately apparent clinically, due to delayed appearance of peritoneal irritation (Motateanu et al. 1992; Contostavlos et al. 1996; Ballard et al. 1997).

Clinical examination is classically falsely negative in 10%– 45% of the cases and confusing in two thirds of patients, with variable combinations of diffuse tenderness, abdominal distension, rigidity, and diminished bowel sounds, no sign taken one by one being specific for bowel perforation (Davis et al. 1976; Hunt et al. 1980; Peitzman et al. 1986; Kearney 1989; Mackersie et al. 1989; Hayes et al. 1991; Hara et al. 1992; Metzger et al. 1995; Talton et al. 1995). However, abdominal tenderness was present on admission in 98% of patients with GI tract injury in whom a reliable examination was possible (Wisner et al. 1990). Indirect clinical markers suggestive of hollow viscus injury should not be neglected: abdominal wall ecchymosis, lumbar vertebral fractures and the presence of solid organ injuries. Skin abrasion of the neck, chest, and abdomen are suggestive of seat belt syndrome, which is likely to produce GI tract injuries (Sivit et al. 1991; Allen et al. 1998).

When patients are in posttraumatic hemodynamic shock, they are rarely bleeding profusely from gastrointestinal injury, except when laceration of large coeliomesenteric vessels is present.

Pharyngeal and oesophageal perforations are particular, as they are often not recognized at admission. Secondary infection from occult perforation may reveal the injury when it had resulted in thoracic complications, such as diffuse mediastinitis, local mediastinal abscess, or pleural empyema. Typical clinical signs and symptoms include dysphagia, odynophagia, chest pain, fever, tachycardia, cyanosis, hypotension, respiratory distress, and occasionally hematemesis (Ghahremani 1993).

Hematuria should be mentioned as a sign which may be associated with blunt small bowel and mesentery injuries. Several studies have shown a relationship between the presence and severity of hematuria and a significantly higher risk of abdominal injuries after blunt trauma (Hunt et al. 1980; Taylor et al. 1988b; Grieshop et al. 1995; Knudson et al. 1992; Frick et al. 1999).

Finally, an inguinoscrotal hernia may be responsible for acute scrotal swelling when its content becomes injured (Mucciolo and Godec 1988). Bowel perforation within a hernia is facilitated by fixation of the bowel segment in the herniated sac (Dauterive et al. 1985).

8.4.2
Diagnostic Peritoneal Lavage

Diagnostic peritoneal lavage (DPL) is not used systematically in blunt trauma and serves primarily as a triage tool in adult patients with multiple system injuries who show signs of hemodynamic instability. The criteria for positive DPL include 10 ml of blood on initial aspiration, red blood cell count >100.000/mm^3, or the presence of food fibers indicating GI perforation. The principal advantages of DPL include its simplicity, its ability to make an early diagnosis of the need for celiotomy, its accuracy, lack of complications, and low cost. Despite a reported sensitivity of 100%, a specificity of 97%, and an accuracy of 99%, disadvantages to the use of DPL in patients with blunt abdominal trauma are regularly stressed, including its oversensitivity, lack of specificity, and failure to detect retroperitoneal duodenal and colon perforation and diaphragmatic injuries (Fischer et al. 1978; Fabian et al. 1986; Feliciano 1991a; Ballard et al. 1997). DPL has been criticized for its relatively invasive complications (1%–2%) and frequency in leading to nontherapeutic laparotomy in 6%–25% (Fischer et al. 1978; Cox 1984; Allen et al. 1998).

Concerning detection of specific GI tract injuries, DPL was found superior to CT with a false negative rate of 6.7%–18% vs. 36%–38% (Talton et al. 1995; Kemmeter et al. 1998) However, the frequently associated liver or spleen injuries are often a source of positive DPL, and consequently the specificity of DPL for bowel rupture remains low (Ballard et al. 1997). Finally, the risk to introduce intraperitoneal air from DPL, even in minimal amounts, may be responsible for false positive CT for bowel perforation (Stapakis and Thickman 1992).

8.4.3
Laboratory Findings

Laboratory tests are of little benefit to identify bowel and mesentery injuries. Base deficit and the presence of hematuria were the only identified consistent laboratory findings. Serum amylase, aspartate aminotransferase, and alanine aminotransferase have not been shown to correlate well with duodenal or small bowel and mesentery injuries, and elevation was noted in only 15% of patients (Barandica and Patel 1997; Frick et al. 1999). Lavage amylase >20 IU/l and lavage alkaline phosphatase >3 IU/l had a positive predictive value of 88% for significant bowel injury (Jaffin et al. 1993; Allen et al. 1998).

8.5
Diagnostic Imaging

8.5.1
Abdominal Radiographs

8.5.1.1
Positive Signs

The radiographic diagnosis of digestive tract perforation is based primarily on the evidence of free air (Schneider and Hauser 1982). Pneumoperitoneum detected on plain radiographs following blunt abdominal trauma is nearly pathognomonic of bowel perforation and usually mandates exploratory laparotomy (Kane et al. 1991) (Fig. 8.1). A large amount of subphrenic air suggests gastric or colon rupture (Fig. 8.2). Retroperitoneal duodenal rupture is suggested by pneumoretroperitoneum in the upper abdomen in a periduodenal location, dilated duodenal loop or segment, and partial obliteration of the upper part or the right psoas muscle. Rupture of the rectum gives extraluminal gas projecting in the presacral space in the pelvis, before dissecting adjacent and remote soft tissue planes. Pharyngeal or esophageal rupture shows dissection by air of soft tissues in the neck, supraclavicular planes, and mediastinum (Han et al. 1985).

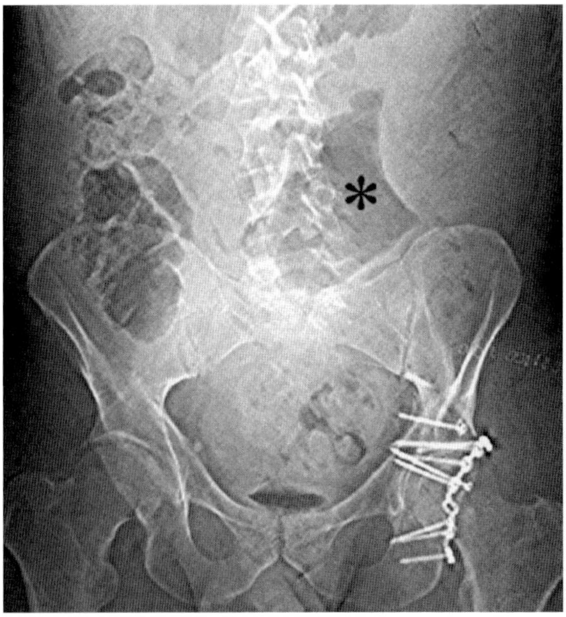

Fig. 8.1. Digitized abdominal radiograph obtained immediately prior to CT scanning shows a large free gas collection (*asterisk*) in the midabdomen, confirmed as pneumoperitoneum on axial slices (see Fig. 8.27)

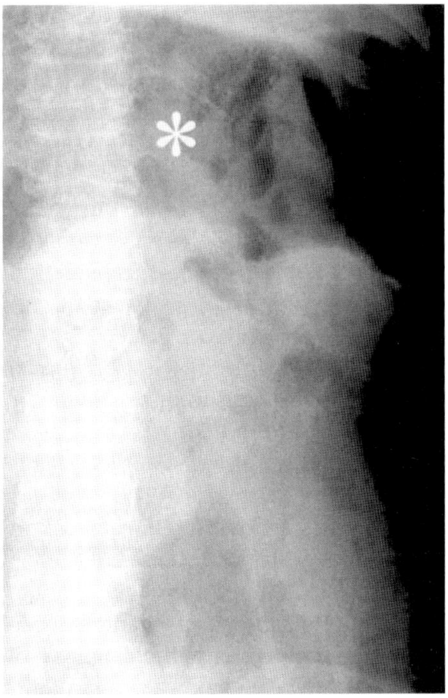

Fig. 8.2. Large left subphrenic gas collection (*asterisk*) on a supine radiograph of the abdomen at admission, indicating gastric rupture after an anterior abdominal stab wound

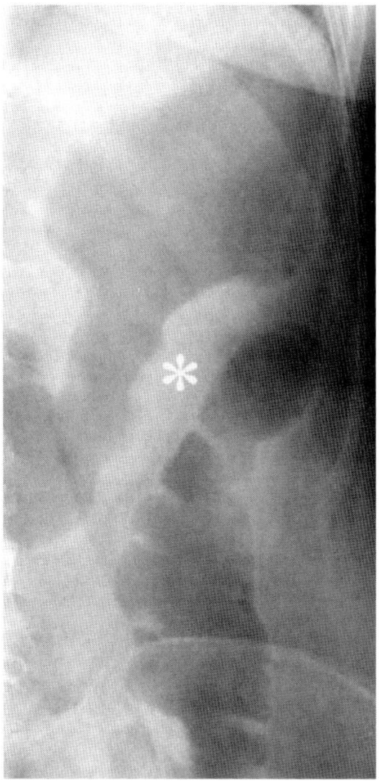

Fig. 8.3. Thickening of the gastrosplenic ligament (*asterisk*) in a patient with gastric wall hematoma and splenic contusion after blunt abdominal injury

Intraperitoneal fluid of whatever nature gravitates to the dependant portions, flank and pelvis, and may cause loss of the normal visceral outline and displacement of adjacent structures.

In addition to pneumoperitoneum and peritoneal fluid, abdominal X-ray may show dilated intestinal or colon segments, irregular contour caused by mural hematoma or displacement of air-filled GI tract segments, or associated spinal or pelvic fractures, site of a bullet or subcutaneous emphysema (Figs. 8.3, 8.4).

8.5.1.2
Pitfalls

Pneumoperitoneum of small amounts may not be demonstrated on plain radiographs, especially during the first hours following trauma (Schneider and Hauser 1982; Diallo et al. 1994). Thoracic air collections may be a possible cause for pneumoperitoneum (Kane et al. 1991).

8.5.1.3
Results

Pneumoperitoneum is seen in only 5% of trauma patients at admission (Kunin et al. 1994). In small

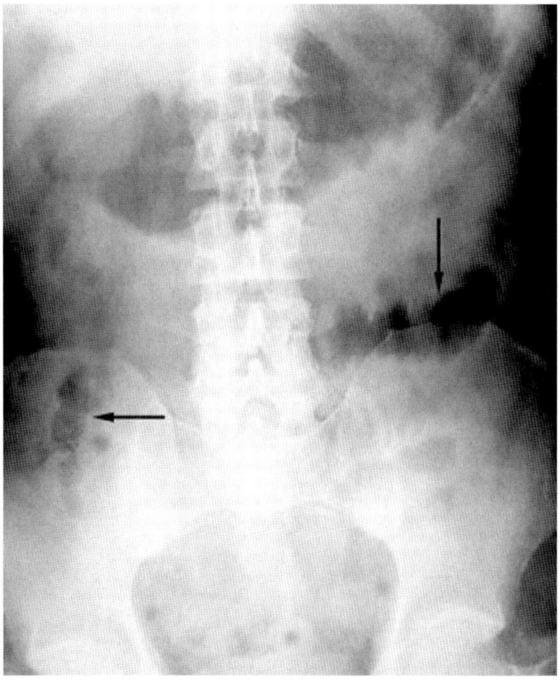

Fig. 8.4. Nonspecific segmental intestinal dilatation with a coarse contour (*arrows*) after blunt abdominal injury

bowel perforation, conventional radiography did not detect free gas in 54%, but showed other indirect signs, such as intraperitoneal free fluid in 71% of the cases (GRASSI et al. 1998). Duodenal rupture is suspected on plain films in 0%–33% of the cases (TOXOPEUS et al. 1972; KELLY et al. 1978).

8.5.2 Luminal Opacification

It is essential to differentiate mural hematoma from perforation, as therapeutic options are different. In the duodenum, the differentiation of perforation from hematoma may remain problematic with CT, when free air in the extraluminal duodenopancreatric space and contrast extravasation are absent. Peroral opacification of the upper GI tract may still be indicated in some circumstances. In the acute phase, duodenography is obtained with iodinated contrast medium through a nasally or orally placed tube into the duodenum under fluoroscopy.

A mural hematoma involves a short segment of the GI tract (10–20 cm in length). In the duodenum, the opacified lumen is narrowed, the mucosal folds have a coarse and thickened appearance proximal to the hematoma and are crowded in a coiled-spring appearance at the level of the hematoma. Incomplete or complete obstruction may be observed. Usually, the radiographic signs subside within a week and have disappeared within 4 weeks (FELSON and LEVIN 1955; MCCORT 1964; WIOT 1966; MORTON and JORDAN 1968; MAUL et al. 1978) (Figs. 8.5–8.8).

In retroperitoneal perforation of the duodenum, oral contrast passing through the wall disruption is far from being the rule and is observed only in the most severe cases of full thickness transsection. Periduodenal air is also inconstant and seen in only 50% of the patients. However, nonspecific signs of obliteration of the right psoas muscle and lumbar scoliosis are present in 90% of the cases (SPERLING and RIGLER 1937; GOULD and THORWARTH 1963; NELSON 1966; MORTON and JORDAN 1968; TOXOPEUS et al. 1972; LUCAS and LEDGERWOOD 1975).

Overall, duodenography, and bowel opacification, in general, have a low sensitivity (around 25%–54%). In patients with suspected blunt injuries they are of minimal utility in the diagnostic evaluation. Specificity is high, the positive radiographic diagnosis of perforation being always confirmed by laparotomy (Figs. 8.31c and 8.12b). Applied to other segments of the GI tract, such as the oesophagus, barium studies can also be falsely negative in 20%–30% of the cases, when a limited mural tear is sealed off by oedema or hematoma (FOLEY et al. 1982; BLADERGROEN et al. 1986; KIM-DEOBALD and KOZAREK 1992).

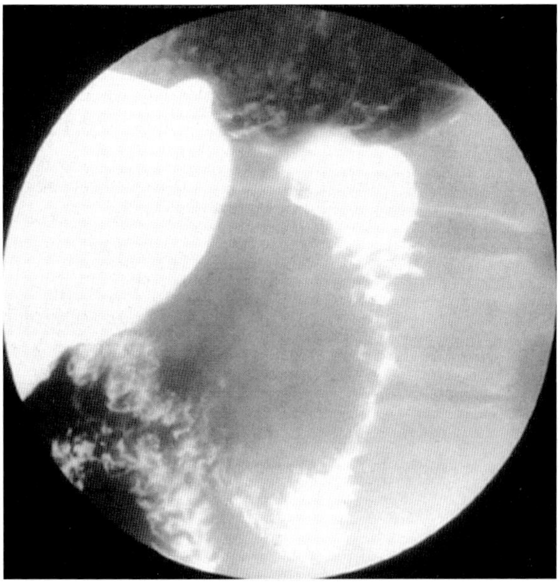

Fig. 8.5. Typical radiographic appearance of a posttraumatic mural hematoma of the second portion of the duodenum: nonobstructive narrowing of the lumen with coarse contour, moderate proximal dilatation of the duodenum and no contrast medium extravasation

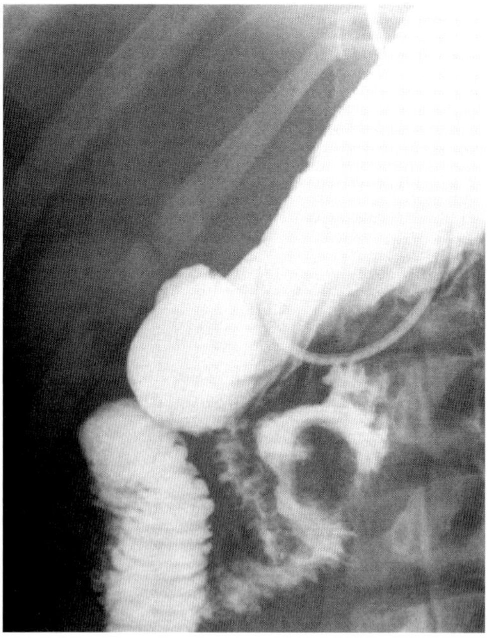

Fig. 8.6. Posttraumatic excentric and limited mural hematoma of the third portion of the duodenum, evidenced on CT at admission (see Fig. 8.14)

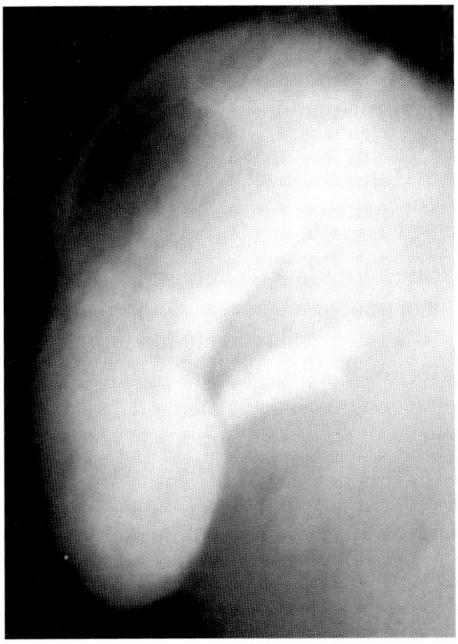

Fig. 8.7. Posttraumatic obstructive mural hematoma of the genu superius of the duodenum, evidenced by CT on admission (see Fig. 8.13)

8.5.3
Ultrasound

8.5.3.1
Positive Signs

Free fluid in the peritoneal cavity is the key finding of GI tract injury on US, but hemoperitoneum can also be caused by extracapsular bleeding of a solid organ, and US findings are not specific for spilling of GI tract luminal content. Mural hematoma has been documented with US in the duodenum and in the mesentery, and shows as a heterogeneous hypoechoic mass with an echoic wall (Foley and Teele 1979; O'Malley and Salem 1979; Fon et al. 1980). Color Doppler study may reveal vascularity at the periphery of the lesion (Zapf et al. 1988; Chao and Kong 1999; Yin et al. 2000). Disruption of the GI tract wall is evidenced only occasionally. Portal venous gas can anecdotally be detected as echoic signals in the small intrahepatic portal branches in an anterior location (Chevallier et al. 2002). Reflecting abdominal foreign bodies having perforated the GI tract are localized with US (Coulier 1997). US also regularly shows posttraumatic intestinal paresis, which is not specific for GI tract injury in polytrauma patients (Grassi et al. 1998).

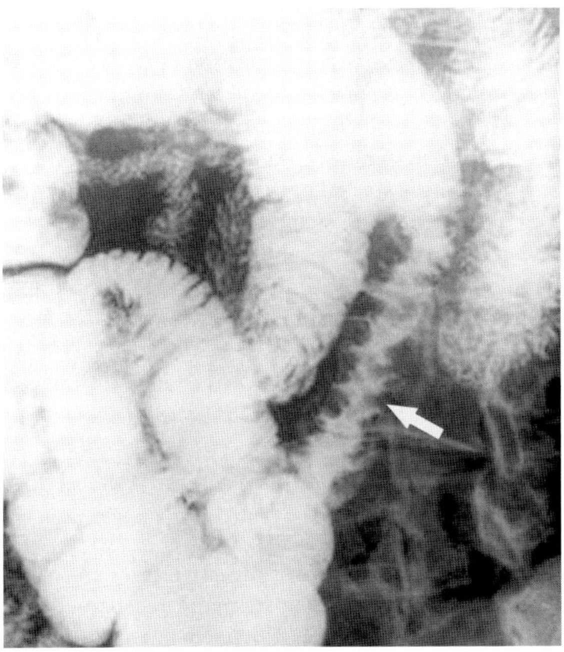

a

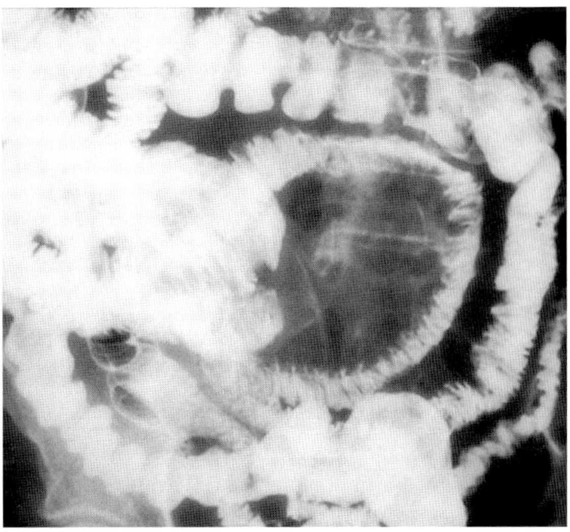

b

Fig. 8.8. (**a**) Posttraumatic mural intestinal hematoma and (**b**) mural and (**a, b**) mesenteric hematoma, in two patients after blunt abdominal injury, managed conservatively (see Fig. 8.15)

8.5.3.2
Pitfalls

Disadvantages of US include the need for at least 70 ml of intraperitoneal fluid for a positive study and a 20%–25% incidence of failure to detect an isoechoic injury to the spleen or liver, particularly when a rapid screening US examination is performed (Feliciano 1991b). Free fluid is not detected in the majority of patients with isolated bowel and mesenteric injury in the early phase (Richards et al. 1999). US is not useful for detecting free gas in the abdomen (Grassi et al. 1998).

8.5.3.3
Results

Although US may provide an overall 80% positive predictive value of blunt GI tract injury, more realistic figures indicate around 35%. It can be concluded that US is unable to diagnose with enough confidence injury to the GI tract or mesentery (Nagel et al. 1991; Sherck et al. 1994; Shih et al. 1995; Yoshii et al. 1998; Frick et al. 1999; Richards et al. 1999). Focused abdominal sonography for trauma (FAST), which is discussed in other chapters, is even less a reliable method for assessing GI tract injury (Stassen et al. 2002). There is a high rate of false negative US findings, as 61% of patients with bowel or mesentery injury had other concomitant abdominal injury, responsible for peritoneal fluid. However, 53% of patients with false negative US had clinical symptoms, such as abdominal tenderness (Richards et al. 1999). Results are also poor in children, where preoperative diagnosis of duodenal and pancreatic injury was established only in 43% with US (Plancq et al. 2000).

8.5.4
Computed Tomography

8.5.4.1
Technique

Optimal CT examination technique is essential for the diagnosis of subtle posttraumatic GI tract injuries. Although oral contrast material is not routinely administered at admission in Europe, bowel opacification might be important for CT evaluation of GI tract injuries in selected patients with a high index of suspicion. A solution of 2%–3% dilated iodinated contrast is given 5–40 min before helical scanning at a concentration of 2%–5% and a total dose of 500–750 ml (Shuman 1997). Intestinal paresis might delay opacification of the small bowel loops. Attention to proper preparation and administration of the contrast material, and more importantly, control of the patient's airway by appropriate tracheal intubation, when necessary, are essential to assure the safety of the procedure (Donohue et al. 1987; Kelly et al. 1989; Feliciano 1991a; Federle et al. 1995, 1997). Opponents claim that oral contrast solutions are unnecessary in the acute CT evaluation of most patients with blunt abdominal trauma, and merely add delay time to CT scanning, as was shown in a randomized controlled study (Stafford et al. 1999). There is agreement however, that intravenous iodinated contrast material is mandatory for evaluation of GI tract and mesenteric injury. When apparently isolated mesenteric hematoma is evidenced, the adjacent bowel should be evaluated by thin slices to rule out mural injury. Scanning should systematically cover the thorax and abdomen down to the perineal floor.

8.5.4.2
Indications

In early times of CT up to the end of the 1980s, scanning was thought less reliable for diagnosis of GI tract than for parenchymal injuries (Sherck and Oakes 1990; Wisner et al. 1990). However, since the early 1980s, several reports in the radiological literature have advocated the use of CT for the detection of blunt GI tract injury (Glazer et al. 1981; Jeffrey et al. 1982). Actually, CT has become the procedure of choice for detecting small bowel and mesentery injury, particularly in patients with unreliable clinical examination caused by diminished level of consciousness. Although systematic repetition of CT for diagnosis of abdominal parenchymal organ contusion is not justified, in case of clinical suspicion of bowel injury, a negative CT should be repeated 4–6 h after abdominal symptoms have started or systematically in nonsymptomatic patients with suspected pancreatic injury or a history of strong deceleration, seat-belt or lap injury, handle bar injury in children, or severe and multiple plain abdominal organ injury (Miyakawa et al. 1992a, b; Catalano 1996; Levine et al. 1997; Grassi et al. 1998; Frick et al. 1999; Richards et al. 1999; Takabe et al. 2000; Pal and Victorino 2002).

8.5.4.3
Positive Signs

Description of CT signs of digestive tract and mesenteric injuries are given in many recent publications and will be discussed here below (Nghiem et al. 1993; Catalano 1996; Sivit 1997; Becker et al. 1998; Frick et al. 1999; Strouse et al. 1999; Pinto et al. 2001):

- Free air in the peritoneal cavity after injury of the GI tract is an almost specific and relatively sensitive sign of perforation of any cause, at any level (Nghiem et al. 1993; Sivit et al. 1994; Furst 2001) (Fig. 8.9). Gas bubbles may accumulate in the area of perforation, or be trapped by adhesions or ligaments, but usually they tend to coalesce rapidly in the right subphrenic or subhepatic space.
- Rupture of the stomach gives massive free air also in the left subhepatic and left subphrenic space.
- Rupture of the rectal wall without laceration of the peritoneum is followed by extraperitoneal air accumulation, dissecting the pelvic fat planes without tendency to coalesce and without pneumoperitoneum.
- Retroperitoneal air around or posterior to the duodenal loop indicates duodenal rupture (Nghiem et al. 1993).
- Rupture of the pharyngeal wall, during blast injury, shows air bubbles located in the soft tissues in front of the cervical spine, that may dissect downwards into the mediastinum (Schwartz et al. 1988)
- Free intra-abdominal fluid, originating from bowel or mesentery, when of small amount, shows as „mesenteric triangles" or „polygons," before accumulating in the perivesical space (Nghiem et al. 1995; Levine et al. 1997) (Figs. 8.10, 8.11). Fluid may be of low density (<20 HU), if it is extravasated from the small bowel, or of intermediate density (>25 HU), in case of hemoperitoneum, or very high density (>150 HU), when iodinated oral contrast material has extravasated in the peritoneal cavity (Nghiem et al. 1993). Small bowel fluid is largely composed of secretions, bile and pancreatic fluid. Density values of intraperitoneal fluid are not specific of bowel content and may correspond to diluted blood, bile, urine, and pancreatic juice. Inhomogeneous fluid is an indicator of bowel contents mixed with blood (Kloppel et al. 1997). Isolated peritoneal fluid or fluid accumulating preferentially or only in the mid abdominal compartments or small bowel mesentery is a strong indicator for intestinal or mesenteric injury (Nghiem et al. 1993; Levine et al. 1995). Similarly, a large volume of isolated peritoneal fluid without visible solid organ injury is an important

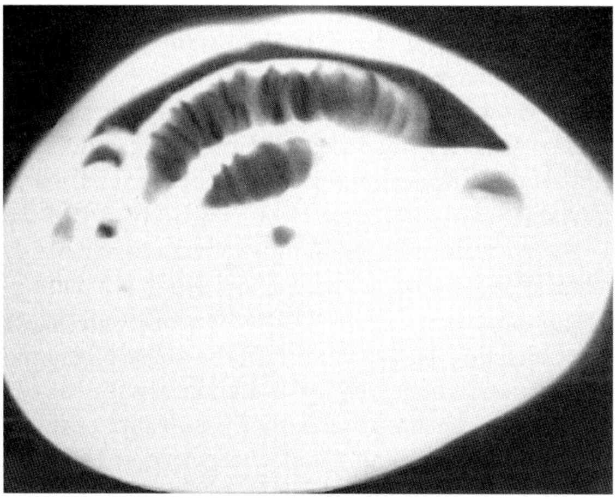

Fig. 8.9. Massive pneumoperitoneum after blunt rupture of the sigmoid colon

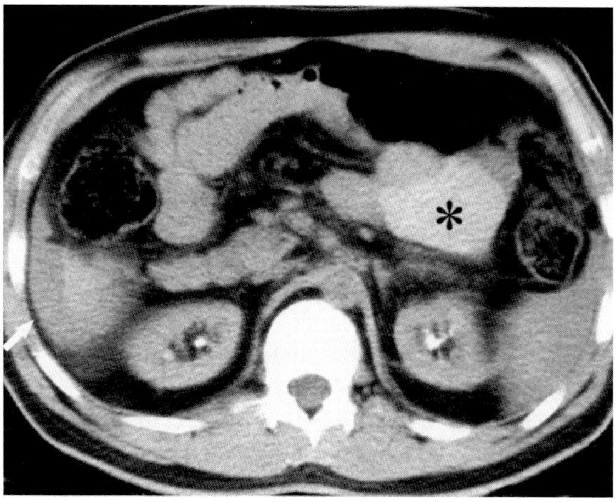

Fig. 8.10. Spontaneous hyperdense polygonal shaped hematoma in the mesentery (*asterisk*) and diluted hypodense blood in the right paracolic gutter (*arrow*)

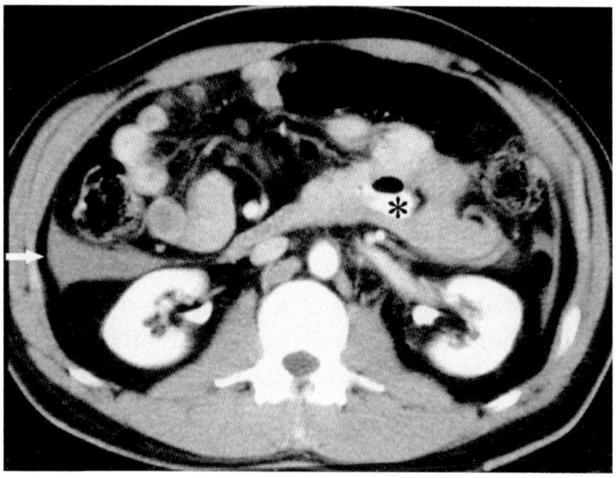

Fig. 8.11. Repeated CT examination 6 h after CT at admission for blunt abdominal injury. Polygonal shaped mesenteric hematoma isolating an intestinal loop, which contains contrast medium (*asterisk*) resulting from a previous contrast enhanced CT: the intravenously injected contrast medium was secreted by the biliary system. Notice diluted hemoperitoneum in the right paracolic gutter (*arrow*)

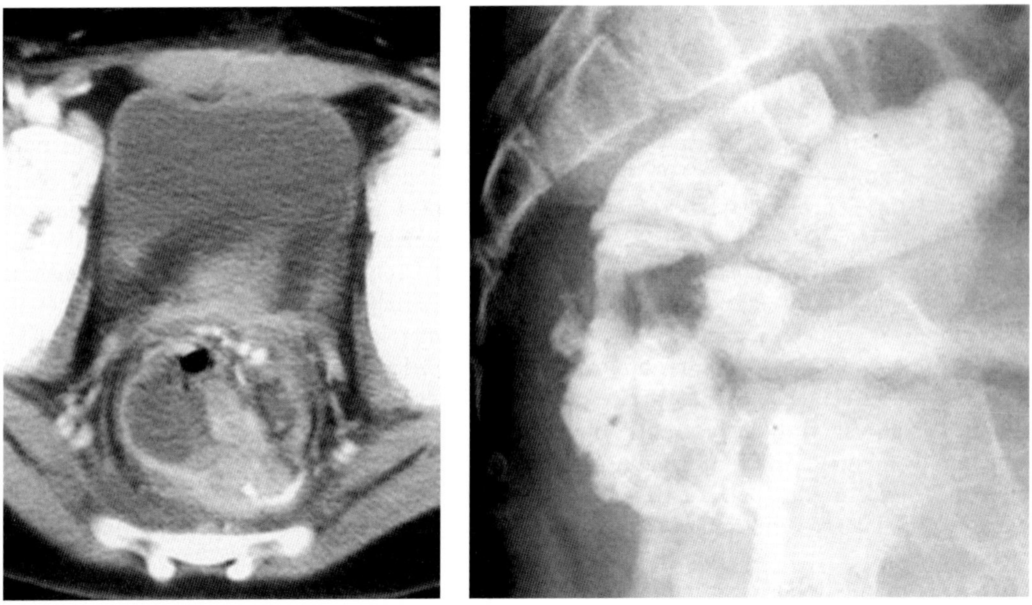

a b

Fig. 8.12. Self-inflicted perforation of the rectum with a foreign body. CT at (**a**, **b**) admission: (**a**) nonrecognition of the left anterior limit of the rectal wall, irregular thickening of the posterior aspect and diffuse infiltration of the perirectal tissue without free extrarectal air. (**b**) confirmation of rectal rupture by enema with iodinated contrast medium

sign of bowel or mesenteric injury (Bulas et al. 1989; Breen et al. 1997; Levine et al. 1997).

- Bowel wall discontinuity can be shown by CT when the site of wall laceration is large enough (Rizzo et al. 1989; Breen et al. 1997) (Fig. 8.12).
- Extravasation of oral contrast medium is not frequent, but virtually pathognomonic for bowel wall perforation, even more when an otherwise unexplainable pneumoperitoneum or pneumoretroperitoneum is associated (Hofer and Cohen 1989; Miyakawa et al. 1992a; Kunin et al. 1993; Ballard et al. 1997; Levine et al. 1997; Tsang et al. 1997; Strouse et al. 1999).
- Intramural hematoma results rather in eccentric than circumferential thickening of the bowel wall. It is dumbbell shaped when of large amount, and not enhanced after i.v. contrast injection. Spontaneous high densities of a mural mass, that may distribute inside the margin of the hemorrhage as a „ring sign," represent acute hematoma. (Jeffrey et al. 1982; Yoshino 1987; Rizzo et al. 1989; Nghiem et al. 1993). Hematoma can be isolated or suggestive of associated bowel laceration, when associated with low density fluid (Schmidt et al. 1994). A massive hematoma may give signs of localized distended loop or GI obstruction (Hughes and Brogdon 1986). Chronic hematoma changes into cyst-like densities over time (Figs. 8.13–8.17).
- Simultaneous interruption of progress of bowel contrast medium, and observation of extra luminal gas and fluid are pathognomonic for bowel rupture (Hofer and Cohen 1989).
- Intense enhancement of the bowel wall by i.v. contrast injection accompanied by bowel wall thickening and free intraperitoneal fluid strongly suggest perforation of the bowel, without being specific (Hara et al. 1992; Nghiem et al. 1993; Brody et al. 2000). Significance of bowel wall enhancement in case of perforation still demands clarification.
- Absence of enhancement or decreased enhancement of the bowel wall indicates bowel ischemia, caused by arterial and/or venous injury leading to devascularization.
- Persistent bleeding from GI tract or mesenteric vessels is demonstrated by intramural, endoluminal or peritoneal extravasation of contrast material (Sitoh and Sitoh 1998) (Figs. 8.18, 8.19, 8.21, 8.22b). Contrast medium that oozes outside the GI tract wall, in contact with a bowel loop is a pathognomonic sign of mural or mesenteric wall origin of bleeding. Early scanning at the phase of arterial mesenteric opacification is mandatory.
- Intestinal pneumatosis is shown as round or linear intramural gas and should be considered as part of an acute injury of the bowel in trauma patients. Other common diagnoses include ischemia of other origin, and infection (Wittenberg et al. 2002).

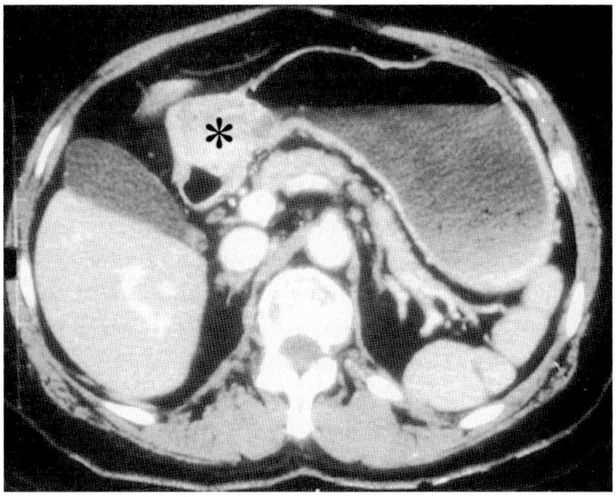

Fig. 8.13. Same patient as in Fig. 8.7. Obstructive posttraumatic hematoma (*asterisk*) of the first portion of the duodenum. Notice gastric distension

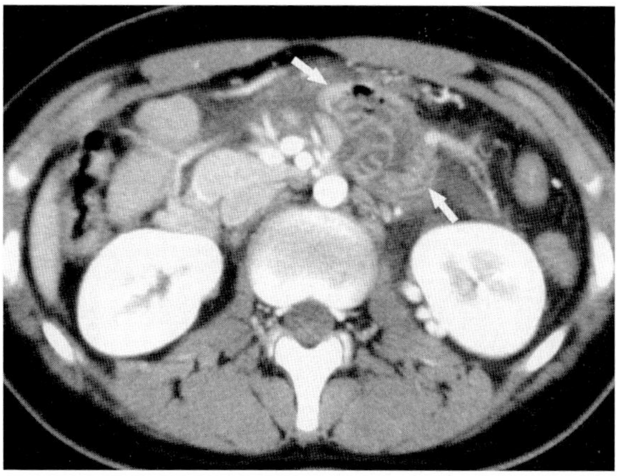

Fig. 8.14. Same patient as in Fig. 8.6. Nonobstructive duodenal hematoma shown as thickening of the wall of the third portion of the duodenum (*arrows*), and periduodenal fluid, without extraluminal gas

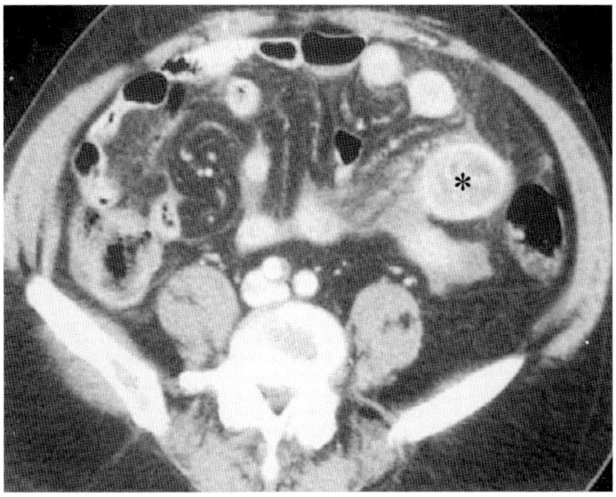

Fig. 8.15. Same patient as in Fig. 8.8b. Thickening of an intestinal loop (*asterisk*) and blurring of the adjacent mesentery after blunt abdominal trauma

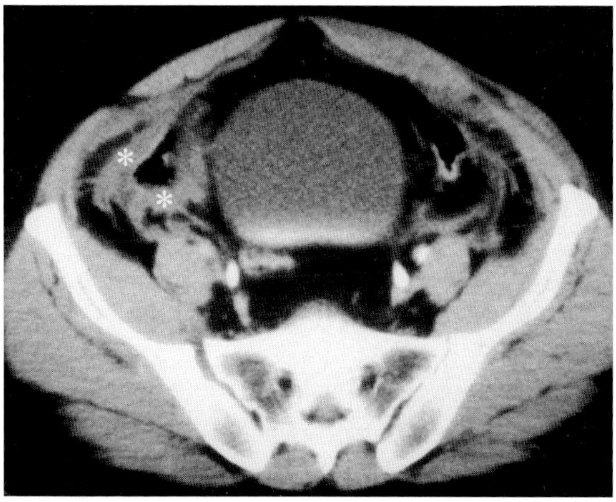

Fig. 8.16. Nonenhanced posttraumatic mural hematoma of the wall of the right colon (*asterisks*) (see Fig. 8.23)

- Hepatic portal venous gas is a sign of severe bowel injury involving bowel wall and veins (Aikawa et al. 1994; Muscari et al. 1999). Air is washed to the intrahepatic portal vein branches and accumulates preferentially in the nongravity-dependant small intrahepatic portal veins in the left lobe when the patient lies supine (Friedman et al. 1991).
- A mesenteric hematoma shows as a mass with solid or more elevated densities that is located adjacent to the bowel wall or more centrally in the mesentery, and remains unenhanced after intravenous contrast medium injection. A large hematoma may exert significant mass effect on adjacent bowel loops. The presence of a mesenteric „sentinel clot" should prompt a careful search for any evidence of gastrointestinal perforation or laceration of mesenteric vasculature (Rizzo et al. 1989; Shanmuganathan et al. 1995; Dowe et al. 1997) (Figs. 8.20–8.22).
- Blurring of fat plans or strands that dissect the peri-intestinal fat or „streaking" of the mesentery correspond to infiltration by limited, noncollected hemorrhage (Hagiwara et al. 1995; Breen et al. 1997; Dowe et al. 1997) (Fig. 8.23).
- In children, and also in adults, the bowel may be affected by hemodynamic shock and show pronounced enhancement of the bowel wall, due to reduced perfusion transit by vasoconstriction

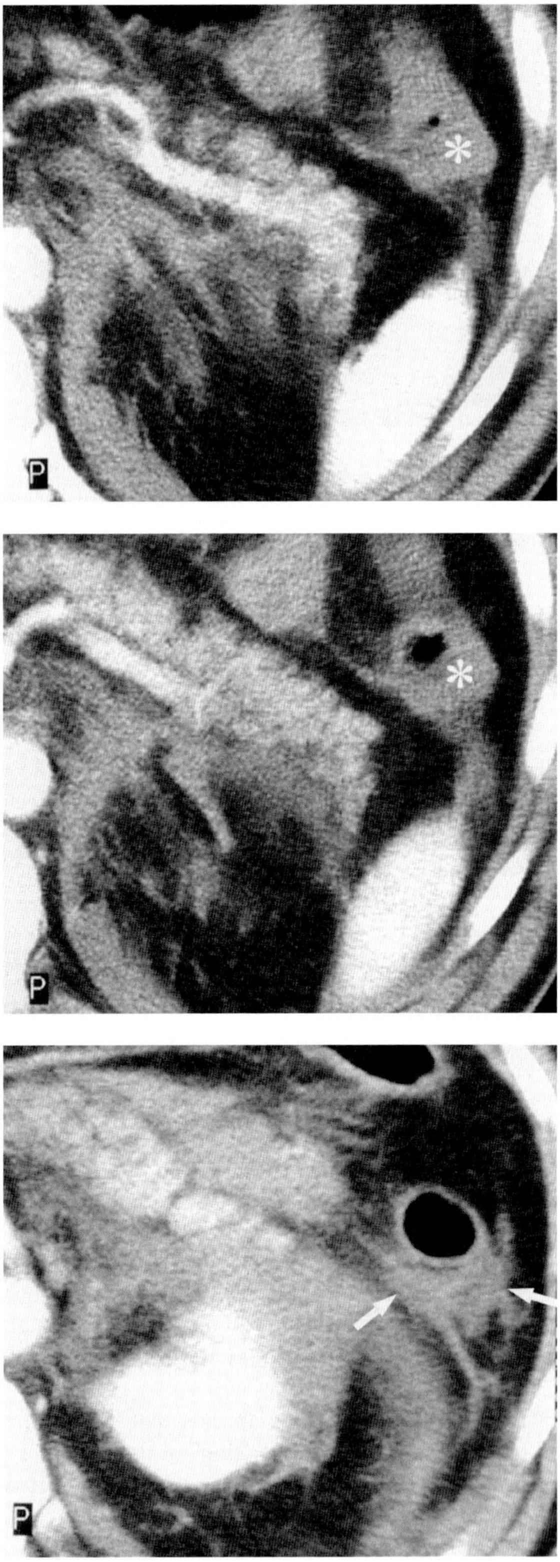

a

b

c

Fig. 8.17. Blunt injury to the left side of the abdomen (**a, b**). Eccentric mural (**a, b, c**) thickening of the left colon (*asterisk*) reducing the lumen and (**c**) localized pericolic hematoma (*arrows*) extending caudally. Notice also left perirenal hematoma

and bowel wall oedema (Figs. 8.24, 8.25). Persistent hyperdensity is part of the hypovolemic or hypoperfusion complex and is due to decreased microcirculation. The aorta and the IVC are also of small diameter (Taylor et al. 1987; Hara et al. 1992; Sivit et al. 1992; Mirvis et al.1994). In addition to staining of contrast, diffuse thickening of the small bowel (mean 11 mm), and fluid-filled, dilated small bowel loops, while colon is normal, is suggestive of hypoperfusion-shock bowel (Sivit et al. 1992; Mirvis et al. 1994).

Association of these individual signs is of value to reach a definite diagnosis or strengthen suspicion and eventually indicate repetition of CT, 4–12 h later.

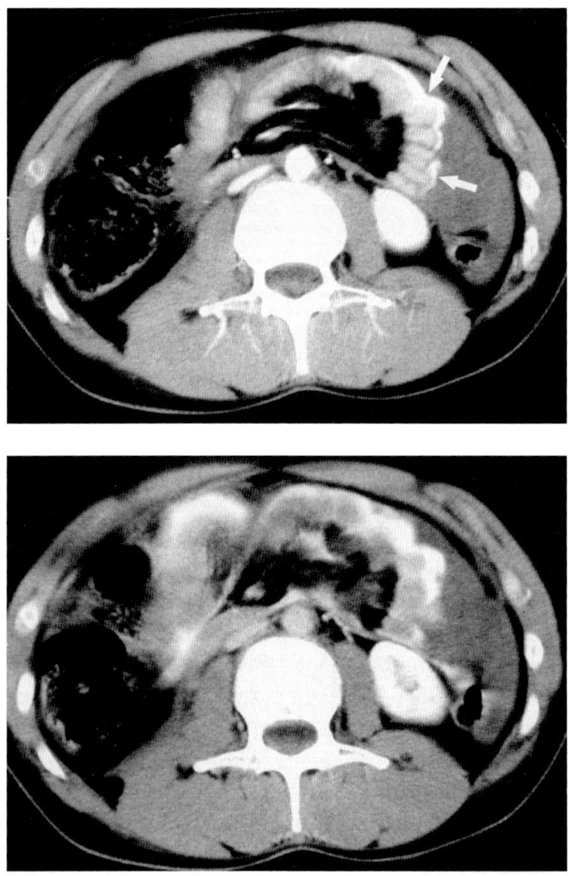

a

b

Fig. 8.18. Contrast-enhanced CT, arterial phase (**a**): massive extravasation of (**a, b**) contrast medium, in contact with the antimesenteric border of the small bowel (*arrows*) which has not yet diluted in the hemoperitoneum. (**b**) Progressive dilution of contrast in the hemoperitoneum at later phase

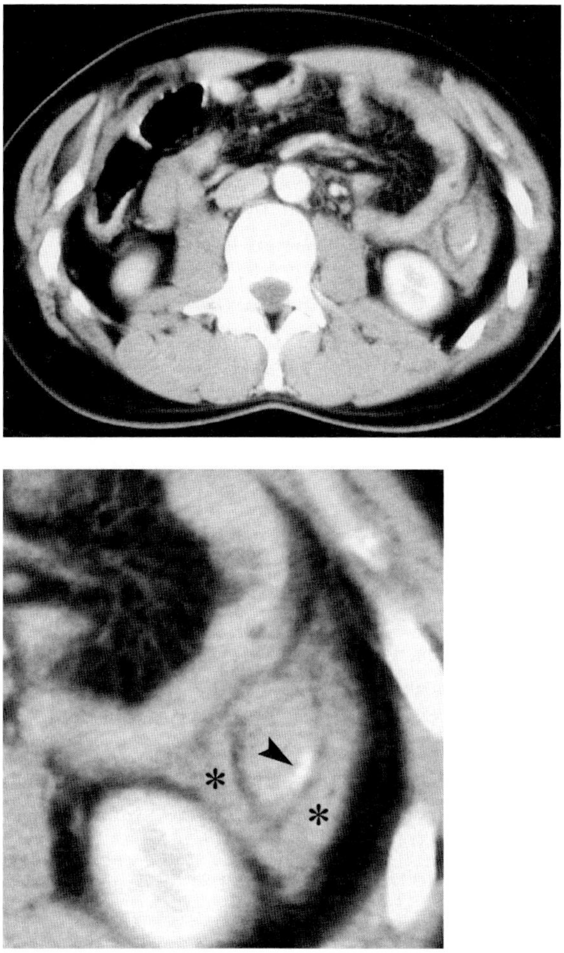

Fig. 8.19. Left colon mural and pericolic hematoma (*asterisks*), intramural (**a**, **b**) contrast accumulation of contrast medium (*arrow*), indicating ongoing hemorrhage

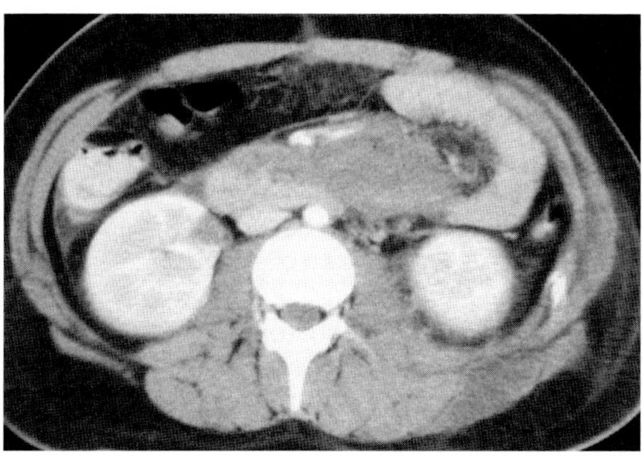

Fig. 8.20. Nonenhanced, well-circumscribed mesenteric hematoma

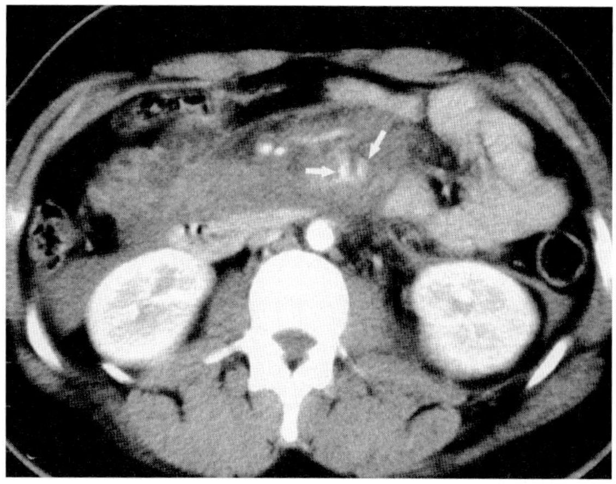

Fig. 8.21. Diffuse mesenteric hematoma with two small foci of contrast medium extravasation (*arrows*), demonstrating ongoing hemorrhage

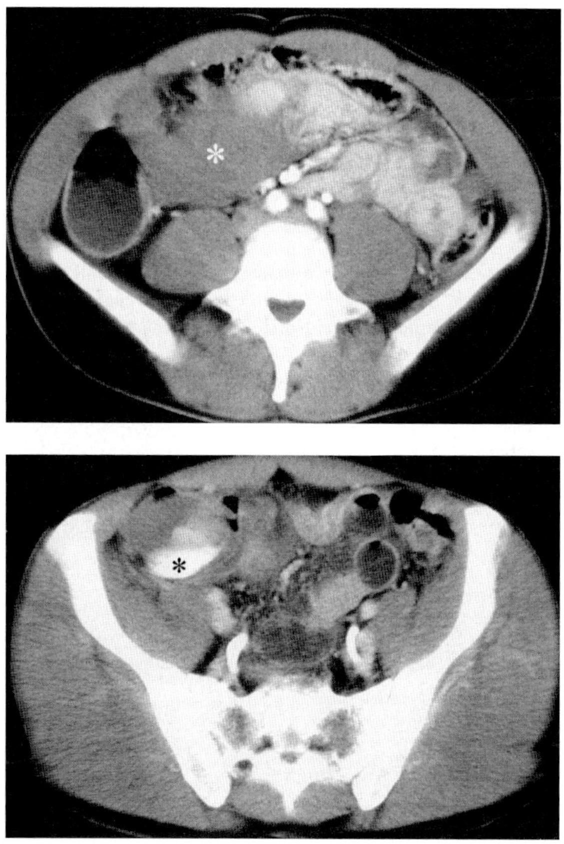

Fig. 8.22. Mesenteric hematoma extending in the right mesenterico-colic space (a, **b**) (**a**) without enhancement (*asterisk*) on the cranial slices; (**b**) extravasated contrast medium sedimentates (*asterisk*) on the most caudal slices

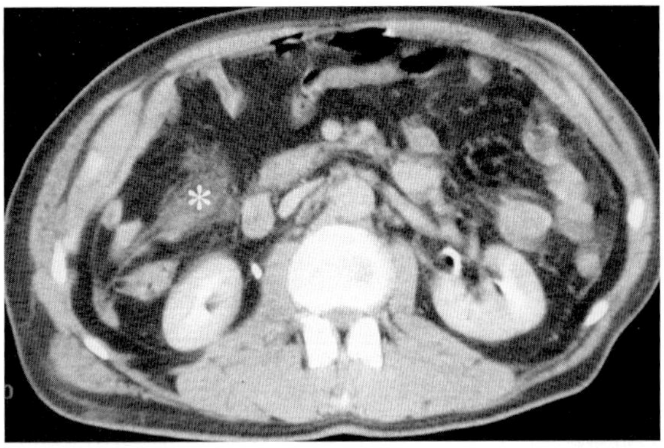

Fig. 8.23. Same patient as in Fig. 8.16. Streaking blurring of the mesentery (*asterisk*) adjacent to a hematoma of the wall of the ascending colon, shown in Fig. 8.16

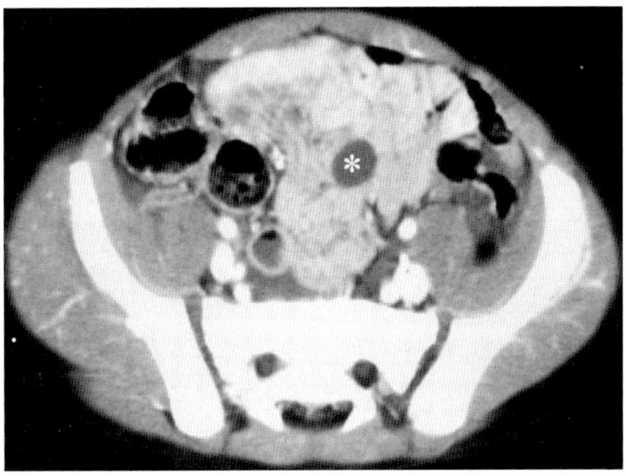

Fig. 8.24. Intense contrast enhancement of the wall of the small bowel in a 10-year-old boy in hemodynamic shock caused by splenic rupture. Notice a small mesenteric hematoma (*asterisk*)

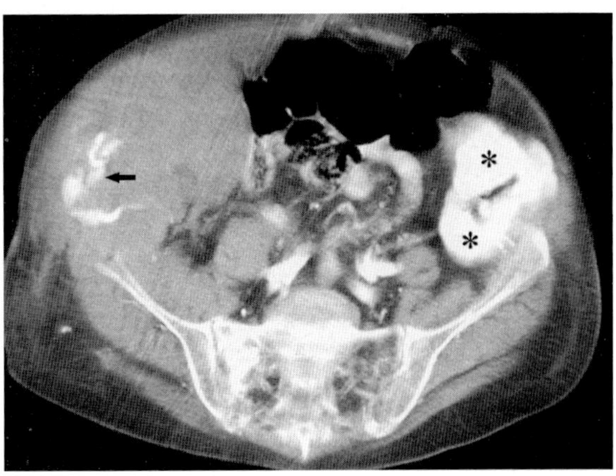

Fig. 8.25. Intense staining of contrast in the wall of the small bowel (*asterisk*) in a patient with ongoing hemorrhage (*arrow*) in a tense hematoma of the abdominal wall associated with pelvic bone fractures

8.5.4.4 Pitfalls

Potential pitfalls were discussed in detail in a recent publication (Brody et al. 2000).

- CT may be falsely negative for GI tract injury in the early posttraumatic phase, either because subtle signs were missed or perforation of the small bowel occurred with delay. In jejunal perforation, CT may remain negative within 12 h following trauma (Cook et al. 1986; Nghiem et al. 1993; Sivit et al. 1994). In patients developing signs of fever or peritonitis, CT should be repeated systematically, keeping in mind that other non-traumatic delayed complications may also induce bowel necrosis (Nghiem et al. 1993).
- Pneumoperitoneum does not necessarily indicate hollow viscus injury, but may be explained either by microperforation of the bowel without clinical significance, or tension pneumothorax, mechanical ventilation, or air introduced during DPL, through the genital tract or by a catheter introduced in a ruptured urinary bladder (Bulas et al. 1989; Kane et al. 1991; Hamilton et al. 1995) (Fig. 8.26). Free intraperitoneal air is seen only in one third to half of all bowel perforations (Jamieson et al. 1996; Roberts 1996).
- Free peritoneal fluid without a known source of parenchymal bleeding, may be suggestive, but is not specific of intestinal injury (Miyakawa et al. 1992b).
- Massive pneumoperitoneum and peritoneal fluid forms an air fluid level that may simulate distended bowel loop (Fig. 8.27).
- Retroperitoneal air should not be mistaken for pneumoperitoneum (Figs. 8.28, 8.29)
- Confidently diagnosing cystic pneumatosis in the antidependent bowel wall is challenging because it can be mimicked by gas bubbles at the top of intramural fluid. Most challenging is differentiating dependently located gas bubbles in the caecum and ascending colonic wall from gas trapped between fecal debris and mucosa. Using thin slices or repositioning and rescanning the patient may be helpful (Wittenberg et al. 2002).
- Portal venous gas does not necessarily indicate bowel necrosis in blunt trauma patients, as it can be produced by a sudden increase in the intra-abdominal pressure with concomitant mucosal disruption, forcing intraluminal gas into the portal circulation (Pal and Victorino 2002). Intraportal air may also be observed several days after blunt trauma and then result from postischemic bowel wall necrosis without previous posttraumatic rupture.

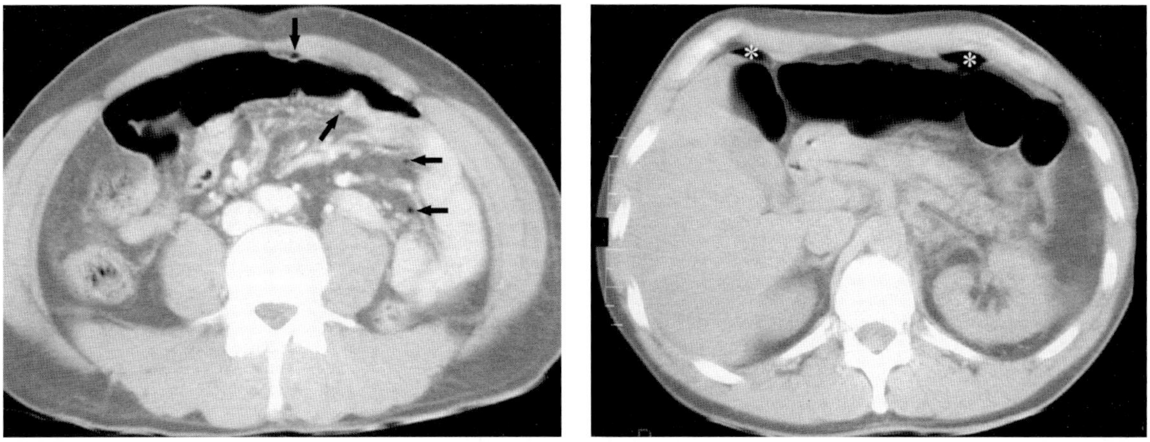

a b

Fig. 8.26. CT obtained at admission after blunt abdominal injury showed. (**a**) minute gas bubbles (*arrows*) in the peritoneal cavity, (**b**) accumulating (*asterisks*) on more cranial slices. No clinically significant bowel perforation became evident during follow-up

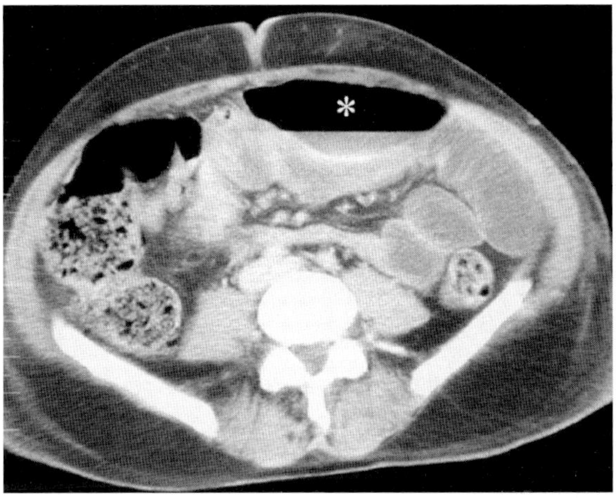

Fig. 8.27. Same patient as in Fig. 8.1. Large pneumoperitoneum and peritoneal fluid may simulate a small bowel segment distended by air (*asterisk*) and fluid

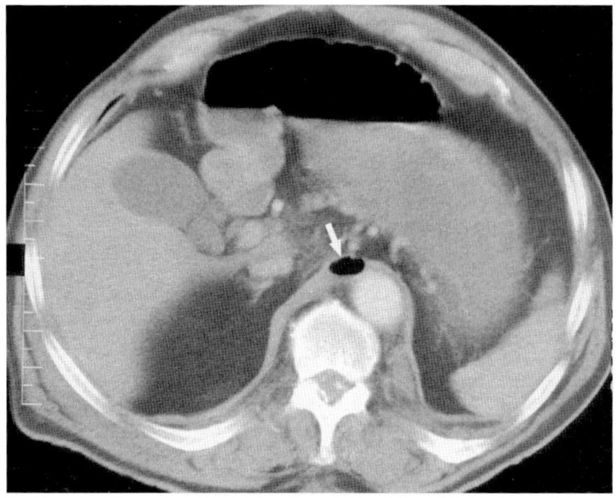

Fig. 8.28. A gas bubble (*arrow*), resulting from posttraumatic pneumomediastinum, dissects the right crus of the diaphragm

Occasionally, air bubbles introduced during emergency venous catheterization may be found in the nondependent hepatic veins and should not be confused with portal vein gas (Fig. 8.30).

- In complex and severe injuries, when intraluminal and intravenous contrast was given, it might be difficult to differentiate wall perforation from arterial bleeding, the oral and intravenously given and extravasated contrast showing similar densities (Kwauk et al. 1995) (Fig. 8.11).
- Duodenal perforation cannot always be distinguished from duodenal hematoma, as the CT findings of periduodenal fluid or wall thickening may be found in both entities (Kunin et al. 1993; Barandica and Patel 1997).
- Preexisting inflammatory bowel disease, such as Crohn's disease may be responsible for wall thickening, which can be erroneously mistaken for bowel wall or mesenteric hematoma (Kwauk et al. 1995) (Fig. 8.31).
- Bowel injury may be confused with hypoperfusion complex on CT. In patients with hypotension and hypoperfusion, the small bowel may show diffuse bowel wall thickening, suggesting posttraumatic injury (Sivit et al. 1992, 1994; Frick et al. 1999).

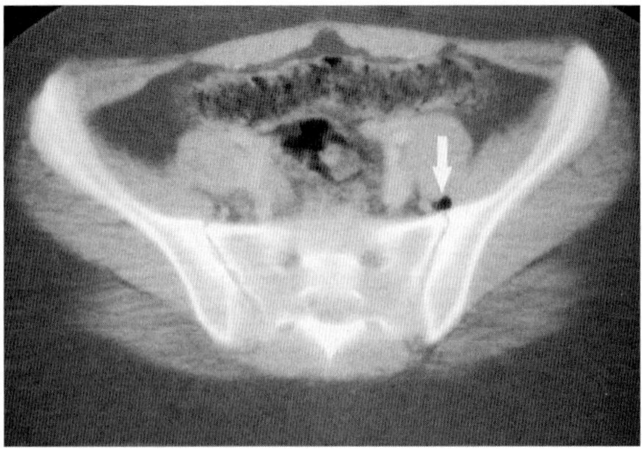

Fig. 8.29. Small gas bubble (*arrow*), which are frequently seen after blunt abdomino-pelvic trauma in front of the sacroiliac joints, should not be mistaken for a sign of colon or rectal perforation

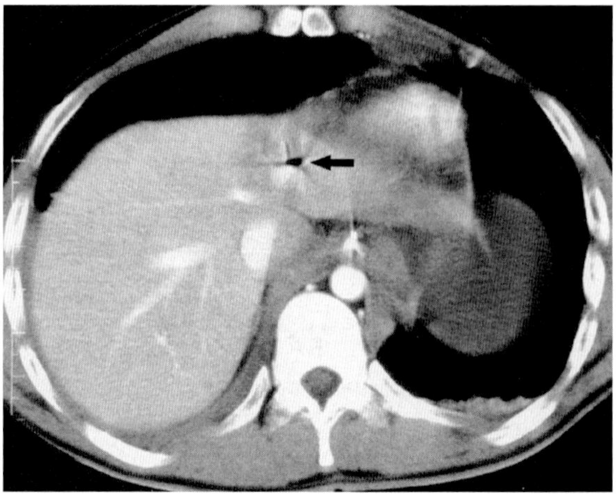

Fig. 8.30. Small air bubble in the left hepatic vein, resulting from venous catheter insertions during resuscitation, should not be confused with intraportal gas

a 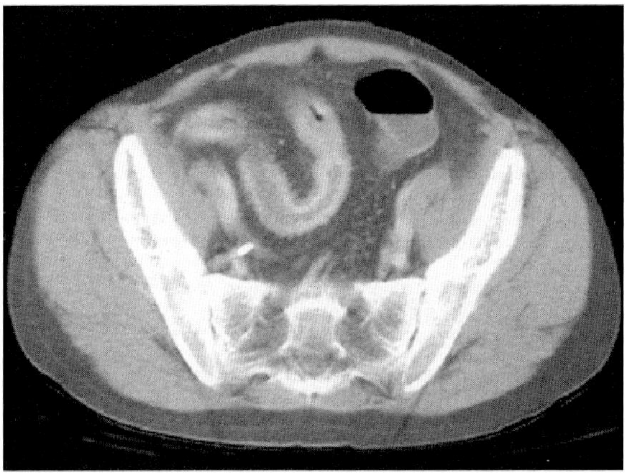

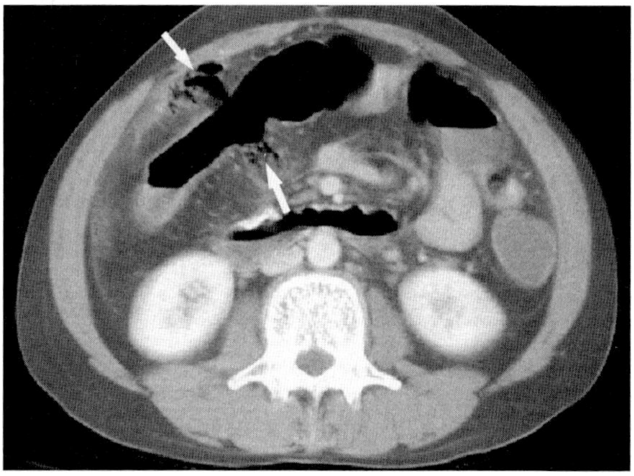 b

c 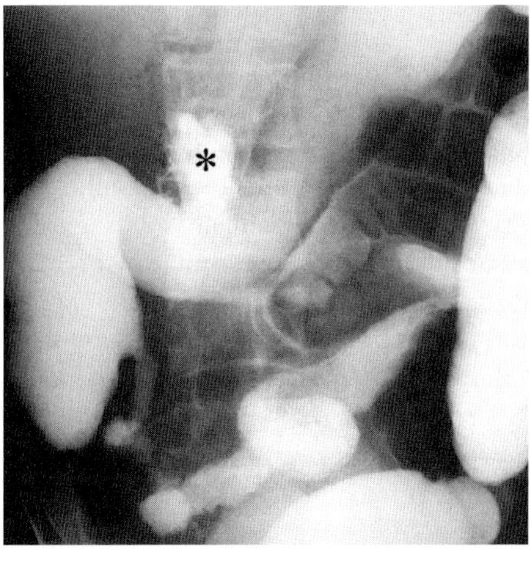

Fig. 8.31. A patient with Crohn's disease was kicked in the abdomen with an iron stick. (**a**) Thickening of a small bowel loop, suggestive of Crohn's disease. (**b**) Free gas bubbles (*arrows*) have accumulated adjacent the transverse colon, dilated with air. (**c**) Enema with iodinated contrast agent confirms extensive ileal and colon Crohn's disease and massive extravasation of contrast material (*asterisk*)

8.5.4.5 Results

Initial reports were focused on duodenal injuries and suggested the usefulness of CT in the diagnosis of duodenal rupture, although the classic pathognomonic findings of duodenal perforation are present in only a minority of cases (Glazer et al. 1981; Karnaze et al. 1981).

In later studies, extending to small bowel and colon, CT was shown to be diagnostic or suggestive of bowel injury in 69%–95% of cases and specific in 94%–100%, largely contributing in the selection of operative or conservative management (Rizzo et al. 1989; Mirvis et al. 1992; Sherck et al. 1994; Ballard et al. 1997; Frick et al. 1999; Lotti et al. 2000; Jarayaman et al. 2001; Pal and Victorino 2002). However, the individual CT signs are present with variable frequency: bowel wall thickening (75%), pneumoperitoneum (32%–56%) and extravasated oral contrast material (12%) (Rizzo et al. 1989; Breen et al. 1997; Levine et al. 1997; Tsang et al. 1997). Catalano found intraperitoneal air, intraperitoneal fluid, or extraluminal contrast present in 61% of the cases, a combination of intraperitoneal air and fluid present in 29%, and gas only in 16% of the cases (Catalano 1996). Breen found for bowel wall thickening a sensitivity of 50% and specificity of 84%; for bowel wall discontinuity, a sensitivity of 58% and a specificity of 95%. Extraluminal air was 44% sensitive and 100% specific. Mesenteric hematoma was 54% sensitive and 94% specific and isolated mesenteric streaking 77% sensitive and 44% specific (Breen et al. 1997).

In children with blunt abdominal trauma, in whom CT showed pneumoperitoneum, only 44% had a ruptured bowel. The remaining 66% had pneumoperitoneum from sources other than bowel wall perforation, including pneumomediastinum dissecting to the abdomen, urinary bladder rupture and previous DPL (Bulas et al. 1989).

Comparative studies of CT and DPL showed a respective false negative rate of 33%–80% for CT and 0%–13% for DPL in the diagnosis of bowel perforation (Federle et al. 1982; Fabian et al. 1986; Kearney 1989; Wisner et al. 1990; Meredith et al. 1992). Opponents to the use of CT to diagnose GI tract injury argue that its false negative rate is at best 3%–26%, as obtained with single detector row technology, and conclude that its utility is limited compared with serial clinical examination and DPL (Marx et al. 1985; Fischer et al. 1988; Kearney et al. 1989; Meyer et al. 1989; Sherck and Oakes 1990; Hamilton et al. 1995; Albanese et al. 1996; Bloom et al. 1996; Allen et al. 1998).

Sensitivity of CT is increased from 73%–100% when performed after 4 h following injury (Miyakawa et al. 1992 b).

There is general agreement on the significantly higher sensitivity of CT compared with conventional radiography. In addition, CT is invaluable for investigation of plain abdominal organ injury and therefore, despite its limitation in depicting early posttraumatic injury to the GI tract, remains the cornerstone in blunt abdominal trauma.

8.5.5 Angiography

Angiography has a limited diagnostic role in the assessment of acute GI tract and mesenteric injuries, as posttraumatic bleeding from the GI tract and large mesenteric vessels requires systematic surgical repair. Expected signs in the mesenteric circulation are vessel displacement, arterial spasm, localized flow interruption, pseudoaneurysm, contrast extravasation, reduced flow and staining in the mesenteric venous return (Osborn et al. 1973). The primary indication for arteriography is the evaluation of ongoing hemorrhage of solid intra-abdominal organs and retroperitoneal or pelvic arterial bleeding in patients with pelvic fractures. Accurate anatomical location allows a choice of either surgical management or transcatheter embolization and thus decreases time consumption for precise bleeding site identification (Gilliland et al. 1982; Strouse et al. 1999) (Fig. 8.32).

In patients in whom conservative nonsurgical management or hemostatic arterial embolization is the therapeutic option, GI tract perforation or mesenteric vascular lesions must be ruled out.

8.5.6 Magnetic Resonance Imaging

Magnetic Resonance Imaging (MRI) has no role in the acute assessment of posttraumatic injuries of the GI tract. In a later phase, MRI contributes to confirm the diagnosis of a mural hematoma and is particularly useful in demonstrating phrenic rupture, complicated by transdiaphragmatic bowel herniation (Mirvis et al. 1988; Daum-Kowalski et al. 1991; Boulanger et al. 1992; Boulos et al. 1997; Wataya et al. 1997; Ramos et al. 2000)

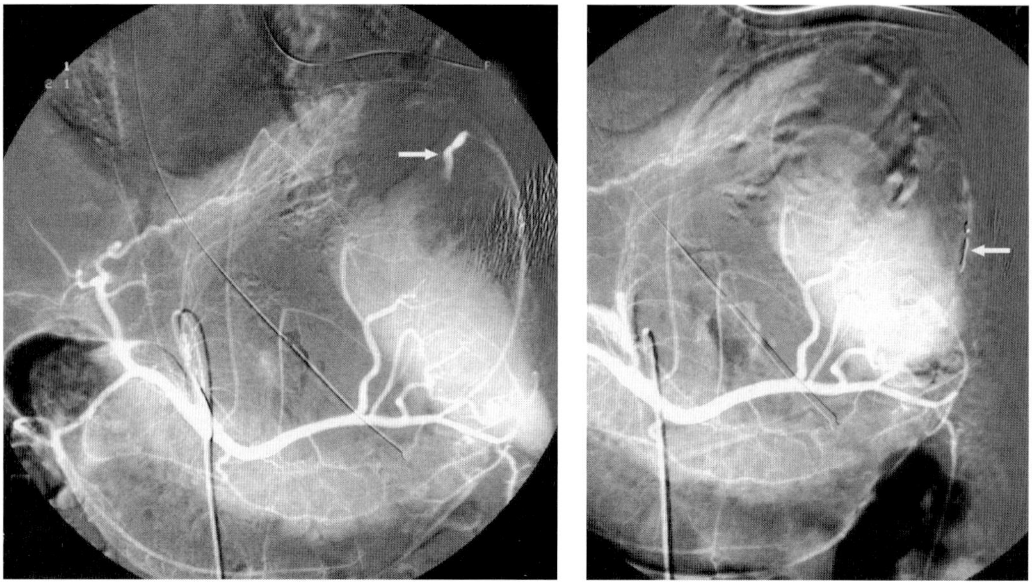

Fig. 8.32. Patient admitted after a knife wound to the abdomen. CT showed (**a**, **b**) gastric perforation and perigastric contrast extravasation. (**a**) Arteriography confirmed bleeding from a branch of the splenic artery (*arrow*). (**b**) Temporizing selective hemostatic embolization with a microcoil (*arrow*) allowed operation on other more severely injured trauma victims first

8.6 Management

8.6.1 Surgical

Studies that have attempted to demonstrate optimal preoperative diagnostic approaches have shown varying results and no clear algorithms for patient care have emerged (Browstein et al. 2000). CT permits adequate planning of emergency surgery and helps to select the cases for follow-up, intensive care, and conservative treatment (Salzano et al. 2000).

In blunt trauma, hemodynamic instability, perforation of the bowel wall, mesenteric desinsertion, vascular injuries, ischemic bowel infarction, massive gas in the portal vein, massive peritoneal fluid without parenchymal contusion, ongoing intraperitoneal hemorrhage, fever, and peritonitis, uncertain imaging results, and all prompt laparotomy and surgical repair (Mackersie et al. 1989; Feliciano 1991a; Brasel et al. 1998; Shilyansky et al. 1997; Cunningham et al. 1998; Hugues 1999; Strouse et al. 1999; Kilgus et al. 1999; Muscari et al. 1999). Other less critical injuries, including nonobstructive mural hematoma, or isolated mesenteric hematoma without mass effect or limited free fluid in an asymptomatic patient can be treated conservatively, when rupture of the GI tract was ruled out (Donohue et al.1987; Salzano et al. 2000).

In penetrating abdominal trauma, there is a high probability of GI tract injuries. Gunshot wounds with obvious traverse of the abdominal cavity cause visceral or vascular injuries in 96%–98% of patients and are a clear indication for urgent coeliotomy (Feliciano 1991a) (Fig. 8.33). In stab wounds penetrating the abdomen, CT now plays a definite preoperative role, as negative predictive value for peritoneal injury is close to 100%.

Indications for delayed laparotomy include delayed diagnosis of hollow visceral injury (perforation, peritonitis, or obstruction) (Bensard et al. 1996). Most GI tract perforations, including duodenal injuries, particularly minor or isolated, are treated with simple surgical repair (Adkins and Keyser 1985; Shorr et al. 1987; Grosfeld et al. 1989; McKenney et al. 1996). Duodenopancreatic resection is performed only in the most severe forms of combined duodenal and pancreatic, ampullary and bile duct injury in stage surgery combining damage control repair and planned reoperation (Feliciano et al. 1987; Carillo et al. 1996). Mural hematoma in the duodenum may regress spontaneously, but the majority of the cases of colonic hematoma may need operation, including a laparoscopic approach in both locations (Maemura et al. 1999; Yin et al. 2000). Vascular coeliomesenteric injury is corrected surgically during urgent coeliotomy (Zeybek et al. 2001).

Mortality, directly related to blunt GI tract injury, is low (2%–6%) after surgical treatment (Cogbill et al. 1990; Carillo et al. 1996; Fang et al. 1999;

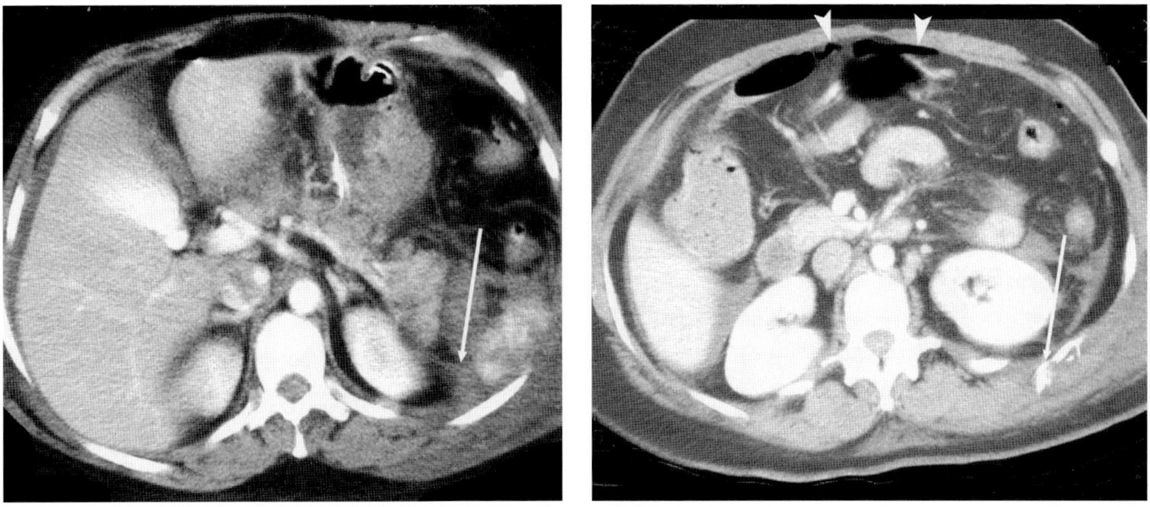

a b

Fig. 8.33. CT at admission after a gunshot wound at the left abdomen. The (**a, b**) bullet transected the tail of the pancreas (*arrow*), (**b**) and fractured a posterior rib at the exit site (*arrow*). Pneumoperitoneum (*arrowheads*) indicated left colon rupture, which was confirmed at surgery

Hugues et al. 2002). Mortality rates of 10%–33% have been reported for small bowel and mesentery injury, and increased mortality with associated injuries was noted by some (Frick et al. 1999). A missed diagnosis of a bowel injury has a significantly increased risk of morbidity (Browstein et al. 2000).

8.6.2 Conservative

The danger inherent to nonoperative management of patients with blunt abdominal injury to solid organs is that concomitant gastrointestinal disruption will escape timely diagnosis and repair (Ulman et al. 1996). The risk of missing significant bowel injury is a permanent thread when reducing the risk of unnecessary laparotomy (Fischer et al. 1988; Bensard et al. 1996; Pinto et al. 2001). Only patients without suspicion of GI tract perfusion or with isolated trace amounts of free fluid or limited mesenteric infiltration can be safely observed (Brasel et al. 1998) (Figs. 8.10, 8.11). Oh the other hand, a patient with free fluid in more than one location has a 50% chance of bowel injury and should be operated upon (Hulka et al. 1998) (Fig. 8.34). Only fully cooperative patients with no signs of GI tract injury and minimal clinical signs should be treated conservatively (Hugues 1999).

GI tract wall hematoma, particularly in a duodenal location, when isolated, is basically treated conservatively, as 50% resolve nonoperatively (Touloukian 1983; Levison et al. 1984; Welling and Reilly 1986; Donohue et al. 1987; Jewett et al. 1988; Fasolini et al. 1994; Shilyansky et al. 1997; Lotti et al. 2000) (Figs. 8.5, 8.6, 8.8). Operative therapy is indicated when a duodenal intramural hematoma does not resolve after 5–10 days or significantly obstructs the bowel lumen (Fischer et al. 1988; Thoms and Ricketts 1988) (Figs. 8.7, 8.13, 8.14).

In the absence of vascular erosion, the conservative measures of oesophageal perforation with a foreign body consists of foreign body removal, intravenous antibiotics, and discontinuing of oral nutrition (Kerschner et al. 2001).

8.6.3 Radiological Treatment

There is a definitive but reduced place for angiographic hemostatic embolization of posttraumatic bleeding in the GI tract, but indications are few at admission (Fig. 8.32). More patients are treated in the recovery phase for postoperative vascular injury than at admission. Pseudoaneurysm, or arteriovenous fistula of visceral arteries are responsible for endoluminal or peritoneal bleeding (Freeman et al. 1985; Hassantash et al. 1995; Reichert et al. 1995). Continuous bleeding in a mural or mesenteric hematoma can result in a tense hematoma, confirmed by increase in size on serial CT examinations or clinical signs of obstruction. Rapid selective embolization of a bleeding branch may reduce the need for blood transfusion and the risk of perforation or secondary bleeding from a pseudoaneurysm

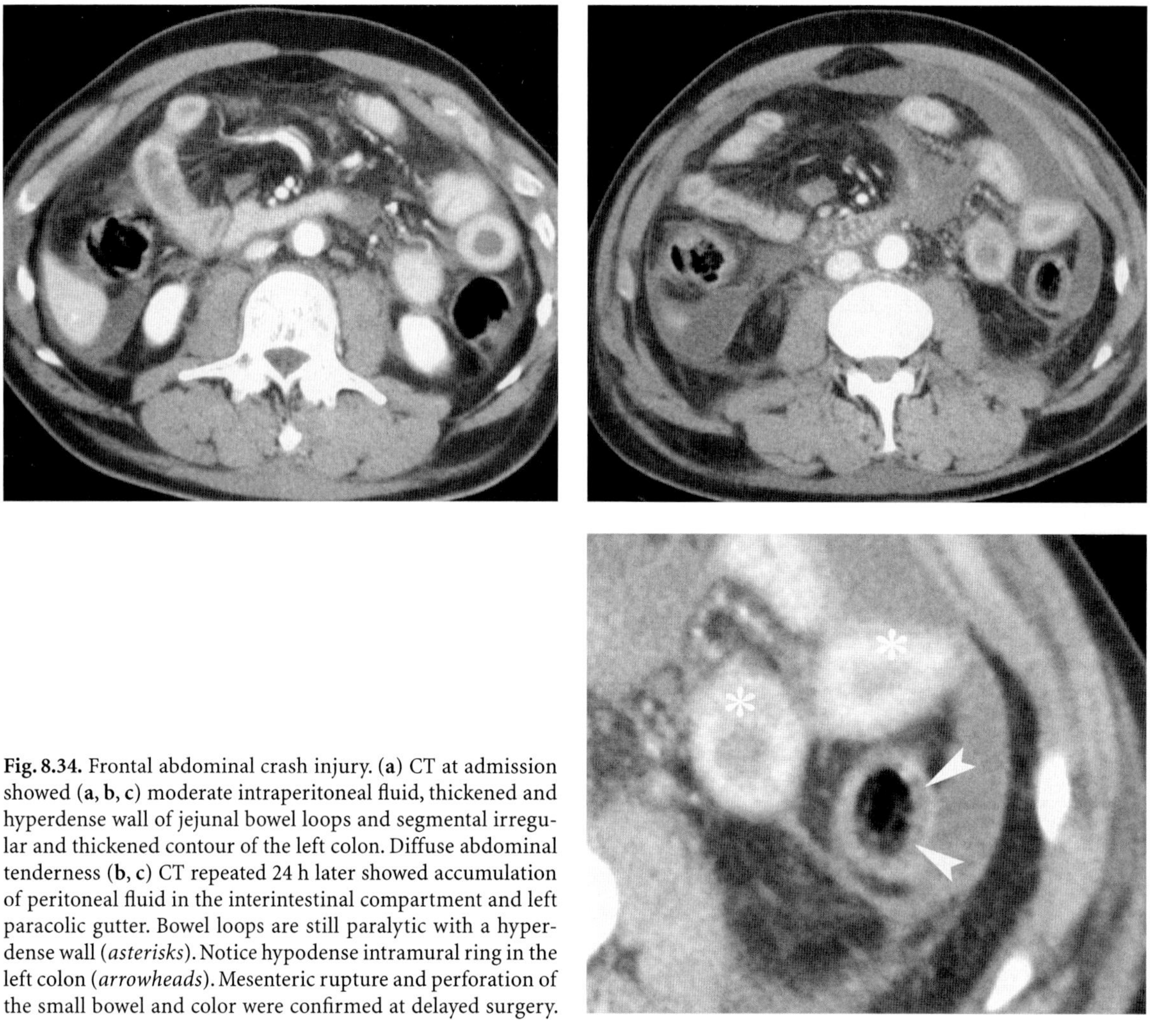

Fig. 8.34. Frontal abdominal crash injury. (**a**) CT at admission showed (**a**, **b**, **c**) moderate intraperitoneal fluid, thickened and hyperdense wall of jejunal bowel loops and segmental irregular and thickened contour of the left colon. Diffuse abdominal tenderness (**b**, **c**) CT repeated 24 h later showed accumulation of peritoneal fluid in the interintestinal compartment and left paracolic gutter. Bowel loops are still paralytic with a hyperdense wall (*asterisks*). Notice hypodense intramural ring in the left colon (*arrowheads*). Mesenteric rupture and perforation of the small bowel and color were confirmed at delayed surgery.

(Marra and Sclafani 1999). Posttraumatic immature false aneurysms are particularly fragile structures that may rupture during embolization (Lina et al. 1979). An extremely cautious embolization technique is mandatory. Filling of the aneurysmal sac with coils is prohibited as secondary rupture followed by catastrophic bleeding is a recognized complication.

8.7 Complications

8.7.1 Vascular

Delayed posttraumatic vascular injuries of the mesenteric circulation are rarely reported (Rosenthal et al. 1987). Most result from penetrating injury. The hemorrhage can remain masked, because of the tamponade in the mesentery during penetrating abdominal injury and initial surgery, and the late complication of false aneurysm comes on the scene only in the follow-up (Zeybek et al. 2001). Pseudoaneurysm may rupture at any time in the peritoneal cavity or induce gastrointestinal hemorrhage. High flow arteriovenous communication can be responsible for dynamic portal hypertension, or intestinal ischemia by arterial flow diversion.

Radionuclide studies (Tc 99 m labeled red blood cells) may evidence such aneurismal or arteriovenous lesions. CT and MRI are able to precisely locate these lesions down to a certain size, provided the radiologist is aware of such a possibility. The largest lesions are easily demonstrated with Doppler studies. Selective angiography is the optimal diagnostic modality, allowing for vaso-occlusive intervention in the feeding vessel, mainly with microcoils or particulate agents (Desai et al. 1987; Rosenthal et al. 1987; Taylor et al. 1988a; Lautin et al. 1999).

8.7.2 Nonvascular

8.7.2.1 Infection and Fistulae

Postoperative infection accounts for much more significant morbidity and mortality following penetrating than blunt abdominal trauma. Complications occur predominantly in patients with delayed intervention, beyond 24–48 h, among which pancreatic or duodenal fistulas and abscess carry a mortality of 30% (Jones et al. 1985; Feliciano et al. 1987; Coleman and Dietz 1990; Allen et al. 1998) (Fig. 8.35). The delayed diagnosis of hollow viscus injury is invariably responsible for increased morbidity and mortality for blunt trauma patients, reaching a 30 day mortality after surgery for blunt GI tract injury of 33%–35% (Hunt et al. 1980; Robbs et al. 1980; Strate and Grieco 1983; Talton et al. 1995; Contostavlos et al. 1996; Hugues et al. 2002).

In particular, delay in the diagnosis of gastric and colon perforation prolongs the periods of peritoneal contamination, and contributes to sepsis and intra-abdominal abscess, which is often extensive, recurrent, and difficult to treat (Nghiem et al. 1993; Croce et al. 1998). The incidence of fistulas and extensive retroperitoneal abscess formation after blunt duodenal injury was reported to be in a rage of 4%–28%, and is extremely common in patients with delayed diagnosis (Fang et al. 1999). Death rate may vary from 9.3%–31% and is often related to associated severe vascular injuries (Matolo et al. 1975; Novikov et al. 1998).

Percutaneous catheter drainage is an alternative to surgical drainage in most patients with postoperative abdominal abscess. Mesenteric hematomas, which are not regressing or exerting a mass effect on bowel loops causing obstruction are also amenable to percutaneous catheter drainage (Kortbeek et al. 1997).

8.7.2.2 Ischemic Intestinal Stenosis

Posttraumatic ischemic stenosis is exceedingly rare, and although certainly not all minor undiagnosed mesenteric injuries lead to stricture formation, all represent a risk (Shalaby-Rana et al. 1992; Hirota et al. 1995; Breen et al. 1997; De Backer et al. 1999). Posttraumatic intestinal or colon stenosis subsequent to a mesenteric tear should be included in the differential diagnosis in a patient with a history of blunt abdominal trauma and signs of intestinal obstruction. An increasing number of late intestinal obstruction is reported after a seat-belt injury (Junghanns 1978). Injury may cause partial thickness ischemia of the bowel wall, with mucosal ulceration and sub-

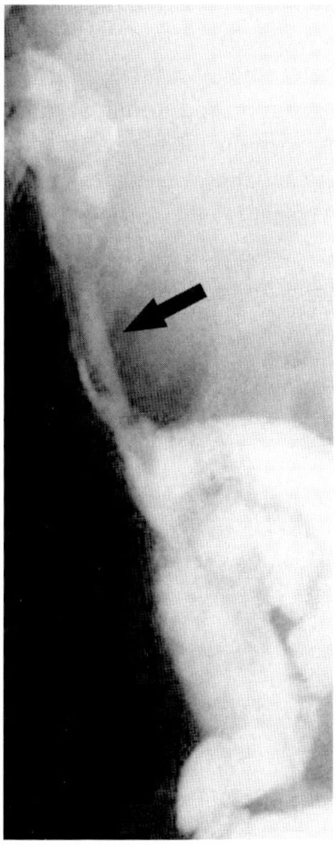

a

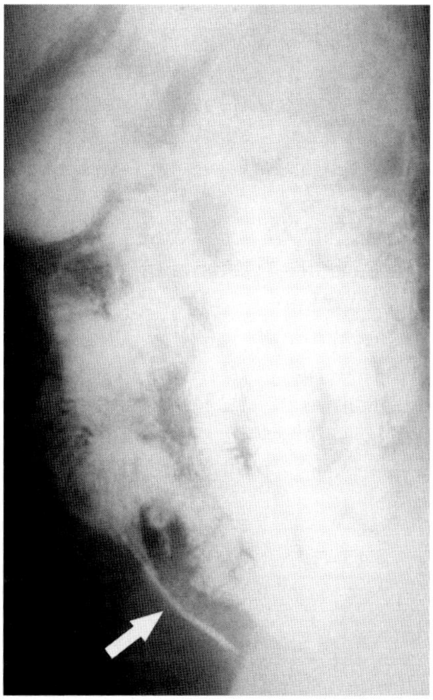

b

Fig. 8.35. Postoperative fistulae (*arrow*) after repair of small bowel rupture in (**a**, **b**) two patients

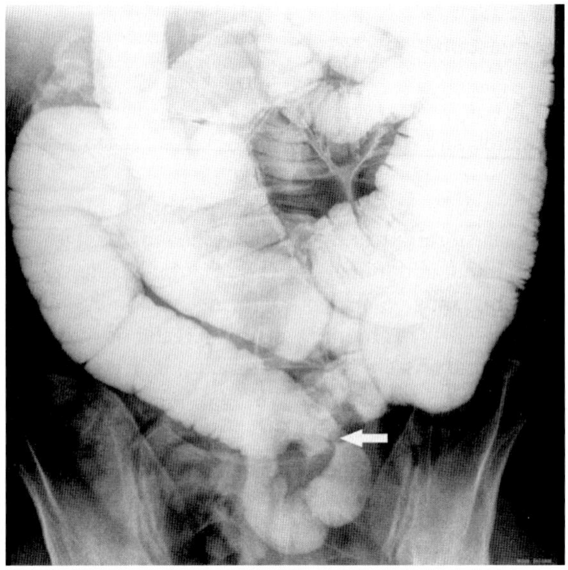

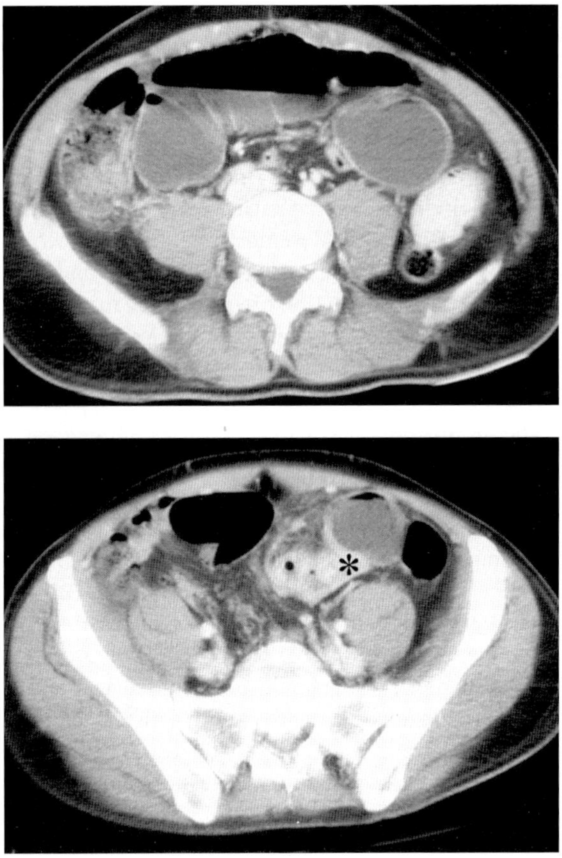

Fig. 8.36. This patient presented with intestinal obstruction 2 months after blunt abdominal trauma. No previous history of abdominal surgery. (**a**) CT showed intestinal obstruction, (**b**) a short segmental narrowing at the transition zone with the normal distal bowel (*asterisk*) without other abnormality. (**c**) Enteroclysis confirmed CT findings consistent with ischemic posttraumatic intestinal stenosis, confirmed at surgery

mucosal inflammation, and fibrosis, or full thickness ischemia with fibrosis of all layers. In either case, this scarring leads to stricture formation and obstruction that typically presents approximately one month following injury or later. Enhanced CT clearly demonstrates a stenotic ileal loop with mural thickening, which may be associated with mesenteric hematoma or isolated at time of diagnosis (Tsushima et al. 2001) (Fig. 8.36). Intramural hematoma, in particular in the duodenum, or occurring occasionally in the colon or other locations, may evolve into a chronic form and result in secondary, or sometimes late obstruction (Giubilei et al. 1983; Yin et al. 2000). An intramural duodenal hematoma can lead to biliary obstruction and pancreatitis, which proved fatal in some cases.

8.8 Conclusion

Bowel and mesenteric injuries from blunt trauma are difficult to diagnose clinically, as the physical and laboratory findings may be subtle and are often overshadowed by other injuries in patients with multisystem trauma. CT represent a proven modality in the evaluation of bowel and mesenteric injuries: careful inspection and technique are required to detect often subtle findings. In patients with surgically confirmed bowel and mesenteric injuries, the presence of mesenteric hematoma and peritoneal fluid were the more frequent CT signs. CT has also been found sensitive in separating surgical and nonsurgical trauma patients.

References

Absun HJ, Irani H, Roe EJ, Bloch JH (1990) Intra-abdominal seatbelt injury. J Trauma 30:189–93

Adkins RB Jr, Keyser JE 3rd (1985) Recent experiences with duodenal trauma. Am Surg 51:121–131

Aikawa H, Mori H, Miyake H, et al. (1994) Imaging and clinical significance of hepatic portal venous gas seen in adult patients. Nippon Shokakibyo Gakkai Zasshi 91:1320–1327

Albanese CT, Meza MP, Gardner MJ, Smith SD, Rowe MI, Lynch JM (1996) Is computed tomography a useful adjunct to the clinical examination for the diagnosis of pediatric gastrointestinal perforation from blunt abdominal trauma in children? J Trauma 40:417–421

Allen GS, Moore FA, Cox CS Jr, Mehall JR, Duke JH (1998) Delayed diagnosis of blunt duodenal injury: an avoidable complication. J Am Coll Surg 187:393–399
Anderson PA, Rivara FP, Maier RV, Drake C (1991) The epidemiology of seatbelt-associated injuries. J Trauma 31:60–67
Appleby JP, Nagy AG (1989) Abdominal injuries associated with the use of seatbelts. Am J Surg 157:457–458
Arajarvi E, Santavirta S, Tolonen J (1987) Abdominal injuries sustained in severe traffic accidents by seatbelt wearers. J Trauma 27:393–397
Asensio JA, Feliciano DV, Britt LD, et al. (1993) Management of duodenal injuries. Curr Probl Surg 30:1023
Ballard RB, Badellino MM, Eynon CA, Spott MA, Staz CF, Buckman RF Jr (1997) Blunt duodenal rupture: a 6-year statewide experience. J Trauma 43:229–232
Barandica R, Patel M (1997) Pediatric duodenal perforation missed on computed tomography. Ann Emerg Med 30: 545–547
Becker CD, Mentah G, Schmidlin F, Terrier F (1998) Blunt abdominal trauma in adults: role of CT in the diagnosis and management of visceral injuries. Part 2: Gastrointestinal tract and retroperitoneal organs. Eur Radiol 8:772–780
Bensard DD, Beaver BL, Besner GE, Cooney DR (1996) Small bowel injury in children after blunt abdominal trauma: is diagnostic delay important? J Trauma 41:476–483
Bernhardt J, Ptok H, Wilhelm L, Ludwig K (2002) Caustic acid burn of the upper gastrointestinal tract: first use of endosonography to evaluate the severity of the injury. Surg Endosc 16:1004–1006
Bladergroen MR, Lowe JE, Pohstlethwait RW (1986) Diagnosis and management of oesophageal perforation and rupture. Ann Thorac Surg 42:235–239
Bloom AI, Rivkind A, Zamir G, et al. (1996) Blunt injury of the small intestine and mesentery–the trauma surgeon's Achilles heel? Eur J Emerg Med 3:85–91
Bogan ML, Conces DJ JR (1989) CT evaluation of esophageal perforation following endoscopic sclerotherapy. Comput Med Imaging Graph 13:341–342
Boulanger BR, Mirvis SE, Rodriguez A (1992) Magnetic resonance imaging in traumatic diaphragmatic rupture: case reports. J Trauma 32:89–93
Boulos I, Chaoui M, Borocco A, Gruner M, Ducou Le Pointe H (1997) Post-traumatic hematoma of the duodenum. A case in a young child. J Radiol 78:61–64
Brasel KJ, Olson CJ, Stafford RE, Johnson TJ (1998) Incidence and significance of free fluid on abdominal computed tomographic scan in blunt trauma. J Trauma 44:889–892
Breen DJ, Janzen DL, Zwirewich CV, Nagy AG, et al. (1997) Blunt bowel and mesenteric injury: diagnostic performance of CT signs. J Comput Assist Tomogr 21:706–712
Brody JM, Leighton DB, Murphy BL, et al. (2000) CT of blunt trauma bowel and mesenteric injury: typical findings and pitfalls in diagnosis. Radiographics. 20:1525–1537
Brown RA, Bass DH, Rode H, Millar AJ, Cywes S (1992) Gastrointestinal tract perforation in children due to blunt abdominal trauma. Br J Surg 79:522–524
Browstein RM, Bunting T, Meyer AA, Fakhry SM (2000) Diagnosis and management of blunt small bowel injury: a survey of the membership of the American Association for the Surgery of Trauma. J Trauma 48:402–407
Buckman RF Jr, Piano G, Dunham CM, et al. (1988) Major bowel and diaphragmatic injuries associated with blunt spleen or liver rupture. J Trauma 28:1317–1321
Bulas DI, Taylor GA, Eichelberger MR (1989) The value of CT in detecting bowel perforation in children after blunt abdominal trauma. AJR 153:561–564
Carillo EH, Richardson D, Miller FB (1996) Evolution in the management of duodenal injuries. J Trauma 40:1037–1045
Catalano O (1996) Computed tomography in the study of gastrointestinal perforation. Radiol Med 91:247–252
Cerise EJ, Scully JH Jr (1970) Blunt trauma to the small intestine. J Trauma 10:46–50
Chan SC, Chen HY, Ng SH, Lee CM, Tsai CH (1999) Hepatic abscess due to gastric perforation by ingested fish bone demonstrated by computed tomography. J Formos Med Assoc 98:145–147
Chao HC, Kong MS (1999) Sonographic diagnosis of mesenteric hematoma. J Clin Ultrasound 27:284–286
Cheung YC, Ng SH, Tan CF, Ng KK, Wan YL (2000) Hepatic inflammatory mass secondary to toothpick perforation of the stomach: triphasic CT appearances. Clin Imaging 24:93–95
Chevallier P, Peten E, Souci J, Chau Y, Padovani B, Bruneton JN (2002) Detection of portal venous gas on sonography, but not on CT. Eur Radiol 12:1175–1178
Chiang WK (1993) Isolated jejunal perforation from nonpenetrating abdominal trauma. Am J Emerg Med 11: 473–475
Chihombori A, Hoover EL, Phillips T, Sclafani S, Scalea T, Jaffe BM (1991) Role of diagnostic techniques in the initial evaluation of stab wounds to the anterior abdomen, back, and flank. J Natl Med Assoc 83:137–140
Cocke WM, Meyer KK (1964) Retroperitoneal duodenal rupture: proposed mechanism–review of the literature and report of a case. Am J Surg 108:834
Cogbill TH, Moore EE, Feliciano DV, et al. (1990) Conservative management of duodenal trauma: a multicenter perspective. J Trauma 30:1469–1475
Coleman EJ, Dietz PA (1990) Small bowel injuries following blunt abdominal trauma. Early recognition and management. N Y State J Med 90:446–449
Contostavlos DL, Sohn M, Callery RT, Tobin JG (1996) Traumatic seromuscular rupture of intestine: the acute and chronic forms. J Trauma 41:525–529
Cook DE, Walsh JW, Vick CW, Brewer WH (1986) Upper abdominal trauma: pitfalls in CT diagnosis. Radiology 159:65–69
Cotton PB, Leman G, Vennes J, et al. (1991) Endoscopic sphincterotomy complications and their management. Gastrointest Endosc 37:383–393
Coulier B (1997) Diagnostic ultrasonography of perforating foreign bodies of the digestive tract. J Belge Radiol 80:1–5
Cox EF (1984) Blunt abdominal trauma. A 5-year analysis of 870 patients requiring celiotomy. Ann Surg 199:467–474
Cranston PE, Bergeron PM, Carlton FB Jr (1993) Evaluation of alimentary tract foreign body: clinical and imaging review of 100 consecutive cases. South Med J 86:1119–1125
Croce MA, Fabian TC, Patton JH Jr, et al. (1998) Impact of stomach and colon injuries on intra-abdominal abscess and the synergistic effect of hemorrhage and associated injury. J Trauma 45:649–655
Cunningham MA, Tyroch AH, Kaups KL, Davis JW (1998) Does free fluid on abdominal computed tomographic scan after blunt trauma require laparotomy? J Trauma 44:599–602; discussion 603
Daum-Kowalski R, Shanley DJ, Murphy T (1991) MRI diagnosis of delayed presentation of traumatic diaphragmatic hernia. Gastrointest Radiol 16:298–300

Dauterive AH, Flancbaum L, Cox EF (1985) Blunt intestinal trauma. A modern-day review. Ann Surg 201:198–203
Davis JJ, Cohn I Jr, Nance FC (1976) Diagnosis and management of blunt abdominal trauma. Ann Surg 183:672–678
De Backer AI, De Schepper AM, Vaneerdeweg W, Pelckmans P (1999) Intestinal stenosis from mesenteric injury after blunt abdominal trauma. Eur Radiol 9:1429–1431
De Vries RA, Kremer-Schneider MM, Otten MH (1991) Intramural hematoma of the esophagus caused by minor head injury 6 h previously. Gastrointest Radiol 16:283–285
Desai SB, Modhe JM, Aulack BG, Ravi R, Sukthankar RU, Pardiwalla BB (1987) Percutaneous transcatheter steel-coil embolization of a large proximal prosttraumatic superior mesenteric arteriovenous fistula. J Trauma 27: 1091–1094
Diallo G, Fournier L, Gignoux M (1994) Value of CT scan in the diagnosis of small pneumoperitoneum. Ann Chir 48: 470–472
Diner WC (1988) Duodenal perforation during intubation for small bowel enema study. Radiology 168:39–41
Donohue JH, Federle MP, Griffiths BG, Trunkey DD (1987) Computed tomography in the diagnosis of blunt intestinal and mesenteric injuries. J Trauma. 27:11–17
Dowe MF, Shanmuganathan K, Mirvis SE, et al. (1997) CT findings of mesenteric injury after blunt trauma: implications for surgical intervention. AJR 168:425–428
Dupont Le Priol PR, Leroux SB, Aquilina CF, Boyer LB, Lointier PH, Michel JL (1992) Rupture of the distal thoracic esophagus by closed trauma. Gastroenterol Clin Biol 16: 362–364
Eldridge TJ, McFall TM, Peoples JB (1993) Traumatic incarceration of the small bowel: case report. J Trauma 35: 960–961
Fabian TC, Mangiante EC, White TJ, Patterson CR, Boldreghini S, Britt LG (1986) A prospective study of 91 patients undergoing both computed tomography and peritoneal lavage following blunt abdominal trauma. J Trauma 26: 602–608
Fang JF, Chen RJ, Lin BC (1999) Surgical treatment and outcome after delayed diagnosis of blunt duodenal injury. Eur J Surg 165:133–139
Fasolini F, Lichtenhahn P, Aeberhard P (1994) Intramural duodenal hematoma after blunt abdominal injury in childhood. Case report. Helv Chir Acta 60:823–826
Federle MP, Crass RA, Jeffrey RB, Trunkey DD (1982) Computed tomography in blunt abdominal trauma. Arch Surg 117:645–650
Federle MP, Peitzman A, Krugh J (1995) Use of oral contrast material in abdominal trauma CT scans: is it dangerous? J Trauma 38:51–53
Federle MP, Yagan N, Peitzman AB, Krugh J (1997) Abdominal trauma: use of oral contrast material for CT is safe. Radiology 205:91–93
Feliciano DV, Martin TD, Cruse PA, et al. (1987) Management of combined pancreatoduodenal injuries. Ann Surg 205: 673–680
Feliciano DV (1989) Abdominal trauma. In: Schwartz SI, Ellis H (eds) Maingot's abdominal operations. Appleton & Lange, East Norwalk, CT, pp 457–512
Feliciano DV (1991a) Diagnostic modalities in abdominal trauma. Peritoneal lavage, ultrasonography, computed tomography scanning, and arteriography. Surg Clin North Am 71:241–256
Feliciano DV (1991b) Immediate and follow-up management of hepatic trauma. Compr Ther 17:51–56
Felson B, Levin EJ (1955) Intramural hematoma of duodenum: diagnostic Roentgen sign. Radiology 63:823–831
Fernandez ET, Hollabauch R, Hixon SD, Whitington G (1988) Late presentation of gastrocolic fistula after percutaneous gastrostomy. Gastrointest Endosc 34:368–371
Fischer RP, Beverlin BC, Engran LH, Benjamin CI, Perry JF (1978) DPL: 14 years and 2586 patients later. Am J Surg 136:701–704
Fischer RP, Miller-Crotchett P, Reed Rl 2nd (1988) Gastrointestinal disruption: the hazard of nonoperative management in adults with blunt abdominal injury. J Trauma 28:1445–1449
Flint LM, McCoy M, Richardson JD, et al. (1980) Duodenal injury: Analysis of common misconceptions in diagnosis and treatment. Ann Surg 191:697
Foley CL, Teele RL (1979) Ultrasound of epigastric injuries after blunt trauma. AJR 132:593–598
Foley MJ, Ghahremani GG, Rogers LF (1982) Reappraisal of contrast media used to detect upper gastrointestinal perforations. Comparison of ionic water-soluble media with barium sulfate. Radiology 144:231–237
Fon GT, Hunter TB, Haber K (1980) Utility of ultrasound for diagnosis of mesenteric hematoma. AJR 134:381–384
Freeark RJ (1969) Role of angiography in the management of multiple injuries. Surg Gynecol Obstet 128:761–771
Freeark RJ, Love L, Baker RJ (1968a) The role of aortography in the management of blunt abdominal trauma. J Trauma 8:557–471
Freeark RJ, Shoemaker WC, Baker RJ (1968b) Aortography in blunt abdominal trauma. Arch Surg 96:705–711
Freeman MP, Tisnado J, Cho SR (1985) Transcatheter embolization of the dorsal pancreatic artery to control massive postoperative bleeding. Am J Gastroenterol 80: 185–187
Frick EJ Jr, Pasquale MD, Cipolle MD (1999) Small-bowel and mesentery injuries in blunt trauma. J Trauma 46:920–926
Friedman D, Flancbaum L, Ritter E, Trooskin SZ (1991) Hepatic portal venous gas identified by computed tomography in a patient with blunt abdominal trauma: a case report. J Trauma 31:290–292
Furst G (2001) Radiological acute diagnosis in suspected perforation of the large intestine. Kongressbd Dtsch Ges Chir Kongr 118:307–310
Garfinkle SE, Matolo NM (1976) Gastric necrosis from blunt abdominal trauma. J Trauma 16:405–407
Ghahremani GG (1993) Radiologic evaluation of suspected gastrointestinal perforations. Radiol Clin N Am 31:1219–1234
Gilliland MG, Ward RE, Flynn TC, Miller PW, Ben-Menachem Y, Duke JH Jr (1982) Peritoneal lavage and angiography in the management of patients with pelvic fractures. Am J Surg 144:744–747
Giubilei D, Cicia S, Mascioli G, Nardis P (1983) Duodenal stenosis from retroperitoneal fibrosis secondary to traumatic retroperitoneal hematoma: a case report. Ital J Surg Sci 13:293–298
Glazer GM, Buy JN, Moss AA, et al. (1981) CT detection of duodenal perforation. AJR 137:333–337
Goff JS, Thompson JS, Pratt CF, Tomasso GI, Penn I (1982) Jejunal rupture caused by a Sengstaken-Blakemore tube. Gastroenterology 82:573–575

Gonzalez JG, Gonzalez RR, Patino JV, Garcia AT, Alvarez CP, Pedrosa CS (1988) CT findings in gastrointestinal perforation by ingested fish bones. J Comput Assist Tomogr 12:88–90
Gonzalez R, Heiss WH, Rauh W (1987) Blunt abdominal trauma caused by child abuse. Monatsschr Kinderheilkd 135:692–695
Gould RJ, Thorwarth WT (1963) Retroperitoneal rupture of duodenum due to blunt, nonpenetrating abdominal trauma. Radiology 80:743–747
Grass RA, Tranbaugh RF, Kudsk KA, et al. (1981) Colorectal foreign bodies and perforation. Am J Surg 142:85–88
Grassi R, Pinto A, Rossi G, Rotondo A (1998) Conventional plain-film radiology, ultrasonography and CT in jejuno-ileal perforation. Acta Radiol 39:52–56
Grieshop NA, Jacobson LE, Gomez GA, Thompson CT, Solotkin KC (1995) Selective use of computed tomography and diagnostic peritoneal lavage in blunt abdominal trauma. J Trauma 38:727–731
Griswold RA, Collier HS (1961) Collective review: blunt abdominal trauma. Surg Gynecol Obstet 112:309–329
Grosfeld JL, Cooney DR (1975) Pancreatic and gastrointestinal trauma in children. Pediatr Clin North Am 22:365–377
Grosfeld JL, Rescorla FJ, West KW, Vane DW (1989) Gastrointestinal injuries in childhood: analysis of 53 patients. J Pediatr Surg 24:580–583
Guzman C, Bousvaros A, Buonomo C, Nurko S (1998) Intraduodenal hematoma complicating intestinal biopsy: case reports and review of the literature. Am J Gastroenterol 93:2547–2550
Hagiwara A, Yukioka T, Satou M, et al. (1995) Early diagnosis of small intestine rupture from blunt abdominal trauma using computed tomography: significance of the streaky density within the mesentery. J Trauma 38:630–633
Hamilton P, Rizoli S, Mclellan B, Murphy J (1995) Significance of intra-abdominal extraluminal air detected by CT scan in blunt abdominal trauma. J Trauma 39:331–333
Han SY, Mcelvein RB, Aldrete JS, Tishler JM (1985) Perforation of the esophagus: correlation of site and cause with plain film findings. AJR 145:537–540
Hara H, Babyn PS, Bourgeois D (1992) Significance of bowel wall enhancement on CT following blunt abdominal trauma in childhood. J Comput Assist Tomogr 16:94–98
Hassantash SA, Mock C, Maier RV (1995) Traumatic visceral artery aneurysm: presentation as massive hemorrhage from perforation into an adjacent hollow viscus. J Trauma 38:357–360
Hayes CW, Conway WF, Walsh JW, Coppage L, Gervin AS (1991) Seat belt injuries: radiologic findings and clinical correlation. Radiographics 11:23–36
Hernandez EJ, Ellington RT, Harford WV (1999) Isolated transverse mesocolon laceration during routine colonoscopy. J Clin Gastroenterol 28:46–48
Hirota C, Iida M, Aoyagi K, et al. (1995) Posttraumatic intestinal stenosis: clinical and radiographic features in four patients. Radiology 194:813–815
Hofer GA, Cohen AJ (1989) CT signs of duodenal perforation secondary to blunt abdominal trauma. J Comput Assist Tomogr 13:430–432
Howell HW, Bartizal JF, Freeark RJ (1976) Blunt trauma involving the colon and rectum. J Trauma 16:624–627
Hughes JJ, Brogdon BG (1986) Computed tomography of duodenal hematoma. J Comput Tomogr 10:231–236
Hugues TM (1999) The diagnosis of gastrointestinal tract injuries resulting from blunt trauma. Aust N Z J Surg 69: 770–777
Hugues TM, Leton C, Hitos K, Perez JV, McDougall PA (2002) Intra-abdominal gastrointestinal tract injuries following blunt trauma: the experience of an Australian trauma center. Injury 33:617–626
Hulka F, Mullins RJ, Leonardo V, Harrison MW, Silberberg P (1998) Significance of peritoneal fluid as an isolated finding on abdominal computed tomographic scans in pediatric trauma patients. J Trauma 44:1069–1072
Hulyalkar AR, Ayd JD (1993) Low risk of gastroesophageal injury associated with transesophageal echocardiography during cardiac surgery. J Cardiothorac Vasc Anesth 7:175–177
Hunt KE, Garrison RN, Fry DE (1980) Perforating injuries of the gastrointestinal tract following blunt abdominal trauma. Am Surg 46:100–104
Jacobson G, Carter R (1951) Small instestinal rupture due to nonpenetrating abdominal injury: roentgenological study. AJR 66:52–64
Jaffin JH, Ochsner MG, Cole FJ, Rozycki GS, Kass M, Champion HR (1993) Alkaline phosphatase levels in diagnostic peritoneal lavage fluid as a predictor of hollow visceral injury. J Trauma 34:829–833
Jamieson DH, Babyn PS, Pearl R (1996) Imaging gastrointestinal perforation in pediatric blunt abdominal trauma. Pediatr Radiol 26:188–194
Jarayaman MV, Mayo-Smith WW, Movson JS, Dupuy DE, Wallach MT (2001) CT of the duodenum: an overlooked segment gets its due. Radiographics 21:S147–S160
Jeffrey RB, Federle MP, Stein SM, Crass RA (1982) CT demonstration of intramural hematoma of the cecum following blunt trauma. J Comput Assist Tomogr 6:404–405
Jewett TC, Caldarola V, Karp MP, et al. (1988) Intramural hematoma of the duodenum. Arch Surg 123:54–57
Jones RC, Thal ER, Johnson NA, Gollihar LN (1985) Evaluation of antibiotic therapy following penetrating abdominal trauma. Ann Surg 201:576–585
Junghanns K (1978) Seat belt related abdominal injuries. Langenbecks Arch Chir 347:373–776
Kallmeyer I, Morse DS, Body SC, Collard CD (2000) Case 2-2000. Transesophageal echocardiography-associated gastrointestinal trauma. J Cardiothorac Vasc Anesth 14: 212–216
Kane NM, Francis IR, Burney RE, Wheatley MJ, Ellis JH, Korobkin M (1991) Traumatic pneumoperitoneum. Implications of computed tomography diagnosis. Invest Radiol 26:574–578
Karnaze GC, Sheedy PF, Stephens DH, McLeod RA (1981) Computed tomography in duodenal rupture due to blunt abdominal trauma. J Comput Assist Tomogr 5:267–269
Kearney PA (1989) Blunt trauma to the abdomen. Ann Emerg Med 18:1322–1325
Kearney PA Jr, Vahey T, Burney RE, Glazer G (1989) Computed tomography and diagnostic peritoneal lavage in blunt abdominal trauma. Their combined role. Arch Surg 124: 344–347
Kelly G, Norton L, Moore G, Eiseman B (1978) The continuing challenge of duodenal injuries. J Trauma 18:160–165
Kelly J, Raptopoulos V, Davidoff A, Waite R, Norton P (1989) The value of noncontrast-enhanced CT in blunt abdominal trauma. AJR 152:41–48
Kemmeter PR, Senagore AJ, Smith D, Oostendorp L (1998) Dilemmas in the diagnosis of blunt enteric trauma. Am Surg 64:750–754

Kerschner JE, Beste DJ, Conley SF, Kenna MA, Lee D (2001) Mediastinitis associated with foreign body erosion of the esophagus in children. Int J Pediatr Otorhinolaryngol 59:89–97

Kihara S, Mizutani T, Shimizu T, Toyooka H (1999) Bleeding from a tear in the gastric mucosa caused by transoesophageal echocardiography during cardiac surgery: effective haemostasis by endoscopic argon plasma coagulation. Br J Anaesth 82:948–950

Kilgus M, Platz A, Trentz O (1999) Duodenal injuries in abdominal trauma Swiss Surg 5:251–255

Kim-Deobald J, Kozarek RA (1992) Esophageal perforation: an 8-year review of a multispecialty clinic's experience. Am J Gastroenterol 87:1112–1119

Kinoshita Y, Udagawa H, Kajiyama Y, et al. (1999) Cologastric fistula and colonic perforation of percutaneous endoscopic gastrostomy. Surg Laparosc Endosc Percut Tech 9:220–223

Kirks DR (1983) Radiological evaluation of visceral injuries in the battered child syndrome. Pediatr Ann 12:888–893

Kloppel R, Brock D, Kosling S, Bennek J; Hormann D (1997) Spinal computerized tomography diagnosis of abdominal seat belt injuries in children. Aktuelle Radiol 7:19–22

Knudson MM, Mc Aninch JW, Gomez R, Lee P, Stubbs HA (1992) Hematuria as a predictor of abdominal injury after blunt trauma. Am J Surg 164:482–486

Kortbeek JB, Brown M, Steed B (1997) Percutaneous drainage of a duodenal haematoma. Injury 28:419–420

Kos X, Trotteur G, Dondelinger RF (1998) Delayed esophageal hemorrhage caused by a metal stent: treatment with embolization. Cardiovasc Intervent Radiol 21:428–430

Kuhlman JE, Fishman EK, Milligan FD, Siegelman SS (1989) Complications of endoscopic retrograde sphincterotomy: computed tomographic evaluation. Gastrointest Radiol 14: 127–132

Kunin JR, Korobkin M, Ellis JH, Francis IR, Kane NM, Siegel SE (1993) Duodenal injuries caused by blunt abdominal trauma: value of CT in differentiating perforation from hematoma. AJR Am J Roentgenol 160:1221–1223

Kunin N, Letoquart JP, La Gamma A, Chaperon J, Mambrini A (1994) Intestinal-mesenteric lesions of closed abdominal traumas. J Chir (Paris) 131:129–134

Kwauk S, Wallace K, Hyde P (1995) Gastrointestinal perforation or vascular injury? A diagnostic dilemma for computed tomography in blunt abdominal trauma. Can Assoc Radiol J 46:57–59

Lam PY, Marks MK, Fink AM, Oliver MR, Woodward A (2001) Delayed presentation of an ingested foreign body causing gastric perforation. J Paediatr Health 37:303–304

Latham P, Hodgins LR (1995) A gastric laceration after transesophageal echocardiography in a patient undergoing aortic valve replacement. Anesth Analg 81:641–642

Lautin JL, Wahl SI, Cynamon J (1999) Emergency management of gastrointestinal hemorrhage. Emerg Radiol 6:227–231

Leddy JE, Frew EM (1977) Complete transection of the body of the stomach resulting from blunt trauma. Can J Surg 20: 264–266

Legier JF (1992) Traumatic seromuscular rupture of intestine. Am J Forensic Med Pathol 13:253–254

Levey JM (2002) Intestinal perforation in a parastomal hernia by a migrated plastic biliary stent. Surg Endosc 16: 1636–1637

Levine CD, Gonzalez RN, Wachsberg RH (1997) CT findings in bowel and mesenteric injury. J Comput Assist Tomogr 21:974–979

Levine CD, Patel UJ, Wachsberg RH, Simmons MZ, Baker SR, Cho KC (1995) CT in patients with blunt abdominal trauma: clinical significance of intraperitoneal fluid detected on a scan with otherwise normal findings. AJR 164:1381–1385

Levison MA, Petersen SR, Sheldon GF, Trunkey DD (1984) Duodenal trauma: experience of a trauma center. J Trauma 24:475–480

Lina JR, Jaques P, Mandell V (1979) Aneurysm rupture secondary to transcatheter embolization. AJR 132:553–556

Lotti R, Gaetano Perri S, Gola P, Leardi S, Cianca G, Citone G (2000) An intramural hematoma of the duodenum. Ann Ital Chir 71:519–523

Love L (1975) Radiology of abdominal trauma. JAMA 231: 1377–1380

Lucas CE, Ledgerwood AM (1975) Factors influencing outcome after blunt duodenal injury. J Trauma 15:839–846

Maatman TJ, Bigham D, Stirling B (2002) Simplified management of post-prostate biopsy rectal bleeding. Urology 60:508

Maccabee DL, Dominitz JA, Lee SW, Billingsley KG (2000) Acute presentation of transverse colon injury following percutaneous endoscopic gastrostomy tube placement: case report and review of current management. Surg Endosc 14:296

Mackersie RC, Tiwary AD, Shackford SR, Hoyt DB (1989) Intra-abdominal injury following blunt trauma. Identifying the high-risk patient using objective risk factors. Arch Surg 124:809–813

Maemura T, Yamaguchi Y, Yukiolka T, Matsuda H, Shimazaki S (1999) Laparoscopic drainage of an intramural duodenal hematoma. J Gastroenterol 34:119–122

Margolis IB, Carnazzo AJ, Finn MP (1976) Intramural hematoma of the duodenum. Am J Surg 132:779–783

Marra JM, Sclafani SJA (1999) Embolotherapy for expanding duodenal hematoma. Emerg Radiol 6:193–196

Marx JA, Moore EE, Jorden RC, Eule J Jr (1985) Limitations of computed tomography in the evaluation of acute abdominal trauma: a prospective comparison with diagnostic peritoneal lavage. J Trauma 25:933–937

Matolo NM, Cohen SE, Fontanetta AP, Wolfman EF (1975) Traumatic duodenal injuries: an analysis of 32 cases. Am Surg 41:331–336

Maul KI, Fallahzadeh H, Mays ET (1978) Selective management of posttraumatic obstructing intramural hematoma of the duodenum. Surg Gynecol Obstet 146:221–224

McCort JJ (1964) Radiographic examination in blunt abdominal trauma. Radiol Clin North Am 2:121–143

McKenney MG, Nir I, Levi DM, Martin L (1996) Evaluation of minor penetrating duodenal injuries. Am Surg 62:952–955

McKenzie AD, Bell GA (1972) Nonpenetrating injuries of the colon and rectum. Surg Clin North Am 52:735–741

McLaughlan J (1839) Fatal false aneurismal tumours occupying nearly the whole of the duodenum. Lancet 2:203–205

Meredith JW, Ditesheim JA, Stonehouse S, Wolfman N (1992) Computed tomography and diagnostic peritoneal lavage. Complementary roles in blunt trauma. Am Surg 58:44–48

Metzger J, Von Flue M, Babst R, Harder F (1995) Small bowel injuries in blunt abdominal trauma–a diagnostic problem! Swiss Surg 5:222–225

Meyer DM, Thal ER, Weigelt JA, Redman HC (1989) The role of abdominal CT in the evaluation of stab wounds to the back. J Trauma 29:1226–1228

Meyers MA, Ghahremani GG (1975) Complications of fiberoptic Endoscopy. II. Colonoscopy. Radiology 115: 301–307

Millar AJ, Numanoglu A, Mann M, Marven S, Rode H (2001) Detection of caustic oesophageal injury with technetium 99m-labelled sucralfate. J Pediatr Surg 36:262–265
Mirvis SE, Gens DR, Shanmuganathan K (1992) Rupture of the bowel after blunt abdominal trauma: diagnosis with CT. AJR 159:1217–1221
Mirvis SE, Keramati B, Buckman R, Rodriguez A (1988) MR imaging of traumatic diaphragmatic rupture. J Comput Assist Tomogr 12:147–149
Mirvis SE, Shanmuganathan K, Erb P (1994) Diffuse small-bowel ischemia in hypotensive adults after blunt trauma (shock bowel): CT findings and clinical significance. AJR 163:1375–1379
Mitani M, Hirata K, Fukuda M, Kanedo M (1996) Endoscopic ultrasonography in corrosive injury of the upper gastrointestinal tract by hydrochloric acid. J Clin Ultrasound 24: 40–42
Miyakawa K, Kaji T, Ashida H, et al. (1992a) Evaluation of non-contrast-enhanced CT in blunt abdominal trauma. Nippon Igaku Hoshasen Gakkai Zasshi 52:300–307
Miyakawa K, Kaji T, Wakabayashi M, et al. (1992b) CT of intestinal injuries following blunt trauma. Nippon Igaku Hoshasen Gakkai Zasshi 52:1653–1660
Morton JR, Jordan GL (1968) Traumatic duodenal injuries. Review of 131 cases. J Trauma 8:127–137
Motateanu M, Mirescu D, Schwieger AF, Laverriere C (1992) Computed tomography of retroperitoneal duodenal rupture in blunt abdominal trauma. Eur J Radiol 15:163–165
Mucciolo RL, Godec CJ (1988) Traumatic acute incarcerated scrotal hernia. J Trauma 28:715–716
Muscari F, Suc B, Lagarrigue J (1999) Hepatic portal venous gas: is it always a sign of severity and surgical emergency. J Chirurgie 124:69–72
Nagel M, Saeger HD, Massoun H, Buschulte J (1991) Injuries of the small and large intestine in the traumatized abdomen. Unfallchirurg 94:105–109
Nance ML, Keller MS, Stafford PW (2000) Predicting hollow visceral injury in the pediatric blunt trauma patient with solid visceral injury. J Pediatr Surg 35:1300–1303
Nance ML, Peden GW, Shapiro MB, Kauder DR, Rotondo MF, Schwab CW (1997) Solid viscus injury predicts major hollow viscus injury in blunt abdominal trauma. J Trauma 4:618–623
Nelson JF (1966) The roentgenologic evaluation of abdominal trauma. Radiol Clin North Am 4:415–437
Nelson RL, Abcarian H, Prasad ML (1982) Iatrogenic perforation of the colon and rectum. Dis Colon Rectum 25: 305–308
Newman KD, Bowman LM, Eichelberger MR, et al. (1990) The lap belt complex: Intestinal and lumbar spine injury in children. J Trauma 30:1133–1139
Nghiem HV, Jeffrey RB Jr, Mindelzun RE (1993) CT of blunt trauma to the bowel and mesentery. AJR 160:53–58
Nghiem HV, Jeffrey RB Jr, Mindelzun RE (1995) CT of blunt trauma to the bowel and mesentery. Seminars US, CT, MRI 16:82–90
Novikov AS, Urakcheev SHK, Bogdanov SV (1998) Injuries of the duodenum. Vestn Khir Im I I Grek 157:49–53
O'Malley BP, Salem S (1979) Abdominal hematomas in unusual locations–contribution of ultrasound. J Can Assoc Radiol 30:182–183
Osborn DJ, Glickman MG, Graja V, Ramsby G (1973) The role of angiography in abdominal nonrenal trauma. Radiol Clin North Am 11:579–592
Ott DJ, Gelfand DW, Chen YM, Munitz HA (1985) Colonoscopy and the barium enema: a radiologic viewpoint. South Med J 78:1033–1035
Pal JD, Victorino GP (2002) Defining the role of computed tomography in blunt abdominal trauma: use in the hemodynamically stable patient with a depressed level of consciousness. Arch Surg 137:1029–1033
Peitzman AB, Makoroin MS, Slasky BS, et al. (1986) Prospective study of CT in initial management of blunt abdominal trauma. J Trauma 26:585–591
Perniceni T, Gayet B (1995) Les traumatisms de l'oesophage. In: Les monographies de l'association française de chirurgie. Rapport présenté au 97è congrès français de chirurgie. Arnette, Paris; pp 67–78
Petit P, Bret PM, Lough JO, Reinhold C (1992) Risks associated with intestinal perforation during experimental percutaneous drainage. Invest Radiol 27:1012–1019
Pinto A, Magliocca M, Grassi R, Scaglione M, Romano L, Angelelli G (2001) Role of computerized tomography in the diagnosis of peritoneo-intestinal lesions resulting from closed trauma. Experience at 2 emergency departments. Radiol Med (Torino) 101:177–182
Plancq MC, Villamizar J, Ricard J, Canarelli JP (2000) Management of pancreatic and duodenal injuries in pediatric patients. Pediatr Surg Int 16:35–39
Pokorny WJ, Brandt ML, Harberg FJ (1986) Major duodenal injuries in children: diagnosis, operative management, and outcome. J Pediatr Surg 21:613–616
Polhamus CD, Werth TE, Clement DJ, Keogh M, Lewis P (1993) Gastrointestinal bleeding complicating transesophageal echocardiography. Endoscopy 25:198–199
Porcu A, Dessanti A, Feo CF, Dettori G (1999) Asymptomatic gastric perforation by a toothpick. A case report. Dig Surg 16:437–438
Rabinovici R, Ovadia P, Mathiak G, Abdullah F (1999). Abdominal injuries associated with lumbar spine fractures in blunt trauma. Injury 30:471–474
Ramos CT, Koplewitz BZ, Babyn PS, Manson PS, Ein SH (2000) What have we learned about traumatic diaphragmatic hernias in children? J Pediatr Surg 35:601–604
Reichert V, Monig SP, Walter M, Dollken W (1995) Traumatic aneurysm of the superior mesenteric artery as the cause of massive upper gastrointestinal hemorrhage. Leber Magen Darm 25:221–222
Richards JR, McGahan JP, Simpson JL, Tabar P (1999) Bowel and mesenteric injury: evaluation with emergency abdominal US. Radiology 211:399–403
Rioux M, Langis P (1994) Sonographic detection of clinically unsuspected swallowed toothpicks and their gastrointestinal complications. J Clin Ultrasound 22:483–490
Rizzo MJ, Federle MP, Griffiths BG (1989) Bowel and mesenteric injury following blunt abdominal trauma: evaluation with CT. Radiology 173:143–148
Robbs JV, Moore SW, Pillay SP (1980) Blunt abdominal trauma with jejunal injury: a review. J Trauma 20:308–311
Roberts JL (1996) CT of abdominal and pelvic trauma. Semin Ultrasound, CT, MR 17:142–169
Root HD, Hauser CW, Mc Kinley CR (1965) Diagnostic peritoneal lavage. Surg 57: 633
Rosenthal D, Ellison RG Jr, Luke JP, Clark MD, Lamis PA (1987) Traumatic superior mesenteric arteriovenous fistula: report of a case and review of literature. J Vasc Surg 5:486–491

Rouse T, Collin J, Daar A (1984) Isolated injury to the intestine from blunt abdominal injury. Injury 16:131–133
Rutledge R, Thomason M, Oller D, et al. (1991) The spectrum of abdominal injuries associated with the use of seat belts. J Trauma 31:820–825
Salzano A, De Rosa A, Rossi E, et al. (2000) The radiological diagnostic and clinical approach to the patient with stab and cut wounds of the chest. The authors' personal experience. Radiol Med 100:24–28
Scalea T, Godstein A, Phillips T, et al. (1986) An analysis of 161 falls from a height: the „jumper syndrome." J Trauma 26: 706–712
Schmidt U, Maull KI, Gould H, Frame S (1994). Value of computerized tomography in diagnosis of small intestine injuries after blunt abdominal trauma Unfallchirurg 97:54–56
Schneider PA, Hauser H (1982) Diagnosis of alimentary tract perforation by CT. Eur J Radiol 2:197–201
Schumpelick V, Amabcher T, Riesener KP (1999) Current therapy of injuries of the colon and retroperitoneum. Chirurg 70:1269–1277
Schwartz JM, Holliday RA, Breda SD (1988) CT diagnosis of pyriform sinus perforation. J Comput Assist Tomogr 12: 869–870
Shah P, Applegate KE, Buonomo C (1997) Stricture of the duodenum and jejunum in an abused child. Pediatr Radiol 27:281–283
Shalaby-Rana E, Eicherlberger M, Kerzner B, et al. (1992) Intestinal stricture due to lap-belt injury. AJR 158:63–64
Shanmuganathan K, Mirvis SE, Reaney SM (1995) Pictural review: CT appearance of contrast medium extravasations associated with injury sustained from blunt abdominal trauma. Clin Radiol 50:182–187
Sherck J, Shatney C, Sensaki K, Selivanov V (1994) The accuracy of computed tomography in the diagnosis of blunt small-bowel perforation. Am J Surg 168:670–675
Sherck JP, Oakes DD (1990) Intestinal injuries missed by computed tomography. J Trauma 30:1–5
Shih HC, Liu M, Wu JK, et al. (1995) Blunt gastrointestinal injury in trauma patients. Am J Emerg Med 13:82–84
Shilyansky J, Pearl RH, Kreller M, Sena LM, Babyn PS (1997) Diagnosis and management of duodenal injuries in children. J Pediatr Surg 32:880–886
Shorr RM, Greaney GC, Donovan AJ (1987) Injuries of the duodenum. Am J Surg 154:93–98
Shuck JM, Lowe RJ (1978) Intestinal disruption due to blunt abdominal trauma. Am J Surg 136:668–673
Shuman WP (1997) CT of blunt abdominal trauma in adults. Radiology 205:297–306
Siegle RL, Rabinowitz JG, Sarasohn C (1976) Intestinal perforations secondary to nasojejunal feeding tubes. AJR 126:1229–1232
Sitoh YY, Sitoh MP (1998) Spiral computed tomography demonstration of active haemorrhage in blunt abdominal trauma. Singapore Med J 39:32–33
Sivit CJ, Taylor GA, Newman KD, et al. (1991) Safety-belt injuries in children with lap-belt ecchymosis: CT findings in 61 patients. AJR 157:111–114
Sivit CT, Taylor GA, Bulas DI, Kushner DC, Potter BM, Eichelberger MR (1992) Posttraumatic shock in children: CT findings associated with hemodynamic instability. Radiology 182:723–726
Sivit CJ, Eichelberger MR, Taylor GA (1994) CT in children with rupture of the bowel following blunt trauma: Diagnostic efficacy and comparison with hypoperfusion complex. AJR 163:1195–1198
Sivit CJ (1997) Gastrointestinal emergencies in older infants and children. Radiol Clin North Am 35:865–877
Snyder WH III, Weigelt JA, Watkins WL, et al. (1980) The surgical management of duodenal trauma. Arch Surg 115:422
Sperling L, Rigler LG (1937) Traumatic retroperitoneal rupture of duodenum. Radiology 29:521–524
St Pierre J, Fortier LP, Couture P, Hebert Y (1998) Massive gasrointestinal hemorrhage after transoesophageal echocardiography probe insertion. Can J Anaesth 45:1196–1199
Stafford RE, McGonigal MD, Weigelt JA, Johnson TJ (1999) Oral contrast solution and computed tomography for blunt abdominal trauma: a randomized study. Arch Surg 134: 622–626; discussion 626–627
Stapakis JC, Thickman D (1992) Diagnosis of pneumoperitoneum: abdominal CT vs. upright chest film. J Comput Assist Tomogr 16:713–716
Stassen NA, Lukan JK, Carrillo EH, Spain DA, Richardson JD (2002) Abdominal seat belt marks in the era of focused abdominal sonography for trauma. Arch Surg 137:718–723
Strate RG, Grieco JG (1983) Blunt injury to the colon and rectum. J Trauma 23:384–388
Strouse PJ, Close BJ, Marshall KW, Cywes R (1999) CT of bowel and mesenteric trauma in children. Radiographics 19: 1237–1250
Takabe K, Ohtani T, Muto I, et al. (2000) Computed tomography (CT) findings of gastric rupture after blunt trauma. Hepatogastroenterology 47:901–903
Talton DS, Craig MH, Hauser CJ, Poole GV (1995) Major gastroenteric injuries from blunt trauma. Am Surg 61:69–73
Taylor DW Jr, Babchuk WI, Walz DJ, Vemuri BR (1988a) Gastrointestinal hemorrhage from fistula between traumatic pseudoaneurysm of the right hepatic artery and the duodenum. Clin Nucl Med 13:337–338
Taylor GA, Eichelberger MR, Potter BM (1988b) Hematuria: a marker of abdominal injury in children after blunt trauma. Ann Surg 208:688–693
Taylor GA, Fallat ME, Eichelberger MR (1987) Hypovolemic shock in children: abdominal CT manifestations. Radiology 164:479–481
Thoms CA, Ricketts RR (1988) Intramural duodenal hematoma in children: reappraisal of current management. South Med J 81:985–988
Ting YM, Reuter SR (1973) Hollow viscus injury in blunt abdominal trauma. AJR 119:408–413
Touloukian RJ (1983) Protocol for the nonoperative treatment of obstructing intramural duodenal hematoma during childhood. Am J Surg 145:330–334
Toxopeus MD, Lucas CE, Krabbenhoft KL (1972) Roentgenographic diagnosis in blunt retroperitoneal duodenal rupture. AJR 115:281–288
Toyonaga T, Shinohara M, Miyatake E, et al. (2001) Penetration of the duodenum by an ingested needle with migration to the pancreas: report of a case. Surg Today 31:68–71
Tsang BD, Panacek EA, Brant WE, et al. (1997) Effect of oral contrast administration for abdominal computed tomography in the evaluation of acute blunt trauma. Ann Emerg Med 30:7–13
Tsushima Y, Yamada S, Aoki J, Endo K (2001) Ischaemic ileal stenosis following blunt abdominal trauma and demonstrated by CT. Br J Radiol 74:277–279
Tyburski JG, Dente CJ, Wilson RF, Shanti C, Steffes CO, Carlin A

(2001) Infectious complications following duodenal and/or pancreatic trauma. Am Surg 67:227–231
Udobi KF, Rodriguez A, Chiu WC, Scalea TM (2001) Role of ultrasonography in penetrating abdominal trauma: a prospective clinical study. J Trauma 50:475–479
Ulman I, Avanoglu A, Ozcan C, Demircan M, Ozok G, Erdener A (1996) Gastrointestinal perforation in children: a continuing challenge to nonoperative treatment of blunt abdominal trauma. J Trauma 41:110–113
Walker CW, Purnell GL, Diner WC (1989) Complications from extravasated retroperitoneal barium: case report and review of the literature. Radiology 173:618–620
Wataya H, Tsuruta N, Takayama K, Mitsudomi T, Nakanishi Y, Hara N (1997) Delayed traumatic hernia diagnosed with magnetic resonance imaging. Nihon Kyobu Shikka Gakkai Zasshi 35:124–128
Weiss M, Dreiling DA (1968) Small-bowel perforation in blunt trauma. Its relationship to previous laparotomy. Am J Gastroenterol 50:279–288
Welling RE, Reilly PS (1986) Nonoperative treatment of a traumatic intramural hematoma of the ascending colon. South Med 79:1309–1310
Westcott JL, Smith JR (1975) Mesenteric and colon injuries secondary to blunt trauma. Radiology 114:597–600
Wilkinson AE (1989) Injuries of the stomach. An analysis of 95 cases. S Afr J Surg 27:59–61
Williams DB, Karl RC (1981) Intestinal injury associated with low-voltage electrocution. J Trauma 21:246–250
Williams RD, Sargent FT (1963) The mechanism of intestinal injury in trauma. J Trauma 3:288–296
Williams SM, Harned RK (1991) Recognition and prevention of barium enema complications. Curr Probl Diagn Radiol 20:123–151
Wiot JF (1966) Intramural small intestinal hemorrhage–a differential diagnosis. Semin Roentgenol 1:219–233
Wisner DH, Blaisdell FW (1992) Visceral injuries. Arch Surg 127:687–693
Wisner DH, Chun Y, Blaisdell FW (1990). Blunt intestinal injury. Keys to diagnosis and management. Arch Surg 125: 1319–1323
Wittenberg J, Harisinghani MG, Jhaveri K, Varghese J, Mueller PR (2002). Algorithmic approach to CT diagnosis of the abnormal bowel wall. Radiographics 22:1093–1109
Yajko RD, Seydel F, Trimble C (1975) Rupture of the stomach from blunt abdominal trauma. J Trauma 15:177–183
Yin WY, Gueng MK, Huang SM, Chen HT, Chang TM (2000) Acute colonic intramural hematoma due to blunt abdominal trauma. Int Surg 85:51–54
Yoshii H, Sato M, Yamamoto S, et al. (1998) Usefulness and limitations of ultrasonography in the initial evaluation of blunt abdominal trauma. J Trauma 45:45–51
Yoshino MT (1987) Duodenal hematoma: CT demonstration of the ring sign. Gastrointest Radiol 12:330–332
Zapf S, Duber C, Kuhn FP, Lauff V (1988) Diagnosis of duodenal wall hematoma. Roentgenblatter 41:27:30
Zeybek N, Tas H, Kaymakcioglu N, Cetiner S, Ozal E, Sen D (2001) Gastrointestinal hemorrhage due to traumatic superior mesenteric artery aneurysm (case report). Ulus Travma Derg 7:274–276
Zinelis SA, Hershenson LM, Ennis Mf, Boller M, Ismail-Beigi F (1989) Intramural duodenal hematoma following upper gastrointestinal endoscopic biopsy. Dig Dis Sci 34: 289–291
Zingg U, Vorburger S, Metzger U (2000) Perforation of Meckel's diverticulum by a toothpick. Chirurg 71:841–843

9 Injuries of the Diaphragm

A. Nchimi, D. Szapiro, R. F. Dondelinger

CONTENTS

- The diaphragm lies at the furthermost bounds of the thoracic and abdominal cavities and should be imaged as a full part of both cavities, in thoracic and abdominal trauma.
- Awareness and knowledge of phrenic injuries are mandatory for accurate management of trauma patients.
- Blunt diaphragmatic injuries may be overlooked at admission, in the absence of herniation of abdominal viscera. Positive signs of phrenic rupture can be subtle on axial cross section images.
- Undiagnosed diaphragmatic tear evolves into potentially disastrous complications.

A. Nchimi, MD
Department of Medical Imaging, University Hospital Sart Tilman, Domaine Universitaire du Sart Tilman B35, 4000 Liège, Belgium
D. Szapiro, MD
Professor and Chairman, Department of Medical Imaging, University Hospital Sart Tilman, Domaine Universitaire du Sart Tilman B35, 4000 Liège, Belgium
R. F. Dondelinger, MD
Professor and Chairman, Department of Medical Imaging, University Hospital Sart Tilman, Domaine Universitaire du Sart Tilman B35, 4000 Liège, Belgium

9.1 History

The first comprehensive description of diaphragmatic hernia was given during the first half of the 16th century by Sennertus (Schneider 1956). Posttraumatic phrenic rupture was described by Paré in a French soldier who survived a gunshot wound to the lower chest. The patient died 8 months later, following necrosis of hollow viscus herniated through a fingertip phrenic defect (Paré 1579). Diagnosis of phrenic hernia in a living patient was made during the second half of the 19th century (Bowditch 1853) and successful surgical repair was reported by Riolfi during the same period (Hedblom 1925). Thereafter, posttraumatic phrenic tears were reported as incidental surgical or necropsy findings with a heavy left predominance attributed to the protective effect of the liver for the right side. Advances in roentgenology increased the number of reports of posttraumatic phrenic hernias during the first half of the 20th century, as sequelae of World War I (Waxman 1922). Late complications were almost always fatal, urging clinicians and radiologists to be aware of this condition (Carter et al. 1951; Hill 1972; Tan et al. 1973; Gourin and Garzon 1974; Fataar and Schulman 1979). Reports of phrenic trauma on large series provided by urban trauma centres have appeared during the past 5 decades.

9.2 Incidence

Although the real incidence is unknown, because of the proportion of asymptomatic patients in which the injury may remain undiagnosed, the prevalence of diaphragmatic trauma is increasing for both blunt and penetrating trauma. In autopsy series of polytrauma victims, phrenic injuries are found in 5–17% (Estrera et al. 1979; Puffer and Gaebler 1991). In the past, variations from 3/1 to 1/8 were found in the ratio of penetrating and blunt trauma to the diaphragm, penetrating trauma being more frequent in the USA than in Europe. These variations reflected the geographic and socio-economic status of the regions served by trauma centres. However, during the last 5 decades, lifestyle and urban violence tended to standardization in developed countries. It is currently admitted that penetrating phrenic trauma is approximately two times more frequent than blunt trauma (Estrera et al. 1985; Chen and Wilson 1991; Calhoon et al. 1992; Asensio et al. 1999). Phrenic injury occurs in 0.8–5.8% of patients with blunt abdominal trauma and in 3–8% of patients undergoing emergency coeliotomy after blunt injury. Motor vehicle collision is responsible for approximately 90% of the cases (Beauchamp et al. 1984; Morgan et al. 1986; Kearney et al. 1989; Voeller et al. 1990; Brandt et al. 1992; Boulanger et al. 1993; Meyers and McCabe 1993; Lee et al. 1994; Shah et al. 1995). Although only few studies are available, incidence in exclusively paediatric age groups seems to be similar to adult groups (Myers 1964; Radhakrishna et al. 1969; Sharma et al. 1977; Adeyemi and Stephens 1981; Brandt et al. 1992; Ramos et al. 2000).

Penetrating diaphragmatic injuries occurred in 10–75% of patients experiencing stab or gunshot wounds to the thoracoabdominal area (Feliciano et al. 1988; Mariadason et al. 1988; Madden et al. 1989; Ochsner et al. 1993; Ivatury et al. 1993; Nel and Warren 1994; Uribe et al. 1994; Spann et al. 1995; Leppaniemi et al. 1996; Martinez et al. 2001). The incidence increases to 90% of patients with left-side thoracic penetrating trauma (Moore et al. 1980; Murray et al. 1997).

In blunt trauma, a similar predominance is found for the left side (Tan et al. 1973; Wise et al. 1973; Gourin and Garzon 1974; Fataar and Schulman 1979). The considerable changes in epidemiology and awareness have increased recognition of right-sided injuries and the left/right ratio is currently believed to be 1/1 for penetrating and 3/1 for blunt trauma (Morgan et al. 1986; Kearney et al. 1989; Mueller and Pendravis 1994; Shanmuganathan et al. 2000). Posttraumatic pericardial, bilateral and ipsilateral double diaphragmatic ruptures are found in less than 1% of patients who reach the hospital alive (Shah et al. 1995; Sharma 1999; Schumpelick et al. 2000).

Immediate posttraumatic deaths directly related to diaphragmatic injury are probably rare. However, overall immediate mortality rates, varying from 17% to 42%, have been reported, due to associated potentially life-threatening injuries that are present in 70–100% of cases (Desforges et al. 1957; Lucido and Wall 1963; Estrera et al. 1979; Waldschmidt and Laws 1980; Niville et al. 1983; Troop et al. 1985; Morgan et al. 1986; Rodriguez-Morales et al. 1986; Smithers et al. 1991; Rizoli et al. 1994). Diaphragmatic rupture must therefore be considered as a confident marker of injury severity (Van der Werken et al. 1983; Meyers and McCabe 1993; Reber et al. 1998). However, due to the diverted attention by other obvious organ injuries and diagnostic difficulties, diaphragmatic rupture, in nonoperatively managed patients, remained undiagnosed in 10–60% of cases (Hood 1971; Wise et al. 1973; Gourin and Garzon 1974; McCune et al. 1976; Ball et al. 1982; Estrera et al. 1985; Wiencek et al. 1986; Kearney et al. 1989; Guth et al. 1995; Shah et al. 1995). These patients, surviving their multiple injuries, may subsequently develop, a few days to years after trauma, complications that have fatal outcomes in 10–66% of cases (Carter et al. 1951; Grage et al. 1959; Gourin and Garzon 1974; Miller et al. 1984; Cruz and Minagi 1994; Groskin 1992; Reber et al. 1998).

9.3 Anatomy of the Diaphragm

The diaphragm is a half-dome-shaped flat musculotendinous structure separating the abdominal and thoracic cavities. The center of the diaphragm is the central tendon, presenting its largest expansion in the transverse plane, with a cloverleaf appearance of one anterior and two lateral leaves. The heart depresses the cranial face of the central tendon. The right and left dome lie lateral to the heart, the right being approximately one intercostal space higher than the left. The foramen of the inferior vena cava, which is the only constant anatomic defect of the central tendon, is located right to the midline. Both the inferior vena cava and pericardium are firmly attached to the central tendon by fibrous tissue. The central tendon is peripherally in continuation with the muscular diaphragm, which can be divided into three parts:

- The posterior part rises from the crura and the lumbocostal arches, containing the apertures of the abdominal aorta and the oesophagus;
- The costal part originates from the six caudal rib cartilages;
- The sternal part originates from the posterior aspect of the xiphoid appendix and the rectus abdominalis sheath.

The cranial face of the diaphragm is covered by the pleura and pericardium, delineating the lung and heart base, while its caudal face is covered by peritoneum delineating the liver, stomach and spleen. The posteroinferior extraperitoneal aspect of the diaphragm is in contact with the adrenal glands and kidneys.

The anterior parasternal (Morgagni's), posterior costovertebral (Bochdalek's), hiatal, paracaval and septal apertures are small congenital defects or weaknesses of the diaphragm, closed by peritoneopleural or peritoneopericardial membranes, from which abdominal organs can bulge into the thorax, covered by a hernial sac (Schumpelick et al. 2000). These defects may enlarge with age (Caskey et al. 1989).

The major role of the diaphragm is respiration. Despite individual variations, the right dome is at the level of the 4th anterior intercostal space at rest, and at the level of 6th anterior intercostal space at the end of maximal inspiration (Simon et al. 1969). The phrenic nerves that originate from the cervical medulla and run vertically, lateral to the middle mediastinum in the thorax, provide innervation of the diaphragm (Fell 1998). The diaphragm also contains lymphatics of both pleural and peritoneal cavities, which drain into the anterior pericardiophrenic and posterior retrocrural lymph nodes (Li et al. 1996; Ohtani and Ohtani 1997; Shao et al. 1998).

Pericardiophrenic arteries, musculophrenic arteries, superior phrenic arteries and small direct aortic branches afford blood supply to the cranial face of the diaphragm, while the caudal face of the diaphragm is supplied by inferior phrenic arteries, which are the first branches of the abdominal aorta. The common origin at the anterior aspect of the aorta, right inferior diaphragmatic artery rising from the celiac trunk or of one of its branches, or of the right renal artery are the most common anatomic variations of these arteries, which are the most important for blood supply to the diaphragm. Phrenic veins have a parallel course to the arteries.

9.4 Mechanism

By definition, diaphragmatic rupture is a loss of the continuity of muscular or tendinous fibres of the diaphragm, leaving in communication the thoracic and abdominal cavity.

9.4.1 Common Causes

The most common cause of penetrating injury are stab and gunshot wounds (Rosati 1998). Of the penetrating injuries in the lower thoracic area, 1/6 patients with stab wounds and half of patients with gunshot wounds had diaphragmatic rupture (Broos et al. 1989). Diaphragmatic perforation may occur from any wound in which the trajectory reaches the fourth and fifth intercostal spaces superiorly and the level of the twelfth rib inferiorly (BORLASE et al. 1989; ORTEGA et al. 1996; VELMAHOS et al. 1997). In most cases, penetrating injuries cause small ruptures, while blunt diaphragmatic injuries are usually associated with larger defects. Blunt traumatic diaphragmatic rupture is due to a car or motorcycle accident in more than 90% of cases. Other modes of injury do not commonly result in diaphragmatic rupture (MCELWEE et al. 1984). Three mechanisms may be involved:

- During a severe blunt abdominal injury, subdiaphragmatic pressure may increase, due to forces exerted on the abdominal wall and simultaneous diaphragmatic contraction against a closed glottis (DE LA ROCHA et al. 1982). It has been calculated that the required sudden increase of pressure must reach at least 100 mmHg to exceed the elasticity of the diaphragm (SAUR and LUTZ 1976). Rupture preferentially occurs on the less elastic central tendon or starts at the congenitally weakest parts of the diaphragm, running radially towards the oesophageal hiatus, which is exceptionally involved. The costolumbar or posterolateral transition zone predominates in some series, while the sternocostal or anteromedial transition zone predominates in others (HARDY 1966; ANDRUS and MORTON 1970; LUCIDO and WALL 1963; SUTTON et al. 1967; EBERT et al. 1967; POMERANTZ et al. 1968; VOELLER et al. 1990). If ruptures were related solely to a homogenous increase in abdominal pressure, right hemidiaphragmatic rupture will be the exception, due partly to the protection afforded by the liver and partly to the congenital strength of the right hemidiaphragm compared to the left (ANDRUS and MORTON 1970; BEKASSY et al. 1973). However, right diaphragmatic tears occur with an increasing prevalence. Therefore, it is not a uniform increase in abdominal pressure that occurs in most cases, due to the orientation of the impact and the position of passengers inside vehicles. Lateral torso impact was found three times more likely to result in diaphragmatic rupture than frontal impact, presumably because there is less dispersion of energy from a side impact, as cars are primarily designed to resist frontal collision (KEARNEY et al. 1989). Subsequently, right diaphragmatic ruptures were found to predominate in both right- and left-side drivers or passengers who have undergone a trauma to their right side, as well as an equal prevalence for backside impacts (KEARNEY et al. 1989; THAKORE et al. 2001). Car security devices have been reported as responsible for the increase of intra-abdominal pressure, associated with diaphragmatic rupture for seatbelts (MUKERJEA and NAIR 1978; BERGQVIST et al. 1978) and pericardiophrenic ruptures for front airbags (SHARMA 1999).
- A violent thoracoabdominal blunt trauma may initiate reflex contractions of the diaphragm. These contractions may be strong enough to result in an avulsion of peripheral attachments of the muscle.
- Protruding fractured ribs may lacerate the diaphragm (SHANMUGANATHAN et al. 2000), as suggested by reports of non-traumatic diaphragmatic laceration, caused by costal exostosis (SIMANSKY et al. 1997). This mechanism explains phrenic rupture occurring at atypical sites such as the oesophageal hiatus and the crus.

9.4.2 Uncommon Causes

Comparison of collective reviews showed in earlier reports that falls from a height, impalement, crush injuries in mines or by vehicles and kicks by a horse or a cow were more prominent than in later series (HOOD 1971; SHARMA 1989).

9.4.2.1 Iatrogenic Injury

Special attention should be focused on the cases in which medical devices may injure the diaphragm, since these injuries are increasing in incidence. Disruption of a counterincision made to repair hiatal hernia is not uncommon (COPPINGER 1960). Incidental perforation of the diaphragm during laparoscopic cholecystectomy has been reported (ALOISE et al. 1994; BAUTZ and KNOTTENBELT 1994; SEILER et al. 1995; NEUMEYER et al. 1996; DAWSON and FERGUSON 1997; ARMSTRONG et al. 1999). Other rarely reported causes in the literature include:

- Surgical interventions in the thoracoabdominal area such as coronary artery bypass, aortic aneurysm repair, lung, heart and liver transplantation, or nephrectomy
- Percutaneous procedures in the thoracoabdominal area such as liver, lung, kidney or adrenal biopsy or catheter drainage of abscesses
- Chest tube insertion
- Ambulatory peritoneal dialysis
- Subxiphoid pericardiocentesis

- Epicardial pacemaker insertions (SWARTZ et al. 1984; STEIGER et al. 1984; KAINUMA and SHIMADA 1988; MAJID 1990; WALLER et al. 1992; MEYERS and MCCABE 1993; NAUNHEIM 1998; GOMEZ-ARNAU et al. 1999; PROKESCH et al. 2000; POTTER et al. 2001)

9.4.2.2 Spontaneous Rupture

Spontaneous rupture is defined by sudden herniation of abdominal content into the thorax, in patients without a medical history suggesting a penetrating or a major blunt trauma. A few cases have been reported in the literature. The authors claimed that these ruptures complicated congenital diaphragmatic eventration or weakness after a minor trauma or another non-traumatic mechanism increasing abdominal pressure such as epidural anaesthesia, emergence from anaesthesia, vomiting, cough, defecation, heavy exercise, pregnancy, childbirth, dancing and lifting, jet flight deceleration, sexual intercourse, or respiratory physiotherapy after lung transplantation (BERNHARDT and LAWTON 1966; SALOMON et al. 1969; DAVE et al. 1973; BEKASSY et al. 1973; MANINGES et al. 1983; HENZLER et al. 1988; RUBIO 1990; EL NAKADI and VANDERHOEFT 1990; MITCHELL et al. 1994; CAMERON and MIRVIS 1996; FAHEEM and FAYAD 1999; FLICK et al. 1999; GOMEZ-ARNAU et al. 1999; KALLAY et al. 2000).

9.4.2.3 Secondary Rupture

Healing of a repaired diaphragm is almost always complete and definitive. Few cases of diaphragmatic rupture occurring after a first successful repair have been reported (HOOD 1971; KAMELGARD et al. 1999).

9.4.3 Associated Injuries

The close relationship of the diaphragm to adjacent intra-abdominal and intrathoracic organs nearly always accounts for associated injuries. Isolated diaphragmatic ruptures may occur in a small proportion of injuries, including iatrogenic trauma, stab wounds and spontaneous ruptures. Associated injuries, including sites other than thorax and abdomen, vary from 50% to 100%, depending on the mechanism of trauma.

9.4.3.1 Abdominal Injuries

Splenic injury is the most common abdominal injury associated with left-sided diaphragmatic rupture, occurring in 20–70% of the cases. Laceration of the left lobe of the liver, hollow viscus perforation, particularly the stomach, mesenteric and epiploic tear, and distal pancreatic contusion are other abdominal organ injuries that may be associated with left-sided penetrating diaphragmatic rupture.

Contusion of hollow viscus, mesenteric haematoma or desinsertion and pancreatic head injury may occur in association with blunt diaphragmatic rupture in 2–10% of cases.

With an estimated incidence of 93%, liver laceration is the most common intra-abdominal injury associated with right-sided diaphragmatic rupture (BOULANGER et al. 1993). Complete dislocation of a liver lobe, trauma to the biliary tract, particularly the gallbladder, hepatic vein desinsertion and tear of portal vein and retrohepatic vena cava are classic observations (COLN et al. 1980; IVATURY et al. 1984; SIMPSON et al. 2000).

Kidney and urinary tract injuries are also frequently reported for both penetrating and blunt diaphragmatic rupture, with an incidence varying between 5% and 15%. Cases of complete avulsion of the vascular pedicle of a herniated kidney were reported (SUTTON et al. 1967; HEEB et al. 1971; STYLIANOS et al. 1991). Association of a perirenal haematoma and diaphragmatic rupture on the same side may prompt the suspicion of renal vascular injury (LEVY et al. 1988; PEITZMAN and UDEKWU 1989).

Other abdominal vascular injuries include direct trauma to major retroperitoneal vessels in penetrating trauma, which often resulted in a fatal outcome, as well as indirect vascular lacerations, frequently associated with genitourinary tract injuries in severe pelvic trauma.

9.4.3.2 Thoracic Injuries

Their real incidence has not been assessed, but various intrathoracic injuries are associated with diaphragmatic rupture, especially when rib fractures are present. Haemothoraces, pneumothoraces, lung atelectasis, lacerations and contusions are frequently reported in both blunt and penetrating phrenic rupture. Thoracic wall vessels in contact with diaphragmatic attachments may be injured during phrenic avulsion. Heart and pericardial injuries are common in patients who died before reaching the hospital and are observed in less than 1% of patients surviving their trauma (Shah et al. 1995; Sharma 1999; Schumpelick et al. 2000). Trachea and main stem bronchi that may be associated with phrenic injuries in blunt anterior thoracic trauma have a mortality as high as 30% (Reuter 1996). Associated ruptures of the thoracic aorta occur in up to 15% of the cases in small series, but their real incidence may be approximately 5%, as found in large series of both dead and surviving subjects (Estrera et al. 1979; Meyers and McCabe 1993; Duverger et al. 2001). It has been stated that direction and strength of the necessary force may be the same to disrupt thoracic aorta and diaphragm (Schroder Hansen et al. 2001). Oesophageal perforation associated with diaphragmatic rupture is a rare occurrence (Cherry 1961). There is one report of phrenic nerve section associated with diaphragmatic rupture in a child who had sustained a stab wound by scissors (Ramos et al. 2000).

9.4.3.3 Extra-truncal and Skeletal Injuries

Although very common, lower rib fractures in blunt trauma should raise the suspicion of diaphragmatic rupture and associated intra-abdominal injuries, since bone edges may lacerate adjacent organs. Other immediate complications such as flail chest and massive pleural effusion occur in up to 50% of cases and may distract attention away from the diaphragm. Pelvic fractures are found almost exclusively associated with blunt diaphragmatic rupture. Strength to open the pelvic ring may be similar to the forces necessary to disrupt the diaphragm or the thoracic aorta. Considering the high incidence of pelvic fractures in blunt diaphragmatic ruptures, it is admitted that after a blunt trauma, when a ruptured diaphragm is present, a pelvic fracture is also present in nearly half of the cases. Although the reverse association is less common, attention must be paid to the diaphragm when a pelvic fracture is found (Grage et al. 1959; Fataar and Schulman 1979).

Proximal long-bone fractures are common with blunt phrenic rupture.

Spine injuries are associated with both blunt and penetrating phrenic rupture. In blunt injury, they predominantly involve the cervical spine. Gunshot wounds to the back involving the thoracic spine are particularly frequent.

Head injuries are associated with blunt diaphragmatic rupture in 30–60% of the cases and are responsible for immediate death in up to half of cases. Respiratory distress resulting from head trauma may mask an underlying diaphragmatic rupture.

9.5 Natural History of Diaphragmatic Injury

The natural history of the injured diaphragm is crucial for understanding the potential complications. Although reported in animal experimental models, healing of a diaphragmatic rupture has never been reported to occur spontaneously in humans, due partly to uninterrupted respiratory motions, as suggested by reports of fetal spontaneous healing (Longaker et al. 1991; Zierold et al. 2001). The existing pleuroperitoneal pressure gradient of 7–22 cm H_2O, favoured by deep inspiration, high intra-abdominal pressure and increased intrapleural pressure, act as a hydrodynamic force, which favours herniation of intra-abdominal content into the chest (Marchand 1957). Many variables determine the time from injury to herniation, the volume of its contents and its consequences.

- Orientation of the defect determines its evolving potential. Due to radial forces, a defect oriented longitudinally to phrenic fibres is likely to extend through the fibre axis, while a defect oriented transversally will not enlarge (Carter et al. 1951)
- The size of the defect varies with the mechanism of trauma: larger defects are found for blunt trauma and smaller ones for penetrations. The minimal size necessary to induce herniation depends on the size of the organ to herniate, since small defects are unlikely to be crossed by large organs. However, constriction induced by smaller defects is more likely to alter the blood supply to herniated organs, endangering them more (Sullivan 1966).
- The side of the defect determines the size of the organs to herniate. Due to the protection afforded by the size of the liver, no herniation may occur through a small right-sided diaphragmatic defect, contrary to the left side, which covers smaller intra-abdominal organs. However, some congenital and acquired conditions may facilitate right-sided herniation through small defects such as anterior colic interposition and atrophy of the right hepatic lobe.
- The location of the defect is of importance, since for those located on the retroperitoneal part of the diaphragm, the transdiaphragmatic pressure

gradient is lower than for those located on its peritoneal part.

These observations suggest that when a defect through the diaphragm exists, the rule is herniation of abdominal contents into the thoracic cavity. Herniation may be delayed for days to years, and in some instances the patient never becomes symptomatic, as for right-sided diaphragmatic injuries from a penetrating wound (McConnel and Trunkey 1990; Guth et al. 1995).

A classification based on these facts has gained wide acceptance. Three phases during posttraumatic phrenic injuries are considered, according to the natural history.

- Phase 1 includes phrenic injuries diagnosed immediately following trauma or during the recovery phase.
- Phase 2 includes those injuries diagnosed on the basis of symptoms or incidentally during the period following the recovery phase.
- Phase 3 includes injuries diagnosed after apparent recovery from the injury, because of acute ischemia or perforation of one of the herniated organs (Carter et al. 1951). Existing adhesions between herniated viscus and serosa and an increase in intra-abdominal pressure may play a role in moving from the second to the third phase.

9.6 Complications

9.6.1 Hernia

The most commonly herniated organs are the stomach, colon, spleen and omentum for a left-sided phrenic rupture, followed by the small intestine, left lobe of the liver, pancreatic tail and the left kidney. In right-sided hernias, the liver, stomach, omentum and colon are the most frequently involved organs, followed by the right kidney and the small intestine. Only the stomach, transverse colon, liver, omentum and exceptionally the jejunum are reported to herniate through pericardiophrenic ruptures (Table 9.1).

9.6.1.1 Herniation of Hollow Viscus

Herniation of the omentum, or part or entire hollow viscus such as the stomach through a large diaphragmatic defect may be of little consequence, as also seen in large hiatal hernias. Two types of complications may occur for herniation of hollow viscus through smaller defects: incarceration with gastrointestinal obstruction or alteration of blood supply to these organs, resulting in severe wall ischemia, which may manifest as a localized or extensive ischemic necrosis that subsequently perforates. When evisceration occurs after a penetrating trauma, hollow organs herniated through the diaphragm and the thoracic wall lead to additional risk of infection.

Gastrointestinal Obstruction and Strangulation

Obstruction and strangulation in diaphragmatic hernia were found to occur nine times more frequently for traumatic than for congenital defects, due to the smaller size of posttraumatic tears (Carter and Giuseffi 1948). The time interval between injury and strangulation may be extremely variable: as short as one day or as long as years, the longest published delay being 48 years (Johnson 1988). In more than 80% of cases, strangulation occurred within 3 years of the injury (Pomerantz et al. 1968). The acute attack generally begins abruptly and pain is a ubiquitous symptom. Vomiting is frequent and may be bloody for gastric hernias. Other signs of obstruction are not constant and depend on the content of hernia; constipation occurs for colic and small intestine hernia, rarely for gastric and omental hernia. Constipation may precede the onset of an acute attack. In such cases, it probably represents a precipitating factor, since it increases the intra-abdominal pressure. As for constipation, abnormal peristaltic activity and abdominal distension may be confusingly absent when stomach or omentum alone is herniated (Carter et al. 1951, Schulman and van Gelderen 1996b).

Table 9.1. Relative frequency of herniation of intra-abdominal organs through diaphragmatic defects

Herniated organ	Left phrenic rupture	Cardiophrenic rupture	Right phrenic rupture
Stomach	+++	+++	+
Colon	+++ (left angle)	++ (transverse)	++ (right angle)
Spleen	+++	–	–
Liver	+ (left lobe)	+ (left lobe)	+++
Gallbladder	–	–	++
Greater omentum	+++	++	+++
Small intestine	++	±	+
Kidney	+ (left)	–	+ (right)

+++ common; ++ rare; + exceptional; – not observed

Gastrointestinal non-mechanical obstruction may occur in association with diaphragmatic rupture, with or without herniation. This condition is almost always related to other associated injuries.

Gastric Volvulus

Unless the oesophageal hiatus is included in the phrenic defect, during intrathoracic herniation of the stomach, the cardia remains in its normal position. This supposes by definition a volvulus (Hood 1971). According to the mobility of the pylorus, two types of gastric volvulus may be encountered:

- A part of the stomach may be herniated into the thoracic cavity, with a longitudinal rotation of the organ axis, the cardia and the pylorus remain fixed. The resulting obstruction is described as organo-axial volvulus. This type represents 65% of gastric volvulus and may be associated with congenital or acquired diaphragmatic defects. Strangulation or gangrene occur in up to 30% of cases (Carter et al. 1980). Borchart's triad, consisting of retching, abdominal pain and failure to pass a nasogastric tube, is related to this condition (Cameron and Mirvis 1996).
- The mesenteric-axial volvulus represents 35% of gastric volvulus and results from herniation of part of the greater curvature of the stomach, associated with mobilization of the pylorus and a horizontal axis rotation of the stomach, with subsequent obstruction of the mobile pylorus. Volvulus may be partial with spontaneous detorsion and recurrent acute episodes. A nasogastric tube passes easily into the stomach. Although less frequent than organoaxial volvulus, most of the posttraumatic diaphragmatic hernias of the stomach, complicated by gangrene are of the mesenteric-axial type (Borsari et al. 1989; Jayanthi et al. 1994; Cameron and Mirvis 1996; Schulman and van Gelderen 1996a; Gibbons and McGuigan 1997)

9.6.1.2 Herniation of Solid Organs

Solid organ hernia usually results in few consequences. However, as for hollow viscus and omentum, tightening or torsion of their vasculature may lead to massive necrosis or functional impairment. Consequently, hepatic insufficiency due to diaphragmatic rupture has been reported (Negre et al. 1986). Documented splenic infarction and ischemic pancreatitis were sporadically reported. Renal necrosis results rather from vascular pedicle avulsion than from its tightening through a diaphragmatic defect.

9.6.2 Pulmonary Complications

Large phrenic defects alter respiratory function, since loss of function of one hemidiaphragm results in a 25–50% decrease in the lung capacity (Shah et al. 1995). Moreover, associated massive herniation and pleural effusion further reduce lung capacity. Severe respiratory trouble may result, especially in infants that have lower respiratory reserve and accessory respiratory muscle function (Karnak et al. 2001). Pneumonia is likely to occur as an infectious consequence of underlying lung collapse. Complicated hollow-organ herniation may result in closed increase of their volume, which may be sufficient to cause tension hemithorax (Ordog et al. 1984).

Large pleural effusions are likely to occur with diaphragmatic injuries. Pneumothoraces are in most cases explained by chest-wall and lung trauma. However, they may be caused by a complication of hollow viscus or omental hernia. Large haemothorax may be related to injury of thoracic wall vessels by diaphragmatic avulsion, and has also been reported in association with intrathoracic migration of the kidney and avulsion of the vascular pedicle (Stylianos et al. 1991). Similar mechanisms were found to cause large urinothorax, while the renal pelvis was avulsed (Lahiry et al. 1978). Posttraumatic pleuro-biliary fistula commonly presents as a small pleural effusion, with a great tendency for infection (Schwegler and Endrei 1975; Ivatury et al. 1984; Ramnarine et al. 2001). Following diaphragmatic rupture, fistulization of pancreatic ducts into the thoracic cavity classically involves the left pleural space and manifests as pleural effusions. Intrathoracic pseudocysts (Sharma et al. 1988) and broncho-pancreatic fistula (Cox et al. 1977) have been reported.

When complicated intrathoracic hernia of hollow viscus goes undiagnosed, altered blood supply to the wall causes visceral wall necrosis that subsequently perforates, causing or aggravating existing pleural effusion. Life-threatening tension pneumothorax occurring as a complication of diaphragmatic rupture is likely associated with colon perforation (Brun and Curt 1987; Hahn and Watson 1990; Mattei et al. 1992; Lacayo et al. 1993; Murray et al. 1997; Seelig et al. 1999), rarely with stomach or small bowel involvement (Montresor et al. 1997). Iatrogenic perforation of the diaphragm, following subphrenic drainage of an infected abdominal collection has also been found to result in tension pneumothorax (KAINUMA and SHIMADA 1988).

The most common cause of pleural empyema associated with diaphragmatic injury is intrathoracic perforation of the colon, which may occur also after surgical correction (DAS 1977; PRICE et al. 1983; SEELIG et al. 1999). Pleural empyema may occur as a complication of intrathoracic perforation of the stomach, small bowel or gallbladder.

9.6.3 Cardiovascular Complications

A large spectrum of complications that in fine alters the cardiac function may complicate a diaphragmatic injury. Hypovolemic shock may result from bleeding injuries, associated with diaphragmatic rupture or as a consequence of intrathoracic necrosis of abdominal contents, which have obvious toxic and infectious properties. Although it has been shown in porcine models that phrenic injury alone or even complicated by gastric herniation is well tolerated haemodynamically unless there is an abrupt increase of intra-abdominal pressure, some specific consequences of diaphragmatic injury alter directly the cardiovascular function (ALI and QI 1992).

9.6.3.1 Cardiac Tamponade

Two mechanisms may explain cardiac tamponade in pericardiophrenic rupture:

- Exiguity of the pericardial cavity is responsible for cardiac tamponade, when intra-abdominal organs herniate through a pericardiophrenic defect, even for small hernias. Massive intrapericardial hernia leading to acute cardiac insufficiency related to heart luxation has been reported (BOGERS et al. 1986). However, not all cardiac luxations lead to functional impairment (DE ROOIJ and HAARMAN 1993).
- In a few cases, the heart may herniate through the defect into the peritoneal cavity, where the pressure exceeds the pericardium, causing tamponade (SHARMA 1999).

Although coexisting with phrenic rupture in some instances, haemopericardium is a rare complication of phrenic rupture. Pneumopericardium complicating phrenic injury is more frequently reported as a consequence of intrapericardial perforation of hollow viscus (RASHID et al. 1999).

9.6.3.2 Central Venous Obstruction

Massive herniation of abdominal contents into the thoracic cavity on one side increases the concerned intrapleural pressure, leading to a mediastinal shift that may cause obstruction of the superior vena cava. However, no case of complete interruption of the superior vena cava related to posttraumatic diaphragmatic hernia has been reported, but an elevated central venous pressure has been found in a large majority of patients with posttraumatic diaphragmatic hernia, even without shock (WILSON et al. 1977; RODRIGUEZ-MORALES et al. 1986). Right liver lobe herniation may be responsible for a twist of the inferior vena cava, with subsequent obstruction, especially in infants (LEE et al. 1995; KARNAK et al. 2001). Delayed posttraumatic Budd-Chiari syndrome due to the same causes has also been reported in adults (CLAY and MUNRO 1971; FERNANDEZ-GONZALEZ et al. 1994).

9.6.4 Other Complications

Other complications of phrenic injuries include wound infection in penetrating trauma, abdominal or intrathoracic splenosis, occurring in left diaphragmatic injuries, thromboembolism, renal failure and multiple organ failure, which are commonly the consequence of the associated injuries rather than the injury to the diaphragm itself.

9.7 Clinical Symptoms and Findings

9.7.1 Clinical Phases

Clinical observations in left diaphragmatic hernia were established in the 19th century and consisted in prominence and immobility of the left hemithorax with absent breath sounds and tympanism, displacement of the area of cardiac dullness to the right, and audible bowel sounds in the left chest (BOWDITCH 1853). Since, a variety of other symptoms and physical findings have been found associated with diaphragmatic rupture (Tables 9.2 and 9.3). Acute diaphragmatic injury may be isolated and is unlikely to be symptomatic without herniation. However, it is commonly associated with other critical injuries that account for the symptoms and mortality during the acute phase (Drews et al. 1973). Although not common, acute posttraumatic diaphragmatic hernia can result in immediate death, when cardiorespiratory dynamics fail (Andrus and Morton 1970). Most often, symptomatic patients show evidence of shock, severe pain in the upper abdomen which may irradiate to the chest or the shoulder (Kehr's sign). Dyspnea and cyanosis may occur, depending on the size of the hernia, haematemesis related to pinching of gastric vessels and haemoptysis related to haemothorax (Carter et al. 1951).

Pericardiophrenic injuries represent a challenging diagnosis at the acute phase, since except bowel sounds that may be audible over the cardiac area, the symptoms mimic those of acute tamponade or left ventricular aneurysm (Galindo Gallego et al. 1996). As the diaphragmatic defect is small, resulting in no acute injury, it may remain occult for many years and manifests as visceral obstruction or strangulation. During the interval phase, patients are most often asymptomatic and the diagnosis was almost always fortuitously made on a chest radiograph (Carter et al. 1951). Patients during this phase may present with confusing chronic and recurrent histories of basal chest or upper abdominal pain, of abrupt onset, which may irradiate to the shoulder, initiated by large meals or constipation, and stimulating peptic ulcer, coronary disease, gallbladder disease, or subacute intestinal obstruction.

Relief of pain by vomiting or by assuming an upright sitting position, nausea, vomitus, melena, flatulence, hiccup and difficulty belching have been reported. Visceral incarceration and strangulation have clinical features described as a thoracoabdominal complex consisting of distinctive gastrointestinal and cardiorespiratory symptoms that may allow earlier diagnosis and treatment (Carter and Brewer 1971).

The abdominal manifestations include sudden excruciating abdominal pain. In this situation, early nausea and vomiting should alert to the possible incarceration of the stomach. However, closed loop obstruction of the stomach in organoaxial volvulus results in hiccupping and retching without vomiting. Incarceration of the small bowel and the colon results in symptoms and signs of intestinal obstruction, characterized by colicky abdominal pain and distension or tympanitic abdomen with peristaltic rushes (Mansour 1997).

Table 9.2. Symptoms of diaphragmatic injury

Difficulty in breathing
Chest pain
Upper abdominal pain
Shoulder pain (Kehr's sign)
Nausea and vomiting
Haematemesis
Haemoptysis
Heartburn
Constipation
Hiccup
Gas and belching
Melaena

Table 9.3. Clinical signs of diaphragmatic injury

Phase 1	Chest wall contusion	
	Abdominal wall contusion	
	Specific signs for other organs injuries	
	Tenderness over ribs	
	Loss of consciousness	Pericardiophrenic hernia
	Hypotension, shock	
	Crepitus	
	Pericardial rub	
	Bowel sounds over the cardiac area	
	Changes in haemodynamics according to the patient's position	
	Morel-Lavallée sound	
	Splashing heart murmur	
	Dyspnea	Phases 2 and 3
	Coughing	
	Cyanosis	
	Mediastinal shift	
	Peristaltic sounds in chest	
	Dullness at percussion	
	Hyper-resonance	
	Abdominal distension	
	Hyperperistalsis	
	Absent bowel sounds	

The thoracic manifestations are characterized by severe chest pain irradiating to the shoulder or neck, sometimes with dyspnea and cyanosis that results from decreased pulmonary function and mediastinal shift produced by massive distension from herniated viscera, pleural effusion or both. At that time, clinical examination of the chest may reveal dullness, tympany or evidence of pleural fluid at one thoracic base, intestinal sounds within the chest and mediastinal shift.

Other conditions than phrenic injury, such as gallbladder and pancreatic diseases, intestinal obstruction, peptic ulcer, cardiopathies, pneumothorax or haemothorax, can mimic these findings. Bowel sounds audible from the chest, which is the most specific clinical sign of diaphragmatic hernia, is found only in 5–7% of cases (Holm et al. 1988; Toh et al. 1991). Thus, in the majority of cases, the diagnosis of diaphragmatic rupture is made by means other than clinical history and physical examination.

9.7.2 Digital Exploration of the Diaphragm

When applicable, digital exploration of the diaphragm under local anaesthesia can be attempted for penetrating trauma to the lower chest or upper abdomen. This technique showed 96–100% sensitivity and 83–94% specificity for the detection of phrenic injury (Restrepo and Cano 1987; Morales et al. 2001). In a recent series, phrenic injury was detected by digital exploration in two-thirds of 82 stable patients with penetrating thoracoabdominal trauma requiring no further surgical intervention; only six patients had inconclusive digital exploration of the diaphragm (Morales et al. 2001).

9.7.3 Other Findings

Patients with posttraumatic diaphragmatic hernia may have positive diagnostic peritoneal lavage (DPL). However, diaphragmatic rupture is one of the most common abdominal injuries with false-negative DPL (Soderstrom et al. 1980; Brotman et al. 1981).

Other findings indicating phrenic injury include palpation of abdominal viscera during chest tube placement, peritoneal lavage fluid or bilious fluid exiting a chest tube, or inability to pass a nasogastric tube (Rosati 1998). Haemodynamic changes according to the patient's position and electrocardiographic signs of myocardial contusion or pericardial effusion are reported as suggestive of pericardiophrenic rupture (Galindo Gallego et al. 1996). Although intra-abdominal injuries from penetrating trauma to the chest without diaphragmatic or peritoneal violation have been described, evidence of abdominal injury after thoracic penetration and the inverse are clinical findings highly suggestive of phrenic injury (Kennedy et al. 1991).

9.7.4 Hazards of Mismanagement

Clinical evidence of lower thoracic injuries in many cases prompts insertion of a chest tube. Careful digital palpation of the chest wall should avoid perforation or laceration of herniated organs in cases of unsuspected diaphragmatic hernia. Direct blind trocar insertion should be avoided in any case (Panagiotis 1989; Zieren et al. 1999). The same precautions are of value during emergency pericardiocentesis for posttraumatic cardiac tamponade (Langley and Innes 1975).

9.8 Imaging

9.8.1 Chest Radiograph

Full inspiration chest radiographs should be obtained in each patient who has experienced blunt or penetrating trauma to the trunk after insertion of a nasogastric tube. The signs of phrenic injury are visible on decubitus anteroposterior views, expiratory, erect or Trendelenburg views, in which intra-abdominal pressure is increased. Horizontal beam lateral decubitus views and chest fluoroscopy may also be useful in selected cases, to better distinguish air-containing abdominal viscera from pneumothorax or appreciate phrenic excursion. However, these projections should not be applied routinely for potentially unstable patients.

9.8.1.1 Positive Signs

The first substantial description of chest radiographic findings in patients with diaphragmatic injury was given in the middle of the 20th century. It was stated that the most significant positive findings are:

- An arch-like shadow resembling an abnormally high diaphragm (the so-called pseudodiaphragm sign)
- Extraneous shadows extending above the anticipated level of the diaphragm
- Shift of the heart and mediastinum away from the injured side
- Areas of discoid atelectases in the lung bases (Carter et al. 1951)

Recently, dividing radiographic signs of diaphragmatic rupture into two groups has been proposed, including a diagnostic or highly suggestive group and a suggestive group (Pikoulis et al. 2000) (Table 9.4). Abnormal cardiac shadow, including enlargement of the lower mediastinum and dislodgement of the heart, suggesting pericardiophrenic rupture, must be added to these signs.

Table 9.4. Radiographic signs of diaphragmatic injury (modified from PIKOULIS et al. 2000)

Diagnostic or highly suggestive signs	Suggestive signs
Air or fluid containing viscera above the diaphragm	Diaphragm elevated less than 6 cm in the absence of atelectasis
Tip of the nasogastric tube above the diaphragm	Obscuration of the diaphragm
Diaphragm elevated more than 6 cm	Mediastinal shift, pleural effusion, abnormal heart shadow

9.8.1.2 Pitfalls

Visualization of air containing viscera and tip of the nasogastric tube above the diaphragm are unequivocal signs of herniation of abdominal contents into the chest. Loculated pneumothorax, gastric dilatation or posttraumatic pneumatocele may simulate air containing viscera above the diaphragm; otherwise, unknown congenital hernias, which require no surgical management, may radiographically simulate posttraumatic hernia (HUMPHREYS and ABBUHL 1991). All phrenic ruptures are not accompanied by herniation, nor do all herniated viscera contain air. Furthermore, partial gastric herniation may present without elevation of the nasogastric tube (Fig. 9.1). Elevation of the diaphragm, even of more than 6 cm, may be found in various pathological conditions, including brain, cervical spine and phrenic nerve injuries (Fig. 9.2). There is a wide range in the respective position and movement of both hemidiaphragms in a normal individual (SIMON et al. 1969). Thus, this finding has to be interpreted cautiously with regard to the other injuries present.

Obscuration of the diaphragm, mediastinal shift, abnormal heart shadow and pleural effusion are also found in various pathological conditions of other origin. Taken alone, none of these signs establishes the diagnosis, but increases suspicion and should prompt other investigations.

9.8.1.3 Results

No prospective evaluation of the diagnostic value of initial chest radiographs is available in the literature. In one study in which 50 patients were reviewed, preoperative diagnosis was not made at initial interpretation in 8 patients, despite obvious positive signs of diaphragmatic rupture on chest radiographs (GELMAN et al. 1991). The proportion of intubated patients at initial chest radiographs, with positive pressure respiratory assistance, that is proved to prevent immediate hernia, is probably a factor that explains false-negative diagnosis (VOELLER et al. 1990; SHAPIRO et al. 1996; KARMY-JONES et al. 2002). Interpretation of the data from the literature suggests that although nonspecific in approximately half of the cases, anomalies are found on initial chest radiograph in more than 85% of cases (HUMPHREYS and ABBUHL 1991).

Only a few studies have specifically investigated the value of chest X-ray in patients with surgically proved phrenic injury (Table 9.5). Combined sensitivities of both diagnostic and suggestive signs for diaphragmatic rupture on initial chest radiograph exceed 70% for left-sided ruptures and is lower than 50% for right-sided ruptures. Thus variations in the published diagnostic values of initial chest radiographs for diaphragmatic rupture may reflect both variations in the left-to-right ratio of injuries among series and variations in the retrospective data analysis. A normal or a nonspecific abnormal chest radiograph does not rule out diaphragmatic rupture. Pathologic findings at the lung bases must prompt repetition of the chest radiograph and the implementation of other imaging techniques, in order to rule out the diagnosis when surgical exploration is not required (Fig. 9.3).

9.8.2 Computed Tomography

Computed Tomography (CT) has gained widespread acceptance in the evaluation of suspected chest or abdominal injuries related to blunt trauma (TRUPKA et al. 1997). The first reports of CT diagnosis of blunt diaphragmatic rupture were made using sequential scanning. The early series evidenced difficulties in the evaluation of the diaphragm, explained by its anatomic disposition, resulting in tangential or oblique scanning, especially for the dome (HEIBERG et al. 1980). Increasing experience of radiologists with the technique and improvement of technology may actually allow the diagnosis of blunt diaphragmatic rupture with a great sensitivity on scans that are performed at admission. Intravenous contrast injection is routine. Oral contrast media may be useful; however, proof has not been established that it increases diagnostic sensitivity of blunt phrenic injury.

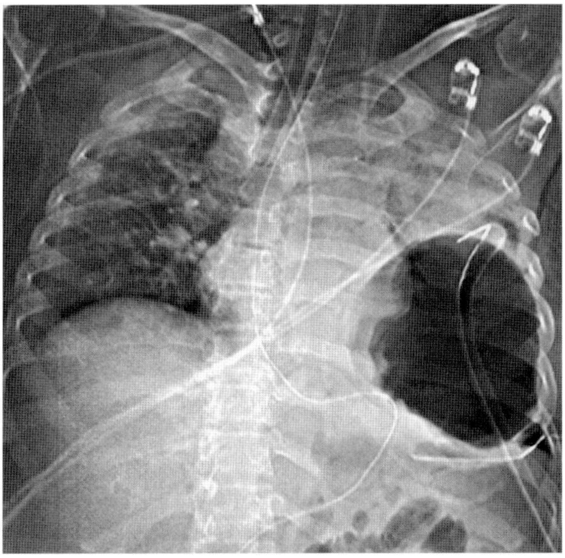

a

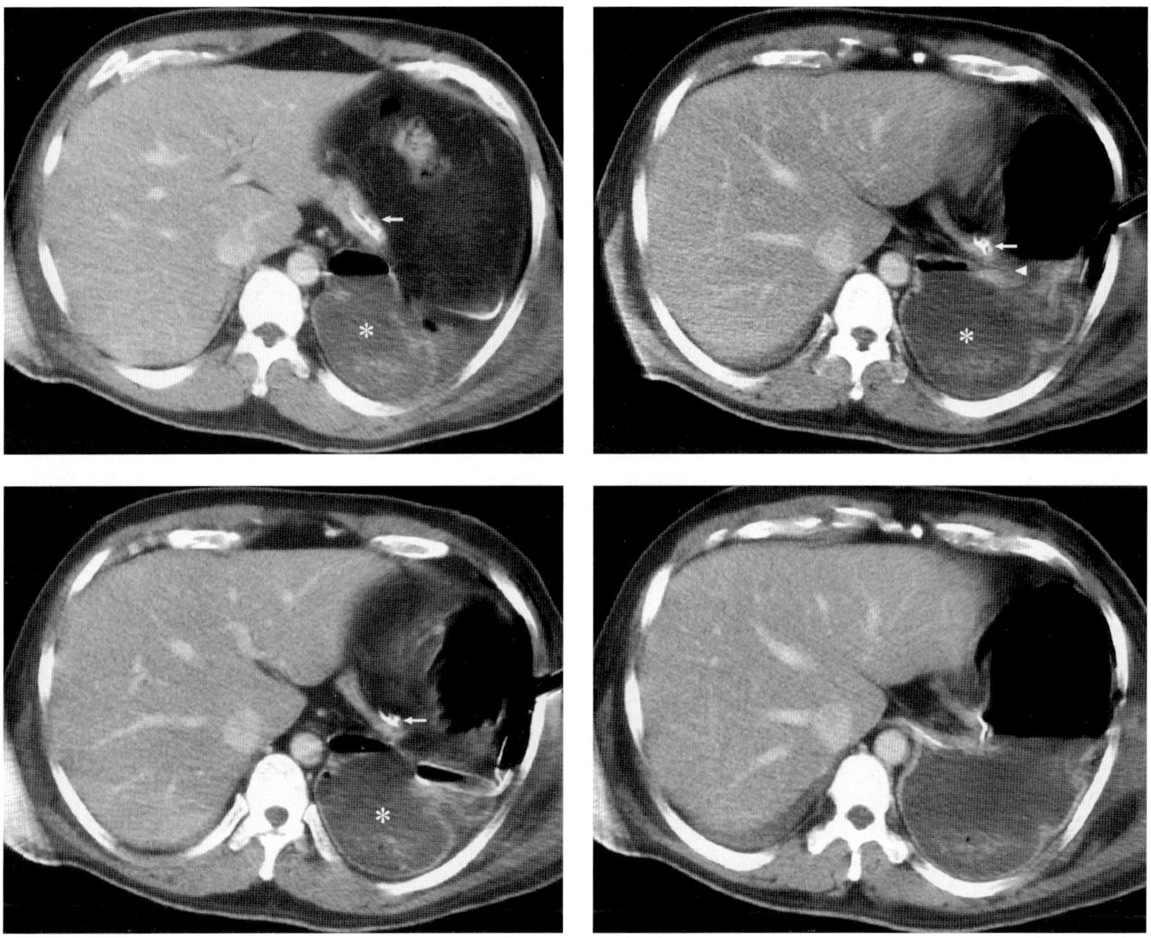

b c d e

Fig. 9.1a–e. A 42-year-old male was admitted after a violent car crash with severe respiratory distress that necessitated intubation. (**a**) Scout view of the chest showed diffuse consolidation of the left lung, obscuration of the diaphragm and air-containing viscera located above the anticipated level of the left diaphragm and below the chest tube. Normal course of the nasogastric tube (**b, c, d**). Spiral CT after IV enhancement on contiguous craniocaudal axial images (**b–d**) showed the nasogastric tube within a flattened stomach (*arrow*). The left hemidiaphragm was almost invisible, and a dilated air and fluid-containing part of the stomach (*asterisk*) was herniated inside the thorax, abutting the chest tube and the posterior thoracic wall. Both parts of the stomach were separated by a focal constriction, resulting of the rotation of the gastric pedicle (*arrowhead*). (**e**) Normal upper abdominal anatomy

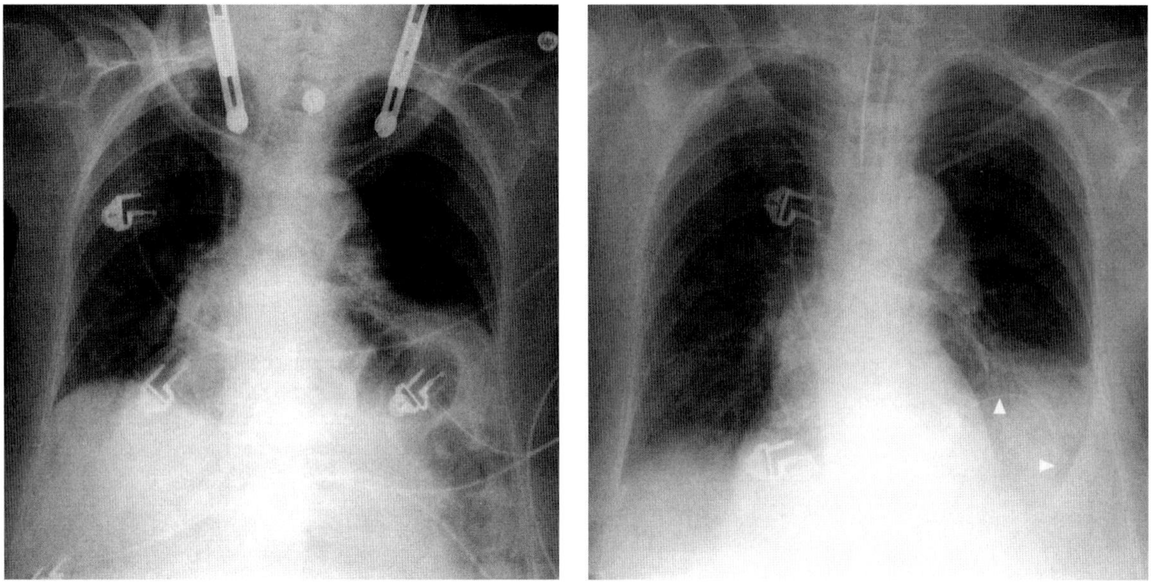

a b

Fig. 9.2a, b. A 93-year-old female was admitted after a fall, secondary to a massive intracranial haemorrhage. **a** At admission, chest radiograph showed an elevated left hemidiaphragm and splenic flexure of the colon. (**b**) Repeated chest radiograph after tracheal and nasogastric intubation showed coiling of the nasogastric tube (*arrowheads*) and basal consolidation of the left lung, suggesting left-sided phrenic rupture. Autopsy showed no phrenic injury

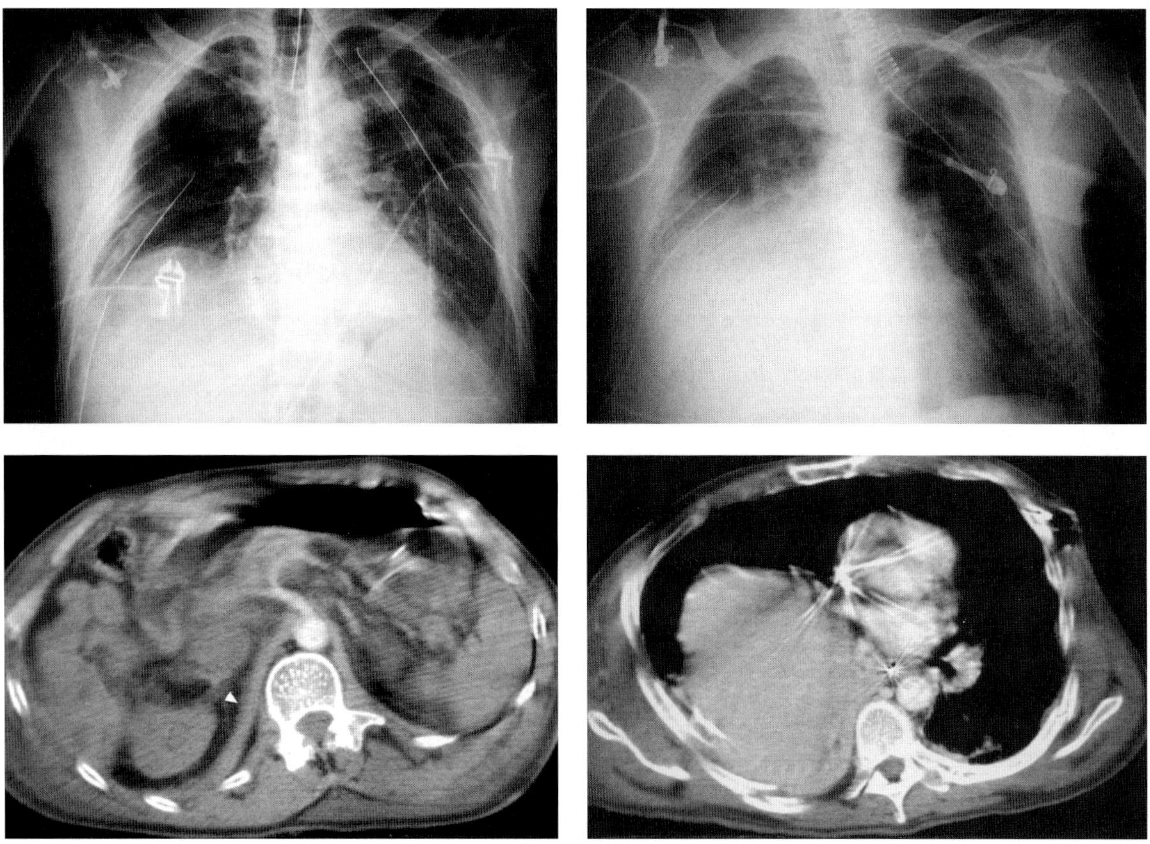

a b c d

Fig. 9.3a–d. A 50-year-old male was admitted after a frontal car crash collision. **a** Initial chest radiograph revealed a slight elevation of the right hemidiaphragm. The patient became shocked and required intensive resuscitation. (**b**) A repeat chest radiograph 1 h later showed a marked elevation of the anticipated level of an obscured right hemidiaphragm. (**c**) The diagnosis of right-sided phrenic rupture was shown by CT and laparotomy. Notice thickening of the right crus of the diaphragm (*arrow*) and (**d**) intrathoracic location of the liver

Table 9.5. Sensitivity of chest radiographs for the diagnosis of blunt diaphragmatic rupture

Reference	Left-sided			Right-sided		
	Suggestive signs	Diagnostic or highly suggestive signs	Frequency of at least suggestive signs (%)	Suggestive signs	Diagnostic or highly suggestive signs	Frequency of at least suggestive signs (%)
Gelman et al. (1991)	6/44	28/44	77	1/6	1/6	33
Willsher and Cade (1991)	2/14	11/14	93	3/4	1/4	100
Guth et al. (1995)	18/44	24/44	72	5/11	0/11	45
Shapiro et al. (1996)	NS	NS	71	NS	NS	0
Pikoulis et al. (2000)	2/15	13/15	100	NS	NS	100

NS, not specified

9.8.2.1 Positive Signs

The positive signs for phrenic injury are often subtle at CT:

- Complete absence of visualization of one hemidiaphragm
- Direct visualization of a diaphragmatic defect
- Herniation of abdominal organs into the thoracic cavity through a defect
- With or without a waist-like area of constriction, the so-called collar sign
- Thickening of the diaphragmatic leaflet, the so-called curled diaphragm sign
- Absence of interposition of lung parenchyma between the cephalic part of the upper abdominal organs and the posterior thoracic wall, the so-called dependent viscera sign (Gurney et al. 1985; Demos et al. 1989; Low and Kelsey 1990; Holland and Quint 1991; Leung et al. 1999; Sadeghi et al. 1999; Koplewitz et al. 2000; Bergin et al. 2001)
- Thoracic fluid abutting the intra-abdominal viscera or the inverse
- Presence of both pneumothorax and pneumoperitoneum
- Presence of both haemothorax and haemoperitoneum (Murray et al. 1996)

9.8.2.2 Pitfalls

As for chest radiographs, any condition that increases pleural pressure such as positive pressure ventilation tends to prevent herniation through a phrenic defect, thus making the diagnosis difficult on CT (Voeller et al. 1990; Shapiro et al. 1996; Karmy-Jones et al. 2002).

The normal diaphragm appears as a linear and regular soft-tissue density structure overlying the upper abdominal organs. Thus the portions of the diaphragm adjacent to the spleen and the liver may go undetected in patients who have little or no fatty tissue interposition below the diaphragm. This fact probably accounts for some of the undiagnosed diaphragmatic ruptures. Interposition of fluid on both sides of the diaphragm may blur its muscular part at CT, leading to false-positive and false-negative diagnosis of rupture.

There are great variations concerning the most sensitive sign of diaphragmatic rupture at CT, which is a phrenic defect (Fig. 9.4). Diaphragmatic defects lying on the posterolateral aspect of the diaphragm are found in up to 11% of healthy adults, and their incidence increases with ageing (Caskey et al. 1989). Except the knowledge of their existence and position, no reliable mean can differentiate these congenital defects from posttraumatic defects (Fig. 9.5).

Diaphragmatic thickening may represent either retraction of the leaves of the torn diaphragm or haematoma (Fig. 9.6). Furthermore, ageing patients may develop focal diaphragm muscle thickening, alone or in association with defects. Thus this sign must be interpreted cautiously in trauma patients (Fig. 9.7).

9.8.2.3 Results

In initial series reporting the value of CT for the diagnosis of blunt diaphragmatic rupture, 50–100% of injuries were missed and CT was said to lack sensitivity (Demos et al. 1989; Voeller et al. 1990; Gelman et al. 1991). Among recent series, using faster spiral scanning techniques, overall sensitivities of 42% and 22% were reported, respectively (Voeller et al. 1990; Nau et al. 2001). It was not specified if the results were those of the initial interpretation or if the initial scans were retrospectively reviewed by blinded independent readers, as for other studies that reported combined sensitivities of 57–90%

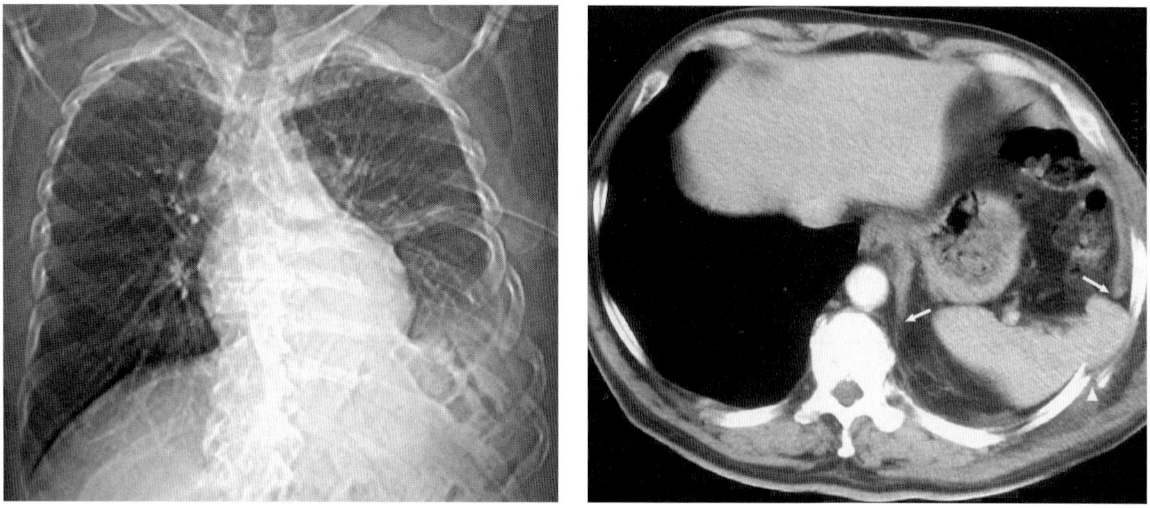

a b

Fig. 9.4. a,b A 32-year-old male was admitted after a left lateral impact from a car crash. (**a**) CT scout view of the thorax showed left elevation of hemidiaphragm, basal lung consolidation and rib fractures. (**b**) IV contrast-enhanced CT showed a large left-sided posterior diaphragmatic defect (*between arrows*) with spleen abutting the posterior chest wall and herniating partially through a lateral defect caused by a fractured rib (*arrowhead*)

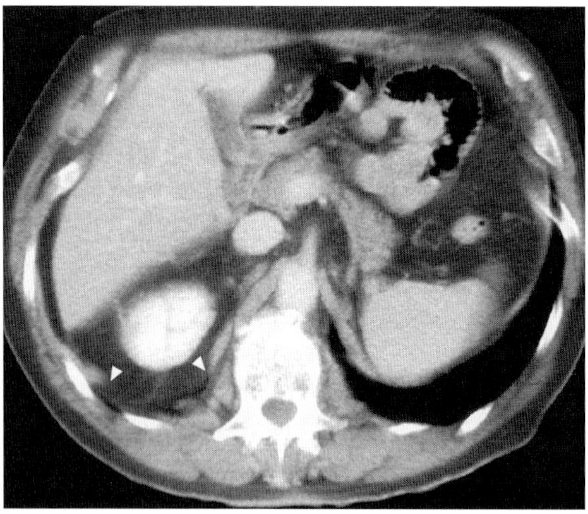

Fig. 9.5. A 64-year-old male admitted after a car crash with thoracic impact had multiple rib fractures. IV contrast-enhanced CT revealed a right posterolateral defect of the diaphragm (*arrowheads*) without herniation and simulating a phrenic injury. In this aged patient, the non-visibility of the diaphragm was a normal finding, and the recovery was uneventful

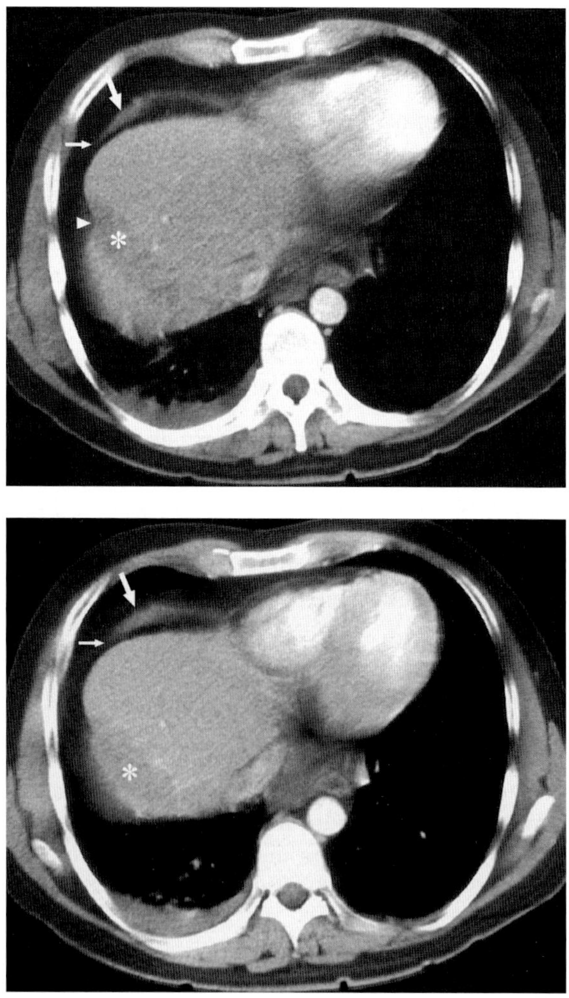

a b

Fig. 9.6 a,b. A 32-year-old male was admitted after a frontal ▷ impact during a car crash, with multiple rib and pelvic fractures (**a, b**). IV contrast-enhanced CT revealed a lateral defect of the right hemidiaphragm (*small arrow*). The liver was partially herniated, with a focal area of constriction through the defect (*arrowhead*). The anterior leaf of the ruptured diaphragm was retracted and thickened (*large arrow*). Note also the liver contusion (*asterisk*) and right pleural effusion

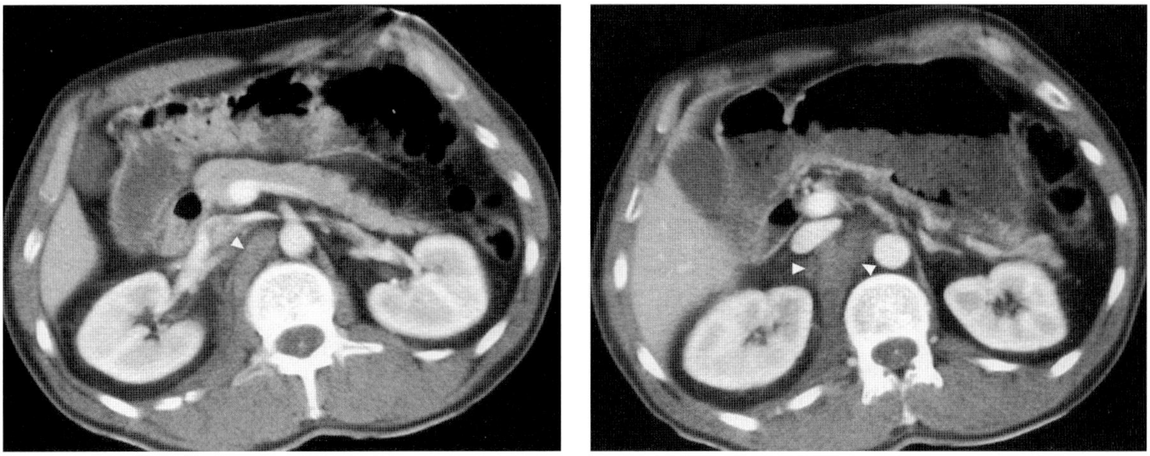

a b

Fig. 9.7a, b. A 52-year-old male was found comatose in his car after a collision with a tree; he had multiple facial fractures and a dissection of the left internal carotid artery (**a, b**). IV contrast-enhanced CT revealed a marked thickening of the postero-medial aspect of the right hemidiaphragm (*arrowheads*), without defect. The patient deceased and a right hemidiaphragmatic haematoma was found at autopsy, without full thickness rupture

and 87–100% specificities (Table 9.6) (Worthy et al. 1995; Murray et al. 1996; Shapiro et al. 1996; Killeen et al. 1999; Leung et al. 1999; Koplewitz et al. 2000; Bergin et al. 2001). Most authors agreed that at the time of review it remained unclear why either positive or negative cases were wrongly diagnosed at initial interpretation (Worthy et al. 1995). Large variations in the interobserver agreement were also reported (Murray et al. 1996).

The single detector spiral technique allows reliable sagittal and coronal reconstruction. Although rarely used during the acute setting of a traumatized patient, coronal reconstructions may be useful in selected cases, in order to visualize the diaphragm in a plane perpendicular to the tangential or oblique planes obtained with axial scanning (Killeen et al. 1999). Decreasing the slice thickness from 10 to 3 mm or less is another factor that enabled improvement of the diagnostic value of CT, even for defects smaller than 5 mm (Killeen et al. 1999). Thus recent multislice scanners, which scan faster with thinner and almost isotropic voxels, allowing anatomic and artefact-free coronal reconstructions, will probably give the diagnosis of blunt diaphragmatic rupture in almost all cases (Fig. 9.8). This technique may also play a role in the future in penetrating trauma that causes smaller diaphragmatic defects, as it has been shown that actual CT technology is unreliable in this indication (Rehm et al. 1989).

Table 9.6. Sensitivity of CT for the diagnosis of blunt diaphragmatic rupture

Reference	Sensitivity Right-sided	Left-sided	Overall (%)
Worthy et al. (1995)	2/3	7/8	82
Murray et al. (1996)	2/3	7/8	82
Shapiro et al. (1996)	NS	NS	42
Killeen et al. (1999)	3/6	14/18	70
Leung et al. (1999)	1/1	5/7	75
Koplewitz et al. (2000)	NS	NS	57
Bergin et al. (2001)	5/6	4/4	90

NS, not specified

9.8.3 Ultrasound

Ultrasound (US) is largely available and is used at the patient' bed for the evaluation of intraperitoneal or pleural fluid (Doust et al. 1975; Landay and Harless 1977). Focused assessment with sonography for trauma patients (FAST) has actually replaced peritoneal lavage, in particular for haemodynamically unstable patients (Boulanger et al. 1998, 2001; Bode et al. 1999; Dondelinger et al. 2002). The first reported US diagnosis of penetrating diaphragmatic rupture was made on a patient in clinical phase 3 (Ammann et al. 1983).

Advantages of US include multiplanar capacity and high spatial resolution. Disadvantages are poor reproducibility, limited use for imaging air or calcium-containing and deep structures.

The in vivo sonographic appearance of the diaphragm is made of a variable number of echoic lines, strongly related to the reflectivity of the peridiaphragmatic structures. Isolated phrenic models appear as a regular and continuous echoic thin line at the level

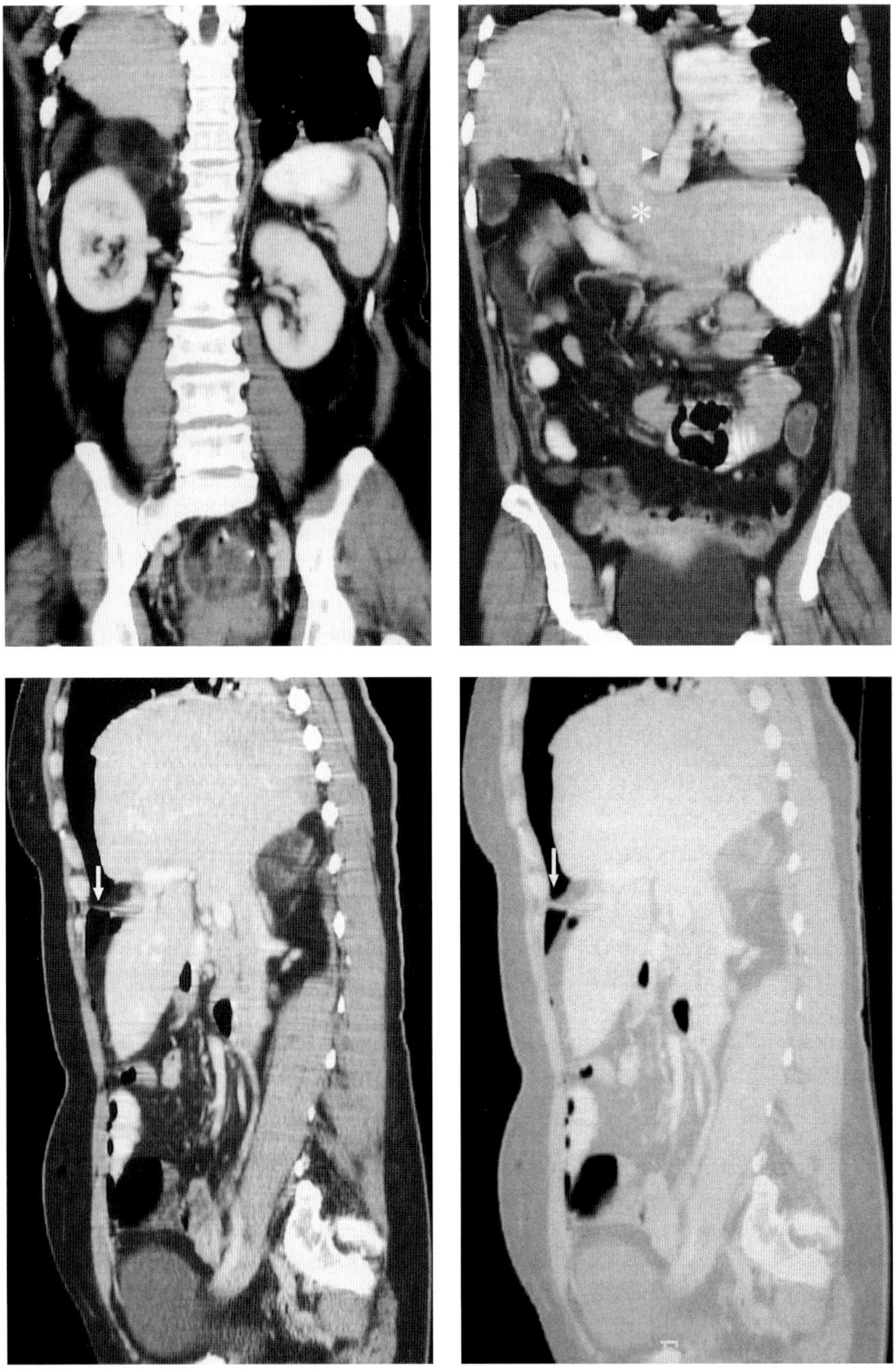

a b

c d

Fig. 9.8a–d. A 43-year-old female was admitted after a fall from a height of 3 m. Body CT after IV and oral contrast was performed during a 15-s breath hold with a multiple-detector spiral scanner and 3-mm-thick slices (**a**): coronal reformatting revealed absence of the posteromedial aspect of the right hemidiaphragm (**b**), associated with herniation of the right lobe of the liver. The upward movement of the right lobe of the liver resulted in a focal tightening of the segment IV (*asterisk*) and displacement of the inferior vena cava (*arrowhead*) (**c**). On sagittal reformatting, the anterior thickened part of the diaphragm was visible (*arrow*) (**d**). The patient had both a pneumoperitoneum and pneumothorax. Both air collections were seen above and below the diaphragm (*arrow*) of the central tendon, while the muscular part is represented by two close parallel echoic lines, both representing interfaces with adjacent fluid, separated by a hypoechoic line representing the muscle (Verschakelen et al. 1989). Thus, the more pleural fluid there is, the more US is effective.

9.8.3.1 Positive Signs

As for the other cross-section imaging techniques, direct signs of diaphragmatic rupture include discontinuity of the diaphragm, non-visualized floating diaphragm, and direct visualization of the intrathoracic herniated organs (Fig. 9.9).

9.8.3.2 Pitfalls

Although not described in the literature, discontinuities of the diaphragm as a variation in the normal ageing patient are a potential source of false-positive US screening. Anisotropic artefact is another source of potential misdiagnosis in phrenic US.

If air-containing lung abuts the diaphragm, it may become impossible to distinguish the diaphragm

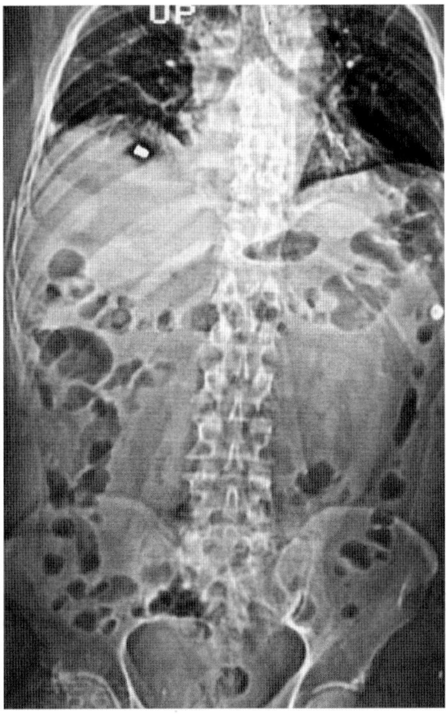

a

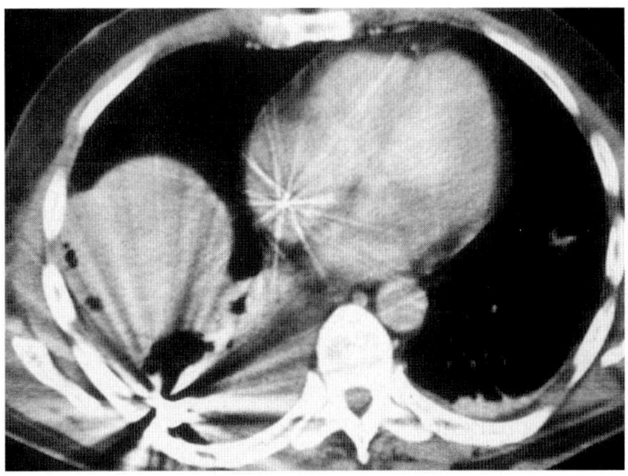

b

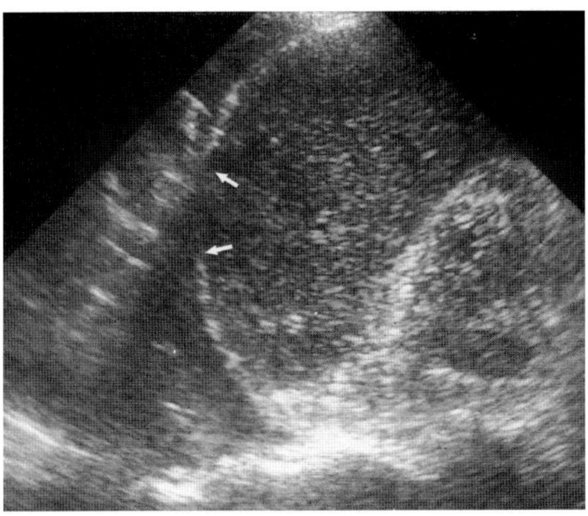

c

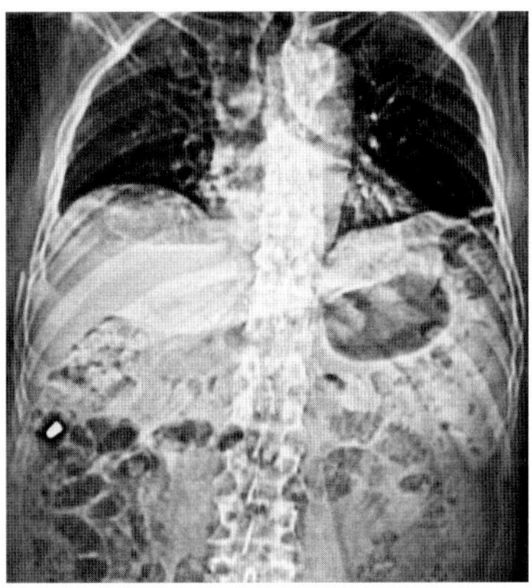

d

Fig. 9.9a–d. A 55-year-old male was transferred after having been shot in the right lower thorax 3 days earlier. (**a**) CT scout view showed right rib fractures and a bullet projecting over the right lobe of the liver. (**b**) CT showed the bullet located in the posterior costophrenic sulcus associated with pleural fluid. (**c**) US showed a normal appearance of the liver and a localized interruption of the right hemidiaphragm (*arrows*), suggesting a diaphragmatic tear without liver herniation of the liver. (**d**) CT scout view obtained 2 days later showed that the bullet has migrated in the abdominal cavity were it appeared located in the right paracolic gutter on axial cuts (not shown). (Courtesy of Professor J. Pringot) from the underlying lung and thus to identify discontinuity of the diaphragm. Pneumothorax, subcutaneous emphysema, chest-wall and abdominal pain, bandages as well as gas within the stomach and the splenic flexure are occurrences that may limit the use of US (Kim et al. 1997).

9.8.3.3 Results

Only case reports and limited series in the literature have illustrated the usefulness of US, regardless of the clinical phase of the patients (Ammann et al. 1983; Newman and Davis 1989; Fung and Vickar 1991; Kim et al. 1997). The examination is rarely performed at admission, where use of CT prevails. The sensitivity of US in detecting rupture of the diaphragm seems to be almost perfect on both sides, with an unknown specificity.

9.8.4 Magnetic Resonance Imaging

The first report of an injury of the diaphragm diagnosed by magnetic resonance Imaging (MRI) was published in the late 1980s (Mirvis et al. 1988). The advantage of MRI is multiplanar imaging capacity, allowing direct sagittal and coronal scanning planes, high tissue contrast resolution, cardiac and respiratory gating possibilities and obviously the lack of ionizing radiation. High-gradient machines allow almost real-time imaging of the diaphragmatic motion. The main disadvantage is limited accessibility for monitored patients, which prevents its use in acutely traumatized patients.

The normal diaphragm appears as a continuous arch-like flat structure, with the same signal as parietal muscles in all sequences. Thus the diaphragm may be of low signal compared to the underlying fat and abdominal organs and of high signal compared to air-filled lungs on T1- and T2-weighed sequences. Lung consolidation and pleural effusion have a higher signal intensity than the diaphragm on T2-weighted images.

Adequate scanning parameters for imaging of the diaphragm includes 5–10 mm slice thickness in axial, sagittal and coronal planes. Spin-echo T1-weighted (repetition time: ±500 ms) or T2-weighted (repetition time: >1500 ms) technique may be used. However, respiratory and cardiac gating is mandatory, since this technique requires long scanning times. Fast gradient-echo pulse acquisitions shorten the repetition time to a few milliseconds and overall scanning time, to allow examinations in a breath-hold of a few seconds without cardiac gating. Intravenous contrast administration is superfluous for imaging the diaphragm.

9.8.4.1 Positive Signs

Positive signs of phrenic injury include constant discontinuity of the diaphragm in all imaged planes and fat or visceral herniation through a phrenic defect, and loss of the homogeneity of the hemidiaphragm (Mirvis et al. 1988) (Fig. 9.10).

9.8.4.2 Pitfalls

A theoretical risk of imaging a so-called pseudo-diaphragm arising from a circumferential chemical-shift artefact is related to the use of fast gradient-echo pulse technique. Although this artefact is unlikely to alter the interpretation of the integrity of the diaphragm, knowledge is mandatory to avoid misdiagnosis. Otherwise, fat suppression inherent to gradient-echo images may impair the visualization of the diaphragm. Thus, when possible, spin-echo sequences should be preferred.

9.8.4.3 Results

The literature concerning MRI for diagnosis of phrenic injuries is made of case reports and few selected cases within large series (Mirvis et al. 1988; Newman and Davis 1989; Daum-Kowalski et al. 1991; Boulanger et al. 1992; Carter et al. 1996; Sadeghi et al. 1999). In a series of 16 patients with suspicious findings of left diaphragmatic hernia on chest radiographs, a sensitivity and a specificity of 100% were found (Shanmuganathan et al. 1996).

9.8.5 Opacifications of the Gastrointestinal Tract

Before the advent of section imaging techniques, opacifications of the gastrointestinal tract were the most useful to confirm or to supply chest radiographic findings when diaphragmatic injury was suspected. Nowadays, they may still be useful in selected cases, and are quickly and easily performed through a nasogastric tube with hydrosoluble contrast agents in acutely injured patients. Barium opacifications

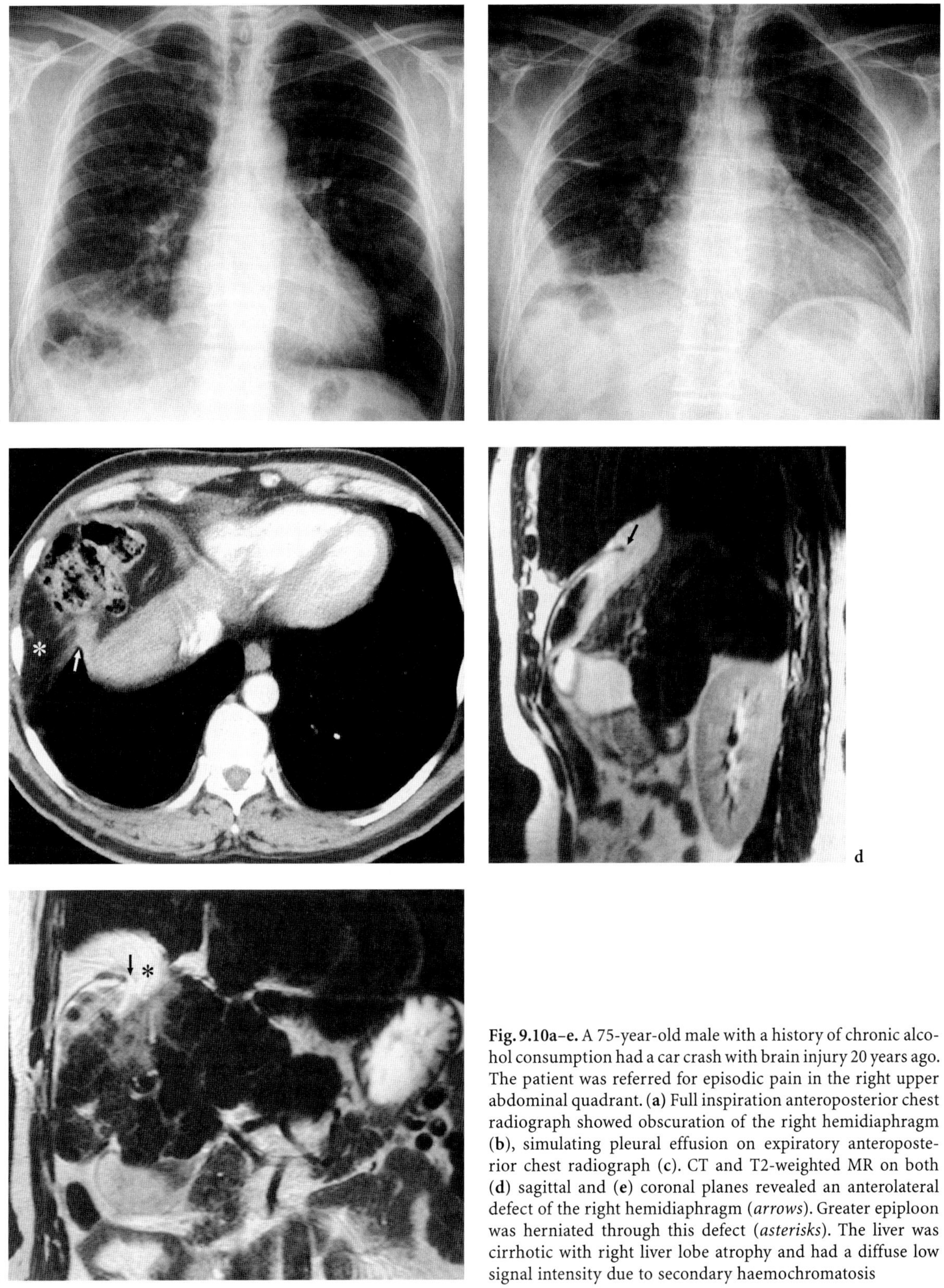

Fig. 9.10a–e. A 75-year-old male with a history of chronic alcohol consumption had a car crash with brain injury 20 years ago. The patient was referred for episodic pain in the right upper abdominal quadrant. (**a**) Full inspiration anteroposterior chest radiograph showed obscuration of the right hemidiaphragm (**b**), simulating pleural effusion on expiratory anteroposterior chest radiograph (**c**). CT and T2-weighted MR on both (**d**) sagittal and (**e**) coronal planes revealed an anterolateral defect of the right hemidiaphragm (*arrows*). Greater epiploon was herniated through this defect (*asterisks*). The liver was cirrhotic with right liver lobe atrophy and had a diffuse low signal intensity due to secondary haemochromatosis

and air insufflation should be reserved for patients in clinical phase 2. Relative frequency of herniation of hollow viscus implies that rectal opacification should not be performed unless oral opacification is negative or there are evident signs of large-bowel obstruction. Follow-through examination of the small intestine and enteroclysis should be avoided, since the small bowel as the only hollow viscus herniated is an uncommon occurrence.

9.8.5.1 Positive Signs

With digestive tract opacifications, the most typical diagnostic appearance in phrenic injuries is a contrast-filled loop of bowel, herniated through the diaphragm, with approximation and narrowing of its afferent and efferent limbs as they pass through the tear (Fataar and Schulman 1979) (Fig. 9.11). However, the efferent limb may be narrowed so as to prevent contrast medium getting into the herniated loop. The efferent limb may be narrowed enough to prevent contrast medium going beyond the loop (Carter et al. 1951).

9.8.5.2 Pitfalls

Even when phrenic injury is suspected by means of clinical or radiographic findings, stomach and colon would be normal in the absence of herniation. Large diaphragmatic defects that are frequently encountered in blunt and crush injuries may lead to a false-negative, since they produce no approximation of limbs.

Herniation of the gastric fundus alone is a particular occurrence that may lead to false-negative opacifications, since this part of the stomach is a blind alley that may not be opacified in decubitus. In these cases, if tilting the patient head down results in only a short projection pointing towards the gastric fundus, hernia must be suspected on the basis of the so-called amputated fundus sign (Fataar and Schulman 1979).

9.8.5.3 Results

Few collective data exist in the literature on the value of gastrointestinal tract opacification in the diagnosis of diaphragmatic injuries, since they are used only in selected cases. In 49 patients with phrenic injuries diagnosed intraoperatively, regardless of the causative agent and the clinical phase, chest radiographs were normal in 2 of the 25 patients who had herniation and 8 of the remaining 24 who had no herniation. In all cases with normal chest radiographs, the diagnosis was not established by gastrointestinal tract opacification. However, in this series, opacifications were shown to be sensitive for patients with nonspecific chest radiograph anomalies and to be specific for phrenic injuries (Fataar and Schulman 1979).

9.8.6 Peritoneography

The following group of imaging tests is based on the visualization of the intrathoracic migration of a contrast agent introduced in the peritoneal cavity.

9.8.6.1 Technique

Iodinated Contrast Peritoneography

Although it was not primarily designed for the diagnosis of diaphragmatic rupture, iodinated peritoneography was successfully used in this indication (Efron and Hyde 1967). However, due to poor acceptance, this technique has disappeared from the diagnostic test armamentarium.

Diagnostic Pneumoperitoneum

Diagnostic pneumoperitoneum was described as a preoperative diagnostic test for phrenic injuries in the middle of the 20th century (Clay and Hanlon 1951). The technique requires performance of an erect chest radiograph after instillation of 300–500 ml of air inside the peritoneal cavity, by the same hole used for diagnostic peritoneal lavage, after having ensured that the former is negative. The technique has its main disadvantages in the possible creation of a tension pneumothorax or abdominal viscus perforation, and intensification of abdominal symptoms or shoulder pain (Brooks 1978).

Radioisotopes

Intraperitoneal instillation of radioisotopes for the diagnosis of diaphragmatic rupture was first used in animal models (Pecoraro et al. 1985; Rappaport et al. 1988; Halldorsson et al. 1992). The technique was successfully applied in humans by instillation of 800 μCi of Tc-99 through a peritoneal lavage catheter (Cesani et al. 1996).

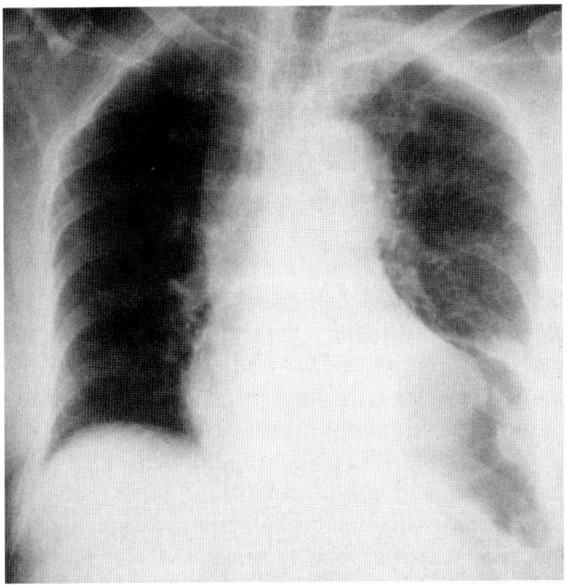

a

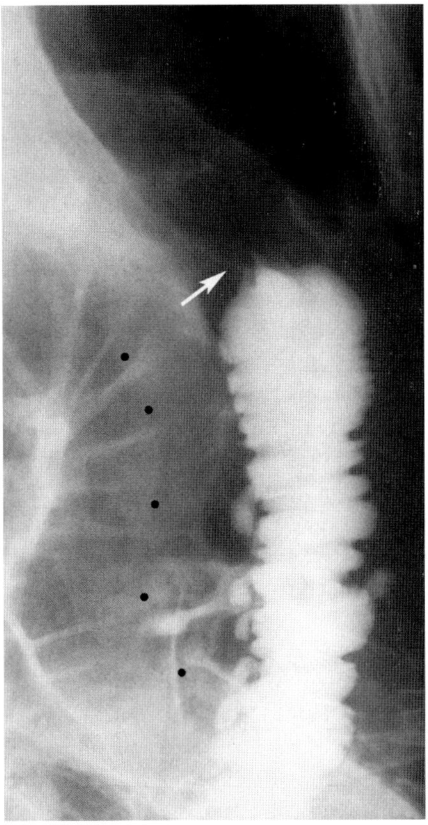

b

Fig. 9.11a, b. A middle aged female with a medical history of blunt thoracoabdominal trauma was admitted for acute bowel obstruction. (**a**) Chest radiograph showed an elevated left hemidiaphragm and dilated bowel projecting over the left hemithorax. (**b**) Water-soluble contrast enema showed the distal end of an incarcerated transdiaphragmatic colon hernia (*arrow*) and the dilatation of the proximal colon (*dots*). (Courtesy of Professor J. Pringot)

MR Peritoneography

In this technique, saline or isotonic glucose solution is instilled inside the peritoneal cavity before scanning with heavily T2-weighted sequences (Prokesch et al. 2000).

9.8.6.2 Positive Signs

For all the above-described techniques, the only sign of diaphragmatic rupture on postinstillation imaging is the intrathoracic detection of the marker instilled inside the peritoneal cavity.

9.8.6.3 Pitfalls

In conventional radiographic and magnetic resonance peritoneographs, it is mandatory to image first the chest to detect the presence of already present pneumothorax or pleural effusion, which are frequent in traumatized patients. Overlooking these conditions may lead to a false-positive results, unless the difference between the pre- and postinstillation volumes of pleural fluid has been accurately assessed and found significant.

Patients with diaphragmatic rupture in clinical phase 2 may develop adhesions between herniated organs and the pleura, which may prevent intrathoracic migration of peritoneal contrast or radio-isotope. Furthermore, small defects of the diaphragm may be covered by an abdominal viscus, with subsequent prevention of the intrathoracic migration of the peritoneal marker into the chest, leading to false-negative peritoneographs, particularly on the right side. Incomplete coverage of these defects leads to slow intrathoracic migration. In these instances, early postinstillation imaging will be falsely negative and late imaging, with more than 1 h delay, may be useful in selected cases (Cesani et al. 1996).

Obviously, retroperitoneal ruptures of the diaphragm are unlikely to be detected by peritoneographs.

9.8.6.4 Results

Although successful for the diagnosis of diaphragmatic rupture in all cases reported, the real sensitivity and specificity of peritoneographs are unknown.

9.8.7
Arteriography

Angiography may be indicated at admission or later, when CT has shown contrast extravasation originating or accumulating in the vicinity of the diaphragm. Inferior phrenic arteries may bleed rarely, but profusely, but rarely in blunt or penetrating phrenic injuries. Haemorrhage may also be related to injury to other arteries such as the phrenic branches of the internal mammary artery or intercostal arteries. In the past, angiography was said to be indicated when cross-section imaging remained dubious (Wenz and Reinhold 1982).

Displacement of main arterial feeders or of an entire organ in the thorax was able to confirm transphrenic herniation of abdominal visceral content. Interruption of arterial supply or stagnant venous flow is suggestive of strangulation. Today, angiography is restricted to haemostatic indications.

9.8.8
Other Techniques

Cases of incidental positive diagnosis of diaphragmatic rupture, made by endoscopy, transsternal or transoesophageal echocardiography or angiography have been reported, while these examinations were performed in patients presenting symptoms of tamponade, low-grade bowel obstruction or abdominal bleeding (Larrieu et al. 1980; Reinbold et al. 1987; Fleyfel et al. 1994; Colliver et al. 1997; Junk et al. 2001).

Liver scintigraphy alone or combined with lung scintigraphy have also been reported to be successful in demonstration of liver hernia, with a band-like photon-deficient collar through right-sided diaphragmatic defects (Bockslaff and Brase 1975; Blumenthal et al. 1984).

9.9
Management

In traumatized and haemodynamically unstable patients, phrenic injuries are discovered at time of surgery, unless there are suggestive signs on chest radiographs, focused abdominal US or both. These diagnostic tests are, with an increasing uniformity, the most recommended for unstable patients after truncal trauma, in order to identify potential life-threatening effusions and to guide surgery by identifying the internal cavity in which there is ongoing bleeding.

For haemodynamically stable patients who are unlikely to undergo surgery, the natural history of the injured diaphragm implies that surgical treatment should be applied as soon as the diagnosis is made. Patients in this condition may allow the use of less invasive surgical techniques. With an incidence as high as 75%, patients with penetrating trauma to the lower chest or the upper abdomen have a high index of suspicion index of phrenic injuries. Thus, although selective nonoperative management has been proposed, based on the site of penetration, and on clinical or US and CT findings, surgery remains indicated in most of these cases, even with negative radiographic findings (Velmahos et al. 1997; Chiu et al. 2001). Overall, due to multiplicity of surgical techniques and clinical conditions, there is actually no consensus in the surgical literature concerning the management of phrenic injuries.

9.9.1
Open Surgery

9.9.1.1
Clinical Phase 1

Laparotomy is the leading life-saving procedure in haemodynamically unstable polytraumatized patients. Life-threatening injuries associated with phrenic injuries occur commonly in the upper abdomen. Laparotomy is the most commonly used surgical technique for both the diagnosis and the treatment of clinical phase 1 patients (Pagliarello and Carter 1992; Lee et al. 1994; Shah et al. 1995).

In this group, when imaging and clinical signs of severe thoracic organ injury are present without evidence of bleeding abdominal organ injury, thoracotomy replaces laparotomy as a gold standard for both diagnosis and treatment of phrenic injuries. However, since thoracotomy explores only one hemidiaphragm, there is a theoretical risk of missing a phrenic injury on the opposite side.

With open surgery, herniated organs are most often reintegrated easily into the abdomen and diaphragmatic defects are closed by direct non-resorbable sutures. In a few cases, the size of the defect requires interposition of a prosthesis, or plicature (Waldhausen et al. 1966; Slim et al. 1998). Intraoperative difficulties include reinsertion of irregular avulsed costal attachments on fractured ribs and posterior right-sided diaphragmatic ruptures. With this technique, secondary diaphragmatic ruptures after surgical cure are rare occurrences (Hood 1971;

KAMELGARD et al. 1999). Suturing leaves of the torn diaphragm to abutting organs was proposed as an alternative surgical cure; however, this technique is no longer in use, since it has been shown that more than one-third of patients presented relapse soon after operation (HEDBLOM 1925).

Subsequent thoracotomy may be indicated during a life-saving laparotomy and vice versa, or a primary thoracoabdominal approach may be indicated. In a series of 86 patients with diaphragmatic injuries, subsequent thoracotomy occurred in 1 out of 65 laparotomies, while subsequent laparotomy occurred in 7 out of 15 thoracotomies (WALDSCHMIDT and LAWS 1980).

9.9.1.2
Clinical Phases 2 and 3

In these phases, abdominal organ injuries do not exist or have been corrected. Diaphragmatic hernias are associated with the risk of adhesions between herniated organs and the pleural cavity, which make the reduction by laparotomy difficult and require extensive dissection. Thus thoracotomy should be the preferred technique in this patient group (MANSOUR 1997; NAUNHEIM 1998). The same rule is of value for pericardiophrenic ruptures, as shown in a collective review: 25 out of 35 patients (71%) managed by an abdominal approach were diagnosed in clinical phase 1; conversely, 18 out of the 24 patients (75%) managed by a thoracic approach were diagnosed in clinical phases 2 or 3 (REINA et al. 2001).

9.9.2
Video-Assisted Surgery

Laparoscopic and thoracoscopic surgery have now gained wide acceptance. They were first used in trauma patients in the 1970s (GAZZANIGA et al. 1976; CARNEVALE et al. 1977); nowadays, they may be successfully used in both penetrating and blunt truncal trauma patients to replace open surgical techniques in selected indications (ADAMTHWAITE 1984; IVATURY et al. 1993; OCHSNER et al. 1993; WONG et al. 1995; LEPPANIEMI and ELLIOTT 1996; ORTEGA et al. 1996; ZANTUT et al. 1997; ABOLHODA et al. 1997; MURRAY et al. 1998; MINEO et al. 1999; MATZ et al. 2000; MARTINEZ et al. 2001; FREEMAN et al. 2001). The most consensual point of these indications is that haemodynamic stability of the patient is mandatory.

Intraoperative difficulties are similar to those of open surgical techniques; laparoscopy is the preferred technique for clinical phase 1 patients and thoracoscopy for clinical phase 2 and 3 patients. However, insufficient pneumoperitoneum, which is described as a relatively frequent difficulty for laparoscopy in the presence of a phrenic injury, and large diaphragmatic desinsertions, which classically do not favour thoracoscopic treatment, are among factors leading to conversion in open surgery (LANG-LAZDUNSKI et al. 1997).

Missed heterolateral diaphragmatic rupture and associated injuries (especially intestinal and retroperitoneal injuries) are theoretical limitations for thoracoscopy and laparoscopy, respectively. Relative contraindications for laparotomy include patients with altered cardiac function, elevated intracranial pressure and multiple previous abdominal operations (HO et al. 1993; JOSEPHS et al. 1994). Those for thoracoscopy include inability for patients to tolerate single lung ventilation and obliteration of the pleural space by adhesions (SIMON and IVATURY 1995).

Mortality related to endoscopic surgical procedures vary from 0% to 1.5%; many of these deaths are not related directly to the procedure itself (BERCI 1993; ORLANDO et al. 1993). In a few cases, laparoscopic procedures may be complicated during material insertion and insufflation by preperitoneal insufflation, tension pneumothorax, vascular and intestinal injuries, CO_2 embolism and cardiac dysrhythmias. These intraoperative complications are related to the surgeon's learning curve and seem to occur more frequently in laparotomies than in thoracotomies (SIMON and IVATURY 1995; LEPPANIEMI and ELLIOTT 1996).

9.9.3
Nonsurgical Management

Rather than indicating a possibility of nonoperative management, spontaneous healing of small penetrating injuries to the diaphragm in animal models suggests that some patients with similar undiagnosed injuries might have healed spontaneously (ZIEROLD et al. 2001). However, potential complications of such injuries implies treating them as diagnosis is made. In one reported case of posttraumatic diaphragmatic crus rupture, nonoperative management was successful; however, follow-up imaging findings were not specified (SHANMUGANATHAN et al. 1996). Although rarely mentioned in the literature, not all phrenic injuries result in full-thickness rupture. Single intramuscular haematomas that do not require surgery may be even more frequent than ruptures in blunt trauma. These observations could be of importance, as imaging techniques may actually reflect the type and location of the diaphragmatic injury and promote expectant nonoperative management in selected cases.

9.10 Outcome

9.10.1 Postsurgical Complications

Postsurgical mortality is related to associated injuries rather than to the surgical cure of phrenic injury. Classic postoperative complications include multiple organ failure, pulmonary embolism, pleural empyema, pneumonia, peritoneal abscess and sterile effusions.

Postoperative complications may occur relatively more commonly for cardiophrenic ruptures. In a review of the literature, seven postoperative deaths occurred from underlying associated injuries or multiple organ failure out of 81 patients, yielding a 9.4% morbidity for patients that had pericardiophrenic ruptures (Reina et al. 2001). Classic postoperative complications include pericardial effusions (Laric et al. 1989; Valestaqui and Mehran 1999); however, tamponade is a rare occurrence (Le Treut et al. 1981).

9.10.2 Grading of Injuries and Predictors of Outcome

9.10.2.1 Grading of Injury

The Organ Injury Scaling Committee of the American Association for the Surgery of Trauma has graded diaphragm injuries into five grades, from simple contusion (grade I) to laceration with tissue loss >25 cm^2 (grade V) (Moore et al. 1994).

This classification is anatomic and does not include pericardiophrenic ruptures. No attempt in the current literature has been made to correlate this classification to the trauma severity and the outcome.

9.10.2.2 Predictors of Outcome

In phase I patients, the Injury Severity Scale (ISS) score related to diaphragmatic injury alone is 9, which correlates with a survival coefficient of 0.99 (Baker et al. 1974). However, the high incidence of associated life-threatening injuries alters both the ISS and survival (Simpson et al. 2000). For penetrating trauma, the effects of the wounding agent may be an important factor conditioning survival, as it influences the severity of associated injuries. As for patients in other clinical phases, the prognosis is related to the mortality and morbidity of acute gastrointestinal obstruction that may be fatal in up to 60% of cases (Carter et al. 1951; Grage et al. 1959; Gourin and Garzon 1974; Miller et al. 1984; Cruz and Minagi 1994; Groskin 1992; Reber et al. 1998).

9.11 Conclusion

Diaphragmatic injuries have entered the new millennium as one of the most unrecognized and undiagnosed. Morbidity and mortality of diaphragmatic injuries implies that a high index of suspicion should be maintained in patients who have sustained severe blunt trauma, especially those with lateral torso impacts, multiple rib and pelvic fractures.

Similarly, the same index of suspicion should be kept with patients sustaining penetrating thoracoabdominal trauma, with entrance near the nipple line, with abnormal chest radiographs. Accurate clinical set up of these patients may provide additional positive findings, and the index should be kept elevated until the injury is ruled out by adequate imaging or surgical revision. If the injury is searched for, chest radiograph and computed tomography may allow the diagnosis in most patients in the acute setting. MRI is useful for patients in a subacute or chronic setting and patients with a high index of suspicion and negative CT.

References

Abolhoda A, Livingston DH, Donahoo JS, Allen K (1997) Diagnostic and therapeutic video-assisted thoracic surgery (VATS) following chest trauma. Eur J Cardiothorac Surg 12: 356–360
Adamthwaite DN (1984) Traumatic diaphragmatic hernia: a new indication for laparoscopy. Br J Surg 71:315
Adeyemi SD, Stephens CA (1981) Traumatic diaphragmatic hernia in children. Can J Surg 24:355–357
Ali J, Qi W (1992) The cardiorespiratory effects of increased intra-abdominal pressure in diaphragmatic rupture. J Trauma 33: 233–239
Aloise F, Rossi EM, Cadregari F et al (1994) Errors in digestive surgery. A case of tension pneumothorax during laparoscopic cholecystectomy. Minerva Chir 49:841–842

Ammann AM, Brewer WH, Maull KI, Walsh JW (1983) Traumatic rupture of the diaphragm: real-time sonographic diagnosis. AJR 140:915–916

Andrus CH, Morton JH (1970) Rupture of the diaphragm after blunt trauma. Am J Surg 119:686–693

Armstrong PA, Miller SF, Brown GR (1999) Diaphragmatic hernia seen as a late complication of laparoscopic cholecystectomy. Surg Endosc 13:817–818

Asensio JA, Demetriades D, Rodriguez A (1999) Injury to the diaphragm. In: Mattock KL, Feliciano DU, Moore EE (eds) Trauma. McGraw-Hill, New York, pp 603–631

Baker SP, O'Neill B, Haddon W Jr, Long WB (1974) The injury severity score: a method for describing patients with multiple injuries and evaluating emergency care. J Trauma 14: 187–196

Ball T, McCrory R, Smith JO, Clements JL Jr (1982) Traumatic diaphragmatic hernia: errors in diagnosis. AJR 138: 633–637

Bautz PC, Knottenbelt JC (1994) Diaphragmatic injury – a source of hazard in laparoscopy. Injury 25:401–402

Beauchamp G, Khalfallah A, Girard R, Dube S, Laurendeau F, Legros G (1984) Blunt Diaphragmatic rupture. Am J Surg 148:292–295

Bekassy SM, Dave KS, Wooler GH, Ionescu MI (1973) „Spontaneous“ and traumatic rupture of the diaphragm: long-term results. Ann Surg 177:320–324

Berci G (1993) Elective and emergent laparoscopy. World J Surg 17:8–15

Bergin D, Ennis R, Keogh C, Fenlon HM, Murray JG (2001) The "dependent viscera" sign in CT diagnosis of blunt traumatic diaphragmatic rupture. AJR 177:1137–1140

Bergqvist D, Dahlgren S, Hedelin H (1978) Rupture of the diaphragm in patients wearing seatbelts. J Trauma 18:781–783

Bernhardt LC, Lawton BR (1966) Pregnancy complicated by traumatic rupture of the diaphragm. Am J Surg 112: 918–922

Blumenthal DH, Raghu G, Rudd TG, Herman CM (1984) Diagnosis of right hemidiaphragmatic rupture by liver scintigraphy. J Trauma 24:536–538

Bockslaff H, Brase A (1975) Demonstration of a post-traumatic, transdiaphragmatic liver prolapse by combined hepatic and lung scans (author's translation). ROFO 123:400–403

Bode PJ, Edwards MJ, Kruit MC, van Vugt AB (1999) Sonography in a clinical algorithm for early evaluation of 1671 patients with blunt abdominal trauma. AJR 172:905–911

Bogers AJ, Zweers DJ, Vroom EM, Huysmans HA (1986) Cardiac subluxation in traumatic rupture of diaphragm and pericardium. Thorac Cardiovasc Surg 34:132–134

Borlase BC, Moore EE, Moore FA, Metcalf RK (1989) Penetrating wounds to the posterior chest: analysis of exigent thoracotomy and laparotomy. J Emerg Med 7:445–447

Borsari A, Villa EM, Caleffi A, Poletti G, Ambrosino A (1989) Post-traumatic intrathoracic gastric volvulus. Presentation of a clinical case. Minerva Chir 44:2275–2279

Boulanger BR, Mirvis SE, Rodriguez A (1992) Magnetic resonance imaging in traumatic diaphragmatic rupture: case reports. J Trauma 32:89–93

Boulanger BR, Milzman DP, Rosati C, Rodriguez A (1993) A comparison of right and left blunt traumatic diaphragmatic rupture. J Trauma 35:255–260

Boulanger BR, Brenneman FD, Kirkpatrick AW, McLellan BA, Nathens AB (1998) The indeterminate abdominal sonogram in multisystem blunt trauma. J Trauma 45:52–56

Boulanger BR, Kearney PA, Tsuei B, Ochoa JB (2001) The routine use of sonography in penetrating torso injury is beneficial. J Trauma 51:320–325

Bowditch HI (1853) Diaphragmatic hernia. Buffalo Med J 9: 1, 65, 94

Brandt ML, Luks FI, Spigland NA, Dilorenzo M, Laberge JM, Ouimet A (1992) Diaphragmatic injury in children. J Trauma 32:298–301

Brooks JW (1978) Blunt traumatic rupture of the diaphragm. Ann Thorac Surg 26:199–203

Broos PL, Rommens PM, Carlier H, van Leeuwen JE, Somville FJ, Gruwez JA (1989) Traumatic rupture of the diaphragm. Review of 62 successive cases. Int Surg 74:88–92

Brotman S, Shatney CH, Cowley RA (1981) False negative peritoneal lavage. Am Surg 47:309–310

Brun RC, Curt JR (1987) A case of traumatic diaphragmatic hernia presenting as acute tension pneumothorax. Injury 18:355–356

Calhoon JH, Grover FL, Trinkle JK (1992) Chest trauma. Approach and management. Clin Chest Med 13:55–67

Cameron EW, Mirvis SE (1996) Ruptured hemidiaphragm: unusual late presentation. J Emerg Med 14:53–58

Carnevale N, Baron N, Delany HM (1977) Peritoneoscopy as an aid in the diagnosis of abdominal trauma: a preliminary report. J Trauma 17:634–641

Carter BN, Giuseffi J (1948) Strangulated diaphragmatic hernia. Ann Surg 128:210–225

Carter BN, Giuseffi J, Felson B (1951) Traumatic diaphragmatic hernia. AJR 65:56–72

Carter EA, Cleverley JR, Delany DJ, Lea RE (1996) Case report: cine MRI in the diagnosis of a ruptured right hemidiaphragm. Clin Radiol 51:137–140

Carter R, Brewer LA III (1971) Strangulating diaphragmatic hernia. Ann Thorac Surg 12:281–290

Carter R, Brewer LA III, Hinshaw DB (1980) Acute gastric volvulus. A study of 25 cases. Am J Surg 140:99–106

Caskey CI, Zerhouni EA, Fishman EK, Rahmouni AD (1989) Aging of the diaphragm: a CT study. Radiology 171:385–389

Cesani F, Zuckermann JA, Patange VB, Briscoe EG (1996) Peritoneoscintigraphy using Tc-99m MAA for diagnosis of diaphragmatic disruptions in trauma patients. Clin Nucl Med 21:290–292

Chen JC, Wilson SE (1991) Diaphragmatic injuries: recognition and management in sixty-two patients. Am Surg 57: 810–815

Cherry JE (1961) Traumatic hernia of the diaphragm and spontaneous perforation of the esophagus. Hawaii Med J 20:341

Chiu WC, Shanmuganathan K, Mirvis SE, Scalea TM (2001) Determining the need for laparotomy in penetrating torso trauma: a prospective study using triple-contrast enhanced abdominopelvic computed tomography. J Trauma 51: 860–869

Clay MG, Munro AI (1971) Bilateral diaphragmatic hernia from blunt injury causing a Budd-Chiari syndrome: use of liver and spleen scan in demonstrating the defects. Ann Surg 173:321–324

Clay RC, Hanlon CR (1951) Pneumoperitoneum in the differential diagnosis of diaphragmatic hernia. J Thorac Cardiovasc Surg 21:57

Colliver C, Oller DW, Rose G, Brewer D (1997) Traumatic intrapericardial diaphragmatic hernia diagnosed by echocardiography. J Trauma 42:115–117

Coln D, Crighton J, Schorn L (1980) Successful management of hepatic vein injury from blunt trauma in children. Am J Surg 140:858–864
Coppinger WR (1960) Rupture of the diaphragm following hiatal hernia. Arch Surg 80:998
Cox CL Jr, Anderson JN, Guest JL Jr (1977) Bronchopancreatic fistula following traumatic rupture of the diaphragm. JAMA 237:1461–1463
Cruz CJ, Minagi H (1994) Large-bowel obstruction resulting from traumatic diaphragmatic hernia: imaging findings in four cases. AJR 162:843–845
Das PB (1977) Penetrating injury of the diaphragm with herniated colon leaking into the left pleural space. Int Surg 62: 463–464
Daum-Kowalski R, Shanley DJ, Murphy T (1991) MRI diagnosis of delayed presentation of traumatic diaphragmatic hernia. Gastrointest Radiol 16:298–300
Dave KS, Bekassy SM, Wooler GH, Ionescu MI (1973) "Spontaneous" rupture of the diaphragm during delivery. Br J Surg 60:666–668
Dawson R, Ferguson CJ (1997) Life-threatening tension pneumothorax during laparoscopic cholecystectomy. Surg Laparosc Endosc 7:271–272
De la Rocha AG, Creel RJ, Mulligan GW, Burns CM (1982) Diaphragmatic rupture due to blunt abdominal trauma. Surg Gynecol Obstet 154:175–180
Demos TC, Solomon C, Posniak HV, Flisak MJ (1989) Computed tomography in traumatic defects of the diaphragm. Clin Imaging 13:62–67
De Rooij PD, Haarman HJ (1993) Herniation of the stomach into the pericardial sac combined with cardiac luxation caused by blunt trauma: a case report. J Trauma 34: 453–454
Desforges G, Strieder JW, Lynch JP, Maddoff IM (1957) Traumatic rupture of the diaphragm: clinical manifestations and surgical treatment. J Thorac Surg 34:779–797
Dondelinger RF, Trotteur G, Ghaye B, Szapiro D (2002) Traumatic injuries: radiological hemostatic intervention at admission. Eur Radiol 12:979–993
Doust BD, Baum JK, Maklad NF, Doust VL (1975) Ultrasonic evaluation of pleural opacities. Radiology 114:135–140
Drews JA, Mercer EC, Benfield JR (1973) Acute diaphragmatic injuries. Ann Thorac Surg 16:67–78
Duverger V, Saliou C, Le P et al (2001) Blunt force rupture of the thoracic aorta and diaphragm: an unusual association. Ann Chir 126:339–345
Ebert PA, Gaertner RA, Zuidema GD (1967) Traumatic diaphragmatic hernia. Surg Gynecol Obstet 125:59–65
Efron G, Hyde I (1967) Non-penetrating traumatic rupture of the diaphragm. Clin Radiol 18:394-398
El Nakadi B, Vanderhoeft P (1990) Effort rupture of the diaphragm. Thorax 45:715
Estrera AS, Platt MR, Mills LJ (1979) Traumatic injuries of the diaphragm. Chest 75:306–313
Estrera AS, Landay MJ, McClelland RN (1985) Blunt traumatic rupture of the right hemidiaphragm: experience in 12 patients. Ann Thorac Surg 39:525–530
Faheem M, Fayad A (1999) Diaphragmatic rupture after epidural anesthesia in a patient with diaphragmatic eventration. Eur J Anaesthesiol 16:574-576
Fataar S, Schulman A (1979) Diagnosis of diaphragmatic tears. Br J Radiol 52:375–381
Feliciano DV, Cruse PA, Mattox KL et al (1988) Delayed diagnosis of injuries to the diaphragm after penetrating wounds. J Trauma 28:1135–1144
Fell SC (1998) Surgical anatomy of the diaphragm and the phrenic nerve. Chest Surg Clin North Am 8:281–294
Fernandez-Gonzalez AL, Llorens R, Herreros JM, Cato J, Lecumberri F, Longo J (1994) Blunt traumatic rupture of the right hemidiaphragm and Budd-Chiari syndrome. Ann Thorac Surg 58:559–561
Fleyfel M, Ferreira JF, Gonzalez de Linares H, Merlier O, Harchaoui A (1994) Cardiac tamponade after intrapericardial diaphragmatic hernia. Br J Anaesth 73:249–251
Flick RP, Bofill JA, King JC (1999) Pregnancy complicated by traumatic diaphragmatic rupture. A case report. J Reprod Med 44:127-130
Freeman RK, Al-Dossari G, Hutcheson KA (2001) Indications for using video-assisted thoracoscopic surgery to diagnose diaphragmatic injuries after penetrating chest trauma. Ann Thorac Surg 72:342–347
Fung HM, Vickar DB (1991) Traumatic rupture of the right hemidiaphragm with hepatic herniation. Real-time ultrasound demonstration. J Ultrasound Med 10:295–298
Galindo Gallego M, Lopez-Cambra MJ, Fernandez-Acenero MJ et al (1996) Traumatic rupture of the pericardium. Case report and literature review. J Cardiovasc Surg (Torino) 37: 187–191
Gazzaniga AB, Stanton WW, Bartlett RH (1976) Laparoscopy in the diagnosis of blunt and penetrating injuries to the abdomen. Am J Surg 131:315–318
Gelman R, Mirvis SE, Gens D (1991) Diaphragmatic rupture due to blunt trauma: sensitivity of plain chest radiographs. AJR 156:51–57
Gibbons JR, McGuigan J (1997) Delayed infarction of the stomach following diaphragmatic injury. Injury 28:690–692
Gomez-Arnau J, Novoa N, Isidro MG, Plaza A, Galindo F, Ezquerro C (1999) Ruptured hemidiaphragm after bilateral lung transplantation. Eur J Anaesthesiol 16:259–262
Gourin A, Garzon AA (1974) Diagnostic problems in traumatic diaphragmatic hernia. J Trauma 14:20–31
Grage TB, MacLean LD, Campbell GS (1959) Traumatic rupture of the diaphragm. Surgery 46:669
Groskin SA (1992) Selected topics in chest trauma. Radiology 183:605–617
Gurney J, Harrison WL, Anderson JC (1985) Omental fat simulating pleural fluid in traumatic diaphragmatic hernia: CT characteristics. J Comput Assist Tomogr 9:1112–1114
Guth AA, Pachter HL, Kim U (1995) Pitfalls in the diagnosis of blunt diaphragmatic injury. Am J Surg 170:5–9
Hahn DM, Watson DC (1990) Tension hydropneumothorax as delayed presentation of traumatic rupture of the diaphragm. Eur J Cardiothorac Surg 4:626–627
Halldorsson A, Esser MJ, Rappaport W et al (1992) A new method of diagnosing injury using intraperitoneal technetium. J Trauma 33:140–142
Hardy KH (1966) Closed traumatic rupture of the diaphragm. A review of the Royal Melbourne Hospital patients 1953–63. Aust N Z J Surg 35:222–225
Hedblom CA (1925) Diaphragmatic hernia. JAMA 85:947–953
Heeb MA, Dupont JR, Critchlow WC (1971) Complete avulsion of kidney into chest complicated by hypofibrinogenemia. Surgery 69:932–935
Heiberg E, Wolverson MK, Hurd RN, Jagannadharao B, Sundaram M (1980) CT recognition of traumatic rupture of the diaphragm. AJR 135:369–372

Henzler M, Martin ML, Young J (1988) Delayed diagnosis of traumatic diaphragmatic hernia during pregnancy. Ann Emerg Med 17:350–353
Hill LD (1972) Injuries of the diaphragm following blunt trauma. Surg Clin North Am 52:611–624
Ho HS, Saunders CJ, Corso FA, Wolfe BM (1993) The effects of CO_2 pneumoperitoneum on hemodynamics in hemorrhaged animals. Surgery 114:381–388
Holland DG, Quint LE (1991) Traumatic rupture of the diaphragm without visceral herniation: CT diagnosis. AJR 157:17–18
Hood RM (1971) Traumatic diaphragmatic hernia. Ann Thorac Surg 12:311–324
Holm A, Bessey PQ, Aldrete JS (1988) Diaphragmatic rupture due to blunt trauma: morbidity and mortality in 42 cases. South Med J 81:956–562
Humphreys TR, Abbuhl S (1991) Massive bilateral diaphragmatic rupture after an apparently minor automobile accident. Am J Emerg Med 9:246–249
Ivatury RR, O'Shea J, Rohman M (1984) Post-traumatic thoracobiliary fistula. J Trauma 24:438–442
Ivatury RR, Simon RJ, Stahl WM (1993) A critical evaluation of laparoscopy in penetrating abdominal trauma. J Trauma 34:822–828
Jayanthi V, Vidyanathan V, Mathai V, Muthusami JC, Jesudason SB (1994) Traumatic eventration of diaphragm complicated by mesenteroaxial volvulus of the stomach. Trop Gastroenterol 15:169–172
Johnson CD (1988) Blunt injuries of the diaphragm. Br J Surg 75:226–230
Josephs LG, Cordts PR, Diedwardo CL, Lamorte WW, Menzoian JO (1994) Do infected inguinal lymph nodes increase the incidence of postoperative groin wound infection? J Trauma 36:815–819
Junk S, Zegarski W, Bilinski PJ (2001) Rupture of diaphragm involving herniated viscera following a blunt trauma diagnosed by gastrofiberoscopy. Endoscopy 33:296
Kainuma M, Shimada Y (1988) Tension pneumothorax following spontaneous rupture of diaphragm by a subphrenic drain in septic peritonitis. Crit Care Med 16:568
Kallay N, Crim L, Dunagan DP, Kavanagh PV, Meredith W, Haponik EF (2000) Massive left diaphragmatic separation and rupture due to coughing during an asthma exacerbation. South Med J 93:729-731
Kamelgard JI, Harris L, Reardon MJ, Reardon PR (1999) Thoracoscopic repair of a recurrent diaphragmatic hernia four years after initial trauma, laparotomy, and repair. J Laparoendosc Adv Surg Tech A 9:171–175
Karmy-Jones R, Carter Y, Stern E (2002) The impact of positive pressure ventilation on the diagnosis of traumatic diaphragmatic injury. Am Surg 68:167–172
Karnak I, Senocak ME, Tanyel FC, Buyukpamukcu N (2001) Abnormal esophageal anatomy associated with a congenital diaphragmatic hernia: report of a case. Surg Today 31: 1005–1007
Kearney PA, Rouhana SW, Burney RE (1989) Blunt rupture of the diaphragm: mechanism, diagnosis, and treatment. Ann Emerg Med 18:1326–1330
Kennedy FR, Fleming AW, Scott RS (1991) Splenic injury from gunshot wounds to the chest without diaphragmatic or peritoneal violation: case reports. J Trauma 31:1561–1562
Killeen KL, Mirvis SE, Shanmuganathan K (1999) Helical CT of diaphragmatic rupture caused by blunt trauma. AJR 173: 1611–1616
Kim HH, Shin YR, Kim KJ et al (1997) Blunt traumatic rupture of the diaphragm: sonographic diagnosis. J Ultrasound Med 16:593–598
Koplewitz BZ, Ramos C, Manson DE, Babyn PS, Ein SH (2000) Traumatic diaphragmatic injuries in infants and children: imaging findings. Pediatr Radiol 30:471–479
Lacayo L, Taveras JM III, Sosa N, Ratzan KR (1993) Tension fecal pneumothorax in a postpartum patient. Chest 103: 950–951
Lahiry SK, Alkhafaji AH, Brown AL (1978) Urinothorax following blunt trauma to the kidney. J Trauma 18:608–610
Landay M, Harless W (1977) Ultrasonic differentiation of right pleural effusion from subphrenic fluid on longitudinal scans of the right upper quadrant: importance of recognizing the diaphragm. Radiology 123:155–158
Lang-Lazdunski L, Mouroux J, Pons F et al (1997) Role of videothoracoscopy in chest trauma. Ann Thorac Surg 63:327–333
Langley JR, Innes BJ (1975) Traumatic nonpenetrating diaphragmatic hernia: report of 5 cases with a brief review of the literature. Am Surg 41:409–412
Laric MJ, Roger M, Broude HB (1989) Intrapericardial diaphragmatic hernia. A case report. S Afr J Surg 27:100–102
Larrieu AJ, Wiener I, Alexander R, Wolma FJ (1980) Pericardiodiaphragmatic hernia. Am J Surg 139:436–440
Lee HK, Kim IO, Kim WS, Chung JW, Yeon KM (1995) Stenosis of the inferior vena cava caused by a traumatic diaphragmatic hernia: case report. Pediatr Radiol 25:S175–S177
Lee WC, Chen RJ, Fang JF et al (1994) Rupture of the diaphragm after blunt trauma. Eur J Surg 160:479–483
Leppaniemi AK, Elliott DC (1996) The role of laparoscopy in blunt abdominal trauma. Ann Med 28:483–489
Leppaniemi AK, Cederberg A, Tikka S (1996) Truncal gunshot wounds in Finland, 1985 to 1989. J Trauma 40:S217–S222
Le Treut YP, Herve L, Cardon JM, Boutboul R, Bricot R (1981) Blunt traumatic rupture of the right ventricle, with intrapericardial rupture of the diaphragm: successful surgical repair. Injury 13:66–68
Leung JC, Nance ML, Schwab CW, Miller WT Jr (1999) Thickening of the diaphragm: a new computed tomography sign of diaphragm injury. J Thorac Imaging 14:126–129
Levy IG, Saadia R, Boffard KD (1988) Right-sided diaphragmatic rupture with herniation of the kidney presenting as an uncontrolled haemothorax – a case report. Injury 19:293
Li J, Zhao Z, Zhou J, Yu S (1996) A study of the three-dimensional organization of the human diaphragmatic lymphatic lacunae and lymphatic drainage units. Anat Anz 178:537–544
Longaker MT, Whitby DJ, Jennings RW et al (1991) Fetal diaphragmatic wounds heal with scar formation. J Surg Res 50:375–385
Low V, Kelsey P (1990) CT demonstration of traumatic ventral hernia and diaphragmatic rupture. A case report. Australas Radiol 34:172–174
Lucido JL, Wall CA (1963) Rupture of the diaphragm due to blunt trauma. Arch Surg 86:989–999
Madden MR, Paull DE, Finkelstein JL et al (1989) Occult diaphragmatic injury from stab wounds to the lower chest and abdomen. J Trauma 29:292–298
Majid AA (1990) Hemorrhage from the diaphragm: an unusual cause of hemothorax after percutaneous liver biopsy. Am J Gastroenterol 85:104–105
Maninges PA, Di Jullo MA, Dronen SC (1983) Diaphragmatic rupture during G-manœuvres in a T33 jet trainer. Aviat Space Environ Med 54:1037–1038

Mansour KA (1997) Trauma to the diaphragm. Chest Surg Clin North Am 7:373–383
Marchand P (1957) A study of the forces productive of gastroesophageal regurgitation and herniation through the diaphragmatic hiatus. Thorax 12:189–191
Mariadason JG, Parsa MH, Ayuyao A, Freeman HP (1988) Management of stab wounds to the thoracoabdominal region. A clinical approach. Ann Surg 207:335–340
Martinez M, Briz JE, Carillo EH (2001) Video thoracoscopy expedites the diagnosis and treatment of penetrating diaphragmatic injuries. Surg Endosc 15:28–33
Mattei P, Wiebke E, Lipsett P (1992) Tension pneumothorax as a presentation of traumatic diaphragmatic hernia. South Med J 85:847–850
Matz A, Landau O, Alis M, Charuzi I, Kyzer S (2000) The role of laparoscopy in the diagnosis and treatment of missed diaphragmatic rupture. Surg Endosc 14:537–539
McConnel DB, Trunkey DD (1990) Nonoperative management of abdominal trauma. Surg Clin North Am 70: 677–688
McCune RP, Roda CP, Eckert C (1976) Rupture of the diaphragm caused by blunt trauma. J Trauma 16:531–537
McElwee TB, Myers RT, Pennell TC (1984) Diaphragmatic rupture from blunt trauma. Am Surg 50:143–149
Meyers BF, McCabe CJ (1993) Traumatic diaphragmatic hernia. Occult marker of serious injury. Ann Surg 218:783–790
Miller L, Bennett EV Jr, Root HD, Trinkle JK, Grover FL (1984) Management of penetrating and blunt diaphragmatic injury. J Trauma 24:403–409
Mineo TC, Ambrogi V, Cristino B, Pompeo E, Pistolese C (1999) Changing indications for thoracotomy in blunt chest trauma after the advent of videothoracoscopy. J Trauma 47:1088–1091
Mirvis SE, Keramati B, Buckman R, Rodriguez A (1988) MR imaging of traumatic diaphragmatic rupture. J Comput Assist Tomogr 12:147–149
Mitchell TE, Ridley PD, Forrester-Wood CP (1994) Spontaneous rupture of a congenital diaphragmatic eventration. Eur J Cardiothorac Surg 8:281–282
Montresor E, Mangiante G, Lupi A et al (1997) Diagnosis and treatment of traumatic diaphragmatic hernia with delayed presentation. Minerva Chir 52:919–925
Moore EE, Malangoni MA, Cogbill TH et al (1994) Organ injury scaling. IV. Thoracic vascular, lung, cardiac, and diaphragm. J Trauma 36:299–300
Moore JB, Moore EE, Thompson JS (1980) Abdominal injuries associated with penetrating trauma in the lower chest. Am J Surg 140:724–730
Morales CH, Villegas MI, Angel W, Vasquez JJ (2001) Value of digital exploration for diagnosing injuries to the left side of the diaphragm caused by stab wounds. Arch Surg 136: 1131–1135
Morgan AS, Flancbaum L, Esposito T, Cox EF (1986) Blunt injury to the diaphragm: an analysis of 44 patients. J Trauma 26:565–568
Mueller CF, Pendravis RW (1994) Traumatic injury of the diaphragm: report of seven cases and extensive literature review. Emerg Radiol 1:118–132
Mukerjea SK, Nair KK (1978) Seat-belt injury causing pneumothorax with rupture of diaphragm, stomach, and spleen. Lancet 2:1044–1045
Murray JA, Demetriades D, Cornwell EE III et al (1997) Penetrating left thoracoabdominal trauma: the incidence and clinical presentation of diaphragm injuries. J Trauma 43: 624–626
Murray JA, Demetriades D, Asensio JA et al (1998) Occult injuries to the diaphragm: prospective evaluation of laparoscopy in penetrating injuries to the left lower chest. J Am Coll Surg 187:626–630
Murray JG, Caoili E, Gruden JF, Evans SJ, Halvorsen RA Jr, MacKersie RC (1996) Acute rupture of the diaphragm due to blunt trauma: diagnostic sensitivity and specificity of CT. AJR 166:1035–1039
Myers NA (1964) Recurrent volvulus of the sigmoid colon in a young patient. Aust N Z J Surg 33:189–193
Nau T, Seitz H, Mousavi M, Vecsei V (2001) The diagnostic dilemma of traumatic rupture of the diaphragm. Surg Endosc 15:992–996
Naunheim KS (1998) Adult presentation of unusual diaphragmatic hernias. Chest Surg Clin North Am 8:359–369
Negre J, Teerenhovi O, Autio V (1986) Hepatic coma resulting from diaphragmatic rupture and hepatic herniation. Arch Surg 121:950–951
Nel JH, Warren BL (1994) Thoracoscopic evaluation of the diaphragm in patients with knife wounds of the left lower chest. Br J Surg 81:713–714
Neumeyer DA, Locicero J III, Pinkston P (1996) Complex pleural effusion associated with a subphrenic gallstone phlegmon following laparoscopic cholecystectomy. Chest 109:284–286
Newman B, Davis PL (1989) Sonographic and magnetic resonance imaging of an anterior diaphragmatic hernia. Pediatr Radiol 20:110–112
Niville EC, Himpens JM, Bruos PL, Gruwez JA (1983) The use of laparotomy in the treatment of recent diaphragmatic rupture due to blunt trauma. Injury 15:153–155
Ochsner MG, Rozycki GS, Lucente F, Wherry DC, Champion HR (1993) Prospective evaluation of thoracoscopy for diagnosing diaphragmatic injury in thoracoabdominal trauma: a preliminary report. J Trauma 34:704–710
Ohtani Y, Ohtani O (1997) Obliteration of the lymphatic trunks draining diaphragmatic lymph causes peritoneal fluid to enter the pleural cavity. Arch Histol Cytol 60:503–510
Ordog GJ, Wasserberger J, Balasubramaniam S (1984) Tension gastrothorax complicating post-traumatic rupture of the diaphragm. Am J Emerg Med 2:219–221
Orlando R III, Russell JC, Lynch J, Mattie A (1993) Laparoscopic cholecystectomy. A statewide experience. The Connecticut laparoscopic cholecystectomy registry. Arch Surg 128:494–499
Ortega AE, Tang E, Froes ET, Asensio JA, Katkhouda N, Demetriades D (1996) Laparoscopic evaluation of penetrating thoracoabdominal traumatic injuries. Surg Endosc 10:19–22
Pagliarello G, Carter J (1992) Traumatic injury to the diaphragm: timely diagnosis and treatment. J Trauma 33:194–197
Panagiotis NS (1989) Chest drainage tubes. Surg Clin North Am 69:41–46
Pecoraro JP, Shea LM, Tenorio LE, Graham AD, Watkins GM (1985) Radioisotope-assisted diagnosis of traumatic rupture of the diaphragm. Am Surg 51:687–689
Peitzman AB, Udekwu AO (1989) Left-sided perinephric hematoma associated with rupture of the left hemidiaphragm: a marker for renal artery injury. Surgery 106:33–36
Pikoulis E, Delis S, Scandalakis P et al (2000) Reliability of initial chest radiographs in the diagnosis of blunt diaphragmatic rupture. Ann Chir Gynaecol 89:10–13

Pomerantz M, Rodgers BM, Sabiston DC Jr (1968) Traumatic diaphragmatic hernia. Surgery 64:529–534
Potter SR, Kavoussi LR, Jackman SV (2001) Management of diaphragmatic injury during laparoscopic nephrectomy. J Urol 165:1203–1204
Price BA, Elliott MJ, Featherstone G, Blesovsky A (1983) Perforation of intrathoracic colon causing acute pneumothorax. Thorax 38:959–960
Prokesch RW, Schima W, Schober E, Vychytil A, Fabrizii V, Bader TR (2000) Complications of continuous ambulatory peritoneal dialysis: findings on MR peritoneography. AJR 174:987–991
Puffer P, Gaebler M (1991) Traumatic diaphragmatic rupture in a forensic medicine autopsy sample. Beitr Gerichtl Med 49:149–152
Radhakrishna C, Dickinson SJ, Shaw A (1969) Acute diaphragmatic hernia from blunt trauma in children. J Pediatr Surg 4:553–556
Ramnarine IR, Mulpur AK, McMahon MJ, Thorpe JA (2001) Pleuro-biliary fistula from a ruptured choledochal cyst. Eur J Cardiothorac Surg 19:216–218
Ramos CT, Koplewitz BZ, Babyn PS, Manson PS, Ein SH (2000) What have we learned about traumatic diaphragmatic hernias in children? J Pediatr Surg 35:601–604
Rappaport WD, Lee S, Coates S et al (1988) Diagnosis of diaphragmatic injury using intraperitoneal technetium. Am Surg 55:621–624
Rashid MA, Wikstrom T, Ortenwall P (1999) Pneumopericardium and pneumoperitoneum after penetrating chest injury. Eur J Surg 165:278–279
Reber PU, Schmied B, Seiler CA, Baer HU, Patel AG, Buchler MW (1998) Missed diaphragmatic injuries and their long-term sequelae. J Trauma 44:183–188
Rehm CG, Sherman R, Hinz TW (1989)The role of CT scan in evaluation for laparotomy in patients with stab wounds of the abdomen. J Trauma 29:446–450
Reina A, Vidana E, Soriano P et al (2001) Traumatic intrapericardial diaphragmatic hernia: case report and literature review. Injury 32:153–156
Reinbold WD, Kirchner R, Dinkel E, Kropelin T (1987) Roentgen diagnosis in diaphragmatic trauma. Radiologe 27:407–413
Restrepo J, Cano F (1987) Digital exploration for diagnosis of diaphragmatic injuries. Rev Col Cirurgia 11:41–44
Reuter M (1996) Trauma of the chest. Eur Radiol 6:707–716
Rizoli SB, Brenneman FD, Boulanger BR, Maggisano R (1994) Blunt diaphragmatic and thoracic aortic rupture: an emerging injury complex. Ann Thorac Surg 58:1404–1408
Rodriguez-Morales G, Rodriguez A, Shatney CH (1986) Acute rupture of the diaphragm in blunt trauma: analysis of 60 patients. J Trauma 26:438–444
Rosati C (1998) Acute traumatic injury of the diaphragm. Chest Surg Clin North Am 8:371–379
Rubio PA (1990) Unusual cause of traumatic diaphragmatic hernia in a 12-year-old boy. South Med J 83:260–261
Sadeghi N, Nicaise N, Debacker D, Struyven J, van Gansbeke D (1999) Right diaphragmatic rupture and hepatic hernia: an indirect sign on computed tomography. Eur Radiol 9: 972–974
Salomon J, Feller N, Levy MJ (1969) A case of spontaneous rupture of the diaphragm. J Thorac Cardiovasc Surg 58:221–224
Saur K, Lutz W (1976) Traumatic rupture of the diaphragm: diagnosis, treatment, and late results (author's translation). Unfallheilkunde 79:349–357
Schneider CF (1956) Traumatic diaphragmatic hernia. Am J Surg 91:290–297
Schroder Hansen K, Vage V, Morild I (2001) Vertical shear forces and their influence on disruption of the diaphragm and thoracic aorta. Eur J Surg 167:548–551
Schulman A, van Gelderen F (1996a) Bowel hernitation through the torn diaphragm: I. Gastric hernitation. Abdom Imaging 21:395-399
Schulman A, van Gelderen F (1996b) Bowel hernitation through the torn diaphragm: II. Intestinal hernitation. Abdom Imaging 21:400-403
Schumpelick V, Steinau G, Schluper I, Prescher A (2000) Surgical embryology and anatomy of the diaphragm with surgical applications. Surg Clin North Am 80:213–239
Schwegler N, Endrei E (1975) Gallstone in the lung. Radiology 115:541–542
Seelig MH, Klingler PJ, Schonleben K (1999) Tension fecopneumothorax due to colonic perforation in a diaphragmatic hernia. Chest 115:288–291
Seiler C, Glattli A, Metzger A, Czerniak A (1995) Injury to the diaphragm and its repair during laparoscopic cholecystectomy. Surg Endosc 9:193–194
Shah R, Sabanathan S, Mearns AJ, Choudhury AK (1995) Traumatic rupture of diaphragm. Ann Thorac Surg 60: 1444–1449
Shanmuganathan K, Mirvis SE, White CS, Pomerantz SM (1996) MR imaging evaluation of hemidiaphragms in acute blunt trauma: experience with 16 patients. AJR 167:397–402
Shanmuganathan K, Killeen K, Mirvis SE, White CS (2000) Imaging of diaphragmatic injuries. J Thorac Imaging 15: 104–111
Shao XJ, Ohtani O, Saitoh M, Ohtani Y (1998) Development of diaphragmatic lymphatics: the process of their connection to the peritoneal cavity. Arch Histol Cytol 61:137-149
Shapiro MJ, Heiberg E, Durham RM, Luchtefeld W, Mazuski JE (1996) The unreliability of CT scans and initial chest radiographs in evaluating blunt trauma induced diaphragmatic rupture. Clin Radiol 51:27–30
Sharma LK, Kennedy RF, Heneghan WD (1977) Rupture of the diaphragm resulting from blunt trauma in children. Can J Surg 20:553–556
Sharma OM (1999) Pericardio-diaphragmatic rupture: five new cases and literature review. J Emerg Med 17:963–968
Sharma OP (1989) Traumatic diaphragmatic rupture: not an uncommon entity – personal experience with collective review of the 1980's. J Trauma 29:678–682
Sharma S, Puri S, Chaturvedi P, Kulshreshtha R, Baijal VN (1988) Mediastinal pancreatic pseudocyst following traumatic rupture of diaphragm. Pediatr Radiol 18:337
Simansky DA, Paley M, Werczberger A, Bar Ziv Y, Yellin A (1997) Exostosis of a rib causing laceration of the diaphragm: diagnosis and management. Ann Thorac Surg 63: 856–857
Simon G, Bonnell J, Kazantzis G, Waller RE (1969) Some radiological observations on the range of movement of the diaphragm. Clin Radiol 20:231–233
Simon RJ, Ivatury RR (1995) Current concepts in the use of cavitary endoscopy in the evaluation and treatment of blunt and penetrating truncal injuries. Surg Clin North Am 75:157–174
Simpson E, Macateer E, Visram A (2000) Review of paediatric trauma admissions at the Royal London Hospital (February 98 to February 99). Paediatr Anaesth 10:696–697

Slim K, Bousquet J, Chipponi J (1998) Laparoscopic repair of missed blunt diaphragmatic rupture using a prosthesis. Surg Endosc 12:1358–1360
Smithers BM, O'Loughlin B, Strong RW (1991) Diagnosis of ruptured diaphragm following blunt trauma: results from 85 cases. Aust N Z J Surg 61:737–741
Soderstrom CA, Dupriest RW JR, Cowley RA (1980) Pitfalls of peritoneal lavage in blunt abdominal trauma. Surg Gynecol Obstet 151:513–518
Spann JC, Nwariaku FE, Wait M (1995) Evaluation of video-assisted thoracoscopic surgery in the diagnosis of diaphragmatic injuries. Am J Surg 170:628–631
Steiger Z, Wilson RF, Nelson RM, Huang CL, Jacobs LA (1984) Iatrogenic hiatal and diaphragmatic hernias. Am Surg 50: 217–221
Stylianos S, Bergman KS, Harris BH (1991) Traumatic renal avulsion into the chest: case report. J Trauma 31:301–302
Sullivan RE (1966) Strangulation and obstruction in diaphragmatic hernia due to direct trauma. Report of two cases and review of the English literature. J Thorac Cardiovasc Surg 52:725–734
Sutton JP, Carlisle RB, Stephenson SE Jr (1967) Traumatic diaphragmatic hernia. A review of 25 cases. Ann Thorac Surg 3:136–150
Swartz D, Livingston C, Tio F, Mack J, Trinkle JK, Grover FL (1984) Intrapericardial diaphragmatic hernia after subxiphoid epicardial pacemaker insertion. J Thorac Cardiovasc Surg 88:633–635
Tan GC, Hamilton SG, Gibson P, Simpson JA (1973) Ruptured diaphragm: experience in a major accident centre over a ten-year period. Aust N Z J Surg 43:163–168
Thakore S, Henry J, Todd AW (2001) Diaphragmatic rupture and the association with occupant position in right-hand drive vehicles. Injury 32:441–444
Toh CL, Yeo TT, Chua CL, Low CH (1991) Diaphragmatic injuries: why are they overlooked? J R Coll Surg Edinb 36: 25–28
Troop B, Myers RM, Agarwal NN (1985) Early recognition of diaphragmatic injuries from blunt trauma. Ann Emerg Med 14:97–101
Trupka A, Kierse R, Waydhas C et al (1997) Shock room diagnosis in polytrauma. Value of thoracic CT. Unfallchirurg 100:469–476
Uribe RA, Pachon CE, Frame SB, Enderson BL, Escobar F, Garcia GA (1994) A prospective evaluation of thoracoscopy for the diagnosis of penetrating thoracoabdominal trauma. J Trauma 37:650–654
Valestaqui R, Mehran RJ (1999) Traumatic hernia of the pericardium. J Trauma 46:513–514
Van der Werken C, Lubbers EJ, Goris RJ (1983) Rupture of the diaphragm by blunt trauma as a marker of injury severity. Injury 15:149–152
Velmahos GC, Demetriades D, Foianini E et al (1997) A selective approach to the management of gunshot wounds to the back. Am J Surg 174:342–346
Verschakelen JA, Marchal G, Verbeken E, Baert AL, Lauweryns J (1989) Sonographic appearance of the diaphragm: a cadaver study. J Clin Ultrasound 17:222–227
Voeller GR, Reisser JR, Fabian TC, Kudsk K, Mangiante EC (1990) Blunt diaphragm injuries. A five-year experience. Am Surg 56:28–31
Waldhausen JA, Kilman JW, Helman CH, Battersby JS (1966) The diagnosis and management of traumatic injuries of the diaphragm including the use of Marlex prostheses. J Trauma 6:332–343
Waldschmidt ML, Laws HL (1980) Injuries of the diaphragm. J Trauma 20:587–592
Waller DA, Satur CM, Mitchell IM, Sivanathan VM (1992) Iatrogenic peritoneopericardial hernia following coronary artery bypass surgery. Eur J Cardiothorac Surg 6:156–157
Waxman HE (1922) Diaphragmatic hernia as late sequel of war wound of chest. JAMA 79:123–124
Wenz W, Reinbold WD (1982) Diagnostic and therapeutic results of angiography of blunt abdominal trauma. Radiologe 22:117–121
Wiencek RG Jr, Wilson RF, Steiger Z (1986) Acute injuries of the diaphragm. An analysis of 165 cases. J Thorac Cardiovasc Surg 92:989–993
Willsher PC, Cade RJ (1991) Traumatic diaphramgatic rupture. Aust N Z J Surg 61:207-210
Wilson RF, Murray C, Antonenko DR (1977) Nonpenetrating thoracic injuries. Surg Clin North Am 57:17–36
Wise L, Connors J, Hwang YH, Anderson C (1973) Traumatic injuries to the diaphragm. J Trauma 13:946–950
Wong NA, Dayan CM, Virjee J, Heaton KW (1995) Acute respiratory distress secondary to Morgagni diaphragmatic herniation in an adult. Postgrad Med J 71:39–41
Worthy SA, Kang EY, Hartman TE, Kwong JS, Mayo JR, Muller NL (1995) Diaphragmatic rupture: CT findings in 11 patients. Radiology 194:885–888
Zantut LF, Ivatury RR, Smith RS et al (1997) Diagnostic and therapeutic laparoscopy for penetrating abdominal trauma: a multicenter experience. J Trauma 42:825–831
Zieren J, Enzweiler C, Muller JM (1999) Tube thoracostomy complicates unrecognized diaphragmatic rupture. Thorac Cardiovasc Surg 47:199–202
Zierold D, Perlstein J, Weidman ER, Wiedeman JE (2001) Penetrating trauma to the diaphragm: natural history and ultrasonographic characteristics of untreated injury in a pig model. Arch Surg 136:32–37

10 Injuries of the Kidney, Ureter, and Adrenal Gland

M. Bezzi, G. Andreoli, V. Miele, C. Andreoli

CONTENTS

M. Bezzi, MD
Department of Radiology, University of Rome "La Sapienza", Policlinico Umberto I, Viale Regina Elena n. 324, 00161 Rome, Italy
G. Andreoli, MD
Department of Radiology, University of Rome "La Sapienza", Policlinico Umberto I, Viale Regina Elena n. 324, 00161 Rome, Italy
V. Miele, MD
Department of Radiology, Ospedale S. Camillo, Via Portuense 332, 00149 Rome, Italy
C. Andreoli, MD
Department of Radiology, University of Rome "La Sapienza", Policlinico Umberto I, Viale Regina Elena n. 324, 00161 Rome, Italy

- Renal trauma should be suspected when there is gross hematuria, or in patients with clear urine or microscopic hematuria when there are signs of shock or multiorgan injury.
- In patients with no evidence of systemic injury or shock, microscopic hematuria alone does not justify radiological evaluation.
- CT is performed in the corticomedullary phase, 60–70 s after contrast medium injection. In order to detect urinary extravasation, delayed scans must be obtained after 3–8 min.
- The grading of renal injury is a valid instrument to measure the seriousness of renal trauma in terms of requirement for conservative or operative management. When adequately performed and interpreted, CT is the best way to provide accurate staging in most cases of renal trauma.

10.1 History

Renal trauma has occurred as a result of accident, violence, and war. The famous Roman author and physician Celsus was convinced that a physician had little chance of saving the life of a man with injured kidneys and wrote: "...servare non potest cui renes vulnerati sunt" (Desnos 1972). One of the first recorded cases of penetrating renal trauma was observed by Ambroise Paré, who had observed a patient presenting with a gunshot wound through the chest and abdomen. The man passed large amounts of blood in the urine. Not understanding the significance of the injury, Paré observed him for a few days before death resulted from hemorrhagic shock and infection (Packard 1921). Among the first scientific observations on the mechanism of blunt trauma, the work of the French surgeon Marcille should be mentioned. Marcille observed some 100 years ago that "by falling on the knob of a cane, one could split a kidney into two parts without causing an externally appreciable wound" (Desnos 1972). In those days, nephrectomy was the recommended treatment for renal trauma. In the last 30 years, however, the concept of nonoperative management of blunt renal trauma has steadily evolved, as investigators recognized that the nephrectomy rate was higher in patients who underwent operative exploration than in patients who were simply observed (Bergren et al. 1987). Today, radiological imaging plays a major role in surgical decision-making. At the beginning of the new millennium, it is widely recognized that accurate grading of renal trauma, obtained with imaging studies, is one of the most important variables in predicting the need for renal surgery or conservative treatment (Santucci and McAninch 2000; Santucci et al. 2001).

10.2 Incidence and Mechanism

The incidence of renal trauma has been reported to include 1 in 3000 hospital admission in the United States (Mertz et al. 1963), 3% of patients hospitalized for trauma (Krieger et al. 1984) and 8%–10% of all abdominal trauma (Bretan et al. 1986). Discussion of renal trauma diagnosis and management should deal separately with blunt and penetrating injuries. This distinction by etiology is relevant because of the differing renal and associated nonrenal injuries and complications.

10.2.1 Penetrating Injuries

In Europe, blatant violence such as shooting and stabbing remains much rarer than in urban areas of the United States. Therefore penetrating lesions to the kidney make up less than 5% of the upper urinary trauma cases seen in our hospital. This initial remark underlines the important role that regional factors play in the incidence and modality of injury. In large European cities and industrial areas such as Basel, 80% of renal injuries are observed in patients whose trauma, and often polytrauma, had been caused by traffic and industrial accidents (Rutishauser 1982).

On the contrary, penetrating trauma accounted for 84% of the 185 renal injuries that underwent surgery at Parkland Memorial Hospital in Dallas, Texas (Sagalowsky et al. 1983). The great majority of penetrating renal injuries were due to gunshot wounds (79%) and the remainder were due to stabbings (21%). In this series, every patient with penetrating injuries from a gunshot wound had other abdominal or thoracic injuries, with the liver, small bowel, stomach, and colon being the organs most commonly involved. Life-threatening aortic or vena caval lesions were seen, respectively, in 4% and 7% of renal gunshot injuries. In the same series, stab wounds were less frequently associated with nonrenal injuries (77% of cases), with liver trauma being the most frequent association. This association has remained stable over the years, since an earlier series from the same institution reported that 83% of penetrating renal traumas also had nonrenal injuries (Bright and Peters 1977).

How often is penetrating abdominal trauma associated with renal injury? Carlton et al., in a series of 181 patients seen at Ben Taub Hospital in Houston, reported that renal lesions were seen in approximately 6%–8% of patients with abdominal gunshot wounds and stabbing (Carlton 1978). In this series the distribution and association of nonrenal lesions was similar to that reported in the above-mentioned series of Sagalowsky. When also other series are considered, renal injuries are present from 6%–14% of all penetrating abdominal wounds (Mertz et al. 1963; Scott et al. 1969; Tynberg et al. 1973; Tunberg and Jona 1985). The mechanism of injury from penetrating trauma is the obvious tissue disruption to the parenchyma, collecting system, and vasculature caused by a foreign body. In patients with gunshot wounds, missile velocity and blast effect must be considered as well. High-velocity bullets generally penetrate and exit from the body. Such high-speed bullets carry a high kinetic energy and radiate energy along their trajectory, thus generating a current of injury known as blast effect. This may cause delayed tissue necrosis, bleeding, and fistula formation in areas that appeared uninjured when the wound was sustained.

Penetrating renal injuries are often complicated by infection. By definition, a knife or a bullet that has penetrated the patient's skin is no longer sterile; thus, the likelihood of renal or perinephric infection is high, also because blood or urine that may surround the injured kidney forms an excellent growth medium for bacteria. In addition, both the retroperitoneum and the peritoneum may be violated, and this increases the possibility of retroperitoneal contamination by visceral contents.

Invasive maneuvers, such as biopsy, nephrostomy, and nephrolithotomy may cause trauma to the kidney that should be classified among the penetrating injuries. The most common abnormality that may result after such maneuvers is a vascular alteration.

Vascular lesions are common biopsy-related complications in native and transplanted kidneys. Their incidence ranges between 1% and 17%, depending on the modality of follow-up and the imaging tests employed (Ekelund and Lindholm 1971; Hubsch et al. 1990; Orons and Zajko 1995). Arteriovenous fistulas (AVFs) occur more frequently (1%–16%) than pseudoaneurysms (2%–3%) or arteriocalyceal fistulas (Benoit et al. 1984; Hubsch et al. 1990; Orons and Zajko 1995).

10.2.2 Blunt Trauma

The common mechanisms of blunt renal trauma are well known: blunt force applied directly to the abdomen or flank or sudden deceleration of the human body. Deceleration or crush injuries may thrust the kidney internally against the rib cage or vertebral bodies or externally against the steering wheel or the dashboard of a vehicle, as it is seen in a head-on automobile accident. A direct blow to the abdomen or flank, such as a kick, occurring during athletics or fighting is another common cause of blunt renal trauma. In such cases, of more importance than the description of the mechanism involved is understanding of the topographical situation of the kidney and surrounding bony structures. The kidney rests on the tough dorsal body wall, which is only partially made by the ribs; in case of direct anterior blow, the kidney is pushed against and bent over the twelfth rib, which acts as a fulcrum. Medially and posteromedially lie the upper lumbar vertebral body and transverse process, which may lacerate or contuse the renal parenchyma, depending on the direction of the blunt force. Renal parenchymal lacerations transect the organ in the transverse plane. This is because the kidney consists of parallel, radially directed units held together by loose connective tissue, the cortical capillary network, and the fibrous capsule. The injury begins on the border of the cortex and moves into the medulla and collecting system as it increases in severity. The deeper the laceration, the greater the likelihood of bleeding from major renal vessels of the central area. In patients with a preexisting renal abnormality, relatively minor trauma may cause disproportionate damage that brings the patient to medical attention. Such underlying conditions include renal calculi with chronic inflammation and/or obstruction, renal tumors, renal cysts, polycystic disease, and some congenital conditions including ureteropyelic junction obstruction and horseshoe kidney (Brower et al. 1978; Kawashima et al. 1997; Klein et al. 1999). Hemorrhage due to such preexisting disorders is more common in children than in adults (Brower et al. 1978; Rhyner et al. 1984). In addition, patients who receive anticoagulant therapy may present renal bleeding even after trivial trauma. Because acute bleeding may obscure the presence of a renal mass, a follow-up CT study after an interval of 3–4 weeks is advisable whenever such a condition is suspected.

Another mechanism of renal injury is the contrecoup mechanism; this occurs when there is sudden cessation of violent movement in a craniocaudal direction, e.g., falling on buttocks from a height or crashing with a hang glider during landing. These injuries are known as deceleration injuries and may cause damage to the renal pedicle, with renal arterial intimal tearing and thrombosis and/or disruption of the UPJ. Children are prone to sustaining the latter injury owing to the greater mobility of the longitudinal spinous ligament, which permits hyperextension injuries in the pediatric population. When the renal artery undergoes excessive stretch, the intimal arterial layer ruptures and this initiates thrombus formation which can cause partial or total arterial occlusion and renal ischemia. The stretch injury can happen at the level of the main renal artery, which is a single artery in 80%–85% of cases, or at the level of segmental branches. More severe injuries can rupture the muscularis and adventitia and lead to a laceration or avulsion of the vessels. The junction of the renal artery and aorta is fixed and characteristically the occlusion is seen 1–2 cm from the origin of the artery, the site of maximum angulation and traction. Venous injuries are less common and tend to be tears and laceration rather than thrombosis (Cass 1989).

Disruption of the UPJ from blunt trauma is rare and is more commonly found in children, with approximately only one-third of the cases involving adults (Mulligan et al. 1998). The right side is involved three times more often than the left side (Howerton and Norwood 1991).

Blunt renal trauma is far more common than penetrating injuries. Miller and McAninch (1995) report that among 2254 patients seen at the San Francisco General Hospital over a 15-year period, 2024 had blunt and 230 had penetrating injury (respectively, 89.8% and 10.2%). As most blunt renal injuries occur in patients suffering from multisystem trauma, the association of renal and nonrenal injuries is common. Patients with blunt trauma have a higher incidence of spleen and liver injuries and lesser occurrence of bowel injury as compared with patients with penetrating trauma (Sagalowsky et al. 1983).

As for the degree of injury, McAninch and Federle (1982) estimated that 75%–80% of all patients with blunt renal trauma have minor isolated renal injury (see 10.4, "Classification" for grading of injury). This rate has been confirmed in earlier series where 87.5% of patients with adult blunt trauma had minor injuries: grades I–II injuries, according to the classification of the American Association for Surgery in Trauma (AAST) (Miller and McAninch 1995).

10.3 Clinical Symptoms and Findings

10.3.1 History

The historic details of the injury can provide significant information about potential renal involvement. Deceleration injuries from high-speed vehicular accidents or falls from heights are associated with major vascular or parenchymal damage (Knudson et al. 2000) The severe nature of the trauma should alert the physician to possible renal injury in these cases. With penetrating trauma, knowledge of the length of the knife or other sharp object may help to determine the depth of penetration and hypothesize the extent of damage and the organs involved.

10.3.2 Symptoms and Signs

It is well accepted that significant renal injury does not occur without gross hematuria, signs of shock, or multisystem trauma (Rosen and McAninch 1994; Nash et al. 1995). Gross hematuria is defined as more than 50 red blood cells per high power field (RBC/HPF). Microhematuria is between 3 and 49 RBC/HPF. Evaluation of the patient with radiological studies is not needed unless there is gross hematuria, hypotension, or clinical findings such as severe flank tenderness, crepitus, clot colic, or a rigid abdomen (Fallon et al. 1984; Nicolaisen et al. 1985; Hardeman et al. 1987; Mee et al. 1989; Nash et al. 1995). A lower rib fracture, a flank mass, or multisystem trauma should also prompt evaluation of possible renal injury (Goldman and Sandler 1998).

The most important sign and the first indicator of renal trauma is hematuria, but the degree of hematuria does not correlate with the severity of renal damage. Hematuria with more than 50 RBC/HPF or positive results on dipstick testing, should initiate a renal trauma work-up. All series emphasize that hematuria is a relevant finding, but a nonspecific one, and that it does not correlate with the grade of injury. This concept has remained constant in the last 3 decades (Bright et al. 1978; Miller and McAninch 1995). It is also accepted by most urologists that in the absence of signs of systemic injury or shock, microscopic hematuria alone does not justify radiological evaluation (Eastham et al. 1991). In a series of 1230 patients with suspected renal trauma, all studied with imaging tests, 1038 (84%) had no gross hematuria and no signs of major multisystem trauma; only one minor trauma was found in this group (Buchberger et al. 1993). Clear urine may be present in mild and major renal trauma. In 10% of patients without hematuria there is either obstruction below the level of injury, clot, hemolysis or a renal pedicle injury. In a recent multicenter report on major renovascular injuries (grade IV–V, according to the AAST classification), hematuria was absent in 18%, present on a microscopic level in 27%, and gross in 42%. The remaining 13% of patients were in severe shock. In nearly 90% of cases, there were injuries in other regions of the body, that, even in absence of hematuria, led to the hypothesis of major renal trauma (Knudson et al. 2000). Anuria is a nonspecific sign. It may be caused by the rupture of a solitary kidney or hemorrhagic shock, or by simple obstruction of the urinary pathway by blood clots or a lesion of the lower urinary tract. Whatever the cause, anuria is alarming and should prompt further investigation. Nonetheless, no catheter should be inserted in the bladder in a patient with anuria before obtaining information about the condition of the lower urinary tract, in order to avoid iatrogenic damage to the urethra, thus causing a permanent injury. If there is blood at the urethral meatus, a retrograde urethrogram must be done prior to catheterization in order to prevent conversion of a partial tear to complete disruption (Peters and Sagalowsky 1997).

If the patient is conscious, symptoms may vary from no pain to colic, flank pain, or abdominal pain, but these are frequently masked by concomitant injuries. They usually have abdomen tenderness, lower rib fractures, vertebral body fractures and flank contusions. A palpable abdominal mass with associated shock may be indicative of a rapidly developing retroperitoneal hematoma from a major renal parenchyma or renal vascular injury. Rapid deceleration injuries usually involve multiple organ systems and patients are often in shock and unconscious.

Stab wounds to the kidneys generally have their entrance points in the lower thorax, flank area, or upper abdomen. The size of the entrance wound has little correlation with the extent of the injury and the depth of penetration. Hematuria, most often gross, is usually present with major parenchymal injuries. Abdominal examination may reveal marked tenderness and generalized rigidity, indicating bowel perforation. Hemorrhagic shock is a common presenting sign, and reestablishment of circulatory volume is of prime importance in the initial treatment.

10.4 Classification

In the past several decades, classifications of renal trauma, either blunt or penetrating, have been proposed by many authors (FEDERLE et al. 1981; NEY and FRIEDENBERG 1981; GUERRIERO 1982; BRETAN et al. 1986; MARBERGER 1988; CARROL and MCANINCH 1989; FEDERLE 1989; MEE and MCANINCH 1989; MOORE et al. 1989; FANNEY et al. 1990; LENT 1996). The degrees of severity of the injuries range from a minimum of two to a maximum of six.

The renal injury scale established by the Organ Injury Scaling committee of the American Association for the Surgery of Trauma (AAST) is a practical classification that can be easily adapted to radiological assessment of renal trauma and is the classification used in our institution (MOORE et al. 1989). Categorization of renal injuries according to their severity helps in selecting the most appropriate therapy and in predicting the results of the treatment. Categorization of injuries does not mandate per se operation or observation but should be used by the surgeon as an aid in deciding on the best care of renal trauma patients. In addition, this classification may help in standardizing the literature and facilitating clinical research and is presently the grading system adopted in most scientific papers. The grading system of the AAST is reported below (Fig. 10.1):

- Grade I: a contusion or nonexpanding subcapsular hematoma without laceration
- Grade II: nonexpanding perirenal hematoma, confined by perirenal peritoneum, or a laceration less than 1 cm deep without extravasation of urine
- Grade III: a laceration that extends into the cortex more than 1 cm without extravasation of urine
- Grade IV: a laceration extending through the corticomedullary junction and into the collecting system. An injury of a main renal artery or vein with contained hemorrhage
- Grade V: completely shattered kidney or avulsion of the renal pedicle, which devascularizes the kidney

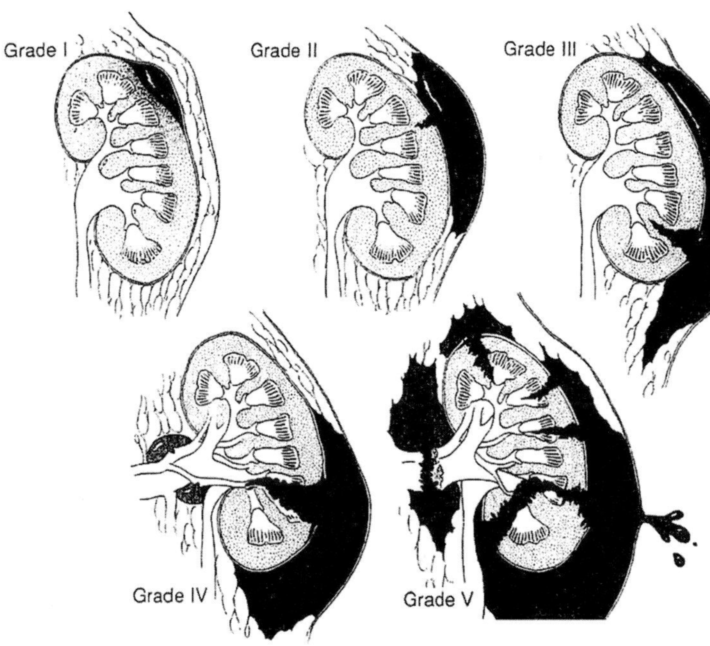

Fig. 10.1. Schematic representation of the renal injury scale established by the Organ Injury Scaling committee of the American Association for the Surgery of Trauma

A classification that has been widely used, both in the radiological and surgical literature, is the classification originally proposed by Federle (1989; Federle et al. 1981):

- Category I lesions: contusion and small laceration of the parenchyma that does not communicate with the collecting system
- Category II lesions: deep parenchymal laceration that communicates with the renal collecting system, leading to urine leakage and/or deep lacerations in the medulla
- Category III lesions: shattered kidney and/or main vascular pedicle injury
- Category IV lesions: avulsion and laceration of the pelvis or UPJ

An interesting classification has been proposed by Lent (1996). To take into consideration all criteria that may be important for the outcome of renal trauma, Lent developed a classification that includes the pathogenesis of the trauma (*P* factor, blunt or penetrating), the locations of the damage with their degrees of injury, scaled from 0 to 9 (*L* factor, parenchyma, vessels, renal pelvis), and the symptoms of the injury, with their degrees of severity, graded from 0 to 3 (*S* factor, hemorrhage, urinary extravasation, damage of renal function). The so-called PLS classification, according to this author, has the advantage of identifying in a single grading system the pathogenesis of the trauma, the extent of damage to the three major components of the kidney, and the severity of symptoms, which can be used as a prognostic factor.

10.5 Imaging

10.5.1 Computed Tomography

Computed tomography (CT) is the imaging modality of choice in the evaluation of renal trauma, as it provides information about renal morphology, vasculature, and function in one examination. The same amount of information could only be obtained by combining several other imaging modalities such as ultrasound, intravenous pyelography (IVP), or angiography.

10.5.1.1 Technique

Nonhelical scanners should be abandoned in the study of trauma patients. Helical CT acquisition minimizes artifacts due to breathing and patient movements, and permits rapid evaluation of the whole kidney during the phase of contrast enhancement and during urine excretion. Helical scanning allows for high-quality multiplanar reconstructions and postprocessing, which are increasingly used for displaying the relationships between the different renal components, parenchyma, vessels, collecting system, and provide useful information for the surgeon. Michel et al. (1996) reported their technique of 3D CT reconstruction in a pilot investigation and demonstrated that high-quality 3D images can be obtained within a few minutes after acquisition and are used by the surgeons in their decision process. Urologic surgeons consider this a useful tool that "may more accurately mimic what they find at renal exploration and may provide a unique 'window' to the surgical anatomy of the patient" (Safir and McAninch 1999). CT arteriography can be used to display the main and segmental renal arteries and is best performed on multiple row detector CT (Fig. 10.2).

a

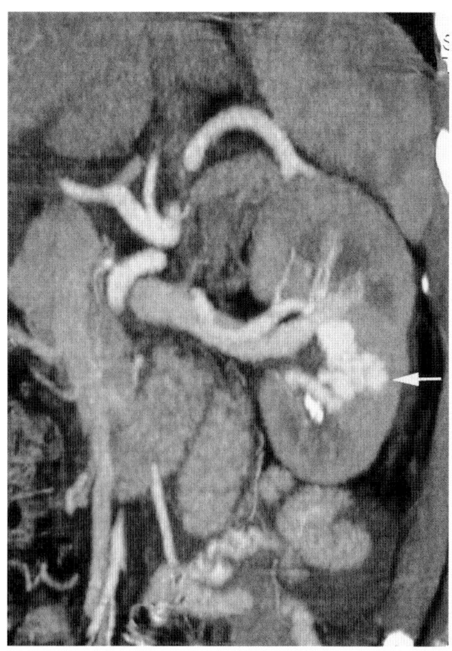

Fig. 10.2a →→

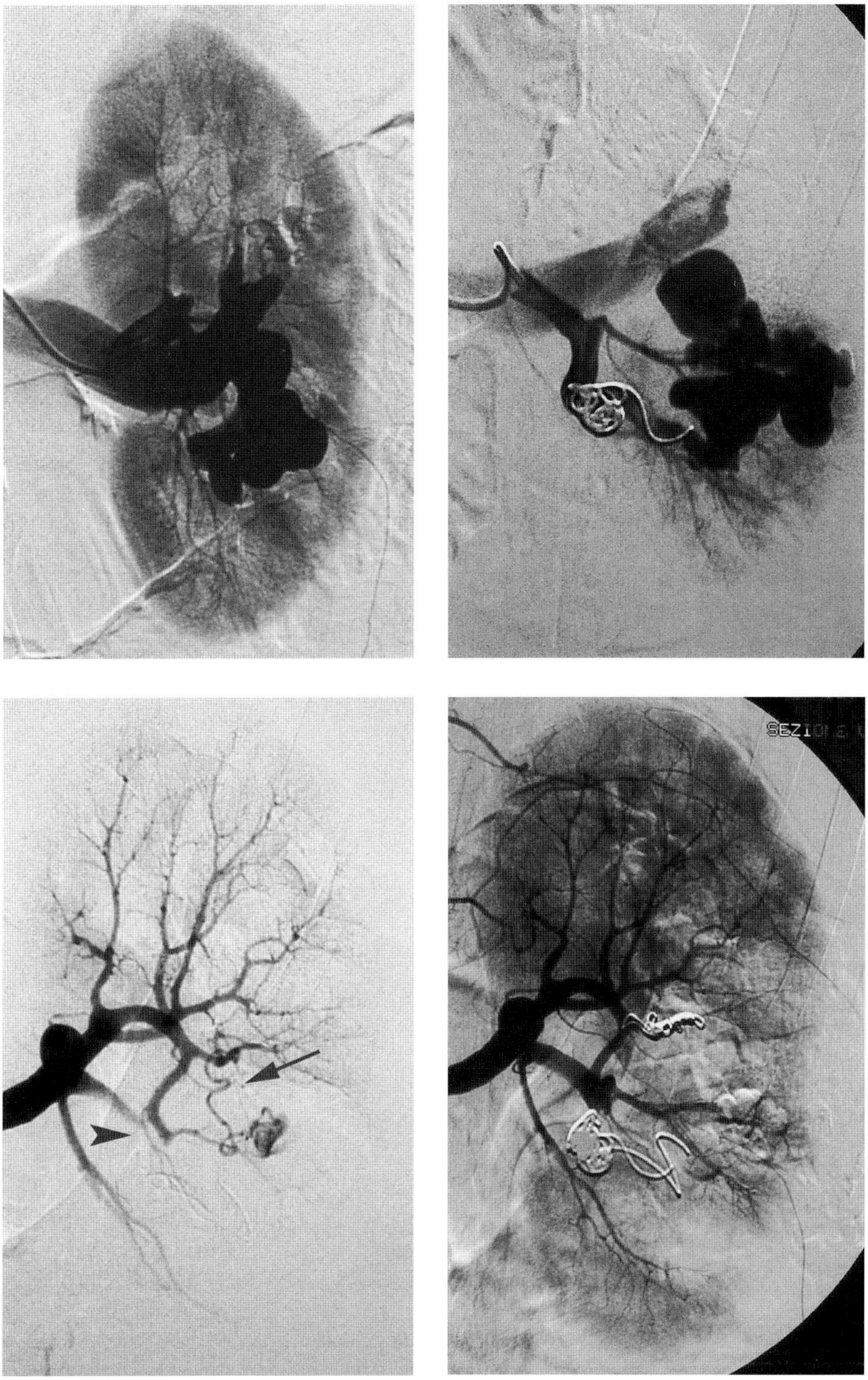

b c d e

Fig. 10.2a–e. AV fistula after penetrating trauma. Coronal MPR of contrast-enhanced CT obtained with multi-detector CT (**a**) shows a large AV fistula of the left kidney (*arrow*). Selective angiography performed before embolization confirms the CT finding (**b**). After superselective catheterization of the segmental branch feeding the AV fistula, several 8- to 10-mm coils were deployed (**c**). Control angiogram after embolization (**d**) shows occlusion of the major feeder (*arrowhead*) and presence of a small arterial feeder from the mid pole of the kidney, unrecognized on the initial angiogram. Final arteriogram after superselective embolization of the lesser feeder (**e**) shows occlusion of the fistula; there are two areas of infarction distal to the two areas of embolization

The CT study should include the upper abdomen and pelvis, from the dome of the diaphragm to the pubic symphysis, unless thoracic trauma is also suspected. Unenhanced scans are obtained to provide information on preexisting high attenuation structures, such as stones and calcifications, and to detect high attenuation values in fluid collections that indicate hemorrhage (40–90 UH). In the setting of abdominal trauma, CT is performed to screen the entire abdomen and pelvis; therefore the urinary tract is studied in most cases with a standard imaging protocol (Becker et al. 1998). At our institution, postcontrast scans are obtained after injection of 120–150 ml of iodinated contrast medium, infused by an automatic injector at a rate of 2–3.5 ml/s; slice collimation is usually 5 mm, reconstruction 5 mm, pitch 1.5–2. With a multiple row detector CT, we use a slice thickness of 3 mm or 1 mm, which allows excellent multiplanar reformatting and MIP processing for CT angiography (Fig. 10.3a). If the patient is intubated and ventilated, breathing can be momentarily suspended by the anesthesiologist, in order to improve image quality. Images are acquired in the corticomedullary phase, approximately 60–70 s after injection, and are suitable to evaluate the renal parenchyma and the renal vessels; the cortical nephrographic phase at 30 s is usually not necessary. This relatively short scan delay time provides improved vascular and parenchymal enhancement, but often fails to identify injuries to the renal collecting system (Brown et al. 1998). In order to detect urinary extravasation, delayed scans must be obtained; the optimal interval between the parenchymal phase and the excretory phase is approximately 2–3 min, according to some authors, and 5–8 min according to others (Mirvis 1996; Mulligan et al. 1998). In our institution, the CT protocol includes delayed scans after 5 min (Fig. 10.3b). In some cases, disruption of the UPJ manifested on delayed scans obtained at 48 h (Mulligan et al. 1998). The rapid acquisition of modern helical scanners, therefore, should not induce the radiologist to move to another study before all proper imaging phases have been obtained in the trauma patient.

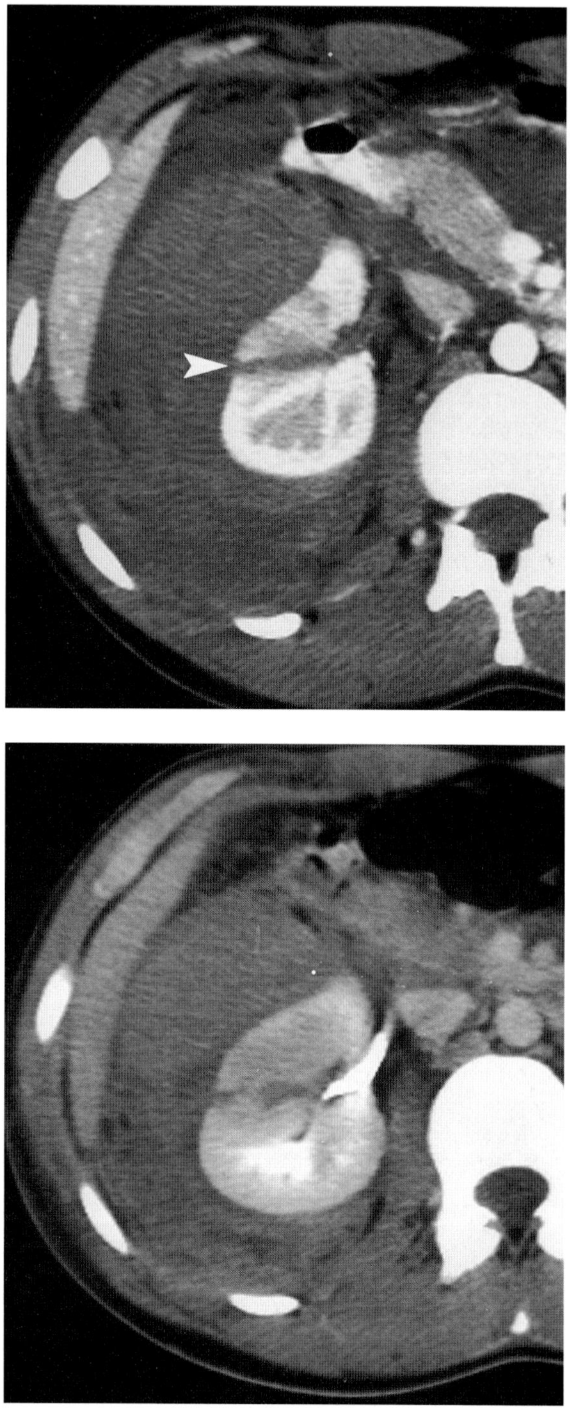

a

b

Fig. 10.3a, b. Renal laceration, >1 cm deep, without involvement of the collecting system after blunt abdominal trauma (AAST grade III). Contrast-enhanced CT demonstrates a deep laceration of the lateral aspect of the right kidney (*arrowhead*), associated with large perinephric collection (**a**). Images obtained in the corticomedullary phase do not permit assessment of extension into collecting system. On delayed images obtained after 8 min (**b**) it is demonstrated that there is no extravasation of urine and that the perirenal collection is a hematoma and not a urinoma

10.5.1.2 Findings

Besides the classification of the AAST, a classification that can be advantageously used in describing and reporting the CT findings in renal trauma is the one proposed by Fanney et al. (1990), who divided the trauma findings into Categories 1, 2, and 3. Both classifications, whose grades partly overlap, are reported below with the corresponding CT finding. Most of the morphological criteria on which the AAST classification is based may be readily applied to CT scans.

- AAST grade I. Category 1. This group includes minor injuries. Renal contusion is diagnosed when one kidney presents global or segmental delayed excretion of contrast medium, due to edema that compresses the tubules. Contusions may also cause disruption of the collecting tubules which appears on delayed images or follow-up scans as an area of focal staining due to intraparenchymal extravasation of urine, so called intravasation (MIRVIS 1996) (Fig. 10.4). Intrarenal hematoma may be appreciated on unenhanced scans as an area of high attenuation within the normal parenchyma, due to interstitial blood extravasation. After contrast medium injection, the hematoma does not enhance to the same degree as the surrounding renal tissue. Segmental infarction due to occlusion of intrarenal arterial branches are hypodense after contrast medium injection and may be differentiated from hematoma by their well marginated wedge or hemispheric shape (Fig. 10.5). A delayed sign of infarction is the cortical rim sign, a peripheral region of cortical enhancement due to collateral circulation, which may be apparent immediately after trauma or may take up to 8 h to become apparent (WONG et al. 1984; LUPETIN et al. 1989; KAMEL and BERKOWITZ 1996) (Figs. 10.6 and 10.7). The infarcted area will later appear as a scar. In small subcapsular hematomas the hemorrhage is confined by the renal capsule and often has a lenticular or crescent shape.

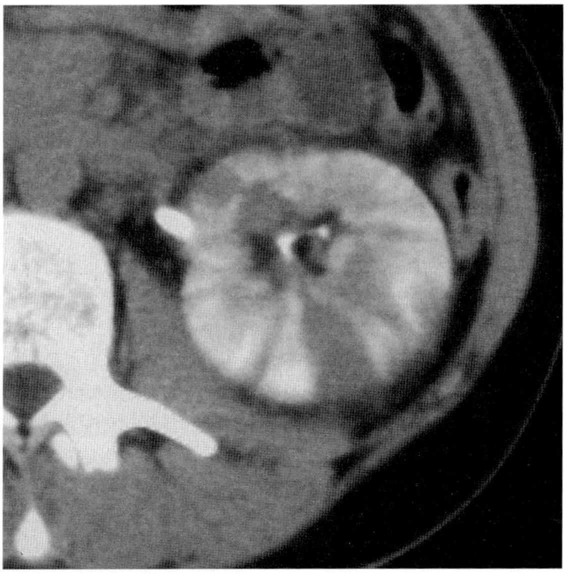

Fig. 10.4. Renal contusion after blunt trauma. On delayed contrast-enhanced CT scan there is persistent opacification of the renal parenchyma with delayed excretion of contrast medium, due to edema that compresses the tubules (so-called striated nephrogram)

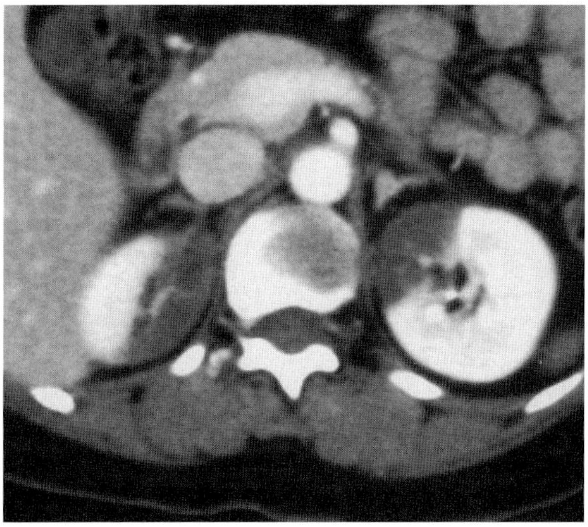

Fig. 10.5. Bilateral segmental renal infarctions at the level of the upper poles after blunt trauma. Contrast-enhanced CT shows two hypodense sharply marginated hemispheric areas consistent with segmental infarction

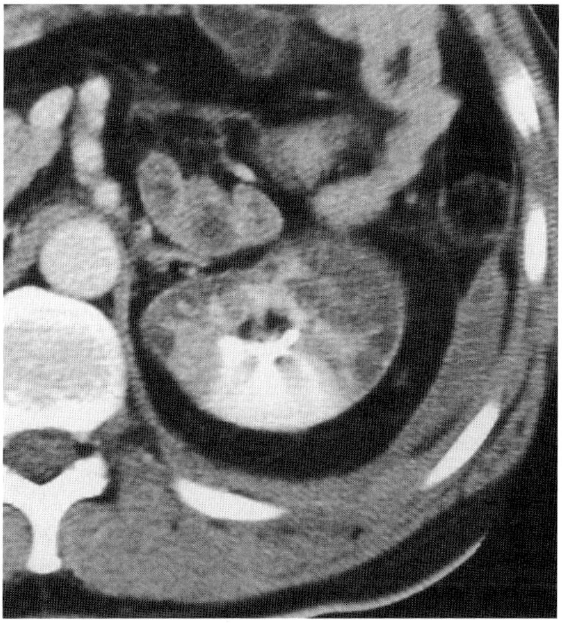

Fig. 10.6. Multiple renal infarctions in the upper pole of the left kidney after blunt trauma. CT shows a cortical rim of enhancement throughout most of the upper pole, while the infracted parenchyma is mainly hypodense. The sign is typical of infarction

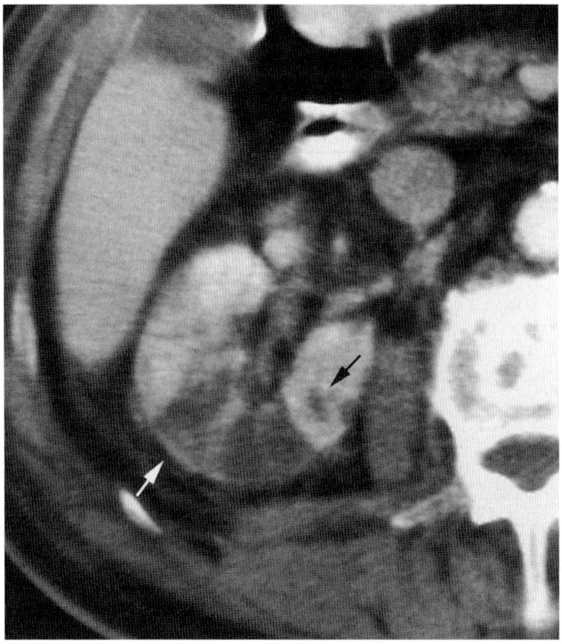

Fig. 10.7. Multiple small hematomas and areas of infarction seen on contrast CT after blunt trauma. Hematomas are seen as hypodense ill-defined areas (*black arrow*). Sharply marginated hypodense areas with cortical rim sign, a peripheral region of cortical enhancement, most likely represents segmental infarctions (*white arrow*)

- AAST grade II and III. Category 2. Large subcapsular hematoma and perirenal hematoma are larger high-attenuation fluid collections which are still confined to the perirenal space (Fig. 10.8). Chronic hematomas may have low attenuation values, and rarely may become infected. Hematomas that compress a large portion of the kidney or surround the whole organ may cause secondary hypertension, although posttraumatic hypertension may also be caused by vascular injury (Massumi et al. 1964; Sufrin 1975; Freed and Tavel 1976; Spirnak and Resnick 1987). Corticomedullary lacerations are parenchymal tears that start on the capsular margin and extend centrally without reaching the collecting system (AAST grade II if less than 1 cm in depth, AAST grade III if more than 1 cm in depth) (Figs. 10.3 and 10.9). Approximately 75%–90% of renal injuries belong to AAST grades I–II (Santucci et al. 2001) and are usually managed conservatively. In a recent survey on 2467 patients with renal trauma, the rate of surgery was 0% in grade I lesions, and 13.8% in grade II lesions, with no nephrectomies performed in either group (Santucci et al. 2001). In the same series, 76.5% of patients with grade III lesions underwent surgical repair or nephrectomy.

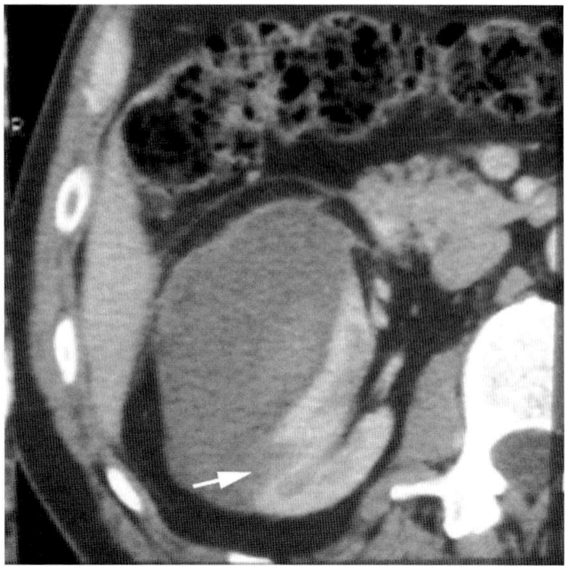

Fig. 10.8. Subcapsular hematoma after blunt abdominal trauma (AAST grade II). Contrast-enhanced CT demonstrates a subcapsular fluid collection flattening the anterior contour of the right kidney. There is minimal cortical laceration (*arrow*)

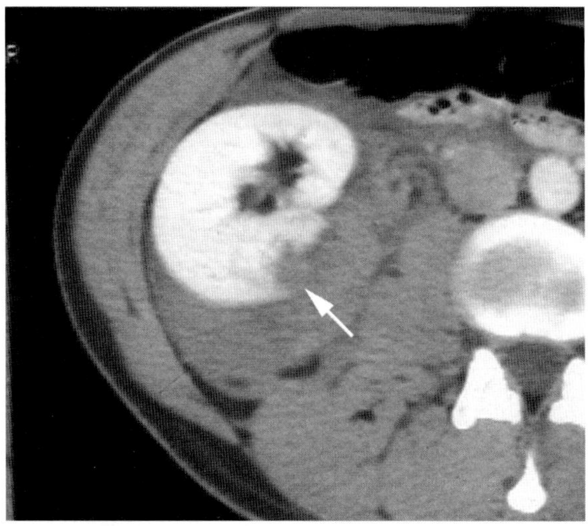

Fig. 10.9. Renal laceration, approximately 1 cm deep, without involvement of the collecting system after blunt abdominal trauma (AAST grade II). Contrast-enhanced CT demonstrates a laceration of the posterior aspect of the right kidney (*arrow*) associated with large perinephric hematoma

- AAST grade IV. Category 2. Complete renal laceration is a laceration that extends into the collecting system and causes urinary extravasation. Diagnosis is made on CT by detecting the increased depth of the parenchymal tear and by showing extravasation of iodinated contrast medium on

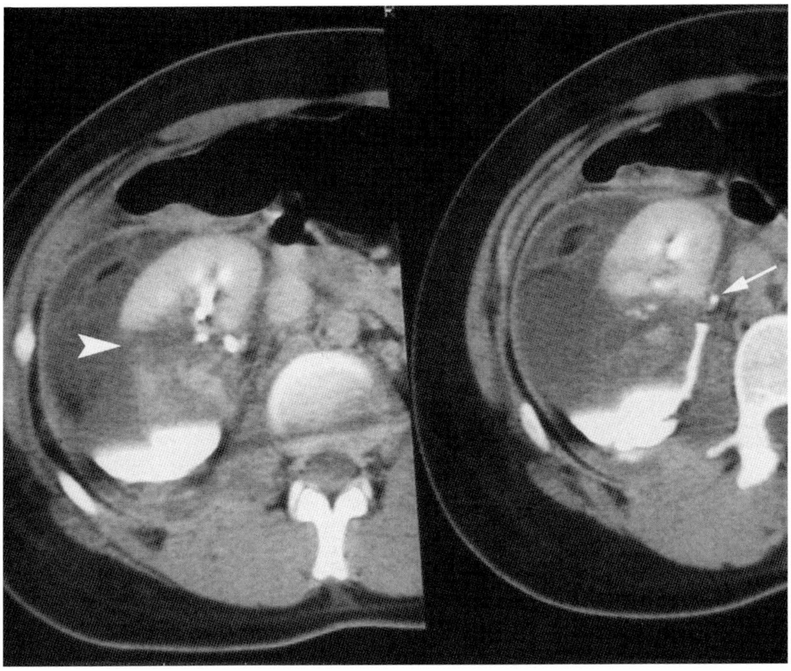

Fig. 10.10. Major renal laceration involving the collecting system after blunt trauma (AAST grade IV). Contrast-enhanced delayed-phase CT shows a major laceration of the mid pole of the right kidney (*arrowhead*) with extravasation of contrast material. There is antegrade filling of the ureter (*arrow*)

delayed scans (Fig. 10.10). Renal fracture is represented by a tear that transects the kidney from its lateral to its medial border, accompanied by extravasation of opacified urine (Fig. 10.11). Disruption of the UPJ is included in this category and may occur without or with major parenchymal injury (Fig. 10.12). For the diagnosis, thin slices are acquired on the delayed phase to precisely point out the level of extravasation. Renal vein injury include tears that require surgical treatment or thrombosis which may be managed conservatively (Fig. 10.13). In grade IV injuries, the rate of surgery is 78%, similar to grade III injuries, but the number of nephrectomies is three times higher (10% vs 3.4%). Despite the high operation rate, mortality for grade IV traumatism may be as low as 0% (Knudson et al. 2000). This observation confirms that grade IV represents a more severe injury and actually validates the AAST grading that separates grades III and IV. On the contrary, the CT classification proposed by Fanney places mild and major injuries that have a completely different outcome in Category 2.

- AAST grade V. Category 2. A shattered kidney with contained fragments is demonstrated at CT as multiple lacerations of the kidney with an intact renal capsule. According to some authors, this type of injury may sometimes be treated conservatively (Fanney et al. 1990; Knudson et al. 2000).

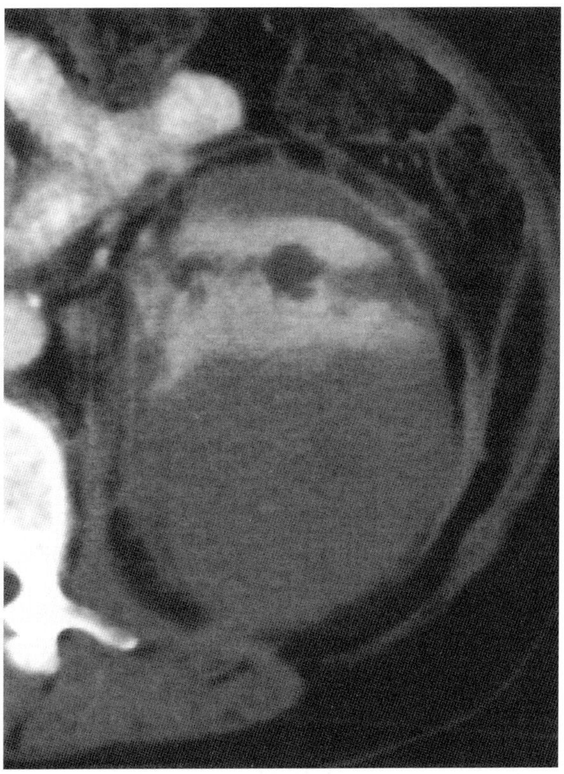

Fig. 10.11. Renal fracture. CT shows a tear that transects the kidney from its lateral to its medial border. In this case the tear is not accompanied by extravasation of opacified urine, since it runs through the lower pole. There is a large perirenal hematoma

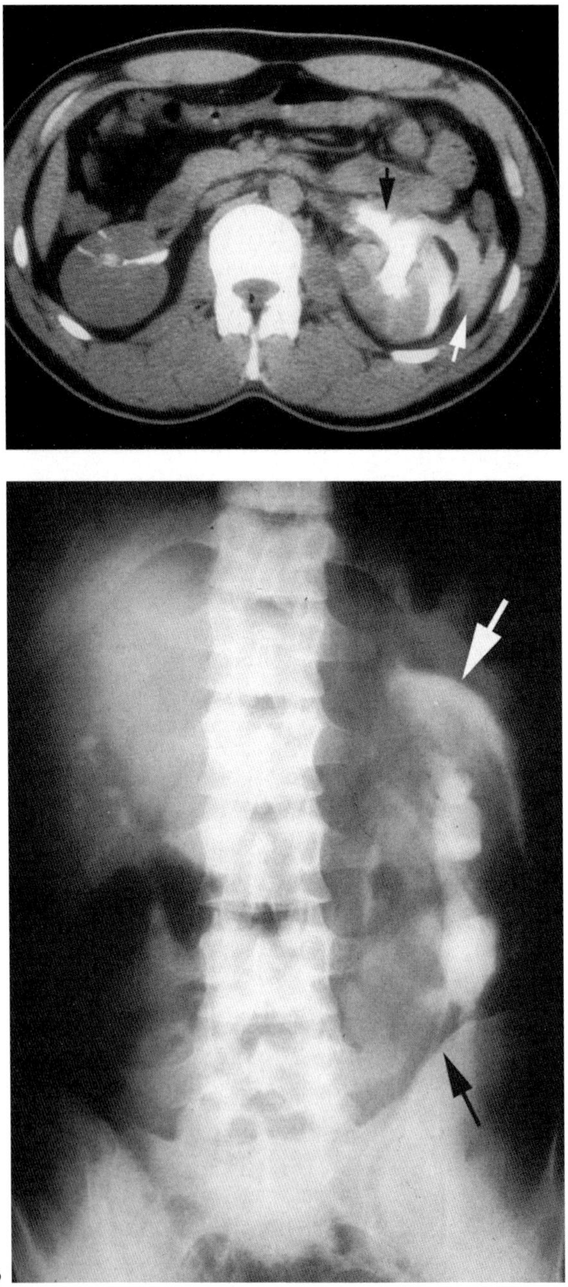

a

b

Fig. 10.12a, b. Laceration of the renal pelvis in a 27-year-old man with malrotated kidney. Unenhanced CT (**a**) performed 6 h after contrast-enhanced study revealed no signs of trauma. There is extravasation of urine at the level of the anterior wall of the renal pelvis (*black arrow*) which extends in the perirenal and pararenal spaces (*white arrow*). The focal areas of striation with contrast staining seen within the right kidney represent intrarenal contusions (the striation is probably due to intravasation). Intravenous pyelography (**b**) confirms extravasation (*white arrow*) with a normal-caliber ureter (*black arrow*), a finding that indicates that ureteral continuity has been maintained. The left kidney is malrotated, a condition that increases the likelihood of renal injury after blunt trauma

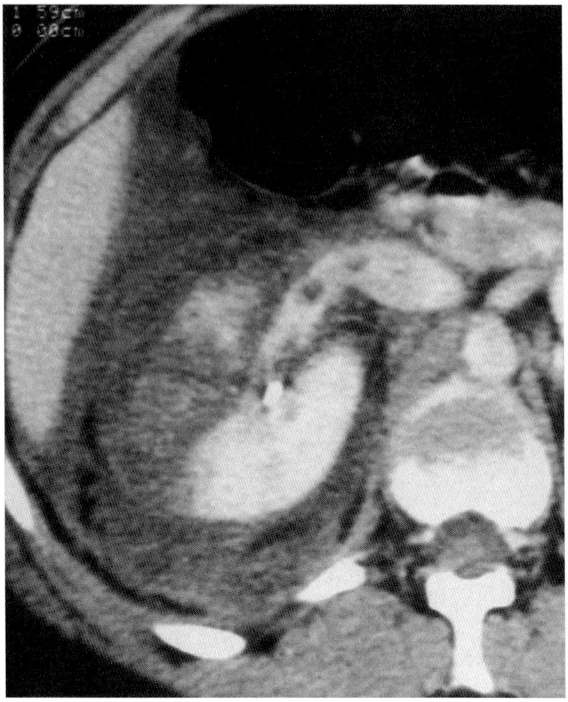

Fig. 10.13. Thrombosis of right renal vein after blunt trauma. Contrast-enhanced CT shows clots within the main renal vein in a patient with AAST grade IV renal trauma (same patient shown in Fig. 10.10)

- AAST grade V. Category 3. A shattered kidney with disrupted fragments results when the capsule is no longer intact and pieces of parenchyma are separated from the structures of the renal sinus; a large retroperitoneal hematoma is often present. Sometimes CT may detect active arterial extravasation in these major traumas (Kawashima et al. 2001) (Fig. 10.14). Both renal artery occlusion and renal artery avulsion are often caused by deceleration injuries. When the artery thromboses, either partially or totally, CT may show a nonenhancing kidney with little perirenal hematoma. When there is vascular avulsion, the kidney enhances much less than the uninjured site, but there is a large retroperitoneal hematoma due to active bleeding from the ruptured vessel (Fig. 10.15). Grade V lesions are surgically treated in 85%–90% of cases, with nephrectomy being the most commonly performed operation (Knudson et al. 2000; Santucci et al. 2001). Mortality in this group of patients varies from 6% to 22% and is largely due to the associated multisystem injuries (Cass 1989; Knudson et al. 2000).

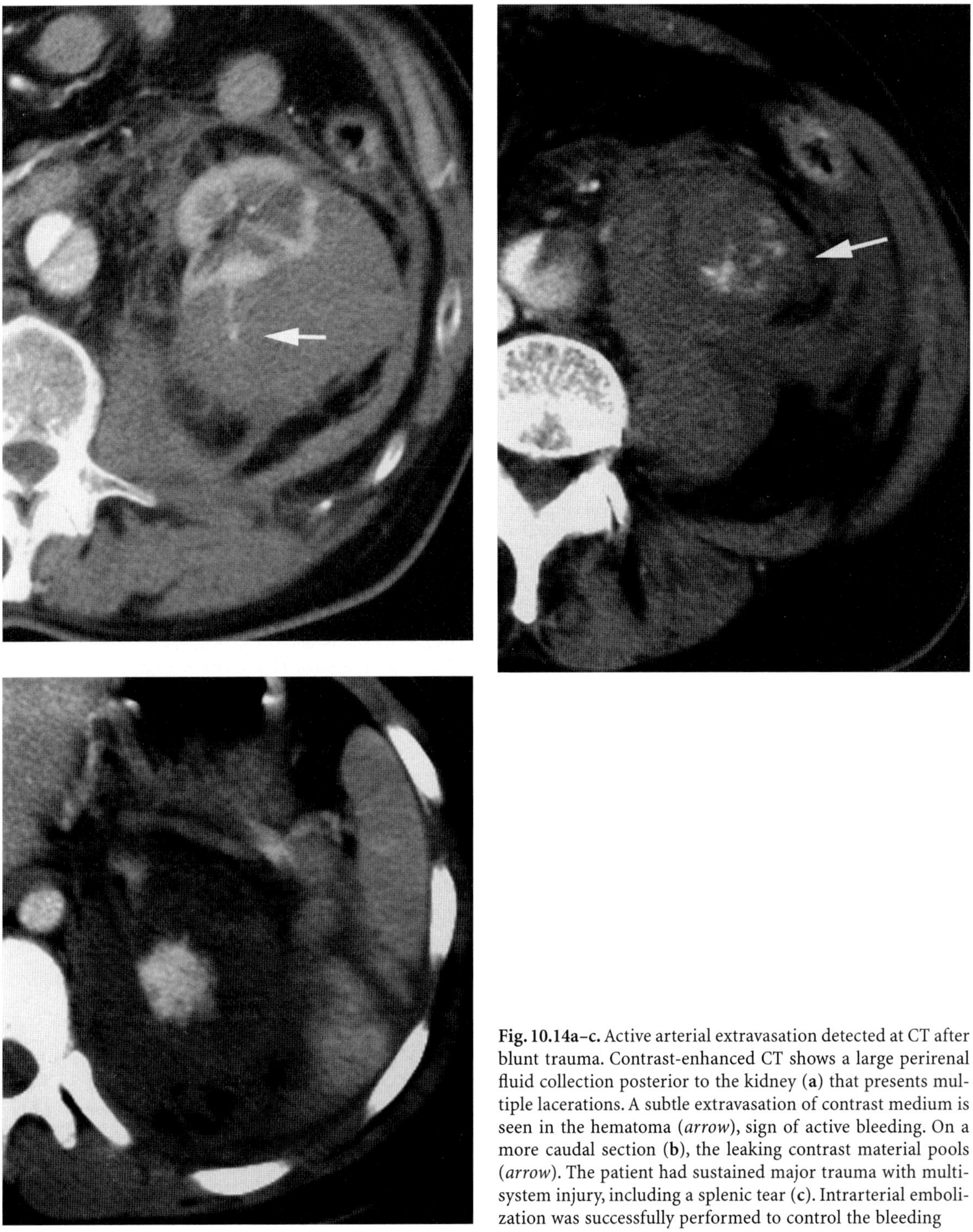

a b c

Fig. 10.14a–c. Active arterial extravasation detected at CT after blunt trauma. Contrast-enhanced CT shows a large perirenal fluid collection posterior to the kidney (**a**) that presents multiple lacerations. A subtle extravasation of contrast medium is seen in the hematoma (*arrow*), sign of active bleeding. On a more caudal section (**b**), the leaking contrast material pools (*arrow*). The patient had sustained major trauma with multisystem injury, including a splenic tear (**c**). Intrarterial embolization was successfully performed to control the bleeding

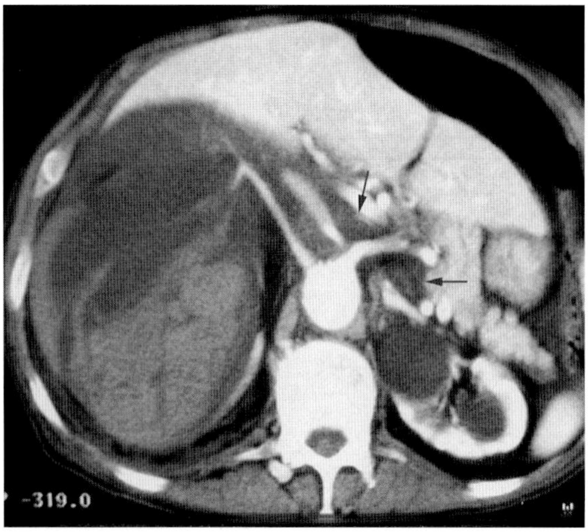

Fig. 10.15. Vascular avulsion of the main right renal artery (AAST grade V) after blunt trauma. Contrast-enhanced CT in corticomedullary phase shows huge perirenal hematoma with enhancement of some portion of the right renal artery, but no appreciable enhancement of the whole kidney. The presence of the hematoma is indicative of avulsion rather than simple traumatic occlusion. Note extension of the hematoma across the midline (*arrows*)

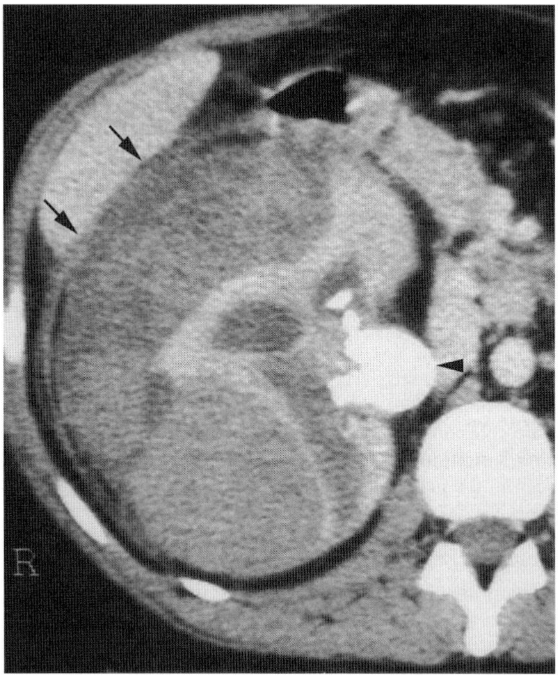

Fig. 10.16. Large subcapsular hematoma in a patient with staghorn calculus after minor blunt trauma. Contrast-enhanced CT demonstrates a subcapsular fluid collection (*arrows*) deforming the lateral contour of the right kidney, with medial displacement of the normal parenchyma. There is a large staghorn calculus (*arrowhead*)

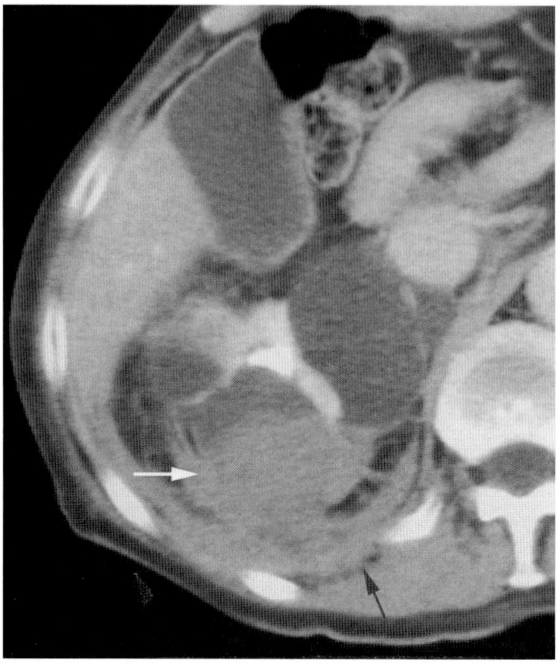

Fig. 10.17. Intraparenchymal and perirenal hemorrhage after blunt trauma in a patient with multiple renal cysts. Contrast-enhanced CT shows hemorrhage within a posterior cyst (*white arrow*) with extension of the hemorrhage in the posterior pararenal space (*black arrow*)

In patients with a preexisting renal abnormality, minor trauma may cause disproportionate injury. Such underlying conditions can usually be demonstrated by CT (Figs. 10.16 and 10.17). One should always remember that acute bleeding from minor trauma can be due to an undiagnosed renal tumor (Fig. 10.18).

10.5.1.3
Results

The usefulness of CT for the assessment of renal trauma was already established during the 1980s (McAninch and Federle 1982; Bretan et al. 1986). However, it is over the past decade that CT has assumed an increasingly important role in patient management. Since most of the anatomical criteria on which the different injury classifications are based may be easily obtained with a contrast-enhanced CT, the main role of this imaging technique is to gather precise data, which are used in establishing the degree of injury.

Despite this widespread use of CT, there are not many recent prospective studies that assess the accuracy of CT in the diagnosis of renal trauma. In a

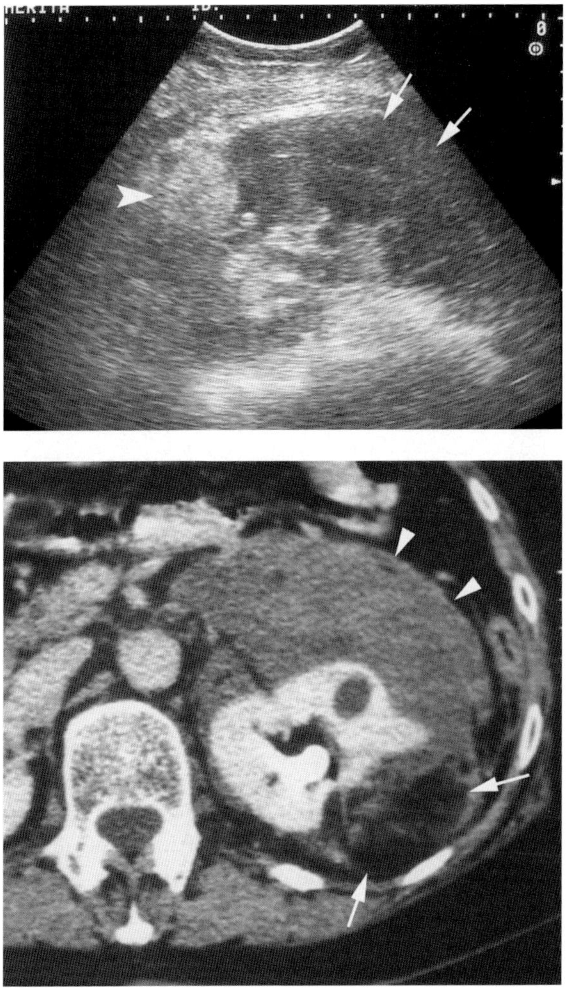

a

b

Fig. 10.18a, b. Perirenal hemorrhage in patient with angiomyolipoma. Ultrasound (**a**) demonstrates a fluid collection anterolateral to the kidney (*arrows*) and a round hyperechoic mass (*arrowhead*) in the upper pole. Contrast-enhanced CT (**b**) confirms the presence of a large hematoma in the left anterior pararenal space (*arrowheads*) and a mass with negative CT values in the posterior aspect of the mid-upper polar region (*arrows*). The patient had sustained minor blunt trauma

prospective series consisting of 85 patients, Bretan reported that CT was more accurate than IVP in staging the degree of renal trauma (Bretan et al. 1986). In 33 out of 85 patients, the CT findings were compared to surgical exploration; there were no false positive or false negative diagnoses. The follow-up of the patients confirmed that no major trauma had been missed by CT imaging. Buchberger et al., in a retrospective study on 1230 patients, had a similar experience and reported that CT was correct in the diagnosis and staging of all cases with mild and major renal injuries (Buchberger et al. 1993).

For most trauma urologists, CT is the imaging modality of choice in the evaluation of renal injury, as it provides information about morphology, vasculature, and the collecting system in one examination. The same amount of data could only be obtained by using a combination of several other imaging modalities, such as ultrasound, IVP, or angiography. Urologists consider the CT findings inferior only to surgical exploration in the assessment of injury grade (Santucci et al. 2001).

10.5.2 Intravenous Pyelography

Although CT has largely replaced intravenous pyelography (IVP) for the evaluation of renal trauma in recent times, IVP with nephrotomography has been the initial imaging test performed for many years (Miller and McAninch 1995). Hessel and Smith analyzed the available literature from the pre-CT era and reported that IVP provided sufficient information for patient management in 90% of patients with renal injury (Hessel and Smith 1974).

10.5.2.1 Technique

There are several factors which may limit the accuracy of IVP in the trauma setting, the most important one being hypotension, therefore high-dose urography is usually carried out. An adequate dose of iodinated contrast medium is 1.5–2.0 ml/kg of 60% nonionic contrast medium or 150 ml in an adult patient. The dose for a child would be 2–3 ml/kg. A plain film of the abdomen is acquired before injection, then a film of the renal region is taken immediately after injection in order to image the maximally dense nephrogram, since an intact renal contour in this phase is one of the most important findings to exclude renal trauma. Additional films are taken at 5, 10 and 15 min and are completed by tomograms in order to reduce the interference of bowel gas and stools. Ureteral compression is not used since it may initiate or increase urine extravasation. Oblique films and adequate views of the ureters and bladder are also an important completion to the study.

Hemodynamically unstable patients with gross hematuria requiring urgent surgery for whatever reason undergo an abbreviated IVP with filming at 1, 3, and 5 min after injection of 100–150 ml of 60% contrast medium. This study may be done in the operating room and, though technically of limited quality, establishes if there is bilateral renal function, should prompt surgical exploration of one kidney be necessary. In addition, this study can be performed with minimal disruption to the surgical team's efforts to stabilize the patient, and in one study safely obviated renal exploration in 32% of patients (Morey et al. 1999). A prerequisite for the performance of an IVP is adequate renal blood flow with good glomerular filtration, which is present when a mean arterial pressure of roughly 80–90 mmHg can be maintained (Pollack and Wein 1989). It is usually possible to obtain this in most cases by infusion of blood, plasma expanders, or vasopressors.

10.5.2.2
Findings

A kidney which homogeneously impregnates with contrast at IVP, has well-defined, regular margins, and which excretes iodinated urine into an intact and nondistorted collecting system is either normal or has sustained no major injury (grades I–II AAST classification). Without oblique views, however, small parenchymal lacerations of the anterior or posterior surface may be missed.

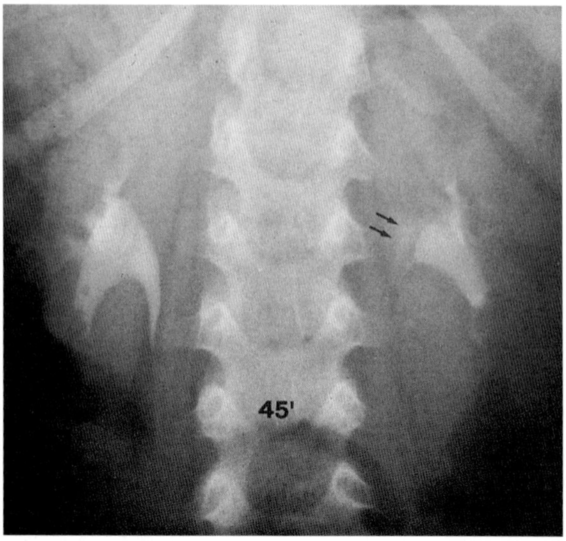

Fig. 10.19. Urinary extravasation demonstrated at intravenous pyelography (IVP) after blunt trauma. The film was taken 45 min after contrast-medium injection. There is subtle extravasation of iodinated urine medially to the left renal pelvis (*arrows*)

- Renal contusion may be seen as a nephrogram of reduced density and reduced excretion of iodinated urine as compared to the uninjured site (Class and Luxenberg 1984). More rarely a striated nephrogram is seen as a result of contusion (Rubin and Schliftman 1979). A nephrogram of reduced density is a nonspecific sign and may be due to parenchymal lacerations or even a shattered kidney. In these cases, however, perirenal hemorrhage is present, a condition not always appreciated on IVP.
- Renal parenchymal laceration appears as a focal abnormality of the contour of the kidney, an intrarenal mass with displacement of the collecting system, or as a defect in the nephrogram.
- The term "renal fracture" usually indicates a deep laceration with separation of two renal poles by a hypodense area, which represents a hematoma. A laceration that involves the collecting system causes extravasation of urine and implies a potentially serious injury (grade IV AAST classification) (Fig. 10.19). Extravasation may remain within the kidney, extend to perinephric fat, or diffuse widely throughout the retroperitoneal space. Laceration of the renal collecting system with little renal parenchymal damage is more common in penetrating trauma than in blunt trauma. When seen in blunt trauma, it is usually associated with major parenchymal lacerations and perirenal hemorrhage. Massive accumulation of iodinated urine, particularly when the renal parenchyma appears intact and the ureter fails to opacify, should suggest avulsion of the UPJ.
- Unilateral absence of nephrogram and excretion at IVP is an indicator of a severe injury, such as pedicle injury or shattered kidney (Stables 1976). In most cases, a nonvisualized kidney will result from thrombosis of the renal artery or less commonly vascular avulsion (grade V AAST classification).

It is important to keep in mind that an absent nephrogram may be caused by nontraumatic conditions, such as preexisting kidney disease, renal ectopia, or congenitally absent kidney.

10.5.3
Ultrasound

Ultrasound (US) is less popular in screening patients with renal trauma than it is in the evaluation of patients with suspected intraabdominal injury (Pearl and Todd 1996). This is due to the retroperitoneal location of the kidneys and to the absence of a specific sign for retroperitoneal injury, such as the intraperitoneal fluid is for of intraabdominal trauma. Some published series assessing the efficacy of US in the trauma setting actually exclude patients with hematuria or suspected retroperitoneal injury from their analysis (BOULANGER et al. 1995; MCKENNEY et al. 1996). Sonography in renal trauma patients is used more in Europe than in the United States.

10.5.3.1
Findings

US signs of renal injury include enlargement of the kidney, changes in echotexture with one or more areas of distorted renal architecture, and alteration of the renal contour. In minor trauma, focal areas of hemorrhage and edema may be seen as hypoechoic ill-defined zones or as hyperechoic areas according to the age of the intrarenal bleeding (Figs. 10.20, 10.21). Perirenal fluid may be hypoechoic if it contains urine, but is more often hyperechoic and indicates the presence of blood (Figs. 10.22, 10.23). A large acute collection containing clear fluid with no internal echoes usually represents a urinoma. A large hematoma may displace the kidney anteriorly or medially, thus pushing the kidney away from the ultrasonic probe and rendering the evaluation of the renal architecture difficult. Chronic hematomas may be completely anechoic (Fig. 10.24). Laceration of the

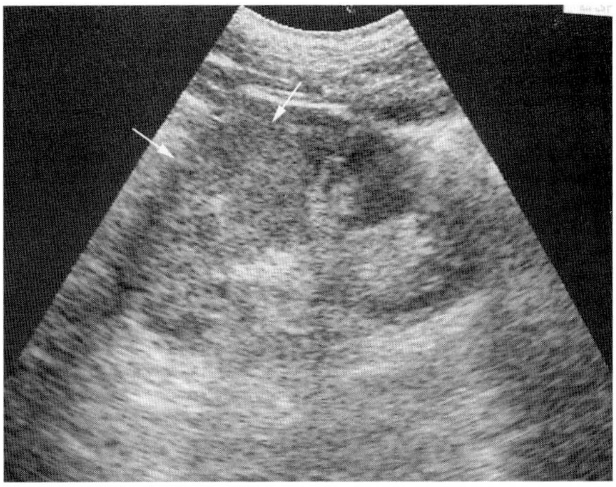

Fig. 10.20. Ultrasound of intrarenal hematoma. There is a large hyperechoic area that replaces the upper portion of the left kidney (*arrows*). The normal renal architecture is not recognized in this area

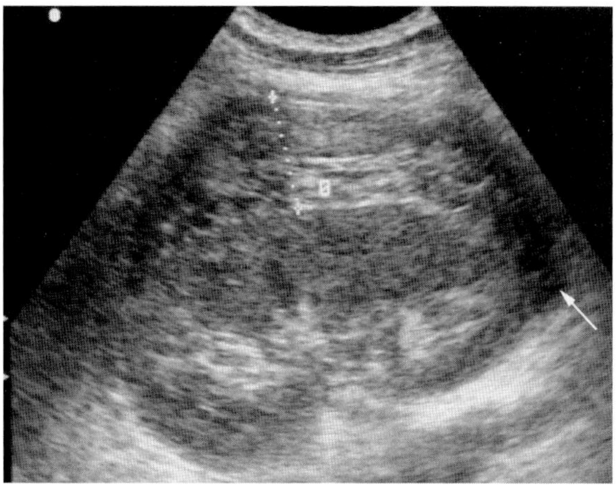

Fig. 10.22. Large perirenal hematoma. Ultrasound, after blunt trauma, shows a large fluid collection containing low-level echoes (*area within calipers*) as well as more fluid portions (*arrow*). The hyperechoic appearance is diagnostic of fresh blood within the retroperitoneal fat

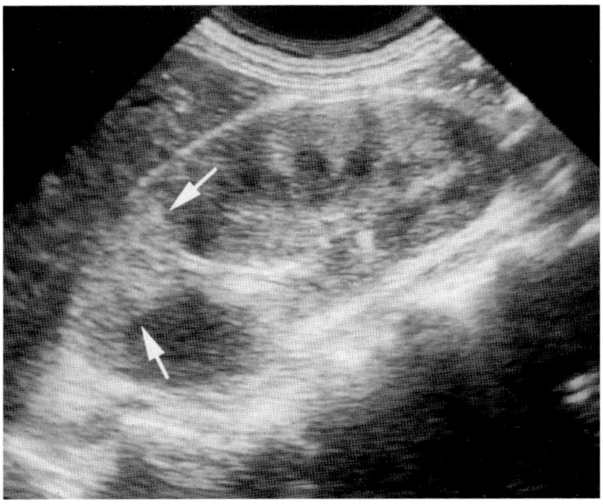

Fig. 10.21. Small upper pole hematoma on ultrasound. There is a small hyperechoic area in the upper pole of the right kidney (*arrows*). The absence of perirenal fluid bespeaks an intact capsule

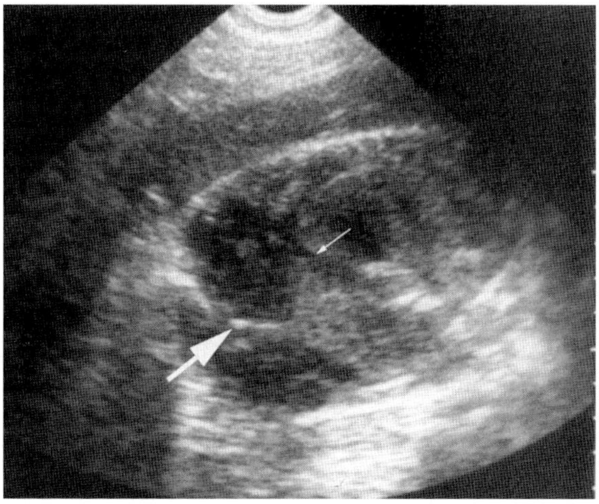

Fig. 10.23. Perirenal hematoma. Ultrasound, after blunt trauma, shows a small fluid collection containing low-level echoes and septations (*large arrow*). An area of discontinuity in the renal capsule is seen (*small arrow*) and represents a laceration

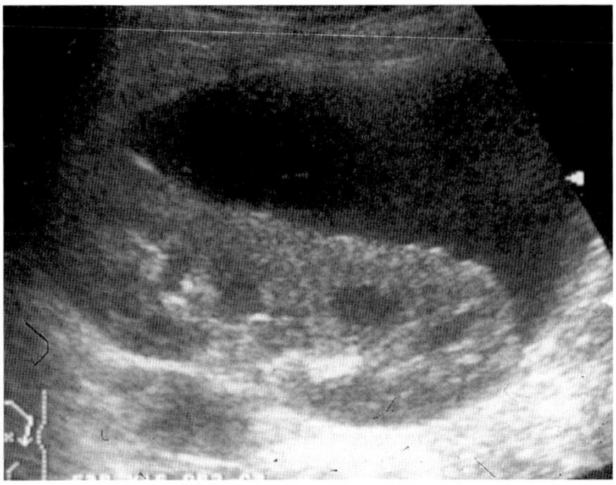

Fig. 10.24. Chronic perirenal hematoma. Ultrasound shows a large fluid collection with no internal echoes in this patients 5 weeks after blunt renal trauma

renal contour are seen only when there is excellent visualization of the whole kidney, a condition that is not always given in the acute trauma setting. Dilation of the collecting system may be present in case of obstruction of the UPJ or ureter by blood clots. Low level echoes within the renal calices and pelvis usually represent hemorrhage. Color Doppler and power Doppler should always be used, if available, since they provide useful information and add little time to the study in the hands of experienced operators. Using pulsed and color Doppler, one should search for the major vascular structure of the renal hilum. Detection of an unequivocal Doppler signal from the main renal artery and vein excludes the possibility of severe vascular injury. Color Doppler may also be used to evaluate the complications due to percutaneous biopsy in allografts and native kidneys (Gainza et al. 1995).

Contrast agents are being increasingly used in US. Two preliminary reports investigated the use of US contrast agents in experimental models of renal trauma, respectively in rabbits and pigs. The use of contrast agents increased the confidence in diagnosis in one study and allowed for the detection of small intraparenchymal hematomas in the other study (Schmiedl et al. 1999; Hochmuth et al. 2000). The US study should be extended to the abdominal cavity, since some patients may have free intraabdominal fluid as a sign of renal trauma. In one study, 35% of patients with renal injuries had free fluid in the abdomen, whereas no free fluid was seen in 65% of cases. All patients with free fluid had moderate or severe renal injuries as a result of multisystem trauma (McGahan et al. 1999).

10.5.3.2
Results

The reports on the use of US in the setting of renal trauma are rather skeptical if they originate from the United States and moderately enthusiastic if they come from European authors. McGahan et al. (1999) assessed the use of emergent US examination in acute traumatic renal injuries over a 3-year period. Thirty-two patients with 37 renal injuries were studied, and renal parenchymal abnormalities were identified on US in only 8 of 37 (22%) injured kidneys. The abnormalities were detected more commonly in cases of severe injury (60%). In their experience, the US study of the kidney was often normal in renal trauma, but it was more likely to be abnormal with severe (grade II or greater) renal injuries. The authors conclude that a negative US examination does not exclude renal injury, and, depending on clinical and laboratory findings, other imaging procedures such as CT should be performed.

The low diagnostic yield of US was confirmed by another study in 46 children with blunt trauma. IVP had a diagnostic accuracy of 80.8% while US was diagnostic in only 41% of cases (Mayor et al. 1995). It has been observed that US may also be negative in cases of major renal trauma (Perry et al. 1997). This latter observation is also confirmed by Lopez Cubillana et al. (1998) who observed that the sensitivity of US decreases as the severity of the trauma increases (75% for grade I, 88.9% for grade II, 73.3% for grade III, and 0% for grade IV), while that of IVP remains high for all degrees of severity (100% for grade I, 92% for grade II, 100% for grade III, and 100% for grade IV). Buchberger et al. (1993), in their retrospective experience with 1230 cases of renal trauma studied with urinalysis, IVP, US, and CT, found 95 patients with mild and major renal trauma (>grade II AAST classification). CT was performed in 45 of these patients and correctly diagnosed and staged all cases. IVP established the correct diagnosis in 72% and US in 85%. However, when IVP and US were combined, the sensitivity for clinically relevant trauma, such as lacerations and pedicle injuries, was 98% with a specificity of 99%. The authors concluded by suggesting that US should be used as a screening modality in flank trauma with suspected renal injury and that additional urography is performed in case US detects intra- or perirenal hematoma (Buchberger et al. 1993). Other authors share the same opinion that US should be the technique of choice for the initial workup of blunt renal trauma (Jakse et al. 1987; Furtschegger et al. 1988; Rosales et al. 1992). Interestingly, US is considered ideal in the setting of mass casualties, when accurate diagnostic information is necessary for purposes of rapid triage on a larger number of patients, such as after an earthquake (NORDENHOLZ et al. 1997). In a report on 400 patients studied in 72 h, physician-performed ultrasound examination discovered trauma-associated pathology in 12.8% of patients, including cases with psoas muscle hematoma and renal injury (SARKISIAN et al. 1991). We should remember that we live in a wealthy society were high-tech medical care, such as helical CT, is available to most patients, while in other regions of the world, such as equatorial Africa, there are emergency units with only modest technical support. In these situations, US may be a very useful and often sufficient tool for accurate diagnosis (N'GOAN et al. 1997).

10.5.4 Magnetic Resonance Imaging

There is limited experience with magnetic resonance imaging (MRI) in renal trauma (MCGEHEE et al. 1993; LEPPANIEMI et al. 1995, 1997; MARCOS et al. 1998; SARKISIAN et al. 1991). This is due to the fact that MRI is not used as a first-line imaging test in body trauma. MRI has several limitations in the evaluation of patients with renal trauma, such as the need for patient immobility during the examination, difficult access to patient monitoring, reduced anatomical coverage (abdomen and pelvis) in examination time longer than helical CT, and lack of 24-h staffing. In one study, MRI was considered as effective as CT in assessing renal parenchymal lacerations, with MRI being useful for its ability to provide direct coronal and sagittal images (LEPPANIEMI et al. 1995). Some authors suggest using MRI when the CT findings are equivocal or show serious injuries (grade III–IV) with lacerations and renal fragmentation that need to be assessed in the coronal or sagittal plane, in a stable and cooperative patient (LEPPANIEMI et al. 1997). In addition, MRI can be used in cases where there is a contraindication to the use of iodinated contrast medium, and in the follow-up of renal trauma in order to reduce the amount of X-ray exposure (Fig. 10.25).

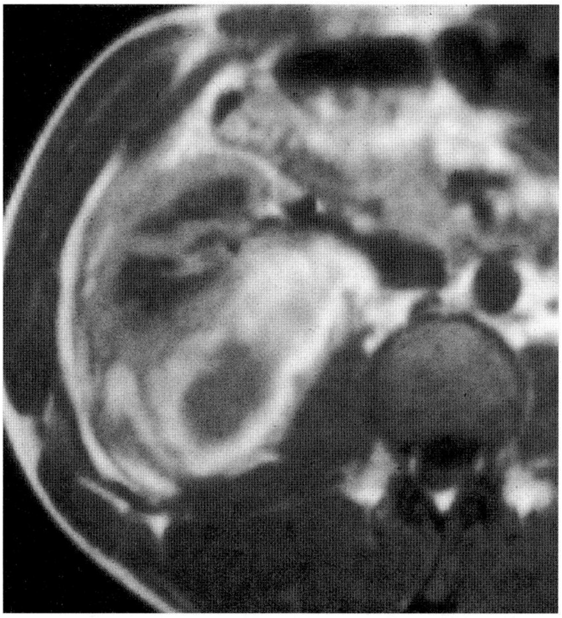

Fig. 10.25. MR after blunt renal trauma. T2-weighted axial MR image shows large hematoma in the posterior pararenal space with anterior displacement of the right kidney

10.5.5 Arteriography

The role of arteriography in renal trauma has diminished since the advent of CT as the diagnostic test of choice. Nowadays, the indications of arteriography in blunt trauma can be summarized as follows:

- Persistent primary or secondary bleeding; angiography may be combined with embolization in such cases.
- Suspected arterial injuries or vascular abnormalities (e.g., tumors, aneurysms, fistulas) not clarified with CT. The latter indication is less common.

In a recent survey of 137 patients who underwent angiography to localize intraperitoneal and retroperitoneal sources of bleeding, renal trauma accounted for only 12 cases (8.7%) (VELMAHOS et al. 2000). Arteriography is contraindicated when the patient is hemodynamically unstable or when there is no enhancement of the injured kidney at CT, a pathognomonic sign of renal artery thrombosis. In such cases, arteriography is not needed to confirm the diagnosis and actually prolongs the time between diagnosis and treatment, thus increasing the warm ischemia time (KANTOR et al. 1989). It is known that renal revascularization is most likely to be successful within 2 h of injury (HOFFMAN et al. 1974). There is more inclination toward the use of arteriography in cases of penetrating injuries. Renal trauma caused by penetration is more likely to result in arterial lacerations and arteriovenous fistulae because of the nature of the mechanism of injury. Arteriography may be indicated in most patients with penetrating trauma to the back whose CT shows active bleeding, renal laceration, large retroperitoneal hematoma, or who have persistent gross hematuria or hypertension (Federle et al. 1987; Kantor et al. 1989) (Fig. 10.26).

In any case, the arteriogram is performed with the double intent of making a diagnosis and providing definitive treatment by embolization of the bleeding site. Selective occlusion of the injured renal vessel without damaging, to a large extent, the surrounding normal parenchyma is the goal of transcatheter therapy. Recent improvements in coaxial systems and guidewires have made it possible to superselectively catheterize 1- to 2-mm vessels, thus minimizing the area of tissue loss (Fig. 10.27). The results are excellent, with cessation of bleeding in 83%–100% of cases (Kantor et al. 1989; Huppert et al. 1993; Dorffner et al. 1998; Kramer et al. 1998). Embolization may not be successful when there are large AV fistulas (Kantor et al. 1989). Transcatheter management is particularly appropriate after iatrogenic penetrating trauma, either in native or transplanted kidneys, due to biopsy, nephrostomy or other percutaneous procedures (Huppert et al. 1993; Dorffner et al. 1998) (Fig. 10.28). The use of a combined CT and angiographic suite allows making the diagnosis of

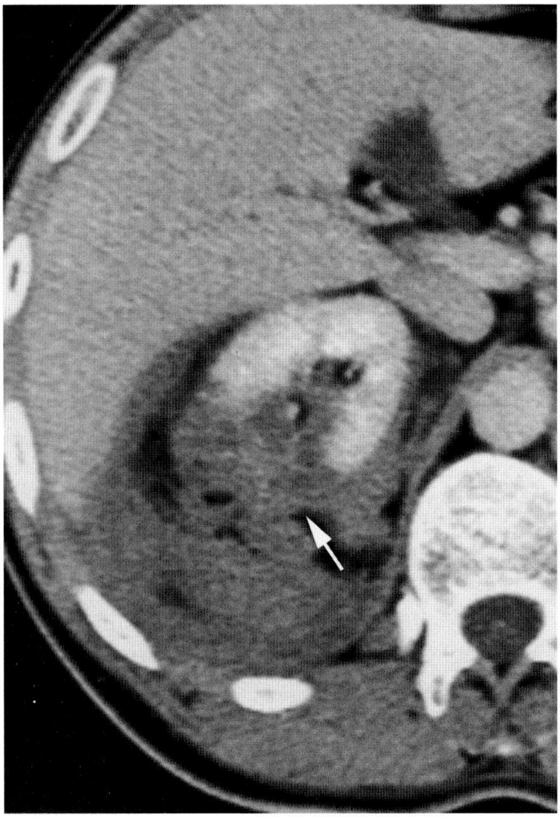

a

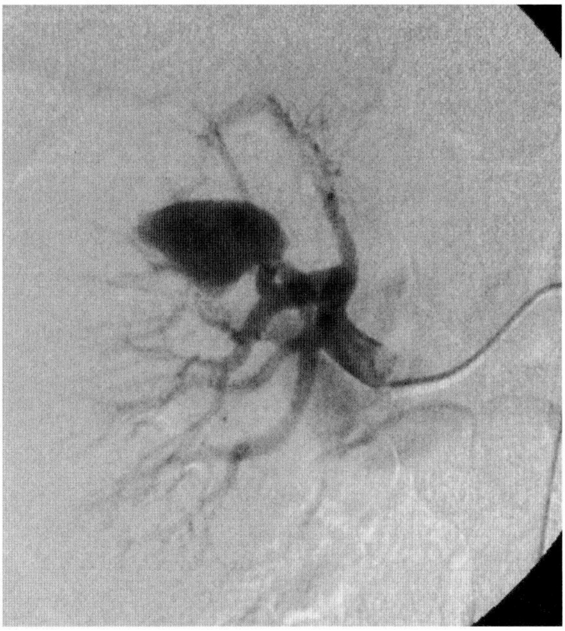

b

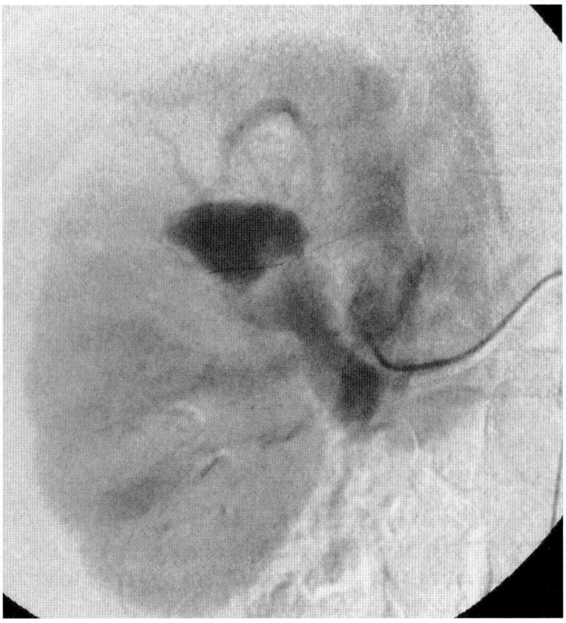

c

Fig. 10.26a–c. Penetrating trauma with AV fistula. Contrast-enhanced CT (**a**) shows an area of parenchymal laceration (*arrow*) after stabbing to the back. Patient refused treatment. After 7 days, due to persistent hematuria, angiography was performed and demonstrated a large AV fistula (**b** and **c**)

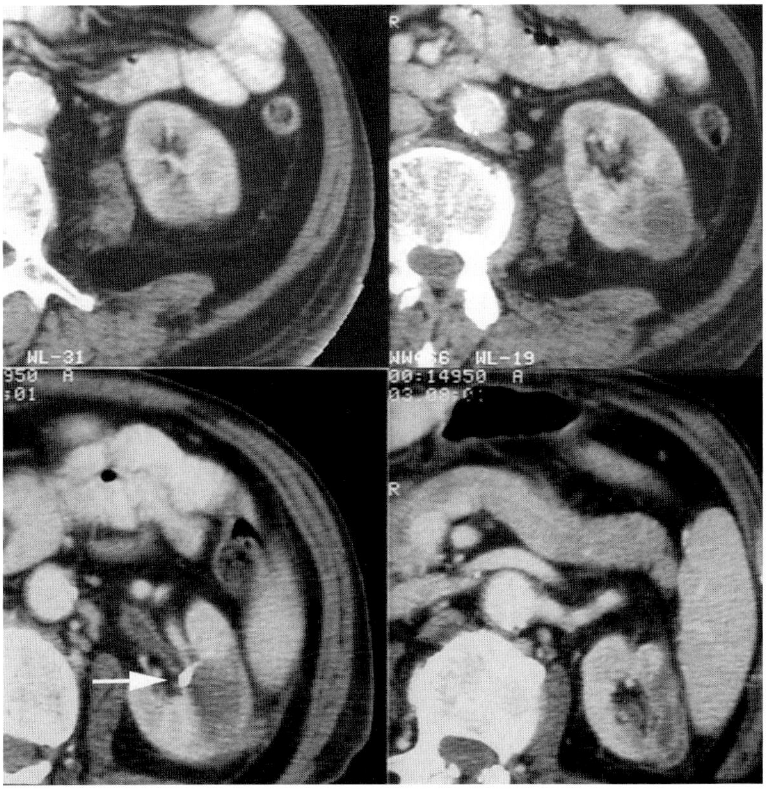

Fig. 10.27. Postembolization infarction. Patient had sustained a stab wound to the back and had undergone transcatheter embolization for progressive hematuria with placement of a metallic coil (*arrow*). There is a sharply demarcated area of decreased attenuation in the interpolar region of the right kidney due to infarction, with limited loss of functioning tissue

a

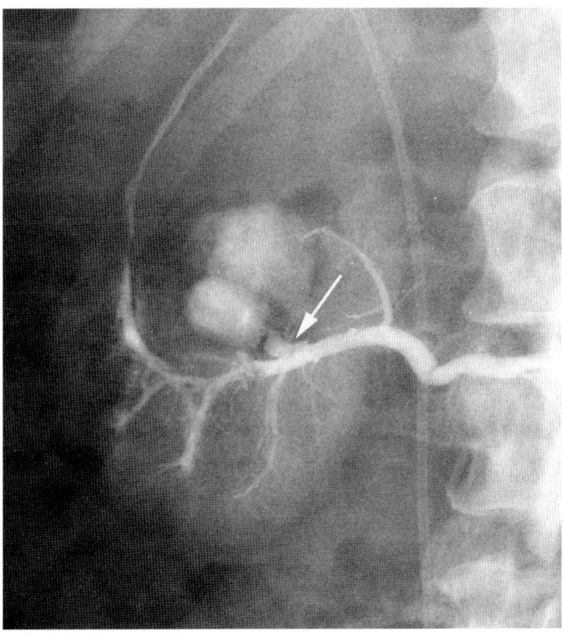

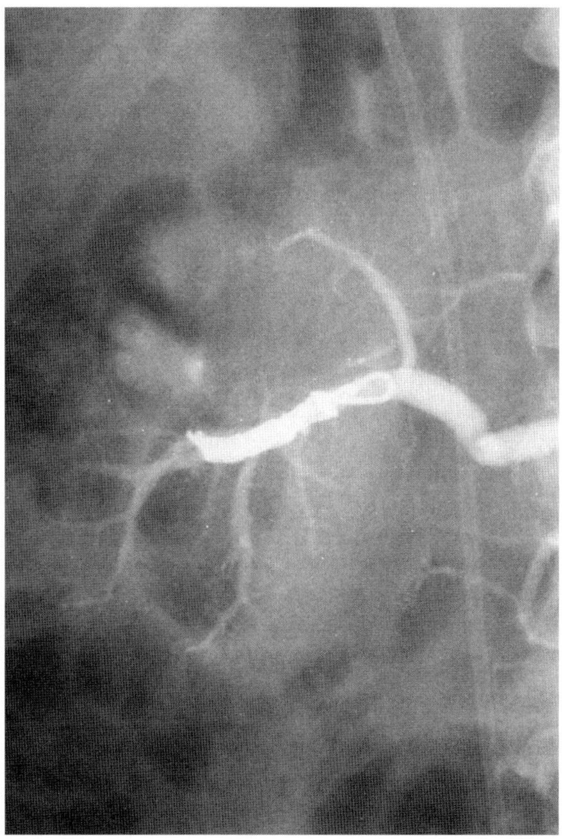

b

Fig. 10.28a, b. Bleeding after extracorporeal shockwave lithotripsy. Selective arteriogram (**a**) of right lower pole artery shows of two large pseudoaneurysmal cavities in the central portion of the kidney, the point of extravasation is shown by the *arrow*. The area of extravasation was embolized with 6-mm diameter coil. Postembolization arteriogram (**b**) shows occlusion of the site of bleeding trauma on spiral CT and managing the active bleeding by transcatheter embolization without transferring the patient. This saves precious time and is particularly useful when the patients are intubated and monitored (Kos et al. 1999). In case of arterial injury, attempts at revascularization will almost always be fruitless if the treatment delay exceeds 12 h. Even under the best circumstances, however, the success rate with relatively early surgery is low (Haas et al. 1998; Knudson et al. 2000). Endovascular repair of an injured renal artery, so far, is mostly reflected in case reports but is a promising less invasive mean of renal artery reconstruction (Goodman et al. 1998; Paul et al. 1999; Lutkevich et al. 2000). Since the most common form of major vascular injury, particularly in the pediatric age group, is dissection or thrombosis due to intimal flap rather than avulsion, renal artery stenting, if performed early after trauma and in absence of other major injuries that demand nephrectomy, may be a way of preserving the injured organ (Goodman et al. 1998; Paul et al. 1999).

10.6 Management

The treatment of renal trauma has been the subject of controversy over recent years. The treatment options depend upon whether a blunt or penetrating injury has occurred and on the degree of injury based upon adequate radiological staging (Matthews and Spirnak 1995). Conservative management of blunt renal trauma has evolved over the past 30 years. The main reason for conservative management lies in the fact that more than 90% of renal trauma patients have minor injuries (AAST grades I and II). More recently, investigators realized that even in case of more serious injuries, the nephrectomy rate was lower in patients who were managed expectantly than in patients who underwent operative exploration. In a series reported by Bergen et al. (1987), the overall nephrectomy rate was 12.6% but was 35% among patients who were explored. Therefore, patients who have sustained blunt renal trauma rarely require surgical exploration, with most reports indicating operation rates lower than 10% (McAninch and Carroll 1989). Most urologists nowadays attempt to manage all renal injuries expectantly. However, some indications for immediate surgical exploration exist. These include patients with AAST grade V renovascular injury as in renal pedicle avulsion, in whom the risk of exsanguination is high, and patients with persistent, life-threatening bleeding, usually associated with an expanding retroperitoneal hematoma (Santucci and McAninch 2000). In addition, if there is clear evidence of pedicle avulsion, then early exploration and repair may improve renal tissue salvage and decrease the length of the hospital stay when compared to patients who are treated conservatively and have subsequent delayed exploration (Husmann and Morris 1990). Other authors prefer to lower the threshold for surgical exploration and suggest that also major laceration with involvement of the collecting system (AAST grade IV) should undergo surgical exploration when there is significant urine extravasation (Cheng et al. 1994). This view is supported by the evidence that while conservative management of renal lacerations not involving the collecting system is successful, with morbidity and subsequent nephrectomy rates equivalent to patients who undergo surgery, patients with significant extravasation have a worse outcome with a conservative approach than with surgery (Husmann and Morris 1990; Husmann et al. 1993; Cheng et al. 1994).

The absolute and relative indications for surgical exploration in patients with blunt renal trauma may be summarized as follows (Knudson and Maull 1999; Meng et al. 1999; Santucci and McAninch 2000):

- Major renovascular injury (AAST grade V)
- Renal laceration with gross extravasation of urine (AAST grade IV)
- Persistent life-threatening renal bleeding with expanding retroperitoneal hematoma (after attempt at endovascular embolization in stable patients)
- Renal parenchymal necrosis
- Development of renovascular hypertension after trauma
- Incomplete injury staging, when a major injury is suspected

There is a strong correlation between the degree of injury and the need for renal exploration. Santucci et al. (2001), in a statistical analysis of 2467 patients, confirmed this correlation both with the need for surgery (AAST grade I, 0%; grade II, 15%; grade III, 76%; grade IV, 78%; grade V, 93%) and for nephrectomy (AAST grade I, 0%; grade II, 0%; grade III, 3%; grade IV, 9%; grade V, 86%). Logistic regression analysis indicated that the odds of surgery increased 15-fold for every increase in injury grade. The authors concluded that staging provided by imaging is of paramount importance in determining the management of renal trauma patients. Surgical exploration, on the contrary, is much more often necessary in patients with penetrating renal trauma. While penetrating injury is rare, and occurs in approximately 8% in a series from North America, up to 60% of these injuries are associated with significant renovascular damage (CARROLL and MCANINCH 1985). Patients with gunshot wounds have an increased likelihood of undergoing surgery as compared to blunt trauma patients with the same degree of injury: this is due to associated vascular injury. In the above-mentioned study of SANTUCCI et al. (2001), when the mechanism of injury was factored in the statistical analysis (blunt, stab, gunshot), the odds of having surgery for every increase in injury grade were higher for penetrating trauma. Gunshot wounds showed the largest increase per increase in injury grade (45-fold), followed by stab wounds (15-fold) and blunt trauma (10-fold) (SANTUCCI et al. 2001). This last observations underscores the fact that blunt and penetrating trauma differ in incidence, etiology, management, and outcome.

10.7 Complications

Failure to recognize and treat major renal lacerations or major disruptions of the collecting system can lead to early or delayed complications, occurring, respectively, before and after the first 4 weeks after injury.

10.7.1 Early Complications

Delayed Renal Bleeding. Delayed renal bleeding is generally manifested 5–20 days after major renal parenchymal laceration. The patient may present with gross hematuria, flank pain, due to obstructing clots or large perinephric hematoma, or hypovolemic shock. Imaging such patients is dictated by the acuteness of the situation and by the availability of prior studies. Patients in hypovolemic shock not responding to fluid replacement may need surgical exploration. For patients who are stable, a repeated contrast-enhanced CT is the procedure of choice and usually is able to depict the cause of bleeding. Delayed bleeding after penetrating trauma should be studied with angiography because of the high incidence of AV fistula, particularly after stab wounds (KANTOR et al. 1989).

Prolonged or Delayed Urinary Extravasation. Gunshot wounds pose a special risk of delayed urinary extravasation because blast injury to the ureter is not always evident at the time of initial exploration. A high index of suspicion of urinary leakage should be maintained when there is persistent fever, ileus, or worsening abdominal or flank tenderness (PETERSON 1989). The diagnosis can be achieved by IVP, sometimes combined with retrograde ureterogram, and CT. Urinomas must be drained and further leakage should be minimized by draining the kidney with a percutaneous nephrostomy.

Retroperitoneal Abscess. This complication is the result of infection of an undrained urinoma or hematoma. The probability of abscess formation is higher if the collection has been seeded during the surgical exploration or if there is concomitant bowel injury. Acute abscesses will be manifested 5–7 days after injury and will cause spiking fever, flank tenderness, ileus, and occasionally flank erythema. Chronic abscesses may cause weight loss, anorexia, fatigue, and even lethargy in children. CT is the diagnostic modality of choice and percutaneous drainage through a retroperitoneal route is the first line treatment.

10.7.2 Late Complications

Hypertension. Hypertension consequent to renal trauma is renin-mediated. Renin secretion by the acutely injured kidney can range from three to eight times the normal values (VON KNORRING et al. 1981; MONTGOMERY et al. 1998; HAAS et al. 1998). Appropriate management of renal trauma lowers the plasma renin activity and relieves the hypertension (KOSSOW 1980). If hypertension persists several weeks after the trauma has healed, one should suspect renal artery injury, AV fistula, perinephric hematoma or scarring (GRANT et al. 1971; MONTGOMERY et al. 1998; HAAS et al. 1998). Hypertension may develop even after occult, clinically not evident renal trauma (MONTGOMERY et al. 1998).

Hydronephrosis and Calculus Formation. These may result from an unrecognized injury to the collecting system, calcification of a retained blood clot or fibrosis in a periureteral hematoma. Diagnosis is made by clinical symptoms and imaging (IVP and CT).

10.8 Ureteral Trauma

Iatrogenic ureteral injury may occur during various types of abdominal, pelvic and lumbar spine surgery or radiological interventions (Fry et al. 1983).

Ureteral injuries from external trauma represent approximately 3% of all genitourinary injuries (Fried and Rutledge 1995). The mobility and anatomical characteristics of the ureter protect it from blunt trauma; its narrow diameter and deep retroperitoneal location close to the spine make it an unlikely target in case of penetrating injury. When the largest series are taken into account, blunt trauma is the cause of ureteral injury in 7.6% of cases, while penetrating trauma is involved in 92.4% of cases (81.4% gunshot wounds, 11% stab wounds) (Carlton et al. 1971; Bright and Peters 1977; Presti et al. 1989; Campbell et al. 1992; Brandes et al. 1994; Armenakas 1999). In case of gunshot wounds, the bullet does not need to transect the ureter to cause significant damage. If its course is simply close to the ureter, the temporary cavitation created by the missile can produce significant tissue destruction, delayed necrosis, and ureteral injury (Armenakas 1999).

Penetrating ureteral injuries are almost always associated with multiple organ injuries, the most common sites being the small bowel, colon, liver, and iliac vessels (Eickenberg and Amin 1976; Holden et al. 1976; Pitts and Peterson 1981; Rober et al. 1990). Ureteral injuries from blunt trauma are rare and usually occur in children during rapid deceleration, causing excessive hyperextension of the vertebral column and disruption of the UPJ. They, too, are almost always associated with multiple organ injuries.

The diagnosis is made difficult by the presence of multisystem trauma and by the absence of clinical findings and signs specific for ureteral trauma. Hematuria is absent in approximately 30% of ureteral injuries (Carlton et al. 1971; Bright and Peters 1977; Liroff et al. 1977; Pitts and Peterson 1981; Presti et al. 1989; Campbell et al. 1992; Brandes et al. 1994). These limitations frequently result in a delayed diagnosis, which is associated with complications such as urinoma, fistula formation, and, eventually, sepsis. To avoid this additional morbidity, it is imperative that the emergency room physician maintain a high level of suspicion based on the injury mechanism and location. Essentially, any patients with penetrating trauma to the abdomen should be suspected of having a ureteral injury. Similarly, all children and young adults with major blunt trauma and multiple associated injuries should undergo ureteral imaging regardless the findings on urinalysis (Armenakas 1999).

Hemodynamically unstable patients can be imaged in the resuscitation suite with an abbreviated IVP with filming at 1, 3, and 5 min after injection of 100–150 ml of 60% contrast medium. This study may show contrast extravasation, which sometimes can be seen only faintly or may demonstrate mild ureteral distention proximal to the area of injury. With the widespread use of CT for the evaluation of the polytrauma patient, ureteral injuries are now being diagnosed mainly by using this imaging technique. Extravasation of contrast medium confined to the periureteral space is a common finding. Extravasation is mainly confined to the medial aspect of the ureter (Kenney et al. 1987; Kawashima et al. 1997). It is imperative to assess the ureter with delayed films, since the acquisition in the corticomedullary phase is not adequate to disclose injuries to the UPJ or ureter (Kawashima et al. 1997; Mulligan et al. 1998). If the results of IVP and CT are inconclusive, then a retrograde ureterogram is indicated. This test, however, is impractical in the acute trauma setting, and is usually performed once the acute phase of the trauma has settled and the patient is stable.

Ureteral injuries are classified as follows on the basis of the Organ Injury Scaling System of the America Association for the Surgery of Trauma (Moore et al. 1992):

Grade I:	Hematoma, contusion, or hematoma without devascularization
Grade II:	Laceration, <50% transection
Grade III:	Laceration, >50% transection
Grade IV:	Laceration, complete transection with 2 cm of devascularization
Grade V:	Laceration, avulsion with >2 cm of devascularization

Selection of the appropriate management option depends on the patient's condition, the site and extent of damage, and the time of diagnosis. In most cases of penetrating injuries, the ureter is surgically exposed, in order to assess the real extent of the injury. General principles of surgical ureteral reconstruction include careful debridement, creation of a watertight tension-free anastomosis, isolation of the anastomosis from associated injuries with an omental flap, and adequate ureteral and retroperitoneal drainage. Minor injuries (AAST grades I–II) can be managed, in the nonacute setting, by retrograde endoscopic maneuvers and ureteral double-J stenting.

10.9 Adrenal Trauma

Adrenal hemorrhage after blunt abdominal trauma in adults is rare with a 2% and 3% overall incidence in hospital reviews and random autopsies, respectively, whereas the overall incidence is not known (Greendyke 1965; Burks et al. 1992). There is a reported incidence of 7%–26% in patients who sustain severe trauma and this is confirmed also by postmortem studies of trauma victims (Sevitt 1955; Porter et al. 1995; Wilms et al. 1987). The association with severe multisystem trauma was confirmed in one series where adrenal injury was associated in 95% of cases with ipsilateral thoracic, abdominal, or retroperitoneal injuries (Burks et al. 1992). Most injuries occur on the right side in 85%, but trauma can be bilateral in 20% of cases (Sevitt 1955; Wilms et al. 1987; Murphy et al. 1988; Rao et al. 1989; Burks et al. 1992). The cause of posttraumatic adrenal hemorrhage may be multifactorial. Several mechanisms have been proposed. These include direct compression of the gland between the spine and liver by direct trauma to the upper abdomen and flank, shearing of small vessels that perforate the adrenal capsule because of deceleration forces, and a short-term rise in intraadrenal venous pressure due to compression of the inferior vena cava. Support for direct compression or shearing of the gland as a mechanism of injury is found in the high frequency of associated ipsilateral intraabdominal (61%) and intrathoracic (44%) injuries. The adrenal glands are located deep in the abdominal cavity and are protected by the surrounding solid viscera and vertebra. These adjacent structures are also likely to be injured by external blunt force that is severe enough to injure the adrenal gland. The right adrenal is more prone to injury than the left, possibly because of its close relation to the liver, inferior vena cava, and the spine. A susceptibility to massive intraglandular bleeding is probably related to the complex vascular supply of the adrenal glands. They have a rich vascular supply coming from branches of the inferior phrenic artery, the aorta, and the renal artery. Each adrenal gland is drained by a single central vein that emerges from the hilum as a single adrenal vein. Therefore, any acute increase in adrenal venous pressure would result in hemorrhage into the gland (Wolveson and Kannegiesser 1985; Sivit et al. 1992; Valls et al. 1992). Support for a short-term rise in intraadrenal venous pressure from compression of the inferior vena cava as a mechanism of injury is found in the more frequent occurrence of hemorrhage in the right adrenal gland (86%). The right adrenal vein drains directly into the inferior vena cava while the left adrenal vein drains into the left renal vein. As a result, it is speculated that the right adrenal gland would be more affected by a sudden rise in intracaval pressure than would the left.

Traumatic adrenal hemorrhage on CT results in a rounded mass, which is of high density on unenhanced scans (50–75 HU) and becomes hypodense relative to the liver, spleen, and kidneys on post-contrast images (Fig. 10.29). At microscopy, blood is found in the medulla, stretching the surrounding cortex. Occasionally, the splayed adrenal limbs are observed surrounding a central hematoma. Periadrenal manifestations include strand-like hemorrhage infiltrating the adjacent fat or a focal periadrenal hematoma that may also extend to the pararenal space or to the psoas muscle (Burks et al. 1992); pseudo-thickening of the ipsilateral diaphragmatic crus by retroperitoneal blood is a frequent secondary finding. Adrenal hemorrhage usually resolves slowly over weeks to months.

Patients with a round hematoma or a mass replacing the whole gland may present a decrease in size and attenuation values of the mass. In small hematomas, complete resolution may be observed, while large adrenal hematomas may present as adrenal cysts after healing (Wilms et al. 1987; Burks et al. 1992).

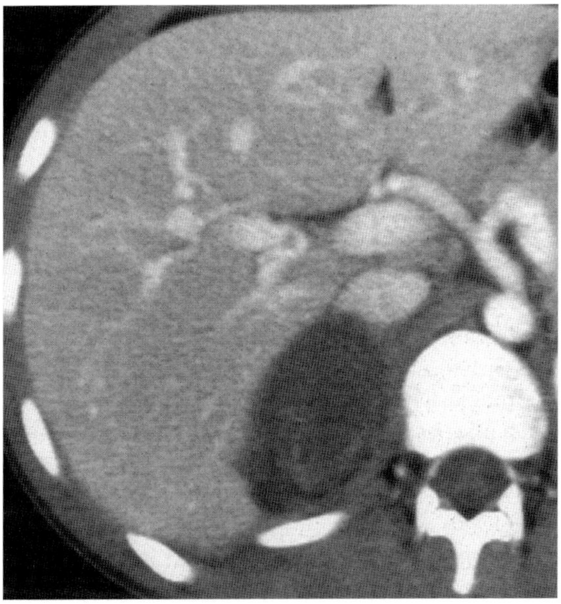

Fig. 10.29. Adrenal hematoma after blunt trauma. Contrast-enhanced CT shows a large hypodense hematoma that replaces the whole right adrenal gland

Adrenal injuries are classified as follows on the basis of the Organ Injury Scaling System of the America Association for the Surgery of Trauma (MOORE et al. 1996):

Grade I:	Contusion
Grade II:	Laceration involving only cortex (<2 cm)
Grade III:	Laceration extending into medulla (>2 cm)
Grade IV:	>50% parenchymal destruction
Grade V:	Total parenchymal destruction (including massive intraparenchymal hemorrhage; avulsion from blood supply

Clinical manifestations of adrenal hemorrhage are rare. Bilateral adrenal hemorrhage may present with acute adrenal insufficiency, which can be managed by administration of corticosteroids (FEUERSTEIN and STREETEN 1991; BURKS et al. 1992). Right-side hematoma may cause compression of the inferior vena cava with thrombus formation (BURKS et al. 1992). In addition, adrenal hematomas, as with any hematoma, should be considered as a source of possible delayed infection.

Distinguishing between an adrenal hematoma resulting from blunt trauma and a posttraumatic hemorrhage in a preexisting unsuspected adrenal mass has obvious clinical implications. The differential diagnosis can be made only with follow-up CT scans. On the contrary, the presence of a discrete adrenal mass after minor blunt trauma, without associated CT findings of periadrenal hematoma or concurrent ipsilateral thoracic or abdominal injuries, should raise the suspicion of a preexisting mass.

10.10 Conclusion

The past 20 years have witnessed the progress in renal trauma imaging and management. CT is well established as an accurate noninvasive technique for the diagnosis and staging of the entire spectrum of renal injuries, and close correlation between CT findings and surgical staging has been demonstrated. The result has been fewer operations and decreased morbidity and mortality coupled with increased renal preservation. The radiologist should have adequate knowledge of the mechanisms of renal trauma as well as the classifications of injury so that he or she is able to provide information of paramount importance for patient management.

References

Armenakas NA (1999) Current methods of diagnosis and management of ureteral injury. World J Urol 17:78–83

Becker CD, Mentha G, Schmidlin F, Terrier F (1998) Blunt abdominal trauma in adults: role of CT in the diagnosis and management of visceral injury, part 2. Gastrointestinal tract and retroperitoneal organs. Eur Radiol 8:772–780

Benoit G, Charpentier B, Roche A et al (1984) Arteriocalyceal fistula after grafted kidney biopsy. Successful management by selective catheter embolization. Urology 24:487–490

Bergren CT, Chan TN, Bodzin JH (1987) Intravenous pyelogram results in association with renal pathology and therapy in trauma patients. J Trauma 27:515–518

Boulanger BR, Brenneman FD, McLellan BA et al (1995) A prospective study of emergent abdominal sonography after blunt trauma. J Trauma 39:325–330

Brandes SB, Chelsky MJ, Buckman RF, Hanno PM (1994) Ureteral injuries from penetrating trauma. J Trauma 36: 766–769

Bretan PN, McAninch JW, Federle MP, Jeffrey RB Jr (1986) Computerized tomographic staging of renal trauma: 85 consecutive cases. J Urol 136:561–565

Bright TC, Peters PC (1977) Ureteral injuries due to external violence: 10 years experience with 59 cases. J Trauma 17: 616–620

Bright TC, White K, Peters PC (1978) Significance of hematuria after trauma. J Urol 120: 455–460

Brower P, Paul J, Brosnam SA (1978) Urinary tract abnormalities presenting as result of blunt abdominal trauma. J Trauma 18:719–722

Brown SL, Hoffman DM, Spirnak JP (1998) Limitation of routine spiral computerized tomography in the evaluation of blunt renal trauma. J Urol 160:1979–1981

Buchberger W, Penz T, Wicke K, Eberle J (1993) Diagnosis and staging of blunt kidney trauma. A comparison of urinalysis i.v. urography, sonography and computed tomography. ROFO 158:507–512

Burks DW, Mirvis SE, Shanmuganathan K (1992) Acute adrenal injury after blunt abdominal trauma: CT findings. AJR 158: 503–507

Campbell EW Jr, Filderman PS, Jacobs SC (1992) Ureteral injury due to blunt trauma. Urology 40:216–220

Carlton CE Jr (1978) Injury of the kidney and ureter. In: Harrison JH et al (eds) Campbell's urology, 4th edn. Saunders, Philadelphia, pp 1192–1245

Carlton CE Jr, Scott R Jr, Guthrie AG (1971) The initial management of ureteral injuries: a report of 78 cases. J Urol 105.335–340

Carrol PR, McAninch JW (1985) Operative indication in penetrating renal trauma. J Trauma 25:587–589

Carrol PR, McAninch JW (1989) Staging of renal trauma. Urol Clin North Am 16:193–201

Cass AS (1989) Renovascular injuries from external trauma. Urol Clin North Am 16:213–220

Cheng DL, Lazan D, Stone N (1994) Conservative treatment of type III renal trauma. J Trauma 36:491–498

Class AS, Luxenberg M (1984) Unilateral nonvisualization on excretory urography after external trauma. J Urol 132: 225–227

Desnos E. (1972) The history of urology, part 1. Thomas, New York, pp 223–234

Dorffner R, Thurnher S, Prokesch R et al (1998) Embolization of iatrogenic vascular injuries of renal transplants: immediate and follow-up results. Cardiovasc Intervent Radiol 21: 129–134

Eastham JA, Wilson TG, Ahlering TE (1991) Radiographic assessment of blunt renal trauma. J Trauma 31:1527–1528

Eickenberg H, Amin M (1976) Gunshot wounds to the ureter. J Trauma 16:562–565

Ekelund L, Lindholm T (1971) Arteriovenous fistulae following percutaneous renal biopsy. Acta Radiol 11:38–48

Fallon B, Wendt JC, Hawtrey CE (1984) Urological injury and assessment in patient with fractured pelvis. J Urol 131: 712–714

Fanney DR, Casillas J, Murphy BJ (1990) CT in the diagnosis of renal trauma. Radiographics 10:29–40

Federle M (1989) Evaluation of renal trauma. In: Pollacck HM (ed) Clinical urography. Saunders, Philadelphia, pp 1472–1494

Federle MP, Kaiser JA, McAninch JW, Brooke Jeffrey R, Mall JC (1981) The role of computed tomography in renal trauma. Radiology 141:455–460

Federle MP, Brown TR, McAninch JW (1987) Penetrating renal trauma: CT evaluation. J Comput Assist Tomogr 11: 1026–1030

Feuerstein B, Streeten DH (1991) Recovery of adrenal function after failure resulting from traumatic bilateral adrenal. Ann Intern Med 115:785–613

Freed TA, Tavel FR (1976) Diagnosis and surgical treatment of Page kidney. Urology 7:330–337

Fried FA, Rutledge R (1995) A statewide, population-based analysis of the frequency and outcome of genitourinary injury in a series of 215,220 trauma patients. J Urol 153: 314A

Fry DE, Milholen L, Harbrecht PJ (1983) Iatrogenic ureteral injury. Options for management. Arch Surg 118:454–457

Furtschegger A, Egender G, Jakse G (1988) The value of sonography in the diagnosis and follow-up of patients with blunt renal trauma. Br J Urol 62:110–116

Gainza FJ, Minguela I, Lopez-Vidaur I, Ruiz LM, Lampreabe I (1995) Evaluation of complications due to percutaneous renal biopsy in allografts and native kidneys with color-coded Doppler sonography. Clin Nephrol 43:303–308

Goldman SM, Sandler CM (1998) Upper urinary tract trauma – current concepts. World J Urol 16:62–68

Goodman DN, Saibil EA, Kodama RT (1998) Traumatic intimal tear of the renal artery treated by insertion of Palmaz stent. Cardiovasc Intervent Radiol 21:69–72

Grant RP, Gifford RW Jr, Pudvan WR et al (1971) Renal trauma and hypertension. Am J Cardiol 27:173–176

Greendyke RM (1965) Adrenal hemorrhage. AJR 43:215–231

Guerriero WG (1982) Trauma to the kidney, ureters, bladder, and urethra. Surg Clin North Am 62:1047–1074

Haas CA, Dinchman KH, Nasrallah PF, Spirnack JP (1998) Traumatic renal artery occlusion: a 15-year review. J Trauma 45:557–561

Hardeman SW, Husmann DA, Chinn HKW, Peters PC (1987) Blunt urinary tract trauma: identifying those patients who require radiological diagnostic studies. J Urol 138:99–101

Hessel SJ, Smith EH (1974) Renal trauma: a comprehensive review and radiological assessment. CRC Crit Rev Clin Radiol Nucl Med 5:251–293

Hochmuth A, Fleck M, Hauff P, Reinhardt M et al (2000) First experiences in using a new ultrasound mode and ultrasound contrast agent in the diagnosis of blunt renal trauma: a feasibility study in an animal model. Invest Radiol 35:205–211

Hoffman RM, Stieper PD, Johnson RW, Belzer FO (1974) Renal ischemic tolerance. Arch Surg 109:550–551

Holden S, Hicks CC, O'Brien DP et al (1976) Gunshot wounds to the ureter: a 15-year review of 63 consecutive cases. J Urol 116:562–564

Howerton RA, Norwood SN (1991) Proximal ureteral avulsion from blunt abdominal trauma. Military Med 156:311–316

Hubsch PJ, Mostbeck G, Barton PP et al (1990) Evaluation of arteriovenous fistulas and pseudoaneurysms in renal allografts following percutaneous needle biopsy. J Ultrasound Med 9:95–100

Huppert PE, Duda SH, Erley CM et al (1993) Embolization of renal vascular lesion: clinical experience with microcoils and tracker catheters. Cardiovasc Intervent Radiol 16: 316–367

Husmann DA, Morris JS (1990) Attempted nonoperative management of blunt renal laceration extending through the corticomedullary junction: the short-term and long-term sequelae. J Urol 143:682–684

Husmann DA, Gilling PJ, Perry MO et al (1993) Major renal laceration with a revitalized fragment following blunt abdominal trauma: a comparison between nonoperative (expectant) versus surgical management. J Urol 150: 1774–1777

Jakse G, Furtschegger A, Egender G (1987) Ultrasound in patients with blunt renal trauma managed by surgery. J Urol 138:21–23

Kamel IR, Berkowitz JF (1996) Assessment of the cortical rim sign in posttraumatic renal infarction. J Comput Assist Tomogr 20:803–806

Kantor A, Sclafani SJA, Scalea T et al (1989) The role of interventional radiology in the management of genitourinary trauma. Urol Clin North Am 16:255–265

Kawashima A, Sandler CM, Corriere JN et al (1997) Ureteropelvic junction injuries secondary to blunt abdominal trauma. Radiology 205:487–492

Kawashima A, Sandler CM, Corl FM et al (2001) Imaging of renal trauma: a comprehensive review. Radiographics 21: 557–574

Kenney PJ, Panicek DM, Witanowski LS (1987) Computer tomography of ureteral disruption. J Comput Assist Tomogr 11:480–484

Klein AJP, Kozar RA, Kaplan LJ (1999) Traumatic hematuria in patients with polycystic kidney disease. Am Surgeon 65: 464–466

Knudson MM, Maull KI (1999) Nonoperative management of solid organ injuries. Surg Clin North Am 79:1357–1371

Knudson MM, Harrison PB, Hoyt DB, Shatz DV et al (2000) Outcome after major renovascular injuries: a western trauma association multicenter report. J Trauma 49:1116–1122

Kos X, Fanchamps JM, Trotteur G, Dondelinger RF (1999) Radiologic damage control: evaluation of a combined CT and angiographic suite with pivoting table. Cardiovasc Intervent Radiol 22:124–129

Kossow AS (1980) Hypertension complicating blunt renal trauma. Urology 16:84–86

Kramer SC, Gorich J, Rilinger N, Gottfried HW et al (1998) The percutaneous transarterial embolization therapy of traumatic kidney hemorrhages. ROFO 169:297–301

Krieger JN, Algood CB, Mason JT et al (1984) Urological trauma in the Pacific Northwest. J Urol 132:70–73

Lent V (1996) What classification is appropriate in renal trauma? Eur Urol 30:327–334
Leppaniemi AK, Lamminen A, Tervhartiala P et al (1995) Comparison of high-field magnetic resonance imaging with computer tomography in the evaluation of blunt trauma. J Trauma 38:420–427
Leppaniemi A, Lamminen A, Tervahartiala P et al (1997) MRI and CT in blunt renal trauma: an update. Semin Ultrasound 18:129–135
Liroff SA, Pontes JE, Pierce JM Jr (1977) Gunshot wounds to the ureter: 5 years of experience. J Urol 118:551–553
Lopez Cubillana P, Rigabert Montiel M, Nicolas Torralba JA et al (1998) Ultrasonography and intravenous urography in the diagnosis of blunt renal trauma. Arch Esp Urol 51: 669–672
Lupetin A, Mainwaring B, Daffner R (1989) CT diagnosis of renal artery injury caused by blunt abdominal trauma. AJR 153:1065–1068
Lutkevich C, Hall JR, Lewis JV et al (2000) Percutaneous transluminal angioplasty of an acute traumatic renal artery occlusion. Tenn Med 93:140–141
Marberger H (1988) Blunt injuries of the kidney. In: Cass AS (ed) Genitourinary trauma. Blackwell Scientific, Boston, pp 11–35
Marcos HB, Noone TC, Semelka RC (1998) MRI evaluation of acute renal trauma. J Magn Reson Imaging 8:989–990
Massumi RA, Andrade A, Kramer N (1964) Arterial hypertension in traumatic subcapsular perirenal hematoma (Page kidney). Am J Med 46:635–639
Matthews LA, Spirnak JP (1995) The nonoperative approach to major blunt renal trauma. Semin Urol 13:77–82
Mayor B, Gudinchet F, Wicky S, Reinberg O, Schnyder P (1995) Imaging evaluation of blunt renal trauma in children: diagnostic accuracy of intravenous pyelography and ultrasonography. Pediatr Radiol 25:214–218
McAninch JW, Carroll PR (1989) Renal exploration after trauma. Indications and reconstructive techniques. Urol Clin North Am 16:203–211
McAninch JW, Federle MP (1982) Evaluation of renal injuries with computer tomography. J Urol 128:456–460
McGahan JP, Richards JR, Jones CD, Gerscovich EO (1999) Use of ultrasonography in the patient with acute renal trauma. J Ultrasound Med 18:207–213
McGehee M, Kier R, Chon SM et al (1993) Comparison of MRI with postcontrast CT for the evaluation of acute abdominal trauma. J Comput Assist Tomogr 17:410–413
McKenney MG, Martin L, Lent K et al (1996) 1000 consecutive ultrasound for blunt abdominal trauma. J Trauma 40: 607–612
Mee SL, McAninch JW (1989) Indication for radiographic assessment in suspected renal trauma. Urol Clin North Am 16:187–192
Mee SL, McAninch JW, Robinson AL et al (1989) Radiographic assessment of renal trauma: a 10-year prospective study of patient selection. J Urol 141:1095–1098
Meng MV, Brandes SB, McAninch JW (1999) Renal trauma: indication and techniques for surgical exploration. World J Urol 17:71–77
Mertz JH, Wishard WN Jr, Nourse MH (1963) Injury of the kidney in children. JAMA 183:730–737
Michel LA, Lacrosse M, Decanniere L et al (1996) Blunt renal traumas: contribution of spiral CT with three dimensional reconstruction to the surgical decision process. Int Surg 81: 377–381
Miller KS, McAninch JW (1995) Radiographic assessment of renal trauma: our 15-year experiences. J Urol 154:352–355
Mirvis SE (1996) Trauma. Radiol Clin North Am 34:1225–1257
Montgomery RC, Richardson JD, Harty JI (1998) Posttraumatic renovascular hypertension after occult renal injury. J Trauma 45:106–110
Moore EE, Shackford SR, Pachter HL et al (1989) Organ injury scaling: spleen, liver, and kidney. J Trauma 29:1664–1666
Moore EE, Cogbill TH, Jurkovich GJ et al (1992) Organ injury scaling. III: chest wall, abdominal vascular, ureter, bladder and urethra. J Trauma 33:337–339
Moore EE, Malangoni MA, Cogbill TH et al (1996) Organ injury scaling. VII: cervical vascular, peripheral vascular, adrenal, penis, testis and scrotum. J Trauma 41:523–524
Morey AF, McAninch JW, Tiller BK, Duckett CP, Carroll PR (1999) Single shot intraoperative excretory urography for the immediate evaluation of renal trauma. J Urol 161: 1088–1092
Mulligan JM, Cagiannos I, Collins JP, Millward SF (1998) Ureteropelvic junction disruption secondary to blunt trauma: excretory phase imaging (delayed films) should help prevent a missed diagnosis. J Urol 159:67–70
Murphy J, Casillas J, Yrizarry J (1988) Traumatic adrenal hemorrhage: radiologic findings. Radiology 169:701–703
Nash PA, Bruce JE, McAninch JW (1995) Nephrectomy for traumatic renal injuries. J Urol 153:609–611
Ney C, Friedenberg M (1981) Trauma to the kidney. In: Ney C (ed) Radiographic atlas of the genitourinary system. Lippincott, Philadelphia, pp 457–514
N'Goan AM, Aguehounde C, N'Gbesso RD et al (1997) Ultrasound scanning of abdominal contusions in children: experience at the Yopougon CHU (Ivory Coast). Santé 7: 300–302
Nicolaisen GS, McAninch JW, Marshall JA et al (1985) Renal trauma: re-evaluation of indication for radiographic assessment. J Urol 133:183–187
Nordenholz KE, Rubin MA, Gularte GG, Liang HK (1997) Ultrasound in the evaluation and management of blunt abdominal trauma. Ann Emerg Med 29:357–366
Orons PD, Zajko AB (1995) Angiography and interventional aspects of renal transplantation. Radiol Clin North Am 33: 461–471
Packard FR (1921) The life and times of Ambroise Paré. Hoeber, New York, p 213
Paul J, Otal P, Perreault P et al (1999) Treatment of posttraumatic dissection of the renal artery with endoprosthesis in 15-year-old girl. J Trauma 47:169–172
Pearl WS, Todd KH (1996) Ultrasonography for the initial evaluation of blunt abdominal trauma: a review of prospective trials. Ann Emerg Med 27:353–361
Perry MJ, Porte ME, Urwin GH (1997) Limitations of ultrasound evaluation in acute closed renal trauma. J R Coll Surg Edinb 42:420–422
Peters PC, Sagalowsky AI (1997) Genitourinary trauma. In: Harrison JH et al (eds) Campbell's urology, 7th edn. Saunders, Philadelphia, pp 3119–3151
Peterson EN (1989) Complications of renal trauma. Urol Clin North Am 16:221–236
Pitts JC, Peterson NE (1981) Penetrating injuries of the ureter. J Trauma 21:978–982
Pollack HM, Wein AJ (1989) Imaging of renal trauma. Radiology 172:279–308
Porter JM, Muscato K, Patrick JR (1995) Adrenal hemorrhage:

a comparison of traumatic and nontraumatic deaths. J Natl Med Assoc 87:569–571
Presti JC Jr, Carroll PR, McAninch JW (1989) Ureteral and renal pelvic injuries from external trauma: diagnosis and management. J Trauma 29:370–374
Rao RH, Vagnucci AH, Amico JA (1989) Bilateral massive adrenal hemorrhage: early recognition and treatment. Ann Intern Med 110:227–235
Rhyner P, Federle MP, Jeffrey RB (1984) CT of trauma to the abnormal kidney. AJR 142:747–750
Rober PE, Smith JB, Pierce JM Jr (1990) Gunshot injuries of the ureter. J Trauma 30:83–86
Rosales A, Arango O, Coronado J et al (1992) The use of ultrasonography as the initial diagnostic exploration in blunt renal trauma. Urol Int 48:134–137
Rosen MA, McAninch JW (1994). Management of combined renal and pancreatic trauma. J Urol 152:22–25
Rubin BE, Schliftman R (1979) The striated nephrogram in renal contusion. Urol Radiol 1:119–121
Rutishauser G (1982) Nierenverletzungen. Helv Chir Acta 49: 735–746
Safir MH, McAninch JW (1999) Diagnosis and management of trauma to kidney. Curr Opin Urol 9:227–231
Sagalowsky AI, McConnell JD, Peters PC (1983) Renal trauma requiring surgery. J Trauma 23:128–131
Santucci RA, McAninch JW (2000) Diagnosis and management of renal trauma: past, present and future. J Am Coll Surg 191:443–451
Santucci RA, McAninch JW, Safir M et al (2001) Validation of the American association for the surgery of trauma organ injury severity scale for the kidney. J Trauma 50:195–200
Sarkisian AE, Khondkarian RA, Amirbekian NM et al (1991) Sonographic screening of mass casualties for abdominal and renal injuries following the 1988 Armenia earthquake. J Trauma 31:247–250
Schmiedl UP, Carter S, Martin RW et al (1999) Sonographic detection of acute parenchymal injury in an experimental porcine model of renal hemorrhage: gray-scale imaging using a sonographic contrast agent. AJR 173:1289–1294
Scott R Jr, Carlton CE, Goldman M (1969) Penetrating injuries of the kidney. J Urol 101:247–253
Sevitt S (1955) Post-traumatic adrenal apoplexy. J Clin Pathol 8:185–194
Sivit CJ, Ingram DJ, Taylor GA, Bulas DI, Kushner DC, Eichelberer MR (1992) Posttraumatic adrenal hemorrhage in children: CT findings in 34 patients. AJR 158:1299–1302
Spirnak JP, Resnick MI (1987) Revascularization of traumatic thrombosis of the renal artery. Surg Gynecol Obstet 164: 22–26
Stables DP (1976) Unilateral absence of excretion on urography after abdominal trauma. Radiology 121:609–615
Sufrin G (1975) The Page kidney. J Urol 113:450–454
Tunberg T, Jona J (1985) Review of multiple traumatic injuries in an urban pediatric population. Pediatr Emerg Care 1: 116
Tynberg TL, Hoch WH, Persky L et al (1973) The management of renal injuries coincident with penetrating wounds of the abdomen. J Trauma 13:502–508
Valls C, Andia E, Gil I (1992) Bilateral posttraumatic adrenal hemorrhage detected with CT. AJR 159:433–434
Velmahos GC, Chahwan S, Falabella A, Hanks SE, Demetriades D (2000) Angiographic embolization for intraperitoneal and retroperitoneal injuries. World J Surg 24:539–545
Von Knorring J, Fyhrquist F, Ahonen J (1981) Varying course of hypertension following renal trauma. J Urol 126:798–801
Wilms G, Marchal G, Baert A, Adisoejoso B, Mangkuwerdojo S (1987) CT and ultrasound features of post-traumatic adrenal hemorrhage. J Comp Assist Tomogr 11:12–115
Wolverson MK, Kannegiesser H (1985) CT of bilateral adrenal hemorrhage with acute adrenal insufficiency in the adult. AJR 142:311–314
Wong W, Moss A, Federle M, Cochran S, London S (1984) Renal infarction: CT diagnosis and correlation between CT findings and etiologies. Radiology 150:201–205

11 Injuries of the Urinary Bladder and Urethra

D. Rickards

CONTENTS

D. Rickards, FRCR, FFRDSA
University College Hospitals, Imaging Department, The Middlesex Hospital, Mortimer Street, London W1N 8TA, UK

Bladder Trauma

- The distinction between intra- and extraperitoneal bladder rupture is all-important.
- Whether using cystography or CT cystography, adequate distension of the bladder with contrast is crucial. At least 350 ml needs to be instilled.
- Postdrainage films are needed with cystography, but not with CT cystography.
- With penetrating injuries, associated trauma to other structures is almost certain.

Urethra

- Imaging in the acute phase is rarely indicated unless urethral catheterization is contemplated.
- Urethral injury usually results in stricture formation.
- In the majority of cases, ascending and descending studies will be needed to assess the extent of a stricture.
- Accurate localization of any traumatic lesion to the sphincter mechanisms is crucial.
- Female urethras rarely suffer trauma.

11.1 Bladder Injury

11.1.1 Anatomy

In children, the bulk of the bladder is intraperitoneal. In adults, it is extraperitoneal, lying within the pelvis and protected by bone laterally, the symphysis pubis anteriorly. Inferiorly lies the pelvic floor musculature and fascia, posteriorly lies the rectum. The bladder base is firmly anchored, while the body of the bladder is mobile. The superior aspect of the bladder is covered by peritoneum.

11.1.2 History

Homer in the Iliad 3000 years ago described the deaths of two souls whose bladders had been speared by Meriones and the aphorism of Hippocrates that bladder wounds were fatal was firmly believed. It was not until 1648, when a merchant fell with a full bladder onto a cauldron, developed lower abdominal pain and passing only a few drops of bloodied urine that Charles Spon performed paracentesis, despite which the patient succumbed. At autopsy, a tear in the fundus of the bladder was found. A formative step occurred in 1724 when Le Dran distinguished between intra- and extraperitoneal bladder tears and was the first to suggest continuous drainage as a therapeutic option (Le Dran 1774). Perineal urethrostomy was first used by William Walker in Boston in a patient with extraperitoneal rupture (Walker 1845). Although laparotomy and suture of bladder tears was first suggested by Jacob Vogt in 1716, it was not until 1876 that Willet in London performed the procedure, but the patient still died of peritonitis (Willet 1876). Success with this procedure was first achieved by Sir William McCormac in 1885 (McCormac 1886). Over the years, therapeutic options are still those of drainage for extraperitoneal rupture, laparotomy and repair for intraperitoneal tears. Cystography was first suggested in 1931 by Stone and it has proved a reliable diagnostic measure, although Gordon-Taylor as recently as 1953 condemned it as unnecessary and dangerous in a book entitled *Modern Trends in Urology* (Stone 1931; Gordon-Taylor 1953).

11.1.3 Imaging

Conventional cystography is tried, tested and proven, but CT cystography is finding its role, especially in the polytrauma patient.

11.1.3.1 Cystography

Gross hematuria in blunt trauma is an absolute indication for cystography (Fuhrman et al. 1993). Before attempted catheterization, it is crucial to confirm the integrity of the urethra in the male. Female urethral trauma is rare and female urethrography impractical. If intact, urethral catheterization with at least a 10-F catheter is performed and contrast instilled into the bladder under gravity, not with a pump, and under fluoroscopic control. It is unwise to use a Foley catheter unless the balloon is not inflated. When inflated, the balloon can mask ruptures of the bladder base and proximal posterior urethra. In the intensive care situation, spot films can be exposed at regular times during filling and emptying (Fig. 11.1). The bladder should be distended with at least 300 ml, preferably more, and intermittent fluoroscopy performed. A spot of the full bladder is performed and then the bladder be allowed to drain. The postdrainage film is important as extraperitoneal leaks can be missed (Carroll and McAninch 1984). In patients who can be moved around on the fluoroscopy table, oblique and if possible lateral films will increase diagnostic accuracy. The accuracy of cystography in diagnosing bladder rupture lies between 80%–95% (Carroll and McAninch 1983) if a strict protocol is adhered to and adequate distension is paramount. A lack of postvoiding film and less than 250 ml of contrast are responsible for false negative findings on retrograde cystography (Cass 1984). Extraperitoneal rupture is more likely to produce a false negative diagnosis (Cass 1976). Where a catheter cannot be passed, a suprapubic should be inserted under US monitoring,

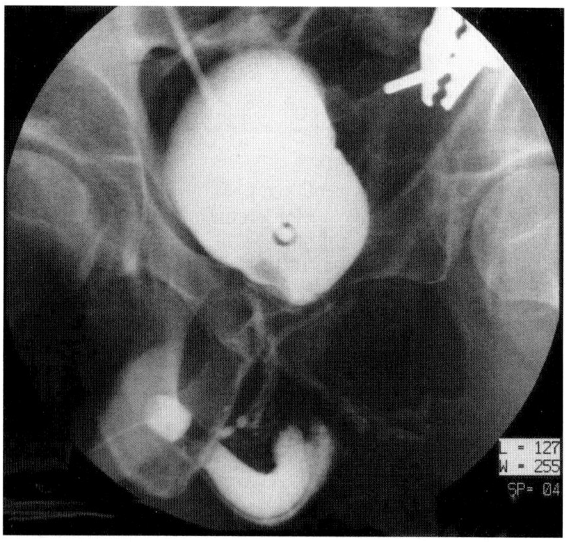

Fig. 11.1. A spot film taken in the intensive care unit of a combined ascending urethrogram and suprapubic cystogram following severe pelvic trauma. Pelvic stability has been achieved with a metal frame, which can impose upon the area of interest. There is complete disruption of the proximal anterior urethra

the bladder filled as above (Fig. 11.2). Diagnosis may be problematic when intestinal loops have obliterated the bladder tear or when no extravasation is seen due to bladder wall dissection without laceration or when a urethral rupture focuses the attention (Nowak and Zielinski 1977).

11.1.3.2
CT Cystography

CT is already the technique of choice in patients with blunt abdominal and pelvic trauma, but its value in assessing bladder trauma has as yet not been fully established (Cass 1990; Sandler and Reed Dunnick 2000). Plain cystography was replaced with CT cystography and small comparative studies with static cystography have been done with no convincing conclusion (Lis and Cohen 1990; Horstman and McClennan 1991). Early attempts to diagnose bladder trauma with CT using i.v. contrast alone was very inaccurate, yielding sensitivities of only 50% (Udekwu et al. 1996; Peng et al. 1999). Delayed imaging at 5 min improved specificity, but is not feasible in a severely injured patient or in a busy department (Mee et al. 1987; Sivit et al. 1995).

Retrograde bladder filling must be done. It is becoming clear that adequate distension on the bladder with at least 350 ml of contrast is essential,

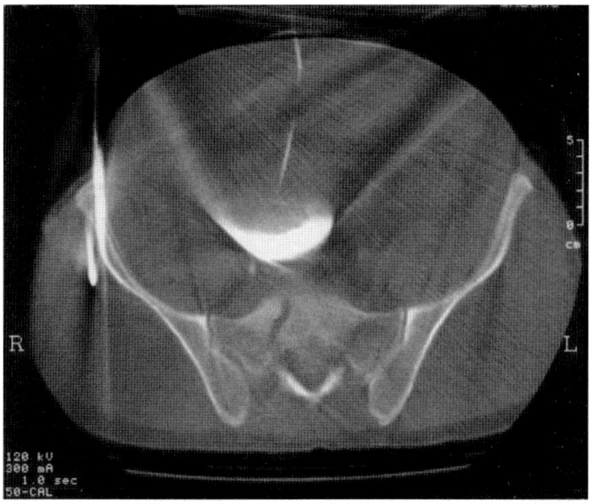

Fig. 11.3. CT cystogram. Via a suprapubic catheter, contrast has been instilled into the bladder, which is displaced superiorly because of pelvic hematoma. Artifacts are caused by the metal work of the stablizing frame. The bladder is intact

as with cystography, and in one series, no injuries were missed (Kane et al. 1989; Sclafani and Becker 1985). Using less will produce false negatives (Spirnark 1988; Vaccaro and Brody 2000). Where urethral catheterization is not possible because of associated urethral injury, a suprapubic will have to be placed under US or CT guidance (Fig. 11.3). Once contrast has been instilled, 5-mm axial sections are obtained. Neither a postdrainage CT or plain abdominal film are required (McConnell et al. 1982).

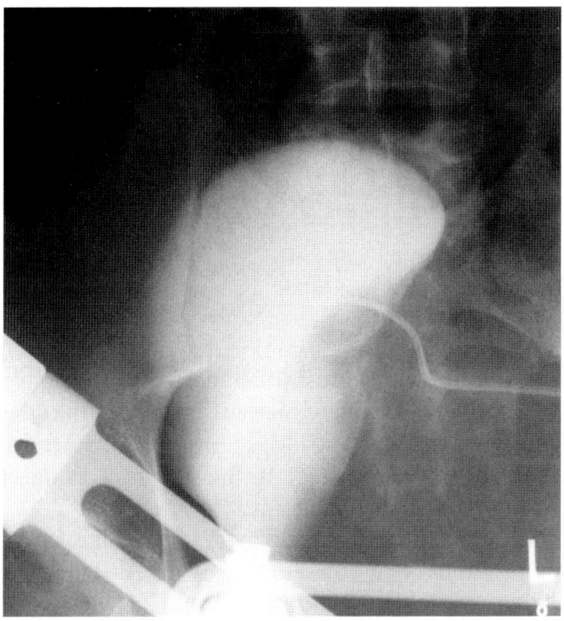

Fig. 11.2. Under ultrasound monitoring, a suprapubic 6-F pigtail catheter has been inserted into the bladder which is grossly displaced superiorly and laterally by pelvic hematoma following massive pelvic injury. There is no extravasation

11.1.3.3
Excretory Urography

Antegrade filling of the bladder at excretory urography has the advantage of outlining the integrity of the ureters and establishing whether there is any obstruction to the upper tracts, but dilution of contrast in the bladder by urine may make visualizing extravasating contrast more difficult to detect. The use of urography clearly depends upon the patient's clinical situation, but it can be very useful (Fig. 11.4).

11.1.4
Mechanism

Bladder trauma occurs as a result of blunt or penetrating trauma or because of iatrogenic reasons. The full bladder is more prone to injury and accurate diagnosis of the type of rupture is essential because it dictates treatment. In the civilian population, blunt

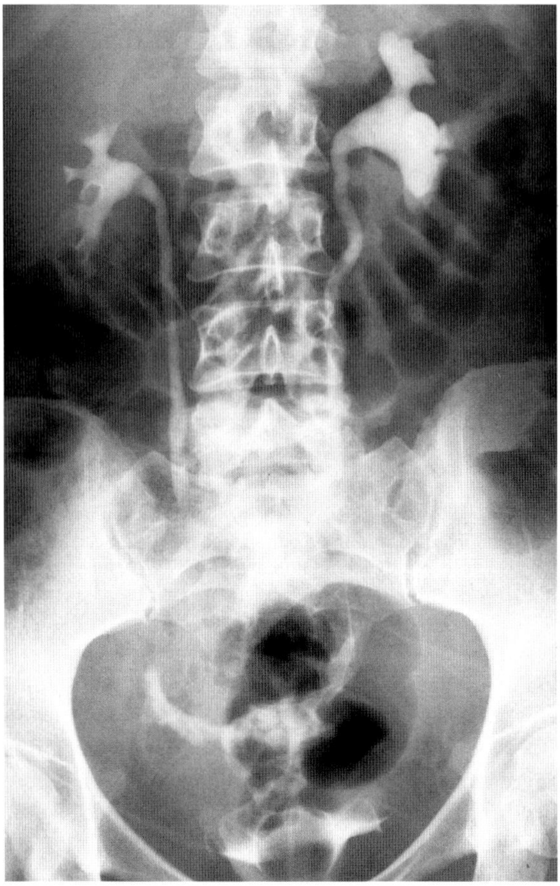

Fig. 11.4. Excretory urogram following blunt pelvic trauma. There is a degree of obstruction to the left ureter, the distal ureters are not seen, there is extravasation of contrast into the extraperitoneal space, but contrast is seen within the bladder. There is both ureteric and bladder injury

trauma accounts for up to 90% of bladder injuries (Brosman and Paul 1976; McConnell et al. 1982). Bladder rupture is a classic consequence of pelvic fracture; particularly the fractured pelvic rami are responsible for bladder injury, mainly extraperitoneal rupture (Lavallee et al. 1979; Taffet 1997). The bladder can occasionally herniate into a diastasis of the pubic symphysis (Cespedes et al. 1995). It must be emphasized that isolated posttraumatic bladder rupture, although uncommon, may result in in recognition being delayed about 5 days (Mokoena and Naidu 1995). Full bladder, alcohol, or drug ingestion may be responsible for bladder rupture, even after minimal trauma (Herd et al. 1994). Sandler described five types related to anatomical location and severity of bladder wall involvement (Sandler et al. 1986).

11.1.4.1 Bladder Contusion (Type 1)

This is the most common form and is an incomplete tear of the mucosa and results in hematuria. No specific treatment is required and the prognosis is excellent. Both cystography and CT cystography will be normal. Minimal trauma with inconsistently occurring hematuria may be observed during repeated excretional forces and abdominal pressure like in marathon runners (Blacklock 1979).

11.1.4.2 Intraperitoneal Rupture (Type 2)

The weakest point of the bladder is the peritoneal surface across the dome (Oliver and Taguchi 1964). A sudden compressive force on the lower abdomen when the bladder is full; for example, the restraining effect of a safety belt, a punch, or a kick are common causes of rupture (Mundy 1983). Anuria should alert even the least wary to this diagnosis, but the ability of the patient to pass urine does not exclude it, sometimes causing a delayed diagnosis (Williams 1976; Brown et al. 1986). The rupture can be intermittently sealed by bowel or omentum, resulting in normal micturition patterns. Eventually, intraperitoneal urine will result in hypernatremia, hyperkalemia and acidosis (Shah et al. 1979; Jerwood and Mason 1995). Unnoticed trauma may occasionally result in urinary ascites, particularly in children (Redman et al. 1979). Hematuria is likely, but physical examination is usually unremarkable until the inflammatory reaction of urine to the peritoneum causes peritonitis. Intraperitoneal leakage of all urine rapidly results in renal failure. Once the diagnosis is established, laparotomy and closure of the rupture is mandatory along with suprapubic and urethral drainage. Early diagnosis and treatment carry an excellent prognosis.

Imaging Findings

- Cystography. Contrast will be seen outlining loops of bowel, intraabdominal viscera, and within the pouch of Douglas (Fig. 11.5). The full bladder might obscure leakage in the pouch of Douglas and postdrainage spot films are important.
- CT Cystography. As with cystography, contrast will be seen around bowel loops, mesenteric folds and in the paracolic gutters.
- Excretory Urography. The ureters will be seen, assuming that there is reasonable renal function and extravasated contrast around abdominal viscera (Fig. 11.6).

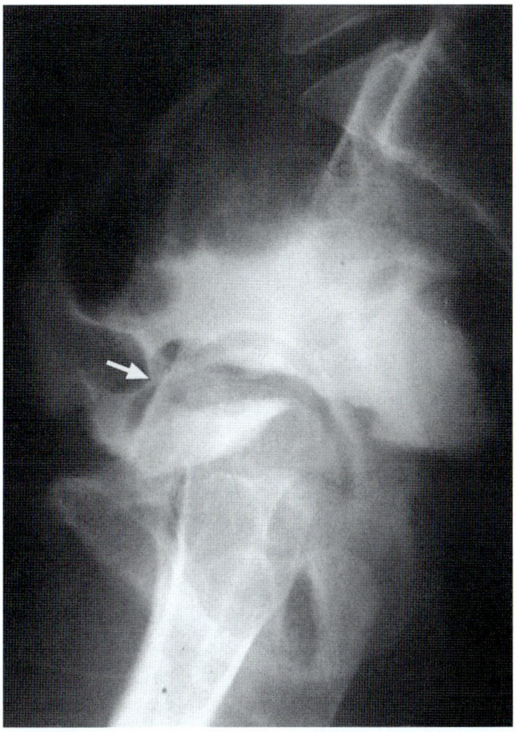

a

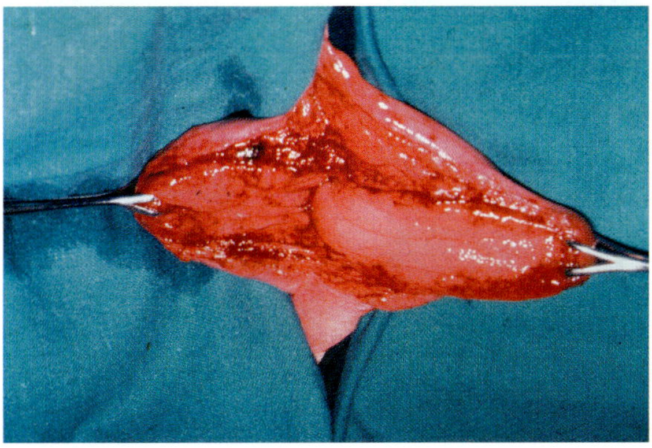

b

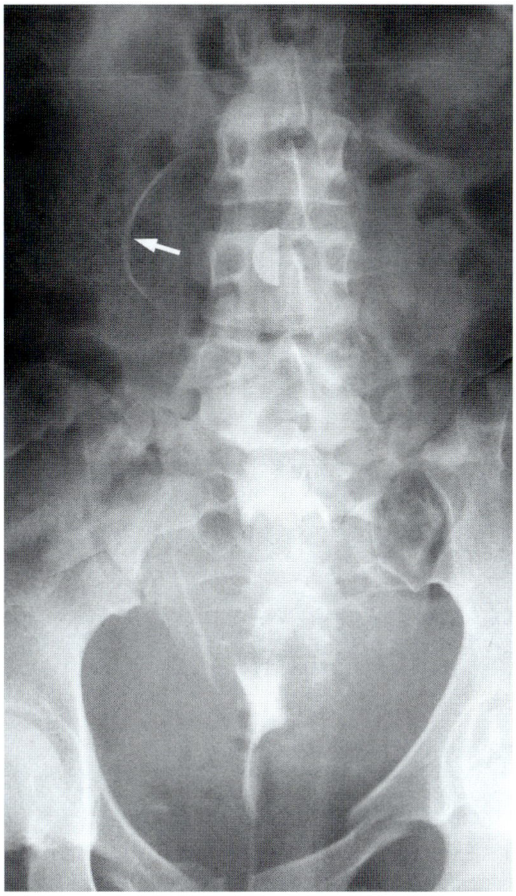

c

Fig. 11.5. **a** Cystography of intraperitoneal bladder trauma. There is intraperitoneal extravasation of contrast (*arrow*). **b** The rupture clearly seen at surgery prior to repair. **c** Following pelvic fracture, the bladder is compressed and elevated due to massive pelvic hematoma; a small amount of extravesical contrast can be seen (*arrow*)

11.1.4.3
Interstitial Bladder Injury (Type 3)

There is a dissecting rupture of the bladder without perforation (Vaccaro and Brody 2000). Normal micturition patterns can be expected with hematuria. Surgical treatment is not required and the prognosis is excellent.

Imaging Findings

- Cystography. Normal findings.
- CT cystography. Usually normal, but rarely intramural contrast without extravasation will be seen (Corriere 1991) (Fig. 11.7).

11.1.4.4
Extraperitoneal Rupture (Type 4)

Extraperitoneal rupture is more common than intraperitoneal rupture in most series and there is associated pelvic fracture in up to 90% of cases (Clark and Prudencio 1972). Direct laceration by bony spicules along the anterolateral aspect with anterior pelvic arch fractures is the usual mechanism, though stress applied to the puboprostatic ligaments associated with diastasis of the symphysis pubis can cause bladder tears (Nowak and Zielinski 1977; Corriere and Sandler 1988).

Simple ruptures are confined to the perivesical space whereas complex ruptures are not. Nevertheless, extraperitoneal ruptures can safely be treated

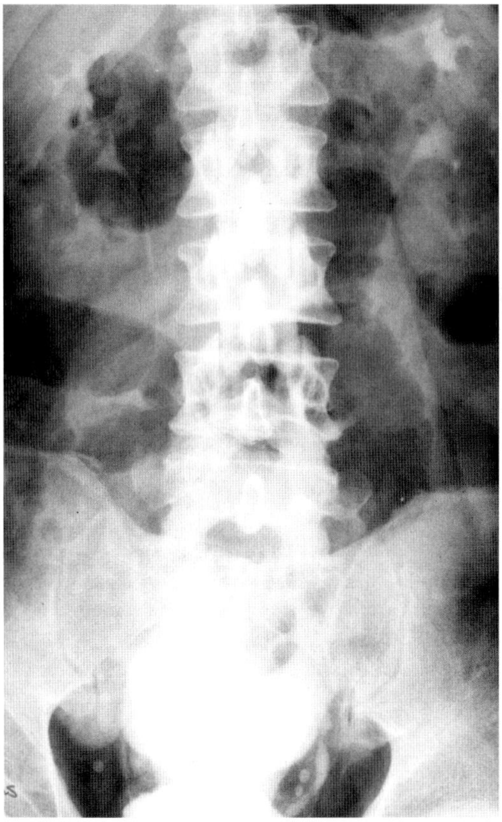

Fig. 11.6. Excretory urogram showing contrast in the paracolic gutter secondary to intraperitoneal bladder rupture

with drainage alone. Where hematuria is gross and clot retention is an issue, surgery should be considered.

Imaging Findings

- Cystography. When simple, contrast will be seen in the perivesical space (Fig. 11.8). When complex, contrast extends beyond the perivesical space into the scrotum, thigh, anterior abdominal wall, or retroperitoneum (Figs. 11.9–11.11).
- CT Cystography. As with cystography, contrast will be seen in the extraperitoneum. CT has the advantage of detailing the relationship of any fractures to the extravasated contrast.

11.1.4.5 Combined Bladder Injury (Type 5)

Both intraperitoneal and extraperitoneal ruptures occur. This can be expected in 0.5% of pelvic fractures and accounts for 5% of all bladder ruptures (Palmer et al. 1983). Micturition patterns are usually abnormal, hematuria very common, and surgical repair is essential. The magnitude of the force responsible for such trauma results in high rate of nonurologic injury and a high mortality rate can be expected.

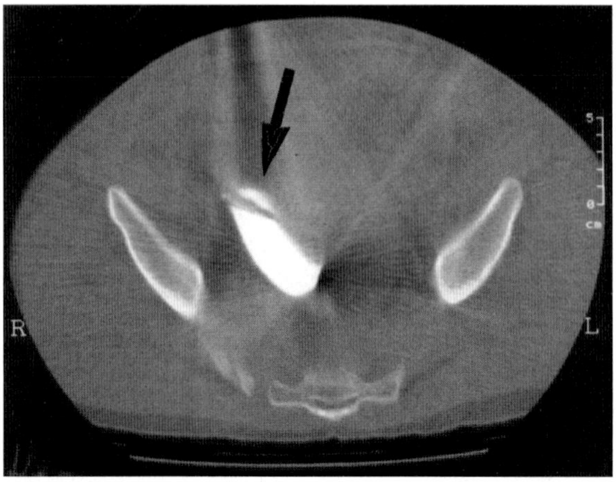

Fig. 11.7. Interstitial extravasation of contrast (*arrow*) at CT cystography

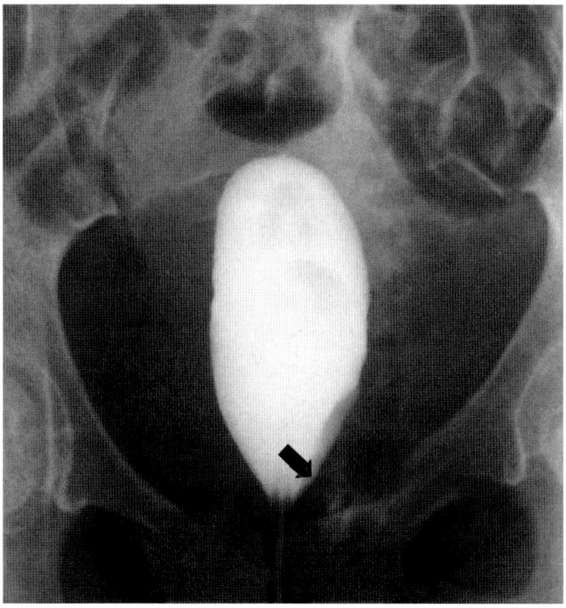

Fig. 11.8. Cystogram showing extraperitoneal bladder rupture (*arrow*) following pelvic fracture. The bladder is compressed and elongated due to hematoma

Imaging Findings

- Cystography. A combination of intra- and extraperitoneal findings may be seen although only one component may be evident (Scott and Porter 1997) (Fig. 11.12).

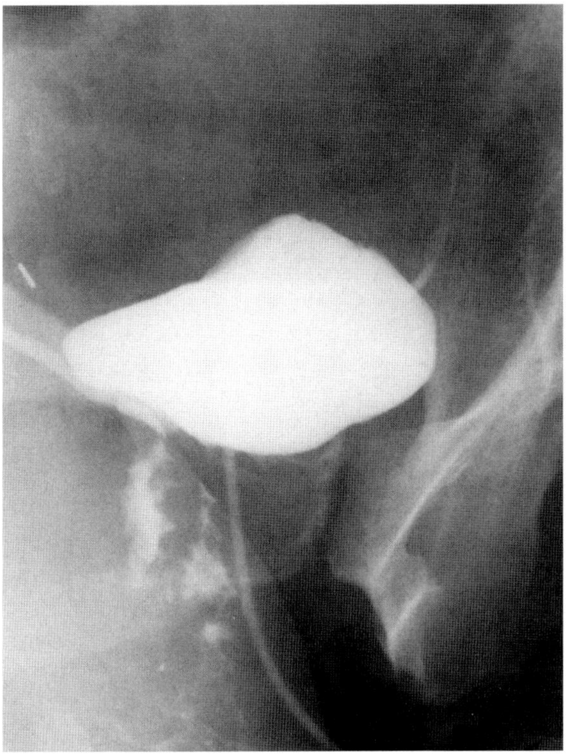

Fig. 11.9. Cystogram showing contrast extravasating beyond the perivesical space

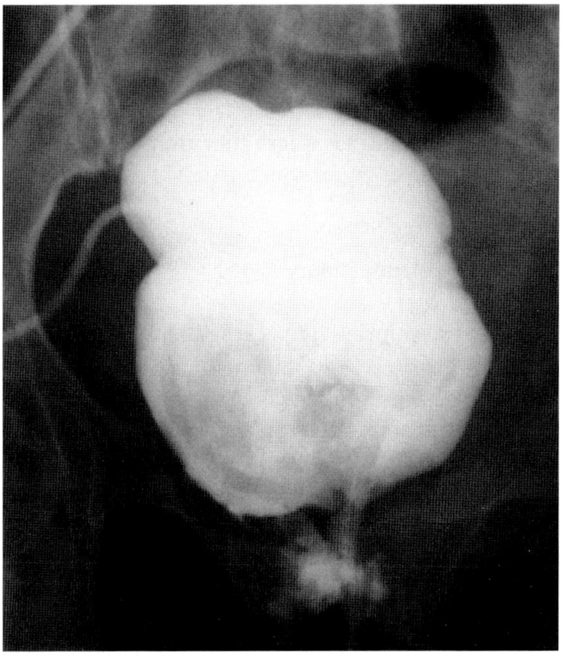

Fig. 11.11. Extraperitoneal bladder rupture with contrast extending into the periprostatic space

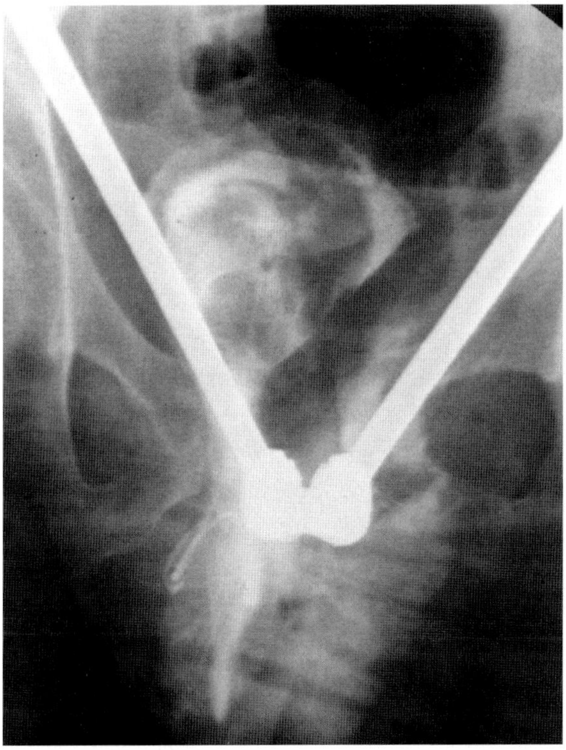

Fig. 11.10. Extraperitoneal bladder rupture at cystography with contrast extravasating into the scrotum

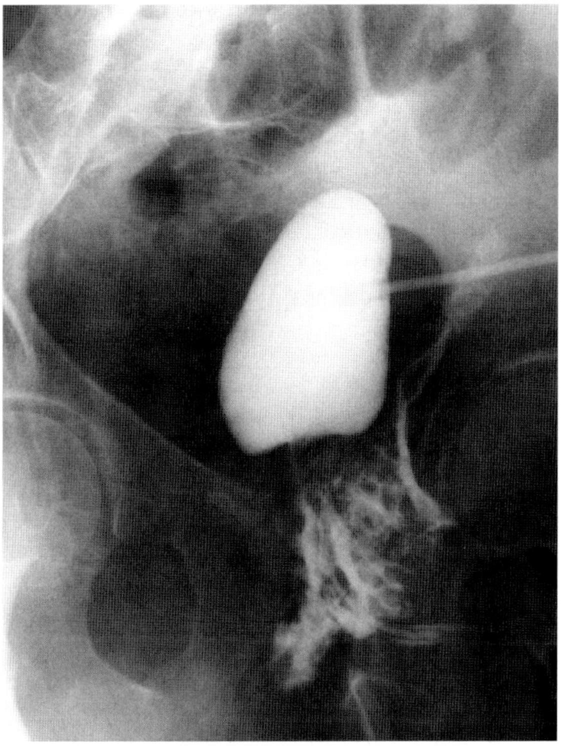

Fig. 11.12. There is extravasation of contrast in both intra- and extraperitoneal spaces following severe pelvic trauma

- CT Cystography. CT will demonstrate patterns of extravasation that are typical for both types of trauma and the extent of pelvic hematoma. It is not always easy to differentiate intra- and extraperitoneal contrast where they may be separated by a thin layer of peritoneum only.

11.1.4.6
Penetrating Bladder Injury

Penetrating injuries are caused by impalement through the lower abdomen, rectum, vagina, or perineum by assaults such as stabbing, shooting, etc. The incidence is low in the civilian population when compared to blunt injuries. The type of bladder trauma depends upon where the missile entered and exited, but any type of bladder injury can result. Associated injuries to surrounding structures is very high, especially with gunshot wounds. If a diagnosis is required prior to surgery, cystography or CT cystography is performed. Where small caliber bullets are responsible, extravasation may not be seen. A bullet may be voided spontaneously after a gunshot wound to the bladder (Sankari and Parra 1993). An intravesical bullet may be eliminated by micturition (Cohen et al. 1975). Although there are units that follow a policy of careful observation and delayed intervention, penetrating injuries to the bladder are surgically dealt with (Sandler et al. 1986; Baniel and Schein 1994). Gas in the urinary bladder is recognized on plain film (Truong et al. 1983). Where there are bladder and rectal injuries, defunctioning colostomy with irrigation of the distal segment and the interposition of an omental flap to prevent the formation of vesicorectal fistula is routine. Combined vaginal and bladder injuries demand the repair of both and an omental flap to prevent fistula. Other causes of bladder injury are perforation of hypogastric artery aneurysm (Verta and Janevicius 1982).

Imaging Findings

- Cystography. Depending upon the path of the bullet or knife, a combination of intra/extraperitoneal extravasation will be seen (Figs. 11.13 and 11.14).
- CT cystography. Because there is such a high incidence of associated injuries, there is usually no time to perform CT, as emergency surgery is needed (McConnell et al. 1982; Theodorakis and Baffes 1985). In one series involving gunshot wounds, the bowel was also involved in 80% of cases, 30% with knife wounds, and major vessels in up to 80%. Where the patient is stable, CT may define associated injuries and locate foreign bodies accurately.

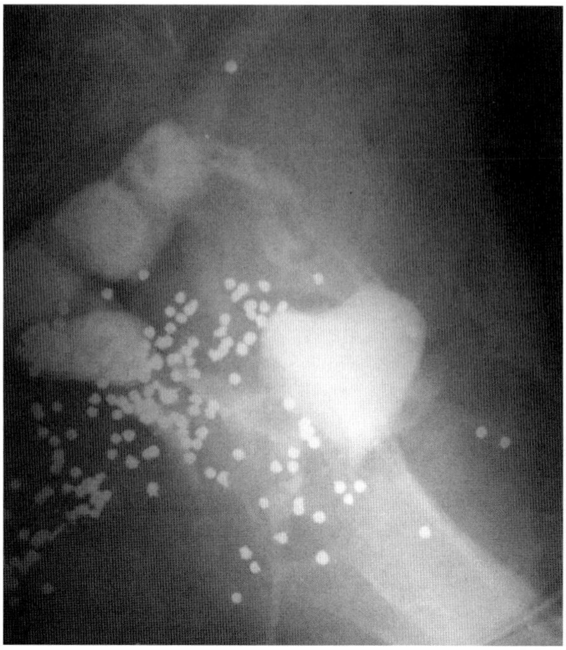

Fig. 11.13. Following a gunshot injury, at cystography, there is extravasation of contrast into the intraperitoneal space; contrast seen within the rectum confirms associated injury

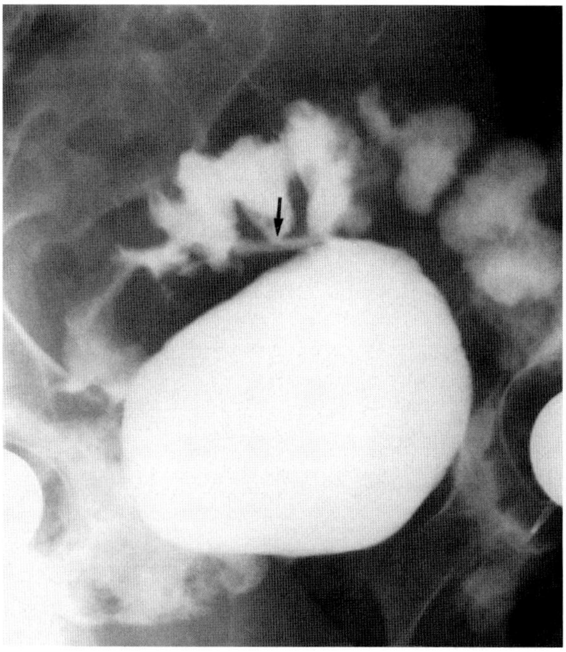

Fig. 11.14. Cystogram following a stab wound. The intraperitoneal connection between the bladder and rectum can be seen (*arrow*)

11.1.4.7
Iatrogenic Injury

There is no endoscopic or open pelvic surgery procedure, including external fixation of pelvic fracture, that is not associated with bladder injury (HUBBARD et al. 1979; CASS and MATSUURA 1983; CASS et al. 1983; SAIDI et al. 1996; POLAT et al. 1997). Vaginal or abdominal hysterectomy with inappropriate dissection between the fascia of the vagina and base of the bladder causes bladder injury, which, if recognized, is repaired, but if not leads to vesicovaginal fistula (BRONITSKY and STUCKEY 1995; LEE et al. 1996; HARRKI-SIREN et al. 1998) (Fig. 11.15). This is more likely after pelvic irradiation. Perforation during hip surgery has been described (COHEN et al. 1977; WHEELER et al. 1983). Endoscopic bladder procedures, including transurethral lithotripsy, may result in perforation (Fig. 11.16), occurring in 0.9% of cases, especially tumor resection and bladder biopsy (MONTIE 1977; KASZTELAN 1983; SUNDNES et al. 1983). Intravesical gas explosion during endoscopic resection was reported (VIVILLE et al. 1984). If recognized and clearly extraperitoneal, no investigation is needed and the perforation seals with a week of catheter drainage. Intraperitoneal perforation can have serious consequences if unrecognized (SPEES et al. 1981). Although the diagnosis can be made cystoscopically, cystography is indicated. Obstetric injury is now rare, bladder laceration can be expected in 0.01% of deliveries and 0.1% to 0.3% of ceaserian sections (FARICY et al. 1978; EISENKOP et al. 1982; BUCHHOLZ et al. 1994; CHUNG et al. 1997; RAJASEKAR and HALL 1997). Stents, drainage catheters, shunts, foreign bodies, or an intrauterine device have all been reported as causes of bladder trauma (KAUFMAN et al. 1983; O'BRIEN and RYCKMAN 1994; SEPULVEDA et al. 1993; CASPI et al. 1996; SAYAN et al. 1996; MATTAR et al. 1997). The bladder wall may rupture after necrosis caused by pelvic artery embolization to control intractable posttraumatic hemorrhage (SIEBER 1994). Finally, idiopathic bladder or rupture occurring after minimal trauma is mentioned (BRERETON et al. 1980; SHUMAKER et al. 1980). Occasionally, foreign bodies such as bullets are voided spontaneously during micturition (ABDELSAYED et al. 1978; DIDOMENICO et al. 1997).

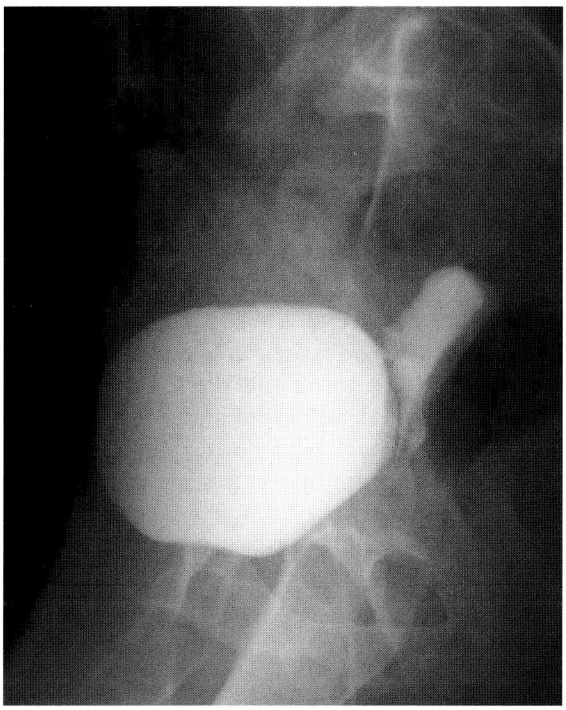

Fig. 11.15. Cystogram demonstrating a vesicovaginal fistula following gynecological surgery

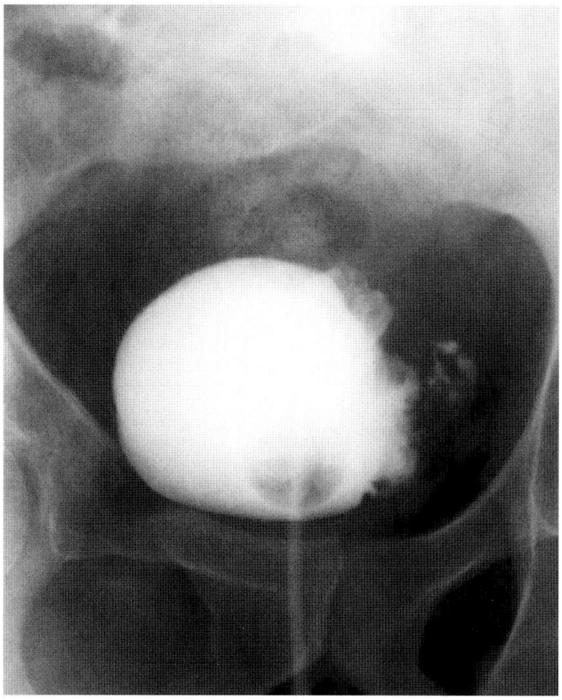

Fig. 11.16. Following resection of a bladder tumor, there is extraperitoneal extravasation of contrast

Imaging Findings

- Cystogrphy. Vesicovaginal fistulae are accurately diagnosed by cystography (Fig. 11.17). Small fistulae may not be evident from simply filling

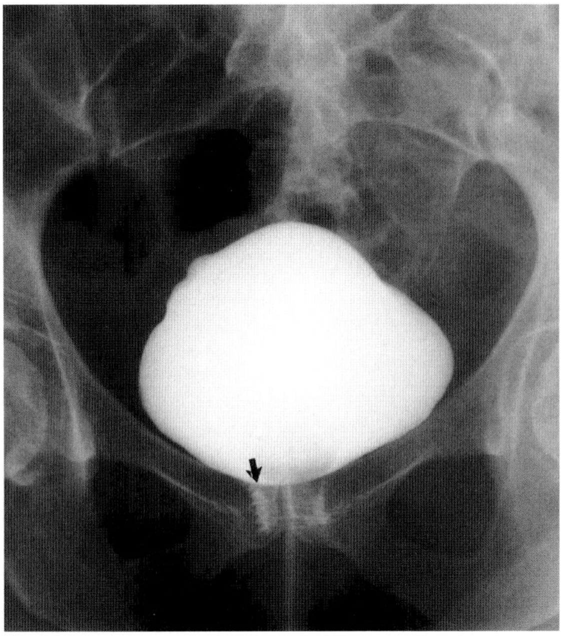

Fig. 11.17. AP radiography at cystography showing contrast within the vagina (*arrow*)

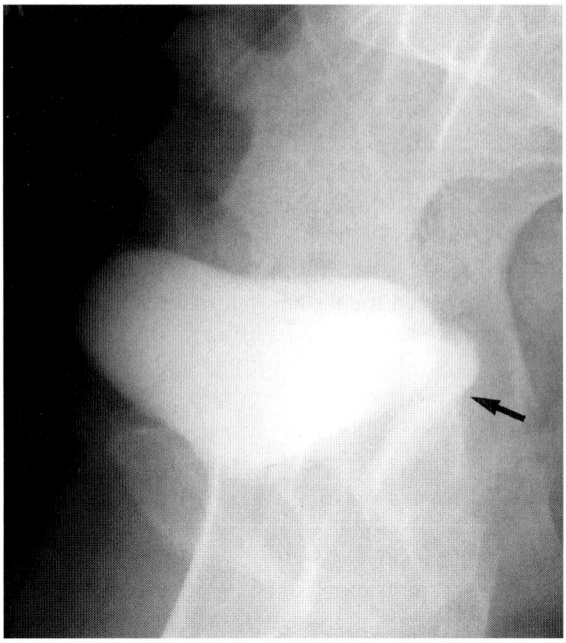

Fig. 11.18. Lateral projection at cystography of a vesicovaginal fistula (*arrow*)

the bladder and lateral or steep oblique screening (Fig. 11.18). The raised intravesical pressure with voiding will precipitate extravasation. It is often not possible to demonstrate the communication between bladder and vagina and it is not necessary to so do, but contrast may enter the vagina normally because of urethrovaginal reflux, which is more common in patients where the urethra is located high up the anterior vaginal wall (Fig. 11.19). Where possible, it is wise to take a rapid sequence of films (2/s) on initiation of voiding to avoid false positive diagnosis. Vesicorectal and vesicovaginorectal fistulas may rarely need an enema study where the cystogram is normal and the index of suspicion high.

11.1.4.8 Radiation Injury

Although not strictly related to external trauma, radiation poses specific problems, of which radiologists need to be aware. Acute radiation cystitis occurs within 6 months of therapy and is characterized by mucosal bleeding, which heals without specific therapy. Radiation cystitis may rupture spontaneously (Addar et al. 1996; Kurizaki and Ishizuka 1997; Steinert and Walter 1997). Gross hematuria up to 12 months after therapy signifies chronic cystitis (Goldberg et al. 1984). The bladder shrinks because of fibrosis, the reduced capacity leading to frequency and nocturia. Urgency and urge incontinence suggest coexistent detrusor instability. Hematuria can be tempered by the installation of 5% formalin or 1% alum (Ostroff and Chenault 1982; Donahue and Frank 1989). Such substances cause denaturation of the tissue protein of superficial cells and a marked reduction in bleeding. They cause pain when instilled and this is generally performed under general anesthesia. It is crucial to prove that there is no vesicoureteric reflux by cystography. Tubular necrosis will occur if these substances do reflux into the collecting system. Postirradiation vesicovaginal fistulae are most commonly seen following radiotherapy for carcinoma of the cervix and present a formidable therapeutic challenge. Repairs must only be carried out on nonmalignant fistulae and omental interposition is crucial to operative success. The availability of omentum can be assessed by CT.

11.2 Urethral Injury

The male urethra accounts for the majority of injuries, but injury is relatively uncommon. Most injuries

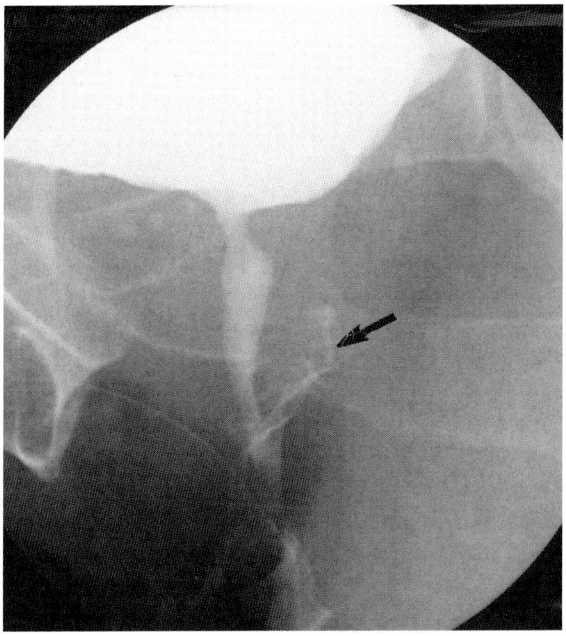

Fig. 11.19. Vesicovaginal reflux. During micturition, contrast can be seen entering the vagina (*arrow*). If not recognized, a misdiagnosis of a fistula will be made

result from blunt or penetrating trauma and iatrogenic injuries are common. The short and well-protected female urethra is rarely injured in trauma, but suffers its fair share of iatrogenic insults.

11.2.1 History

There is literature on urethral rupture and the end result of trauma: stricture. The first successful treatment of rupture was enlightened (Chopart 1791). Verguin in 1757 treated a complete disruption on the bulbar urethra by passing a curved catheter through a well-established suprapubic tract and a second catheter up the anterior urethra. With a finger in the patient's perineal wound suffered at the time of injury, he brought the two into contact and railroaded a second catheter into the bladder with complete recovery of the patient's bladder function. Brikett (1866) at Guy's in London treated a patient who had been kicked in the perineum by a horse. No catheter could be passed so he exposed the urethra and on finding a gap of an inch between the ends, joined them with one silk suture over a catheter with excellent results, the first urethroplasty. Over the years, this technique was refined, but the composition of catheters was then blamed for subsequent stricture formation (Harrison 1883). Rutherford was particularly scathing in regards to their use and recommended suprapubic drainage only after realignment of the urethra (Rutherford 1904). Diagnosis was clinical and inferred after the inability to pass catheters or probes. Urethrography was first described by Cunningham in 1910. He experienced difficulties in outlining the posterior urethra with available contrast media. This problem was solved by Flocks in 1933 by using opaque fluid made viscous by tragacanth (Flocks 1933). When the author first started his consultant career at the Institute of Urology in London in 1985, urethrography was performed using Conray 289 mixed in equal parts with KY jelly and allowed to stand for 1 h to allow the bubbles time to dissipate! Although wonderful images of the urethra were obtained, not surprisingly the sepsis rate was high.

11.2.2 Male Urethral Anatomy

The male urethra is subdivided into four parts based on anatomy and function. The posterior urethra extends from the bladder neck to the distal aspect of the distal sphincter at the urogenital diaphragm and is divided into the prostatic and membranous portions. The anterior urethra extends from the urogenital diaphragm to the external meatus and is subdivided into penile and bulbar portions and is enveloped by corpus spongiosum (Gosling 1979). The penile urethra has little spongiosum around it, whereas the bulbar urethra has more and this accounts for the relative failure of optical urethrotomy in the former. The urogenital diaphragm is inserted anterior-laterally into the pubic arch and ischium and postural into the perineal muscles. The Buck fascia is a dense, elastic layer which envelops the corpora cavernosa and extends into the perineum to envelop the bulbar urethra.

The arterial supply to the urethra has therapeutic implications. Its main supply is from bulbar arteries, which are proximal branches of the internal pudendal (Fig. 11.20). Distally, it is supplied by the dorsal artery, which is a terminal branch of the internal pudendal. The urethra can be detached at either end without compromising its viability.

The sphincter mechanism has three components. The proximal sphincter is the bladder neck and its smooth muscle is quite distinct from the detrusor muscle, but continuous with the prostate capsular musculature. Integrity of the bladder neck is crucial for normal antegrade ejaculation and that is its pri-

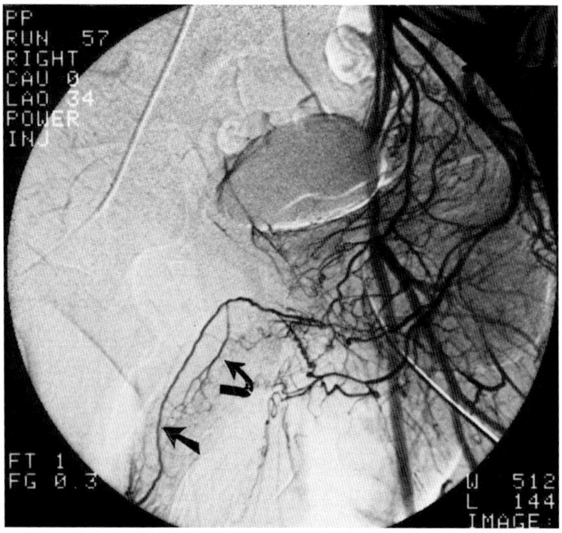

Fig. 11.20. Penile angiogram. The dorsal artery (*straight arrow*) and the bulbar artery (*curved arrow*) are seen

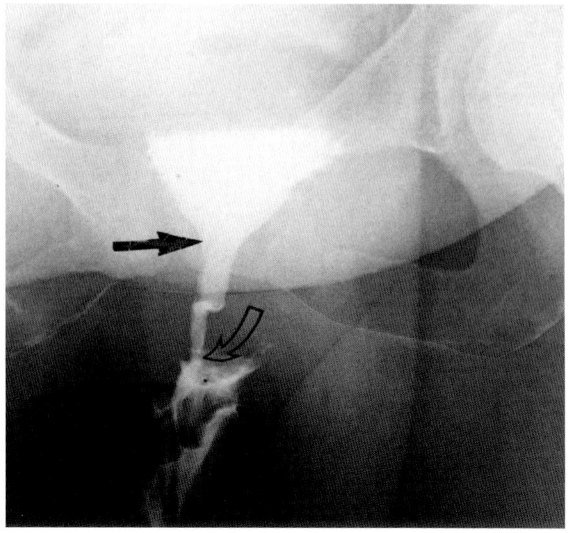

Fig. 11.21. Female micturating cystogram in a normal female extending from the bladder neck (*arrow*) to the external meatus (*open arrow*)

mary function. In the absence of a functioning distal sphincter, urinary continence can be achieved solely at the bladder neck level. Bladder neck function is linked to detrusor activity and involuntary, unstable contractions of the bladder will lead to opening of the bladder neck and where there is a compromised distal sphincter, incontinence will occur. The distal sphincter itself has two components, intrinsic and extrinsic. The intrinsic portion is 2 cm long extending from just cephalad to the veru montanum to the bulbar urethra and is within the wall of the membranous urethra. It is composed of slow-twitch striated muscle and maintains continence. The extrinsic portion abuts the membranous urethra posteriorly and laterally and is composed of fast-twitch striated muscle.

11.2.3 Female Urethral Anatomy

The female urethra is 3.5 cm long and is protected behind the symphysis pubis (Fig. 11.21). Its inferior half is inseparable from the anterior vaginal wall and is supported by pubourethral ligaments and the pelvic floor musculature. Continence depends upon the striated distal sphincter musculature. The female bladder neck is not a sphincter of importance and the bladder neck can be normally open in a symptomatic nulliparous female (Chapple et al. 1989). It is rarely involved in trauma.

11.2.4 Imaging

11.2.4.1 Ascending Urethrography

Ascending urethrography involves the retrograde injection of contrast to distend and outline the anterior urethra. The normal distal sphincter provides a resistance that permits such distension. With an increased force of injection, the resistance afforded by the distal sphincter will be overcome and contrast will pass through the posterior urethra into the bladder. This can be achieved by passing a small Foley catheter into the distal anterior urethra and inflating its balloon with 2–3 ml of air, which should be placed in the navicular fossa. This is not ideal because it causes pain, can injure the urethra, and the catheter is of small caliber. A Knutson's clamp is preferable since it causes no urethral injury and is less painful. If there is a Foley catheter already in place for drainage purposes, a small catheter can be passed alongside it, a clamp component of the Knutson's clamp placed over the distal anterior urethra and activated. This is not ideal as a watertight seal is not possible and adequate distension will be achieved (McLaughlin and Pfister 1974). Contrast should be instilled under fluoroscopic monitoring with the patient supine-oblique on the table (Fig. 11.22). Anterior-posterior projections will cause false negatives because the urethra is foreshortened (Sandler et al. 1981a).

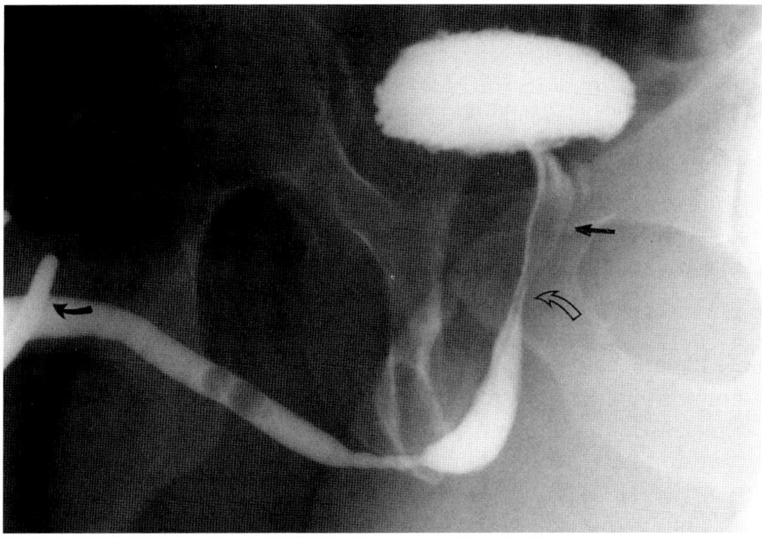

Fig. 11.22. Ascending urethrogram. Contrast is injected via a Knutson's clamp (*curved arrow*). The verumontanum (*arrow*) and distal sphincter (*open arrow*) can be identified. There is a proximal anterior urethral stricture

11.2.4.2
Descending or Micturating Urethrography

Descending or micturating urethrography necessitates instilling contrast into the bladder and the patient micturating. This defines the anatomy of posterior urethra (Fig. 11.23) and, when the patient is asked to interrupt micturition, will define the function of the sphincter mechanisms. This study only needs to be performed when the integrity of the posterior urethra or the sphincter mechanisms is in doubt. Retrograde injection is done via a Knutson's clamp or through a suprapubic catheter. If there is extravasation on an ascending study, the retrograde route must not be used. The bladder needs to be distended until the patient has a strong desire to void. At this stage, fluoroscopy of the bladder will define associated injuries, whether there is vesicoureteric reflux, and what the bladder outline looks like. It also gives some indication as to bladder capacity. With the patient erect and in an oblique position, voiding is requested and when adequate distension of the posterior urethra has been seen, the patient is asked to interrupt micturition and the function of the sphincters observed. Under normal circumstances, the distal sphincter should close, the posterior urethra empty completely with milk-back of contrast into the bladder, and the anterior urethra empty completely. At the end of micturition, the amount of residual urine can be roughly assessed.

11.2.4.3
Ultrasound

Ultrasound has an advantage over urethrography in that it details the anatomy around the urethra, but distension of the urethra is needed by the retrograde injection of saline; in the trauma situation, this is not indicated.

11.2.4.4
Computed Tomography

CT has the advantage of detailing the periurethral anatomy, especially the bony pelvis, but is of limited value in assessing the urethra itself.

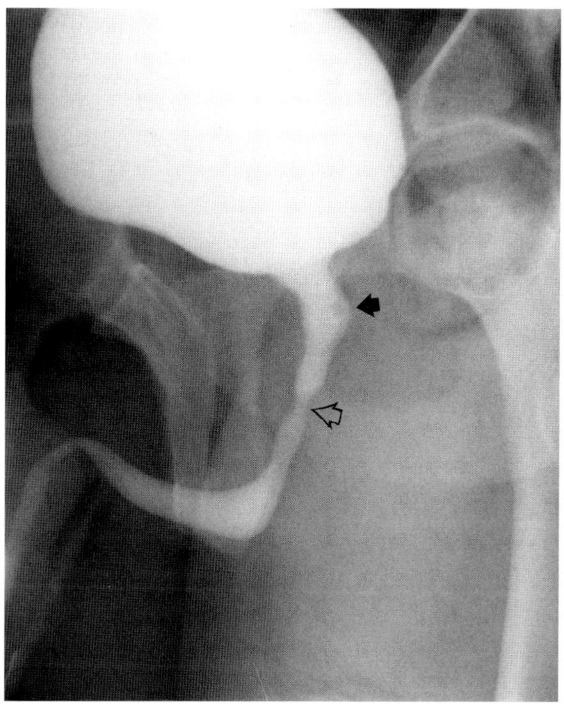

Fig. 11.23. Descending urethrogram. The verumontanum (*arrow*) and distal sphincter area (*open arrow*) are identified

11.2.5 Cause

The common causes are blunt injuries to the perineum, injuries associated with pelvic fracture, as well as penetrating and iatrogenic injuries.

11.2.5.1 Blunt Perineal Injury

Most are due to straddle injuries where the bulbar urethra is compressed against the symphysis pubis as a result of falling astride a blunt object such as railing, gymnasium equipment, etc., but any part of the urethra can be involved. Pelvic fracture may be presentand associated with urethral injury in 3.5% of cases, urinary bladder injury in 9%, and combined injury in 1% (Palmer et al. 1983). The severity of the force determines the extent of injury, but it can be severe enough to transect the urethra (Fig. 11.24). In the vast majority of cases, urethral contusion or incomplete rupture occurs. If Buck's fascia is ruptured, blood will extravasate to produce perineal and scrotal hematoma. If intact, extravasation will be confined to the shaft of the penis.

Findings on ascending urethrography depend upon the severity. With a partial rupture, localized extravasation may be seen, but with the more common urethral contusion, urethrography will be normal. Delayed stricture formation can occur with contusions and follow-up urethrography is advised (Corriere and Harris 1981) (Figs. 11.25 and 11.26). With a partial rupture, urethral continuity is present, but extravasation into the periurethral tissues will be seen often with venous intravasation. With complete ruptures, no contrast will be seen proximal to the injury. Partial and complete ruptures should be treated with suprapubic drainage and are likely to be complicated by stricture formation (Pontes and Pierce 1978). Passing a Foley catheter may make a partial rupture complete. Complete ruptures are best treated by urethroplasty some months following injury. Partial ruptures should be assessed by urethrography after 2 weeks of suprapubic drainage and if no extravasation seen, the patient be allowed to void. The increasing popularity of radical prostatectomy for prostate cancer frequently results in extravasation at the site of the anastomosis of the bladder base to the bulbar urethra, but this is usually self-limiting and most urologists do not ask for urethrography prior to routine catheter removal.

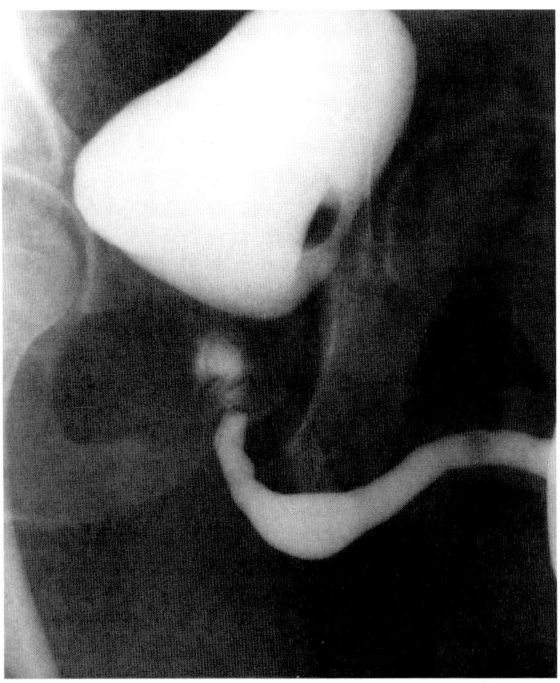

Fig. 11.24. Combined ascending and descending study showing complete transection of the posterior urethra without pelvic fracture, but with localized extravasation of contrast

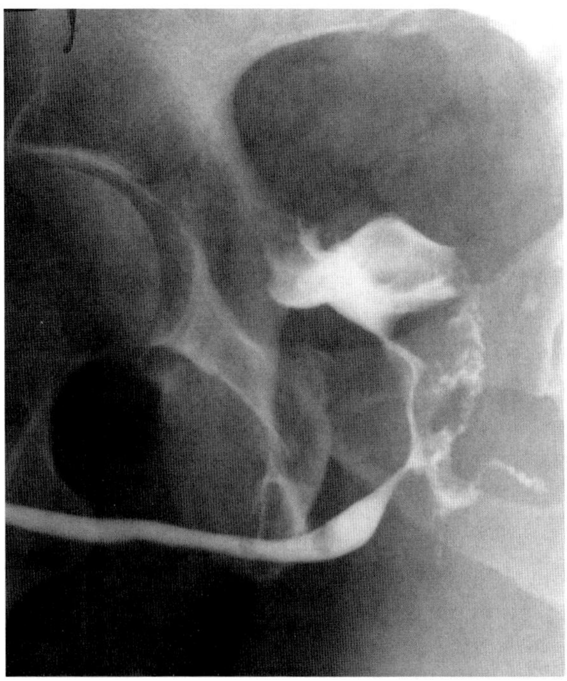

Fig. 11.25. Ascending urethrogram showing a partial rupture of the penile urethra with considerable extravasation and with contrast entering the bladder

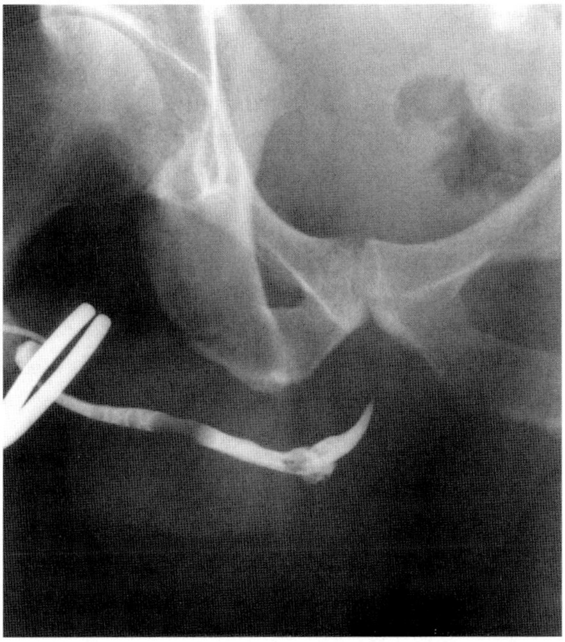
a
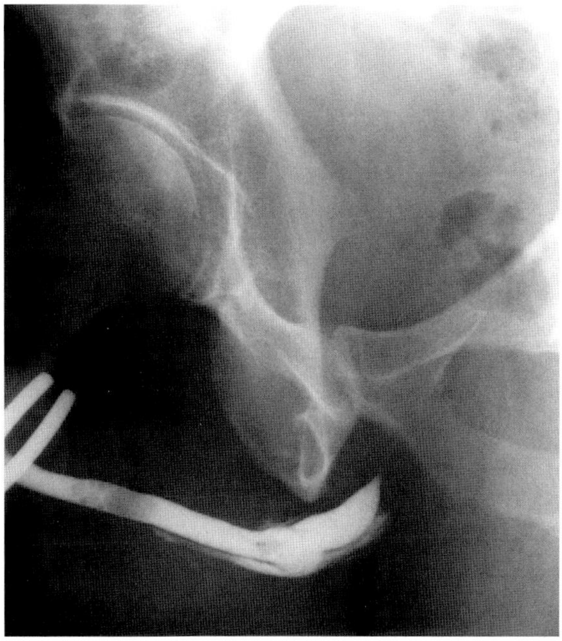
b
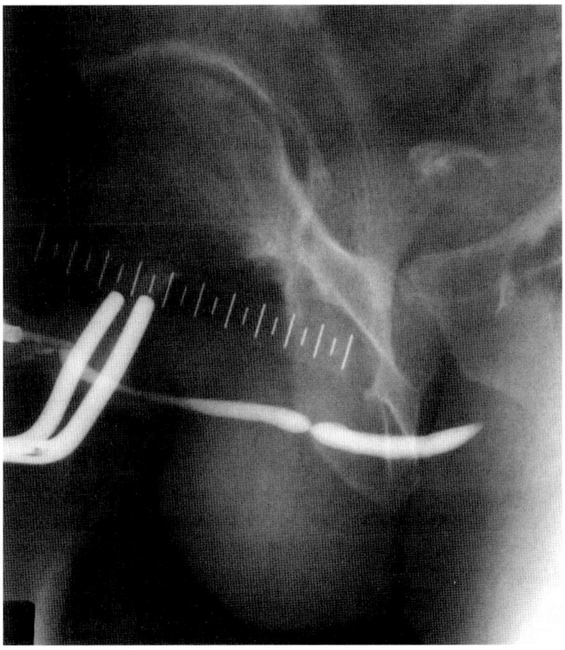
c

Fig. 11.26. **a** Ascending urethrogram following blunt pelvic trauma. There is localized extravasation associated with a filling defect within the urethra due to blood clot. **b** Further injection causes extravasation. The study should be terminated at this point. **c** Ascending urethrogram 6 months later shows a tight stricture

11.2.5.2
Iatrogenic Injury

Iatrogenic injury is the leading cause of minor urethral trauma. The bulbar urethra is most commonly affected because of its angular course (Fig. 11.27). Attempted catheterization can cause contusion or partial tears, especially in the uncooperative patient. The appearance of urine from the end of the catheter does not guarantee that the catheter is with the bladder and the inexperienced can blow the balloon up with 10–20 ml of saline within the urethra.

Trauma due to rigid instrumentation is also most commonly seen at the bulbar urethra, but this is decreasing because of flexible cystoscopy replacing rigid procedures and endoscopes are forward-looking. Meatal (Fig. 11.28) and distal anterior injury can occur as a result of circumcision and because of foreign bodies. Urethrography, where necessary, will show extravasation at the trauma site. Extrava-

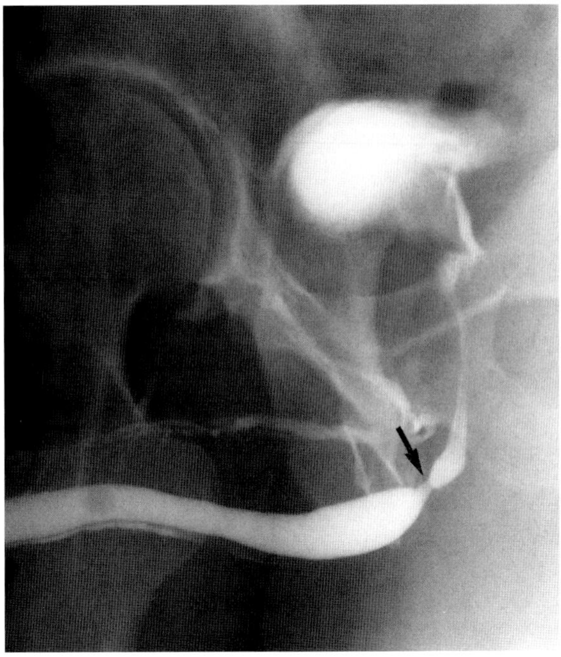

Fig. 11.27. Ascending urethrogram showing a classic bulbar stricture (*arrow*) 2 years following cystoscopy. Note the venous intravasation, a recognized complication of urethrography and one that should be covered by antibiotics

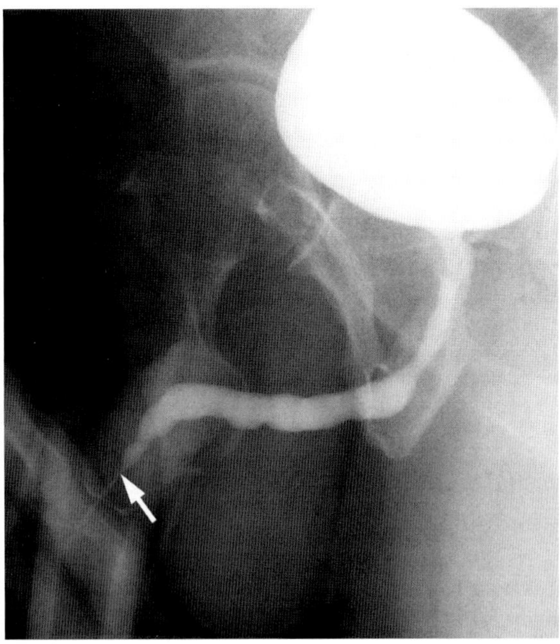

Fig. 11.28. A descending urethrogram showing a short meatal stricture (*arrow*)

sation following transurethral resection of the prostate (TURP) is common with extensive resections (Fig. 11.29).

11.2.5.3
Penetrating Injury

Gunshot and stab wounds are becoming more prevalent in our increasingly violent society. Any part of the urethra can be involved and urethrography will determine the site and extent of injury (Figs. 11.30 and 11.31). Primary repair is the treatment of choice,

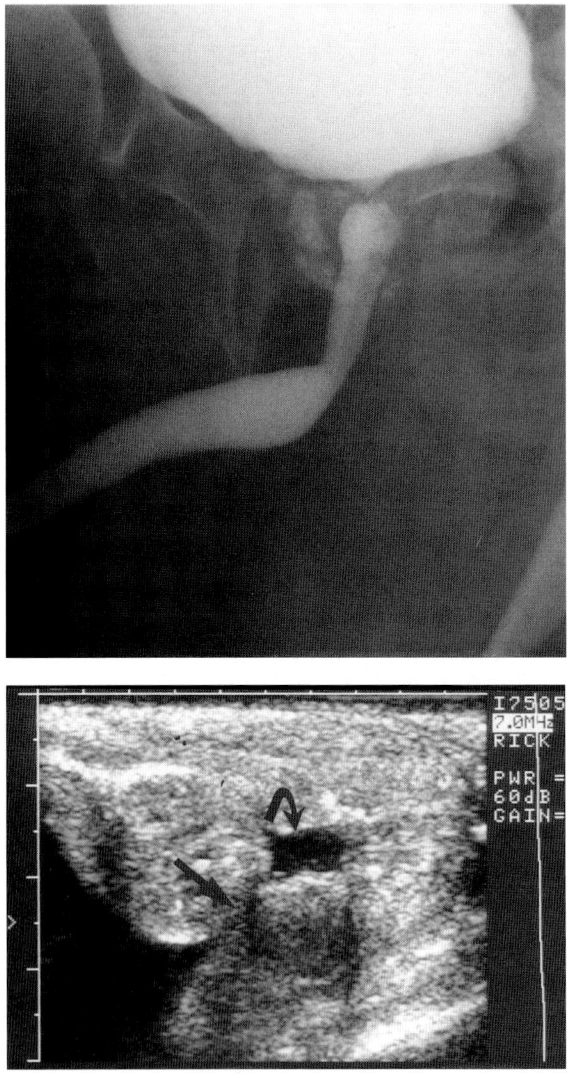

a

b

Fig. 11.29. a An ascending urethrogram showing a bladder neck stricture following a transurethral resection of the prostate (TURP). **b** Transrectal ultrasound using a linear array probe clearly shows the stenosis at the bladder neck (*arrow*). What is left of the TURP cavity (*curved arrow*) especially as surgical exploration is usually needed because of damage to other organs (HUSMANN et al. 1993).

11.2.5.4 Urethral Injury Following Pelvic Fracture

The urinary bladder is involved in 2%–10% and the posterior urethra is involved in 2%–10% of patients who sustain a pelvic fracture (EID 1982; MERLINI et al. 1982; HOCHBERG and STONE 1993). In females, urethral injuries are uncommon (CARTER and SCHAFER 1993). Straddle fracture combined with diastasis of the sacroiliac joint put the bulbomembranous urethra at particular risk of rupture (KORAITIM et al. 1996). Motor vehicle accidents are responsible for the majority of such injuries in the civilian population. Heavy machine workers, miners, and builders are also prone because of the potential of crush injury with such occupations. The severity of the injury varies, but at one end of the spectrum lies urethral contusion requiring no treatment to total urethral distraction requiring major reconstructive surgery. In the latter group, vascular and neural damage will coexist, leading to a high incidence of impotence (PAICK et al. 1993) (Fig. 11.32). If not injured at the time of trauma, reconstructive surgery puts them in jeopardy. It has been shown that erectile dysfunction is more likely when both pubic rami are involved (CRASSWELLER et al. 1977; Mark et al. 1977).

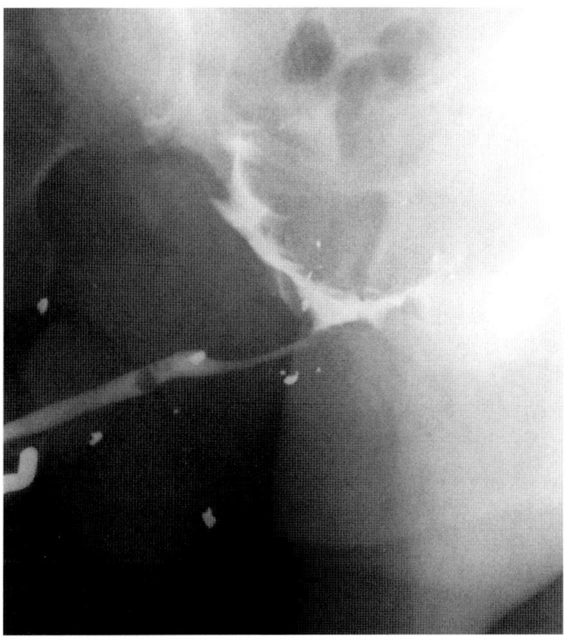

Fig. 11.30. Ascending urethrogram following a gunshot injury. There is complete transection of the urethra with considerable extravasation

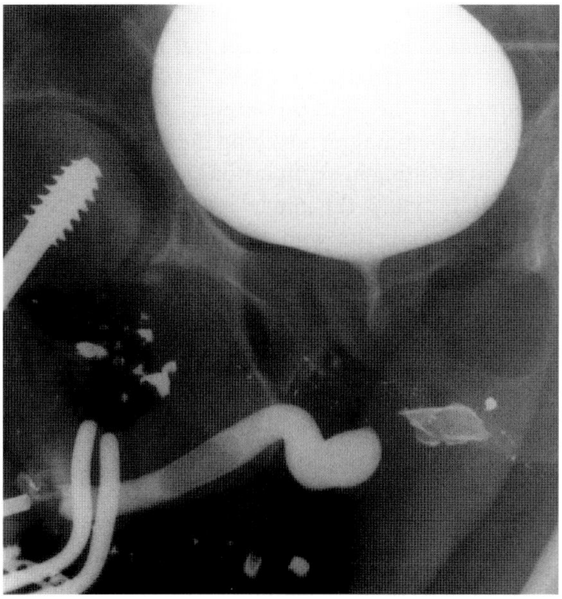

Fig. 11.31. Combined ascending and descending urethrogram 6 months following a gun shot injury. There is complete transection of the urethra and a long defect that includes the distal sphincter mechanism

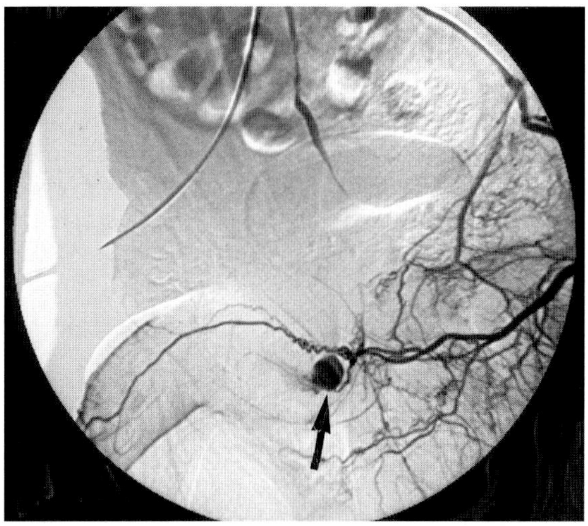

Fig. 11.32. Penile angiogram in a patient with impotence following pelvic fracture. There is an aneurysm visible (arrow)

Based on findings at urethrography in the acute phase, classifications of posterior urethral injury have been proposed. Three types were described by COLAPINTO and MCCALLUM (1977). In type 1, the posterior urethra is elongated because the puboprostatic ligaments rupture, resulting in a large hematoma elevating the bladder, but rarely resulting in rupture (Jones and Kock 1977). In type 2, there is rupture of the posterior urethra superior to the urogenital diaphragm, involving the sphincter active area and resulting in extraperitoneal extravasation of contrast. In type 3, the injury extends inferior to the urogenital diaphragm into the bulbar urethra, resulting in additional extravasation of contrast into the periurethral tissues (Fig. 11.33). In all 3 types, there is fracture of the puboprostatic ligaments, displacing the prostate superiorly with and without rupture of the urogenital diaphragm depending upon the severity of the injury. Type 2 and 3 injuries are associated with either partial or complete rupture; when partial, contrast will be seen entering the bladder. The incidence of partial to complete ruptures varies; in some series partial tears accounting 19%–27%, whereas in others, partial tears account for up to 90% (Sandler et al. 1981b; McAninch 1981; Webster et al. 1983). The discrepancy is probably related to referral patterns where primary treatment involved attempted catheterization converting type 2 into type 3 injuries before definitive specialized treatment could be made available. This classification was added to Goldman to include associated bladder neck injuries, type 4, and anterior urethral injuries, type 5 (Goldman et al. 1997). Bladder neck injuries were reported in females, but it is in males where careful assessment is most important because urinary continence will depend upon a functioning bladder neck where the distal sphincter has been destroyed (Turner Warwick 1977; Perry and Husmann 1992) (Fig. 11.34).

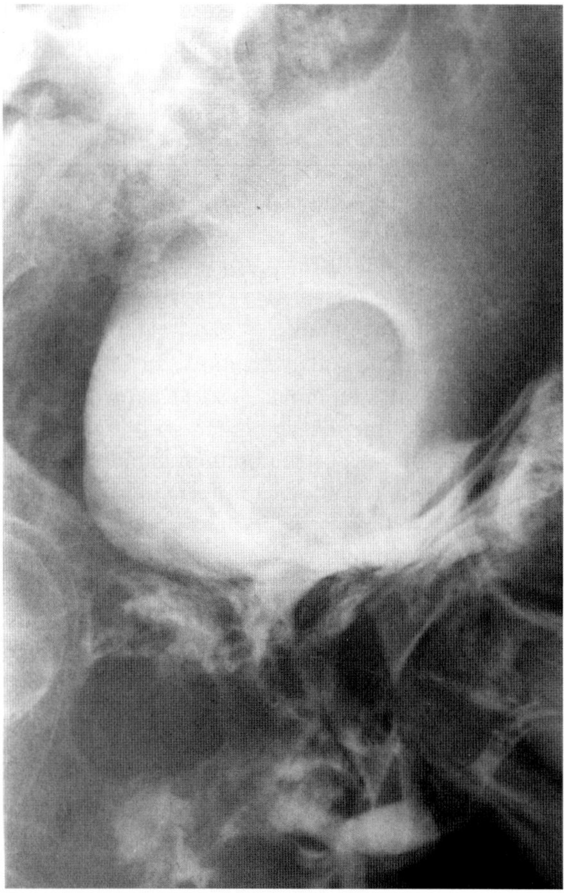

Fig. 11.33. A type 3 pelvic fracture injury. There is continuity of the urethra with contrast seen in the bladder, but there is extravasation above and below the urogenital diaphragm

11.2.6 Diagnosis of Posterior Urethral Injury

Clinically, blood per urethra, a palpable bladder, and an inability to void suggest posterior urethral injury (Mitchell 1968). Inability to void may stem from sphincter spasm, a fortunate coincidence, or urinary extravasation would be more common. The inability to pass a catheter is neither diagnostic nor wise, potentially increasing the severity of the injury and introducing infection (Glass et al. 1978). The inability to pass a catheter can make the diagnosis of concomitant urinary bladder injury difficult (Belis et al. 1979). Associated bladder injury can be expected in 15% of these patients (Mitchell 1968).

Radiologically, ascending urethrography will define the site and severity of the injury. However, primary surgical repair of posterior urethral injuries

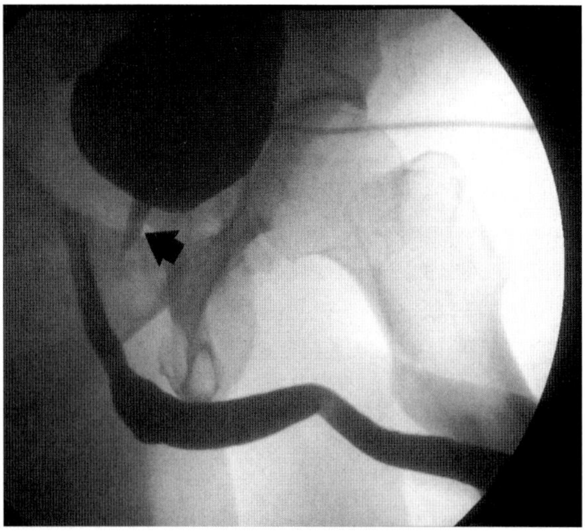

Fig. 11.34. Combined ascending and descending urethrogram. The bladder neck is incompetent with passive filling of the posterior urethra (arrow). There is a large urethral defect which includes the sphincter active area

is rarely performed, leading to a high morbidity that includes a stricture rate of up to 100%, incontinence in 40%, and impotence in 60% (GIBSON 1970; MOREHOUSE et al. 1972; WEBSTER and SIHELNIK 1985). The current trend is for patients to be treated with an attempt to stent the urethra, in order to align the ends or suprapubic drainage for up to 6 months followed by elective surgery that reduces the morbidity rate for stricture to 5%, incontinence to 2%, and impotence to 10% (PONTES 1977; MOREHOUSE and MCKINNIN 1980). There is a small percentage of cases that require immediate surgery (SIMPSON-SMITH 1937). These include those with associated rectal injury in whom evacuation of infected hematoma and fashioning a colostomy are necessary. Where there are type 5 injuries, the bladder neck should be debrided and repaired, improving the chances of continence.

Following a period of suprapubic drainage, ascending and descending urethrography must be performed preoperatively. An ascending study will demonstrate the inferior extent of the disruption. Contrast instilled through the suprapubic invariably causes the patient a great deal of discomfort as the bladder has been decompressed for a significant time. However, the radiologist must persist in encouraging the patient to void, to distend the posterior urethra and define the uppermost level of disruption. It will be possible to assess whether the bladder neck is incompetent and to what extent the distal sphincter is involved (Fig. 11.35). Asking the patient to try and interrupt micturition will give some idea as to residual sphincter activity.

Once reconstructive surgery has been performed, urethral and suprapubic catheters are left in situ for 2 weeks. Before they are removed, a urethrogram needs to be performed to check that there is no extravasation at the operative site. Although this can be done through the suprapubic way with a descending study, it is often difficult for the patient to void around the balloon of the Foley catheter, which obstructs the bladder neck. Passing a small catheter upstream along the urethral catheter and instilling contrast under fluoroscopic observation will provide the information (Fig. 11.36). Where a urethroplasty has failed or other inappropriate surgical procedures have been performed, careful urethrography must be done prior to corrective surgery. Multiple bladder necks and false passages may be seen and it is up to the radiologist to use a descending study to define them and identify the true posterior urethra with its residual sphincter activity (Fig. 11.37). Urethral diverticula and foreign bodies are all complications of failed surgery. Posttraumatic strictures of the posterior urethra are classic complications of injury to the prostatomembranous urethra, requiring reconstructive repair or dilatations and internal urethrotomy (HALLER et al. 1979).

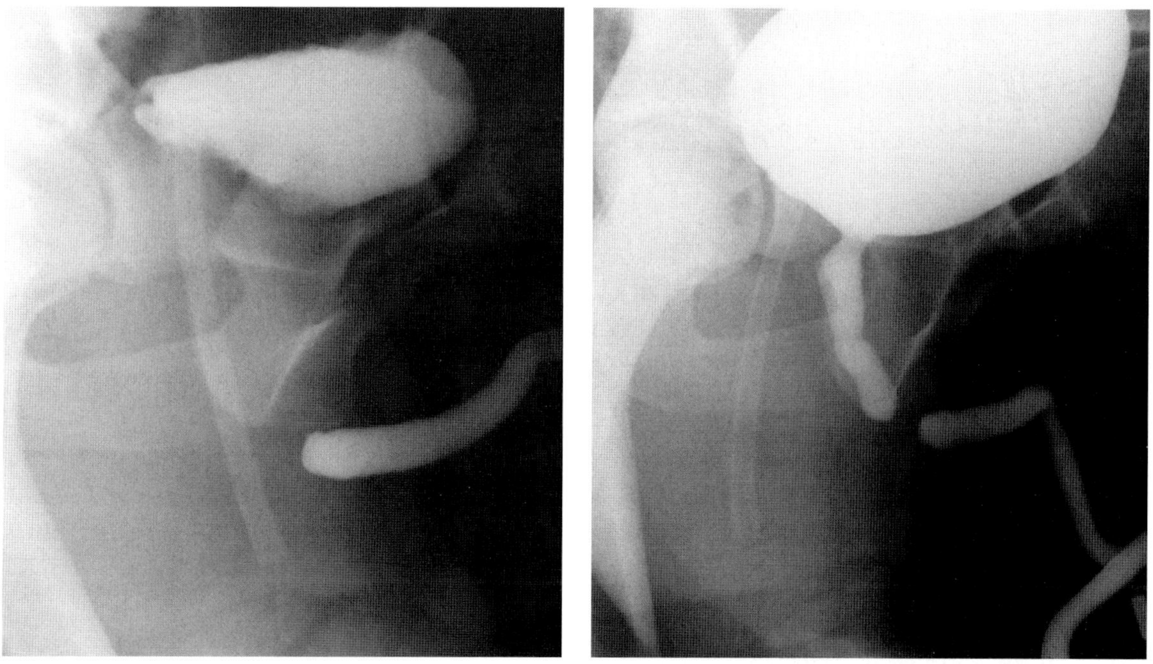

a b

Fig. 11.35. a An ascending study 5 months after pelvic fracture shows the inferior extent of the urethral defect. The bladder neck is closed. **b** With further bladder filling, the patient has opened his bladder neck attempting to void and the proximal extent of the defect is now clearly seen

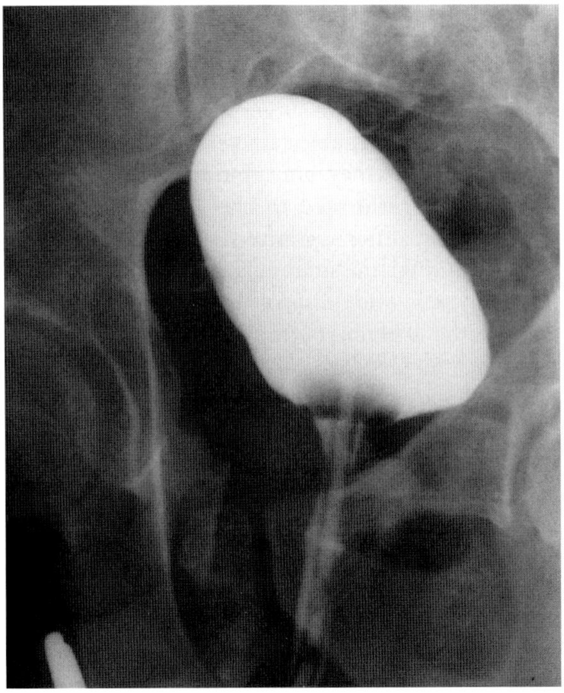

Fig. 11.36. Urethrogram alongside an indwelling catheter following urethroplasty for pelvic fracture stricture shows no extravasation

11.2.7 Female Urethral Injury

These are rare, more common in children, perhaps because adults tend to die more commonly from associated injuries (Blandy 1980; Patel et al. 1982; Venn et al. 1999). Avulsion injuries of the bladder neck are due to rapid deceleration and these are unlikely to be overlooked because of the severity of the trauma that usually causes associated avulsion of the vagina and rectal injury. Less severe injuries, usually longitudinal tears, can go unnoticed, presenting late with extravasation or incontinence. Damage to the innervation may occur alone or in conjunction with an otherwise uncomplicated urethral injury; this can present subsequently with sphincter weakness incontinence. Imaging the female urethra with ascending studies is not warranted. If there is a suprapubic in place, descending studies will demonstrate extravasation in the acute phase and stricture formation (Figs. 11.38 and 11.39) of posttraumatic diverticula (Fig. 11.40).

a

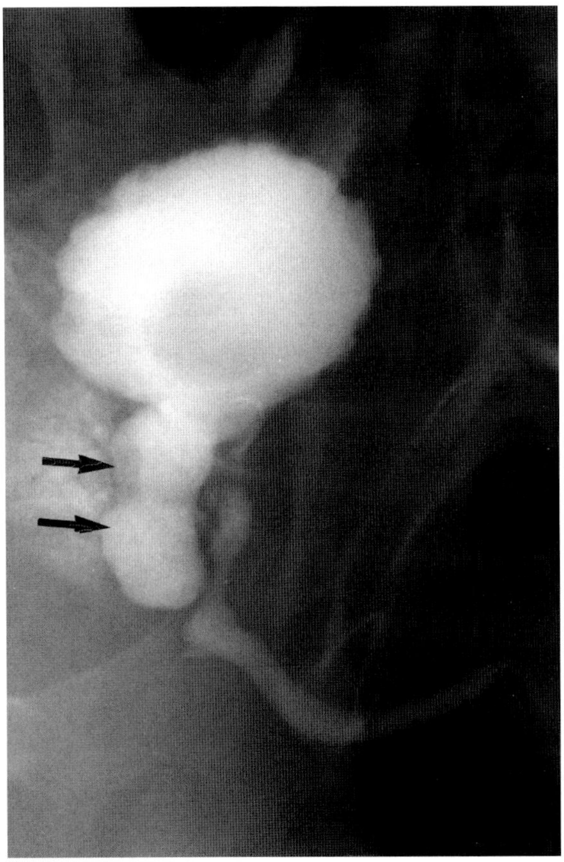

b

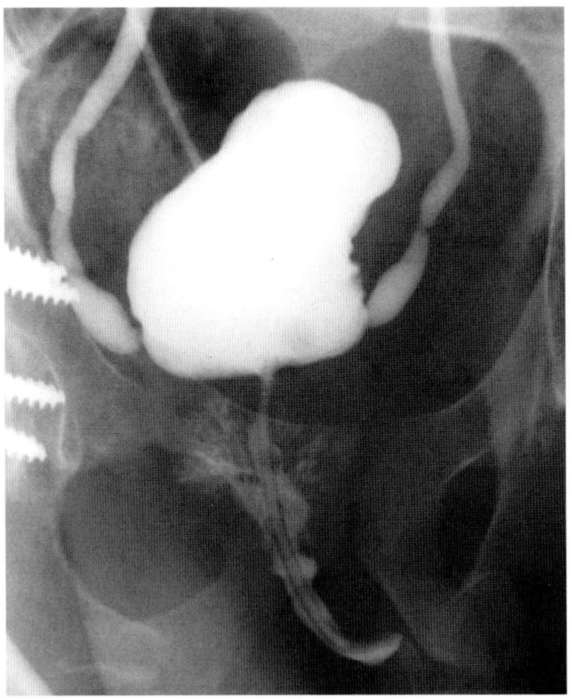

Fig. 11.37. a Ascending urethrogram following pelvic fracture. The true posterior urethra (*arrows*) is not in continuity with the true anterior urethra. **b** Following urethroplasty, a urethrogram alongside a catheter shows no extravasation, but there is intraprostatic reflux

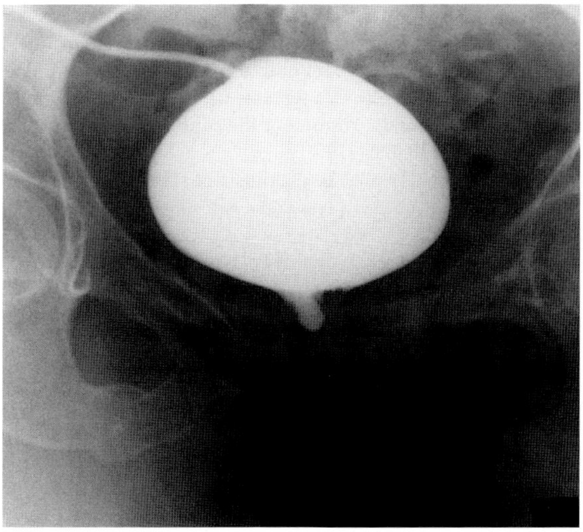

Fig. 11.38. Cystogram via a suprapubic in a female patient 6 month following pelvic fracture shows a complete distal sphincter stenosis

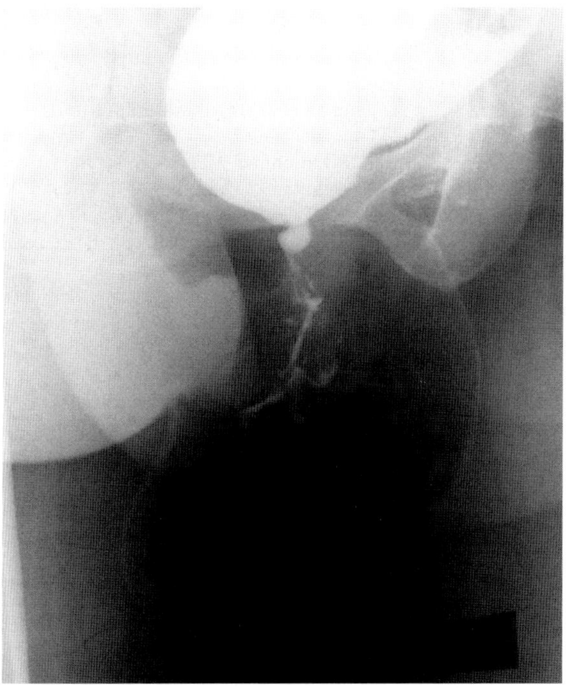

Fig. 11.39. Cystogram in a female patient showing a posttraumatic distal urethral stricture

11.3 Conclusion

There is no complexity in diagnosing trauma to the bladder or urethra. Fluoroscopy with contrast is adequate in most cases, but CT cystography is clearly indicated in bladder trauma, especially where associated injuries are suspected. However, in many countries, availability is an issue. Accurate diagnosis determines treatment in bladder trauma. In most units, surgery for urethral trauma is delayed and the radiologist's task is to accurately determine the site of trauma and its relationship to the sphincter mechanisms. As with all procedures, there is a false negative and false positive rate, but in these instances, it is very low.

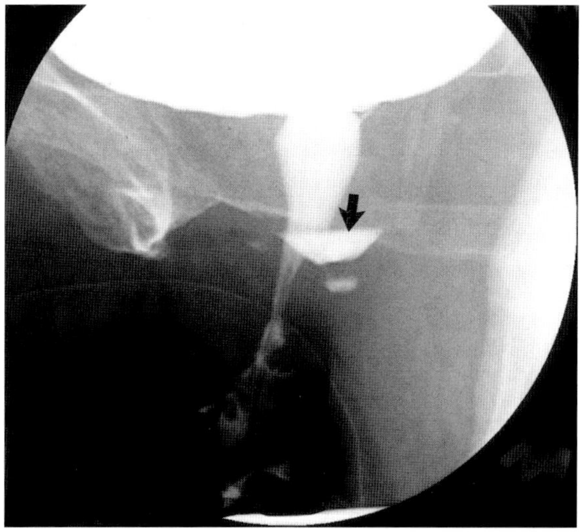

Fig. 11.40. Descending urethrogram in a female patient 2 years following pelvic fracture. A diverticulum is seen (arrow)

References

Abdelsayed MA, Bissada NK, Finkbeiner AE, Redman JF (1978) Spontaneous passage of bullet during voiding. South Med J 71:83–84

Addar MH, Stuart GC, Nation JG, Shumsky AG (1996) Spontaneous rupture of the urinary bladder: a late complication of radiotherapy – case report and review of the literature. Gynecol Oncol 62:314–316

Baniel J, Schein M (1994) The management of penetrating trauma to the urinary tract. J Am Coll Surg 178:417–425

Belis JA, Recht KA, Milam DF (1979) Simultaneous traumatic bladder perforation and disruption of the prostatomembranous urethra. J Urol 122:412–414

Blacklock NJ (1979) Bladder trauma in the long-distance runner. Am J Sports Med 7:239–241

Blandy JP (1980) Urethral stricture. Post Med J 56:383–418

Brereton RJ, Philip N, Buyukpanukcu N (1980) Rupture of the urinary bladder in children. The importance of the double lesion. Br J Urol 52:15–20

Brikett EL (1866) Complete transverse division of the urethra by a kick of a horse in the perineum: perineal section: recovery. Lancet ii:693

Bronitsky C, Stuckey SJ (1995) Complications of laparoscopic-assisted vaginal hysterectomy. J Am Assoc Gynecol Laparosc 2:345–347
Brosman SA, Paul JG (1976) Trauma of the bladder. Surg Gynecol Obstet 142:605–608
Brown D, Magill HL, Black TL (1986) Delayed presentation of intraperitoneal bladder rupture. Paediatr Radiol 16:252–253
Buchholz NP, Daly-Grandeau E, Huber-Buchholz MM (1994) Urological complications associated with caesarian section. Eur J Obstet Gynecol Reprod Biol 56:161–163
Carroll PR, McAninch JW (1983) Major bladder trauma – the accuracy of the cystogram. J Urol 130:887–888
Carroll PR, McAninch JW (1984) Major bladder trauma: mechanisms of injury and a unified method of diagnosis and repair. J Urol 132:254–257
Carter CT, Schafer N (1993) Incidence of urethral disruption in females with traumatic pelvic fractures. Am J Emerg Med 11:218–220
Caspi B, Rabinerson D, Appelman Z, Kaplan B (1996) Penetration of the bladder by a perforating intrauterine contraceptive device: a sonographic diagnosis. Ultrasound Obstet Gynecol 7:458–460
Cass AS (1976) Bladder trauma in the multiple injured patient. J Urol 115:667–669
Cass AS (1984) False negative retrograde cystography with bladder rupture owing to external trauma. J Trauma 24: 168–169
Cass AS (1990) Diagnostic studies in bladder rupture: indications and techniques. Urol Clin North Am 16:267–273
Cass AS, Matsuura JK (1983) Late bladder complications with use of external fixator device for pelvic fractures. Urology 21:616–618
Cass AS, Behrens F, Comfort T, Matsuura JK (1983) Bladder problems in pelvic injuries treated with external fixator and direct urethral drainage. J Trauma 23:50–53
Cespedes RD, Roettger RH, Peretsman SJ (1995) Herniation of the urinary bladder: a complication of traumatic pubic symphysis diastasis. South Med J 88:849–850
Chapple CR, Helm CW, Blease S, Milroy EJG, Rickards D, Osborne J (1989) Asymptomatic bladder neck incompetence in nulliparous females. Br J Urol 64:357–359
Chopart F (1791) Traité des maladies des voies urinaires, vol 2. Paris
Chung CL, Cheng PJ, Liang CC, Chang FH, Lee JD, Soong YK (1997) Obstetrical hysterectomy and placenta previa/accreta: three bladder injury case reports. Changgeng Yi Xue Za Zhi 20:44–51
Clark SS, Prudencio RF (1972) Lower urinary tract injuries associated with pelvic fracture. Surg Clin North Am 52: 183–201
Cohen SP, Varma KR, Goldman SM (1975) Spontaneous expulsion of intravesical bullet. Urology 5:387–389
Cohen MS, Warner RS, Fish L (1977) Bladder perforation after orthopaedic hip surgery. Urology 9:291–291
Colapinto V, McCallum RW (1977) Injury to the male posterior urethra in fractured pelvis: a new classification. J Urol 118: 575–580
Corriere JN (1991) Trauma to the lower urinary tract. In: Gillwater J et al (eds) Adult and paediatric urology, 2nd edn. Mosby Year Book, St Louis, pp 400–513
Corriere JN, Harris JD (1981) The management of urologic injuries in blunt pelvic trauma. Radiol Clin North Am 19: 187–193
Corriere JN, Sandler CM (1988) Mechanisms of injury, patterns of extravasation and management of extraperitoneal bladder rupture due to blunt trauma. J Urol 139:43–44
Crassweller PO, Farrow GA, Robson CJ, Russell JL, Colapinto V (1977) Traumatic rupture of the supramembranous urethra. J Urol 118:770–774
Cunningham JH (1910) The diagnosis of stricture of the urethra by the roentgen rays. Trans Am Assoc Gen Urin Surg 5:369
Didomenico D, Guinan P, Sharifi R (1997) Spontaneous expulsion of an intravesical bullet. J Am Osteopath Assoc 97: 415–416
Donahue LA, Frank IN (1989) Intravesical formalin for haemorrhagic cystitis: analysis of therapy. J Urol 141:809–812
Eid AM (1982) Early urinary complications of fractures of the pelvis. Arch Orthop Trauma Surg 100:99–106
Eisenkop SM, Richman R, Platt LD, Paul RH (1982) Urinary tract injury during cesarian section. Obstet Gynecol 60: 591–596
Faricy PO, Augspurger RR, Kaufman JM (1978) Bladder injuries associated with cesarean section. J Urol 120:762–763
Flocks RH (1933) The roentgen visualisation of the posterior urethra. J Urol 30:711
Fuhrman GM, Simmons GT, Davidson BS, Buerk CA (1993) The single indication for cystography in blunt trauma. Am Surg 59:335–337
Gibson GR (1970) Impotence following fractured pelvis and ruptured urethra. Br J Urol 42:86–88
Glass RE, Flynn JT, King JB (1978) Urethral injury and fractured pelvis. Br J Urol 50:578–582
Goldberg ID, Garnick MD, Bloomer WD (1984) Urinary tract toxic effects of cancer therapy. J Urol 132:1326
Goldman SM, Sandler CM, Corriere JN, McGuire EJ (1997) Blunt urethral trauma: a unified anatomical mechanical classification. J Urol 157:85–89
Gordon Taylor G (1953) Injuries of the urinary tract. In: Riches E (ed) Modern trends in urology. Butterworth, London
Gosling JA (1979) The structure of the bladder and urethra in relation to function. Urol Clin North Am 6:31–44
Haller JO, Kassner EG, Waterhouse K, Glassberg KI (1979) Traumatic strictures of the prostatomembranous urethra in children: radiologic evaluation before and after urethral reconstruction. Urol Radiol 1:43–52
Harrison R (1883) On some points in the treatment of urethral abscess, stricture and extravasation of urine. Lancet 1:57
Harrki-Siren P, Sjoberg J, Tiitinen A (1998) Urinary tract injuries after hysterectomy. Obstet Gynecol 92:113–118
Herd AM, Crofts NG, Lee LM, Girard JV, Sweetland RJ (1994) Isolated bladder rupture after minor trauma in a patient with alcohol intoxication. J Emerg Med 12:409–411
Hochberg E, Stone NN (1993) Bladder rupture associated with pelvic fracture due to blunt trauma. Urology 41:531–533
Horstman WG, McClennan BL (1991) Comparison of computed tomography and conventional cystography for detection of traumatic bladder rupture. Urol Radiol 12:188–193
Hubbard JG, Amin M, Polk JC Jr (1979) Bladder perforations secondary to surgical drains. J Urol 121:521–522
Husmann DA, Boone TB, Wilson WT (1993) Management of low velocity gunshot wounds to the anterior urethra: the role of primary repair versus urinary diversion alone. J Urol 150:70–72
Jerwood DC, Mason NP (1995) Pseudo-renal failure after traumatic bladder rupture. Br J Urol 76:406–407

Jones SJ, Kock MO (1977) Delayed rupture of type 1 posterior urethral injury: case report. J Urol 118:575–580
Kane NM, Francis IR, Ellis JH (1989) The value of CT in the detection of bladder and posterior urethral injures. AJR 153:1243–1246
Kasztelan Z (1983) An analysis of complications following transurethral resection of bladder tumors. Z Urol Nephrol 76:383–387
Kaufman JM, Pai S, Austin TL, McPherson RI (1983) Neonatal bladder injury occurring after umbilical artery catheterization by cutdown. JAMA 250:2968–2970
Koraitim MM, Marzouk ME, Atta MA, Orabi SS (1996) Risk factors and mechanism of urethral injury in pelvic fractures. Br J Urol 77:876–880
Kurizaki Y, Ishizuka O (1997) Spontaneous rupture of the urinary bladder in a woman with radiation cystitis: a case report. Hinyokika Kiyo 43:513–515
Lavallée G, Grégoire A, Laperrière J, Sylvestre J (1979) Lower urinary tract trauma. J Can Assoc Radiol 30:49–52
Le Dran HF (1774) Traité des opérations de chirurgie. Brussels
Lee CL, Kai YM, Soong YK (1996) Management of urinary bladder injuries in laparoscopic assisted vaginal hysterectomy. Acta Obstet Gynecol Scand 75:174–177
Lis LE, Cohen AJ (1990) CT cystography in the evaluation of bladder trauma. J Comput Assist Tomogr 14:386–389
Mark SD, Keane TE, Vandemark RM, Webster GD (1977) Impotence following pelvic fracture urethral injury: incidence, aetiology and management. Br J Urol 75:62–64
Mattar MS, Al-Alfy AA, Dahniya MH, Al-Marzouk NF (1997) Urinary bladder perforation: an unusual complication of neonatal nasogastric tube feeding. Pediatr Radiol 27: 858–859
McAninch JW (1981) Traumatic injuries of the urethra. J Trauma 21:291–297
McConnell JD, Wilkerson MD, Peters PC (1982) Rupture of the bladder. Urol Clin North Am 9:293–296
McCormac W (1886) Some observations on rupture of the urinary bladder with an account of 2 cases of intraabdominal rupture successfully treated by abdominal section and subsequent suture of the vesical rent. Lancet:1118
McLaughlin AP, Pfister RC (1974) Double catheter technique for evaluation of urethral injury and differentiating urethral from bladder rupture. Radiology 110:716–719
Mee SL, McAinnich JW, Federle MP (1987) Computerized tomography in bladder rupture: diagnostic limitations. J Urol 137:207–209
Merlini M, Besson A, von Niederhausern W, Saegesser F (1982) Urethral complications of severe fractures of the pelvis. Sem Hop 58:284–288
Mitchell JP (1968) Injuries of the urethra. Br J Urol 40:649–670
Mokoena T, Naidu AG (1995) Diagnostic difficulties in patients with a ruptured bladder. Br J Surg 82:69–70
Montie J (1977) Bladder injuries. Urol Clin North Am 4:59–67
Morehouse DD, McKinnin KJ (1980) Management of prostatomembranous urethral disruption – 13-year experience. J Urol 123:173–174
Morehouse DD, Belitshy P, McKinnon K (1972) Rupture of the posterior urethra. J Urol 107:255–258
Mundy AR (1983) Injuries of the lower urinary tract. Surgery 1:67–70
Nowak A, Zielinski J (1977) Difficulties in bladder rupture diagnosis. Eur Urol 3:351–354
O'Brien WJ, Ryckman FC (1994) Catheter-induced urinary bladder rupture presenting with pneumoperitoneum. J Pediatr Surg 29:1397–1398
Oliver JA, Taguchi Y (1964) Rupture of the full bladder. Br J Urol 36:224–225
Ostroff EB, Chenault OW (1982) Alum irrigation for the control of massive bladder haemorrhage. J Urol 128:929–930
Paick JS, Donatucci CF, Lue TF (1993) Anatomy of the cavernous nerves distal to prostate: microdissection study in the male cadaver. Urology 42:145–149
Palmer JK, Benson GS, Corriere JN Jr (1983) Diagnosis and initial management of urological injuries associated with 200 consecutive pelvic fractures. J Urol 130:712–714
Patel U, Nesbitt R, Meyer R (1982) Genitourinary tract injuries due to fracture of the pelvis in females: sequelae and their management. Br J Urol 54:32–38
Peng MY, Parisky YR, Cornwell EE, Radin R, Bragin S (1999) CT cystography versus conventional cystography in the evaluation of bladder injury. AJR 172:1269–1272
Perry MO, Husmann DA (1992) Urethral injuries in female subjects following pelvic fractures. J Urol 147:139–143
Polat O, Gul O, Aksoy Y, Ozbey I, Demiral A, Bayraktar Y (1997) Iatrogenic injuries to ureter, bladder and urethra during abdominal and pelvic operations. Int Urol Nephrol 29:13–18
Pontes JE (1977) Urologic injuries. Surg Clin North Am 57: 77–96
Pontes JE, Pierce JM (1978) Anterior urethral injuries: four years of experience at the Detroit General Hospital. J Urol 120:563–564
Rajasekar D, Hall M (1997) Urinary tract injuries during obstetric intervention. Br J Obstet Gynaecol 104:731–734
Redman JF, Seibert JJ, Arnold W (1979) Urinary ascites in children owing to extravasation of urine from the bladder. J Urol 122:409–411
Rutherford H (1904) On ruptured urethra: its treatment by combined drainage. Lancet 11:751
Saidi MH, Sadler RK, Vancaillie TG, Akright BD, Farhart SA, White AJ (1996) Diagnosis and management of serious urinary complications after major operative laparoscopy. Obstet Gynecol 87:272–276
Sandler CM, Reed Dunnick N (2000) Bladder trauma. In: Pollack HW, McClennan BL (eds) Clinical urology, vol 2. Saunders, Philadelphia, pp 1799–1818
Sandler CM, Phillips JM, Harris JD, Toombs BD (1981a) Radiology of the bladder and urethra in blunt pelvic trauma. Radiol Clin North Am 19:195–211
Sandler CM, Harris JR, Corriere JN, Toombs BD (1981b) Posterior urethral injuries after pelvic fracture. AJR 137: 1223–1237
Sandler CM, Hall JT, Rodriguez MB, Corriere JN (1986) Bladder injury in blunt pelvic trauma. Radiology 158:633–638
Sankari BR, Parra RO (1993) Spontaneous voiding of a bullet after a gunshot wound to the bladder: case report. J Trauma 35:813–814
Sayan A, Demircan M, Erikci VS, Celik A, Arikan A (1996) Neonatal bladder rupture: an unusual complication of umbilical catheterization. Eur J Pediatr Surg 6:378–379
Sclafani SJA, Becker JA (1985) Radiologic diagnosis of extraurinary trauma. Urol Radiol 7:201–210
Scott MH, Porter JR (1997) Extraperitoneal bladder rupture – pitfalls in CT cystography. AJR 168:1232
Sepulveda WH, Ciuffardi I, Olivari A, Gallegos O (1993) Sonographic diagnosis of bladder perforation by an intrauterine device. A case report. J Reprod Med 38:911–913

Shah PM, Kim K, Samirez-Schon G (1979) Elevated blood urea nitrogen: an aid to the diagnosis of intraperitoneal rupture of the bladder. J Urol 122:741–743

Shumaker BP, Pontes JE, Pierce JM Jr (1980) Idiopathic rupture of bladder. Urology 15:566–568

Sieber PR (1994) Bladder necrosis secondary to pelvic artery embolization: case report and literature review. J Urol 151: 422

Simpson-Smith A (1937) Traumatic rupture of the urethra: eight personal cases with a review of 381 recorded ruptures. Br J Surg 25:309–332

Sivit CJ, Cutting JP, Eichelberger MR (1995) CT diagnosis and localization of rupture of the bladder in children with blunt abdominal trauma: significance of contrast material extravasation in the pelvis. AJR 164:1243–1246

Spees EK, O'Mara C, Murphy JB, Michigan S, Newton CG (1981) Unsuspected intraperitoneal perforation of the urinary bladder as an iatrogenic disorder. Surgery 89:224–231

Spirnark JP (1988) Pelvic fractures and injury of the lower urinary tract. Surg Clin North Am 68:1057–1069

Steinert M, Walter F (1997) Spontaneous intraperitoneal perforation of the urinary bladder – a rare cause of acute abdomen. 2 case reports. Zentralbl Chir 122:301–303

Stone E (1931) Spontaneous rupture of the bladder. Ann Surg 93:129

Sundnes KO, Vaagenes P, Kvarstein B (1983) An unusual complication of lithotripsy. Anaesthesia 38:666–668

Taffet R (1997) Management of pelvic fractures with concomitant urologic injuries. Orthop Clin North Am 28:389–396

Theodorakis SP, Baffes TG (1985) Penetrating wounds of the pelvis. South Med J 78:782–783

Truong P, Bouchet P, Battistelli JM, Marty F (1983) Posttraumatic pneumobladder. Apropos of a case. J Radiol 64: 433–435

Turner Warwick R (1977) Complex traumatic posterior urethral strictures. J Urol 118:564–570

Udekwu PO, Gurkin B, Oller DW (1996) The use of computed tomography in blunt abdominal injuries. Am Surg 62: 56–59

Vaccaro JP, Brody JM (2000) CT cystography in the evaluation of major bladder trauma. RadioGraphics 20:1373–1381

Venn NS, Greenwell TJ, Mundy AR (1999) Pelvic fracture injuries of the female urethra. Br J Urol Int 83:626–630

Verta MJ Jr, Janevicius RV (1982) Isolated hypogastric artery aneurysms. J Cardiovasc Surg (Torino) 23:432–434

Viville C, De Petriconi R, Bietho L (1984) Intravesical explosion during endoscopic resection. Apropos of a case. J Urol 90: 361–363

Walker WJ (1845) Medical communications to Massachusetts Medical Society, vol 2

Webster GD, Sihelnik S (1985) The management of strictures of the membranous urethra. J Urol 134:469–471

Webster GD, Mathes GL, Selli C (1983) Prostatomembranous urethral injury: a review of the literature and a rational approach to their management. J Urol 130:898–902

Wheeler JS Jr, Babayan RK, Austen G Jr, Krane RJ (1983) Urologic complications of hip arthroplasty. Urology 22: 499–503

Williams NS (1976) Late presentation of intraperitoneal rupture of the bladder. Postgrad Med J 52:246–247

Willett A (1876) Abdominal section in a case of bladder rupture. St Bart's Hosp Report 12:209

12 Injuries of Abdominal Vessels

A. GRAHAM and J. E. JACKSON

CONTENTS

- An understanding of the different ways in which a vessel can respond to trauma is essential as it is usually the type of vascular injury that determines the method of endovascular therapy rather than the organ within which it occurs
- Thorough diagnostic angiography of complex lesions, especially arteriovenous fistulae, must be performed to document the anatomy completely before proceeding with embolization
- The key to successful embolization is the total exclusion of the vascular injury from the circulation

12.1 Introduction

While clinically important injuries to the abdominal organs, especially the kidneys and liver, are relatively common following blunt abdominal trauma, the improvements that have occurred in the initial imaging assessment, particularly by ultrasound and computed tomography, have resulted in a much lesser need for *diagnostic* angiography, as most significant vascular injuries will be identified without recourse to this modality. *Therapeutic* angiographic techniques, however, are well established in the treatment of a small group of patients with abdominal vascular trauma and the indications for these have probably increased over the past decade owing to the excellent results that are often obtained with a consequent reduction in the need for surgery. Individuals suffering from complications of iatrogenic trauma – most commonly biopsies of the liver or kidney – will often proceed directly to angiography and embolization without preliminary cross-sectional imaging. Endovascular methods of treatment in each of the specific vascular territories in the abdomen have been discussed in some detail in each of the foregoing chapters and this chapter will, therefore, mainly con-

A. GRAHAM, MD
Hammersmith Hospital, Du Cane Road, London, W12 0NN, UK
J. E. JACKSON, MD
Consultant Radiologist, Hammersmith Hospital, Du Cane Road, London, W12 0NN, UK

centrate upon techniques of endovascular therapy related to the different types of vascular injury that may occur.

12.2 Angiographic and Embolization Technique

12.2.1 General Principles

While the diagnosis of a significant vascular injury in the stable trauma patient is usually made with noninvasive imaging modalities including ultrasound, Doppler ultrasound, computed tomography (CT) and magnetic resonance imaging (MRI), diagnostic angiography may still be necessary when these studies are negative or equivocal and a strong clinical suspicion of an arterial injury exists. In most instances, however, diagnostic arteriography is performed only as part of a therapeutic procedure when a significant vascular injury has already been identified on cross-sectional imaging. Whatever the indication for the study, however, and whatever the site of presumed vascular injury, the same general principles of diagnostic angiography apply:

- The operator must have a thorough knowledge of arterial and venous anatomy and of the normal variants.

- It is important to obtain good quality angiographic images, as the signs of vascular trauma may be subtle. This is likely to be more difficult in this group of patients than in individuals undergoing elective angiographic procedures due to a combination of their clinical state and the presence of extraneous equipment including, for example, monitoring wires, surgical drains and orthopedic internal and external fixation devices. Images of sufficient quality are possible, however, in almost all individuals under local anesthetic. Images obtained using a digital subtraction arteriographic (DSA) technique (there are now few centers that have the facility to perform conventional film angiographic images) have excellent contrast resolution and will therefore show contrast medium extravasation well but are degraded by movement, which in the abdomen is due to a combination of bowel peristalsis and patient respiration. The former can usually be obliterated by the liberal use of parenteral antiperistaltic agents. Breath-holding may be difficult, though in this group of individuals unless they are anesthetized and intubated, and images will often need to be obtained during normal respiration; the acquisition of numerous mask images obtained during the different phases of respiration before the injection of contrast medium will, however, still allow one to obtain good quality, diagnostic images. Oblique projections will be required to visualize regions obscured on frontal views by the aforementioned surgical and monitoring equipment that may be present.

- It is wise in the majority of cases to begin with nonselective angiograms before directly catheterizing the vessel(s) that is felt on clinical or imaging grounds to be injured. The reasons for this are several, the most important of which is that arteriography performed from a nonselective or proximal position will often allow assessment of the full extent of the vascular injury and its effect upon the surrounding vessels. Errors in diagnosis and subsequent management are less likely if the angiographer has an overview of the whole picture rather than the localized view that might result from proceeding directly to more selective studies. As a simple example, consider the case of a patient with blunt trauma to the abdomen and a large expanding retroperitoneal hematoma surrounding the right kidney associated with cortical renal contusion on CT. Although it is perhaps likely that a vascular injury of the kidney is the cause of the retroperitoneal hematoma, the performance of selective renal arteriography as the initial procedure might miss other sources of bleeding such as a small accessory renal artery branch, a low intercostal artery, a lumbar artery, or an adrenal artery, which would be more likely to be shown on a preliminary abdominal aortogram. A second important reason why selective catheterization is best avoided until images are obtained from a more proximal catheter position, is the possibility of causing further trauma to an already injured vessel with either the catheter or guidewire and/or provoking further arterial hemorrhage or arterial occlusion before the nature of the arterial injury is fully appreciated. A nonocclusive main renal vascular pedicle injury, for example, unrecognized because an abdominal aortogram was not performed first, could be converted to a complete occlusion by attempts at selective catheterization.

- If a source of hemorrhage has not been demonstrated on abdominal aortograms and subsequent selective studies, then superselective studies of the vessels thought most likely to have been injured may be helpful to provoke further bleeding.

- Complications related to angiography are more likely in this group of individuals than in those undergoing an elective procedure for obvious reasons; hypovolemia causing an increased risk of contrast medium nephrotoxicity and altered hemostasis secondary to hemorrhage and subsequent transfusion resulting in puncture site complications are just two examples. Close monitoring of the patient is obviously essential during angiography and clotting parameters should be corrected if possible before or during the procedure.

In addition to the above recommendations regarding diagnostic angiography, there are several general principles of embolization that should be followed in order to reduce the risk of complications, in particular that of occluding arterial branches supplying normal tissue:

- Non-radio-opaque embolic material should be mixed with contrast medium so that it can be clearly visualized during vessel occlusion.

- Embolic material should always be injected or pushed through the catheter during continuous fluoroscopy to avoid misplacement and inadvertent occlusion of non-target vessels.

- Arteriograms should be performed at intervals during embolization to monitor the progress of the procedure and ensure that embolic material is not passing into adjacent normal branches.

- Ischemic complications of embolization in patients with traumatic injuries are more common than in patients undergoing embolization for other indications because of adjacent tissue damage that may have compromised collateral flow. Great care should be taken, therefore, to embolize selectively while preserving as many of the normal surrounding vessels as possible.

12.2.2 Catheters

Numerous preshaped angiographic catheters are available and the choice of these will largely depend upon the vascular territory being imaged and the angiographer's preference. In the abdominal vasculature femorovisceral (Cobra) and femorocerebral I (Sidewinder, Simmons) catheters of 5 F with a lumen of 0.035 in. or 0.038 in. are those that are most commonly used and are suitable in almost all situations. It may occasionally be useful to have the additional stability of a 7-F catheter for catheterization of the visceral vessels, especially when there is tortuosity of the iliac arteries, or when using a coaxial technique. For catheterizing small or tortuous vessels, coaxial catheters, which are now marketed by a number of different companies, are invaluable, especially when embolization is required. Most of these devices have a proximal shaft diameter of 3 F, tapering to approximately 2 F at the tip. Many of these catheters have a hydrophilic coating to aid superselective catheterization.

12.2.3 Embolic Agents

The type of embolic agent used will depend largely on the nature and site of the vascular injury that is being treated. The most commonly utilized agents are absorbable gelatin sponge, polyvinyl alcohol, conventional steel coils and microcoils and the choice of these will often depend upon the experience and personal preference of the angiographer. Detachable coils, which are available in both conventional and microcoil forms, are especially useful when attempting to occlude high-flow arteriovenous fistulae; the greater control that one has when placing these devices, when compared with nondetachable coils, reduces the likelihood of coil migration through an abnormal arteriovenous communication. Detachable balloons may be used in a similar manner. Liquid embolic agents such as alcohol or sodium tetradecyl sulfate, which are potent sclerosants, are rarely required for the treatment of posttraumatic vascular injuries and should generally be avoided; their inappropriate use will often result in tissue infarction. N-butyl-2-cyanoacrylate (glue) is a difficult agent to use but may be invaluable in certain circumstances, especially when very rapid control of brisk contrast medium extravasation is required (Gorich et al. 1993).

12.3 Mechanism

12.3.1 Types of Vascular Injuries

Whatever the site of vascular trauma, vessels can respond in a limited number of ways to an injury and it is worth considering these in detail, rather than discussing the separate abdominal organs, as it is usually the type of injury that determines the method of endovascular therapy rather than the organ within which it occurs. Following trauma there may be:

- A vascular injury with active extravasation of contrast
- A vascular injury with the formation of a pseudoaneurysm
- Adjacent arterial and venous injuries with the formation of an arteriovenous fistula
- Vessel dissection causing reduction of blood flow or complete occlusion

When discussing each of these vascular injuries, it is worthwhile considering two separate vessel types, one of which we will term "vital" and the other "nonvital". A vital vessel is defined as one that, if occluded, will produce symptomatic distal ischemia; an example would include the main renal artery. A non-vital vessel is one that can be safely occluded, as a collateral circulation is likely to develop rapidly and prevent symptomatic distal ischemia; examples in the abdomen would include the gastroduodenal artery and a proximal intrahepatic arterial branch.

12.3.2 Vessel Injury with Active Contrast Medium Extravasation

When this type of injury is seen in a nonvital end artery then occlusion of the injured vessel proximal to the site of extravasation will stop the bleeding. This form of embolization will usually suffice when bleeding occurs from a distal branch of the kidney, for example, because although these vessels are not true end arteries, as there are communications between these vessels and capsular arteries via tiny perforating branches, the anastomoses that are present are of insufficient size to prevent thrombosis of the hemorrhaging vessel. Elsewhere in the abdomen, the potential for the development of a collateral supply to a vessel that has been occluded proximally is so great that definitive embolization will require exclusion of the arterial injury from the circulation by placing embolic material on either side of the arterial defect (Fig. 12.1). It is, therefore, critical that complete occlusion of the vessel beyond the arterial defect is performed prior to proximal embolization; if this is not obtained then contrast medium extravasation is likely to continue. Contrast medium extravasation from a vital vessel will require the placement of a covered endovascular stent across the arterial injury. Alternatively, an occlusion balloon catheter may be inflated across or proximal to the arterial injury to occlude flow, and thereby stop bleeding, while the patient is transferred to the operating room for definitive surgery.

12.3.3 Vessel Injury with Development of a Pseudoaneurysm

This form of injury may develop anywhere in the vascular tree after blunt or penetrating trauma (Collins et al. 1988). All that it represents, in fact, is an injured vessel with an area of contained hemorrhage and embolization is usually performed in the same way as has been discussed in the preceding section when there is active extravasation. The aim of embolization, therefore, is to exclude the arterial injury from the circulation. If the pseudoaneurysm arises from a nonvital vessel, distal and then proximal embolization of the main trunk of the artery on either side of the arterial defect should be performed. This is usually best achieved with metallic coils (Fig. 12.2). As stated in Sect. 12.3.2, it is critical that complete occlusion of the vessel beyond the pseudoaneurysm is achieved before proximal embolization is performed. Placement of metallic coils directly into the aneurysmal sac should be avoided if possible. There are many reasons why this procedure is not recommended: it should be remembered that a pseudoaneurysm lacks a true wall; it is simply an extravascular cavity, often lined with thrombus, which is contained by the surrounding tissues and is, therefore, an extremely weak structure that can easily rupture, as it often does spontaneously. Packing such a cavity with coils is asking for trouble and rupture is likely. The lack of a supporting wall will also mean that any attempt to pack the sac will usually result in a ball of coils considerably larger than the original size of the patent cavity. This will not only act as a space-occupying lesion, but also as an ideal nidus for infection. However, a pseudoaneurysm embolized correctly by its exclusion from the vessel from which it arises as discussed above, will thrombose completely and gradually disappear. Perhaps most importantly, the coil ball that results is unstable if the artery from which the pseudoaneurysm arises is not also occluded, because there is nothing to hold it in place; as the thrombus within the pseudoaneurysm contracts the coils are likely to move away from the vessel wall and rebleeding may occur. A pseudoan-

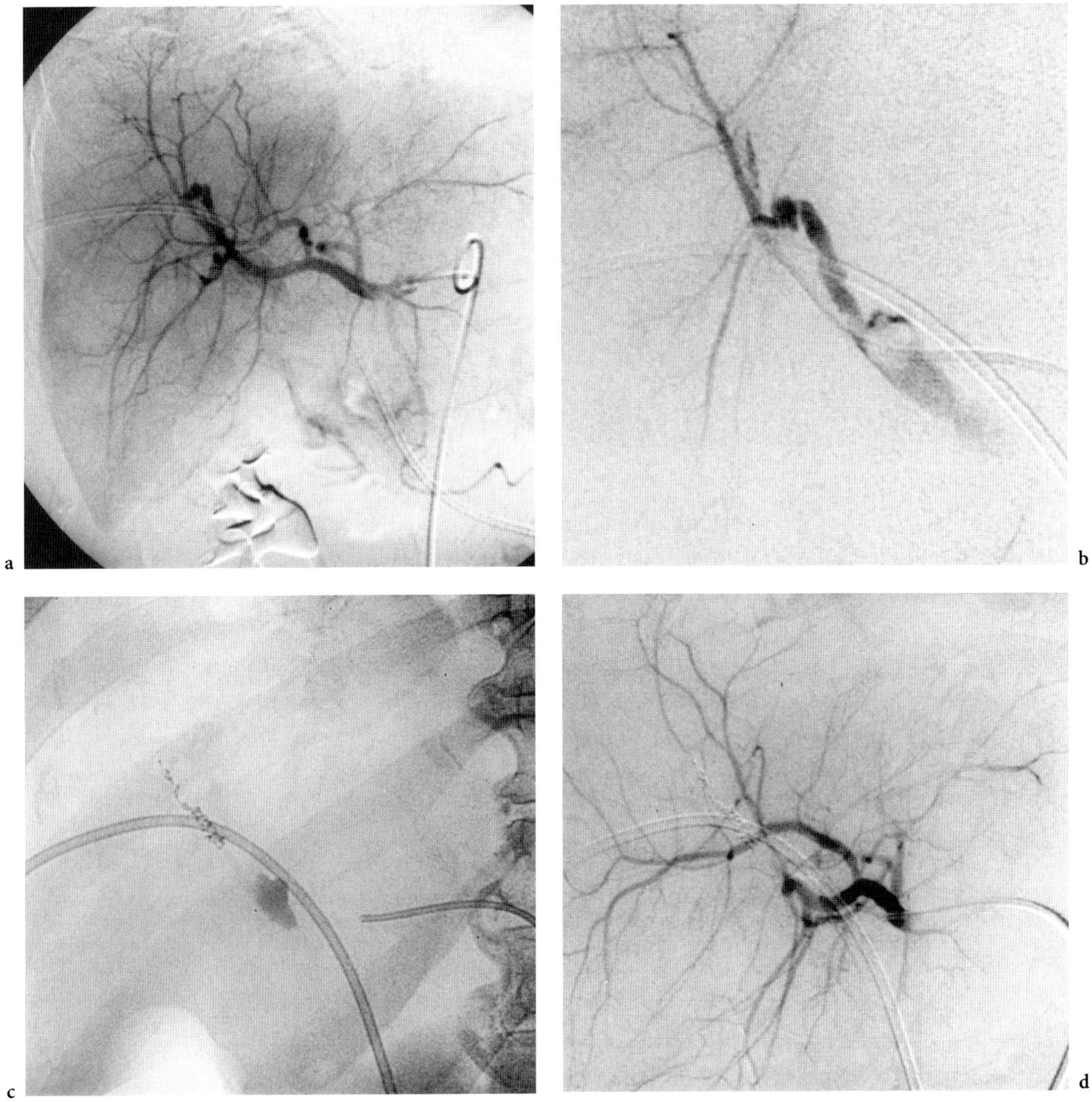

Fig. 12.1a–d. Hemobilia following percutaneous biliary drainage treated by embolization. **a** Selective common hepatic arteriogram demonstrates brisk contrast medium extravasation from a right hepatic arterial branch immediately adjacent to the biliary drainage catheter. **b** The angiographic catheter has been introduced into the traumatized intrahepatic vessel and contrast medium extravasation is seen from this artery into the adjacent bile duct. **c** Embolization coils have been placed both beyond and then proximal to the arterial injury thus excluding it from the circulation. **d** The postembolization arteriogram demonstrates successful embolization with no residual contrast medium extravasation. Note the filling of the hepatic arterial branch distal to the embolization coils that has occurred via intrahepatic collateral vessels, which stresses the importance of achieving occlusion of this artery beyond the injury before performing proximal embolization

eurysm of a vital vessel needs to be isolated from the circulation while maintaining patency of the vessel from which it arises; this will in most instances require the use of a covered stent (Fig. 12.3) and, in situations where this is not possible, operative repair will be necessary.

12.3.4 Arterial and Venous Injury with Development of an Arteriovenous Fistula

There are certain vascular territories including the liver, kidney, and spleen where the formation of an

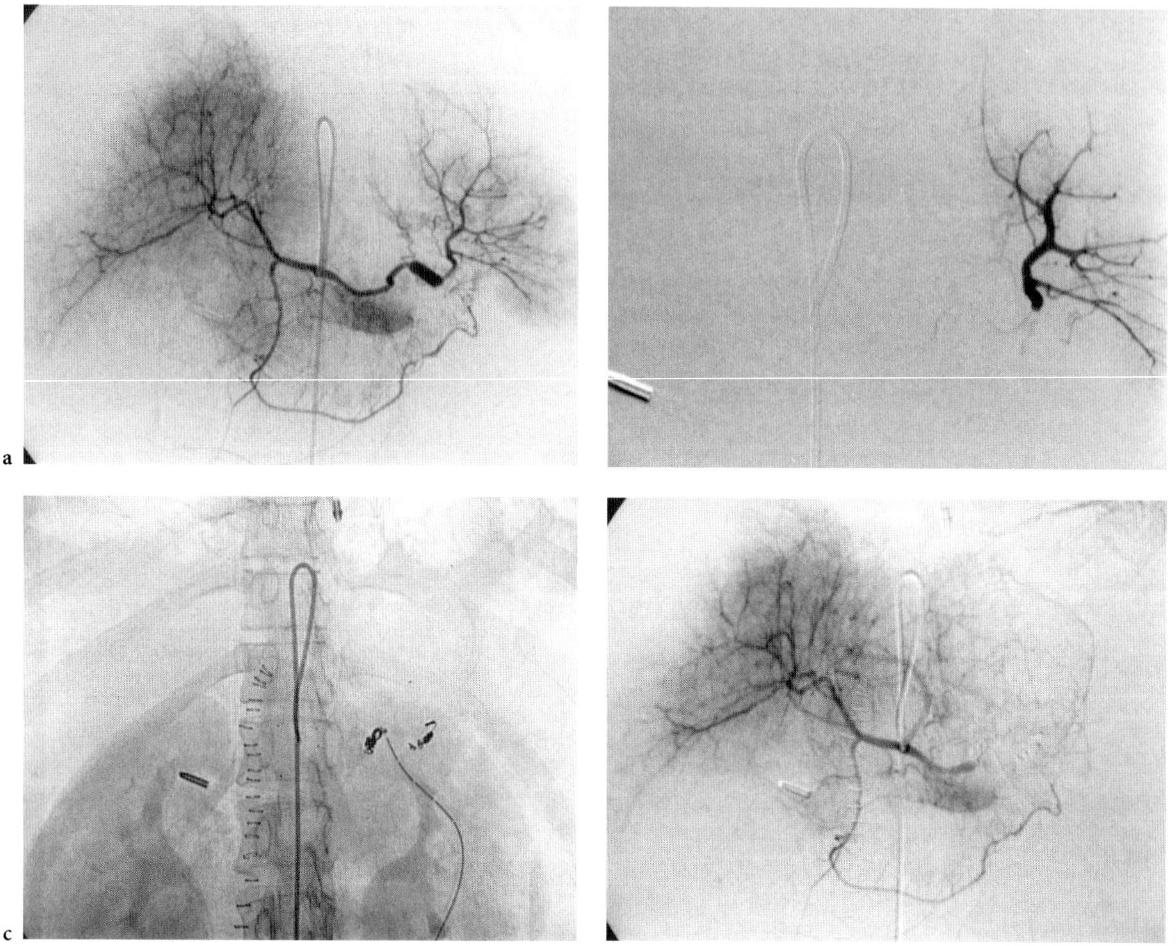

Fig. 12.2a–d. Main splenic artery pseudoaneurysm following surgery causing massive hemorrhage. **a** Coeliac axis arteriogram demonstrates a fusiform aneurysm of the distal main splenic artery. Note the marked attenuation of the vessels due to hypovolemia following recent hemorrhage. **b** The splenic artery beyond the pseudoaneurysm has been selectively catheterized with a coaxial catheter to allow distal embolization. **c** A control film after embolization demonstrates the position of platinum microcoils placed beyond and then proximal to the pseudoaneurysm. **d** Postembolization coeliac axis arteriogram demonstrates the exclusion of the pseudoaneurysm from the circulation and an increase in size of the left gastric artery branches that will be providing a collateral supply to the spleen via short gastric vessels

arteriovenous fistula (AVF) in response to penetrating or blunt trauma is common, presumably due to the close proximity of arteries and veins in these organs (Fig. 12.4). Elsewhere in the abdomen AVF are relatively uncommon; when they do occur they may initially be silent and only present a long time, maybe many years, after an original episode of trauma with symptoms secondary to high flow and venous hypertension (Fig. 12.5). Complete angiographic assessment of the vascular anatomy of these chronic AVF is mandatory before embolization is performed. They are often extremely complex and unless the site and number of the arteriovenous communications and potential feeding vessels (especially those to the "back door" of the fistula) are fully appreciated prior to embolization, then the procedure is unlikely to be successful. The fistula must be excluded from the circulation and this is most commonly achieved from an arterial access but may, in some complex cases, be easier from the venous side or by using a combination of the two approaches (Ben-Menachem 1995). It is important to ensure that embolic material does not pass through the shunt and this may be difficult in the presence of very rapid flow and large arteriovenous communications. In such circumstances, detachable coils are very useful as they may be easily withdrawn from the catheter if they are obviously not stable enough within the AVF to allow safe detachment, or are of an inappropriate size. The use of an occlusion balloon catheter inflated within the vessel

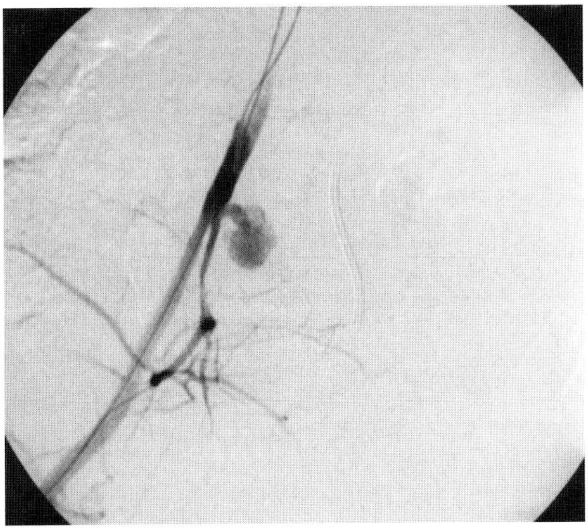
a

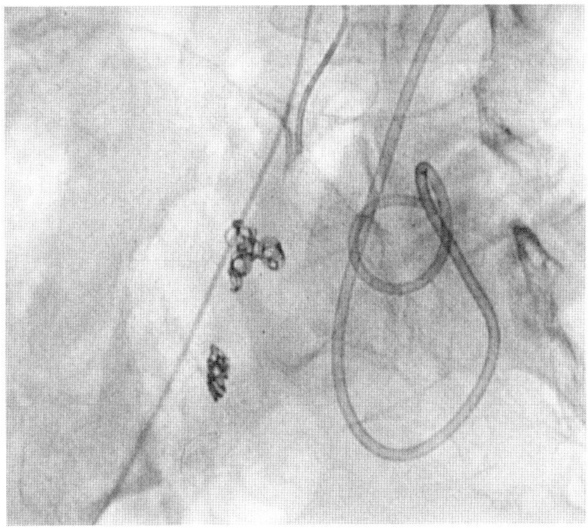
b

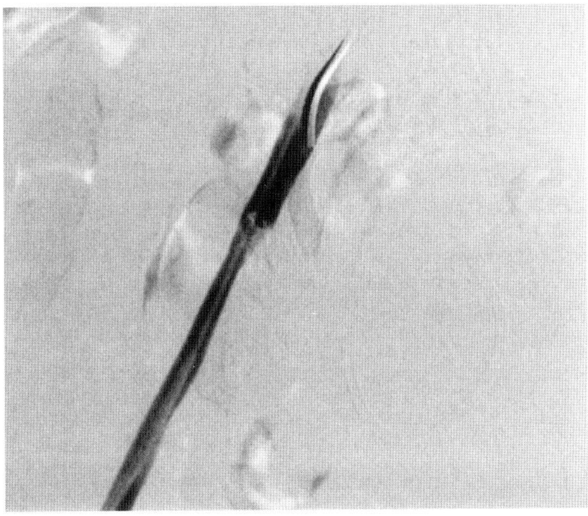
c

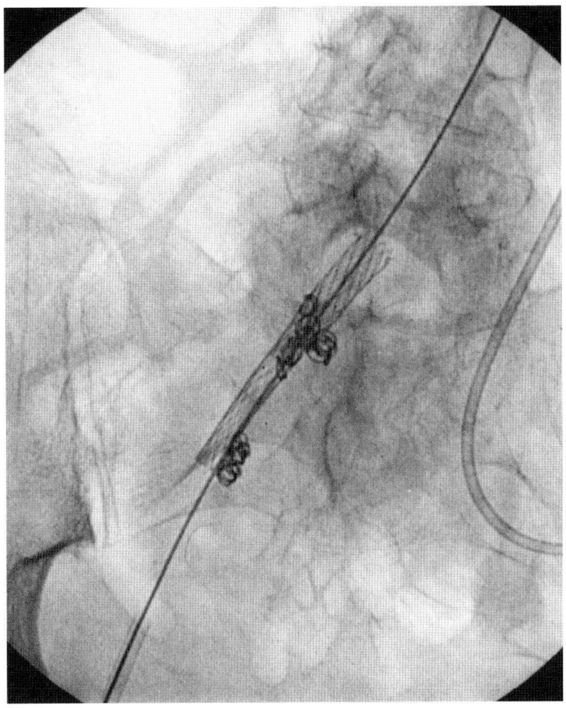
d

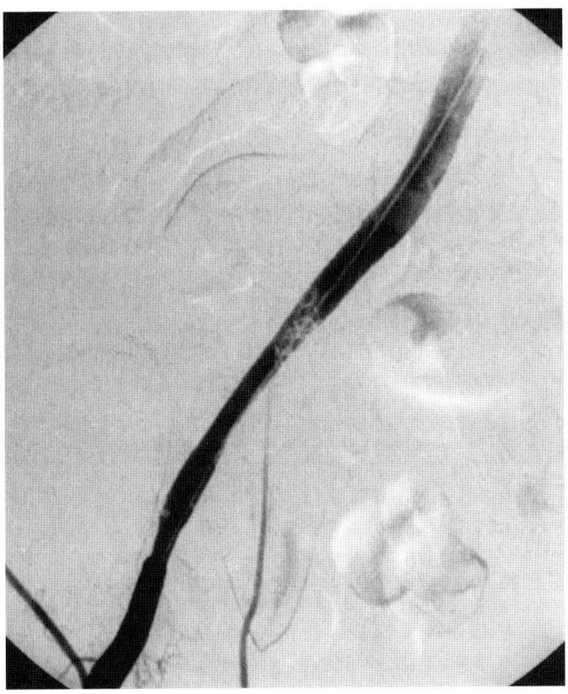
e

Fig. 12.3a–e. A patient with massive retroperitoneal bleeding following pelvic surgery. **a** Right common iliac arteriogram demonstrates a pseudoaneurysm arising from the origin of the internal iliac artery. **b** Control film after embolization demonstrates the position of coils that were first placed in the internal iliac artery beyond the pseudoaneurysm and then across the neck of the arterial injury. A loop of the final coil protrudes into the lumen of the external iliac artery. **c** Common iliac arteriogram after embolization demonstrates the occlusion of the internal iliac artery pseudoaneurysm and the coil protrusion into the lumen of the external iliac artery. **d** In view of the proximity of the pseudoaneurysm to the origin of the internal iliac artery and coil protrusion, a covered stent has been placed within the common and external iliac arteries. **e** A final arteriogram demonstrates wide patency of the iliac vessels and successful exclusion of the pseudoaneurysm

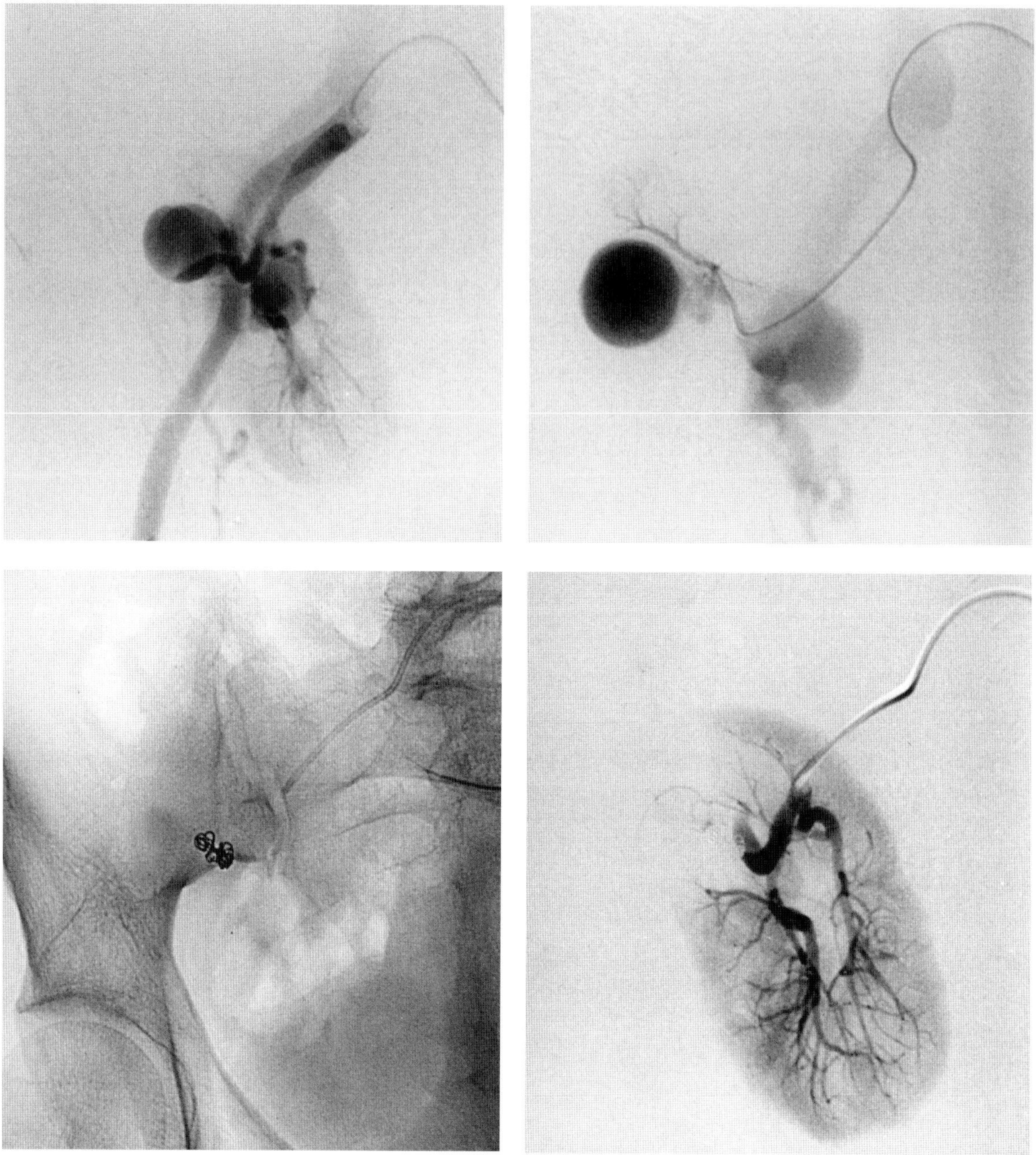

Fig. 12.4a–d. Postbiopsy fistula of a renal transplant causing renal dysfunction. **a** Right common femoral artery angiogram demonstrates a large arteriovenous fistula (AVF) in the superior pole of the renal transplant through which there is rapid AV shunting. Note the faint opacification of the common iliac vein on this early arterial image. **b** The catheter has been introduced into the large vessel supplying the AVF prior to embolization. **c** Detachable coils have been placed at the neck of the AVF. **d** The postembolization arteriogram demonstrates complete occlusion of the AVF with good preservation of normal renal artery branches

Fig. 12.5a–f. Right buttock AVF following severe pelvic trauma many years previously. **a** Axial CT scan with intravenous contrast medium through the pelvis demonstrates an expansile lesion within the right iliac blade containing an eccentric area of contrast medium enhancement. Note also marked enlargement of the right gluteal muscles and the prominent vessel within the superficial fat of the right buttock. **b** An abdominal aortogram demonstrates a massive AVF between the right superior gluteal artery and the adjacent, markedly enlarged, vein. **c** Right internal iliac artery angiogram shows the AVF in more detail. Note that the superior gluteal vein does not communicate with the internal iliac vein as it was occluded at the time of the original injury and there is, therefore, massive venous hypertension within the right buttock. **d** A selective inferior gluteal artery angiogram performed before embolization shows that the superior gluteal artery branches beyond the AVF are filled in their entirety and do not communicate with the abnormal arteriovenous communication. There is, in other words, no "back door" to the AVF. **e** A compact nest of coils has been placed at the site of the AVF. **f** The postembolization internal iliac artery angiogram demonstrates complete occlusion of the AVF

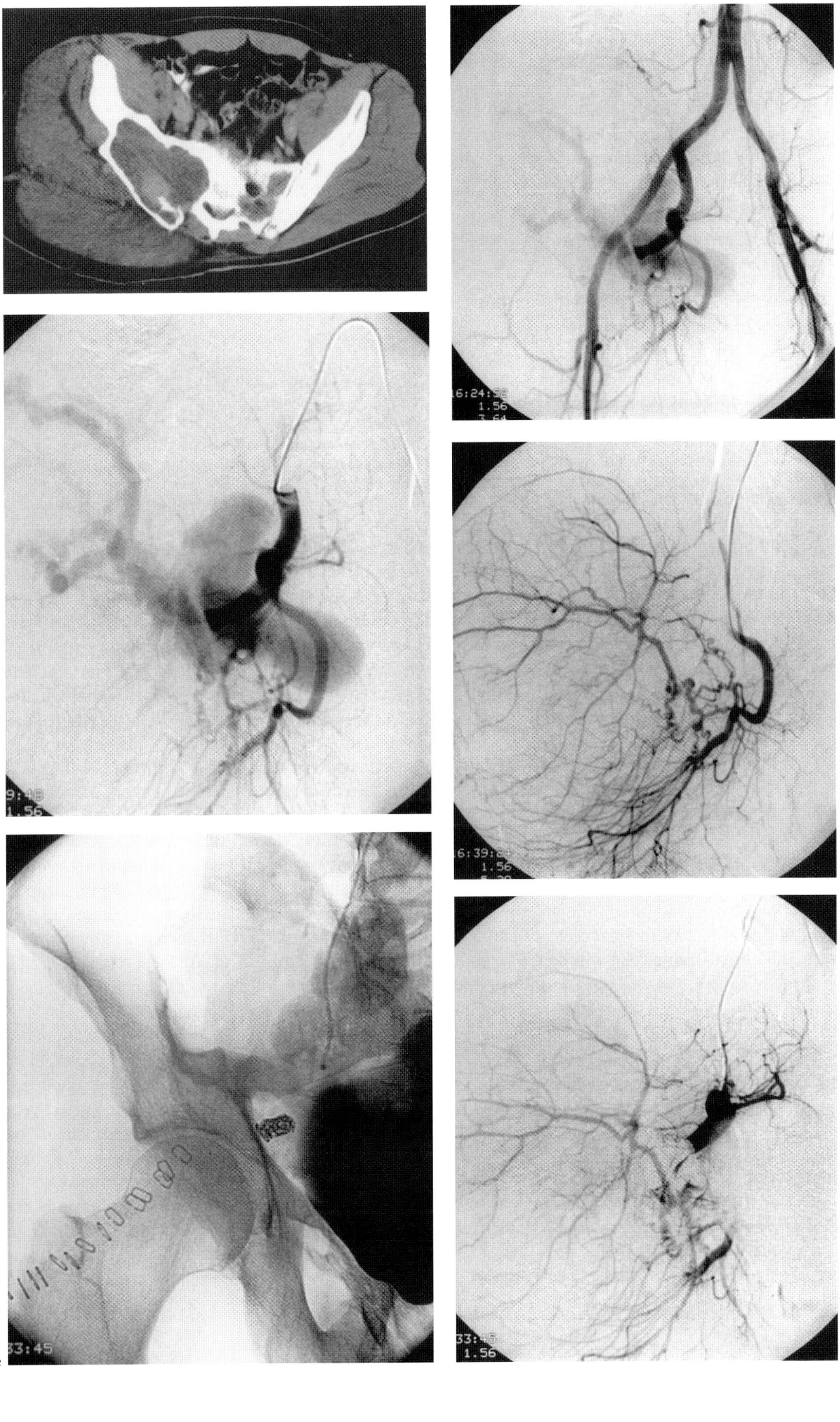

a b c d e f

supplying an AVF may help by reducing or obliterating flow during definitive embolization, which can be performed via the balloon catheter lumen. Glue is a useful agent for the treatment of certain AVF although rapid flow may make it difficult to achieve successful polymerization at the correct site across the arteriovenous communication; once again some form of flow occlusion during its use may be helpful.

12.3.5 Vessel Dissection with Subsequent Reduction of Blood Flow or Complete Occlusion

Dissection of a vessel following trauma may be a localized event, as sometimes occurs at the renal artery origins due to a rapid deceleration injury (Fig. 12.6) or may occur due to extension of an aortic dissection into a visceral artery branch. Both of these are likely to be obvious on cross-sectional imaging and the method of treatment will depend to some extent upon the imaging findings. If flow beyond a dissection is severely compromised to, for example, a kidney or bowel, then urgent therapy is required, which is often surgical in the acute setting. There is a role for endovascular therapy in certain circumstances, however, including arterial stenting and fenestration of the dissection flap, but this subject lies outside the remit of this chapter and will not be discussed further (Williams et al. 1997).

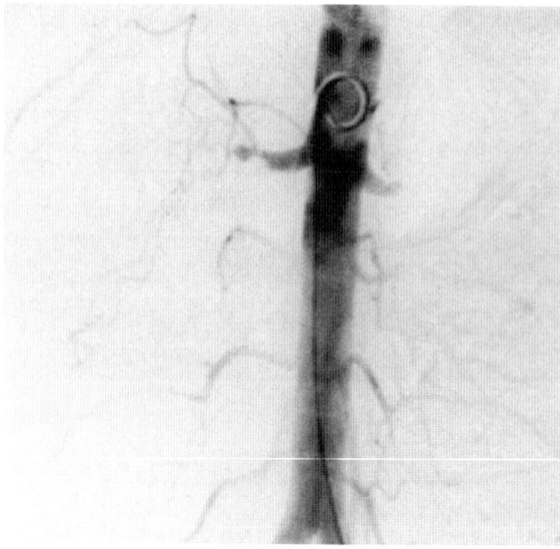

Fig. 12.6. An abdominal aortogram in a young male patient following a severe road traffic accident shows complete transection of both renal arteries

12.4 Injuries to Specific Vascular Territories

The indications for arteriography, the angiographic findings and results of embolization in patients suffering abdominal trauma are discussed in each of the chapters in this book relating to the specific abdominal organs. To avoid repetition, this section will, therefore, be short and will concentrate upon the technique of embolization in certain vascular territories, although some overlap is likely.

12.4.1 Splenic Injuries

As mentioned in Chap. 4, there has been a trend over the past decade towards the nonoperative, conservative management of splenic injuries in patients who are hemodynamically stable. The arguments in favor or against this form of therapy have already been discussed and will not be reiterated. Suffice to say that the debate continues as to the place of splenic arteriography with or without embolization in patients who are shown to have a splenic injury on CT. The general message appears to be that those individuals who are seen on CT to have splenic contrast medium extravasation, or a splenic vascular blush suggestive of a pseudoaneurysm, are at risk of further bleeding and should proceed immediately to angiography with a view to embolization (Hagiwara et al. 1996; Gavant et al. 1997; Davis et al. 1998; Shanmuganathan et al. 2000). The majority of these patients will not require open operative treatment so long as the embolization is technically successful. The absence of these CT signs appears to accurately predict successful nonoperative management (Federle et al. 1998; Starnes et al. 1998). Readers are referred to the chapter on splenic injury for more details on this subject.

The main angiographic findings of significant splenic injury are those of contrast medium extravasation, pseudoaneurysm formation, and arteriovenous fistulae which, when seen, should be occluded selectively, following the guidelines discussed in Sect. 12.3. The splenic artery is often extremely tortuous but selective catheterization of intrasplenic branches can usually be achieved using a coaxial catheter and occlusion of the abnormal vessels is then best performed with platinum microcoils. It has been suggested that proximal occlusion of the main splenic artery with metallic coils may also be helpful in splenic trauma by reducing splenic perfusion pressure (Sclafani et al. 1991, 1995). While this may be of benefit, the technique goes against the general principles of vascular embolization in trauma and must be considered to be the option of second choice and only performed if distal embolization of the abnormal intrasplenic vessels themselves cannot be achieved. If main splenic artery embolization is performed, coils should be placed in the mid portion of the splenic artery between the dorsal pancreatic artery and arteria pancreatica magna. One of the major reasons for attempting to conserve the spleen is because of the known risk of septic complications in patients who have undergone splenectomy. As splenic function is related both to mass and to blood flow (Horton et al. 1982), it is possible that the immune competency of the spleen is not completely preserved after embolization of the splenic artery and this is another reason why this form of therapy should be avoided if possible.

12.4.2 Hepatic Injuries

The liver is commonly injured following blunt and penetrating abdominal trauma, but in patients who are hemodynamically stable after initial resuscitation, nonoperative management has become the standard of care in order to avoid the significant morbidity and mortality associated with surgical management (Croce et al. 1995; Carillo et al. 1998). Those individuals who are unstable will proceed to surgery and in this group the operation performed will depend upon a number of factors, including the type and extent of the hepatic injury, the presence of injuries to other organs, and the experience of the surgeon. Even severe hepatic bleeding can be successfully managed, however, by the temporary placement of packs around the liver with re-laparotomy at a later date (Krige et al. 1992; Marr et al. 2000). In those who continue to bleed despite appropriate packing, an arterial source of hemorrhage is likely, and these individuals should be referred for immediate angiography and embolization.

Persistent severe hemorrhage following iatrogenic liver trauma, such as liver biopsy or percutaneous biliary intervention, is uncommon but is also usually from an arterial source when it does occur and is best treated by embolization (Fig. 12.1). Regardless of the type of trauma, the most commonly encountered angiographic findings are active extravasation of contrast medium into the peritoneum or biliary tree, pseudoaneurysm formation, and arterioportal communications, which may coexist. The arterioportal communications are identified by the opacification of peripheral branches of the portal vein during the early phase of an hepatic arteriogram; although they are often small they are worthwhile noting as they are a useful indicator of the site of significant hepatic trauma. The technique of embolization within the liver should follow the general principles discussed in Sect. 12.3. It is important to remember that the hepatic arterial branches are not end arteries; immediately following the proximal occlusion of an intrahepatic artery with coils, subsequent arteriograms will demonstrate continued opacification of the branch beyond the occlusion by intra- and extrahepatic arterial collaterals (Fig. 12.1). It is clear, therefore, that the only way that one can guarantee that hemorrhage will be controlled by embolization is by occluding the abnormal vessel beyond and then proximal to an area of contrast medium extravasation or pseudoaneurysm formation. Focal injuries are usually best managed in this way with coils; more diffuse hepatic injuries, where there are multiple vessels involved, may require the use of particulate agents such as absorbable gelatin sponge or polyvinyl alcohol injected with contrast medium to obtain a more generalized embolization. This method of embolization is more likely to result in hepatic infarction, however, as the integrity of the portal vein is also likely to have been compromised in this more severe type of injury and it is important, therefore, to embolize as selectively as possible while still achieving hemostasis (Henne-Bruns and Kremer 1992). Trauma to the extrahepatic portion of the right hepatic artery is most commonly iatrogenic and is well recognized after laparoscopic cholecystectomy. A pseudoaneurysm may result and thiys is generally best managed by distal and proximal embolization, as previously discussed.

12.4.3 Mesenteric Vessel Injuries

About 5% of patients undergoing surgery for abdominal trauma have bowel or mesenteric injury. Isolated mesenteric vessel injury, however, is rare and is most commonly the result of penetrating trauma. The majority of patients with this type of injury will be hemodynamically unstable at presentation and require immediate surgery; angiography is rarely necessary unless bleeding recurs. Acute bowel ischemia resulting from a posttraumatic aortic dissection with involvement of the origins of the mesenteric vessels will often require surgical management. When chronic ischemic symptoms occur following a similar arterial injury that compromises visceral arterial flow, there are a number of endovascular techniques that may be of benefit, including fenestration of the dissection flap and/or stent placement (Williams et al. 1997). Arterioportal fistulae between the main trunks or peripheral branches of the superior mesenteric artery and vein are rare, although they have been reported after bowel resection if the artery and vein are ligated together rather than separately. Whether or not such communications are amenable to endovascular therapy will depend upon their site (Fig. 12.7).

12.4.4 Pancreatic Injuries

Arterial abnormalities associated with pancreatic trauma are rare and are usually the result of posttraumatic pancreatitis, particularly in children, causing pseudoaneurysms of the splenic, gastroduodenal, and pancreaticoduodenal arteries. Arterial embolization is the procedure of first choice and is directed at excluding the pseudoaneurysm from the circulation by placing coils beyond and then proximal to its neck.

12.4.5 Renal Injuries

Half of renal vascular injuries are iatrogenic, resulting from damage caused during renal biopsies (Fig. 12.4) or percutaneous renal intervention such as nephrostomy tube placement or nephrolithotomy. Of the noniatrogenic injuries, 95% are caused by blunt trauma, although the percentage caused by penetrating injuries increases in urban environments. Approximately 80% of blunt

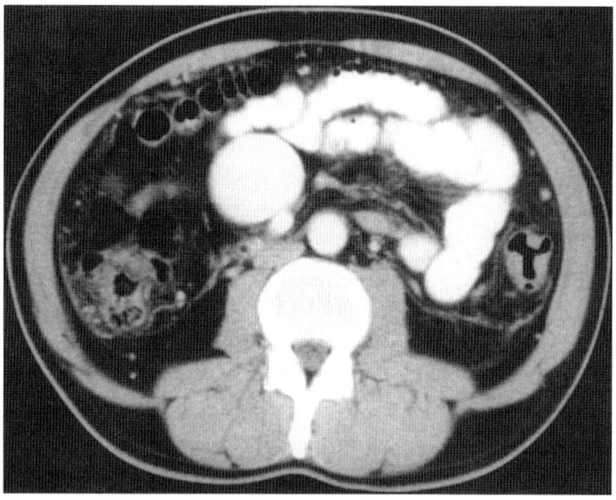

a

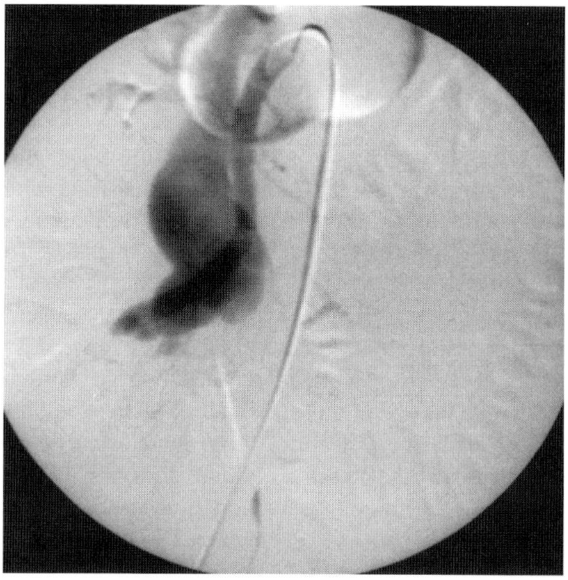

b

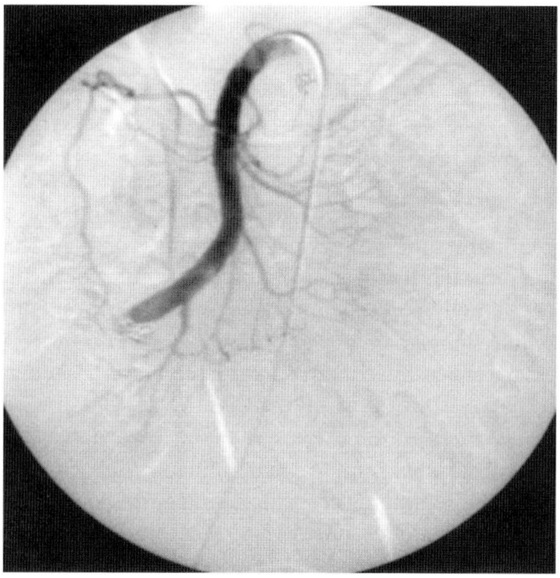

c

Fig. 12.7a–c. Patient presenting with abdominal pain several years following a right hemicolectomy. **a** Axial CT scan performed during the arterial phase of contrast medium enhancement through the mid abdomen demonstrates massive enlargement of the superior mesenteric vein, which is of similar attenuation to the adjacent superior mesenteric artery and aorta, consistent with the presence of an arteriovenous communication. **b** A main superior mesenteric artery angiogram shows a large AVF between the distal superior mesenteric artery and the adjacent vein. Note the very poor filling of the jejunal and ileal arteries due to the steal effect through the AVF. **c** Metallic coils have been placed at the site of the AVF beyond the last ileal artery. The AVF has been occluded and jejunal and ileal artery branch filling is much improved injuries to the kidney result in contusions and minor lacerations that heal spontaneously without intervention. Main renal pedicle injuries will be identified on cross-sectional imaging and will require surgery in most instances. Patients who develop massive bleeding after biopsy or percutaneous renal intervention should undergo angiography with a view to embolization. Pseudoaneurysms, arteriovenous fistulae, and contrast medium extravasation into the pelvicalyceal system or retroperitoneum may be encountered (Swana et al. 1996). As has been mentioned above (Sect. 12.3.2), the kidney is for all intents and purposes an end organ without a significant collateral supply, and embolization will, therefore, lead to tissue loss. Every effort must be made, therefore, to embolize very selectively so as to preserve as much normal renal parenchyma as possible and this is possible in the vast majority of cases by the use of a coaxial catheter. Coils are the simplest embolic agents and these can be placed immediately proximal to the angiographic abnormality to achieve complete occlusion (Beaujeux et al. 1995). Particulate agents such as absorbable gelatin sponge and polyvinyl alcohol are rarely required and when necessary should be used with great care so as to avoid their overspill into normal adjacent renal artery branches.

Aortic dissections with involvement of one or both renal artery origins may be managed, in appropriate circumstances, using similar techniques to those mentioned in Sect. 12.4.3.

12.5 Conclusion

Endovascular techniques play an important role in the management of abdominal vessel trauma, particularly in the control of major hemorrhage; with the increasing trend towards the nonoperative management of solid organ trauma, the role of the vascular interventional radiologist is likely to increase. An understanding of the vascular injuries that may result from trauma and the general principles of embolization of these injuries, regardless of the territory within which they occur, is essential if they are to be treated correctly.

References

Beaujeux R, Saussine C, al-Fakir A et al (1995) Superselective endovascular treatment of renal vascular lesions. J Urol 153:14–17

Ben-Menachem Y (1995) Transvenous approach to salvage incomplete arterial embolization of compound traumatic arteriovenous fistulae. Cardiovasc Intervent Radiol 18:391–395

Carillo EH, Paltz A, Miller FB et al (1998) Non-operative management of blunt hepatic trauma. Br J Surg 85:461–468

Collins PS, Golocovsky M, Salander JM, Champion H, Rich NM (1988) Intra-abdominal vascular injury secondary to penetrating trauma. J Trauma 28:S165–S170

Croce EH, Fabian TC, Menke PG et al (1995) Nonoperative management of blunt hepatic trauma is the treatment of choice for hemodynamically stable patients: results of a prospective trial. Ann Surg 221:744–753

Davis KA, Fabian TC, Croce MA et al (1998) Improved success in nonoperative management of blunt splenic injuries: embolization of splenic artery pseudoaneurysms. J Trauma 44:1008–1013

Federle MP, Courcoulas AP, Powell M, Ferris JV, Peitzman AB (1998) Blunt splenic injury in adults: clinical and CT criteria for management, with emphasis on active extravasation. Radiology 206:137–142

Gavant ML, Schurr M, Flick PA, Croce MA, Fabian TC, Gold RE (1997) Predicting clinical outcome of nonsurgical management of blunt splenic injury: using CT to reveal abnormalities of splenic vasculature. AJR 173:855–856

Gorich J, Brambs HJ, Allmenroder C et al (1993) The role of embolization treatment of acute haemorrhage. ROFO 159: 379–387

Hagiwara A, Yukioka T, Ohta S, Nitatori T, Matsuda H, Shimazaki S (1996) Nonsurgical management of patients with blunt splenic injury: efficacy of transcatheter arterial embolization. AJR 167:159–166

Henne-Bruns D, Kremer B (1992) Injuries of the portal vein and vena cava in severe blunt abdominal trauma. Zentralbl Chir 117:343–347

Horton J, Ogden ME, Williams S et al (1982) The importance of splenic blood flow in clearing pneumococcal organisms. Ann Surg 195:172–176

Krige JE, Bornman PC, Terblanche J (1992) Therapeutic perihepatic packing in complex liver trauma. Br J Surg 79:43–46

Marr JD, Krige JE, Terblanche J (2000) Analysis of 153 gunshot wounds of the liver. Br J Surg 87:1030–1034

Sclafani SJA, Weisberg A, Scalea T et al (1991) Blunt splenic injuries: nonsurgical treatment with CT, arteriography, and transcatheter arterial embolization of the splenic artery. Radiology 181:189–196

Sclafani SJA, Shaftan GW, Scalea TM et al (1995) Nonoperative salvage of computed tomography-diagnosed splenic injuries: utilization of angiography for triage and embolization for haemostasis. J Trauma 39:818–827

Shanmuganathan K, Mirvis SE, Boyd-Kranis R, Takada T, Scalea TM (2000) Nonsurgical management of blunt splenic injury: use of CT criteria to select patients for splenic arteriography and potential endovascular therapy. Radiology 217:75–82

Starnes S, Klein P, Magagna L, Pomerantz R (1998) Computed tomographic grading is useful in the selection of patients for nonoperative management of blunt injury to the spleen. Am Surg 64:743–749

Swana HS, Cohn SM, Burns GA et al (1996) Renal artery pseudoaneurysm after blunt abdominal trauma: case report and literature review. J Trauma 40:459–461

Williams DM, Lee DY, Hamilton BH et al (1997) The dissected aorta: percutaneous treatment of ischaemic complications – principles and results. J Vasc Interv Radiol 8:605–625

13 Blunt Abdominal Trauma in Patients with Preexisting Lesions

S. Ledbetter and D. B. Nunez Jr.

CONTENTS

- Enlarged or otherwise abnormal organs are more susceptible to injury in patients sustaining blunt abdominal trauma
- Recognition of preexisting lesions in injured organs may significantly alter the management of these patients
- A lower threshold for CT imaging is warranted in patients with known abnormal organs

S. Ledbetter, MD
Assistant Director of Emergency Radiology, Department of Radiology, Brigham and Women's Hospital, Harvard Medical School, Boston, MA 02115, USA
D. B. Nunez Jr., MD
Director of Emergency Radiology, Department of Radiology, Brigham and Women's Hospital, Harvard Medical School, Boston, MA 02115, USA

13.1 Introduction

This chapter considers the variety of preexisting lesions that may be detected in blunt trauma patients who undergo helical CT for suspected traumatic visceral injuries and how such lesions may increase the likelihood and severity of injury. Representative cases of benign and malignant diseases, congenital and acquired abnormalities, and other miscellaneous intraabdominal lesions illustrate the importance of recognizing underlying disease in the management of trauma patients. Unsuspected malignant tumors were incidentally discovered during CT obtained for abdominal trauma in 3.6% of cases (Cook et al. 1986).

The mechanism of blunt abdominal trauma strongly influences the severity of injury. Important mechanistic information such as force of impact, e.g., height, speed, use of protective devices, e.g., seatbelt, lap belt, airbag, helmet, and site of injury, e.g., right, left, or midline package, act as gross indicators of the likelihood and severity of injury in the initial assessment of trauma patients prior to imaging. However, given an equal mechanism of trauma, structural and anatomical variations among patients may affect the likelihood or severity of injury sustained and often are not known until after imaging. For example, abnormally positioned or developed organs might not benefit from the normal anatomically protective features of the human body, i.e., the thoracic cage. Enlarged organs are more susceptible to the effects of compression than are normal organs and are therefore more likely to sustain injury. In addition, tumors, infiltrative diseases, and vascular lesions change the intrinsic properties of normal parenchyma. Alterations in elasticity and viscosity of parenchymal tissues in pathological states may adversely affect organ impact resistance and increase the likelihood of traumatic disruption. As such, organs of abnormal size, morphology, location or intrinsic properties may be more susceptible to the forces of blunt trauma than are normal viscera. As an example, preexisting liver disease such as cirrhosis was shown to have an incidence of 0.5% in trauma patients. Hospital stay is increased in trauma patients with cirrhosis up to 36% and mortality by a factor of 5 (Gomez et al. 1994). Imaging can suggest, on the ground of anatomical findings, the diagnosis of diffuse disease such as liver cirrhosis, steatosis, and portal hypertension.

In addition to the increased risk and severity of traumatic injury in patients with preexisting lesions, the presence of these lesions is likely to influence management and may alter the decision between a surgical or a nonsurgical approach to treatment. Intravenous contrast-enhanced helical CT is better suited than other diagnostic modalities: ultrasound, intravenous urography, diagnostic peritoneal lavage, for detecting preexisting pathological conditions as well as for evaluating the extent of injury. CT superbly reveals alterations in visceral morphology, size, and location. CT has the added benefit of demonstrating atypical patterns of organ enhancement or acute physiopathological events such as posttraumatic bleeding, which allows for better detection of preexisting lesions and organ injury, respectively.

13.2 Tumors, Malignant and Benign

13.2.1 Renal

Kidneys with underlying tumors are more susceptible to traumatic injury than are normal kidneys (Rhyner et al. 1984; Cook et al. 1986). At times, the trauma may be incidental, essentially unrecognized by the patient, and in the absence of patient history felt to be a spontaneous hemorrhage. As such, though spontaneous hemorrhage is known to occur, the presumption of spontaneity should remain suspect even in the absence of a trauma history (Fig. 13.1). Bleeding may occur within the tumor, in the adjacent renal parenchyma, or may result in subcapsular or retroperitoneal bleeding, particularly in cases of hypervascular tumors such as renal cell carcinoma (Fig. 13.2). In addition, urine extravasation can occur with relatively minor trauma if predisposing lesions are present, increasing the likelihood and severity of parenchymal injury. Delayed scanning in the pyelographic phase of contrast excretion will enable evaluation of the renal collecting system in these patients.

Angiomyolipomas, also known as renal hamartomas, are benign tumors composed of mature or immature thick-walled blood vessels, fat and smooth

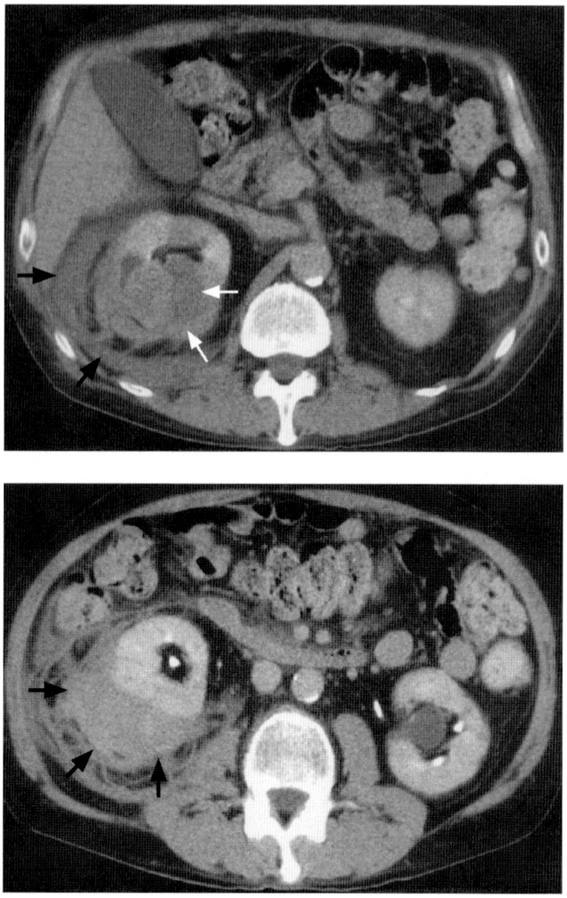

a

b

Fig. 13.1a, b. A 54 year-old man presented with atraumatic right flank pain. **a** Axial CT image shows a large and heterogeneously enhancing mass (*white arrows*) posteriorly in the right kidney. **a, b** There is surrounding high-density perirenal hematoma (*black arrows*) without active arterial extravasation. The patient underwent surgical excision of a renal cell carcinoma

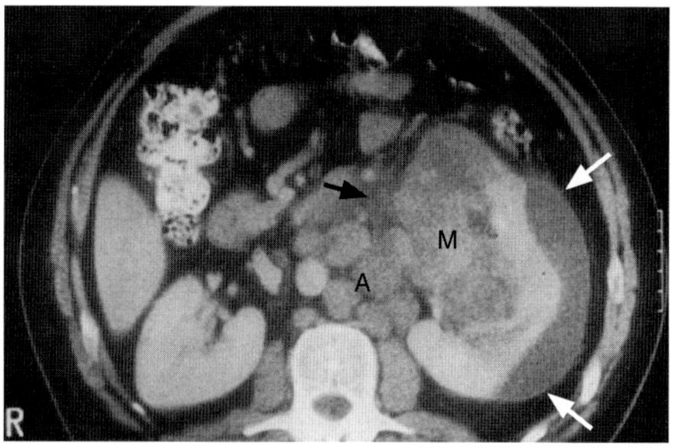

Fig. 13.2. A 55-year-old man with a left renal cell carcinoma was admitted with flank pain and hematuria after falling from standing. Contrast-enhanced axial CT image reveals a large heterogeneous left renal mass (*M*) with associated hilar and retroperitoneal adenopathy (*A*). In addition, there is evidence of a subcapsular hematoma (*white arrow*) and anterior retroperitoneal bleeding (*black arrow*)

muscle elements in varying proportions (Steiner et al. 1993). The presence of fat is a distinguishing and pathognomonic feature of angiomyolipomas, though CT findings may vary depending on the predominance of the different tissue elements. Angiomyolipomas may vary in size from small nodules to bulky masses, but most are hypervascular. Frequently, these lesions are discovered incidentally during abdominal imaging in patients without trauma. Angiomyolipomas may be complicated by hemorrhage, which can be spontaneous or associated with relatively minor or incidental trauma (Lemaitre et al. 1995) (Fig. 13.3). These lesions may be treated surgically or by selective arterial embolization (Fig. 13.4).

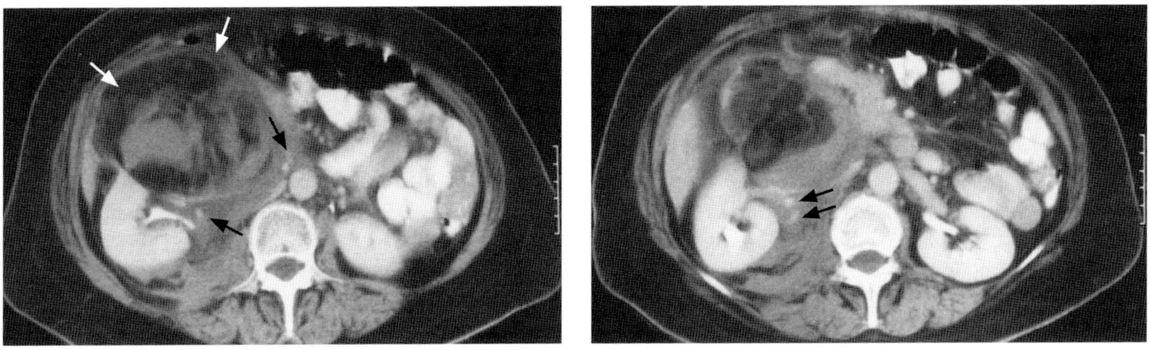

a b

Fig. 13.3a, b. A 33-year-old man with renal angiomyolipoma sustained blunt trauma to the right flank. **a** Axial CT images show a large and heterogeneous, fat-containing mass (*white arrows*) that grows anteriorly from the right kidney. **a, b** There is surrounding high-density collection and focal areas of contrast material extravasation (*black arrows*) representing bleeding sites. Bleeding responded to conservative management

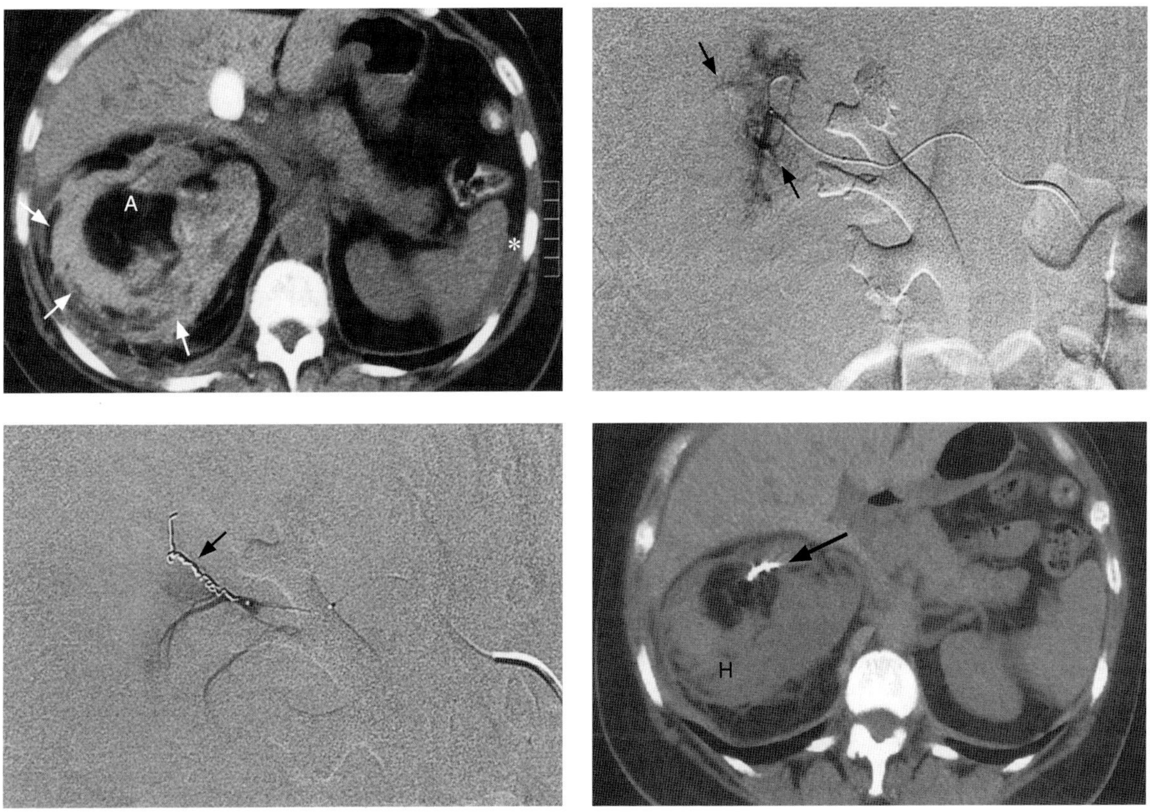

a b c d

Fig. 13.4a–d. A 55-year-old female with right flank and abdominal pain after incidental trauma. **a** Contrast-enhanced axial CT image shows a fat attenuating mass in the right kidney diagnostic of an angiomyolipoma (*A*). Surrounding perinephric high-attenuation stranding is compatible with perirenal hemorrhage (*arrows*). Note also the small amount of hemoperitoneum around the spleen (∗). **b** Selective right renal arteriogram reveals a vascular blush in the region corresponding to the upper pole mass and active hemorrhage from a segmental arterial branch (*arrows*). **c** Selective right renal arteriogram after transcatheter embolization of the bleeding arterial branch and placement of an occluding coil (*arrow*). **d** CT after embolization demonstrating the vascular coil (*arrow*) and stable perinephric hemorrhage (*H*)

13.2.2 Hepatic

Most hepatic hemangiomas are small and asymptomatic and therefore discovered incidentally in patients undergoing imaging for reasons other than trauma. Large hemangiomas can occasionally produce symptoms related to spontaneous hemorrhage or internal thrombosis (Scribano et al. 1996). These lesions can become very large and can rupture following blunt abdominal trauma (Hotokezaka et al. 1996). CT can diagnose a ruptured giant hemangioma (Fig. 13.5) by identifying signs of bleeding such as contrast material extravasation or hemoperitoneum associated with a mass possessing imaging features characteristic of a hemangioma (i.e., scattered calcifications, sustained peripheral nodular enhancement, delayed fill-in). Laparoscopic inspection can rapidly confirm the liver lesions as a source of bleeding and guide further management (Manning et al. 1993).

A bleeding hepatic adenoma must be considered in the differential diagnosis in female patients with a history of oral contraceptive use or in male patients known to use anabolic steroids.

Hepatocarcinomas are known to bleed spontaneously or after contusion of the liver (Nagasue and Inokuchi 1979; Dixon et al. 1982; Kew and Hodkinson 1991). Some hepatocarcinomas, but also adenomas or focal nodular hyperplasia may be pedunculated and hang under the liver, becoming particularly exposed to injury and torsion of the pedicle (Green and Brown 1973). Occult hepatocarcinoma was discovered during CT for abdominal injury in 1.2% (Cook et al. 1986).

a

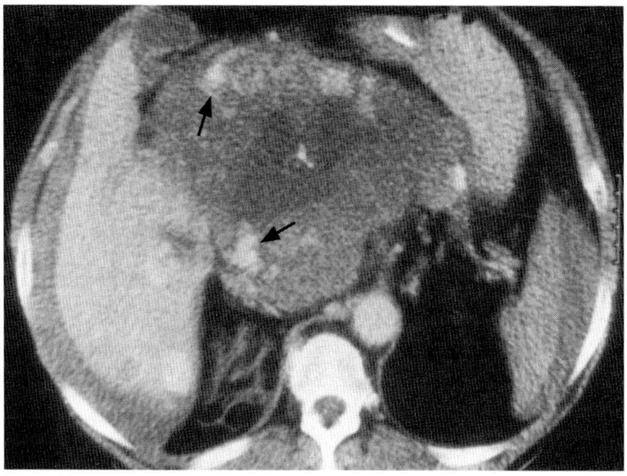

b

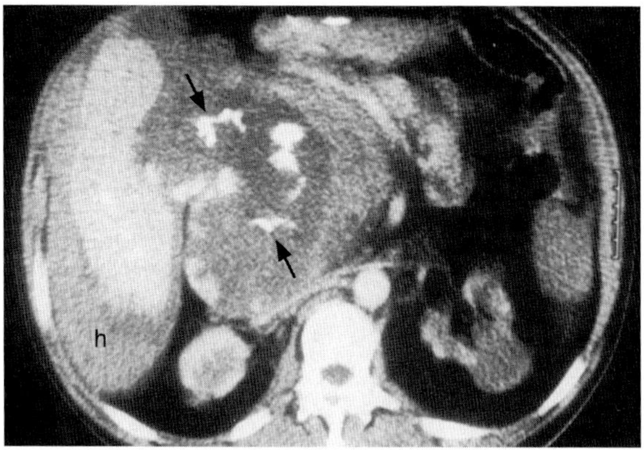

Fig. 13.5a, b. A 72-year-old man with a giant hepatic hemangioma was involved in a motor vehicle accident. **a** Contrast-enhanced CT reveals a large heterogeneous mass arising from the right liver lobe with central low attenuation and scattered high-density areas representing focal extravasation of contrast material (*arrows*). **b** Axial CT image caudal to **a** shows abundant high-density hemoperitoneum (*h*). Note irregular clusters of calcifications (*arrows*) within the tumor. A ruptured giant cavernous hemangioma was found at autopsy

13.2.3 Other (Pancreatic, Splenic, Mesenteric and Intestinal)

Pancreatic tumors are susceptible to injury because of their midline location in the abdomen, which may increase the likelihood of a crushing injury against the vertebral column (Komatsu et al. 1999). Focal hypodense splenic lesions may be seen in patients with myelogenous or other cancers and may represent lymphomatous involvement or metastatic disease (Fig. 13.6). Mesenteric and intestinal tumors

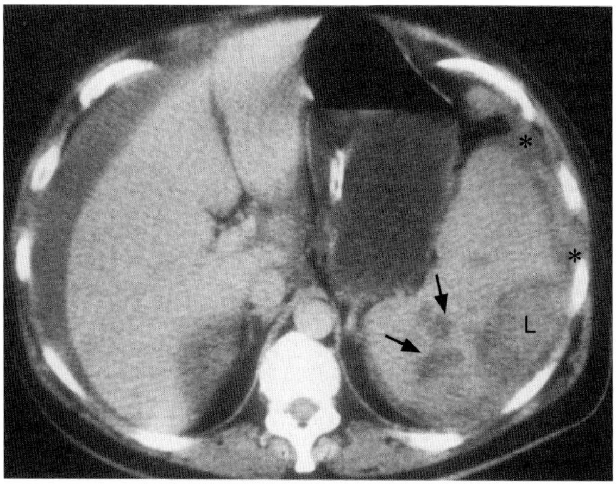

Fig. 13.6. A 67-year-old man with non-Hodgkin's lymphoma and splenomegaly was a victim of assault. Contrast-enhanced axial CT image shows splenomegaly and multiple nonenhancing hypodense nodules representing preexisting lymphomatous lesions (*arrows*) in addition to high-density splenic laceration (*L*) with hemoperitoneum and sentinel clot adjacent to spleen (*). This patient required splenectomy

and inflammatory lesions such as Crohn's disease are vulnerable to the effects of blunt impact, particularly when large (Fig. 13.7). Incidental discovery of a gastric leiomyosarcoma, mistaken for a hematoma, was reported (Cook et al. 1986). Slow intraperitoneal hemorrhage following blunt abdominal trauma may occasionally present as hemorrhagic ascites (Dwivedi et al. 1998).

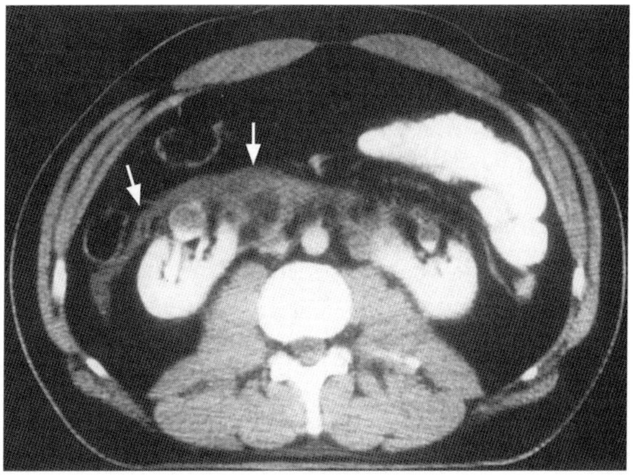

Fig. 13.8. A 39-year-old man with a horseshoe kidney presented with hematuria after blunt trauma. Contrast-enhanced axial CT image shows a poorly enhancing band of soft tissue connecting the kidneys that represents contused renal isthmus with anterior retroperitoneal bleeding (*arrows*) and thickening of the renal fascia

13.3 Congenital Anomalies

13.3.1 Renal

Because of their altered morphology and location, horseshoe kidneys and ectopic kidneys are more susceptible to traumatic injury than are normal kidneys (Rhyner et al. 1984). Horseshoe kidney is the most common renal fusion anomaly and occurs when the inferior portions of each metanephric blastema fuse during abnormal cell migration and create a midline fibrous or parenchymal band called the renal isthmus. CT images will reveal that the inferior poles of the two kidneys are directed medially and fused at midline to create a preaortic renal isthmus, usually at the L4 vertebral body level. At midline, the renal isthmus is vulnerable to compression between the abdominal wall and the vertebral column (Fig. 13.8), particularly in the setting of a midline blunt abdominal force.

Any abnormality in recruiting blood supply or associated abnormalities in the spine may prevent the cephalic migration of the kidneys and result in renal ectopy. The most common form of simple renal ectopy is a pelvic kidney, located either in the true pelvis or adjacent to the sacrum. Though morphology is usually intact, the pelvic kidney is more susceptible to injury because of its close proximity to the pelvic ring, which frequently is disrupted after major trauma (Fig. 13.9). A pelvic kidney also forfeits the normally protective effects of the thoracic cage. CT will also easily detect the congenital absence of one kidney and perhaps lead to more heroic measures to salvage the traumatized single kidney.

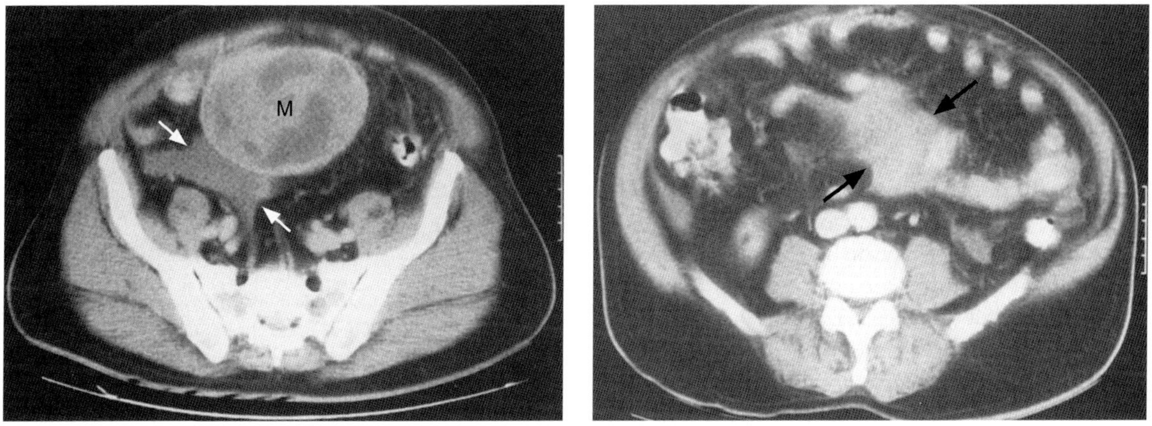

a b

Fig. 13.7a, b. A 63-year-old man with intestinal leiomyosarcoma was admitted with increasing abdominal tenderness and distention after allegedly trivial trauma to the abdomen. **a** Axial CT images show a large heterogeneous mass (*M*) in the mid abdomen. **a, b** There is associated hemoperitoneum (*arrows*) and mesenteric stranding. The patient underwent surgical control of bleeding and tumor resection

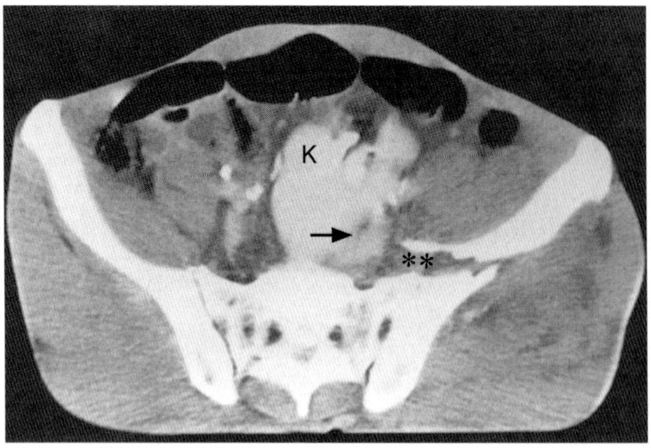

Fig. 13.9. A 65-year-old man with an ectopic pelvic kidney (*K*) sustained pelvic fractures after a high-velocity impact. Axial CT image reveals a displaced iliac bone fracture with sharp edges of bone (*) directed at and lacerating the lateral aspect of the pelvic kidney (*arrow*). Treatment was focused on stabilization of fractures and the renal lesion was managed nonoperatively

13.3.2 Intestinal

Apart from expansile lesions, bowel injury may also occur because of the forces of deceleration against points of bowel fixation, analogous to the mechanism proposed for aortic injury at the site of tethering by the ligamentum arteriosum. The points of fixation may include areas of adhesion or developmental anomalies such as a Meckel's diverticulum. Though space-occupying intestinal tumors may be detected preoperatively, congenital abnormalities such as a Meckel's diverticulum are less likely to be detected. Indeed, it may be difficult if not impossible to discern whether or not the presence of a fixation point is merely coincidental or contributory to the injury (Fig. 13.10).

13.3.3 Other (Liver, Spleen and Pancreas)

Congenital anomalies or variants of the liver, bile ducts, spleen and pancreas are relatively rare. When present, these anomalies typically do not have features that increase risk of injury e.g., enlargement, ectopy, fixation or alter treatment decisions. Rupture of a choledochal cyst may occur spontaneously, or induced by minor trauma, or occasionally lead to hemoperitoneum and bile ascites requiring urgent laparotomy (Battersby 1978; Ando et al. 1995). Traumatic pancreatitis was observed in a patient with pancreas divisum, but this anomaly was not shown to influence the prognosis of pancreatic injury (Portis et al. 1994). The possibility of a pancreatobiliary anomaly should be considered, when interpreting magnetic resonance cholangiopancreatographies or instrumental opacification of the biliary and pancreatic ducts (Sugiyama et al. 1998).

13.4 Organomegaly

13.4.1 Spleen

Of all the abdominal organs, the spleen is at greatest risk for injury following blunt abdominal trauma (Shuman 1998). The presence of splenomegaly increases the risk of sustaining significant injury even after minor trauma. In children, splenomegaly is most

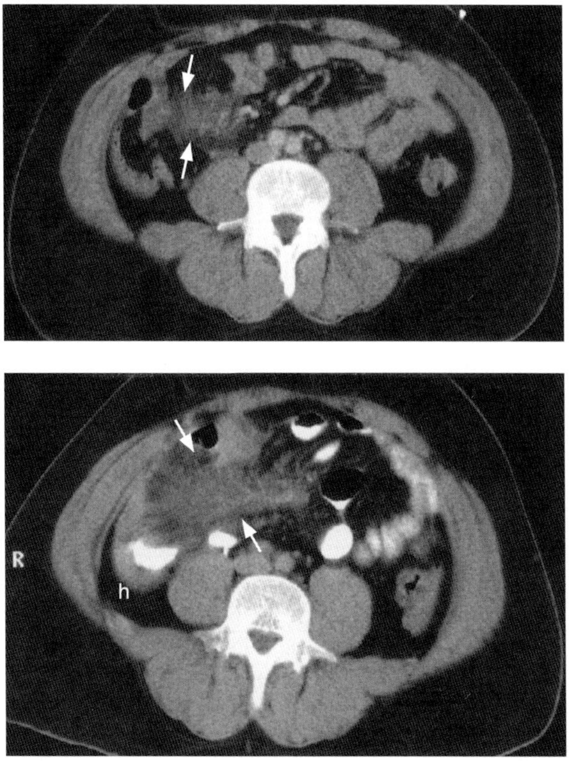

Fig. 13.10a,b. A 36-year-old man suffered significant blunt abdominal trauma. **a** CT at presentation demonstrated a small amount of stranding in the right lower quadrant consistent with mesenteric hematoma (*arrows*). Mesenteric or small-bowel injury was suspected and the patient was managed expectantly. **b** The patient developed worsening pain. Follow-up CT 8 h later demonstrated increased mesenteric stranding (*arrows*) and intraperitoneal hemorrhage (*h*). The patient went to surgery where a mesenteric rent was found involving a Meckel's diverticulum. The diverticulum and mesentery were resected

often the result of infection, specifically mononucleosis. Human immunodeficiency virus (HIV) is the most common infectious cause in adults. However, the most severe cases of splenomegaly are found typically in patients with chronic hematological disorders, including lymphoproliferative and myeloproliferative diseases such as lymphoma and leukemia. Patients with splenic sequestration syndromes also may experience significant splenic enlargement. A special consideration in the trauma patient is splenomegaly resulting from liver cirrhosis and portal hypertension since these patients have a particularly high risk of catastrophic bleeding after splenic injury.

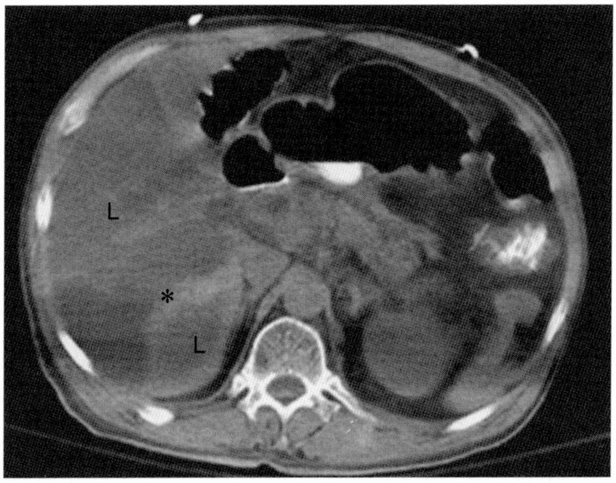

a

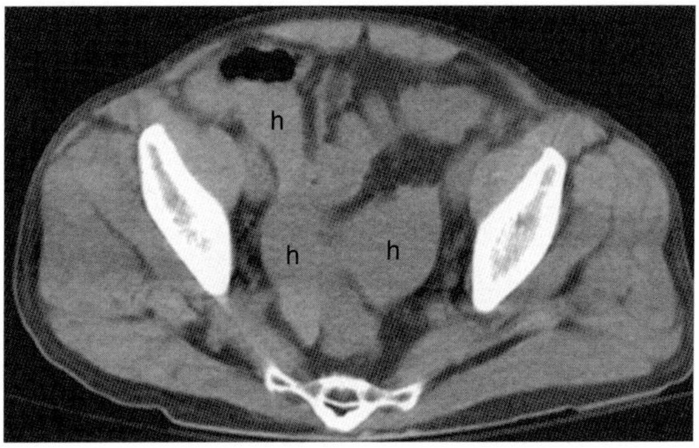

b

Fig. 13.11a, b. A 49-year-old man with a hepatosteatosis sustained a high-velocity impact. **a** Axial CT image reveals a laceration (*) through the right lobe of a fatty liver (*L*). **b** A CT image in the lower pelvis demonstrates a large amount of hemoperitoneum (*h*)

13.4.2 Liver

The more common non-neoplastic causes of hepatomegaly include diffuse fatty infiltration, hepatitis, and passive vascular congestion secondary to right-sided cardiac failure. In addition to organ enlargement, these conditions also alter tissue properties in a way that may adversely affect their resistance to traumatic injury (Fig 13.11). Fatty infiltration is recognized by diffuse low density of the liver parenchyma when compared to the spleen. There are generally no CT findings related to hepatitis apart from hepatomegaly. Distention of the hepatic veins at their confluence with the inferior vena cava suggests right-sided heart failure, though this may be an unreliable finding in trauma patients with a significant alteration in circulating blood volume (blood loss leading to a false negative result or vigorous expansion from i.v. fluids with a false positive result).

Hyper- or hypotrophy of a lobe or segment should be interpreted correctly, as they may become involved in trauma of the liver and gallbladder (Koplewitz et al. 1999).

13.5 Acquired Cystic Disease or Abscess

13.5.1 Renal

Most renal cysts are asymptomatic and complications are rare. Hemorrhage and/or rupture can occur spontaneously or because of trauma, particularly in larger cysts (Redmond and Royle 1985; Papanicolau et al. 1986). Rupture may occur into an adjacent calyx, leading merely to cyst decompression, or into the perirenal space of the retroperitoneum, causing significant perirenal stranding. In trauma patients, CT can diagnose ruptured renal cysts while excluding significant other renal parenchymal injury such as laceration or ureteropelvic junction avulsion. CT can readily show bleeding into the cyst and surrounding tissues, which is more likely to require surgery or intervention for management (Fig. 13.12). Likewise, CT may show merely spillage of the cyst contents into the perirenal space without evidence of hemorrhage, leading only to conservative management without surgery or intervention (Fig. 13.13). Adult polycystic kidney disease (PCKD) serves as an extreme example of renal enlargement secondary to acquired cystic disease and these kidneys are at increased risk of injury during trauma (Amend and Galen 1973; Leslie et al. 2000). Additionally, the liver is commonly affected (~70%) in PCKD, with splenic and pancreatic involvement occurring less frequently (<5%). Closer scrutiny of these organs is warranted in these patients.

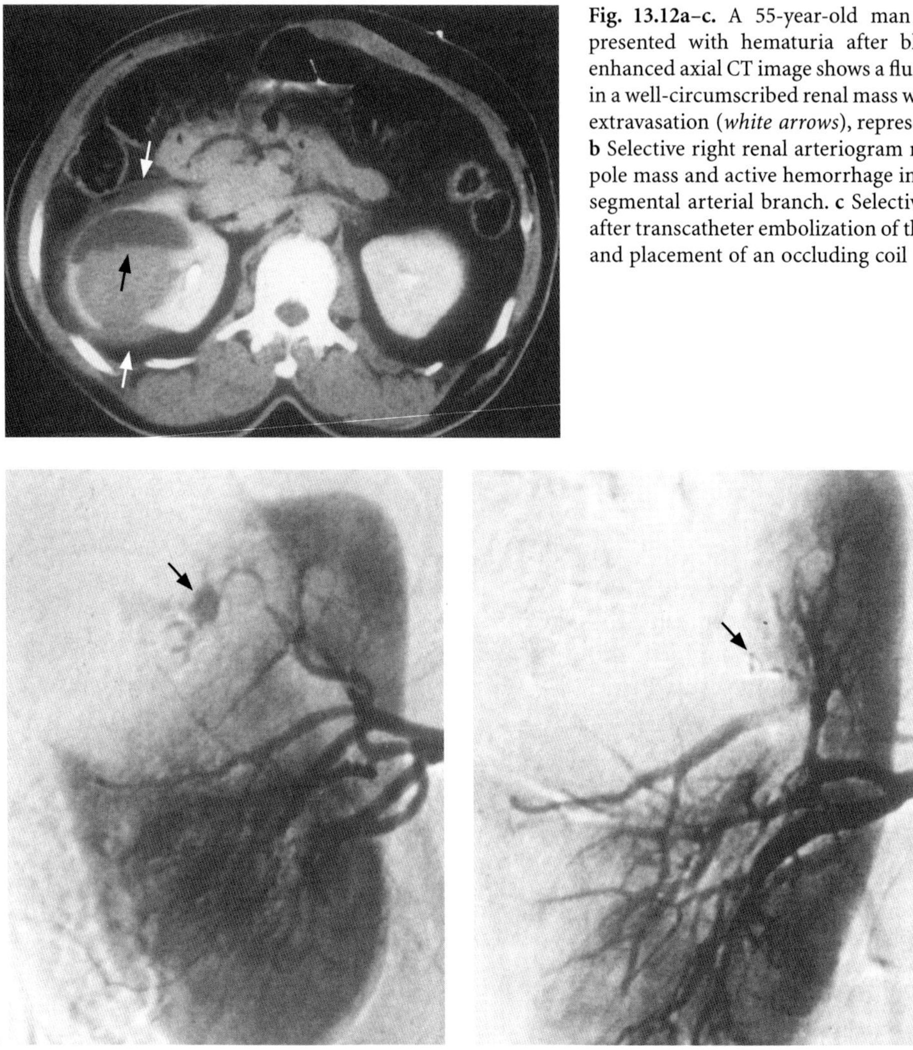

a b c

Fig. 13.12a–c. A 55-year-old man with a right renal cyst presented with hematuria after blunt trauma. **a** Contrast-enhanced axial CT image shows a fluid-fluid level (*black arrow*) in a well-circumscribed renal mass with associated perinephric extravasation (*white arrows*), representing rupture of the cyst. **b** Selective right renal arteriogram reveals an avascular upper pole mass and active hemorrhage into the cyst (*arrow*) from a segmental arterial branch. **c** Selective right renal arteriogram after transcatheter embolization of the bleeding arterial branch and placement of an occluding coil (*arrow*)

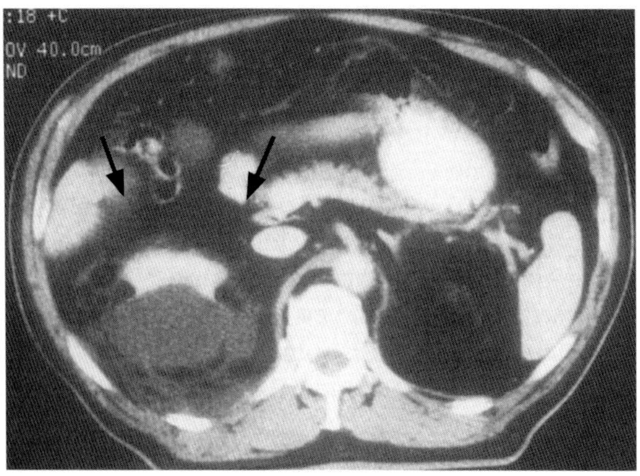

Fig. 13.13. A 43-year-old woman with a right renal cyst was admitted after a motor vehicle collision. CT shows a well-circumscribed fluid density mass in the lower pole of the right kidney with associated perirenal stranding (*arrows*) secondary to retroperitoneal extravasation of cyst contents. The patient was managed without surgery or intervention

13.5.2 Pancreatic

Pancreatic pseudocysts occur in 30–40% of patients following pancreatitis. In up to half of patients, the pseudocyst will resolve. However, approximately 50% do not resolve spontaneously and therefore become the most common cause of pancreatic cystic lesions. They may become quite large space-occupying lesions and susceptible to traumatic injury, particularly given their common midline location (Fig. 13.14). CT is excellent for depicting the sequelae of pancreatitis and any superimposed acute traumatic injury.

13.5.3 Hepatic

Hepatic biliary or parasitic hydatid cysts may enlarge due to intracystic hemorrhage or rupture following abdominal trauma (Berenson et al. 1974; Marti and Rohner 1977; Yokoyama et al. 1984; Leviav and Weissberg 1996; Morano et al. 1996). Posttraumatic rupture of alveolar echinococcus was also reported, with long survival, despite recurrences (Sato et al. 1996). Rupture of a renal hydatid cyst concomitant to liver injury can occur (Teinturier et al. 1960).

Preexisting pyogenic or amebic liver abscess may render the hepatic parenchyma more fragile than cysts, particularly when under tension, and be responsible for diffuse peritonitis following post-traumatic rupture (Goonaratna and Kitulgala 1967; Ramachandran and Edwards 1978). Imaging is particularly puzzling, when liver injury and a residual ruptured abscess cavity coexist.

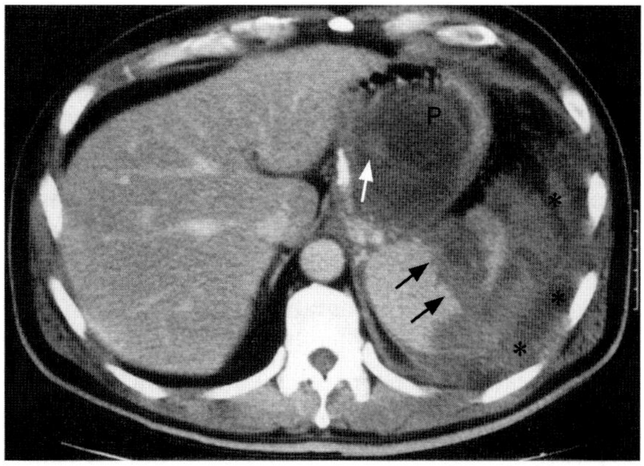

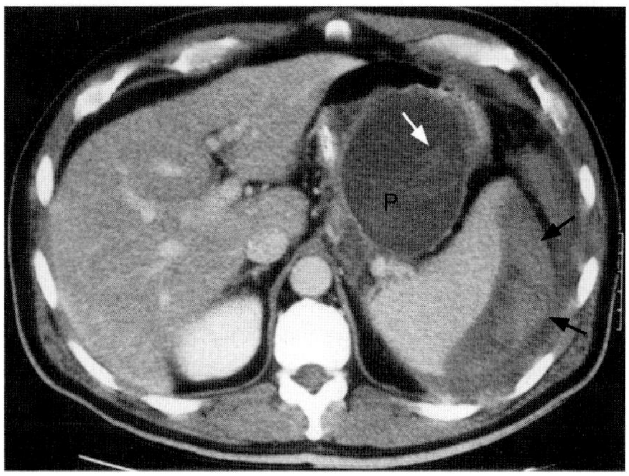

Fig. 13.14a, b. A 45-year-old man with a pancreatic pseudocyst was involved in a car accident. **a** CT images in the upper abdomen reveal a grade IV splenic laceration (*black arrows*) with perisplenic hematoma (*) and evidence of bleeding (*white arrow*) into a pancreatic pseudocyst (*P*). **b** Axial CT image caudal to **a** reveals a large high-density subcapsular hematoma (*black arrows*) of the spleen. Bleeding (*white arrow*) into the pseudocyst (*P*) is also seen. Patient underwent splenectomy and drainage of the pseudocyst

13.6 Aneurysms and Atherosclerosis

Vascular aneurysms, particularly those involving the aorta, may rupture because of abdominal trauma (Bunai et al. 1999). In most cases, contrast-enhanced helical CT clearly depicts these lesions and any associated active arterial extravasation. Ninety percent of abdominal aortic aneurysms are infrarenal and, when large, begin to occupy a more midline position in the lower abdomen. Traumatic aneurysm rupture appears no different from its nontraumatic counterpart and is indicated by the presence of high-attenuation hemorrhage in the retroperitoneum around the aorta with or without active arterial extravasation following intravenous contrast administration. Apart from rupture, trauma to the abdominal aorta may also cause distal embolization of atherosclerotic plaque, resulting in vascular occlusion and tissue ischemia (Tsai et al. 1997).

13.7 Metastatic Spread of Cancer Cells

A great deal of experimental work was published on the potential role of trauma in the spread of malignant cells from an injured malignant tumor, but clinical data remain too scarce to draw meaningful conclusions (Agostino and Cliffton 1965; Rudenstam 1968; Agostino 1969).

13.8 Conclusion

This chapter has considered a variety of preexisting lesions that may be detected in blunt trauma patients who undergo helical CT for suspected traumatic injuries. Such preexisting lesions may affect not only the likelihood and severity of injury, but also the decision of how to treat. Representative cases of benign and malignant diseases, congenital and acquired abnormalities, and other miscellaneous intraabdominal lesions illustrate the importance of recognizing these preexisting lesions, as well as appreciating the consequences they may have for patient management.

References

Agostino D (1969) On the production of metastases following trauma to the tumor. Osp Ital Chir 21:81–96

Agostino D, Cliffton EE (1965) Organ-localization and the effects of trauma on the fate of circulating cancer cells. Cancer Res 25:1728–1732

Amend WJ, Galen M (1973) Polycystic kidney disease and seatbelts. Ann Intern Med 79:287

Ando H, Ito T, Watanabe Y, Seo T, Kaneko K, Nagaya M (1995) Spontaneous perforation of choledochal cyst. J Am Coll Surg 181:125–128

Battersby C (1978) Ruptured choledochal cyst: recognition and management. Aust N Z J Surg 48:515–517

Berenson MM, Freston JW, Koehler PR, Chang F (1974) Traumatic intrahepatic rupture of an echinococcal cyst. J Trauma 14:798–804

Bunai Y, Nagai A, Nakamura I, Ohya I (1999) Traumatic rupture of an abdominal aortic aneurysm associated with the use of a seatbelt. J Forensic Sci 44:1304–1306

Cook DE, Walsh JW, Withley CV, Brewer WH (1986) Upper abdominal trauma: pitfalls in CT diagnosis. Radiology 159: 65–69

Dixon JM, Nirmul D, Eremin O (1982) Haemoperitoneum due to traumatic rupture of a hepatoma in a patient with haemochromatosis. J R Coll Surg Edinb 27:362–363

Dwivedi DN, Srinath C, Pande GK (1998) An unusual cause of haemorrhagic ascites following blunt abdominal trauma. Trop Gastroenterol 19:156–158

Gomez GA, Jacobson LE, Asension JA, Nauta RJ (1994) Preexisting liver disease in the trauma patient. Crit Care Clin 10:555–566

Goonaratna C, Kitulgala DM (1967) Rupture of a left-lobe amoebic liver abscess following a car accident. Ceylon Med J 12:181–182

Green MT Jr, Brown JR (1973) Avulsion of pedunculated focal nodular hyperplasia: an unusual football injury. J La State Med Soc 124:39–42

Hotokezaka M, Kojima M, Nakamura K et al (1996) Traumatic rupture of hepatic hemangioma. J Clin Gastroenterol 23: 69–71

Kew MC, Hodkinson J (1991) Rupture of hepatocellular carcinoma as a result of blunt abdominal trauma. Am J Gastroenterol 86:1083–1085

Komatsu T, Taira S, Matsui O, Takashima T, Note M, Fujita H (1999) A case of ruptured mesenchymal chondrosarcoma of the pancreas. Rodiat Med 17:239–241

Koplewitz BZ, Manson DE, Ein SH (1999) Posttraumatic torsion of accessory lobe of the liver and the gallbladder. Pediatr Radiol 29:799–802

Lemaitre L, Robert Y, Dubrulle F, Claudon M (1995) Renal angiomyolipoma: growth followed up with CT and/or US. Radiology 197:598–602

Leslie CL, Simon BJ, Lee KF, Emhoff TA, Munshi IA (2000) Bilateral rupture of multicystic kidneys after blunt abdominal trauma. J Trauma 48:336–337

Leviav S, Weissberg D (1996) Traumatic rupture of hydatic cysts. Can J Surg 39:293–296

Manning MM, Murray KD, Townsend MC (1993) The laparoscopic diagnosis and treatment of cavernous hemangioma hemorrhage following blunt trauma. J Laparoendosc Surg 3:399–403

Marti MC, Rohner A (1977) Traumatic rupture of an hepatic hydatic cyst. Helv Chir Acta 44:99–102

Morano C, Fornari L, Persico Stella L (1996) Acute abdomen caused by the rupture of a solitary non-parasitic cyst of the liver. Minerva Chir 51:713–716

Nagasue N, Inokuchi K (1979) Spontaneous and traumatic rupture of hepatoma. Br J Surg 66:248–250

Papanicolau N, Pfister RC, Yoder I (1986) Spontaneous and traumatic rupture of renal cysts: diagnosis and outcome. Radiology 160:99–103

Portis M, Meyers P, McDonald JC, Gholson CF (1994) Traumatic pancreatitis in a patient with pancreas divisum: clinical and radiographic features. Abdom Imaging 19:162–164

Ramachandran S, Edwards R (1978) Hepatic trauma and amoebic liver abscess. J Trop Med Hyg 81:40–41

Redmond P, Royle G (1985) Rupture of a calcified renal cyst following blunt abdominal trauma. Br J Radiol 58:683–684

Rhyner P, Federle MP, Jeffrey RB (1984) CT of trauma to the abnormal kidney. AJR 142:747–750

Rudenstam CM (1968) Experimental studies in trauma and metastasis formation. Acta Chir Scand (Suppl) 391:1–83

Sato N, Namieno T, Takahashi H et al (1996) A long-surviving patient with recurrence of hepatic alveolar echinococcosis after traumatic intra-abdominal rupture. J Gastroenterol 31:885–888

Scribano E, Loria G, Ascenti G et al (1996) Spontaneous hemoperitoneum from a giant multicystic hemangioma of the liver: a case report. Abdom Imaging 21:418–419

Shuman WP (1998) CT of abdominal trauma in adults. Radiology 205:297–306

Steiner MS, Goldman SM, Fishman EK, Marshal FF (1993) The natural history of renal angiomyolipoma. J Urol 150: 1782–1786

Sugiyama M, Atomi Y, Naka S, Nagashima Y, Kozawa K, Wada N (1998) Pancreatobiliary anomaly. Hepatogastroenterology 45:1141–1144

Teinturier J et al (1960) Posttraumatic intraperitoneal rupture of a hydatid renal cyst associated with hepatic laceration. Mem Acad Chir 86:398–403

Tsai FC, Wang CC, Fang JF et al. (1997) Isolated common iliac artery occlusion secondary to atherosclerotic plaque rupture from blunt abdominal trauma: case report and review of the literature. J Trauma 42:133–136

Yokoyama T, Myoshi N, Ichikawa T, Okita M (1984) Solitary nonparasitic cyst of the liver in children: two cases of rapid enlarging cyst by minor abdominal injury. Hiroshima J Med Sci 33:595–598

14 Injuries of the Scrotum

B. MARTIN and R. F. DONDELINGER

CONTENTS

B. MARTIN, MD
Institut de Radiologie de Paris, Scanner – IRM Paris Hoche, 31, av. Hoche, 75008 Paris, France
R. F. DONDELINGER, MD
Professor and Chairman, Deptartment of Medical Imaging, University Hospital Sart Tilman, Domaine Universitaire du Sart Tilman B35, 4000 Liège, Belgium

- High-resolution ultrasound and color Doppler is the optimal routine imaging modality in scrotal injury
- Testicular dislocation, testicular fracture, and compressive hematocele must be promptly recognized, for prompt surgical testicular salvage
- Acute torsion of the spermatic cord can occur in case of testicular dislocation and in particular in sports trauma: surgical exploration should not be delayed by an inconclusive ultrasound examination
- Tubular ectasia of the rete testis gives a hypoechoic perihilar net. When recognized correctly in a patient with a history of previous pelvic surgery, unnecessary exploratory surgery can be avoided

14.1 History

The first well-documented case of blunt scrotal trauma was reported in the literature in 1918 and concerned bilateral testicular dislocation (HERBST and POLKEY 1936). The advent of ultrasound (US) has substantially changed the management of closed scrotal trauma, as blunt testicular injury frequently went undiagnosed or surgically ignored, when a large surrounding hematoma was present (MCANINCH et al. 1984).

14.2 Incidence

Traumatic testicular injuries are uncommon, due to size, anatomical location, and mobility of the testis. As blunt scrotal trauma does not represent a life-threatening condition, true incidence remains unknown. It is obvious that in case of multiple and severe abdominal injuries, scrotal injury is usually neglected or underestimated. In these cases, the trauma victim often complains several months later of scrotal symptoms. Testicular pain accounts for 0.5% of total emergency department visits, and posttraumatic injury represents only a small portion of these cases (Blaivas and Sierzenski 2001). In fact, scrotal trauma represents 7.4% of all US examinations performed for acute scrotal pathology (Martin and Conte 1987). However, scrotal and testicular injury accounts for about 10% of all urogenital traumas in a multicenter register (Zink et al. 1990). Scrotal injury is probably increasing in frequency, due to more challenging sports activities on the one hand, but also physical aggressions and particularly bicycle or motorcycle accidents as well as improved diagnostic capabilities. In Europe, blunt injury predominates with 63–90% of the cases, penetrating trauma is consequently less frequent (Bautista Casanovas et al. 1992; Altarac 1994; El Moussaoui et al. 1996; El Kamel et al. 1997). Young males with a mean age of 20–30 are mainly involved. School boys are also involved during sports or leisure injuries or traffic accidents. Testicular injury is unilateral in 92–100%, and bilateral in 0–8% (Altarac 1994; El Kamel et al. 1997). An associated trauma of the lower urogenital tract has been reported in 10–80% of fractures or traumatic luxation of the pelvic ring (De Peretti et al. 1993).

14.3 Mechanism

Because of its superficial location, the scrotum is particularly exposed to injury. Penetrating injury includes knife wounds, gunshots, dog or other animal bites, impalement, urethral catheterization, and self-inflicted injury (Parvey and Patel 1998; Ficarra et al. 1999; Cummings and Boullier 2000). Penetrating scrotal trauma is isolated in over 70% of cases or associated with epididymal, spermatic cord, skin, penile, perineal, urethral, and vascular lesions in the thigh (Lee et al. 1992; Schwarz and Blair 1995; Cline et al. 1998).

Blunt injury may have various causes: a car accident with significant associated abdominal injuries; physical aggression; occupational or sport trauma; a direct astride impact on a bicycle or more often a motorcycle with trauma to the perineum and scrotum on the tank, which is a particularly frequent mechanism of scrotal injury. The gasoline tank, by striking the perineum and the scrotum in the midline, is responsible for an upward and outward dislocation of the testis (Pollen and Funckes 1982; Sparnon et al. 1982; El Moussaoui et al. 1996; Hendry 2000). Mountain bikers are exposed to repeated microtrauma to the scrotum and half of them complain of clinical symptoms (Frauscher et al. 2000). Cyclists are known to develop perineal nodular indurations or so-called accessory testicles, which are postnecrotic pseudocysts involving connective tissue as a result of repeated microtrauma (Vuong et al. 1988). Stretching exercises while wearing restrictive gym shorts may result in scrotal hematoma (Ragozzino 1993). Strangulation of the scrotum by a ring is an anecdotal cause of scrotal injury (Zermann and Schubert 1997). In the neonate, scrotal hematoma may be caused by intraabdominal hemorrhage (Amoury et al. 1982; Meixner 1983; Porcelli et al. 1990). Testicular injury may occur in breech delivery in up to 6.5% (Finan and Redman 1985; Tiwary 1989). Delayed visceral rupture, such as splenic, hepatic, or adrenal rupture may be responsible for scrotal hematoma in the neonate and sometimes in adults (Heydenrich 1974; Henry 1978; Sujka et al. 1986; Skoog and Belman 1986; Karpe and Nybonde 1989; Roback et al. 1996; Koumanidou et al. 2000). It should be mentioned that about 10–15% of testicular tumors are revealed by an episode of scrotal trauma (Tumeh et al. 1991). Finally, a spontaneous hematocele, usually bilateral, may appear within several hours of administration of an overdose of anticoagulants.

14.4 Clinical Findings

14.4.1 Acute Presentation

In acute conditions, the diagnosis of blunt scrotal injury is clinically obvious: the patient presents with an enlarged and painful scrotum. Cutaneous ecchymosis or a hematoma of the superficial layers may be seen with a purple coloration of the swollen scrotum. Clinical examination is highly painful and therefore remains often limited. However, on some occasions, the clinical diagnosis of a shattered testis may be strongly suggested, when the normal palpable shape of the testis cannot be found by palpation (Haas et al. 1999). In rare occasions, one hemiscrotum is found empty on palpation in a patient with no previous history of cryptorchidism. Usually a painful mass is palpable superficially in an inguinal, prepubic, or crural location, corresponding to a testicular dislocation (Gimbergues et al. 1999; Comesana Davila et al. 1999). The presence of an ipsilateral cremasteric reflex, when applicable, virtually rules out the possibility of a testicular torsion and its absence increases suspicion of torsion (Rabinowitz 1984). In bilateral testicular rupture, one testis can remain asymptomatic, despite rupture being present (Warden and Schellhammer 1978). Inguinoscrotal bruising in the neonate may be suggestive of extrascrotal, intraabdominal bleeding (Kirby and Davidson 2000). In fact, most often, the clinical examination remains inconclusive because the swollen and painful scrotum, and the usually associated hematocele, obscures the scrotal content.

14.4.2 Late Presentation

Conversely to the acute condition, scrotal injury that was previously denied by the patient or neglected by the physician represents both a clinical and imaging challenge and its diagnosis can be notoriously difficult. Clinically, the injured scrotum presents as an enlarged, hard, and often painless scrotum. Transillumination of the scrotum is negative, mimicking a testicular tumor, particularly in an elderly patient. On other occasions, a testicular nodule is palpated in a patient who does not remember previous trauma. Delayed posttraumatic malacoplakia of the epididymis has been described (McClure 1980).

14.5 Classification

Testicular and scrotal injuries are classified into five stages in the classic surgical grading system (Moore et al. 1996). In testicular injury, contusion or hematoma is staged grade I; grades II–IV consider laceration of the tunica albuginea and extent of parenchymal loss. Grade V corresponds to avulsion or shattered testis. Scrotal injury is based on a similar grading, considering contusion as grade I, scrotal laceration in grades II and III, and avulsion in grades IV and V. Other similar classifications are available, taking into account results of US examination (Couvelaire and Schimmel 1976; Sauvage et al. 1988; Larsen et al. 1993; El Kamel et al. 1997):

- Shattered testis
- Testicular dislocation (bilateral or unilateral, deep or superficial, with or without torsion of spermatic cord)
- Fracture
  - Incomplete
  - Partial
- Hematoma
  - Subcapsular
  - Perihilar
- Contusion

14.6 Imaging

14.6.1 Ultrasound

Although clinical examination often gives the clue to posttraumatic scrotal abnormality, ultrasound (US) is recognized as the imaging modality of choice in the diagnosis of scrotal injury and other pathologies, particularly in blunt injury (Hendrikx et al. 1997). It is no longer true, that patients with laceration of the scrotum are not referred for ultrasound, as they are treated by emergency surgery (Hricak and Filly 1983). US is also of value in penetrating injury, helping to distinguish less serious injuries such as hematoma, hydrocele, and hematocele from testicular fracture. Intrascrotal foreign bodies are recognized and precisely localized (Learch et al. 1995). Serial clinical examination and careful imaging, related to missile or knife trajectory is of utmost importance to guide management.

14.6.2 Other Techniques

Computed tomography (CT) has little usefulness for specific scrotal injury, but is invaluable in the diagnostic workup of abdominal and pelvic injury and contributes to localization of a pelvic testis, in case of testicular dislocation (Toranji and Barbaric 1994).

Magnetic resonance imaging (MRI) has no effective impact on the diagnosis of the acutely injured scrotum. However, in case of a doubtful intratesticular nodule evidenced on US in the delayed posttraumatic phase, MRI may be useful to differentiate a testicular tumor from a chronic and organized testicular hematoma. Testicular hematoma shows as an intratesticular lesion that has a hyperintense signal on T1-weighted sequences and a mixed signal on T2-weighted images (Schnall 1993).

Nuclear medicine studies had gained some popularity in the United States in the investigation of acute scrotal conditions, particularly for testicular torsion and the spectrum of acute epididymitis, but has a low acceptance in Europe (Holder et al. 1981; Chen et al. 1986; Bockisch et al. 1989; Van Ahlen et al. 1991).

14.6.3 Acute Blunt Injury

14.6.3.1 Ultrasound Examination Technique

High-resolution US, using a 10- to 13-MHz probe, should be the gold standard in ultrasound examination, with the systematic adjunction of color and power Doppler (Hendrikx et al. 1997; Dubinsky et al. 1998). The examination should be performed bilaterally, screening both testicles as well as the other intrascrotal structures: epididymis, hydatids if present, the intrascrotal part of the spermatic cord, tunica vaginalis, its interepididymo-testicular recesses, and the scrotal wall.

Color Doppler should always be set to allow detection of low-velocity flow in the testicular parenchyma. For this purpose, the scale or pulse repetition frequency should be set as low as possible, any wall filter should be set low or removed, the Doppler power output should be maximized, and the color Doppler gate should be set as wide as possible (Herbener 1996). However, now almost all US systems are equipped with optimal automatic settings for any anatomical area; nevertheless, it is often useful to discuss with the US field engineer to optimize this setting package.

The normal sonographic aspects will be briefly reviewed. The testis is ovoid in shape. In the adult it measures around 40 mm in length and 30 mm in width and 20 mm in thickness, with a volume of 15–20 cm^3. The volume is automatically calculated by the US machine. Through our daily experience, the most sensitive parameter for detecting a small degree of hypotrophy is the maximum thickness on the longitudinal section: normal 20 mm or more; 15–20 mm slightly hypotrophic; less than 15 mm severely hypotrophic, with sometimes only several cm^3 of testicular volume. The testicular pattern is moderately echoic and homogeneous. An echoic band is usually seen in the posterolateral aspect of the testis and represents the mediastinum of the testis. It is a thickening of fibrous tissue and a real vascular and tubular crossroads from which vessels, arteries, veins, lymphatics, as well than spermatic tubules enter or leave. With the high-frequency probes, the head and body of the epididymis are always well demonstrated. This is less true for the tail of the epididymis. The normal epididymis is homogeneous, with the same or a slightly more echoic pattern than the testis. The head is seen as a usually triangular-shaped 10–12 mm structure, over the upper pole of the testis. The head normally continues as a thin, sometimes slightly lobulated, 2- to 4-mm body, which may be most often located posteriorly or anteriorly, and in around 10% of the cases it is located close and along the longitudinal axis of the testis. The visibility of the tail is inconstant; it is marked by a small, 3- or 5-mm round structure below the testis.

The spermatic cord is located superior to the testis and the epididymis and extends up into the inguinal canal. It contains all the structures entering or leaving the scrotum, namely the vas deferens, the spermatic, deferential, and cremasteric arteries, the spermatic venous plexus, the lymphatic vessels, and the ligament of Cloquet, which represents the remnant from the obliteration of the peritoneo-vaginal canal. These structures are held together by fatty, cellular, connective tissue. The latter is responsible for the US aspect of the spermatic cord: an echoic bandlike structure less than 1 cm in diameter, through which run fine hypoechoic linear vessels, arteries, and veins, which may be identified by color and power Doppler. Pulsed Doppler normally reveals a low-resistance waveform within the testicular artery and its branches. Consequently, its resistive index in an adult is largely less than 1.00, between 0.48 and 0.72 (Herbener 1996). The cremasteric and deferential arteries usually show a high-resistance waveform with low diastolic flow.

14.6.3.2 Testicular Injury

Any component of the scrotum may be involved in blunt or penetrating injury.

Shattered Testis

The normal testis is no longer recognized, due to multiple fractures. Extruded testicular parenchyma may be evidenced. The fragments of the testis are blurred within a large hematocele. In fact, in this situation, US is often of little value, because the diagnosis is already established clinically and orchidectomy is indicated.

Fractured Testis

In cases of fractured testis, the role of US is crucial to demonstrate the disruption of the tunica albuginea (LEWIS and MICHELL 1991) (Fig. 14.1). In some cases, the diagnosis is obvious, because of a large tear with a disruption of the tunica albuginea and associated evisceration of testicular tissue, which is easily recognizable. In other cases, the sonographic diagnosis may be more difficult if the tear of the tunica albuginea is limited. A localized disruption of the echoic line of the tunica albuginea should be detected. It is often surrounded by a mild, acute hydrohematocele and the regular contour of the testis is lost. A heterogeneous parenchyma and an abnormal contour with indistinct margins strongly suggest testicular rupture (BUCHBERGER et al. 1990). In some cases, a prominent vessel can be mistaken for a fracture plane (LEARCH et al. 1995). Localized or extensive fractures of the testis require prompt surgical intervention, which aims at conservation of the testis. Early surgery reduces the risk of testicular necrosis, abscess formation, and consequently the number of secondary orchidectomies (JEFFREY et al. 1983; LUPETIN et al. 1983; ALTARAC 1994; HRICAK et al. 1995; LIN et al. 1998).

Pseudoaneurysm

To our knowledge, only one case report of intratesticular pseudoaneurysm has been published (DEE et al. 2000). The vascular lesion was detected 3 days after a scrotal trauma with increasing enlargement. A round anechoic, 11-mm mass, with pulsatile high-resistance flow was detected on US. The neck of the pseudoaneurysm was clearly visible and there was no obvious break in the tunica albuginea. Follow-up US showed the spontaneous thrombosis of the pseudoaneurysm 4 days later.

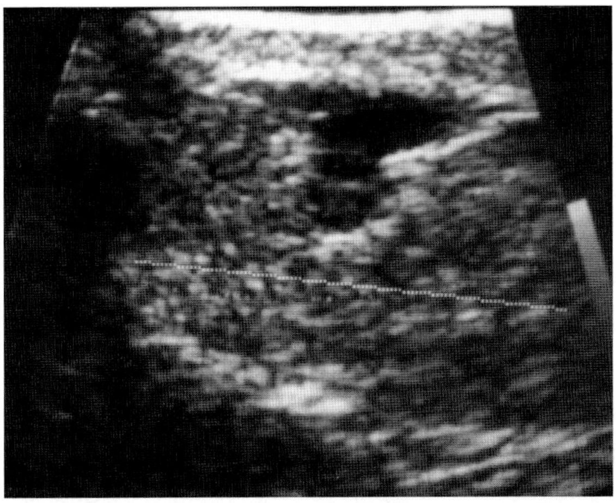

Fig. 14.1. Fractured testis, seen 3 h following trauma. Sagittal section: rupture of the tunica albuginea anteriorly over less than 1 cm. Interruption of its echoic line and testicular tear filled with a small hematocele. Conservative surgical repair was possible

Hematocele

Hematocele is defined as a blood collection located between the two layers of the tunica vaginalis and represents the most frequent posttraumatic injury of the scrotum (SIEGEL 1997). Hematocele may occur as an isolated finding or is associated with an underlying traumatic lesion of the testis. In half of the cases, testicular rupture is associated with a hematocele (MUNTER and FALESKI 1989). In the subacute phase, clots in the hematocele can mask a testicular fracture or rupture. Careful examination should localize the normal testis, which can be displaced to a peripheral location in the scrotum (COHEN et al. 1992). For that reason, US should always be performed as early as possible following trauma. US appearances depend on the age of the hematoma and the degree of liquefaction (Figs. 14.2 and 14.3). Recently clotted blood is hyperechoic, and is often associated with an anechoic fluid-like component. Both a large hematocele or progressive scrotal enlargement are indications for surgery in order to avoid testicular damage by compression. Evacuation of hematocele is advisable to relieve disability and accelerate a return to normal (ALTARAC 1994).

Testicular Hematoma

A hematoma is usually associated with a testicular fracture adjacent to the hematoma. Consequently a careful and detailed examination of the testicular albuginea should be obtained. However, hematoma can also occur as an isolated finding. A testicular hematoma is seen as a rounded, often subcapsular area, which presents various echoic patterns, depending on the age of blood: echoic, mixed, or hypoechoic (Fig. 14.4). No vascular flow is recorded by color Doppler inside a hematoma. A clot may be difficult to distinguish from exteriorized testicular content when the testicular margin is unclear (HERBENER 1996). When present as an isolated finding, no treatment is necessary. Follow-up US examination after several weeks is indicated to exclude an underlying hypovascular testicular tumor: an isolated posttraumatic hematoma should normally progressively decrease in size.

Testicular Dislocation

Dislocation of the testis is an uncommon occurrence. Fewer than 100 cases of testicular dislocation secondary to trauma have been reported

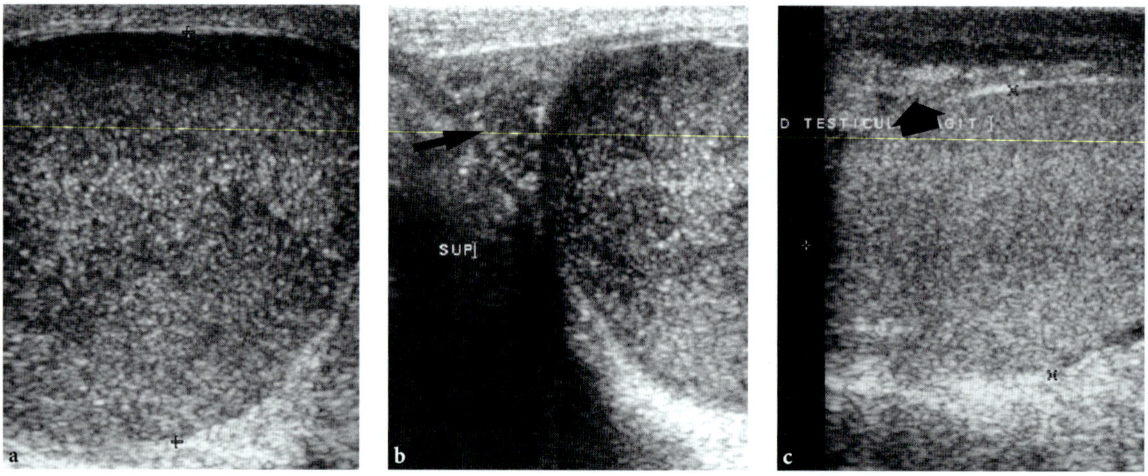

Fig. 14.2a–c. Acute hematocele following a minor trauma in a hemophilic patient. **a** A large hematocele is located in the superior interepididymotesticular recess and shows a highly echoic and homogeneous pattern caused by the presence of fresh blood. **b** The epididymal head (*arrow*) is seen cranial to the hematocele. **c** The testicle shows a normal US pattern and is surrounded by the hematocele extending anteriorly (*arrow*)

a
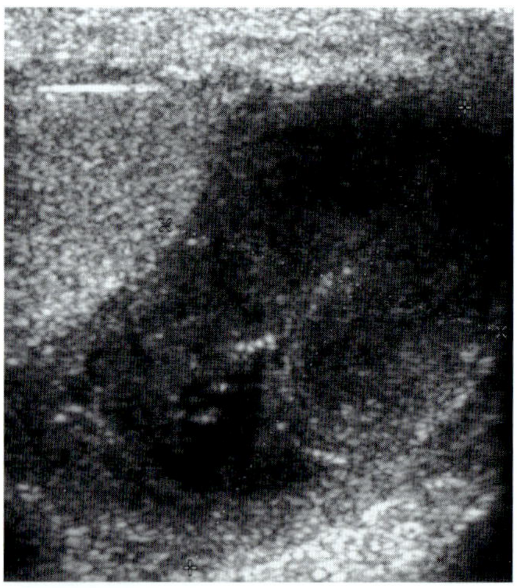

Fig. 14.3a–c. Hematocele seen 2 weeks following a violent trauma. **a** Sagittal section through the lower pole of the testicle: large organized blood collection beneath the testis, situated in the tunica vaginalis. **b** Cranial sagittal section: the entire epididymis appears slightly enlarged and hypoechoic. **c** The testicular vascular map appears unaffected on color Doppler confirming the absence of compression. However, considering the size of hematocele, surgical drainage was performed

b
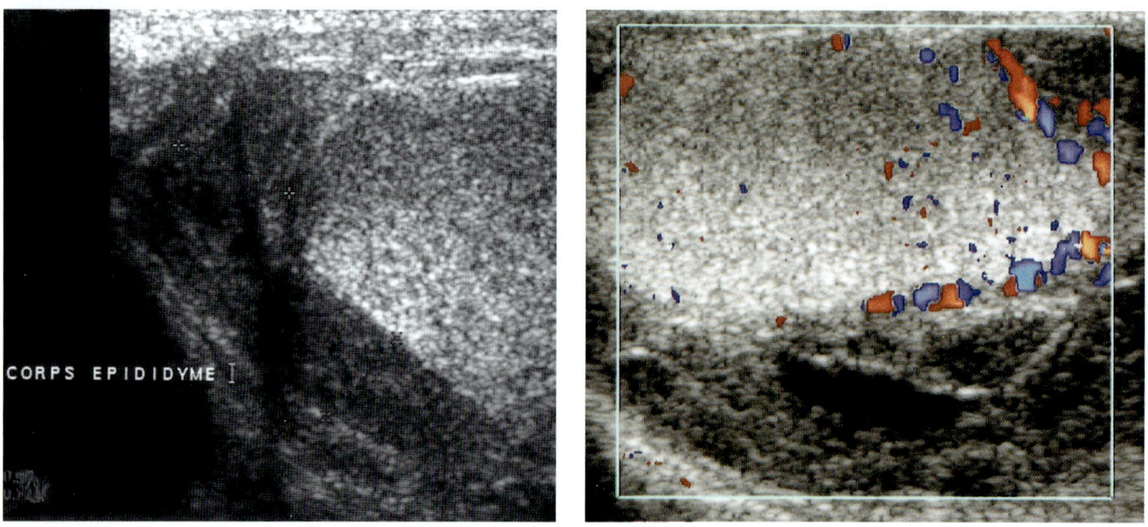

c

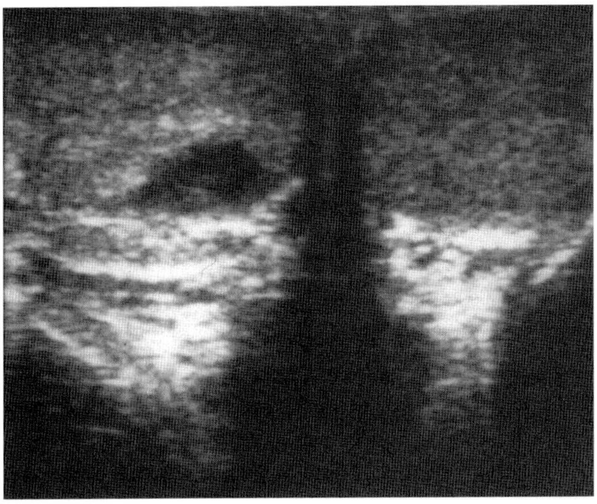

Fig. 14.4. Small subcapsular testicular hematoma diagnosed 3 days following trauma. Bilateral transverse section through the testis. Hematoma is seen as a small elongated hypoechoic subcapsular area located posteriorly in the right testicle. The remaining testicle appears slightly more echoic due to edema and contusion. Clinical and US follow-up showed regression of the hematoma several weeks later

(O'Donnell et al. 1998). Unilateral or bilateral dislocation may occur. Surgical reduction is often required and should be early, as spontaneous reduction is rare (Tan and Lee 1998). Usually posttraumatic testicular dislocation occurs immediately following trauma, but may be progressive over several days (Schwartz and Faerber 1994). Dislocation of the testicle can be noticed by the patient only weeks or months after the trauma (Ishikawa et al. 1990). The dislocated testis can migrate to the abdomen when an inguinal hernia is present (Feder et al. 1991).

14.6.3.3 Epididymal Injury

Injury to the epididymis occurs in about 21% with scrotal trauma and is rarely an isolated finding (Buchberger et al. 1990). The most frequent injury is an incomplete separation from the testis, usually associated with a swelling of the epididymis. In US, this type of lesion may be suspected when an abnormal enlargement of the interepididymal-testicular recess, or a hypoechoic, diffuse enlargement of the whole epididymis are seen. Epididymal hematoma shows as an enlarged hyperechoic epididymis, whereas posttraumatic epididymitis gives a hypoechoic swelling (Buchberger et al. 1990). Color Doppler may show diffuse or sometimes focal epididymal hyperemia, which might be indistinguishable from infectious epididymitis (Gordon et al. 1996). Usually, epididymal injury does not require surgical treatment, but a localized laceration of the epididymis may lead to late fibrotic changes.

14.6.3.4 Spermatic Cord Injury

Hematoma

In cases of blunt testicular trauma, rupture of the spermatic cord is not directly evidenced, but rather a hematoma at the site of laceration. On US, the hematoma is demonstrated by a predominantly hypoechoic rounded collection, located above both the epididymis and the testis. Such a hematoma is usually caused by an injury of the venous plexus. The most important role of US is to confirm, by color Doppler, that there is no significant arterial compression and that the testicular vascularization is unaffected (Fig. 14.5). This is a common observation, because the hematoma is self-limited by the connective tissue of the spermatic cord.

Torsion

Torsion of the spermatic cord may occur in case of scrotal trauma, especially in a young individual, suffering from a testicular dislocation but also in case of an apparently benign sports injury (Yagi et al. 1999; Kochakarn et al. 2000). A history of scrotal trauma is present in 5% of cases of torsion of the testis and in 10% with torsion of the testicular appendages (Elsaharty et al. 1984). Usually the diagnosis is made by clinical examination and search for the cremaster reflex. However, if inconclusive, US is mandatory and is able to confirm the diagnosis, based on the following observations: the most conclusive sign is the frank hypovascularization of the testicle, with a lack of the normal central vascularization, which is well demonstrated by comparison with the normal contralateral testis, using color Doppler. The lack of central blood flow at color Doppler in the affected testis compared with the normal blood flow in the contralateral testis is the key finding (Kass and Lundak 1997; Horstman 1997) (Figs. 14.6–14.9). On the contrary, the presence of central testicular blood in an acute scrotum does not rule out torsion of the spermatic cord. It should be kept in mind that the key finding is the lack of central testicular blood flow and not the waveforms of the spermatic cord arteries, at times confusing because they depend on the severity of the torsion, which may sometimes be incomplete or intermittent.

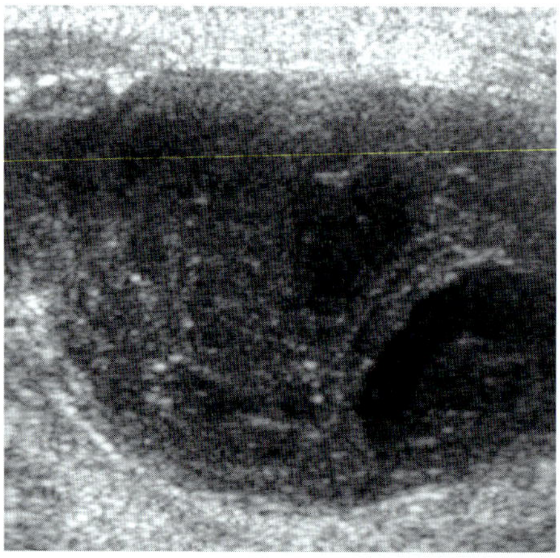

a

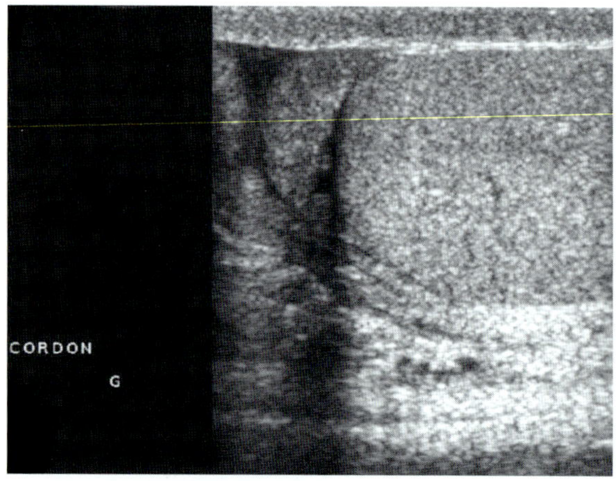

c

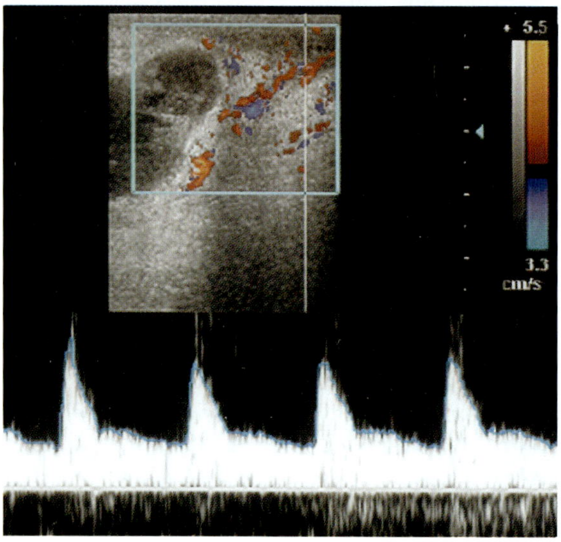

b

Fig. 14.5a–c. Hematoma of the left spermatic cord, seen 3 weeks following blunt scrotal injury. **a** The chronic, organized blood collection is hypoechoic. **b** On the color Doppler, the wave of the spermatic artery is not affected. **c** The left testis and epididymis show a normal appearance on US

The following morphological signs are not always present together, but in our experience, the presence of two of them is enough for establishing the diagnosis of acute or subacute torsion o the spermatic cord:

- Enlargement of the scrotal part of the spermatic cord, which is seen as a 2- or 3-cm-thick, abnormal round or linear echoic structure, traversed by hypoechoic thin structures (vessels) on transverse and longitudinal scans. This structure should be distinguished from the epididymis, which is usually somewhat enlarged and echoic, due to hemorrhagic stasis, but always hypovascular and therefore easily differentiated from an epididymis on color Doppler.

- Abnormal position of the epididymal head and the associated hydatids, which are rotated beneath the testis, in case of a rotation of 180°. Consequently, the head of epididymis will be no longer present above the testis but beneath it, and is shown as an enlarged, echoic, but overall hypovascular structure on color Doppler, sometimes associated with one or two small sessile and pedunculated hydatids.

- A mild hydrohematocele is almost always present, especially in cases with a time interval between onset of torsion to diagnosis. It is due to a hemorrhagic effusion and is shown as a small amount of septated collection in the tunica vaginalis, between the testis and other scrotal layers, which are usually only moderately thickened.

Exploratory orchidotomy should not be delayed, when US is positive.

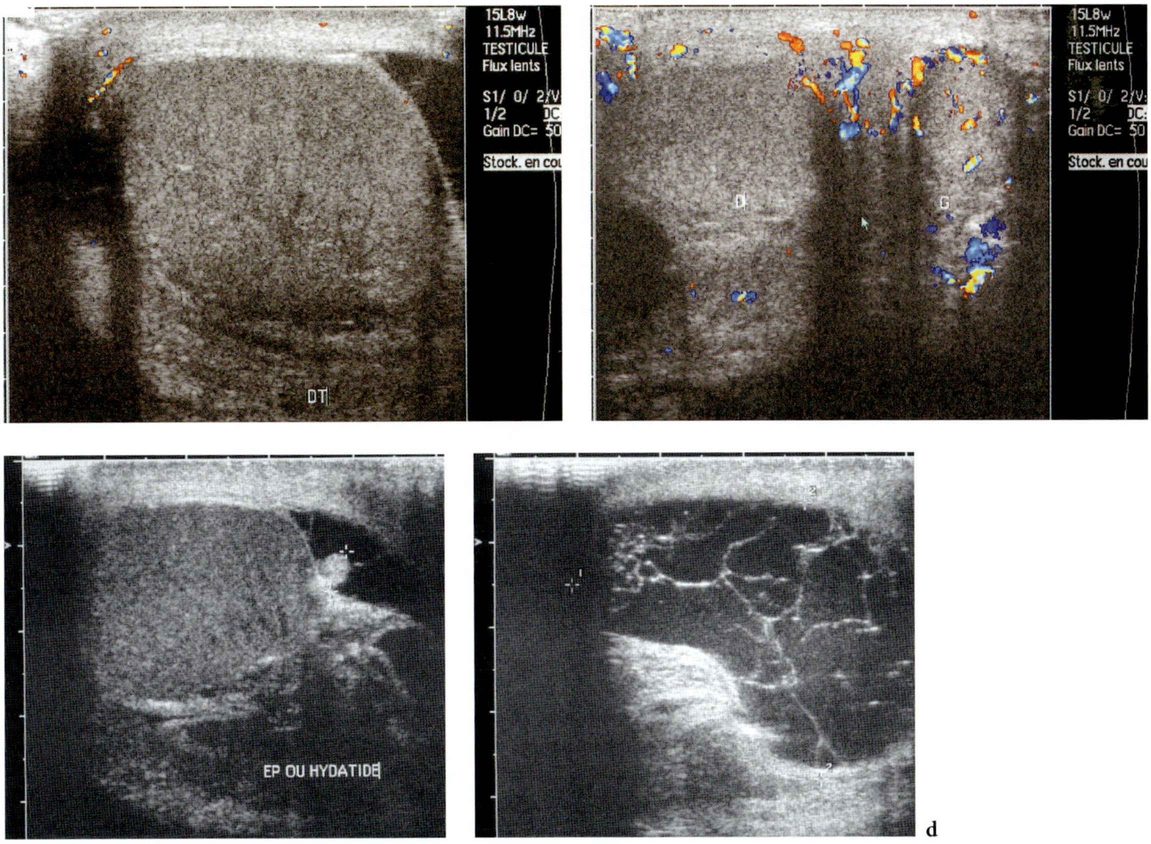

Fig. 14.6a–d. Torsion of the spermatic cord seen at day 12 in a young adult presenting acute scrotal pain after a physical training. **a** Sagittal section of the right testis, with color Doppler: the testis is slightly enlarged and hypoechoic, particularly around the hilum. **b** Transverse section through both testicles, with color Doppler: there is a striking difference between the normal vascular map of the left testis and the totally hypovascular right testis due to ischemia. **c** The head of the epididymis or a hydatid is abnormally located below the lower pole of the testis. **d** Mild hydrohematocele

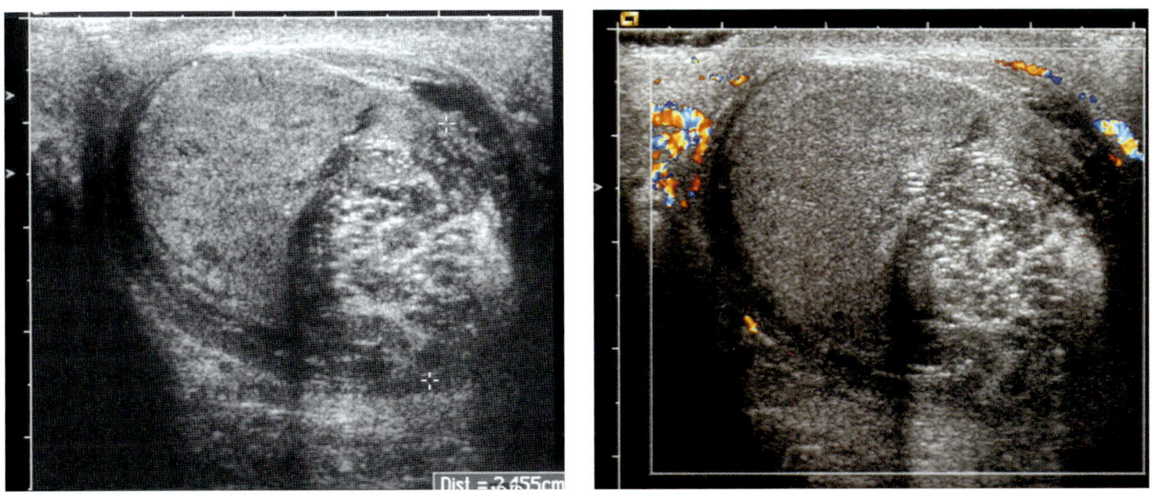

Fig. 14.7a, b. Torsion of the spermatic cord in a 13-year-old patient after a skiing injury, misdiagnosed in the acute phase and seen on US 5 weeks later when the patient complained of an enlarged and painful scrotum. **a** Sagittal sections show a 2- to 3-cm-thick echoic, round structure below the testis, which corresponds to the twisted intrascrotal spermatic cord. The testicle itself above is enlarged and heterogeneous and shows small hypoechoic areas which represent ischemic changes. **b** Color Doppler confirms absence of testicular vascularization. Only peripheral vascularization of the scrotal layers are seen

a
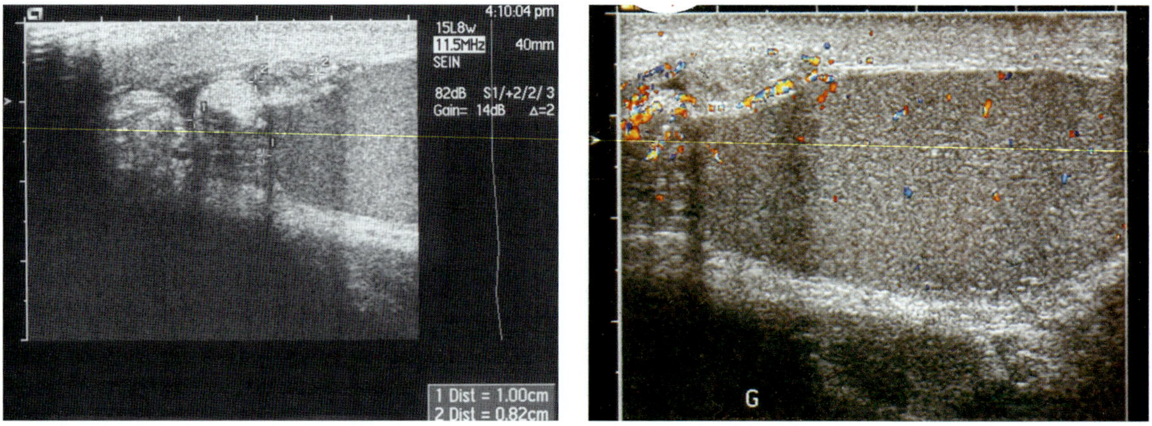

b

Fig. 14.8a,b. Torsion of the hydatid which appeared in a teenager after a rugby workout and was confirmed by surgery. **a** Sagittal section through the upper part of the scrotum demonstrates an abnormal small elongated anterior structure, which is solid and slightly echoic. **b** The same section on color Doppler shows a normal vascular pattern of the testis and peripheral vascularization. The US aspect of the epididymis was unremarkable. The suggested diagnosis of twisted hydatid was confirmed by surgery

a
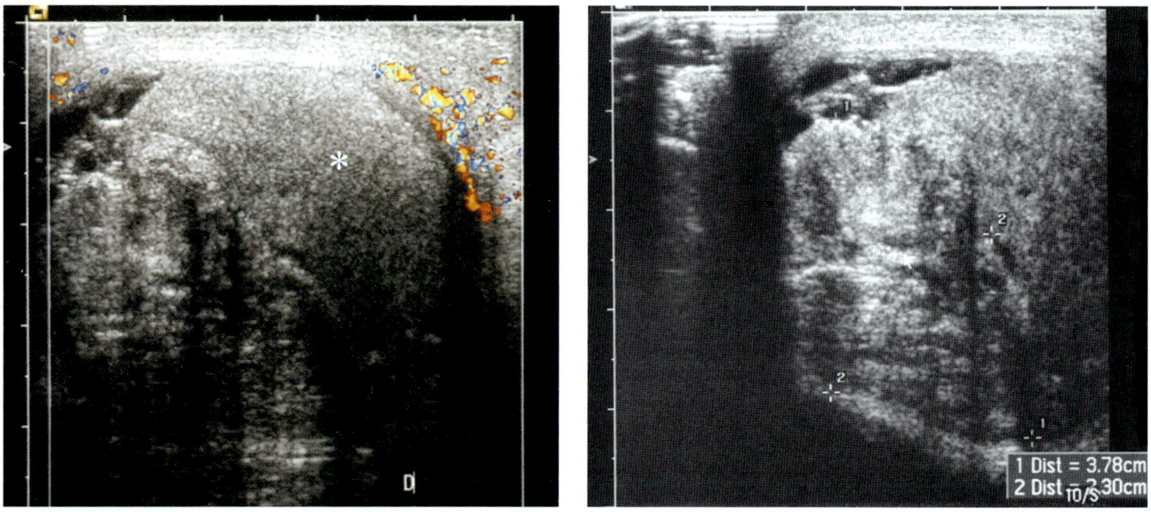

b

Fig. 14.9a,b. Torsion of the spermatic cord seen at the 3rd month. Transverse section through the scrotum. **a** Color Doppler shows an entirely hypovascular testis (*asterisk*) compressed by an enlarged posterior echoic structure which comprises the twisted spermatic cord. **b** The same section shows also a moderate hydrohematocele at the upper pole

14.6.4 Chronic Blunt Injury

As in the acute phase, any component of the scrotum may be involved, but the most worrisome lesion is testicular:

- Testicular atrophy:
  - Diffuse
  - Segmental
- Testicular pseudotumoral hematoma
- Pseudo-tumoral chronic hematocele
- Tubular ectasia of the rete testis

14.6.4.1 Testicular Atrophy

The causative link of a testicular atrophy and a previous injury is established by the history of the patient. A dislocated testis may remain unnoticed for months following injury and undergo atrophy (Ishikawa et al. 1990). Testicular atrophy is a frequent sequela of scrotal trauma and may occur in 50% of patients without surgical repair (Cross et al. 1999) (Fig. 14.10). The usual mechanism is postischemic changes. Post-traumatic testicular atrophy may be severe, leaving a residual testicle less than 1 cm^3. In our experience, if

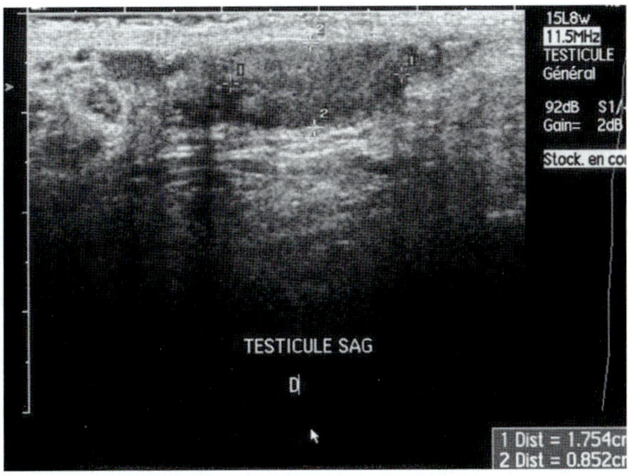

Fig. 14.10. Severe atrophy of the testis following a direct scrotal trauma in childhood. The thickness of the testis is less than 1 cm. A posttraumatic atrophic testis is often moderately heterogeneous, but without a suspicious pseudotumoral hypoechoic nodule seen

the trauma occurred during childhood, the contralateral testis often appears larger than normal (20 cm^3 or more), as if there were a compensatory testicular hypertrophy. The atrophic testis appears slightly heterogeneous, but without a frank hypoechoic nodule or focalized abnormal vascularization, but reduced flow on color Doppler. If a nodule is found, a nonpalpable tumor should be suspected.

14.6.4.2 Fibrous Testicular Degeneration

Fibrous changes within the testicle usually appear secondary to a hematoma or a localized contusion, often in a subcapsular location (Fig. 14.11). They appear as hypoechoic hypovascular bands without a nodular pattern. Diagnosis is easy when a history of trauma is reported, but may be difficult otherwise. The most determinant sonographic finding is a hypoechoic linear band.

14.6.4.3 Chronic Testicular Hematoma

A chronic testicular hematoma may persist if regression is not complete. The clinical presentation and US findings mimic a testicular nodule. However, on US, there is no frank central vascularization, but a perinodular vascular circle. Exploratory surgery is mandatory in many cases for confirmation of the diagnosis. Nevertheless, it is helpful to suggest the diagnosis of hematoma on US to allow a partial orchidectomy. Extemporaneous examination of a testicular biopsy will rule out tumor (Fig. 14.12). Proliferative spindle cell lesions with a pseudotumoral appearance may develop in association with chronic hematoma. These nodules are composed of myofibroblasts and pronounced smooth muscle differentiation (Papadimitriou and Drachenberg 1994). Isolated or multiple calcifications may be observed as a sequela of testicular trauma (Fig. 14.13).

14.6.4.4 Testicular or Epididymal Cyst

Posttraumatic chronic testicular or epididymal cysts are not well known, neither clinically nor on US (Fig. 14.14). It is difficult to differentiate epididymal

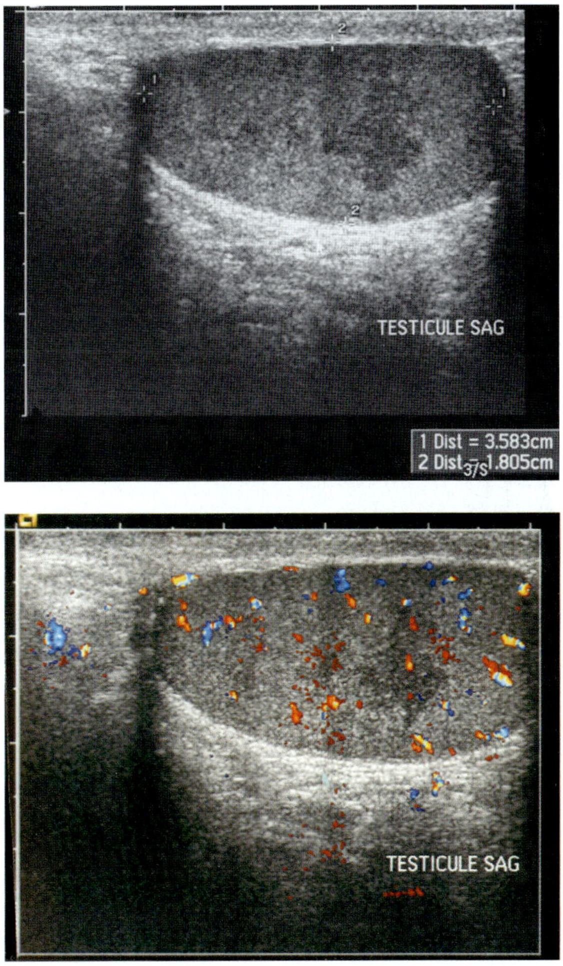

a b

Fig. 14.11a, b. Pseudotumoral fibrotic testicular changes after chronic trauma. **a** Sagittal section shows a hypoechoic intratesticular area presenting a geographical contour without a nodular aspect. **b** Color Doppler shows unaffected testicular vascularization in the hypoechoic area. Surgical biopsy was performed and confirmed intratesticular granulomatous changes

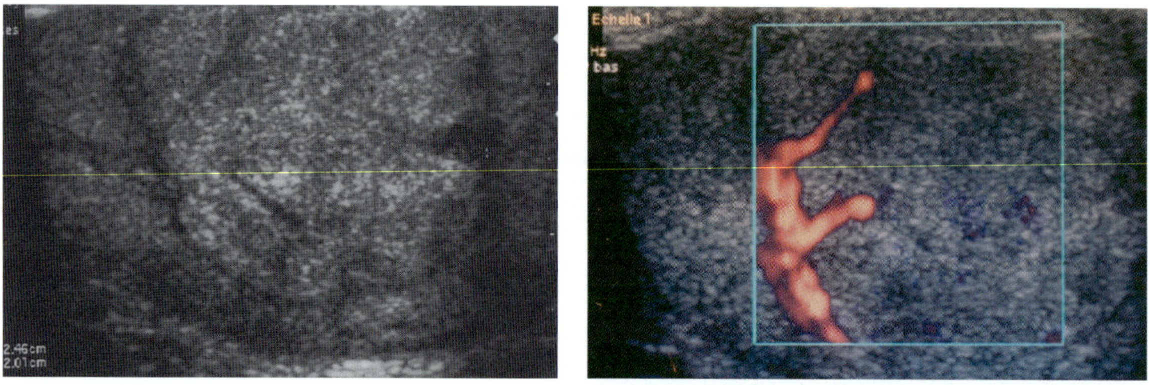

a b

Fig. 14.12a, b. Chronic organized testicular hematoma mimicking a testicular tumor both on clinical examination and US in a 35-year-old man presenting with an enlarged testicle. **a** Transverse section shows a large echoic intratesticular mass surrounded by a thin, smooth hypoechoic line. **b** Power Doppler shows no central vascularization of the mass, but a number of vessels penetrating into the lesion. In the absence of a history of trauma, a testicular tumor could not be ruled out. At surgery, a chronic and well-organized testicular hematoma without associated tumoral lesion was found

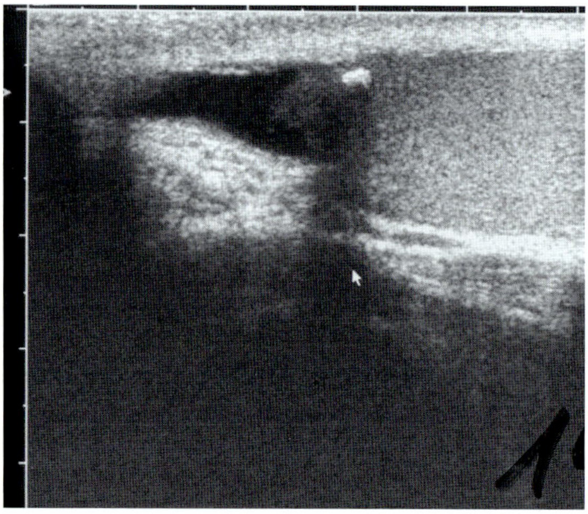

Fig. 14.13. Isolated calcification of the testicular layers following chronic trauma. A unique calcification of 3 mm is demonstrated by US at the junction of the head of the epididymis and the otherwise normal testis (*arrow*)

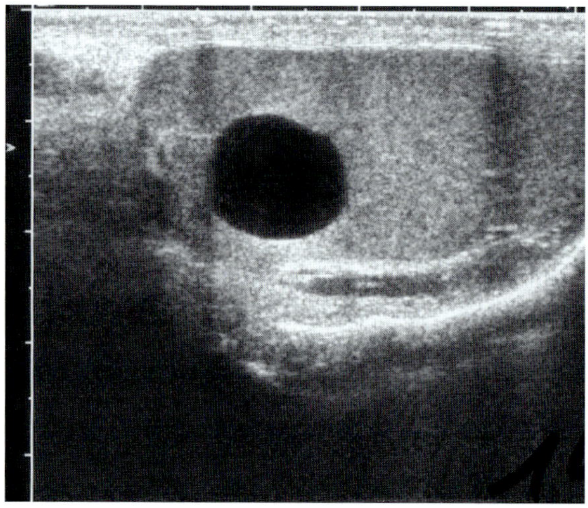

Fig. 14.14. Large isolated cyst of the testis in a 50-year-old patient with a history of severe perineal and scrotal trauma. This posttraumatic cyst was probably caused by a localized parenchymal loss

or paraepididymal cysts from embryonal remnants or congenital cysts or postinfectious cysts.

14.6.4.5 Chronic Hematocele

Persistent chronic hematocele is a rare condition, which is usually observed in elderly patients presenting with an enlarged hard scrotum, mimicking a testicular tumor (Martin 1992). US may not make it easy to separate chronic hematocele from a reactive hydrocele. In many cases, US establishes the correct diagnosis by showing a compressed, normal, or atrophic testis, located deep within a trabecular hypoechoic and hypovascular mass of the tunica vaginalis.

14.6.5 Iatrogenic Injury

We will not go into acute postsurgical complications, which are rare.

14.6.5.1
Pneumoscrotum

Pneumoscrotum is a cause of retroperitoneal air that extends mainly through retroperitoneal pathways to the scrotum. It can be observed with blunt or penetrating scrotal and pelvic injury. Among iatrogenic causes, endoscopic retroperitoneal perforation of the gastrointestinal tract is a frequent cause. Pneumomediastinum may extend to the abdomen, responsible for pneumoscrotum (KLIMACH et al. 1990). Other causes include spontaneous perforation of the retroperitoneal segment of the gastrointestinal tract, gas-producing retroperitoneal infection, necrotizing pancreatitis, and in the past, diagnostic pneumoretroperitoneum (HAN et al. 1985). Among other iatrogenic insults, acute scrotal lesions can occur consecutive to barium peritonitis, through a patent processus vaginalis (GRABLE and MOAZAM 1985). Imaging is not required for the diagnosis. The scrotal air usually does not compress the testicle.

14.6.5.2
Testicular Atrophy

This complication may be observed after an arterial injury. It is usually segmental, the location depending on which testicular arterial branch has been injured (Fig. 14.15). The appearance on US is a hypoechoic well-shaped, often somewhat triangular but never round, subcapsular area with no significant vascularization on Doppler color examination.

14.6.5.3
Fibrous Changes Following Spermatozoid Extraction for Intracytoplasmic Spermatozoid Injection

Fibrous changes for intracytoplasmic spermatozoid injection (ICSI) are usually hypoechoic, but sometimes hyperechoic depending on the setting of the US examination, and located on the needle path (BACKUS et al. 1994; YAGAN 2000). Sometimes, after several months, an isolated microlith may be noted at the site of biopsy (Fig. 14.16). Since this technique is becoming more widespread, US images should be known by radiologists and not be confused with suspicious aspects of cancer in these infertile patients, who have a higher cancer risk than the population at large.

14.6.5.4
Tubular Ectasia

This benign entity is seen more frequently in middle-aged patients, who have undergone previous pelvic surgery, in particular repair of an inguinal hernia. The seminiferous tubules are ectatic in the rete testis (Fig. 14.17). The US aspect should not be confused with a hypoechoic tumor, especially when there is no associated spermatocele (OLDER and WATSON 1994). Similar changes may be observed after vasectomy. The key findings for diagnosis are the following: linear or cystic hypoechoic small areas with multiple echoic interfaces with no Doppler flow, which are located within the scrotal mediastinum and are

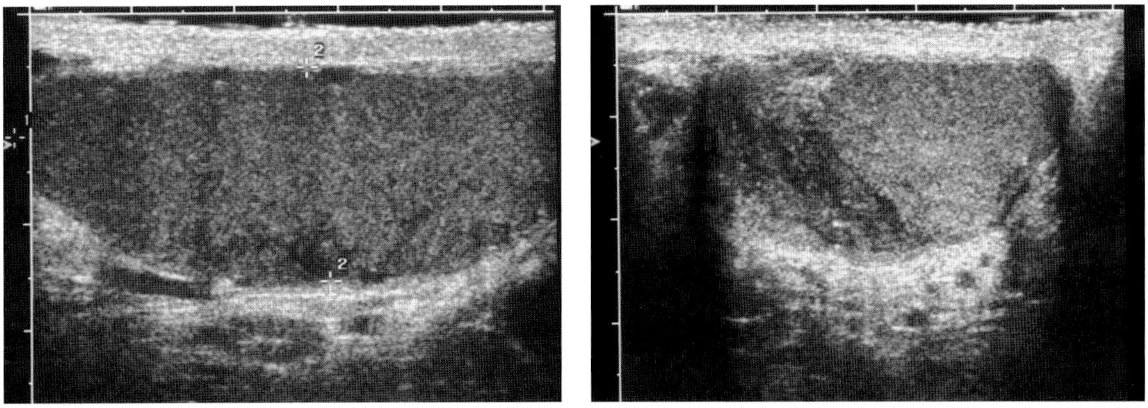

a b

Fig. 14.15a, b. Interlobular fibrosis of the testicle following surgery for cryptorchidism. **a** Sagittal section demonstrates a slightly hypotrophic testicle presenting hypoechoic linear bands stretching from the albuginea to the hilum. Note also, the small hypoechoic structures that represent subalbugineal veins, which are often more obvious after scrotal surgery. **b** Typical aspect of interlobular fibrotic changes along the vascular intratesticular arterioles

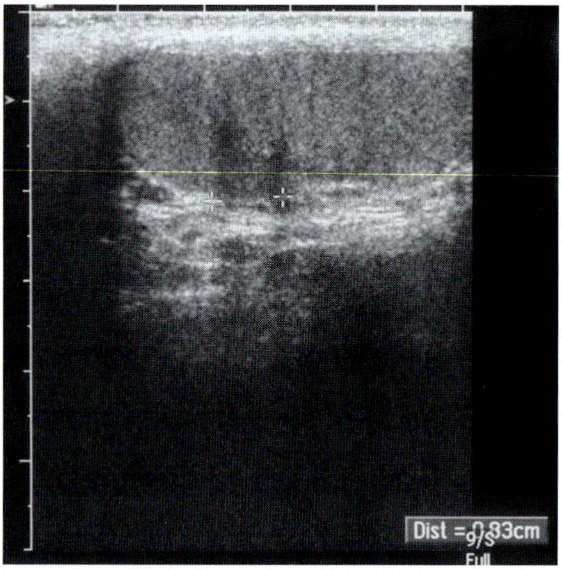

a

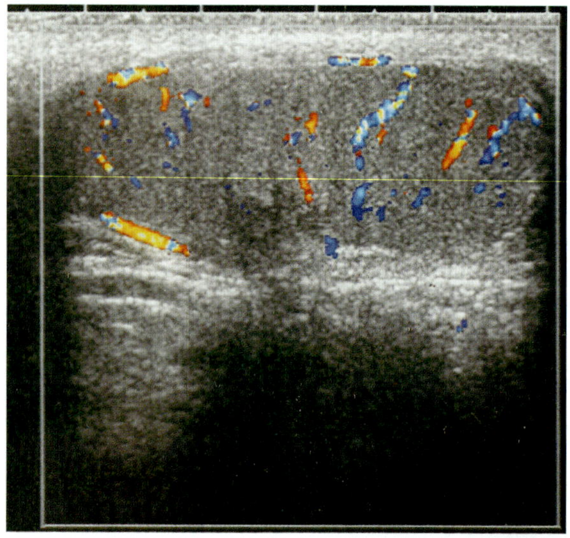

b

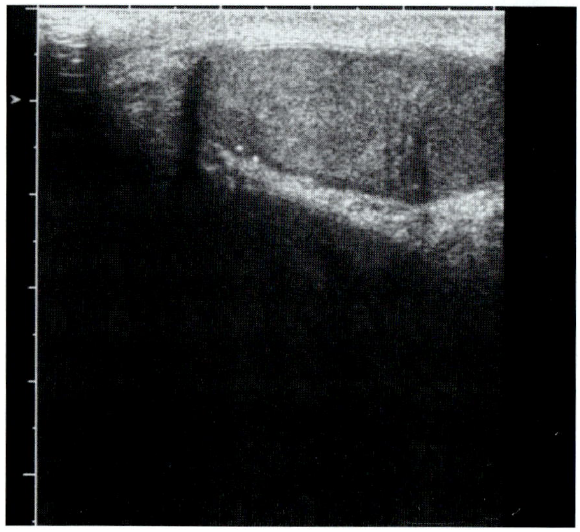

c

Fig. 14.16a–c. Iatrogenic testicular changes after testicular biopsies for spermatozoid extraction in an azoospermic patient. US was obtained 10 months later. **a** On the sagittal section, a well-demarcated hypoechoic area due to the biopsy is shown. **b** Hypovascular appearance on color Doppler. **c** Note the presence of two microliths located posteriorly, on a biopsy path. A preprocedure US was normal

sometimes associated with paraepididymal contiguous cysts or spermatoceles. Ectasia is almost always bilateral but often asymmetrical (Brown et al. 1992; Cho and Kosek 1995; Colangelo et al. 1995). The US aspect is pathognomonic and MRI is not necessary for confirmation of the diagnosis (Tartar et al. 1993) (Fig. 14.18). This entity must be recognized to avoid unnecessary biopsy or surgical exploration.

14.7 Results

Correlative studies between US and surgery showed a close to 100% sensitivity of US for testicular injuries and an 80% specificity for fractures of the tunica albuginea (Sasso et al. 1995). Small fractures of the tunica are not always detected with US (Jeffrey et al. 1983; Kratzik et al. 1989). Tiny fractures of the tunica are clearly shown with MRI, which is able to exquisitely delineate the hypointense line of the tunica albuginea. Early torsion is the greatest provider of false negative results (Fournier et al. 1985). However, with the advent of color and power Doppler, which depict very low flow of blood inside the testis, the results are markedly improved. US had a tendency to understage testicular injury (Sasso et al. 1995). In other studies, staging of trauma severity by US was 100% accurate in gunshot wounds and US is reliable in the diagnosis of testicular rupture, which indicates surgical repair in all cases (Lewis and Michell 1991; Pecori et al. 1991).

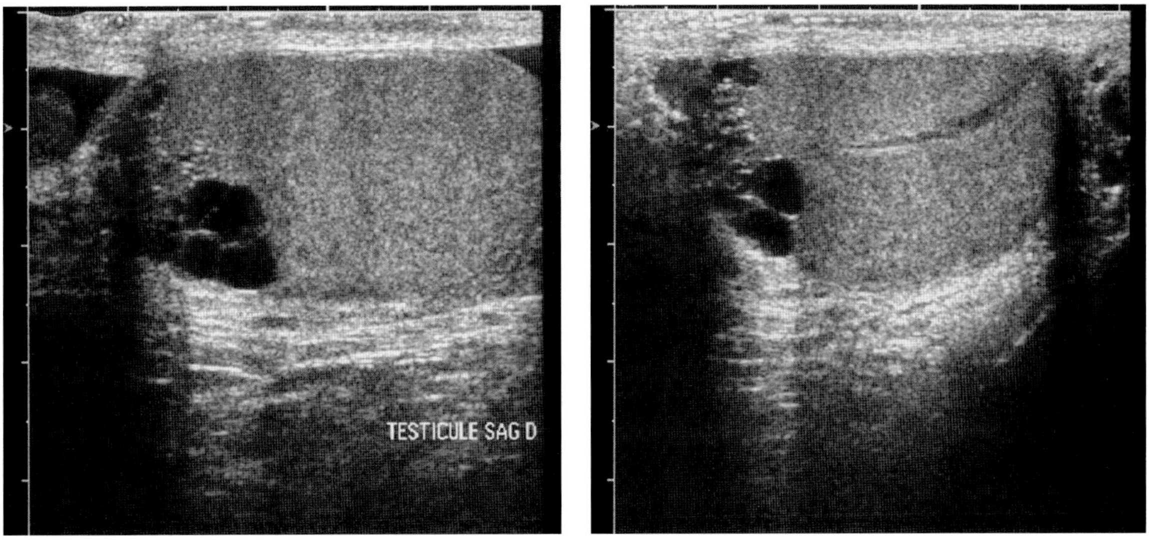

a b

Fig. 14.17a, b. Bilateral tubular ectasia of the rete testis in a 60-year-old patient with a history of rectal surgery. **a, b** Transverse scan through the right testis showing the pathognomonic sonographic aspect of tubular ectasia of the rete testis. A network of tiny linear or round transsonic structures is localized in the testicular hilum. Note also a well-demonstrated transmediastinal artery, which should not be confused with a fracture in case of a history of acute trauma

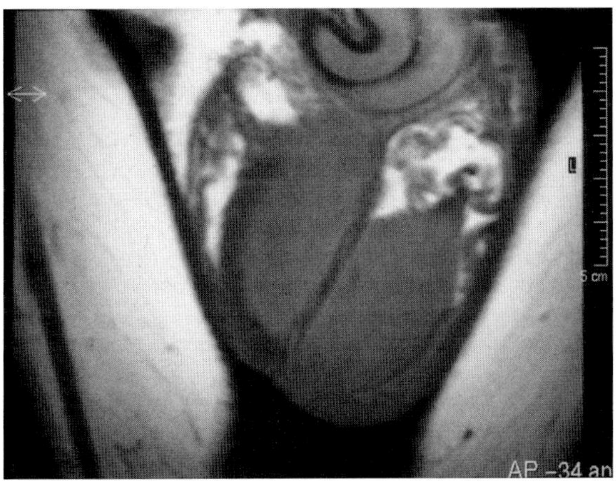

a

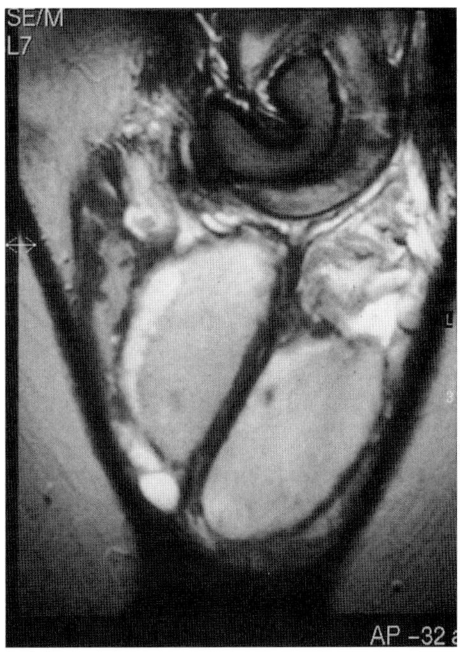

b

Fig. 14.18a, b. Typical tubular ectasia of the rete testis on MRI. **a, b** Both are coronal images through both testes. **a** A T1-weighted image. **b** A T2-weighted image. The tubular ectasia is easily recognizable as a fluid structure along the hilum, hypointense on T1 and hyperintense on T2, with also a tiny associated spermatocele below the otherwise normal testis. Note also the bilateral varicocele

US is particularly valuable in patients with intratesticular hematoma without hematocele and with a reassuring physical examination (Kratzik et al. 1989; Martinez Pineiro et al. 1992). In 65% of the cases, US showed lesions that were unsuspected clinically in blunt contusion (Sellem et al. 1987). A heterogeneous parenchymal echo pattern is the most reliable predictive sign of testicular abnormality, but a large hematoma can obscure the compressed testis. In this case, color Doppler, by showing the testicular vascularization, greatly helps to recognize a compressed but normal testis. US is also particularly valuable to predict conservative management of simple testicular contusion (Patil and Onuora 1994). The differential diagnosis between hematocele, pyocele, or exudative hydrocele may remain problematic theoretically, but in fact, the clinical findings are different and it is usually easy to establish the correct diagnosis. The other diagnoses, such as scrotal hematoma, peritesticular fluid, torsion, posttraumatic epididymitis, epididymal hematoma, and testicular rupture are established with confidence in the vast majority of cases (Schaffer 1985). The main advantage of US is to differentiate testicular from extratesticular pathology with almost error-free confidence (Rifkin et al. 1985).

14.8 Management

Surgical revision is still obtained in the majority of patients with significant scrotal trauma. However, hematoma limited to the scrotal wall or a limited skin penetration does not require revision (Sasso et al. 1994). Early surgical revision should be obtained in case of ruptured testis and hematocele. The decision to operate should be firmly based on clinical findings, aided by US (Table 14.1). Surgical management in the acute posttraumatic phase includes evacuation of a hematoma or a hematocele, or partial or total orchidectomy. Testicular atrophy should be avoided by relieving pressure caused by intratesticular bleeding (Larsen et al. 1993). The testicular salvage rate in penetrating injury is 35%, 97% having been surgically explored (Cline et al. 1998). The testicular salvage rate is greater than 80% when rupture is repaired within 72 h. If surgery is delayed, orchidectomy may be required in more than 50% of the patients (Cass and Luxenberg 1991; Bhandary et al. 1992; Herbener 1996; Martinez Pineiro et al. 1992).

In series with predominantly blunt scrotal injuries, surgery is performed in 81–100% of the cases with a testicular preservation of 80% (Altarac 1994; El Moussaoui et al. 1996). In one report, surgical exploration was obtained in 82% of blunt scrotal contusion, but 50% of patients without surgical revision had orchidectomy (Barthelemy et al. 1992).

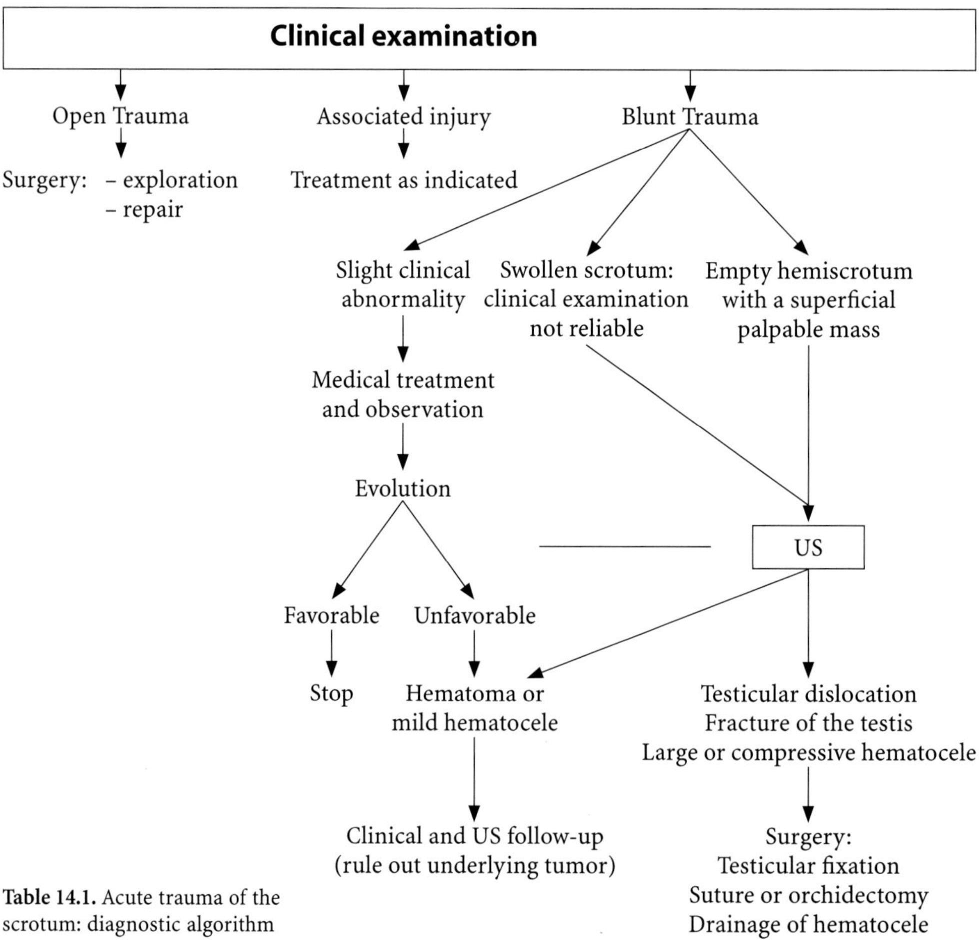

Table 14.1. Acute trauma of the scrotum: diagnostic algorithm

In another report of 17 patients with blunt scrotal injury, but without hematocele in 9 patients with normal palpation, US showed parenchymal lesions in 6, such as subcapsular hematoma or contusion, indicating surgery in 6 (Martinez Pineiro et al. 1992). Nonsurgical management in blunt scrotal injury can now reach 47–73%, depending on severity of injury of the included patients (Anderson et al. 1983; Bautista Casanovas et al. 1992). Intratesticular and small intrascrotal hematoma can be treated conservatively (Kratzik et al. 1989). In one limited series, 9 out of 11 patients with hematoma, hydrocele, or hematocele were treated conservatively (Learch et al. 1995). Anecdotally, a completely severed testis was replanted with microsurgical anastomosis of the sectioned funiculus (Xu et al. 1988). Closed reduction of a dislocated testis may be attempted if the testis is palpable in the upper scrotum, but most often surgical fixation is required (O'Donnell et al. 1998).

14.9 Conclusion

A direct perineal impact and motorcycle fall with direct trauma on the reservoir are classical mechanisms of blunt scrotal injury. Except in cases of the rare testicular dislocation, where one or both hemiscrotum are empty, clinical examination of usually enlarged and painful posttraumatic scrotum is limited. High-resolution US with color Doppler is the most powerful imaging technique to evidence testicular fracture oand/or hematocele. There is general agreement for prompt surgery in order to avoid secondary orchidectomy or testicular atrophy. The value of MRI for scrotal trauma as well as for associated abdominopelvic injuries has to be investigated.

References

Altarac S (1994) Management of 53 cases of testicular trauma. Eur Urol 25:119–123

Amoury RA, Barth GW, Mall RT, Rhodes PG, Holder TM, Ashcraft KW (1982) Scrotal ecchymosis: sign of intraperitoneal hemorrhage in the newborn. South Med J 7:1471–1478

Anderson KA, McAninch JW, Jeffrey RB, Laing FC (1983) Ultrasonography for the diagnosis and staging of blunt scrotal trauma. J Urol 130:933–935

Backus ML, Mack LA, Middleton WD, King BF, Winter TC III, True LD (1994) Testicular microlithiasis: imaging appearances and pathologic correlation. Radiology 192:781–785

Barthelemy Y, Delmas V, Villers A, Baron JC, Sibert A, Boccon-Gibod L (1992) Scrotal trauma. Report of 33 cases. Prog Urol 2:628–634

Bautista Casanovas A, Gonzales AF, Iglesias DIZ JL et al (1992) Scrotal trauma in childhood. An Esp Pediatr 37:477–480

Bhandary P, Abbitt PL, Watson L (1992) Ultrasound diagnosis of traumatic testicular rupture. J Clin Ultrasound 20: 346–348

Blaivas M, Sierzenski P (2001) Emergency ultrasonography in the evaluation of the acute scrotum. Acad Emerg Med 8:85–89

Bockisch A, van Ahlen H, Makarewitsch J, Ruhlemann J, Hotze A, Biersack HJ (1989) The significance of testicular scintigraphy for the differential diagnosis of the acute scrotum. [in German] Nuklearmedizin 28:84–87

Brown DL, Benson LB, Doherty FJ et al (1992) Cystic testicular mass caused by dilated rete testis. Sonographic findings in 31 cases. AJR 158:1257–59

Buchberger W, Furstchegger A, Kastlunger W, Jenewein K, Waldenberger P (1990) The value of sonography in scrotal trauma. ROFO 153:385–389

Cass AS, Luxenberg M (1991) Testicular injuries. Urology 37: 528–530

Chen DC, Holder LE, Kaplan GN (1986) Correlation of radionuclide imaging and diagnostic ultrasound in scrotal diseases. J Nucl Med 27:1774–1781

Cho CS, Kosek J (1985) Cystic dysplasia of the testis: sonographic and pathologic findings. Radiology 156:777–778

Cline KJ, Mata JA, Venable DD, Eastham JA (1998) Penetrating trauma to the male external genitalia. J Trauma 44: 492–494

Cohen HL, Shapiro ML, Haller JO, Glasberg K (1992) Sonography of intrascrotal hematomas simulating testicular rupture in adolescents. Pediatr Radiol 22:296–297

Colangelo SM, Fried K, Hyacinthe L, Fracchia JA (1995) Tubular ectasia of the rete testis: an ultrasound diagnosis. Urology 45:532–534

Comesana Davila E, da Silva EA, Pereiro Alvarez B, Meijide Rico F, Pesqueira Santiago D, Zungri Telo E (1999) Traumatic unilateral testicular dislocation. Arch Esp Urol 52: 278–280

Couvelaire R, Schimmel F (1976) Scrotal contusions. Concours Med 98:6785–6794

Cross JJ, Berman LH, Elliott PG, Irving S (1999) Scrotal trauma: a cause of testicular atrophy. Clin Radiol 54:317–320

Cummings JM, Boullier JA (2000) Scrotal dog bites. J Urol 164: 57–58

Dee KE, Deck AJ, Waitches GM (2000) Intratesticular pseudoaneurysm after blunt trauma. AJR 174:1136

De Peretti F, Cambas PM, Vaneau B, Argenson C (1993) The gasoline tank of motorcycles. Role in severe trauma of the pelvis. Presse Med 22:61–63

Dubinsky TJ, Chen P, Maklad N (1998) Color-flow and power Doppler imaging of the testes. World J Urol 16:35–40

El Kamel R, Atallah R, Rouis M, Mosbah AT (1997) Proposal of a classification of scrotal contusions. J Urol (Paris) 103: 17–19

El Moussaoui A, Jouale A, Benjelloun S (1996) Injuries of the scrotum. Analysis of 25 cases. J Urol (Paris) 102:88–91

Elsaharty S, Pranikoff K, Magoss IV, Sufrin G (1984) Traumatic torsion of the testis. J Urol 132:1155–1156

Feder M, Scchetti A, Myrick S (1991) Testicular dislocation following minor scrotal trauma. Am J Emerg Med 9:40–42

Ficarra V, Caleffi G, Mofferdin A, Zanon G, Tallarigo C, Malos-

sini G (1999) Penetrating trauma to the scrotum and the corpora cavernosa caused by gunshot. Urol Int 62:192–194
Finan BF, Redman JF (1985) Neonatal genital trauma. Urology 25:532–533
Fournier GR Jr, Laing FC, Jeffrey RB, McAninch JW (1985) High-resolution scrotal ultrasonography: a highly sensitive but nonspecific diagnostic technique. J Urol 134:490–493
Frauscher F, Klauser A, Hobisch A, Pallwein L, Stenzl A (2000) Subclinical microtraumatisation of the scrotal contents in extreme mountain biking. Lancet 356:1414
Gimbergues P, Guy L, Boyer L, Boiteux JP (1999) Traumatic dislocation of the testis. Report of three cases. Prog Urol 9:322–326
Gordon LM, Stein SM, Ralls PW (1996) Traumatic epididymitis: evaluation with color Doppler sonography. AJR 166: 1323–1325
Grable MS, Moazam F (1985) Acute scrotal lesion secondary to barium peritonitis in an infant. Urology 25:499–501
Haas CA, Brown SL, Spirnark JP (1999) Penile fracture and testicular rupture. World J Urol 17:101–106
Han SY, Tishler JM, Aldrete JS (1985) Extraperitoneal gas: compartmental localization and identification of source. J Can Assoc Radiol 36:17–21
Hendrikx AJ, Dang CL, Vroegindeweij D, Korte JH (1997) B-mode and colour-flow duplex ultrasonography: a useful adjunct in diagnosing scrotal diseases? Br J Urol 79:58–65
Hendry WF (2000) Testicular, epididymal and vasal injuries. Br J Urol 86:344–348
Henry JJ (1978) Unusual presentation of splenic ruptures. Soc Pediatr Urol Newslett 1:87
Herbener TE (1996) Ultrasound in the assessment of the acute scrotum. J Clin Ultrasound 24:405–421
Herbst RH, Polkey HJ (1936) Luxation testis traumatica and experimental study of mechanism. Am J Surg 34:18–20
Heydenrych JJ (1974) Haemoperitoneum and associated torsion of the testicle in the newborn. S Afr Med J 48:2221
Holder LE, Melloul M, Chen D (1981) Current status of radionuclide scrotal imaging. Semin Nucl Med 11:232–249
Horstman WG (1997) Scrotal imaging. Urol Clin North Am 24: 653–671
Hricak H, Filly RA (1983) Sonography of the scrotum. Invest Radiol 18:112–121
Hricak H, Hamm B, Kim B (eds) (1995) Imaging of the scrotum: textbook and atlas. Raven, New York, pp 49–92
Ishikawa J, Sengoku A, Umezu K, Eto H, Harada M, Kamidono S (1990) Traumatic dislocation of the testis: a case report. Hinyokika Kiyo 36:471–473
Jeffrey RB, Laing FC, Hricak H, McAninch JW (1983) Sonography of testicular trauma. AJR 141:993–995
Karpe B, Nybonde T (1989) Adrenal hemorrhage versus testicular torsion – a diagnostic dilemma in the neonate. Pediatr Surg Int 4:337
Kass EJ, Lundak B (1997) The acute scrotum. Pediatr Clin North Am 44:1251–1266
Kirby CP, Davidson PM (2000) Inguinoscrotal bruising: a sign of neonatal adrenal hemorrhage. Pediatr Emerg Care 16: 179
Klimach OE, Defriend DJ, Foster DN (1990) Pneumoscrotum following endoscopic sphincterotomy. Surg Endosc 4: 230–231
Kochakarn W, Choonhaklai V, Hotrapawanond P, Muangman V (2000) Traumatic testicular dislocation a review of 36 cases. J Med Assoc Thailand 83:208–212
Koumanidou C, Manopoulou E, Pantazis J et al (2000) Scrotal hematocele as an unusual presentation of blunt abdominal trauma in three male infants. J Clin Ultrasound 28:190–193
Kratzik C, Hainz A, Kuber W et al (1989) Has ultrasound influenced the therapy concept of blunt scrotal trauma? J Urol 142:1243–1246
Larsen A, Stamnes O, Majak M (1993) Testicular trauma. Tidsshr Nor Laegeforen 113:1853–1855
Learch TJ, Hansch LP, Ralls PW (1995) Sonography in patients with gunshot wounds of the scrotum: imaging findings and their value. AJR 165:879–883
Lee JY, Cass AS, Streitz JM (1992) Traumatic dislocation of testes and bladder rupture. Urology 40:506–508
Lewis CA, Michell MJ (1991) The use of real time ultrasound in the management of scrotal trauma. Br J Radiol 64:792–795
Lin WW, Kim ED, Quesada ET, Lipshultz LI, Coburn M (1998) Unilateral testicular injury from external trauma: evaluation of semen quality and endocrine parameters. J Urol 159:841–843
Lupetin AR, King W III, Rich PF, Lederman RB (1983) The traumatized scrotum: ultrasound evaluation. Radiology 148:203–207
Martin B (1992) Atlas of scrotal ultrasound. Springer, Berlin Heidelberg New York
Martin B, Conte J (1987) Ultrasonography of the acute scrotum. J Clin Ultrasound 15:37–44
Martinez Pineiro L Jr, Cerero E, Cozar JM, Avellana JA, Moreno JA, Martinez Pineiro JA (1992) Value of testicular ultrasound in the evaluation of blunt scrotal trauma without hematocele. Br J Urol 69:286–290
McAninch JW, Kahn RI, Jeffrey RB, Laing FC, Krieger MJ (1984) Major traumatic and septic genital injuries. J Trauma 24: 291–298
McClure J (1980) A case of malacoplakia of the epididymis associated with trauma. J Urol 124:934–935
Meixner J (1983) Unusual birth injury of the scrotum. Zentralbl Gynakol 105:1326–1328
Moore EE, Malangoni MA, Cogbill TH et al (1996) Organ injury scaling. VII. Cervical, vascular, peripheral vascular, adrenal, penis, testis and scrotum. J Trauma 41:523–524
Munter DW, Faleski EJ (1989) Blunt scrotal trauma: emergency department evaluation and management. Am J Emerg Med 7:227–234
O'Donnell C, Kumar U, Kiely EA (1998) Testicular dislocation after scrotal trauma. Br J Urol 82:768
Older RA, Watson LR (1994) Tubular ectasia of the rete testis: a benign condition with a sonographic appearance that may be misinterpreted as malignant. J Urol 152:477–478
Papadimitriou JC, Drachenberg CB (1994) Posttraumatic spindle cell nodules. Immunohistochemical and ultrastructural study of two scrotal lesions. Arch Pathol Lab Med 118:709–711
Parvey HR, Patel BK (1998) Urethral complications of urinary catheterization presenting as primary scrotal masses: sonographic diagnosis. J Clin Ultrasound 26:261–264
Patil MG, Onuora VC (1994) The value of ultrasound in the evaluation of patients with blunt scrotal trauma. Injury 25: 177–178
Pecori M, Repetti F, di Lascio N et al (1991) Rupture of the testicle: comparison of echographic picture and operative findings. Arch Ital Urol Nephrol Androl 63:135–137
Pollen JJ, Funckes C (1982) Traumatic dislocation of the testes. J Trauma 22:247–249

Porcelli F, Bono S, Mestril L et al (1990) Neonatal scrotal hemorrhage caused by post-traumatic hemoperitoneum. Pediatr Med Chir 12:695–696
Rabinowitz R (1984) The importance of the cremasteric reflex in acute scrotal swelling in children. J Urol 132:89–90
Ragozzino MW (1993) Stretcher's scrotum. N Eng J Med 328: 815
Rifkin MD, Kurtz AB, Pasto ME, Goldberg BB (1985) Diagnostic capabilities of high-resolution scrotal ultrasonography: prospective evaluation. J Ultrasound Med 4:13–19
Roback MG, Battan FK, Koyle M, Meagher DP Jr (1996) Acute scrotal swelling after blunt thoracoabdominal trauma. J Trauma 40:155–156
Sasso F, Gulino G, Destitio A, Speca S, Alcini E (1994) The role of ultrasonography in scrotal traumas. Int Urol Nephrol 26: 209–214
Sasso F, Gulino G, di Pinto A, Alcini E (1995) Correlation between ultrasonography imaging and surgical findings in scrotal trauma. Arch Ital Urol Androl 67:159–162
Sauvage P, Geiss Leculee A, Hideux S (1988) Pediatric testicular injuries. Chir Ped 22:136–141
Schaffer RM (1985) Ultrasonography of scrotal trauma. Urol Radiol 7:245–249
Schnall M (1993) Magnetic resonance imaging of the scrotum. Semin Roentgenol 28:19–30
Schwartz SL, Faerber GJ (1994) Dislocation of the testis as a delayed presentation of scrotal trauma. Urology 43:743–745
Schwarz RJ, Blair GK (1995) Trans-scrotal intra-abdominal injuries: two case reports. Can J Surg 38:374–376
Sellem G, Tobelm G, Economou C, Amer M, Arvis G (1987) The value of echography in scrotal contusions. Personal experience a propos 20 cases. Ann Urol 21:327–330
Siegel MJ (1997) The acute scrotum. Radiol Clin North Am 35: 959–976
Skoog SJ, Belman AB (1986) The communicating hematocele: an unusual presentation for blunt splenic trauma. J Urol 136:1092
Sparnon T, Moretti K, Sach RP (1982) BMX handlebar. A threat to manhood? Med J Aust 2:587–588
Sukja SK, Evans EJ, Nigam A (1996) Delayed rupture of the spleen presenting as a scrotal hematoma. J Trauma 26:85–86
Tan PK, Lee YM (1998) Traumatic dislocation of the testes. Ann Acad Med Singapore 27:269–271
Tartar VM, Trambert MA, Balsara ZN, Mattrey RF (1993) Tubular ectasia of the testicle: sonographic and MR imaging appearance. AJR 160:539–542
Tiwary CM (1989) Testicular injury in breech delivery: possible implications. Urology 34:210–212
Toranji S, Barbaric Z (1994) Testicular dislocation. Abdom Imaging 19:379–380
Tumeh SS, Benson CB, Richie JP (1991) Acute diseases of the scrotum. Semin Ultrasound CT MR 12:115–130
Van Ahlen H, Bokisch A, von Stauffenberg A, Bruhl P (1991) Static and dynamic radionuclide imaging in the diagnosis of the acute scrotum. Urol Int 47:20–24
Vuong PN, Camuzard P, Schoonaert MF (1988) Perineal nodular indurations ("accessory testicles") in cyclists. Fine needle aspiration cytologic and pathologic findings in two cases. Acta Cytol 32:86–90
Warden S, Schellhammer PF (1978) Bilateral testicular rupture: report of a case with an unusual presentation. J Urol 120: 257–258
Xu YM, Wu P, Cai PC, Cheng ZC (1988) Replantation of the testis: report of a case. J Urol 139:596–598
Yagan N (2000) Testicular US findings after biopsy. Radiology 215:768–773
Yagi H, Igawa M, Shiina H, Shigeno K, Yoneda T, Wada Y (1999) Traumatic dislocation of the testis. Urol Int 62: 188–191
Zermann DH, Schubert J (1997) Strangulation of the scrotum. Scand J Urol Nephrol 31:401–402
Zink RA, Muller-Mattheis V, Oberneder R (1990) Results of the West German multicenter study "Urological Traumatology". Urologe 29:243–250

15 Injuries of the Lumbar Spine

D. J. Wilson, G. M. Allen, J. Hillier

CONTENTS

- Fractures in the lumbar region occur most commonly at the thoracolumbar junction
- Spinal fractures are often multiple and careful screening for other lesions is mandatory
- Lumbar hyperflexion is associated with injury to the abdominal viscera
- Stability of a fracture is crucial to management
- Plain films are the workhorses of imaging. CT is a necessary supplement
- MRI is occasionally of value, especially when there is neurological damage

15.1 History

Injuries to the lumbar spine are the result of severe trauma. Car accidents and falls from a height are the common causes, these two comprising over 95% of injuries (Marczynski et al. 1999). In wars, penetrating injuries predominate (Splavski et al. 1998). In the presurgical era patients with spine fractures were often too ill to survive, but improved resuscitation techniques and more rapid transport to the hospital have led to increased survival rates and the need for more aggressive treatment of unstable fractures. Conservative management relies on immobilization but has a significant risk of associated morbidity, for example, pneumonia and pressure sores. Surgical stabilization was introduced to counter these problems but it could only be safely achieved when the type and extent of the injury was demonstrated on radiographs. Approximately 15%–20% of spinal fractures require surgical treatment (Marczynski et al. 1999).

D. J. Wilson, MD
Consultant Radiologist, Department of Radiology, Nuffield Orthopaedic Centre, Windmill Road, Headington, Oxford OX3 7LD, UK
G. M. Allen, MD
Consultant Radiologist, Department of Radiology, Nuffield Orthopaedic Centre, Windmill Road, Headington, Oxford OX3 7LD, UK
J. Hillier, MD
Department of Radiology, Nuffield Orthopaedic Centre, Windmill Road, Headington, Oxford OX3 7LD, UK

Medical imaging since its advent has been a very important tool in the management of spinal injury (Kaye and Nance 1990; Pathria and Petersilge 1991). Conscious patients complain of back pain or tenderness, and those without such symptoms do not need routine thoracolumbar radiography unless associated features mean that they are at particularly high risk of having suffered injury (Meldon and Moettus 1995). In these patients, screening by radiological examination is essential. High-risk groups include those with high-velocity injury, reduced consciousness, associated head injury, and associated pelvic injury (Frankel et al. 1994; Stanislas et al. 1998). Femoral shaft fractures are also associated with thoracolumbar fractures (3.5%) (Rupp et al. 1994). It is prudent to screen the spine for injury clinically and radiologically in all patients who have suffered major trauma (Woodring et al. 1988).

Classification of injury is based on anatomical patterns; these have been inferred by their imaging appearances (Holdsworth 1963; Denis 1983; McAfee et al. 1983; Leventhal 1998). The advent of CT allowed better planning of surgical intervention and this was further enhanced by the development of helical (spiral) CT with image reconstruction in the planes more suited than the axial plane for the assessment of the spinal column (Brandser and El Khoury 1997). In the cervical spine, high-resolution helical CT has been shown to demonstrate a substantial number of fractures that are not visible even on review of the plain films (7 of 12 cases of cervical fracture were visible on CT only) (Jelly et al. 2000).

MRI now allows us to study the soft tissue and bone marrow, further improving our understanding of the results of trauma (Cotler et al. 1989). MR-assisted surgery is in its early stages of development, but is an exciting new technique that is likely to change surgical practice (Verheyden et al. 1999).

15.2 Incidence

Fractures of the lumbar spine are fortunately much less common than injury to the peripheral skeleton. However, they are frequent enough to be considered as part of the routine work of a trauma unit. The axial skeleton is well protected by muscle and is substantial in its nature. Fractures of the normal spine are therefore associated with high energy and have a strong association with severe injury elsewhere. Motor vehicle accidents are the commonest cause of lumbar spine fractures. They are rare in sporting injuries, although horse-riding accidents have a high risk of spinal injury. Multiple injuries are commonly associated with lumbar spine fractures (43% of cases) (Marczynski et al. 1999). There is a strong link with injuries of the abdominal viscera although it is only the minority of patients with lumbar spine fractures who will have suffered damage to the abdominal viscera (10%) (Rabinovici et al. 1999). There is no correlation between fracture type and the incidence of visceral injury (Rabinovici et al. 1999).

In patients with bone-softening disease, the trauma may be minor. Osteoporotic collapse is the commonest form of spinal fracture and it is of epidemic proportion in the aging population. Fracture-inducing osteoporosis is seen mainly in women but may affect men (10:1 ratio). Osteoporotic insufficiency fractures occurring in the thoracolumbar region may compress neural structures but they are less likely to cause neurological damage than in the cervical spine (23% of cases of thoracolumbar fracture) (Thorngren et al. 1981; Heggeness 1993). In chronic alcoholics, osteopenia and vertebral fractures are commonly encountered (36% of cases) (Peris et al. 1995). Metastases to bone are the second most common cause of vertebral collapse followed closely by myeloma. Other bone pathology is much less common but may lead to fracture. In young people, metabolic disorders such as osteogenesis imperfecta and focal lesion such as fibrous dysplasia should be considered. Fractures in children are often contiguous and in the lumbar spine most commonly occur at L2 (Hegenbarth and Ebel 1976).

15.3 Mechanism

15.3.1 Anatomy

The lumbar spine consists of five mobile vertebral segments separated by intervertebral discs. Rotation, flexion, and extension may occur at each interspace limited in part by the facet joints and in part by the extent of stretching and distortion that may take place in the intervertebral disc. Ligamentous structures bind the vertebral segments, principally the posterior and anterior longitudinal ligaments and the interspinous ligaments. Each vertebral body has two transverse processes. Intertransverse ligaments also act as the origin of the psoas muscles, binding the adjacent transverse processes on each side to each other. The strong spinal musculature attaches to the vertebral bodies and acts as a very effective support, especially when trauma occurs. The weakest point in the lumbar region is where the thoracic cage and vertebral column join the lumbar spine: at this point the muscles are less supportive and greater motion may occur. This is why the majority of fractures occur at the thoracolumbar junction. It may be that variation in the alignment of the facet joints between individuals alters the risk of injury at this location (SINGER et al. 1989). In fractures resulting from falls, the most commonly injured vertebrae are T12 (32%) and L1 (37%) (RICHTER et al. 1996).

The conus medullaris is the lowest part of the spinal cord. In the mature adult, its tip is located in the region of the second lumbar vertebral segment. The cauda equina is the collection of lumbar and sacral nerve roots that transit the lumbar canal, emerging through the neural foramina to innervate the lower limbs. These foramina are the narrow bony canals through which the neural structures pass and are common sites for compression, either due to direct disruption of the architecture or due to accelerated degenerative proliferation following trauma. WHITESIDES (1977) reported that the most common cause of neural injury in the thoracolumbar region was the unstable burst fracture. Neurological deficit is less common in injuries of the lumbar spine than it is in thoracic and cervical trauma (RIGGINS and KRAUS 1977), but there remains a significant risk, 25% according to MELDON and MOETTUS (1995) and 10%–38% according to MCCULLEN et al. (1998), rising to 40% if the thoracolumbar junction is involved (FRANKEL et al. 1994). The lower in the lumbar region that the fracture occurs, the less chance there is of neurological deficit. This is because the reduction in spinal canal diameter that is associated with neurological damage is more in the lower spine (T11/12 35%; L1 45%; L2 55%) (MCCULLEN et al. 1998). Soft tissue structures, including the intervertebral discs, the facet joint synovium, and epidural soft tissue, may compress neural tissue. Epidural hematoma may compress neural elements although detection by MR is dependent on pulse sequence selection (SILBERSTEIN and MCLEAN 1995).

The lowest lumbar vertebra articulates with the sacrum. Injuries in the region often involve the sacral segments (DENIS et al. 1988; ALBERT et al. 1993). Fusion of the upper sacral segments and the lower lumbar segments is variable, with a wide range of anatomical variation. Additional mobile segments and full or partial fusion of the lower lumbar segments are common. Incomplete fusion of the lower lumbar and upper sacral neural arches are common and if these are not associated with neural tube deficiency, are normally of no clinical significance. In trauma their importance is one of exclusion. A congenitally defective neural arch should not be confused with a fracture. Rounded edges and tapered segments of bone are the hallmarks of a congenital anomaly.

With age and disease, bone may partially or fully bridge the vertebral segments. This leads to reduced flexibility and increased risk of fracture during trauma. Spondyloarthropathies, such as ankylosing spondylitis (ANDRE et al. 1999) or diffuse idiopathic skeletal hyperostosis (DISH) (HENDRIX et al. 1994; LE HIR et al. 1999), render the vertebral column brittle and especially at risk of fracture with relatively minor trauma. In common with fractures through bone that is abnormal, they are often atypical in their pattern. Transverse shear fractures may occur and as they involve all three columns they are very unstable (FAST et al. 1986; HANSON and MIRZA 2000). These fractures may be occult and difficult to diagnose (FINKELSTEIN et al. 1999). The incidence does not seem to be related to reduced bone density, and the brittle unbending nature of the spine is the major factor (MITRA et al. 2000). Surgical repair is difficult and failure to unite is common, a combined posterior and anterior surgical fusion is recommended (OLERUD et al. 1996).

15.3.2 Classification

In 1949 NICHOLL proposed the concept that spine fractures should be considered stable or unstable, thereby predicting the best management. HOLDSWORTH (1963) expanded this concept, dividing fractures into five types: those that he considered stable (wedge compression and compression burst) and unstable (dislocations, extension fractures and dislocation, and rotational fracture dislocations). The spine was thought to be unstable if the posterior ligament complex was disrupted (i.e., the facet joint capsules, intraspinous and supraspinous ligaments, and the ligamentum flavum). This description is flawed because Holdsworth describes an extension injury as unstable but also says that the anterior ligament complex is disrupted rather than the posterior one! He also did not include the flexion distraction injury. KELLY and WHITESIDES (1968) and WHITESIDES (1977) developed a classification system based on two columns, recognizing the unstable burst fracture as the commonest cause of neural injury in the thoracolumbar region.

Bedbrook looked at the stability of spinal fractures from cadaver work and refuted this concept, saying that the division of the posterior ligamentous complex did not cause instability. Not until the disc and some stripping of the anterior longitudinal ligament occurred did the spine become unstable (Bedbrook 1971).

Perhaps the best-known work on this subject followed when Denis (1983) described the three-column system. Denis noted that Holdsworth's two-column theory indicated that injury to the posterior elements would lead to instability, but added a third or central column to this description, calling it the middle column. A posterior element injury is only unstable if the posterior longitudinal ligament and the posterior annulus fibrosus are damaged as well. He also added the "seat belt" fracture to Holdsworth's list. Biomechanical studies have confirmed the importance of the three-column concept, emphasizing that the middle column is the main determinant of spinal stability (Panjabi et al. 1995). The anterior column includes the anterior longitudinal ligament and anterior vertebral body. The middle column includes the posterior longitudinal ligament, posterior vertebral body, and posterior annulus fibrosis. The posterior column includes the neural arch, ligamentum flavum, facet joints, and interspinous ligaments. This classification, however, was very complex, containing more than 20 divisions, but did not reflect the surgical management, which was the same for all five types of burst fracture. Fergusson and Allen described fractures using the mechanisms by which they were produced (Fergusson and Allen 1984; Capen 1999).

The AO (Arbeitsgemeinschaft für Osteosynthesefragen) classification of spinal fractures has been modified by Magerl and co-workers (1994). They divide fractures into three types: A (vertebral body compression), B (anterior and posterior element injuries with distraction), and C (anterior and posterior element injuries with rotation). Morphological criteria are used for further subdivision of the injuries. This scheme has not gained the widespread usage enjoyed by the AO classification of limb fractures. Doubt has been raised by some workers who found only 67% interobserver agreement when using this system, applying only the principle ABC classification (Blauth et al. 1999).

McAfee used CT to analyze 100 fractures and modified the list to: wedge compression fractures, stable burst fractures, unstable burst fractures, Chance fracture, flexion distraction injuries, and translational injuries (McAfee et al. 1983). This classification does not, however, include a pure extension injury. These are uncommon though, leading to injury to the posterior elements of the vertebral body. An injury is unstable if it involves all three columns. Knowing the column affected in the different fractures will help assess stability (Table 15.1).

Table 15.1. Column involvement by McAfee classification

Type of fracture	Column		
	Anterior	Middle	Posterior
Wedge compression	Yes	No	No
Stable burst	Yes	Yes	No
Unstable burst	Yes	Yes	Yes
Chance	Probable	Probable	Yes
Flexion-distraction	Yes	Yes	Yes
Translational injuries	Yes	Yes	Yes

The major addition to Denis's classification is that McAfee considers a burst fracture stable if the posterior column is not involved. Distraction injuries with subluxation or dislocation of the posterior elements may lead to dislocated or perched facets. This is seen more frequently in the cervical spine where the orientation of the facets and the lack of heavy supporting muscles are increased risk factors.

In 1948 Chance described a transverse fracture pattern that has since been named after him (Chance 1948; Rogers 1971). They commonly occur in lap strap seat belt injuries and are a transverse, distraction fracture. The original description was that of a splitting of the posterior ligaments and neural arch, without involvement of the vertebral body. A complete transverse injury of the vertebral body was then observed, termed a fulcrum fracture (Howland and Curry 1965). It was proposed that the seat belt acted as a fulcrum, shifting the line of shear in the usual hyperflexion injury to the anterior vertebral body, rather then the middle column. The term "Chance fracture" is now used to include transverse fractures involving the posterior elements and facet joints, and/or the vertebral body. They may occur in accidents where seat belts are not used, however (Hall and Robertson 1985). It is important to appreciate that there is a high incidence of intraabdominal trauma in these patients (Dehner 1971; Huelke and Kaufer 1975; Taylor and Eggli 1988; Taylor et al. 1988; Appleby and Nagy 1989; Newman et al. 1990; Reid et al. 1990; Anderson et al. 1991; Saboe et al. 1991; Sivit et al. 1991; Jeanneret and Holdener 1992; Ryan et al. 1994; Huelke et al. 1995; Porter and Zhao 1998; Letts et al. 1999; Rabinovici et al. 1999; Holland et al. 2000).

Minor injuries to the spine include fractures of the articular processes, isolated fractures of the spinous processes and fractures of the transverse processes, which can affect the neural plexus if at the L4/5 level. These classifications take into account the importance of stability. However, biomechanical studies suggest that there can be varied degrees of stability for a given fracture type. Kifune et al. found that while all experimentally induced endplate fractures were stable and all burst fractures were unstable, there was varied stability for wedge compression injuries (Kifune et al. 1995). Whatever system is employed, the clinical team should take all circumstances into account and recognize the considerable biological variation.

15.3.3 Common Mechanisms

These fracture patterns may result from a variety of forces. Each leads to a particular pattern of injury, which will be described below. Complex and especially high-kinetic-energy trauma may lead to a mixed pattern.

15.3.3.1 Hyperflexion

The commonest cause of spinal fracture is hyperflexion (50% fractures) (McCullen et al. 1998). Most injuries involve only the anterior elements of the vertebral columns and are stable. An especially dangerous form of hyperflexion injury is when the body decelerates when held only by a lap belt (Huelke and Kaufer 1975; Legay et al. 1990; Newman et al. 1990; Reid et al. 1990; Anderson et al. 1991; Glassman et al. 1992; Huelke et al. 1995). Aircraft lap belts, some rear seat belts in cars and bus seat belts are of this limited variety. The chest strap of a cross belt in motor vehicles may be loose or poor-fitting, giving the same effect. It is notable that the incidence of these injuries is much lower in Europe where three point seat belts are universal (3.4%) (Jeanneret and Holdener 1992). Signs of injury that are important clinically are seat belt bruising (Sivit et al. 1991) and persisting tachycardia (abdominal injury) (Holland et al. 2000). In rapid deceleration, the spine is flexed over the belt. This type of injury is commonly associated with damage to the abdominal organs (see Chap. 4, 5, and 7 on liver, spleen and pancreas injury) (Letts et al. 1999). Anterior compression of the vertebrae plus tearing of the posterior structures is the likely result. The spinous processes may fracture, but in the lumbar region it is more likely that the interspinous ligaments tear. The posterior longitudinal ligaments are at risk. The posterior damage may not be apparent on plain films and the instability of the injury may be misjudged if account is not taken of the mechanism and the likely soft tissue damage (Fig. 15.1). Forced flexion may also occur when a weight impacts on the upper back and forces the lower body into flexion. If the compression is confined to the anterior vertebral body and leaves the posterior ligaments intact, then these fractures may be stable (Fig. 15.2). In late pregnancy, such hyperflexion injuries may cause the spine to pivot around the fetus; the spine is then more under tension than compression. Such injuries are more likely to be unstable and warrant early consideration of surgical fixation (Tanchev et al. 2000).

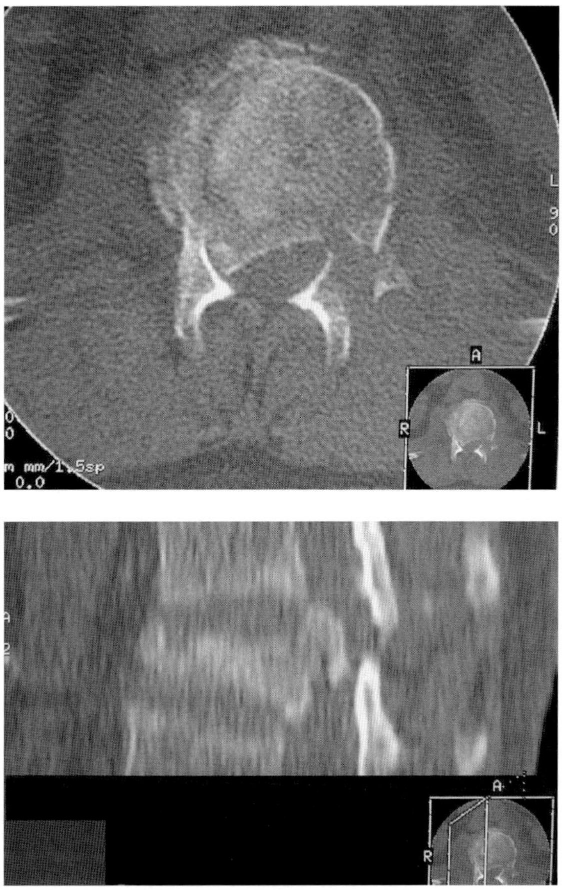

a

b

Fig. 15.1a, b. Unstable burst fracture with sagittal CT reconstruction. Note the retropulsed fragment and the loss of both anterior and middle column integrity. The posterior elements are distracted

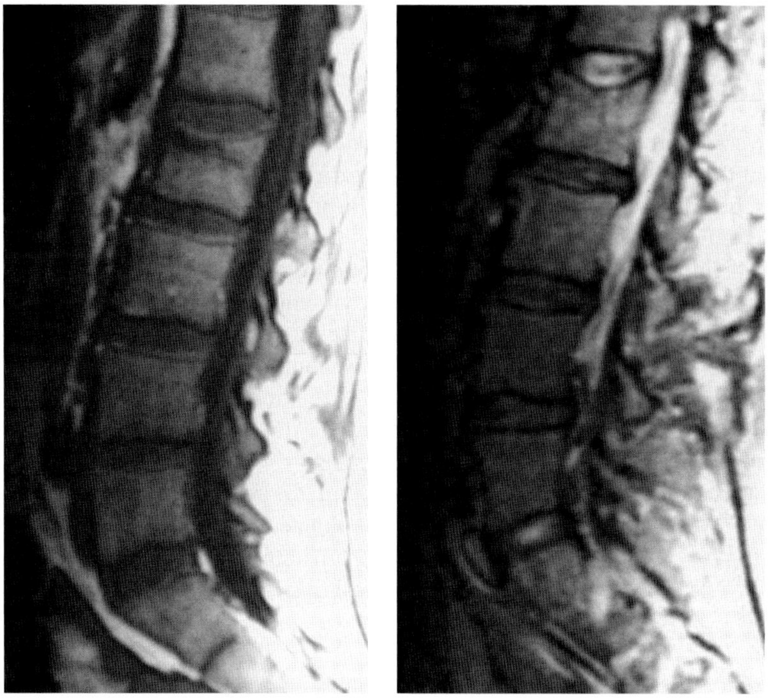

Fig. 15.2. Sagittal T1-weighted spin echo (a) and sagittal T2-weighted fast spin echo (b) MRI of a stable anterior column compression fracture

The most severe result of hyperflexion, perhaps with a rotational element, is fracture dislocation of the lumbosacral spine. There is a very high incidence of neurological damage in this fortunately rare injury (Herron and Williams 1984; Grabe 1988; Steinitz et al. 1997). Facet dislocation may occur and it has a high association with neural damage (76%) (Gellad et al. 1986).

15.3.3.2
Hyperextension

Falling backwards onto an object typifies the rare injury of hypertension (2% of fractures) (McCullen et al. 1998). The forces extend the spine, tearing anterior longitudinal ligaments, splitting the intervertebral discs and compressing the posterior structures. The neural foramina and therefore the nerve roots are commonly affected. Compression fractures of the laminae and facet regions ensue. There may be posterior wedging of the vertebrae, and fragments of bone may be avulsed from the anterior vertebrae by the action of the anterior longitudinal ligament or the insertion of Sharpey's fibers that are at the margin of the discs. Abdominal organs are less at risk with this type of injury. The transverse nature of the injury renders the spine potentially unstable.

15.3.3.3
Axial Compression

A common form of injury is vertical compression. Falls are the most frequent cause of this type of injury (83% of 101 cases) (Richter et al. 1996). Ejection from a fast jet almost inevitably causes vertebral compression fractures; this is really the reverse process to a fall. Compression may include a hyperextension or hyperflexion element. Pure axial loading is seen in a blow to the head and can cause burst fractures of the vertebra. This in turn may lead to splitting of the ring of the pedicles and lamina (Fig. 15.3). This burst injury with splaying of the pedicles is often an unstable fracture (Fig. 15.4). Biomechanical studies show that this is multidirectional instability (Panjabi et al. 1994). Minor degrees of compression are difficult to recognize and often are overlooked on plain films. They may be seen on MR imaging but rarely require other than symptomatic treatment. Endplate injury may lead to premature disc degeneration (Kerttula et al. 2000). Fortunately, it is likely that those not obvious on a lateral radiograph are stable mechanically and warrant symptomatic treatment only. Compression injuries are common after minor or negligible trauma in patients with osteoporosis. There is a high association between compression fractures of the spine and fractures of the calcaneus. There is evidence

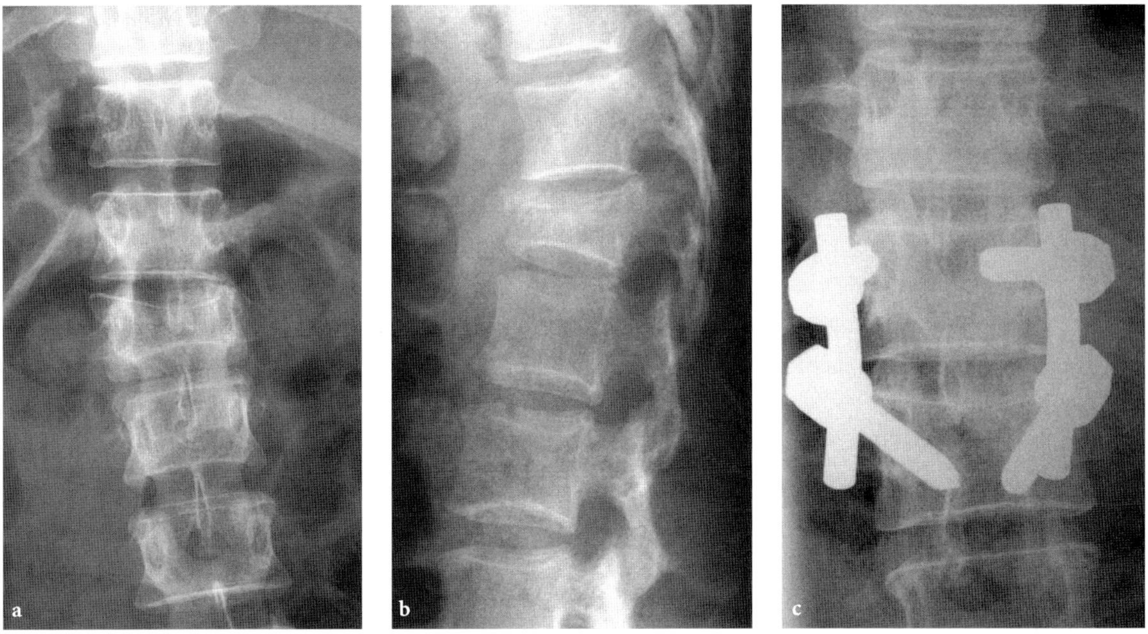

Fig. 15.3a–c. a, b. Anterior and middle column height loss with a short curve scoliosis secondary to the additional height loss on the left. Note the splayed pedicles, indicating a posterior column injury. **c** Fixation is by pedicle screws and posterior instrumentation

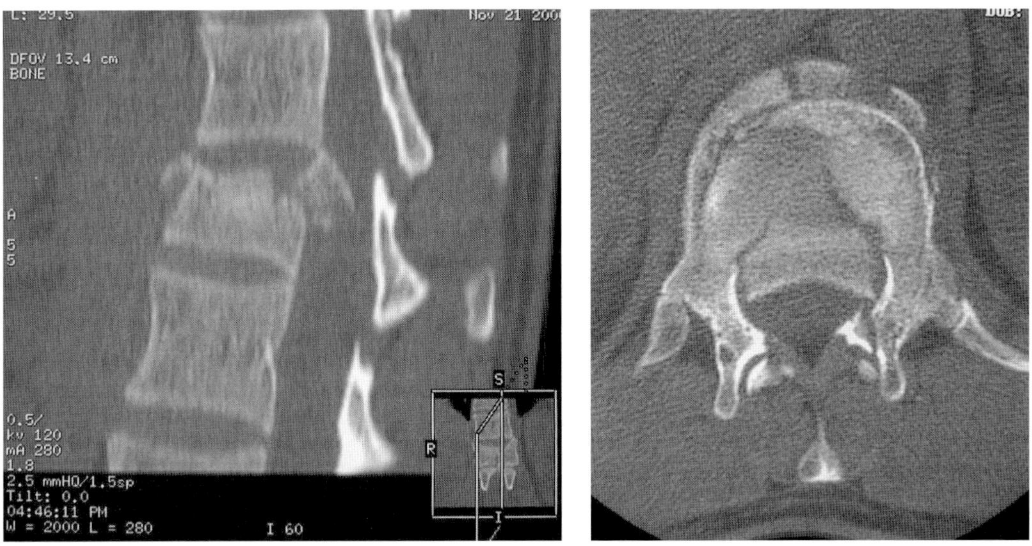

a b

Fig. 15.4a, b. Burst fracture with a large free retropulsed fragment

that Schmorl's nodes may occur acutely as the result of trauma due to axial overloading (FAHEY et al. 1998).

15.3.3.4
Rotation

Twisting components of the force will lead to complex fractures in the posterior elements (laminae, facet joints, pars interarticularis, and the transverse processes). The vertebra may split in a sagittal plane. Neural foraminal compromise is common. Many rotational injuries lead to an unstable fracture complex. This mechanism accounts for around 14% of spinal fractures (MCCULLEN et al. 1998).

15.3.3.5
Shearing

Transverse force that fractures the lumbar spine must be of very high energy. These injuries are associated with complex and multiple injuries that are often life-threatening (10% of fractures) (McCullen et al. 1998). The exception is when the fracture occurs in abnormal bone such as in ankylosing spondylitis or Paget's disease, when minimal force may be catastrophic.

15.3.3.6
Distraction

In these injuries, the force across the vertebra pulls it apart. This occurs in the Chance fracture, where compression is not an element (Fig. 15.5). Flexion distraction may combine to compress the anterior column and tear apart the posterior structures (Gertzbein and Court-Brown 1988). This mechanism accounts for around 5% of spinal fractures (McCullen et al. 1998). Rarely, lateral distraction may injure the spine. Such injuries have a high association with other skeletal and abdominal trauma (Denis and Burkus 1991a). Using the McAfee classification of fractures with addition of extension fractures for completeness, the mechanisms involved can be shown as follows in Table 15.2.

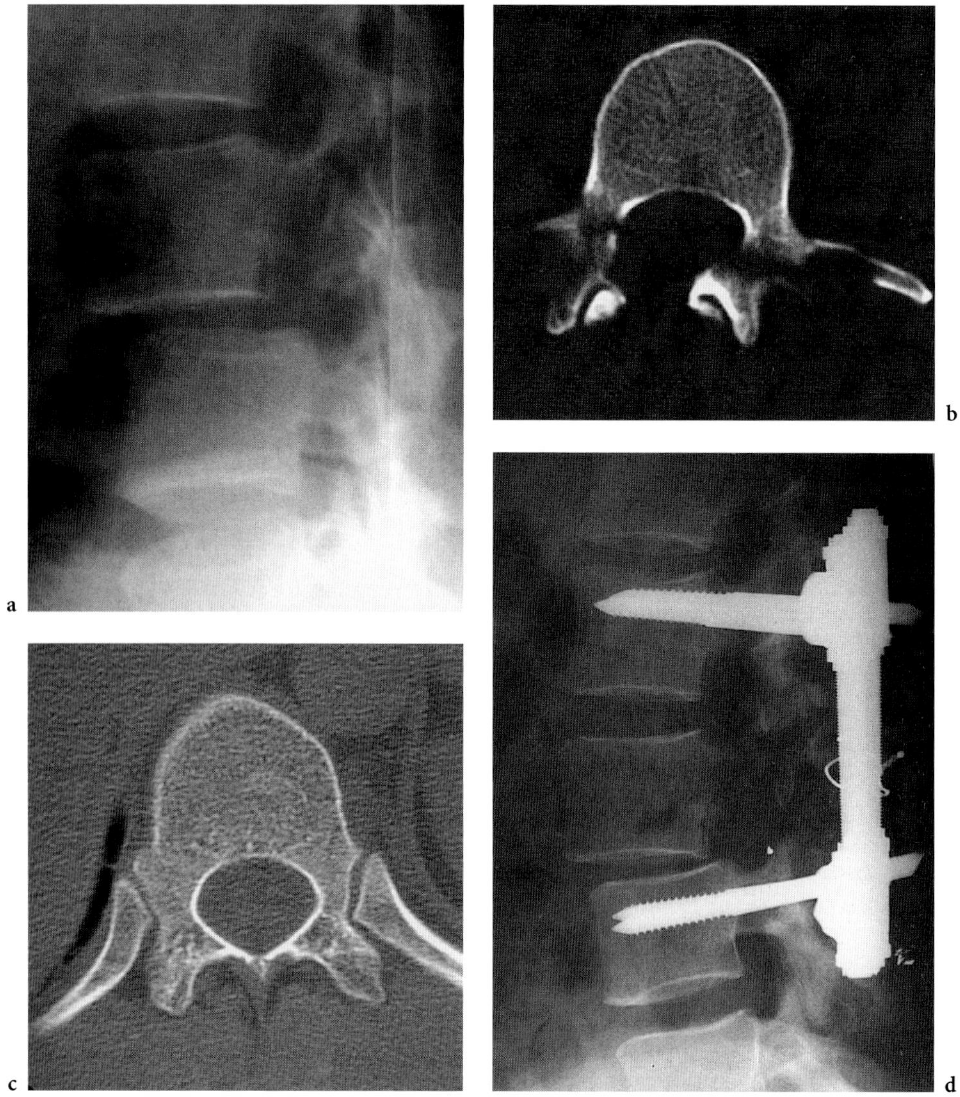

Fig. 15.5a–d. a, b. Chance fracture. **c** CT of a normal level to confirm a location suitable for insertion of a fixation device. **d** Postoperative view with pedicle screw fixation

Table 15.2. A modified version of the McAfee classification including extension fractures

Fracture	Hyperflexion	Hyper-extension	Rotation/shearing	Axial compression	Distraction
Wedge	Yes			Yes	
Stable burst	Probable			Yes	
Unstable burst	Probable			Yes	
Chance					Yes
Flexion-distraction	Yes			Yes	Yes
Translational	Yes		Yes	Yes	
Extension		Yes			

15.3.4 Unusual Mechanisms and Other Injuries

15.3.4.1 Direct Blows

Blunt impact may break the spinous processes or the transverse processes. However, most injuries to the transverse process are a result of avulsion of the insertion of psoas muscles and imply a more complex injury.

15.3.4.2 Stress

Repetitive subcritical trauma may lead to stress fractures. These typically occur in the pars interarticularis. A common mechanism in the UK is fast bowling at cricket.

15.3.4.3 Electric Shock and Convulsions

The muscle spasm and distortion caused by electric shock or epileptic fits (Grabe 1988) may cause muscle insertion avulsion. In the lumbar spine, this is usually limited to the transverse processes. Compression injuries may occur from the same mechanism and will be more striking in the older and more porotic patient (Youssef et al. 1995).

15.3.4.4 Gunshots

In the United States gunshot wounds are the third most common cause of spinal cord injury after road traffic accidents and falls (Heary et al. 1996). The nature of the injury depends on the velocity of the bullet. Military weapons use high-velocity ordnance and lead to massive tissue loss, especially at the exit site (Splavski et al. 1996a). The shock wave may damage the spinal cord (47.6% neurological deficit) (Splavski et al. 1996b). Surgical débridement and exposure is important to remove nonviable tissue and prevent infection. Civilian and police weapons are of low velocity and surgery may not be indicated in spinal injuries and the risk of infection is lower than with high-velocity bullets (Heary et al. 1996) (2% spine, 15% extraspinal) (Velmahos and Demetriades 1994; Velmahos et al. 1995; Isiklar and Lindsey 1997).

15.3.4.5 Dural Tears

Dural tears are an uncommon but important complication of lumbar spine trauma. They occur in 7%–16% of cases that are operated upon. Nerve roots may become entrapped between fracture fragments, and it is important to look for this eventuality during the operation. Myelography is rarely undertaken and blood in the cerebrospinal fluid is not normally detected (Morris et al. 1984). The best means of predicting a tear on imaging is to consider the possibility when there is a lamina fracture (Cammisa et al. 1989; Denis and Burkus 1991b; Kahamba et al. 1998) or a central split of the spinous process (Brandser and El Khoury 1997).

15.3.5 Associated Injuries

The abdominal viscera, spleen, duodenum, and pancreas, are at risk in hyperflexion injuries (Dehner 1971; Saboe et al. 1991). In patients with seat belt injuries, around 65% may have concomitant intraabdominal injury (Anderson et al. 1991). Direct blows to the back may damage the kidneys. The great vessels are well protected in the lumbar region and are rarely affected. Spinal fractures are multiple in a significant number of cases (27%) (MARCZYNSKI et al. 1999). When one is recognized, there should be an immediate search for other fractures, including the cervical, thoracic, and pelvic regions. It is very easy to concentrate on the lesion first seen and to overlook lesions elsewhere that may give fewer symptoms but be more threatening to spinal stability. Pelvic ring fractures are associated with spine fractures; in one study, 26% of those patients with sacral fractures also suffered thoracolumbar fractures (ALBERT et al. 1993). They were also seen in 7% of those with other pelvic injuries. The essential lesson is to look for the other lesion whenever the axial skeleton is injured. It is natural to concentrate on the first injury seen and it is common to overlook the second or third fracture. Anderson et al. found that 23% of thoracolumbar fractures were overlooked at the initial emergency department triage (ANDERSON et al. 1996).

15.3.6 Kummell Phenomenon

Osteonecrosis of the vertebral body may follow trauma. This leads to vacuum phenomena within the bone and vertical collapse that occurs some weeks after the injury: this is termed the Kummell phenomenon and may easily be confused with malignancy or infection (VAN EENENAAM and EL-KHOURY 1993; BHALLA and REINUS 1998).

15.4 Clinical Symptoms and Findings

15.4.1 Pain

Pain is almost universal in spinal fractures and ligament injury. The patient may find the pain elsewhere, which masks the symptoms from an injury that is more threatening in terms of stability. Tenderness may be overlooked at first. The unconscious patient cannot report pain and localization of fractures requires careful clinical and radiological screening. Occasionally, severe and unstable fractures may be surprisingly pain-free and the absence of symptoms does not exclude the diagnosis entirely (MELDON and MOETTUS 1995). When the mechanism of injury suggests spinal trauma, then full screening is indicated. Analgesia and muscle relaxants can inhibit muscle spasm that would normally protect an unstable segment.

15.4.2 Dysfunction

Muscle spasm is a major mediator of pain and restriction of movement. It may mask other complaints and may limit the range of movement required to assess for instability (see flexion–extension views).

15.4.3 Deformity

Indentations and steps in the normal spinal curves are serious signs of a potential fracture. Careful palpation is of value especially in the unconscious patient.

15.5 Imaging

Plain films should be taken in all cases where imaging is clinically indicated. CT is used to study details of recognized fractures and to examine areas difficult to see on the plain films. Most would reserve MR for cases where there is neurological deficit or when the integrity of the posterior ligaments would affect the management (DU MESNIL DE ROCHEMONT et al. 1997).

15.5.1 Plain Films

15.5.1.1 Technique

Whether to investigate with any imaging must be the first decision. There is good evidence that if the patient is alert and there is no tenderness, then spinal injury may be safely excluded, avoiding the need for imaging (SAMUELS and KERSTEIN 1993; DURHAM et al. 1995). When there is pain, tenderness, dysfunction, or altered consciousness levels, plain films are the primary and principal investigation in the assessment of lumbar spine injuries. Good-quality images are essential. Often the patient is necessarily fastened to a spinal board, which will degrade the images. It is easy to sacrifice quality when the pressures of managing an acutely sick patient distract the clinical team. It is the role of the radiographer and radiologist to ensure that technical standards are as high as possible and that all regions are examined adequately. The temptation to accept a clinician's view that the "films will do" should be resisted. The standard examination will vary according to circumstances. In the emergency room or resuscitation area, AP (anterior posterior) and cross-table lateral views will usually suffice for immediate triage of the lumbar region. These images will inevitably be less satisfactory than those taken in the controlled environment of the radiology department. When time and clinical urgency allow, an AP, lateral, and lateral of the lumbosacral junction would be more useful (Fig. 15.1). These films will be part of a more extensive screening of the spine, chest, and pelvis. Additional views may be required when interpretation is difficult. These may include a pair of 45° oblique images, an AP of the sacrum, and occasionally coned views of a small section of the lumbar spine. Conventional plain film tomography still has some advocates but helical CT (HCT) with off-plane reconstruction has virtually supplanted its use (Fig. 15.6). In those units with older conventional CT units, there will be occasions when conventional plain film tomography is of particular value. Flexion–extension lateral plain films may be used to assess for instability after the pain and spasm have settled. Instability is said to exist when there is over 19° of kyphosis or an increase of over 33 mm between the spinous processes. Measurements of over 12° and 20 mm but short of the above measurements are regarded as signs of impending instability (Neumann et al. 1995).

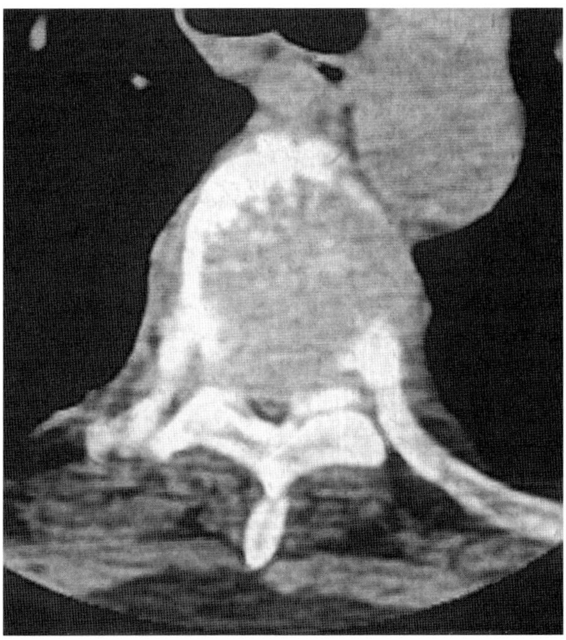

Fig. 15.6. CT of a compression fracture that proved to be pathological through a metastasis

The incidence of noncontiguous injury is high: 4.5% according to Calenoff et al. (1978) and 6.4% according to Keenen et al. (1990a). If there is an indication to investigate for spinal injury it is essential to review the whole spine. Any other areas of discomfort or tenderness should be examined radiologically. In patients with reduced consciousness levels, the whole spine should be radiographed (Pal et al. 1988).

15.5.1.2 Signs and Pitfalls

The L1 vertebral body is commonly slightly wedged anteriorly. This is a normal appearance. Careful review of vertebral body heights is required to detect subtle compression; when there is doubt it is of value to measure the anterior and posterior heights of adjacent vertebral bodies. This can be quickly achieved by marking the margins on a piece of paper. The pedicles are increasingly widely spaced descending the lumbar spine. Excessive widening of the interpeduncular distance at a single level is an important and very sensitive sign of a burst fracture (Martijn and Veldhuis 1991). Paravertebral planes are less clear than in the thoracic region, where air in the lungs aids the detection of soft tissue swelling. However, fat plane displacement may cause asymmetry that might be recognized on the AP film. Transverse process fractures are often overlooked because this area on the films is rather dark. Review of darker films with a bright light should overcome this potential error. Pars interarticularis fractures may be difficult to interpret on the AP and lateral films alone. Even minor degrees of vertebral malalignment or spondylolisthesis should lead to additional imaging (oblique views and sometimes CT). Widening of the interspinous process distance (over 7 mm) on an AP radiograph has a strong association with unstable injuries (Neumann et al. 1999). Fractures and ligament injuries commonly cause local muscle spasm and a secondary scoliosis centered at the level of injury. The posterior structures are complex and overlap on a lateral projection; careful comparison with the AP radiograph is important to increase the chance of detecting occult injury. Avulsion of the ring apophysis may be seen in adolescents or young adults. It is a rare injury but may give rise to a step in the contour of the endplate that becomes permanent (Sward et al. 1993; Martinez Lage et al. 1998).

15.5.2
Ultrasound

Ultrasound (US) is of limited value in trauma to the lumbar spine. By comparison, it is invaluable in examining for injuries to adjacent soft tissue structure and the associated intraabdominal injury. The technique is very sensitive to small quantities of fluid, within the abdomen, which may herald the presence of injuries to the viscera. Occasionally a swelling or mass, perhaps due to a hematoma, may be usefully examined using US to determine its nature (McKenney 1999).

15.5.3
Nuclear Medicine

Isotope bone scintigraphy has been used to detect occult fractures. However, it may be insensitive to occult injury (3 of 38 missed) (Hildingsson et al. 1993). MRI has supplanted the technique in the detection of occult lesions (Amour et al. 1994).

15.5.4
Computed Tomography

15.5.4.1
Technique

Computed tomography (CT) is a radiation-expensive technique and care should be exercised to limit the examination to the affected area only, while including the entire potentially injured region. Plain films are essential in planning the study, although the digital radiograph (scout or pilot view) are a viable alternative when the patient is taken to the CT for other indications (Tress and Hare 1990). If it is likely that stabilizing surgery is to take place, then the examination should include the vertebrae that will be used to hold the fixation device. If a spinal instrument or screw is inserted through a lamina or pedicle that is fractured itself, then the surgery may become very difficult and have considerably increased risk. CT sections through the vertebrae above and below the affected level are of considerable value when planning surgery. Slice thickness and helical CT pitch should be selected to reduce the risk of obscuring fractures by volume averaging. In general, 5 mm is the maximum thickness that should be employed with 1–2 mm in areas where sagittal or coronal reconstructions are needed. A pitch of 1:1 is preferred, although this can be increased to 1:5 with little loss in precision. When using multislice systems, the pitch is less critical and some machines will produce good results with pitches up to 2.0. Transverse fractures may not be seen in the axial plane and thin section reconstructions are important. This is a particular problem in children as the structures are smaller (Taylor and Eggli 1988; Glass et al. 1994). CT is the best means of detecting transverse process fractures. These have a strong association with injury to the abdominal contents (Krueger et al. 1996; Patten et al. 2000). Pars interarticularis fractures are best seen when the gantry is angled so that the initial plane of imaging lies along the pars interarticularis (reverse angle gantry). CT is the method of choice when imaging patients with missile injuries (Splavski et al. 1998). It may be necessary to introduce intrathecal contrast to assess for cord and root compression by fragments of bone or pieces of bullet or shrapnel.

15.5.4.2
Signs

Fractures are best seen on bone window settings, although it is useful to review the study with soft tissue settings to look for swelling and hematoma. Reconstructions are helpful in judging malalignment, but rarely add further information on which parts of the spine are fractured (Fig. 15.7). It is wise to rely principally on the initial axial sections.

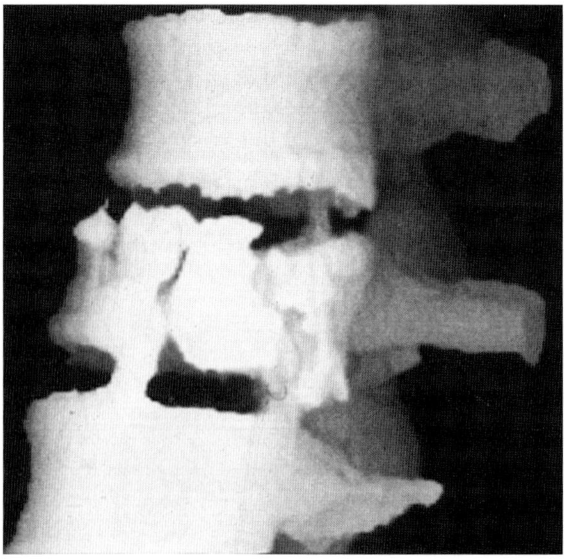

Fig. 15.7. Three-dimensional surface reconstruction of a complex fracture. The computer algorithm has removed more bone than was missing in reality

15.5.4.3
Pitfalls

Undisplaced fractures in the same plane as the axial sections may be overlooked (Glass et al. 1994). A combination of volume averaging and the poorer resolution of reconstruction lead to this problem. Careful attention to technique and review of the plain films are the means to minimize this risk. Perhaps the greatest risk with CT is that the wrong level is examined. There are occasions where the clinical team wrongly assume that as the patient has undergone an unremarkable CT examination, then the whole region must be normal.

15.5.5
Magnetic Resonance Imaging

15.5.5.1
Technique

Magnetic resonance imaging (MRI) systems are available in an increasing number of trauma units and many clinical teams are using them as first line investigation devices for a variety of acute conditions. There are significant practical problems associated with MRI in trauma patients. The geographical location of the MRI system may make examination difficult. With solenoid (tube) design systems, it is difficult to monitor and observe medically unstable patients. Metal equipment and external fixation devices that are not designed for use in a magnetic field are contraindicated. The limited size of the bore of solenoid systems can create problems when the patient cannot lie supine with the legs straight and arms along the sides. Open systems deal with some of these problems (C-shaped or double doughnut design); however, until recently these devices have been of lower field strength and produce images that are less convincing than solenoid systems. Recent technical developments have overcome some of the field strength limitations of open-design MRI systems and the application of MRI in acute trauma is likely to become more widespread and effective over the next few years. The acutely ill patient must be stabilized before entering the MRI scanner and the unit must be established for anesthetic monitoring with MRI safe hardware. Such facilities are not universally available in all MRI units. Patients with implanted pacemakers, intracranial aneurysm clips, and other non-MRI-compliant implants cannot be safely imaged by MRI; however, most orthopedic internal fixation and joint prostheses are not a contraindication to MRI. If there has been an eye injury with the potential for retained metal fragments, then radiographs of the orbits are indicated prior to MR examination.

15.5.5.2
Signs

MRI is not a good technique for examining the cortex of bone and at first sight it would not appear to be a useful method of imaging fractures. However, MRI provides the best contrast of any technique between normal bone and bone with edema. All recent fractures will be surrounded by edema and hemorrhage, so provided that the observer recognizes that this is the cardinal sign, MRI is a very sensitive method. In general, it is wise to perform T1- and T2-weighted images in all cases. There are advantages in selecting different planes, but it may also be helpful to compare identical images with different weighting. T1-weighted images show edema as low-signal (gray or dark), while T2-weighted images show fluid as high-signal (white). Both give a high signal from fat, which is plentiful in bone marrow. To discriminate fluid from fat on T2-weighted images, it helps to use techniques that suppress the signal from fat: radio frequency-selective fat suppression or short tau inversion recovery (STIR), leaving fluid as the only high signal in bone. As different planes and additional imaging techniques add to the accuracy of diagnosis, it is common to perform three or sometimes four different imaging sequences for each examination. This leads to an examination time of around 30–40 min, which may be rather long for a patient in pain or when there are pressing medical priorities.

MRI of the lumbar region is particularly useful in judging whether the spinal canal is compromised and whether the discs and nerve roots are affected. Disc prolapse, root compression, epidural hematoma, and vertebral malalignment are all better imaged with MRI than with older techniques. It is also excellent for seeing the disruption of the spinous ligaments, i.e., the anterior and posterior longitudinal ligaments, which will add important information as to the stability of the injury (Terk et al. 1997; Wilmink 1999).

A normal MRI examination is a very powerful tool and there is a role for MRI in screening for occult disease. As there is no ionizing radiation employed in MRI, it is safe to cover a wide area in each examination. For example, with new technology (phased array surface coils) it is possible and wise to examine the whole spine in high resolution in a relatively short and reasonable period of time, to pick up other occult fractures.

15.5.5.3
Pitfalls

When fractures are established or older and the edema of adjacent bone has settled, it may be difficult to detect the cortical break that would be easily seen on CT. At the other extreme, when the changes due to trauma are extensive, the massive increase in signal may confuse the observer and obscure fracture lines and areas of potential mechanical instability. Most of these potential pitfalls may be overcome by careful review of plain films and the selective use of CT to examine limited areas in detail. MRI is a rapidly developing technique and the advantages described above depend critically on recent and modern equipment. Not all MRI systems are regularly updated and there may be serious limitations using older devices.

15.6
Management

15.6.1
Patient Handling

The decision to use an imaging technique depends on the potential advantage versus the risks and to a lesser extent the cost. Careful transport of the patient is essential and the patient will almost invariably be placed on a spine board or similar immobilization device. There is evidence that spinal traction is not necessary for safe transportation by road or air (Burney et al. 1989). In acute trauma, the first decision is whether the patient is fit to be examined. Hemodynamic stability is the first priority, with the importance of A(irway), B(reathing) and C(irculation) being observed at all times in the assessment of spinal and other injuries. Imaging may be integral in deciding how to deal with blood loss and careful consideration must be given to the timing of the investigation. The lead clinician should be aware of the potential benefit of imaging while understanding the physical and practical constraints of each technique. It is often wise to go straight to the method that will provide the most definitive and convincing result rather than climbing the ladder of increasingly sophisticated methods. This means that there will be occasions when MR should be the first test. One clinician should remain responsible for the patient's well-being while the examination takes place. They may need a large team for support, but the crucial issue is that while the patient is being imaged they should be under observation by that team. While investigating for spinal injury, it must be assumed that there is the risk of mechanical instability, which could lead to permanent neurological damage if the patient is moved inappropriately. Log rolling is not a safe means of moving or nursing patients with potentially unstable spine injuries (McGuire et al. 1987). Spine boards and fixation devices should be used until the combination of clinical assessment and imaging rules out this necessity. This may present particular problems in transferring patients from bed to examination table and also when MRI is used, with the limitation of metal devices. Trauma units who employ MRI should review the metal content of spinal boards, collars, and halo traction devices. All devices can now be obtained with non ferrous (MRI-safe) metal.

15.6.2
Pain Relief

All imaging methods, with the possible exception of ultrasound, require that the patient remain immobile for periods of time. This is particularly true for MRI. Apart from the humanitarian issue, a patient in pain is unlikely to be able to cooperate fully and the imaging may be degraded in accuracy or even impossible to perform. Adequate analgesia is essential. Opiates, local blocks, Entonox, sedation, and anesthesia all have their role. It may be necessary for an anesthetic team to accompany the patient during imaging. When radiation is used, this team should be protected and monitored (lead aprons and film badges). Imaging may be used to assist in pain relief. Local anesthetic blocks may be placed under fluoroscopic, ultrasound, CT, or interventional MRI guidance.

15.6.3
Conservative Management

Nonoperative management usually involves pain relief and immobilization (Weinstein et al. 1987) the stability of the any fractures having been judged by imaging. If there is doubt about that stability then there is a role for serial imaging in selected patients. A view should be taken of the relative risk of radiation if this course is undertaken. If repeated CT is likely, then there are real and significant long-term risks. This may influence the surgeon's decision as to when surgery should take place. Equally, it may be appropriate to switch to MRI for follow-up studies.

The complication rate of conservative management is probably little different from that related to surgery (RECHTINE et al. 1999).

Muscle spasm that occurs immediately after the trauma may mask instability. As this settles, it can be useful to perform spinal flexion–extension views using plain films. These should be performed when it is certain that the potential instability is not critical and does not threaten to transect the cord, when the pain has resolved and when the patient can cooperate. They should be taken at the limits of motion that the patient is prepared to achieve and they should not be forced beyond that limit. If the range of motion achieved is insufficient to be sure that the spine is stable, then the examination was performed too early when the patient was in too much pain. A further period of conservative management should follow.

15.6.4 Surgery

There is no doubt that patients with incomplete neurological damage will benefit from early surgery, but those with complete cord transection in the past were often treated conservatively (YAZICI et al. 1995; SCHLEGEL et al. 1996; GAEBLER et al. 1999). In the last decade it has been recognized that even when there is profound paraplegia, there are advantages in stabilizing surgery to reduce pain, diminish residual deformity, and aid rehabilitation. Spinal surgery for trauma has a significant complication rate but in most practices the advantages are felt to outweigh the risks (JODOIN et al. 1985; OSTI et al. 1987).

Unstable injuries are most often treated by surgery (CHAPMAN and ANDERSON 1994). Posterior instrumentation (RIEBEL et al. 1993) and anterior fusion (PENTA and FRASER 1997) may be employed. There is considerable debate regarding the best form of fusion, with no clear conclusion (FRASER 1995).

Compression of the spinal cord or cauda equina is due to narrowing of the bony spinal canal due to the fracture or dislocation, acute disc prolapse, or epidural hematoma. The aim of surgery is to decompress the spinal canal and to stabilize the segment involved. This may be achieved by distraction with implanted rods or pedicle screws (ROSENTHAL and LOWERY 1980). The fragments are indirectly pulled back into place when the ligamentous structures are pulled taut. Full restoration of the canal diameter is not essential; there is evidence that the resultant cross-sectional measurements are not related to the neurological recovery (DOERR et al. 1991; HERNDON and GALLOWAY 1988). If the diameter is restored to 75% of its original area, then any residual narrowing may safely be ignored (KUNER et al. 1997). Remodeling will improve the diameter with time. The alternative approach is to decompress the spine directly and to stabilize the segment with internal fixation devices, typically by pedicle screws with rods (GAEBLER et al. 1997, 1999; KUNER et al. 1997). There is no clear difference in outcome when anterior and posterior surgical decompression is compared (MCCULLEN et al. 1998). Intraoperative ultrasound has recently been employed to locate displaced fragments in the spinal canal (DEGREIF and WENDA 1998). Cross-sectional imaging may help the surgeon place pedicle screws accurately, as there is a wide variation in the morphology of the pedicles and a significant difference in the approach that should be used in different ethnic groups (HOU et al. 1993).

It is important that any fixation devices used in the spine are held in normal intact bone. Prior to surgery, it is a considerable help if the imaging includes those areas that may be used for fixation. This means that the surgeon and radiologist should discuss the potential treatment options and the radiologist should design the studies to include the areas likely to be involved. This usually means a single CT section through the lamina of any vertebra that may be used to hold the implanted device.

MRI has been used to predict the likely affect of distraction surgery (BRIGHTMAN et al. 1992). If the longitudinal ligaments are ruptured, then distraction is unsafe.

Fluoroscopy is often used in the operating room to assist in the placement of fixation devices. CT-linked guidance systems are used by some in the placement of pedicle screws. A small number of institutions use intraoperative CT and MRI (VERHEYDEN et al. 1999). This may become more frequent with the advent of mobile fluoroscopic CT.

Following surgery, plain films are important to document the procedure and to judge whether there are any complications. Studies have shown that around 10% of pedicle screws do not follow the track of the pedicle. Hooks and rods may detach or snap (FOLEY et al. 1983). These misplacements may be apparent on well-centered and properly aligned AP and lateral films, but they can be difficult to detect if there is any rotation. Fluoroscopy may be the solution but the definitive test is usually CT. Modern CT systems use software that helps to reduce the artifact from metal implants and the screw tracks are usually clear. Volume rendering from multislice data has the advantage of reducing the apparent metal artifact.

Occasionally MR may give better images than CT, but again metal artifact may present problems. The more recent the implants, the fewer artifacts there are on MR. Fast-spin echo images usually give the least artifact. It is worth trying in a different plane if the initial images are too degraded.

Cross-sectional imaging (CT and MRI) is very useful in showing where decompressive surgery took place, deciding whether it adequately achieved the objective, and in looking for complications. In the immediate postoperative period, edema and soft tissue swelling may confuse the picture. These areas will enhance with contrast. This should settle rapidly and if there is doubt and the patient is reasonably stable a follow-up study in a few days may resolve difficult problems. In children, fractures have great potential for remodeling but damage to the growth plates may lead to progressive deformity over time (Hubbard 1976). Poor or failed union of fractures may cause late instability and a combination of imaging may be required in those with new or persisting symptoms (Keene et al. 1988). Rarely nonsurgical osseous bridging of vertebral segments may follow trauma (Osti and Fraser 1992).

15.7 Complications

15.7.1 Neurological Damage

Structures that might be damaged in the lumbar region are the conus medullaris, the cauda equina, and the nerve roots. Any of these may be compressed or transacted at the time of the injury. Similarly, they may be injured by the mechanical instability that results from trauma. Finally, they may be damaged by surgery. High-resolution MR may show transected roots, but it is more common to identify neurological damage by observing the structures that are compressing or transecting the nerve and deducing that the neural pathway is disrupted. Disc prolapse, epidural hematoma, bony intrusion, and impingement by fixation devices are such signs. It is the combination of neurological deficit clinically and the imaging to support the location that leads to the diagnosis. Care should be exercised to exclude other lesions. Injury at another level may coexist and the neurological level of deficit is not as precise in predicting the anatomical level as has been thought in the past. This is particularly true in the early days after injury. A more extensive examination using MR of adjacent regions is valuable.

15.7.2 Defective Union

Malunion of fractures may lead to alignment and structural abnormalities. Flexion, extension, rotation, and scoliosis may result. Unstable segments may lead to a pseudarthrosis.

15.7.3 Infection

Infection may occur as a result of direct implantation at the time of a penetrating injury or secondary to surgery. In the spine, infection is most often centered on the disc space, although with implantation or surgery, the posterior structures and epidural space are more often involved. Plain films may show bony destruction but MRI is more sensitive and will show the extent of involvement of bone and soft tissue in much more detail. MRI is the best means of following progress on antibiotic therapy and it is also the preferred method of planning débridement. Intravenous contrast with MRI may also be important in picking up subtle epidural lesions (Numaguchi et al. 1993).

15.7.4 Dural Tears

Dural tears may be the result of the fracture or surgical intervention (over 7% of operations (Keenen et al. 1990b). They are associated with burst fractures and a neurological defect. Lamina fractures are highly predictive. Contrast introduced into the CSF followed by CT (CT myelography) will show a leak into the epidural space (Morris et al. 1984).

15.8 Conclusion

Plain films are mandatory in patients who have suffered injury to the lumbar spine. Identified injuries may be studied further to assess the need for surgery using CT. MRI is of value in cases of neurological compromise, cases where pain persists without apparent reason and an occult fracture or soft tissue injury is suspected, and in the diagnosis of infection. Care should be taken to handle the patient correctly to avoid catastrophic neurological damage. There are pitfalls in the interpretation of all the possible imaging methods but careful analysis and clinical correlation should provide competent diagnosis and accurate management planning.

References

Albert TJ, Levine MJ, Ah HS, Colter JM, Balderston RA (1993) Concomitant noncontiguous thoracolumbar and sacral fractures. Spine 18:1285–1291

Amour TE, Hodges SC et al (eds) (1994) MRI of the spine. Raven, New York, pp 563–576

Anderson PA, Rivara FP, Maier RV, Drake C (1991) The epidemiology of seatbelt-associated injuries. J Trauma 31:60–67

Anderson S, Biros MH, Reardon RF (1996) Delayed diagnosis of thoracolumbar fractures in multiple-trauma patients. Acad Emerg Med 3:832–839

André V, Le Dreff P, Colin D, André M, Garcia JF (1999) Spinal fractures in ankylosing spondylarthritis. Apropos of 4 cases. J Radiol 80:1575–1578

Appleby JP, Nagy AG (1989) Abdominal injuries associated with the use of seatbelts. Am J Surg 157:457–458

Bedbrook GM (1971) Stability of spinal fractures and fracture dislocations. Paraplegia 9:23–32

Bhalla S, Reinus WR (1998) The linear intravertebral vacuum: a sign of benign vertebral collapse. AJR 170:1563–1569

Blauth M, Bastian L, Knop C, Lange U, Tusch G (1999) Interobserver reliability in the classification of thoraco-lumbar spinal injuries. Orthopäde 28:662–681

Brandser EA, El Khoury GY (1997) Thoracic and lumbar spine trauma. Radiol Clin North Am 35:533–557

Brightman RP, Miller CA, Rea GL, Chakeres DW, Hunt WE (1992) Magnetic resonance imaging of trauma to the thoracic and lumbar spine. The importance of the posterior longitudinal ligament. Spine 17:541–550

Burney RE, Waggoner R, Maynard FM (1989) Stabilization of spinal injury for early transfer. J Trauma 29:1497–1499

Calenoff L, Chessare JW, Rogers LF, Toerge J, Rosen JS (1978) Multiple level spinal injuries: importance of early recognition. AJR 130:665–669

Cammisa FP Jr, Eismont FJ, Green BA (1989) Dural laceration occurring with burst fractures and associated laminar fractures. J Bone Joint Surg Am 71:1044–1052

Capen DA (1999) Classification of thoracolumbar fractures and posterior instrumentation for treatment of thoracolumbar fractures. Instr Course Lect 48:437–441

Chance G (1948) Note on a type of flexion fracture of the spine. Br J Radiol 21:452–453

Chapman JR, Anderson PA (1994) Thoracolumbar spine fractures with neurologic deficit. Orthop Clin North Am 25:595–612

Cotler H, Kulkarni M, Bondurant F, Jia L (1989) Preliminary report on the use of MRI in acute spinal trauma. Zhonghua Wai Ke Za Zhi 27:708–710, 779

Degreif J, Wenda K (1998) Ultrasound-guided spinal fracture repositioning. Surg Endosc 12:164–169

Dehner JR (1971) Seatbelt injuries of the spine and abdomen. AJR 111:833–843

Denis F (1983) The three-column spine and its significance in the classification of acute thoracolumbar spinal injuries. Spine 8:817–831

Denis F, Burkus JK (1991a) Lateral distraction injuries to the thoracic and lumbar spine. A report of three cases. J Bone Joint Surg Am 73:1049–1053

Denis F, Burkus JK (1991b) Diagnosis and treatment of cauda equina entrapment in the vertical lamina fracture of lumbar burst fractures. Spine 16:S433–S439

Denis F, Davis S, Comfort T (1988) Sacral fractures: an important problem. Retrospective analysis of 236 cases. Clin Orthop 227:67–81

Doerr TE, Montesano PX, Burkus JK, Benson DR (1991) Spinal canal decompression in traumatic thoracolumbar burst fractures: posterior distraction rods versus transpedicular screw fixation. J Orthop Trauma 5:403–411

Du Mesnil de Rochemont R, Lanfermann H, Heindel W (1997) Injuries of the spine: current concepts in radiologic diagnosis. Aktuel Radiol 7:1–13

Durham RM, Luchtefeld WB, Wibbenmeyer L, Maxwell P, Shapiro MJ, Mazuski JE (1995) Evaluation of the thoracic and lumbar spine after blunt trauma. Am J Surg 170:681–684

Fahey V, Opeskin K, Silberstein M, Anderson R, Briggs C (1998) The pathogenesis of Schmorl's nodes in relation to acute trauma. An autopsy study. Spine 23:2272–2275

Fast A, Parikh S, Marin EL (1986) Spine fractures in ankylosing spondylitis. Arch Phys Med Rehabil 67:595–597

Ferguson RL, Allen BL Jr (1984) A mechanistic classification of thoracolumbar spine fractures. Clin Orthop 189:77–88

Finkelstein JA, Chapman JR, Mirza S (1999) Occult vertebral fractures in ankylosing spondylitis. Spinal Cord 37:444–447

Foley MJ, Calenoff L, Hendrix RW, Schafer MF (1983) Thoracic and lumbar spine fusion: postoperative radiologic evaluation. AJR 141:373–380

Frankel HL, Rozycki GS, Ochsenr MG, Harviel JD, Champion HR (1994) Indications for obtaining surveillance thoracic and lumbar spine radiographs. J Trauma 37:673–676

Fraser RD (1995) Interbody, posterior, and combined lumbar fusions. Spine 20:167S–177S

Gaebler C, Maier R, Kukla C, Vecsei V (1997) Long-term results of pedicle stabilized thoracolumbar fractures in relation to the neurological deficit. Injury 28:661–666

Gaebler C, Maier R, Kutscha-Lissberg F, Mrkonjic L, Vecsei V (1999) Results of spinal cord decompression and thoracolumbar pedicle stabilisation in relation to the time of operation. Spinal Cord 37:33–39

Gellad FE, Levine AM, Joslyn JN, Edwards CC, Bosse M (1986) Pure thoracolumbar facet dislocation: clinical features and CT appearance. Radiology 161:505–508

Gertzbein SD, Court-Brown CM (1988) Flexion-distraction injuries of the lumbar spine. Mechanisms of injury and classification. Clin Orthop 227:52–60

Glass RB, Sivit CJ, Sturm PF, Bulas DI, Eichelberger MR (1994) Lumbar spine injury in a pediatric population: difficulties with computed tomographic diagnosis. J Trauma 37: 815–819

Glassman SD, Johnson JR, Holt RT (1992) Seatbelt injuries in children. J Trauma 33:882–886

Grabe RP (1988) Fracture-dislocation of the lumbosacral spine during a grand mal epileptic seizure. A case report. S Afr Med J 74:129–131

Hall HE, Robertson WW Jr (1985) Another chance: a non-seatbelt related fracture of the lumbar spine. J Trauma 25: 1163–1166
Hanson JA, Mirza S (2000) Predisposition for spinal fracture in ankylosing spondylitis. AJR 174:150
Heary RF, Vaccaro AR, Mesa JJ, Balderston RA (1996) Thoracolumbar infections in penetrating injuries to the spine. Orthop Clin North Am 27:69–81
Hegenbarth R, Ebel KD (1976) Roentgen findings in fractures of the vertebral column in childhood examination of 35 patients and its results. Pediatr Radiol 5:34–39
Heggeness MH (1993) Spine fracture with neurological deficit in osteoporosis. Osteoporos Int 3:215–221
Hendrix RW, Melany M, Miller F, Rogers LF (1994) Fracture of the spine in patients with ankylosis due to diffuse skeletal hyperostosis: clinical and imaging findings. AJR 162: 899–904
Herndon WA, Galloway D (1988) Neurologic return versus cross-sectional canal area in incomplete thoracolumbar spinal cord injuries. J Trauma 28:680–683
Herron LD, Williams RC (1984) Fracture-dislocation of the lumbosacral spine. Report of a case and review of the literature. Clin Orthop 186:205–211
Hildingsson C, Hietala SO, Toolanen G, Bjornebrink J (1993) Negative scintigraphy despite spinal fractures in the multiply injured. Injury 24:467–470
Holdsworth F (1963) Fractures, dislocations and fracture/dislocations of the spine. J Bone Joint Surg Br 45:6–20
Holland AJ, Cass DT, Glasson MJ, Pitkin J (2000) Small bowel injuries in children. J Paediatr Child Health 36:265–269
Hou S, Hu R, Shi Y (1993) Pedicle morphology of the lower thoracic and lumbar spine in a Chinese population. Spine 18:1850–1855
Howland W, Curry J (1965) Fulcrum fractures of the lumbar spine. JAMA 193:240
Hubbard DD (1976) Fractures of the dorsal and lumbar spine. Orthop Clin North Am 7:605–614
Huelke DF, Kaufer H (1975) Vertebral column injuries and seat belts. J Trauma 15:304–318
Huelke DF, Mackay GM, Morris A (1995) Vertebral column injuries and lap-shoulder belts. J Trauma 38:547–556
Isiklar ZU, Lindsey RW (1997) Low-velocity civilian gunshot wounds of the spine. Orthopedics 20:967–972
Jeanneret B, Holdener HJ (1992) Vertebral fractures and abdominal trauma. A retrospective study based on 415 documented vertebral fractures. Unfallchirurg 95:603–607
Jelly LM, Evans DR, Easty MJ, Coats TJ, Chan O (2000) Radiography versus spiral CT in the evaluation of cervicothoracic junction injuries in polytrauma patients who have undergone intubation. Radiographics 20:251–259
Jodoin A, Dupuis P, Fraser M, Beaumont P (1985) Unstable fractures of the thoracolumbar spine: a 10-year experience at Sacré-Coeur Hospital. J Trauma 25:197–202
Kahamba JF, Rath SA, Antoniadis G, Schneider O, Neff U, Richter HP (1998) Laminar and arch fractures with dural tear and nerve root entrapment in patients operated upon for thoracic and lumbar spine injuries. Acta Neurochir (Wien) 140:114–119
Kaye JJ, Nance EP Jr (1990) Thoracic and lumbar spine trauma. Radiol Clin North Am 28:361–377
Keene JS, Lash EG, Kling TF Jr (1988) Undetected posttraumatic instability of "stable" thoracolumbar fractures. J Orthop Trauma 2:202–211
Keenen TL, Antony J, Benson DR (1990a) Non-contiguous spinal fractures. J Trauma 30:489–491
Keenen TL, Antony J, Benson DR (1990b) Dural tears associated with lumbar burst fractures. J Orthop Trauma 4: 243–245
Kelly RP, Whitesides TE Jr (1968) Treatment of lumbodorsal fracture-dislocations. Ann Surg 167:705–717
Kerttula LI, Serlo WS, Tervonen OA, Paakko EL, Vanharanta HV (2000) Post-traumatic findings of the spine after earlier vertebral fracture in young patients: clinical and MRI study. Spine 25:1104–1108
Kifune M, Panjabi MM, Arand M, Liu W (1995) Fracture pattern and instability of thoracolumbar injuries. Eur Spine J 4:98–103
Krueger MA, Green DA, Hoyt D, Garfin SR (1996) Overlooked spine injuries associated with lumbar transverse process fractures. Clin Orthop 327:191–195
Kuner EH, Schlickewei W, Kuner A, Hauser U (1997) Restoration of the spinal canal by the internal fixator and remodelling. Eur Spine J 6:417–422
Legay DA, Petrie DP, Alexander DI (1990) Flexion-distraction injuries of the lumbar spine and associated abdominal trauma. J Trauma 30:436–444
Le Hir PX, Sautet A, Le Gars L et al (1999) Hyperextension vertebral body fractures in diffuse idiopathic skeletal hyperostosis: a cause of intravertebral fluid-like collections on MR imaging. AJR 173:1679–1683
Letts M, Davidson D, Fleuriau-Chateau P, Chou S (1999) Seat belt fracture with late development of an enterocolic fistula in a child. A case report. Spine 24:1151–1155
Leventhal MR (1998) Fractures, dislocations and fracture-dislocations of spline. In: Canale S (ed) Campbell's orthopaedics. Mosby, St Louis, pp 2704–2790
Magerl F, Aebi M, Gertzbein SD, Harms J, Nazarian S (1994) A comprehensive classification of thoracic and lumbar injuries. Eur Spine J 3:184–201
Marczynski W, Kroczak S, Baranski M (1999) Fractures of thoracic and lumbar spine; treatment and follow-up. Ann Transplant 4:46–48
Martijn A, Veldhuis EF (1991) The diagnostic value of interpediculate distance assessment on plain films in thoracic and lumbar spine injuries. J Trauma 31:1393–1395
Martinez Lage JF, Poza M, Arcas P (1998) Avulsed lumbar vertebral rim plate in an adolescent: trauma or malformation? Childs Nerv Syst 14:131–134
McAfee PC, Yuan HA, Fredrickson BE, Lubicky JP (1983) The value of computed tomography in thoracolumbar fractures. An analysis of one hundred consecutive cases and a new classification. J Bone Joint Surg Am 65:461–473
McCullen G, Vaccaro AR, Garfin SR (1998) Thoracic and lumbar trauma: rationale for selecting the appropriate fusion technique. Orthop Clin North Am 29:813–828
McGuire RA, Neville S, Green BA, Watts C (1987) Spinal instability and the log-rolling maneuver. J Trauma 27:525–531
McKenney KL (1999) Ultrasound of blunt abdominal trauma. Radiol Clin North Am 37:879–893
Meldon SW, Moettus LN (1995) Thoracolumbar spine fractures: clinical presentation and the effect of altered sensorium and major injury. J Trauma 39:1110–1114
Mitra D, Elvins DM, Speden DJ, Collins AJ (2000) The prevalence of vertebral fractures in mild ankylosing spondylitis and their relationship to bone mineral density. Rheumatology (Oxf) 39:85–89

Morris RE, Hasso AN, Thompson JR, Hinshaw DB, Vu LH (1984) Traumatic dural tears: CT diagnosis using metrizamide. Radiology 152:443–446

Neumann P, Nordwall A, Osvalder AL (1995) Traumatic instability of the lumbar spine. A dynamic in vitro study of flexion-distraction injury. Spine 20:1111–1121

Neumann P, Wang Y, Karrholm J, Malchau H, Nordwall A (1999) Determination of inter-spinous process distance in the lumbar spine. Evaluation of reference population to facilitate detection of severe trauma. Eur Spine J 8:272–278

Newman KD, Bowman LM, Eichelberger MR et al (1990) The lap belt complex: intestinal and lumbar spine injury in children. J Trauma 30:1133–1138; discussion 1138–1140

Nicholl E (1949) Fractures of the dorso-lumbar spine. J Bone Joint Surg Br 31:376

Numaguchi YD, Rigamonti D, Rothman MI, Sato S, Mihara F, Sadato N (1993) Spinal epidural abscess with gadolinium-enhanced MR imaging. Radiographics 13:545–560

Olerud C, Frost A, Bring J (1996) Spinal fractures in patients with ankylosing spondylitis. Eur Spine J 5:51–55

Osti OL, Fraser RD (1992) Osseous bridging of lumbar intertransverse processes after trauma. A case report. Spine 17:362–363

Osti OL, Fraser RD, Cornish BL (1987) Fractures and fractures-dislocations of the lumbar spine. A retrospective study of 70 patients. Int Orthop 11:323–329

Pal JM, Mulder DS, Brown RA, Fleiszer DM (1988) Assessing multiple trauma: is the cervical spine enough? J Trauma 28: 1282–1284

Panjabi MM, Oxland TR, Lin RM, McGowen TW (1994) Thoracolumbar burst fracture. A biomechanical investigation of its multidirectional flexibility. Spine 19:578–585

Panjabi MM, Oxland TR, Kifune M, Arand M, Wen L, Chen A (1995) Validity of the three-column theory of thoracolumbar fractures. A biomechanical investigation. Spine 20: 1122–1127

Pathria MN, Petersilge CA (1991) Spinal trauma. Radiol Clin North Am 29:847–865

Patten RM, Gunberg SR, Brandenburger DK (2000) Frequency and importance of transverse process fractures in the lumbar vertebrae at helical abdominal CT in patients with trauma. Radiology 215:831–834

Penta M, Fraser RD (1997) Anterior lumbar interbody fusion. A minimum 10-year follow-up. Spine 22:2429–2434

Peris P, Guanabens N, Pares A et al (1995) Vertebral fractures and osteopenia in chronic alcoholic patients. Calcif Tissue Int 57:111–114

Porter RS, Zhao N (1998) Patterns of injury in belted and unbelted individuals presenting to a trauma center after motor vehicle crash: seat belt syndrome revisited. Ann Emerg Med 32:418–424

Rabinovici R, Ovadia P, Mathiak G, Abdullah F (1999) Abdominal injuries associated with lumbar spine fractures in blunt trauma. Injury 30:471–474

Rechtine GR Jr, Cahill D, Chrin AM (1999) Treatment of thoracolumbar trauma: comparison of complications of operative versus nonoperative treatment. J Spinal Disord 12:406–409

Reid AB, Letts RM, Black GB (1990) Pediatric Chance fractures: association with intra-abdominal injuries and seatbelt use. J Trauma 30:384–391

Richter D, Hahn MP, Ostermann PA, Ekkernkamp A, Muhr G (1996) Vertical deceleration injuries: a comparative study of the injury patterns of 101 patients after accidental and intentional high falls. Injury 27:655–659

Riebel GD, Yoo JU, Fredrickson BE, Yuan HA (1993) Review of Harrington rod treatment of spinal trauma. Spine 18:479–491

Riggins RS, Kraus JF (1977) The risk of neurologic damage with fractures of the vertebrae. J Trauma 17:126–133

Rogers LF (1971) The roentgenographic appearance of transverse or chance fractures of the spine: the seat belt fracture. AJR 111:844–849

Rosenthal RE, Lowery ER (1980) Unstable fracture-dislocations of the thoracolumbar spine: results of surgical treatment. J Trauma 20:485–490

Rupp RE, Ebraheim NA, Chrissos MG, Jackson WT (1994) Thoracic and lumbar fractures associated with femoral shaft fractures in the multiple trauma patient. Occult presentations and implications for femoral fracture stabilization. Spine 19:556–560

Ryan S, Sandler A, Trenhaile S, Ephgrave K, Garner S (1994) Pancreatic enzyme elevations after blunt trauma. Surgery 116:622–627

Saboe LA, Reid DC, Davis LA, Warren SA, Grace MG (1991) Spine trauma and associated injuries. J Trauma 31:43–48

Samuels LE, Kerstein MD (1993) 'Routine' radiologic evaluation of the thoracolumbar spine in blunt trauma patients: a reappraisal. J Trauma 34:85–89

Schlegel J, Bayley J, Yuan H, Fredricksen B (1996) Timing of surgical decompression and fixation of acute spinal fractures. J Orthop Trauma 10:323–330

Silberstein M, McLean K (1995) Fast magnetic resonance imaging in spinal trauma. Aust Radiol 39:118–123

Singer KP, Willen J, Breidahl PD, Day RE (1989) Radiologic study of the influence of zygapophyseal joint orientation on spinal injuries at the thoracolumbar junction. Surg Radiol Anat 11:233–239

Sivit CJ, Taylor GA, Newman KD et al (1991) Safety-belt injuries in children with lap-belt ecchymosis: CT findings in 61 patients. AJR 157:111–114

Splavski B, Vrankovic D, Blagus G, Mursic B, Ivekovic V (1996a) Spinal stability after war missile injuries of the spine. J Trauma 41:850–853

Splavski B, Vrankovic D, Saric G, Blagus G, Mursic B, Rukovanjski M (1996b) Early management of war missile spine and spinal cord injuries: experience with 21 cases. Injury 27:699–702

Splavski B, Saric G, Vrankovic D, Glavina K, Mursic B, Blagus G (1998) Computed tomography of the spine as an important diagnostic tool in the management of war missile spinal trauma. Arch Orthop Trauma Surg 117:360–363

Stanislas MJ, Latham JM, Porter KM, Alpar EK, Stirling AJ (1998) A high-risk group for thoracolumbar fractures. Injury 29:15–18

Steinitz DK, Alexander DI, Leighton RK, O'Sullivan JJ (1997) Late displacement of a fracture dislocation at the lumbosacral junction. A case study. Spine 22:1024–1027

Sward L, Hellstrom M, Jacobsson B, Karlsson L (1993) Vertebral ring apophysis injury in athletes. Is the etiology different in the thoracic and lumbar spine? Am J Sports Med 21:841–845

Tanchev P, Dikov D, Novkov H (2000) Thoracolumbar distraction fractures in advanced pregnancy: a contribution of two case reports. Eur Spine J 9:167–170

Taylor GA, Eggli KD (1988) Lap-belt injuries of the lumbar spine in children: a pitfall in CT diagnosis. AJR 150:1355–1358

Taylor GA, Fallat ME, Potter BM, Eichelberger MR (1988) The role of computed tomography in blunt abdominal trauma in children. J Trauma 28:1660–1664

Terk MR, Hume-Neal M, Fraipont M, Ahmadi J, Colletti PM

(1997) Injury of the posterior ligament complex in patients with acute spinal trauma: evaluation by MR imaging. AJR 168:1481–1486
Thorngren KG, Liedberg E, Aspelin P (1981) Fractures of the thoracic and lumbar spine in ankylosing spondylitis. Arch Orthop Trauma Surg 98:101–107
Tress BM, Hare WS (1990) CT of the spine: are plain spine radiographs necessary? Clin Radiol 41:317–320
Van Eenenaam DP, El-Khoury GY (1993) Delayed post-traumatic vertebral collapse (Kummell's disease): case report with serial radiographs, computed tomographic scans, and bone scans. Spine 18:1236–1241
Velmahos G, Demetriades D (1994) Gunshot wounds of the spine: should retained bullets be removed to prevent infection? Ann R Coll Surg Engl 76:85–87
Velmahos GC, Degiannis E, Hart K, Souter I, Saadia R (1995) Changing profiles in spinal cord injuries and risk factors influencing recovery after penetrating injuries. J Trauma 38:334–337
Verheyden P, Katscher S, Schulz T, Schmidt F, Josten C (1999) Open MR imaging in spine surgery: experimental investigations and first clinical experiences. Eur Spine J 8: 346–353
Weinstein JN, Collalto P, Lehmann TR (1987) Long-term follow-up of nonoperatively treated thoracolumbar spine fractures. J Orthop Trauma 1:152–159
Whitesides TE Jr (1977) Traumatic kyphosis of the thoracolumbar spine. Clin Orthop 128:78–92
Wilmink JT (1999) MR imaging of the spine: trauma and degenerative disease. Eur Radiol 9:1259–1266
Woodring JH, Lee C, Jenkins K (1988) Spinal fractures in blunt chest trauma. J Trauma 28:789–793
Yazici M, Gulman B, Sen S, Tilki K (1995) Sagittal contour restoration and canal clearance in burst fractures of the thoracolumbar junction (T12–L1): the efficacy of timing of the surgery. J Orthop Trauma 9:491–498
Youssef JA, McCullen GM, Brown CC (1995) Seizure-induced lumbar burst fracture. Spine 20:1301–1303

16 Injuries of the Pelvic Bone

F. Portier, E. Mouhsine, N. Theumann, A. Denys, P. Schnyder, J. P. Verdon

CONTENTS

F. Portier, MD
Service de Radiodiagnostic et Radiologie interventionelle, CHUV, Rue du Bugnon, 1011 Lausanne, Switzerland
E. Mouhsine, MD
Service de Chirurgie Orthopédique, CHUV, Rue du Bugnon, 1011 Lausanne, Switzerland
N. Theumann, MD
Service de Radiodiagnostic et Radiologie interventionelle, CHUV, Rue du Bugnon, 1011 Lausanne, Switzerland
A. Denys, MD
Service de Radiodiagnostic et Radiologie interventionelle, CHUV, Rue du Bugnon, 1011 Lausanne, Switzerland
P. A. Schnyder, MD
Professor, Service de Radiodiagnostic et Radiologie interventionelle, CHUV, Rue du Bugnon, 1011 Lausanne, Switzerland
J. P. Verdon, MD
Service de Radiodiagnostic et Radiologie interventionelle, CHUV, Rue du Bugnon, 1011 Lausanne, Switzerland

Isolated Acetabular Fractures

- Function is mainly at stake
- Radiological assessment relies upon good-quality plain films completed by CT imaging in fine slices with multiplanar reconstruction
- Letournel's classification remains the reference
- Re-establishing a joint congruence to prevent early coxarthrosis is the main point

Pelvic Ring Fractures

- Often occur in violent trauma and are associated with visceral lesions, putting vital prognosis at stake
- Radiological assessment must be included in multidisciplinary management
- In case of hemodynamic shock, external fracture stabilization and embolization of pelvic bleeding must be performed as soon as possible
- In other cases, CT imaging allows fast and complete investigation of both visceral and osseous lesions
- Tile/AO classification is the most used today

16.1 Introduction

Pelvic trauma includes a great variety of polymorphous lesions, which differ from each other by their anatomical aspect, context, and therapeutic implications: isolated bone tear needing no particular treatment; acetabular fractures with major functional prognosis or high-energy trauma with pelvic ring disruption, vital lesions, and hemorrhage implying emergency hemostasis. In order to be efficient, the radiologist first has to know the diagnostic value of each radiological technique, in order to suggest the investigation strategy which is the most appropriate to a given clinical situation. Then, he must be able to accurately describe fractures and include them in a classification in agreement with the clinician.

16.2 Incidence

Pelvic ring fractures account for up to 1.5% of all joint fractures (Melton et al. 1981; Mucha and Farnell 1984). Simple fractures without significant displacement mainly affect elderly female patients having sustained low-energy trauma. Severe displaced lesions affect younger, predominantly male patients implicated in a high-energy trauma, which results in multiple trauma in 75% of the cases (Pohlemann et al. 1994; Eastbridge and Burgess 1997; Gansslen et al. 1996). Melton reported 175 pelvic fractures over 10 years, including 84 fragmented and isolated lesions, 71 simple pelvic ring ruptures, and 20 severe fractures (Melton et al. 1981). Among the latter, 48% were provoked by high-energy trauma and 2% by simple falls. The average age of the first group was about 33, while in the second, it was about 69 years. Low-energy trauma provoked fragmented or simple lesions in 95% of cases. The female/male sex ratio was 2:1. Pohlemann reported 200 serious fractures (10.5%) out of a series of 1409 cases within 20 years (Pohlemann et al. 1998). The most frequent causes of pelvic trauma are related to car accidents (50–60%) and car–pedestrian crashes (14–18%) (Cryer et al. 1988; Dalal et al. 1989; Burgess et al. 1990; McIntyre et al. 1993; Vazquez and Garcia 1993). In a recent review of traffic accidents, 4.1% of cases presented pelvic ring lesions. Among these, 47% of cases were car passengers, 31% pedestrians, 12% motorcyclists, and 10% cyclists (Pohlemann et al. 2000). In the same group, only those belt-fastened patients, for whom the speed gradient exceeded 30 km/h, suffered pelvic ring lesions, while the unbelted ones suffered lesions with lower speed gradients.

16.3 Anatomy and Biomechanics

16.3.1 Pelvic Ring

The pelvis is a ring composed of three bones: the sacrum dorsally and two innominate bones front-medially. The sacrum joins the innominate bone by the sacroiliac joints. The two innominate bones join frontally by the symphysis pubis. The innominate bone includes three separate ossification zones: the ilium, the ischium, and the pubis. The posterior stability of the ring is assured by the posterior tension band, which includes the posterior and interosseous sacroiliac ligaments. This ligamentous complex and the sacrotuberous ligaments resist vertical translation between the ilia and the sacrum. The anterior sacroiliac, symphyseal, and sacrospinous ligaments are transversely oriented and resist rotation of the pelvis (Kellam and Browner 1992; Tile 1995) (Fig. 16.1). Pelvic instability is defined by two displacements: rotational and vertical. The forces, caused by rotational displacements, tend either to open and externally rotate the pelvis, or to close and rotate it internally. Vertical instability indicates disruption of the posterior tension band and implies craniocaudal, rotational, and anteroposterior displacement (Kellam and Browner 1992). Three basic mechanisms lead to pelvic ring disruptions (Pennal and Sutherland 1961; Daffner 1990; Hunter et al. 1997). They are based on the direction of the force imparted to the pelvis at the time of injury.

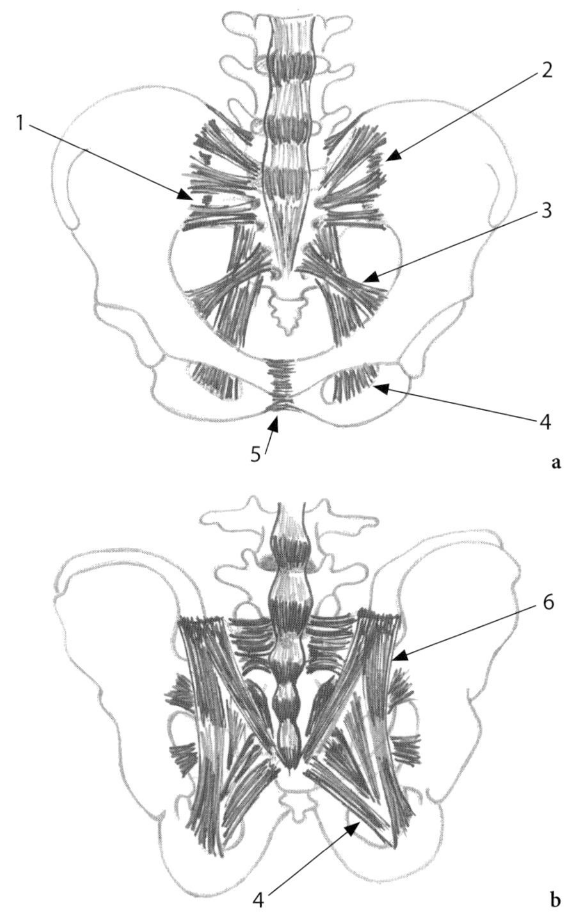

Fig. 16.1a, b. Schematic display of normal pelvic ligaments. **a** Anterior view. **b** Posterior view. *1*, Interosseous sacroiliac ligament; *2*, anterior sacroiliac ligaments; *3*, sacrospinous ligaments; *4*, sacrotuberous ligaments; *5*, symphysis pubis; *6*, posterior sacroiliac ligaments

16.3.1.1
Anteroposterior Compression

The anterior-posterior (AP) compression injury pattern is due to a force directly applied to the pubis or to the posterior pelvis and results in iliac external rotation deformity (Fig. 16.2). The symphyseal separation suggests damage to the ligamentous structures and possible instability. The presence of a vertical obturator ring fracture, a diastasis of both the symphysis pubis and the sacroiliac joint are important points of this pattern and serve as stability hallmarks (Young and Burgess 1987; Daffner 1990; Kellam and Browner 1992; Tile 1995).

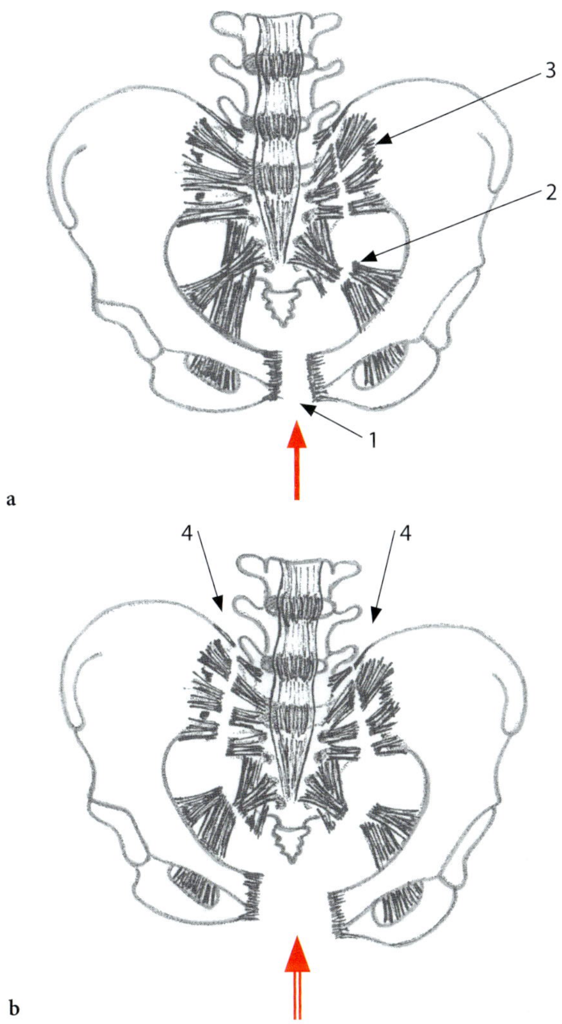

Fig. 16.2a,b. Anteroposterior compression. **a** Low energy. **b** High energy. *1*, Symphysis diastasis; *2*, sacrospinous and sacrotuberous ligament disruption; *3*, anterior sacroiliac ligament disruption, *4*, posterior sacroiliac ligament disruption

16.3.1.2
Lateral Compression

The lateral compression injury pattern or iliac internal rotation injury is the result of a lateral blow to the side of the pelvis (Fig. 16.3). This fracture affects either one or both sides of the pelvic ring. Anteriorly, the fracture fragments frequently override the adjacent fragments. Posteriorly, the fracture fragments are impacted mainly in elderly patients or there is a diastasis of the sacroiliac joint, mainly in the younger patients, and sometimes associated with ligamentous disruption (Young and Burgess 1987; Daffner 1990; Kellam and Browner 1992; Rogers 1992).

16.3.1.3
Vertical Shear

The vertical shear pattern is often an unstable state, when it appears after a vertical axial fall, with presence of anterior and posterior fractures of the pubic rami, fractures of the sacrum, sacroiliac diastasis, or iliac wing fracture (Fig. 16.4). A typical finding is always present as a superior and usually asymmetric displacement of the involved hemi-pelvis secondary to the vertical axial fall (Hunter et al. 1997).

16.3.2
Acetabulum

The acetabulum is composed by two columns: the large anterior column and the small posterior column. An inverted Y is formed by these two columns which sup-

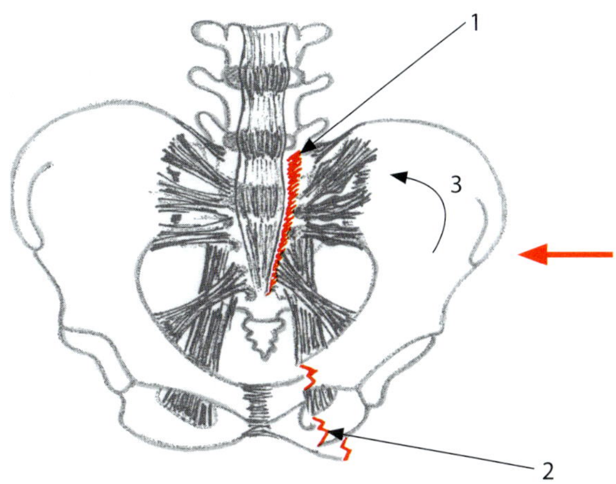

Fig. 16.3. Schematic display of lateral compression. *1*, Impacted fractures of the sacrum; *2*, horizontal overlapping ring fracture; *3*, internal rotation of the left hemipelvis

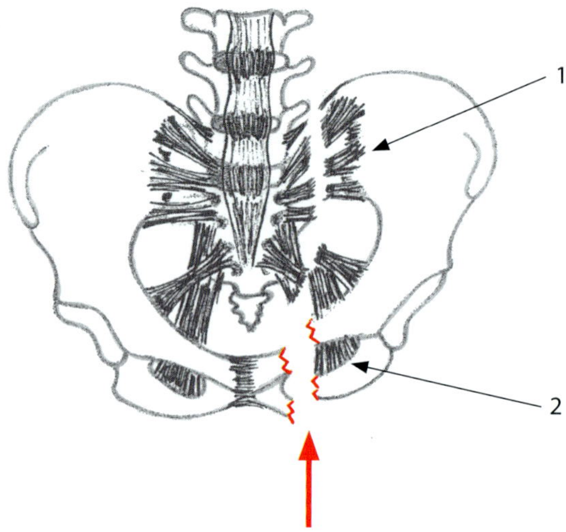

Fig. 16.4. Schematic display of vertical shear pattern. *1*, Note both anterior and posterior ligamentous disruption; *2*, obturator ring fractures

port the hip (Harley et al. 1982; Mayo 1987; Goulet and Bray 1989; Martinez et al. 1992) (Fig. 16.5). The anterior column begins at the inferior pubic ramus and extends above the acetabulum into the iliac wing. The posterior column is shaped by the ischium and extends to the greater sciatic notch and the sacroiliac. The inferior junction of the two columns forms the ischiopubic junction. The quadrilateral plate shapes the medial wall of the acetabulum. It is a thin layer of bone between the hip joint and the pelvis. In addition to the two columns, the bone stability of the hip is increased by the presence of anterior and posterior walls, the latter being larger than the former. Basic fracture mechanisms will be described with the classifications further down.

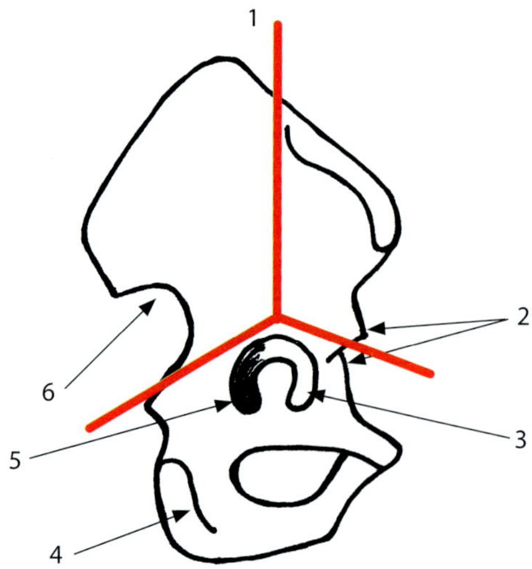

Fig. 16.5. Normal acetabular anatomy. *1*, Inverted Y; *2*, iliopectineal line; *3*, anterior wall; *4*, ischial tuberosity; *5*, posterior wall; *6*, sciatic notch

16.4 Imaging

16.4.1 Plain Films

The anteroposterior view of the pelvis is the basic projection for pelvic trauma. It allows identification of the ilioischial line, the iliopectineal line and the iliopubic line, as well as the anterior and posterior acetabular wall (Fig. 16.6). The iliopectineal line is formed by the anterior structure of the acetabulum. The ilioischial line is formed by posterior structures of the acetabulum (Ersoy et al. 1995). More specifically to each type of fracture, many projections have been evaluated, among which Pennal's are mostly used in pelvic ring investigations and Judet's in acetabulum investigations.

16.4.1.1 Pelvic Ring

Figures 16.7 and 16.8 show projections of the pelvic inlet, with the tube angled 45° caudally, and the pelvic outlet, with the tube angled 45° cephalad, which may be added to the AP view when pelvic fracture is suspected (Fig. 16.7) (Mayo 1987; Daffner 1990; Kellam and Browner 1992; Rogers 1992; Routt 1993). These projections are known as Pennal's projections. The pelvic inlet view proves best for displaying an antero-posterior displacement of the hemi-pelvis as well as horizontal rotation, while an outlet view identifies vertical displacement, superior displacement of the hemi-pelvis thus being evaluated in comparison with the levels of posterior elements. Anteriorly, the symphysis pubis and pubis rami are inspected, whereas posteriorly the iliac crests, the sacrum, sacral foramina, sacroiliac joints, and transverse processes of L5 are evaluated to rule out possible injuries. Particular attention is paid to the sacrogluteal line, which corresponds to the continuation of the iliopectineal line around the greater sciatic notch and onto the body of the sacrum. This hallmark is useful in identifying posterior fractures. The arcuate lines of the sacrum, representing the dense cortical bone between the sacral foramina, should also be examined. A distortion or break here highlights a lesion (McLeod and Powell 1997).

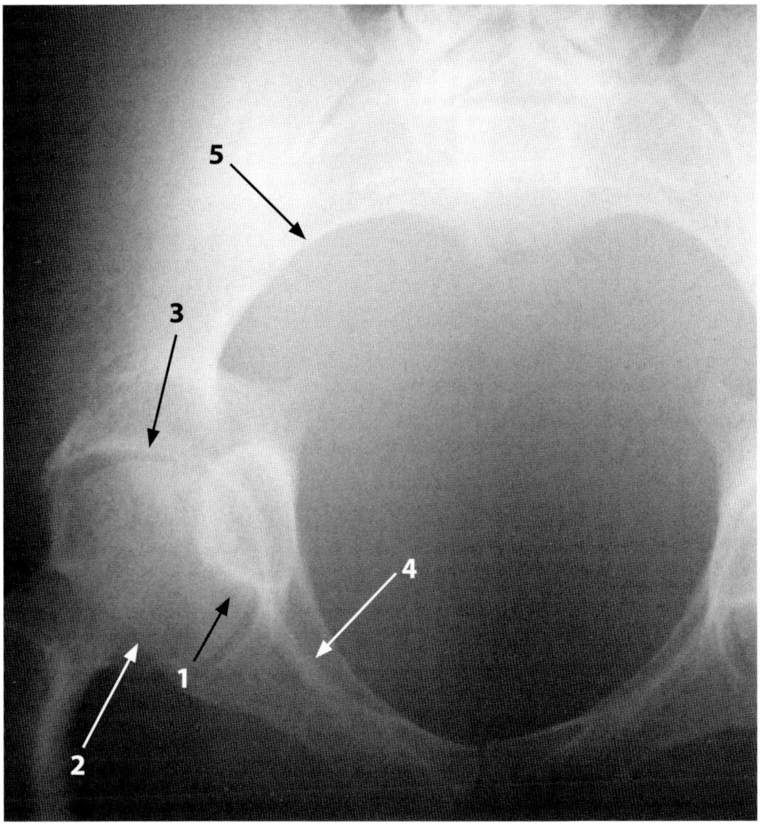

Fig. 16.6. Normal anatomy, anteroposterior view (AP). *1*, Anterior lip; *2*, posterior lip; *3*, Roof; *4*, ilioischial line; *5*, iliopectineal line; *6*, tear drop; *7*, sSacrogluteal line; *8*, arcuate line

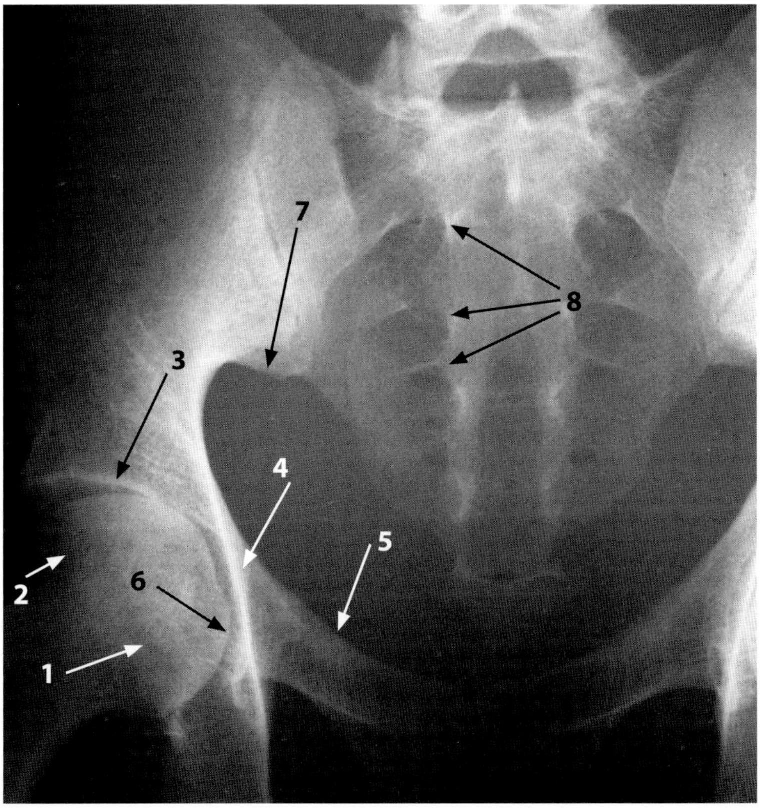

Fig. 16.7. Inlet view. *1*, Anterior lip; *2*, posterior lip; *3*, roof; *4*, iliopectineal line; *5*, anterior border of the sacral

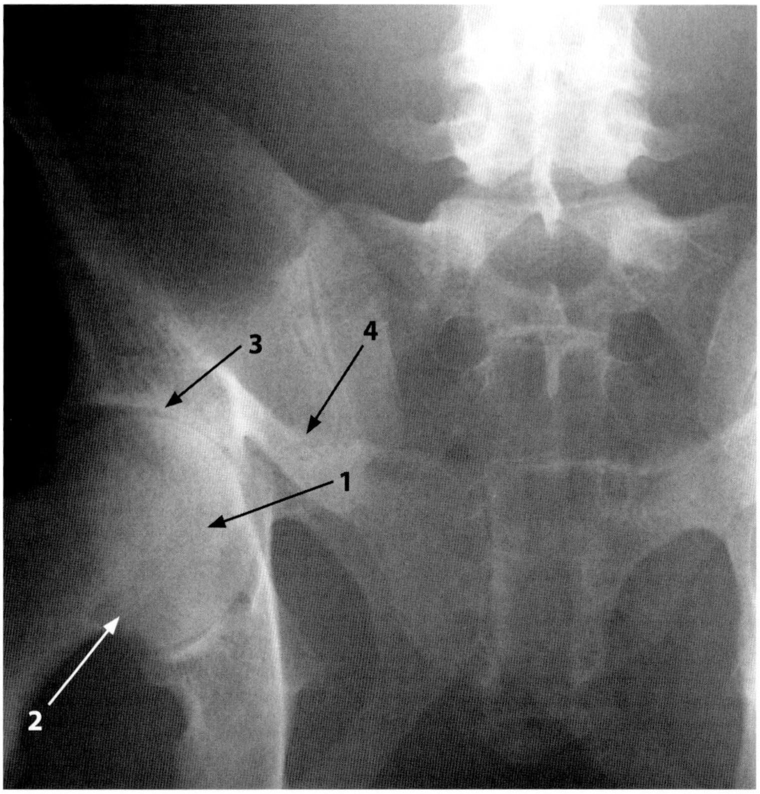

Fig. 16.8. Normal anatomy, outlet view. *1*, Anterior lip; *2*, posterior lip; *3*, roof; *4*, iliopectineal line

16.4.1.2 Acetabulum

If an acetabular fracture is suspected, three more projections are mandatory in addition to the anteroposterior view: an anteroposterior view centered on the injured hip and two oblique views according to Judet, obtained with the patient rotated 45° in a right posterior oblique or oblique iliac view and left posterior oblique or obturator oblique view, in the supine position (Figs. 16.9 and 16.10) (Letournel and Judet 1993). In the majority of cases, these four projections are sufficient for classifying these fractures and to proposing a therapeutic strategy. The two oblique views and the classic anteroposterior view of the hip identify six basic landmarks: the acetabular roof, the acetabular anterior lip, the acetabular posterior lip, the ilioischial line, the iliopectineal or iliopubic line, and the tear drop. The ilioischial line is shaped by posterior parts. The iliopectineal line is shaped by anterior parts of the acetabulum. If a disruption of the landmarks is seen on plain films, the fracture can often be classified properly. The iliac oblique view shows the iliac wing, useful for displaying a fracture that extends above the acetabulum into the iliac wing. The obturator oblique view shows fractures of the obturator ring, of the posterior wall of the acetabulum, and of the greater sciatic notch (Perry and Delong 1997).

16.4.2 Computed Tomography

16.4.2.1 Technique

Several protocols can be applied:

- In case of pelvic trauma, complete pelvis investigation may be performed with 5-mm slices every 5 mm allowing for a wide area investigation, from above the iliac crests down to the ischia, with a sufficient investigation quality. Depending on the mechanism of injury, an intravenous contrast agent injection is useful to investigate visceral lesions. Associated examination of the abdomen seems mandatory as the abdomen and pelvis remain the same traumatic entity (Federle 1995; Chaumoitre et al. 2000). CT acquisition should start at least 60 s after injection of contrast to make sure that a good visceral enhancement is obtained

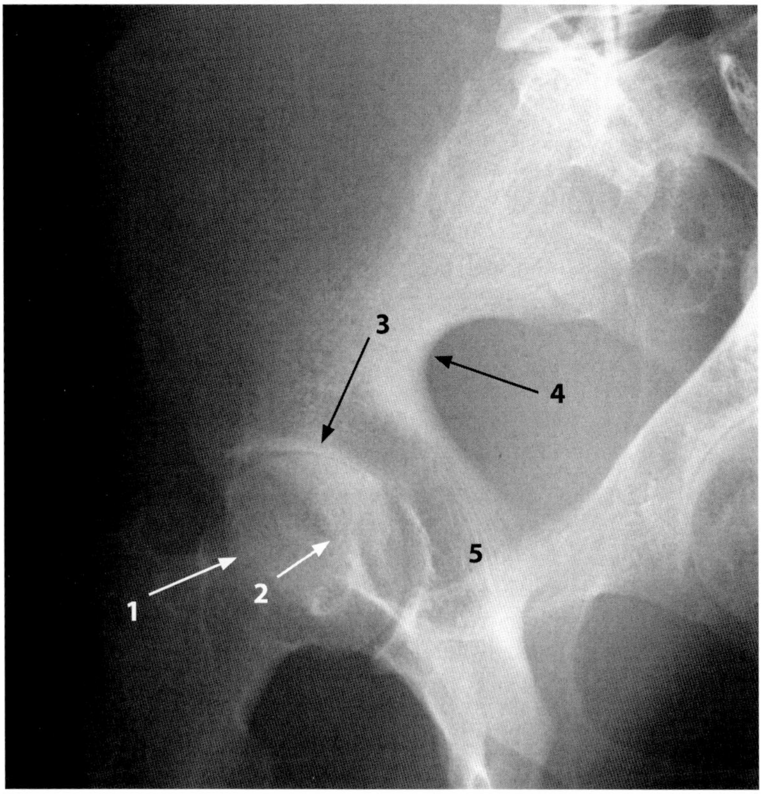

Fig. 16.9. Normal anatomy, iliac oblique view. *1*, Anterior lip; *2*, posterior lip; *3*, roof; *4*, greater sciatic notch; *5*, quadrilateral surface

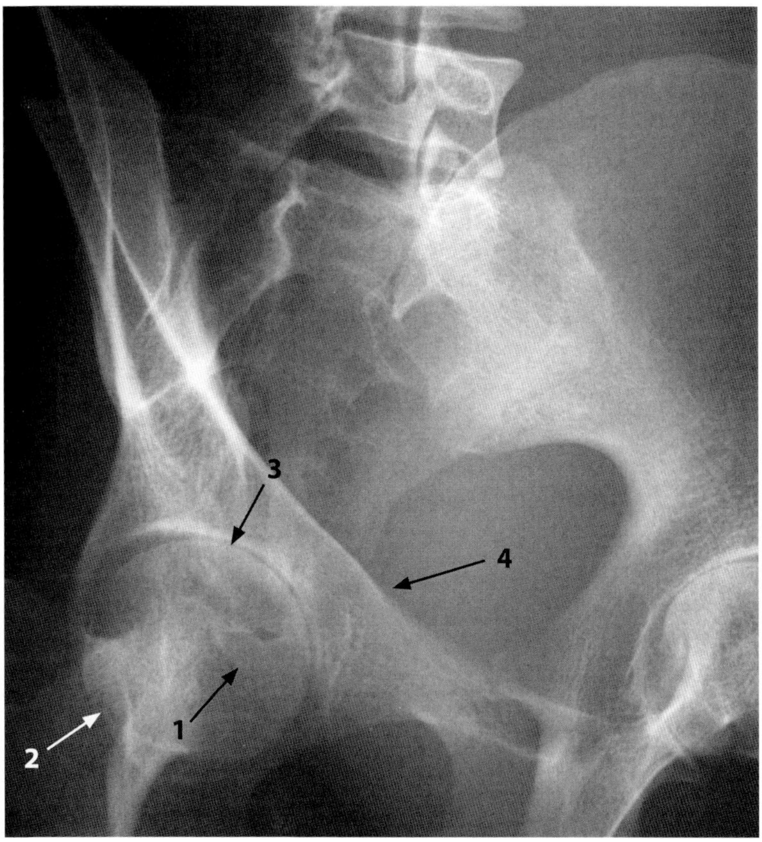

Fig. 16.10. Normal anatomy, obturator oblique view. *1*, Anterior lip; *2*, posterior lip; *3*, roof; *4*, pelvic brim

and mainly to detect an active hemorrhage showing as contrast agent extravasation. Such a protocol makes it possible to evaluate both osseous and visceral lesions.

- If an acetabular lesion is suspected from the clinical examination and plain films or seen on CT, thinner slices from 1–3 mm, joint or overlapping, are mandatory. They allow a better analysis of the lesions and good quality multiplanar reconstructions. If not performed before, a systematic investigation of the entire pelvis with a 5-mm slice thickness is recommended to complete the acetabular examination.
- Multiplanar reconstructions are useful for understanding complex fractures, mainly of the acetabulum. They often need thinner acquisition with 3-mm slice thickness or less and overlapping reconstruction to improve imaging quality. However, even with 5-mm-thick slice acquisitions, multiplanar reconstructions may be of interest. In this case, quality may be improved by overlapping axial slices. Reconstruction in anatomical planes, sacrum plane, or iliac wing plane may be added to the classic sagittal and frontal reconstruction planes.
- 3D reconstruction is favored by surgeons but should only be used as a tool to the understanding of complex fractures, in particular for acetabular fractures or when significant displacements of the fragments have occurred. Reading should always be achieved with axial and/or multiplanar reconstructions, which remain the best analysis tools.
- In case of doubt on sacral lesions, acquisitions in the oblique coronal plane, tilting the gantry parallel to the long sacral axis, often improve imaging quality. But in most cases, multiplanar reconstructions are sufficient.

16.4.2.2 Multislice Computed Tomography

Multidetector technology provides extended possibilities in trauma investigation: a large area of exploration, faster acquisition, thinner thickness of slices, and easy reformatting in the appropriate plane. At our institution, pelvic investigation of multiple trauma patients is systematically included in a complete thoracic, abdominal, and pelvic examination obtained with the multislice technique using 5-mm slices every 5 mm after intravenous contrast injection. Slices may be secondarily reconstructed in 2.5-mm thickness in case of suspected lesion. This protocol has been used in our hospital for more than 1 year, with about 300 patients explored. It allows faster and more accurate detection of visceral and osseous lesions in one examination. Secondary multiplanar and 3D reconstructions with 2.5-mm-thick slices are of great quality even for acetabular fractures. If needed, better quality may be obtained with 1.25- or 1-mm-thick slices in addition to the initial investigation protocol.

16.4.2.3 Indications

Because of its potential, indications of CT are on the rise. For Hunter, they may be detailed as follows: acetabular fractures, dislocations of the hip, all potential or recognized sacral fractures, all potential or recognized sacroiliac injuries, and any question of stability in pelvic fractures (Hunter et al. 1997).

16.4.2.4 Results

CT imaging has become an outstanding tool in pelvis imaging (Geusens et al. 2000). Its technological improvements, helicoidal and multidetector technologies, have recently increased its potentials. In some cases, its performance has proved to be superior to plain films. About 30% of pelvic fractures detected by CT are missed by plain films (Rogers 1992; Berg et al. 1996). In sacral trauma, plain films missed 29% of sacroiliac diastasis, 57% of acetabular rim fractures, and 34% of vertical shearing fractures (Montana et al. 1986). Plain films also missed up to 40% of intraarticular fragments and 50% of femoral head fractures visualized with CT (Harley et al. 1982; Vas et al. 1982). It should be mentioned that detection of additional fractures will change the patient's management (Vas et al. 1982; Gill and Bucholz 1984). CT imaging has limitations. Some authors relate false negatives but comparison with the new-generation CT device might show better results (Young et al. 1986). However, plain films should never be neglected, particularly in the initial evaluation. In acetabular fractures, for instance, CT imaging remains insufficient in the characterization of some fractures while plain films allow better understanding of its findings (Brandser et al. 1995; Mayo 1987). Moreover, CT imaging allows complete investigation of visceral pelvic lesions and of associated thoracic, abdominal and even brain lesions (Killeen and Demeo 1999; Chaumoitre et al. 2000).

16.4.3 Magnetic Resonance Imaging

Some studies have shown its superiority in particular circumstances, such as the detection of intraarticular splinters, evaluation of the femoral head, and detection of hidden fractures, mainly in the elderly (POTTER et al. 1994). However, its use remains of minor importance in pelvic trauma in the acute phase.

16.5 Classifications

16.5.1 Pelvic Ring Fractures

One of the first descriptions of iliac wing fracture was reported by Duverney in 1751 (McLEOD and POWELL 1997). Until the 1950s, classifications of pelvic ring fractures were based only on anatomical descriptions of the lesions. PENNAL and SUTHERLAND (1961) suggested the first mechanistic classification of these fractures. They distinguished several categories of fractures according to the mechanism of lesion: anteroposterior or lateral compression or vertical shearing. Thus were established the bases of most of the classifications established so far. BUCHOLZ (1981) gave a clear definition of the anterior and posterior pelvic ring and insisted on the frequent occurrence of unknown lesions of the posterior ring. They suggested an anatomical classification based on the importance of these lesions of the posterior ring.

In the late 1980s, Tile and Young developed two classifications that have been the most frequently used over the last few years. TILE (1988, 1995) modified Pennal's classification. He introduced the concept that management of these fractures was directly related to the importance and direction of instability. Tile insisted on the importance of the evaluation of stability, but the classification did not include a description of complex fractures. Fractures are classified using their principal elementary lesion. At the same time, Young developed a classification called the Young and Burgess classification, including the mechanism of the lesion and radiographic grading of severity on the AP projection of the pelvic radiograph (Table 16.1). This classification emphasizes the level of energy imparted (YOUNG et al. 1986; BURGESS et al. 1990). They also notified that the mechanism may not always be identified and therefore introduced the category called "combined mechanical injury". Later, Dalal demonstrated that the Young-Burgess classification could be of value in predicting associated injuries and in prioritizing the work-up during resuscitation of an acutely ill patient (Dalal et al. 1989).

However, all classifications remain difficult to apply. On one hand, the link between the mechanism of trauma and anatomical lesions can be difficult to define. On the other hand, the evaluation of lesion stability remains ill defined in emergency cases, as it often relies on incompletely validated radiological criteria. Tile, in association with the thoughts of a working group of the Association for Osteosynthesis (AO), suggested an alphanumerical classification in order to harmonize the therapeutic management and the prog-

Table 16.1. Young-Burgess' classification of pelvic fractures

Fracture type	Classification	Features	Stability
Anterior compression	Antero-posterior compression: type I–III	External rotation or open book injuries Type I: SP disrupted ST, SS, ASI, and PSI spared Type II: SP, ST, SS, and ASI disrupted, PSI spared Type III: SP, ST, SS, ASI, and PSI disrupted	 Type I: stable Type II: R unstable; V and P stable Type III: R, V, and P unstable
Lateral compression	Lateral compression: type I–III	Internal rotation injuries Type I: Ipsilateral sacral compression Type II: type I with associated iliac wing fracture Type III: type I or II with contralateral open book injury (windswept pelvis)	 Type I: stable Type II: R unstable, V stable Type III: R unstable, V stable
Vertical shear	Vertical shear	Disruption of SP, ST, SS, ASI, and PSI Vertical displacement of one hemipelvis Posterior disruption may include sacral or iliac fractures with sparing of ASI and PSI	R, V, and P unstable
Complex	Complex	Variable	Variable

SP, symphysis pubis; *ST*, sacrotuberous ligament; *SS*, sacrospinous ligament; *ASI*, anterior sacroiliac ligaments; *PSI*, posterior sacroiliac ligaments; *R*, rotationally; *V*, vertically; *P*, posteriorly nostic evaluation (Table 16.2) (Müller et al. 1990; Tile 1995, 1996a; Orthopaedic Trauma Association Committee For Coding and Classification 1996). This Tile and AO classification seems to be the most frequently used nowadays and is our reference classification. It describes the mechanisms involved, the elementary lesions, and the therapeutic consequences implied. The Tile and AO classification suggests three subdivided main categories (A, B, C).

16.5.1.1 Type A Fracture

A type A fracture is an incomplete fracture with neither disruption of the pelvic ring nor lesion of the posterior band (Fig. 16.11a).

- Type A1 corresponds to an avulsion fracture of the pelvic ring. It usually concerns teenagers at the end of their growth and may involve the anterior-superior, anterior-inferior or ischial spine. The avulsion of the anterior-superior spine is caused by the sudden contraction of the sartorius, while that of the anterior-inferior spine is caused by the contraction of the rectus femoris; the avulsion of the pubic tubercle is caused by the contraction of the pectineus (Fig. 16.12).
- Type A2.1 corresponds to a stable iliac wing fracture caused by a direct blow to the ilium and does not involve the pelvic ring which, remains stable (Fig. 16.13).
- Type A2.2 relates to a stable, minimal, or undisplaced fracture of the pelvic ring and usually

Table 16.2. Tile/AO classification of pelvic fractures

Mechanism	Classification	Features	Stability
	Type A	A1: apophyseal avulsions A2: stable iliac wing fracture or stable, minimally displaced ring fracture A3: sacrococcygeal fractures	Stable
Anterior compression	Type B1	External rotation or open book injuries B1.1: unilateral anterior sacroiliac disruption B1.2: sacral fracture	Partially stable (complete rupture of anterior arch, incomplete rupture of posterior arch)
Lateral compression	Type B2	Internal rotation injuries B2.1: anterior compression fracture of the sacrum B2.2: partial sacroiliac joint fracture B2.3: incomplete posterior iliac wing fracture	Partially stable (complete rupture of anterior arch, incomplete rupture of posterior arch)
Anterior	Type B3	Bilateral external rotation (bilateral open book) B3.1: bilateral B1 B3.2: B1 and B2 B3.3: bilateral B2	Partially stable (complete rupture of anterior arch, incomplete rupture of posterior arch)
Vertical shear	Type C	C1: complete unilateral rupture C1.1: iliac fracture C1.2: sacroiliac dislocation C1.3: sacral fracture C2: bilateral injury (B + C types) C3: bilateral complete rupture	Unstable (complete rupture of both anterior and posterior arch)

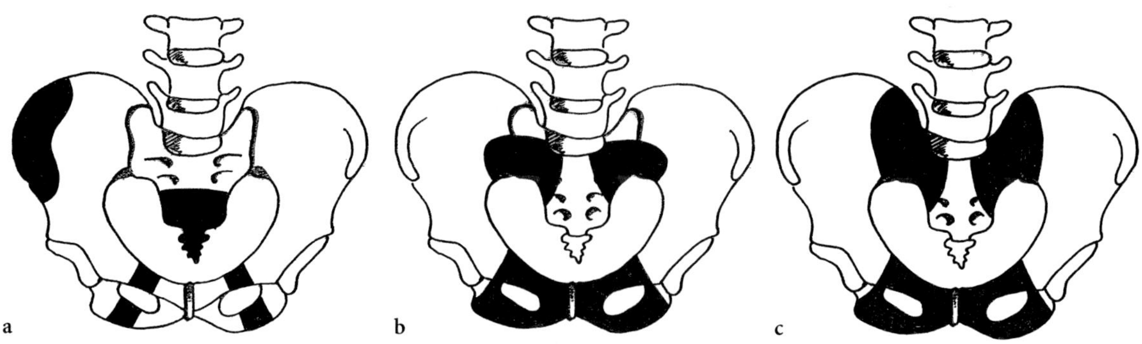
a b c

Fig. 16.11a–c. Tile classification. Black areas represent fracture zones. **a** Lesion sparing (or with no displacement of) posterior arch. **b** Incomplete disruption of posterior arch; partially stable. **c** Complete disruption of posterior arch; unstable affects elderly women with osteoporosis after a fall. The mechanism corresponds to a lateral compression, cracking the pubic rami (Fig. 16.14).

- Type A2.3 relates to anterior ring fractures or four pillar fractures and involves the four pubic rami frontally, without posterior injury. These fractures are caused by a direct blow or by a high-energy trauma of shearing or lateral compression (Fig. 16.15).
- Type A3 fractures are sacral or coccygeal fractures.
- Type A3.1 implies fractures of the coccyx or sacrococcygeal dislocation common after a sitting fall and may be the source of prolonged pain, but no neurological disability is observed. The transverse fractures of the sacrum distal to the gluteal line do not involve the pelvic ring.
- Type A3.2 fractures relate to undisplaced fractures and rarely cause neurological deficit.
- Type A3.3 fractures correspond to displaced and translated fractures with injury to the sacral nerve roots.

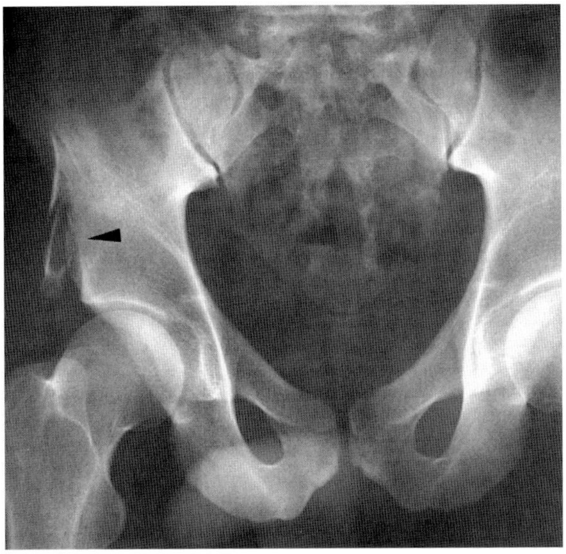

Fig. 16.12. Type A1 fracture. Anteroposterior view. Fracture avulsion of the right anteroinferior iliac spine (*arrowhead*)

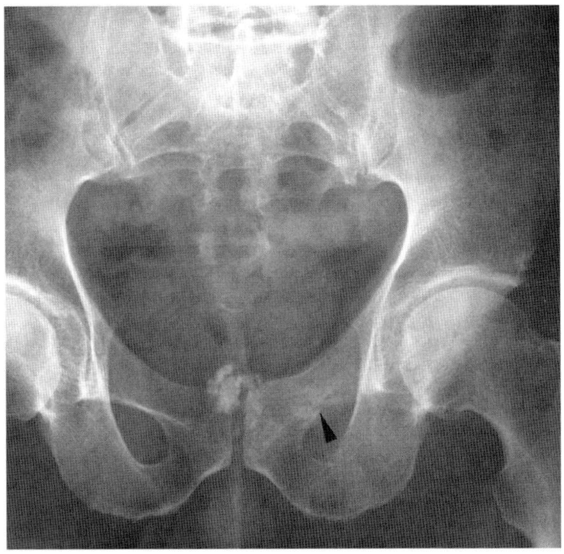

Fig. 16.14. Type A2.2 fracture. AP view. Left unilateral pubic rami fracture (*arrowhead*)

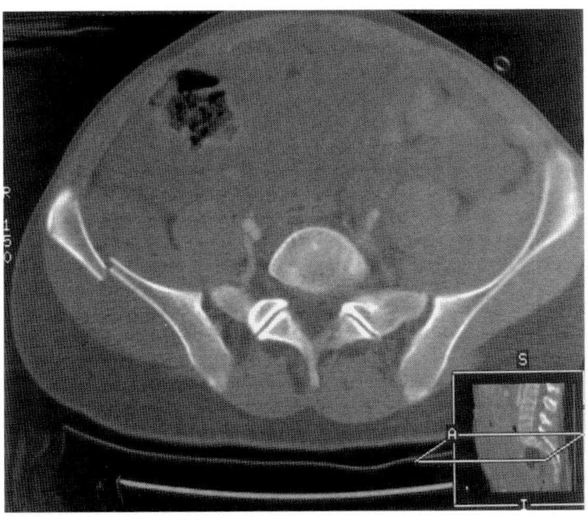

Fig. 16.13. Type A2.1 fracture. Isolated right iliac wing fracture

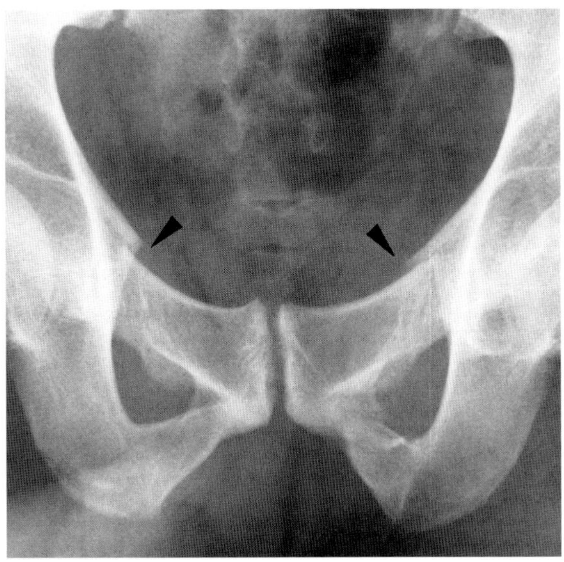

Fig. 16.15. Type A2.3 fracture. AP view. Bilateral pubic rami fractures (*arrowheads*)

16.5.1.2 Type B Fracture

The type B fracture relates to disruption (or fracture) of the symphysis pubis, associated with anterior sacroiliac joint disruption (unilateral or bilateral) (Fig. 16.11b). The posterior sacroiliac ligaments, responsible for the vertical stability, remain untouched. The typical lesion is caused by an anteroposterior compression applied to the anterior-superior iliac spines of the fixed pelvis. A posterior blow against the posterior-superior iliac spines may produce a similar fracture. Displacement of the symphysis pubis is an important feature of this type. If the splitting of the symphysis pubis is smaller than 2.5 cm, it cannot be associated with a disruption of either the pelvic floor or the sacrospinous ligament, but when it is wider than 2.5 cm, it is often associated with a disruption of either the pelvic floor or the sacrospinous ligament. In the latter case, a much higher occurrence of visceral injury can be observed.

Type B1 relates to a unilateral "open book" injury, usually caused by a violent external rotation of one femur. The typical situation is that of the motorcyclist who puts out a leg for balance and gets caught by a stationary object such as a road panel or a tree. The external rotation force usually disrupts the symphysis pubis first, and as the external rotation continues, a disruption of the pelvic floor, the fascia, and the sacrospinous and anterior sacroiliac ligaments follows. The variants include B1.1 (sacroiliac joint anterior disruption) and B1.2 (sacral fractures) (Fig. 16.16).

Type B2 relates to lateral compression injuries characterized by a unilateral partial disruption of the posterior arch maintaining the vertical or posterior stability. The underlying mechanism is an internal rotation. A lateral compressive force directed at the pelvic ring may cause two types of injury, the first in which the anterior and posterior lesions occur on the same side of the pelvis and the second in which the displacement is shown on the opposite side. In the latter case, the relative stability is maintained by the osseous impaction without muscle or ligament tears. Variants include the type B2.1 fracture, corresponding to an anterior crush fracture of the sacrum, the type B2.2 fracture or partial sacroiliac joint fracture and subluxation, and the type B2.3 fracture, which is related to the incomplete iliac fracture (Figs. 16.17 and 16.18.). Type B3 stands for the classic, bilateral open book injury. In spite of the relative stability of the pelvic ring, maintained by the posterior sacroiliac ligaments, the pelvic floor disruption causes visceral injuries. Variants include type B3.1 or bilateral B1, type B3.2 or B1 on one side and B2 on the other side, and type B3.3, which is a bilateral B2 type fracture (Fig. 16.19).

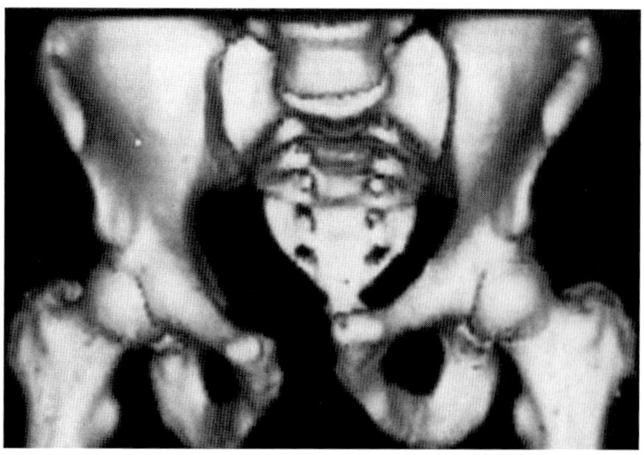

Fig. 16.16. Type B1.1 fracture. Unilateral open book injury. 3D CT scan. Symphyseal disjunction and anterior sacroiliac disruption

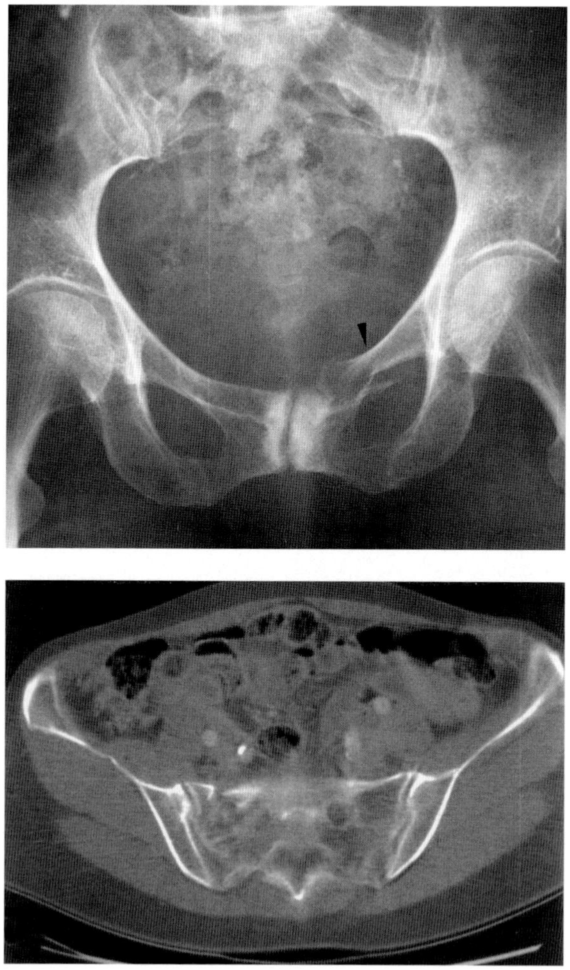

a

b

Fig. 16.17a, b. Type B2.1. Lateral compression, stable fracture. **a** AP view. Left pubic rami fracture (*arrowhead*). **b** CT scan. Anterior compression fracture of right superior sacroiliac joint

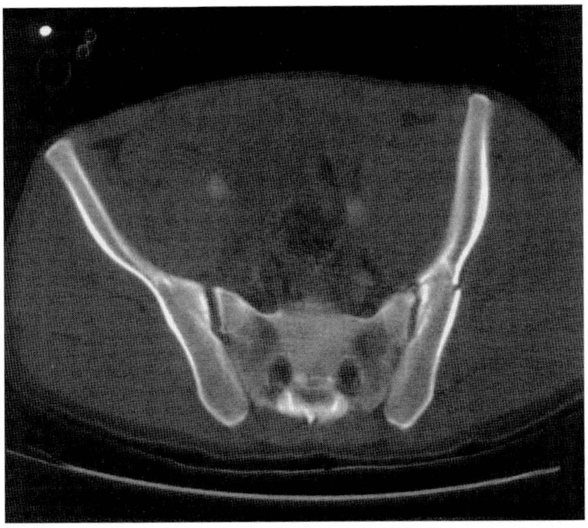

a

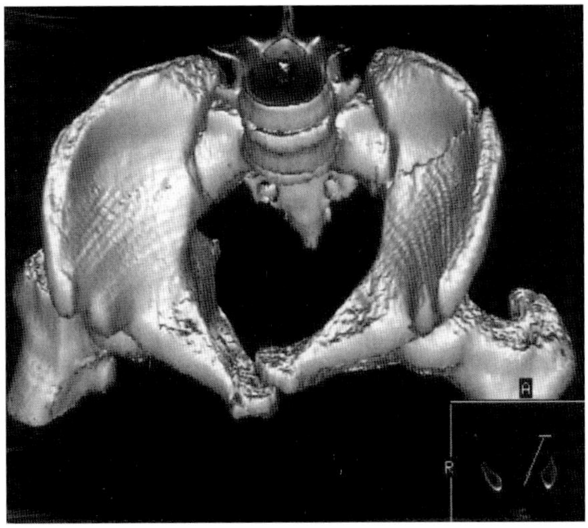

b

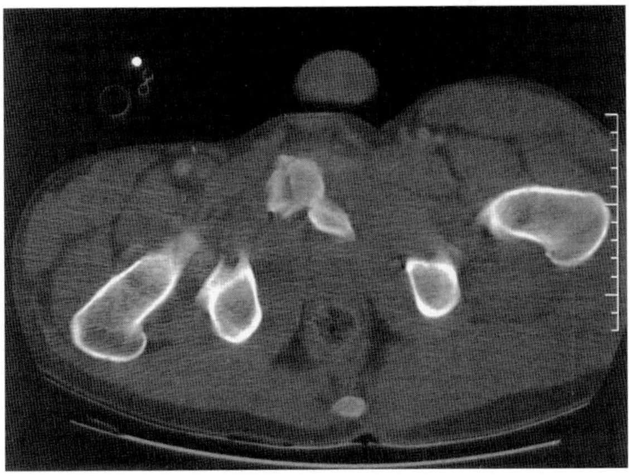

c

Fig. 16.18a–c. Type B2.3. fracture. Lateral compression. Partially stable fracture. **a** CT scan. Partial left iliac wing fracture. **b** CT scan. Internal symphyseal displacement. **c** 3D CT. Left iliac wing fracture, internal rotation of left hemi-pelvis

16.5.1.3 Type C Fracture

The type C fracture relates to unstable injuries with complete disruption of the posterior sacroiliac complex, involving vertical shearing forces. These unilateral or bilateral fractures are almost always caused by severe trauma such as falls from heights, crushing injuries, or motor vehicle accidents. They cause massive disruption of both the pelvic ring and the surrounding soft tissues. Type C1 corresponds to unilateral injuries of the hemi-pelvis. Type C1.1 relates to sheer fractures of the ilium, which begin at the inferior part of the sacroiliac joint and run to the iliac crest at the rear. Type C1.2 stands for sacroiliac dislocations. These fractures can only be associated with extreme violence, as the sacroiliac ligaments are the strongest in the human body. (Fig. 16.20). Type C1.3 deals with fractures of the sacrum caused by high-energy shearing forces. Type C2 stands for bilateral injuries of the pelvic ring in which one side remains partially stable and thus corresponds to a type B injury, for example in sacral fractures, while the opposite relates to an unstable Type C injury, such as an iliac fracture (Fig. 16.21). Type C3 deals with bilateral injuries in which both hemi-pelves are unstable (Fig. 16.22).

16.5.1.4 Incidence

Type A lesions represent up to 52%, type B up to 27%, and type C up to 21% of all cases (Pohlemann et al. 2000). The type B and C lesion percentage increases with the speed implied in the trauma.

16.5.2 Acetabular Fractures

The study of acetabular trauma has to be closely connected to Letournel and Judet's research. After establishing the bases of standard radiography from

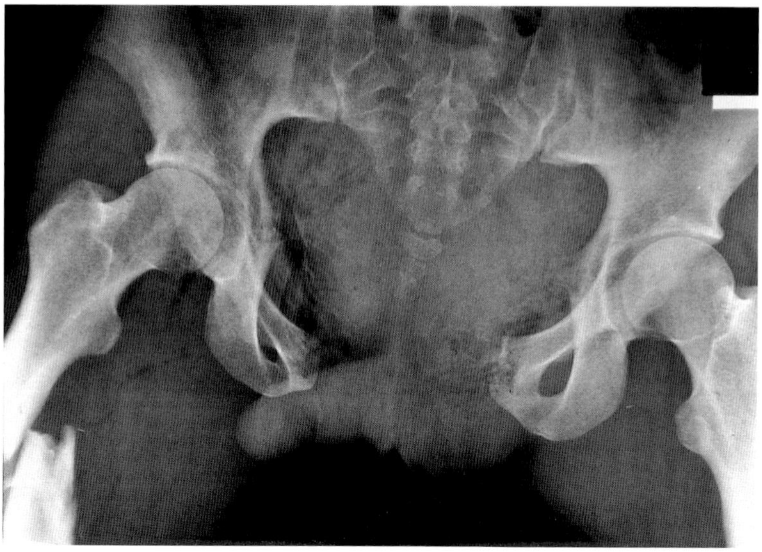

a

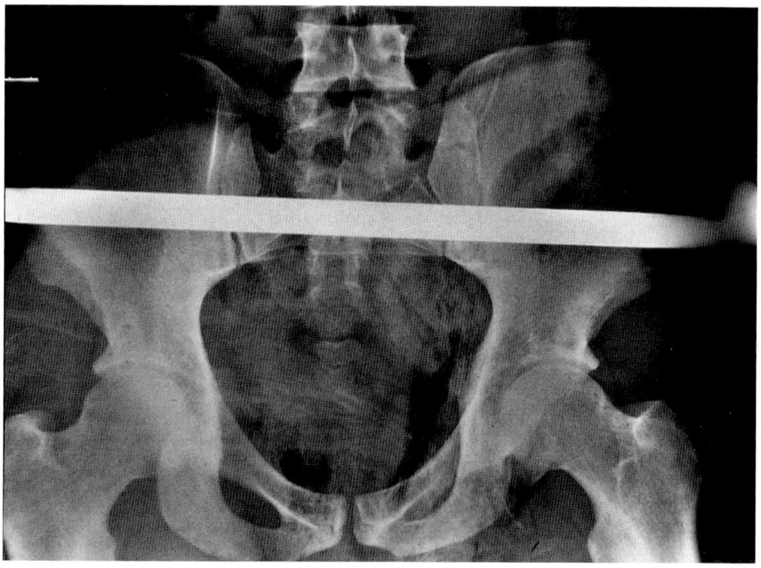

b

Fig. 16.19a, b. Type B3 fracture. **a** AP view. Open book lesion with symphyseal diastasis and bilateral sacroiliac disruption. **b** AP view. Same patient after external fixation and reduction

outstanding anatomical studies which allowed them to introduce the concept of the two columns of the hip bone, they developed a classification of acetabular fractures still in use today (JUDET et al. 1964; LETOURNEL and JUDET 1993). This classification is divided into ten patterns, consisting in five elementary and five associated patterns (Fig. 16.23). Elementary fractures run in a single plane whereas associated fractures are combinations of elementary patterns. Elementary fractures are anterior wall fractures, anterior column fractures, posterior wall fractures, posterior column fractures, and transverse fractures. Associated fractures are T-shaped fractures, complete two-column fractures, transverse and posterior wall fractures, posterior column and posterior wall fractures, and anterior column posterior hemi-transverse fractures, the latter type being uncommon.

Acetabular fractures are uncommon and therefore this classification remains difficult to remember. However, among these ten fracture types, five of them are very common: complete two-column, transverse, T-shaped, transverse with posterior wall and posterior wall fractures constitute about 90% of acetabular fractures. Thus, knowledge of these five types allows correct assessment of 90% of all acetabular fractures (BRANDSER et al. 1995). Grouping the different categories could be another way to simplify this classification. Brandsers uggests three major categories:

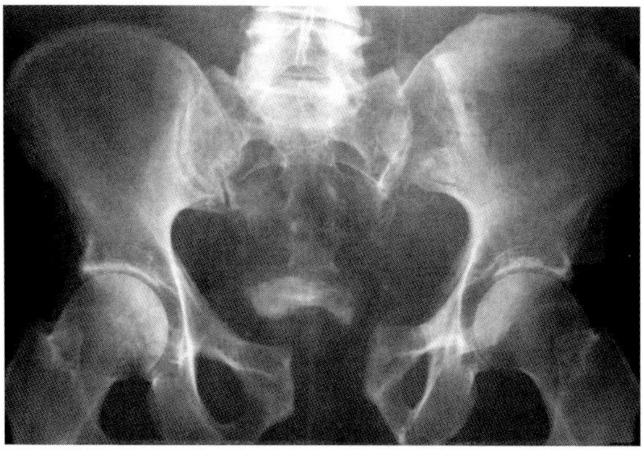
a

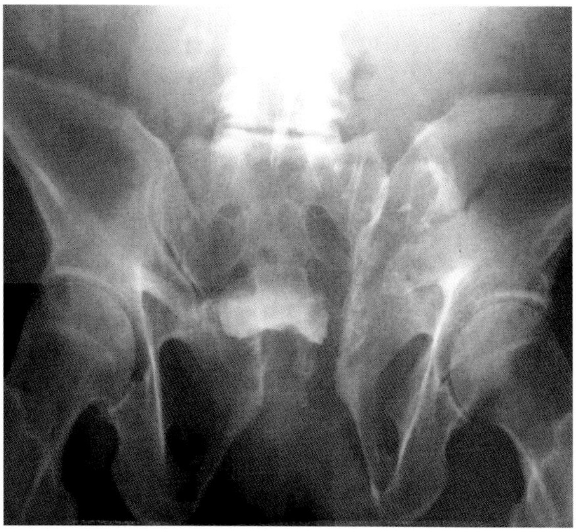
b

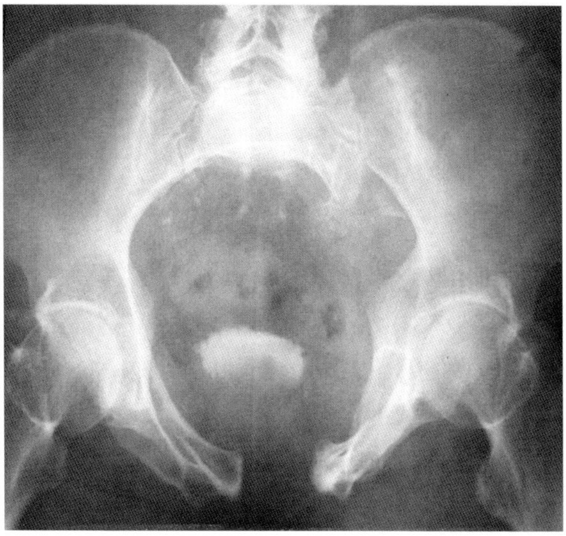
c

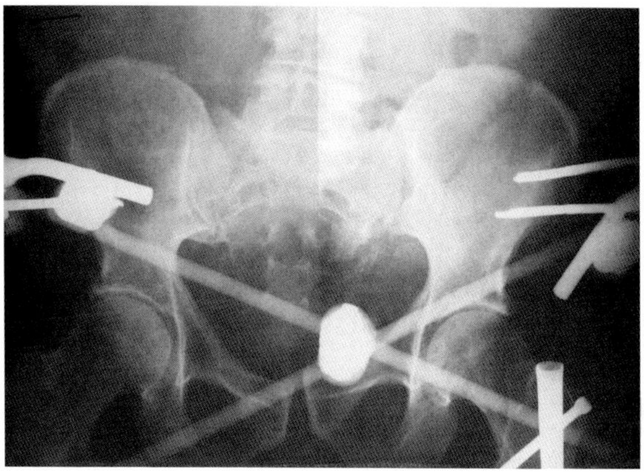
d

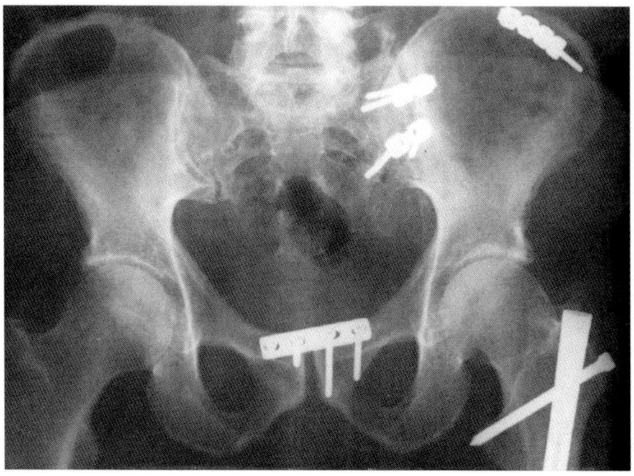
e

Fig. 16.20a–e. Type C1.2. fracture. Major trauma, unstable fracture of pelvic ring. **a** AP view. Symphyseal diastasis, left sacroiliac disruption and iliac wing fracture. **b** Outlet view. Note the ascension of the left hemi-pelvis related to complete posterior ligaments disruption. **c** The inlet view confirms the posterior displacement of the left iliac wing. **d** Same patient after temporary external fixation. **e** Same patient after internal fixation

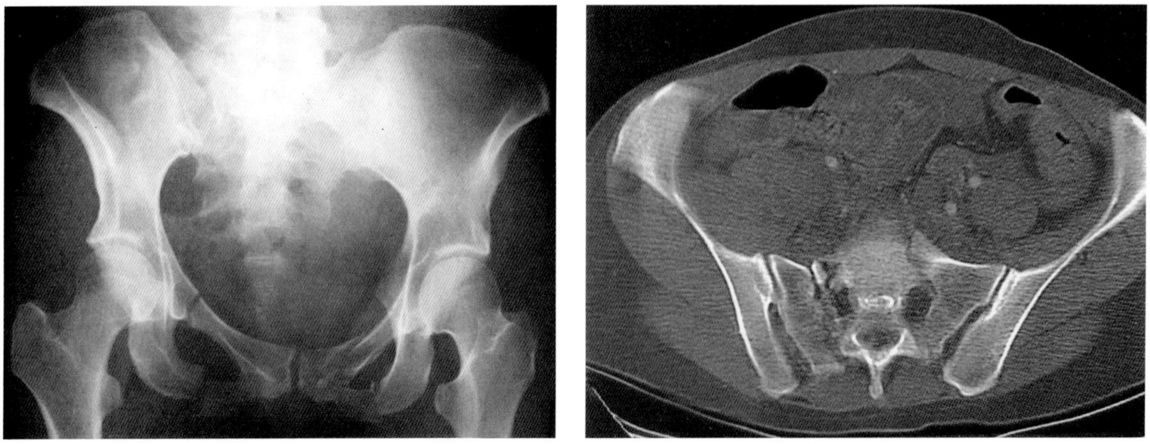

a b

Fig. 16.21a, b. Type C2. fracture. Bilateral sacral fracture complete on the right (unstable) and incomplete on the left side (stable). **a** AP view. Bilateral pubic rami fractures and right sacral fracture. Note the rupture of right arcuate lines. **b** Axial CT scan

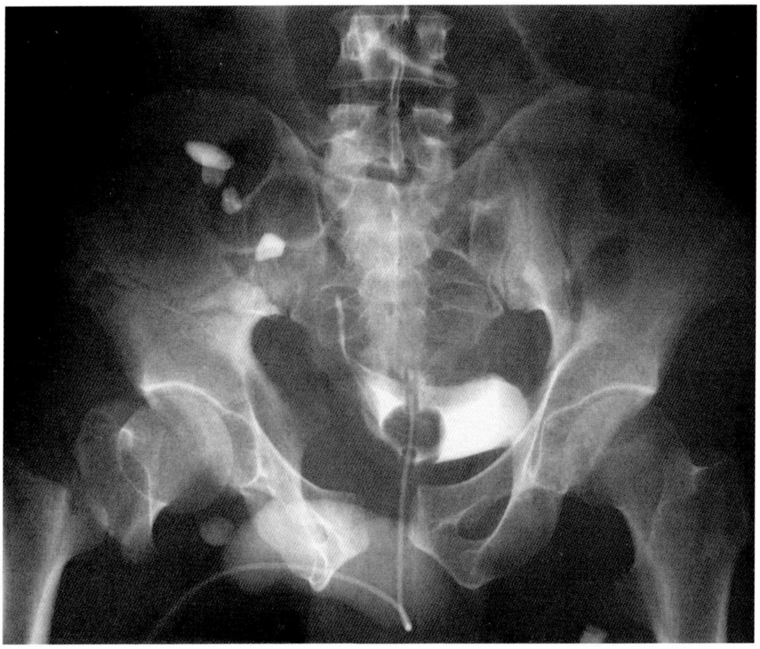

Fig. 16.22. Type C3. fracture. Bilateral instability. AP view. Bilateral iliac wing fractures, symphyseal disjunction

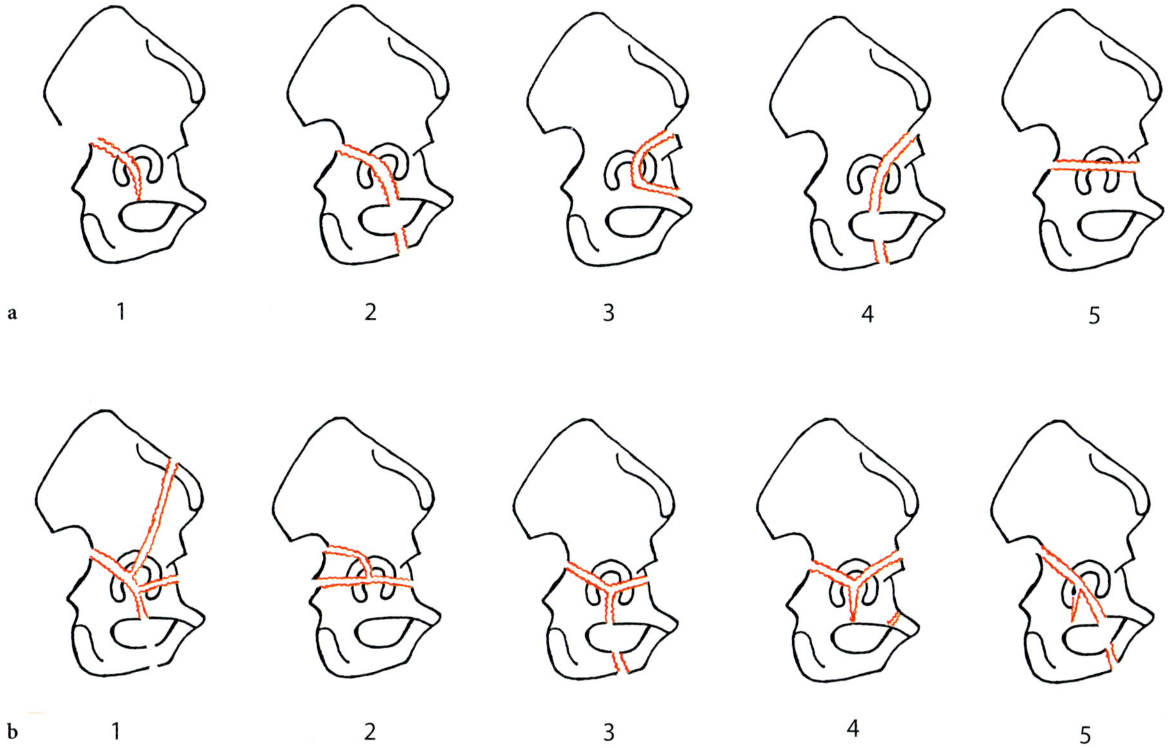

Fig. 16.23a, b. Acetabular fractures. Letournel and Judet's classification. **a** Elementary fractures. *1*, Posterior wall fracture; *2*, posterior column fracture; *3*, anterior wall fracture; *4*, anterior column fracture; *5*, transverse fracture; **b** associated fractures; *1*, two-column fracture; *2*, transverse posterior wall fracture; *3*, T-type fracture; *4*, anterior wall posterior hemi-transverse fracture; *5*, posterior column posterior wall fracture

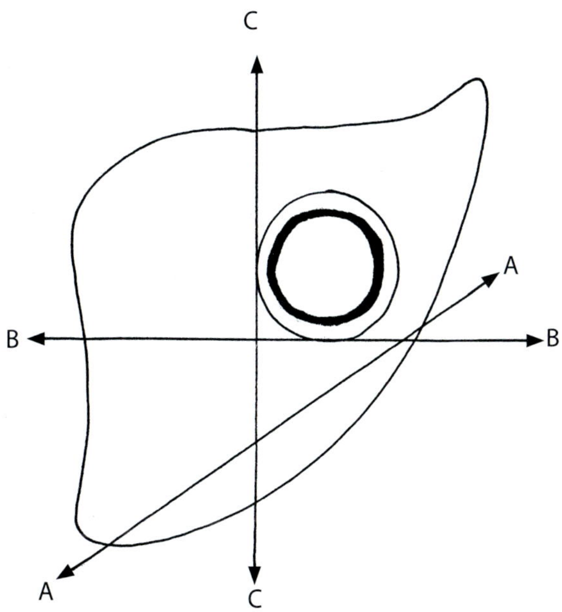

Fig. 16.24. Schematic representation in the axial plane of main fracture orientation depending on fracture type. (Level: roof of the acetabulum). *A* Wall fracture; *B* column fracture; *C* transverse fracture

transverse type fractures, column type fractures, and wall type fractures. CT is helpful in recognizing these three categories, by identifying the main orientation fracture on a slice through the roof of the acetabulum (Lude et al. 1999; Hunter et al. 1997) (Fig. 16.24). We prefer Tile's grouping in anterior, posterior, and transverse fractures. In our experience, these groups are easier both to memorize and to identify from radiological data (Figs. 16.25–16.28).

16.5.2.1 Anterior Fractures

This group includes the anterior wall and the anterior column fractures. They are often associated with a pelvic fracture, and, as such, considered rather as pelvic ring than acetabulum fractures. These injuries are caused by a lateral blow to the greater trochanter when the leg is externally rotated. An anterior hip dislocation is rarely associated; when compared with posterior fracture types, it is almost always associated with posterior hip dislocation. With anterior injury, the complications are less frequent and the

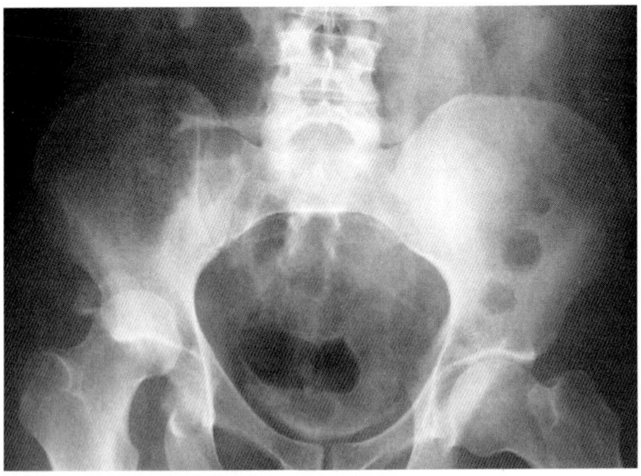

a

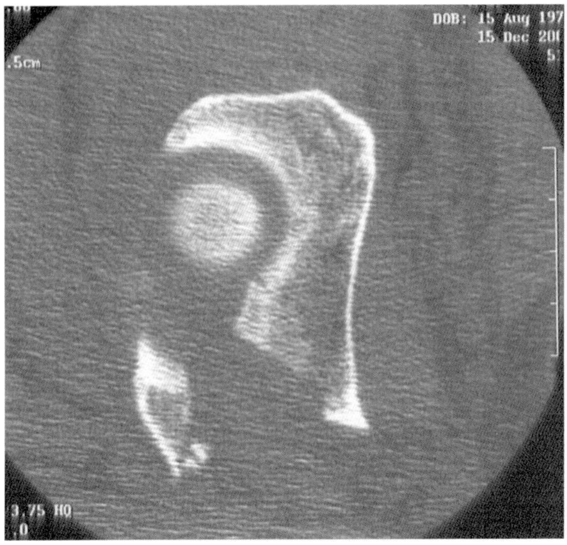

b

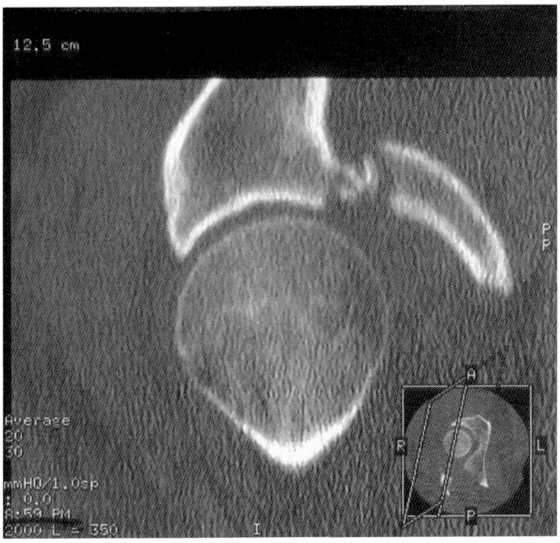

c

Fig. 16.25a-c. Posterior wall fracture. **a** AP view; **b** axial CT scan; **c** CT sagittal reconstruction confirms posterior wall fracture and suggests potential posterior instability

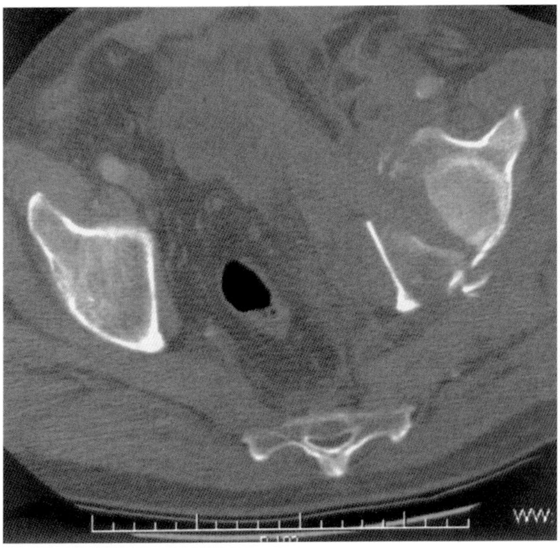

a

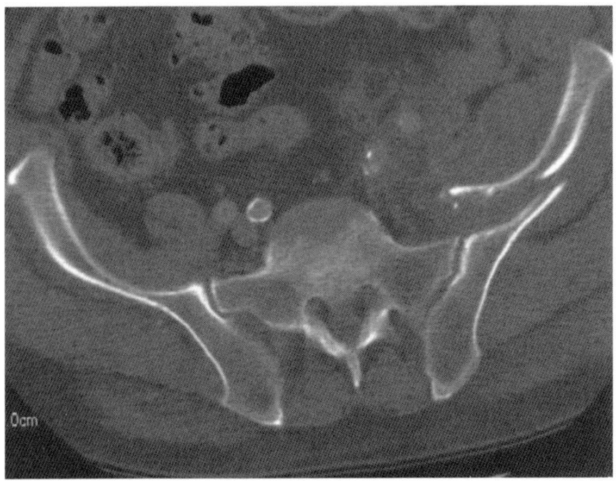

b

Fig. 16.26a, b. Two-column fracture of the acetabulum. **a** Axial CT scan at the level of the roof of the acetabulum; **b** axial CT scan. Extension of the fracture into the iliac wing

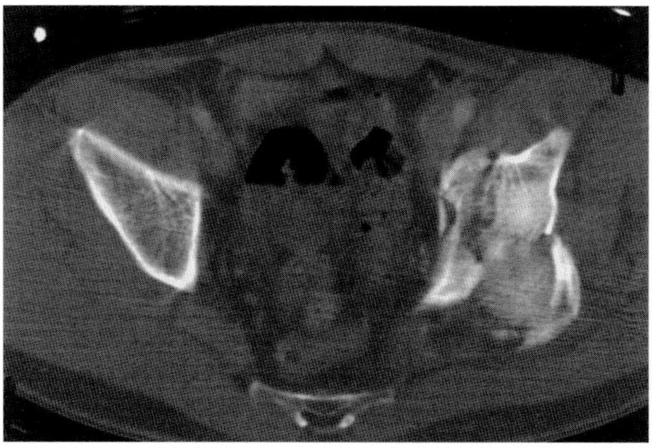

Fig. 16.27. Transverse posterior wall fracture. Axial CT scan. Note the sagittal fracture line and the tear of the posterior wall associated with posterior luxation of the femoral head

a

b

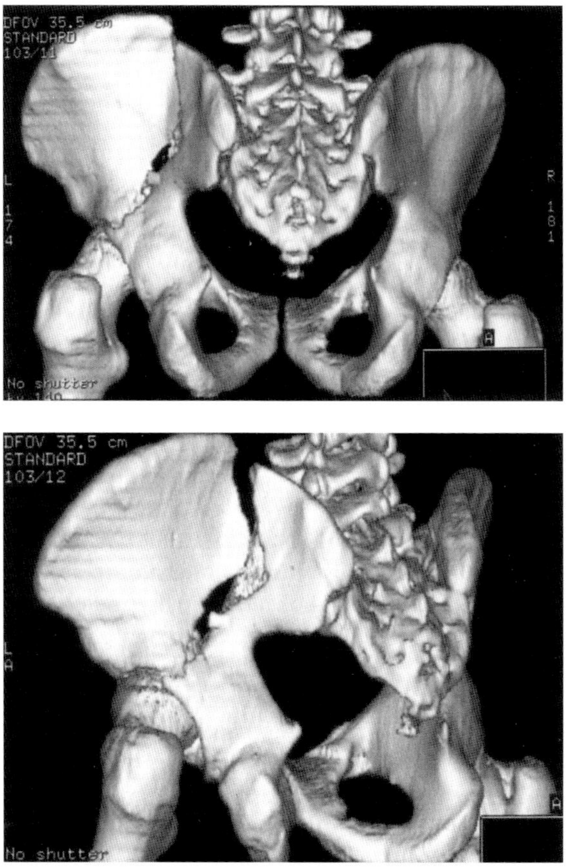

Fig. 16.28a, b. Anterior column fracture. 3D CT scan. **a** Anterior view illustrates the orientation of the fracture. **b** Posterior view demonstrates integrity of posterior column

overall prognosis remains better than in other types (Tile 1995). The anterior wall fracture usually begins at the anterior-inferior iliac spine, passes below through the cotyloid fossa, up to the junction of the articular dome and the superior ramus. The anterior column fracture is characterized by a fracture line that extends from the middle of the pubic ramus to any point above the anterior segment of the iliac crest (Perry and Delong 1997).

16.5.2.2
Posterior Fractures

This group includes the posterior wall and the posterior column fractures. Posterior fractures are usually caused by a blow to the flexed knee, also called dashboard injury and therefore, associated knee injuries are common. Posterior dislocation of the hip is frequent and almost always present when the posterior wall is fractured. This complication affects the prognosis, since the prevalence of vascular necrosis and sciatic nerve lesions is markedly increased (Tile 1995). The posterior wall fracture is identified by a disruption of the posterior border, best seen on the obturator oblique view. The posterior column fracture is completely detached, because it usually originates in the greater sciatic notch, crosses the weight-bearing dome and the obturator foramen. The plain films show medial displacement of the femoral head (Perry and Delong 1997).

16.5.2.3
Transverse and T-type Fractures

Transverse and T-type fractures are commonly caused by high-energy shearing forces. They appear simple but often have the worst prognosis. In a pure transverse fracture, the fracture line extends transversely from the anterior to the posterior column. So the weight bearing dome portion remains attached to the ilium. This type of fracture presents three subdivisions: the transtectal transverse fracture which goes through the weight-bearing dome; the juxtatectal transverse fracture which occurs just above the cotyloid fossa; the infratectal transverse fracture which affects the whole weight-bearing dome. The T-type fracture essentially consists in a transverse fracture with a vertical component, splitting the cotyloid fossa. The posterior column thus becomes a loose fragment (Perry and Delong 1997).

16.6 Management

16.6.1 Clinical Evaluation

Cross-questioning and anamnesis should define the type and mechanism of trauma. A high-energy mechanism relates to crush lesions, traffic accidents, and defenestration, while a typical low-energy mechanism is simple muscular contraction. Defining the initial shock spot leads to a particular mechanism and a certain type of lesion: anteroposterior compression relates to open-book lesions; lateral impact on the great trochanter or iliac wing is associated with rotation lesions; shearing strain in axial trauma on one or both members as they occur follows defenestration or dashboard syndrome and connects with unstable lesions of the posterior ring. Investigation should look for impact lesions or graze on the pelvis, while clinical check-up should look for pain at palpation or pelvic manipulation. The value of this clinical investigation will vary according to the patient's state. In a patient without spinal column lesion, a normal clinical status of the pelvis rules out pelvic ring fracture and thus radiological investigation need not be performed (Salvino et al. 1992; Yugueros et al. 1995). On the other hand, if pain occurs at palpation or manipulation, or if the clinical findings cannot be trusted for sure, as with an unconscious or intoxicated patient or with spinal column lesion, radiological investigation is mandatory. However, one must be careful in pelvic clinical evaluation, which may lead to aggravation of fracture displacement or hemorrhage.

16.6.2 Imaging Strategies

Initial clinical evaluation leads to different situations.

16.6.2.1 Minor Trauma Limited to the Hip

Radiological appraisal must include four basic projections: the anteroposterior pelvic view, front hip view, and oblique views. Normal views of good quality can rule out fractures. In case of doubt or recognized lesion, further exploration with CT is highly advisable. It confirms fractures, defines their characteristics, looks for associated lesions and aids in planning surgical management.

16.6.2.2 Major Trauma

It should be carefully analyzed, whether it is a predominant pelvic trauma or a complex trauma, in a conscious or unconscious patient. In any case, the patient must be considered as polytraumatized with possible hidden visceral or osseous lesions. Radiological assessment must be included in a multidisciplinary approach and correspond to pre-established protocols in order to optimize management.

First, an anteroposterior pelvic view as well as anteroposterior thoracic and profile cervical spine views should be taken in any patient. Inlet and outlet views may complete assessment, systematically or on request. In case of isolated pelvic fracture, indication for angiography with possible hemostatic embolization must be settled, following external pelvic fixation. In case of a stable patient, complete body assessment should be performed. Thoracic, abdominal, and pelvic investigation is advisable in the same examination, with whole body CT as described above. It leads to the more specific and least time-consuming assessment and allows better therapeutic management.

16.6.3 Treatment

The great variety of clinical situations explains the diversity of possible treatments. Some principles can be established, keeping in mind that therapeutic indications rely upon precise lesion assessment (Bonneviale 1996; Tile 1996b). In case of pelvic ring lesions, stabilization of the patient's hemodynamics must first be sought. It may consist in external fracture stabilization, in surgical hemostatic treatment, or in hemostatic embolization. The radiologists have to know the importance of angiography in the management of hemorrhagic blows in pelvic trauma. The external fixation of the fracture is essential for hemodynamic stabilization, contributing to hemostasis (Wolinsky 1997; Yang and Iannacone 1997). A 2-cm symphyseal diastasis can increase pelvic volume in the adult from a normal of 1.5 l to as much as 5 l (Hunter et al. 1997).

After completing hemostasis, the choice of orthopedic management will rely upon the associated neurological, thoracic or abdominopelvic, or osseous lesions. Type A lesions rarely lead to surgical fixing. Type B or C lesions usually need osteosynthesis. Because of the latter's complexity, a clear evaluation of the real advantage implied by surgical fixing must be made. It should consider neurological complications, skin necrosis, and sepsis. If surgery is required, it must be completed within the first 3 weeks of trauma to prevent lesions from fixing or becoming irreducible. If performed, internal fixation allows easier reduction and stabilization of the fracture and facilitates patient mobilization.

For the acetabulum, emergencies consist in the associated displacement of the femoral head, which must be reduced at once. A suspected injury of the gluteal artery with a sciatic notch fracture is also an emergency and has to lead to angiography with possible embolization in mind. In other cases, reduction of an acetabular fracture is not an emergency and best recovers when treated within the 3rd and 7th day after trauma. In all cases, the main preoccupation must lie in the restoration of the articular congruence in order to prevent early coxarthrosis. However, the indications are often difficult to come to terms with, due to fracture complexity, age, osseous potential, associated lesions, etc. In cases of association of pelvic ring and acetabular fractures, priority is given to pelvic ring fracture management.

16.7 Complications

16.7.1 Death Rate

The death rate in pelvic trauma ranges between 5% and 15%, but may reach 50% of cases (Mucha and Farnell 1984; Cryer et al. 1988; Dalal et al. 1989; Burgess et al. 1990; Rogers 1992; Davidson et al. 1993; Gruen et al. 1994; Pohlemann et al. 1998). The cause of death directly relates to pelvic trauma in 12% of cases (Mucha and Farnell 1984). This rate is closely connected to the associated lesions, to the importance of trauma and to the patient's age (Routt 1993; Gustavo Pareira et al. 2000). The Injury Severity Score (ISS) and patient's hemodynamic state seem to be the best prognostic features. The value of the fracture type as a prognostic tool has also been evoked. In Pohlemann's series, death rate amounts to 11.7% in the A, 14.9% in the B, and 23% in the C type fractures (Pohlemann et al. 1994). The best prognostic improvement factors are multidisciplinary management and early fracture fixing (Browner et al. 1987; Philips and Contreras 1990; Riemer et al. 1993). For a single ISS and comparable age group, the death rate can be reduced by a factor of 3 by early fracture management (Bone et al. 1994). In pelvic fractures with intense bleeding, mainly in cases of pelvic ring disruption, transfusion is mandatory in nearly 50% of cases (Cryer et al. 1988). These hemorrhages cause half of the fatalities and may sometimes occur in isolated acetabular lesions (Poole et al. 1991).

16.7.2 Associated Lesions

Associated vascular and visceral lesions are frequent and will be dealt with in other chapters. Briefly, brain lesions occur in 26–55% and abdominal lesions in 15–26% of cases (Emerman 1979; Ben Menachem et al. 1991; Rogers 1992; Siegmeth et al. 2000). Pulmonary lesions are frequent, with aortic isthmus rupture occurrences increased sixfold when associated with pelvis fractures (Conolly and Hedberg 1969; Ochsner et al. 1989, 1992). Lower urinary track lesions are found in 4–17% of cases in the urethra and 5–25% of cases in the bladder (Colapinto 1980; Heare et al. 1989; Werkman et al. 1991; Rogers 1992; McCort and Mindelzun 1994). Urinalysis shows microscopic or gross hematuria in 87% of patients with pelvic fracture (Emerman 1979). Anorectal or gynecological lesions are rare and most often secondary to open trauma. Peripheral nerve lesions represent 10% of cases, mainly complicating sacrum fractures (40% of cases) (Rai et al. 1990). Posterior femoral head dislocation accompanies sciatic lesions in 20% of cases (Lude et al. 1999).

16.8 Conclusion

Pelvic fractures form a polymorphous group. In the isolated acetabular fractures, function is mainly at stake. Radiological assessment relies upon good-quality plain films completed by CT imaging in fine slices with multiplanar reconstruction. Letournel's classification remains the reference. Management consists mainly in re-establishing a joint congruence to prevent early coxarthrosis. Pelvic fractures often occur in violent trauma and are associated with visceral lesions, putting vital prognosis at stake. Radiological assessment must be included in multidisciplinary management and CT imaging is the most complete and least time-consuming device, allowing for investigation of both visceral and osseous lesions. In case of hemodynamic shock, external fracture stabilization and embolization of pelvic bleeding are preponderant. The Tile/AO classification is the most used today. It provides a good description of mechanisms and lesions and more adapted management.

References

Ben Menachem Y, Coldwell DM, Young JW et al (1991) Hemorrhage associated with pelvic fractures: causes, diagnosis and emergent management. AJR 157:1005–1013

Berg EE, Chebuhar C, Bell RM (1996) Pelvic trauma imaging: a blinded comparison of computed tomography and roentgenograms. J Trauma 41:994–998

Bone LB, McNamara K, Shire B et al (1994) Mortality in multiple trauma patients with fractures. J Trauma 37:262–265

Bonneviale P (1996) Ruptures de l'anneau pelvien. Encycl Med Chir, Elsevier, 14-072-A-10

Brandser EA, El-Khoury GY, Marsh JL (1995) Acetabular fractures: A systematic approach to reclassification. Emerg Radiol 2:18–28

Browner BD, Cole JD, Graham JM et al (1987) Delayed posterior internal fixation of unstable pelvic fractures. J Trauma 27:998–1006

Bucholz RW (1981) The pathological anatomy of the Malgaigne fracture dislocation of the pelvis. J Bone Joint Surg 63A:400–404

Burgess AR, Eastbridge BJ, Young JE (1990) Pelvic ring disruption: effective classification system and treatment protocol. J Trauma 30:845–856

Chaumoitre K, Portier F, Petit P et al (2000) CT imaging of pelvic injuries in polytrauma patients. J Radiol 81:111–120

Colapinto V (1980) Trauma to the pelvis: urethral injury. Clin Orthop 151:46–55

Conolly WB, Hedberg EA (1969) Observations on fractures of the pelvis: J Trauma 9:104–111

Cryer HM, Miller FB, Evers BM et al (1988) Pelvic fracture classification: correlation with hemorrhage. J Trauma 28: 973–980

Daffner RH (1990) Pelvic trauma. In: McCort JJ, Mindelzun RE (eds) Trauma radiology. Churchill Livingstone, New York, pp 339–380

Dalal SA, Burgess AR, Siegel JH et al (1989) Pelvic fracture in multiple trauma: classification by mechanism is key to pattern of organ injury, resuscitative requirements, and outcome. J Trauma 29:981–1002

Davidson BS, Simmons GT, Williamson PR et al (1993) Pelvic fractures associated with open perineal wounds: a survivable injury. J Trauma 35:36–39

Eastridge BJ, Burgess AR (1997) Pedestrian pelvic fractures: 5-year experience of a major urban trauma center. J Trauma 42:695–700

Emerman CE (1979) Abdominopelvic injury associated with pelvic fracture. JACEP 8:312–315

Ersoy G, Karcioglu O, Enginbas Y et al (1995) Should all patients with blunt trauma undergo "routine" pelvic X-ray? Eur J Emerg Med 2:65–68

Federle M (1995) Should patients who undergo CT scanning of the abdomen for blunt trauma always have a CT scan of the pelvis as well, regardless of the severity and location of the trauma? AJR 164:762

Gansslen A, Pohlemann T, Paul C et al (1996) Epidemiology of pelvic ring injuries. Injury 27 [Suppl 1]:SA13–SA20

Geusens E, Brys P, Maleux G et al (2000) Imaging in pelvic trauma. J. Belge Radiol 83:173–180

Gill K, Bucholz RW (1984) The role of computerized tomographic scanning in the evaluation of major pelvic fractures. J Bone Joint Surg Am 6:34–39

Goulet J, Bray T (1989) Complex acetabular fractures. Clin Orthop 240:9–19

Gruen GS, Leit ME, Gruen J et al (1994) The acute management of hemodynamically unstable multiple trauma patients with pelvic ring fractures. J Trauma 36:706–713

Gustavo Pareira J, Coimbra R, Raslan S et al (2000) The role of associated injuries on outcome of blunt trauma patients sustaining pelvic fractures. Injury 31:677–682

Harley JD, Mack LA, Winquist RA (1982) CT of acetabular fractures: comparison with conventional radiography. AJR 138:413–417

Heare MM, Heare TC, Gillespy T (1989) Diagnostic imaging of pelvic and chest wall trauma. Radiol Clin North Am 27: 873–889

Hunter J, Braudser E, Tran K (1997) Pelvic and acetabular trauma. Radiol Clin North Am 35:559–590

Judet R, Judet J, Letournel E (1964) Fractures of the acetabulum: Classification and surgical approaches for open reduction. J Bone Joint Surg 46:1615–1646

Kellam JF, Browner BD (1992) Fractures of the pelvic ring. In: Browner BD, Jupiter JB, Levine AM, Trafton PG (eds) Skeletal trauma. Saunders, Philadelphia, pp 849–897

Killeen KL, Demeo JH (1999) CT detection of serious internal and skeletal injuries in patients with pelvic fractures. Acad Radiol 6:224–228

Letournel E, Judet R (1993) Fractures of the acetabulum, 2nd edn. Springer, Berlin Heidelberg New York

Lude F, Puget J, Martimbeau C (1999) Fractures du cotyle. Encycl Med Chir, Elsevier, 14-073-A-10

Martinez C, Di Pasquale T, Helfet D et al (1992) Evaluation of acetabular fractures with two- and three-dimensional CT. Radiographics 12:227–242

Mayo K (1987) Fractures of the acetabulum. Orthop Clin North Am 18:43–57

McCort JJ, Mindelzun RE (1994) Bladder injury and pelvic fractures Emerg Radiol 1:47–51

McIntyre RC Jr, Bensard DD, Moore EE et al (1993) Pelvic fracture geometry predicts risk of life-threatening hemorrhage in children. J Trauma 35:423–429

McLeod M, Powell J (1997) Evaluation of pelvic fractures: clinical and radiologic. Orthop Clin North Am 28:299–319

Melton LJ, Sampson JM, Morrey FB et al (1981) Epidemiologic fractures of pelvic fractures. Clin Orthop 155:43–47

Montana MA, Richardson ML, Kilcoyne RF et al (1986) CT of sacral injury. Radiology 161:499–503

Mucha P, Farnell MB (1984) Analysis of pelvic fracture management. J Trauma 24:379–385

Müller ME, Allgower M, Schneider R et al (1990) Manual of internal fixation, 3rd edn. Springer, Berlin Heidelberg New York

Ochsner MG Jr, Champion HR, Chambers RJ et al (1989) Pelvic fracture as an indicator of increased risk of thoracic aortic rupture. J Trauma 29:1376–1379

Ochsner MG Jr, Hoffman AP, Di Pasquale D et al (1992) Associated aortic rupture pelvic fracture: an alert for orthopedic and general surgeons. J Trauma 33:429–434
Orthopaedic Trauma Association Committee for Coding and Classification (1996) Fracture and dislocation compendium. J Orthop Trauma 10 [Suppl 1]
Pennal GF, Sutherland GO (1961) Fractures of the pelvis. American Academy of Orthopaedic Surgeons Film Library
Perry D, Delong W (1997) Acetabular fractures. Orthop Clin North Am 28:405–417
Philips TF, Contreras D (1990) Timing of operative treatment of fractures in patients who have multiple injuries. J Bone Joint Surg Am 72:784–788
Pohlemann T, Bosch U, Gansslen A et al (1994) The Hanover experience in management of pelvic fractures. Clin Orthop 305:69–80
Pohlemann T, Gansslen A, Stief CH (1998) Complex injuries of the pelvis and acetabulum. Orthopäde 27:32–44
Pohlemann T, Richter M, Otte D et al (2000) Mechanism of pelvic girdle injuries in street traffic. Medical-technical accident analysis. Unfallchirurg 103:267–274
Poole GV, Ward EF, Muakkassa FF et al (1991) Pelvic fracture from major blunt trauma. Outcome is determined by associated injuries. Ann Surg 213:532–539
Potter HG, Montgomery KD, Heise CW et al (1994) MR imaging of acetabular fractures: value in detecting femoral head injury, intraarticular fragments and sciatic nerve injury. AJR 163:881–886
Rai SK, Far RF, Ghovanlou B (1990) Neurologic deficits associated with sacral wing fractures. Orthopedics 13:1363–1366
Riemer BI, Butterfield SI, Diamond DI et al (1993) Acute mortality associated with injuries to the pelvic ring: the role of early patient mobilization and external fixation. J Trauma 35:671–677
Rogers LF (1992) Radiology of skeletal trauma, 2nd edn. Churchill Livingstone, New York, pp 991–1105
Routt ML (1993) Pelvic fractures. In: Hansen ST, Swiontkowski MF (eds) Orthopaedic trauma protocols. Raven, New York, pp 225–236
Salvino CK, Esposito JT, Smith D et al (1992) Routine pelvic x-ray studies in awake blunt trauma patients: a sensible policy? J Trauma 33:413–416
Siegmeth A, Mullner T, Kukla C et al (2000) Associated injuries in severe pelvic trauma. Unfallchirurg 103:572–581
Tile M (1988) Pelvic ring fractures: should they be fixed? J Bone Joint Surg Br 70:1–12
Tile M (1995) Fractures of the pelvis and acetabulum. Williams and Wilkins, Baltimore
Tile M (1996a) Acute pelvic fractures. I. Causation and classification. J Am Acad Orthop Surg 4:143–151
Tile M (1996b) Acute pelvic fractures. II. Principles of management. J Am Acad Orthop Surg 4:152–161
Vas WG, Wolverson MK, Sundaram M et al (1982) The role of computed tomography in pelvic fractures. J Comput Assist Tomogr 6:796–801
Vazquez WD, Garcia VF (1993) Pediatric pelvic fractures combined with an additional skeletal injury is an indicator of significant injury. Surg Gynecol Obstet 177:468–472
Werkman HA, Jansen C, Klein JP et al (1991) Urinary tract injuries in multiply injured patients: a rational guideline for the initial assessment. Injury 22:471–474
Wolinsky PR (1997) Assessment and management of pelvic fracture in the hemodynamically unstable patient. Orthop Clin North Am 28:321–329
Yang AP, Iannacone WM (1997) External fixation for pelvic ring disruptions. Orthop Clin North Am 28:331–344
Young JWR, Burgess AR (1987) Radiological management of pelvis ring fractures. Urban and Schwarzenberg, Baltimore
Young JWR, Burgess AR, Brumbach RJ et al (1986) Pelvic fractures: value of plain radiography in early assessment and management. Radiology 160:44–451
Yugueros P, Sarniento JM, Garcia AF et al (1995) Unnecessary use of pelvic x-ray in blunt trauma. J Trauma 39:722–725

17 Penetrating Abdominal Injuries

S. J. A. Sclafani and S. Sheeran

CONTENTS

S. J. A. Sclafani, MD
Director, Department of Radiology, Kings County Hospital Center, 451 Clarkson Avenue, Brooklyn, NY 11203, USA
Sean Sheeran, MD
Department of Radiology, Kings County Hospital, 451 Clarkson Ave, Brooklyn, NY 11203, USA

- There is no indication for imaging the unstable patient with anterior abdominal penetration
- There is no indication to image the symptomatic patient with abdominal, flank or back penetration
- The primary purpose of imaging penetrating flank and back trauma is to exclude injuries requiring laparotomy
- Diagnosis and exclusion of penetrating colonic injuries should use gastrointestinal, colonic and intravenous contrast administration

17.1 Introduction

Improvements in the care of the injured civilian have often followed modifications in the care of soldiers during armed conflicts. Military surgeons have developed modern treatment modalities in response to the effects of wounding agents and the recognition of the needs for improvements. The recently ended century saw major changes in the management of penetrating vascular and enteric injuries, hospital transport and recognition of multiple organ failure. The advances in the treatment of colonic injuries began with the standardization of treatment of bowel perforations during the Second World War. Clear guidelines for the treatment of colonic injury and recommendations for routine colonic diversion resulted in marked improvements in the outcomes of patients with this devastating wound. The modern management of vascular injuries was a major focus of military surgeons during the Korean conflict in the middle of the century. Vascular repair rather than ligation became the norm. There was a marked improvement in outcomes with a significant decrease in amputations. The recognition and management of the syndromes of acute respiratory distress and multiple organ failure occurred during the Korean War and further evolved in the 1960s and 1970s during the tragic American involvement in Southeast Asia. Modern prehospital evacuation and transport of the injured evolved from methods utilized during the Vietnam War. Helicopters are now used to bring patients from the highways to the trauma centers.

The last half century has been witness to a spread of violence from the battlefield between armed forces to more sporadic and widespread assaults on nonmilitary personnel within the cities. Terrorism, crime and insane behavior have placed at risk an unsuspecting and unprepared public. In the last three decades, the United States has been witness to an unusually high frequency of violent trauma. Fueled by criminal behavior associated with drug trafficking, liberal laws regarding firearm possession, several long and sometimes overlapping economic recessions, and a demographic increase in teenagers, the likely protagonists, violence has wreaked havoc in the cities.

This epidemic of urban violence has created an environment that has been a stimulus similar to warfare in the advances in the treatment of the injured. The same kinds of trauma care innovations and advances usually seen during warfare have occurred in the urban trauma center. Many of these innovations are in imaging and they would not have been possible or applicable on the battlefield because the devices used for them, such as computed tomography units and angiography suites, are big, heavy and require fixed locations. Wounds caused in an urban setting are located in proximity to the tertiary care trauma centers and emergency medical services deliver these patients to facilities that have available all the equipment and staff needed to image and intervene. Because of this proximity to tertiary care hospitals, traumatologists have developed paradigms different from those necessary during warfare, where transport of patients for more definitive care was time-consuming and impractical.

One of the advances resulting from the experiences of urban conflict has been the management of penetrating abdominal trauma. Because the patient arrives at the urban trauma center sooner and in better condition, diagnosis and treatment of many wounds can be more deliberate. Clinical and imaging evaluations of abdominal penetrations enable some of the patients to avoid unnecessary laparotomy. The battlefield surgeon does not have this luxury and is much more likely to treat the patient operatively before additional casualties arrive in the field hospital. These innovations include nonoperative management of some abdominal gunshot and stab wounds, the use of computed tomography for the diagnosis of acute injuries and their complications, and the role of interventional radiology in their management.

Diagnostic imaging and invasive radiology are vital components of the medical response to urban penetrating trauma and have become increasingly important, with recent trends toward nonoperative management. The purpose of this chapter is to review penetrating abdominal trauma including the mechanism and types of injuries, the value of various imaging modalities, and the role of interventional radiology in the management of these patients.

17.2 Mechanism

17.2.1 Gunshot Wounds

The nature and extent of gunshot wounds depends in large part on characteristics of the bullet, the weapon, and the affected tissues (Henneman 1989; Hollerman et al. 1990a). Relevant bullet characteristics include its mass, velocity, caliber, shape, design, and degree of deformation and fragmentation. Weapon characteristics include type – handgun, rifle, or shotgun – spin, and longitudinal velocity. The elasticity, density, and anatomy of the affected tissues are important characteristics effecting wounds.

Two major mechanisms of wounding have been described: tissue crushing, which forms a permanent cavity, and radial stretching of tissue, which forms a temporary cavity (Henneman 1989; Hollerman et al. 1990a). Tissue crushing is related to a number of factors, including bullet yaw – the angle between the long axis of the bullet and its flight – deformation, and fragmentation. As the amount of yaw increases, there is a corresponding increase in the amount of tissue crushing. Deformation of the bullet is another important factor since greater deformation results in increased surface area and more tissue crushing. Fragmentation of the bullet increases the volume of tissue crushed and results in a larger permanent cavity.

Temporary cavitation causes tissue damage primarily by stretching and distortion (Henneman 1989; Hollerman et al. 1990a). The extent of tissue damage by temporary cavitation depends in part on the kinetic energy of the missile and the density and elasticity of the affected tissues. In general, tissue with low elasticity and high density such as bone sustains more damage from a temporary cavity than highly elastic and low-density tissues such as lungs. Similar to tissue crushing, bullet characteristics, including velocity, mass, shape, design, and fragmentation, influence the size and location of the temporary cavity (HENNEMAN 1989).

17.2.2 Shotgun Wounds

Shotgun rounds are composed of numerous pellets or balls of stainless steel or lead, which are contained within a cartridge filled with wadding of cloth or paper. When fired, shotguns deliver this mass as a unit. The type of injury seen depends most importantly upon the distance between the weapon and the victim. Short range effects include a large focal delivery of this round into a small area. When striking at short range, the round is effectively a single blast causing damage by crushing tissue at high velocity. The area of damage is deeper and more discrete. Each pellet contains kinetic energy that is dissipated in the tissues. When delivered at close range, these pellets contain sufficient energy to penetrate bowel and vessels. When fired from afar, this mass of pellets breaks up into a spray of discrete pellets that do not contain sufficient kinetic energy to penetrate deeply. Radiographs can distinguish these scenarios. For example, when the shot pellets are distributed over a small area, then one can infer that the injury was at close range. However, when there is a wide distribution of the pellets, then the weapon was fired from some distance and one can predict that the likelihood of injury diminishes considerably (Fig. 17.1). Radiography, nonetheless, can be very difficult to interpret because these pellets cannot be localized easily because of overlap of the numerous shot. In addition to the pellets of a shotgun, the wounding agent also includes the cartridge, which can penetrate the body as well. This may lead to foreign bodies of wadding and cartridge being embedded within the soft tissues. These nonopaque foreign bodies, sometimes difficult to recognize, can be problematic sources of infectious complications. At times ultrasound (US), computed tomography (CT) and magnetic resonance imaging (MRI) can be of help in evaluating these nonopaque foreign bodies.

17.2.3 Stab Wounds

Stab wounds are most commonly from knives, but may result from other sharp objects such as ice picks and screwdrivers. Glass penetrations may be related to accidental falls against glass windows or from explosions that send secondary missiles of glass. The mechanism of injury from stab wounds is related to direct cutting of tissues from the blade or other sharp objects. The extent of these knife penetrations may be unknown and difficult to estimate. The weapon or object may be unknown to the victim who may not be able to describe its length. The weapon may go straight in and out but it may also extend cephalad or caudad. These factors make estimation of the wounding potential more difficult than a gunshot wound that has an entry and an exit. When imaging stab wounds, one must make worst case estimations

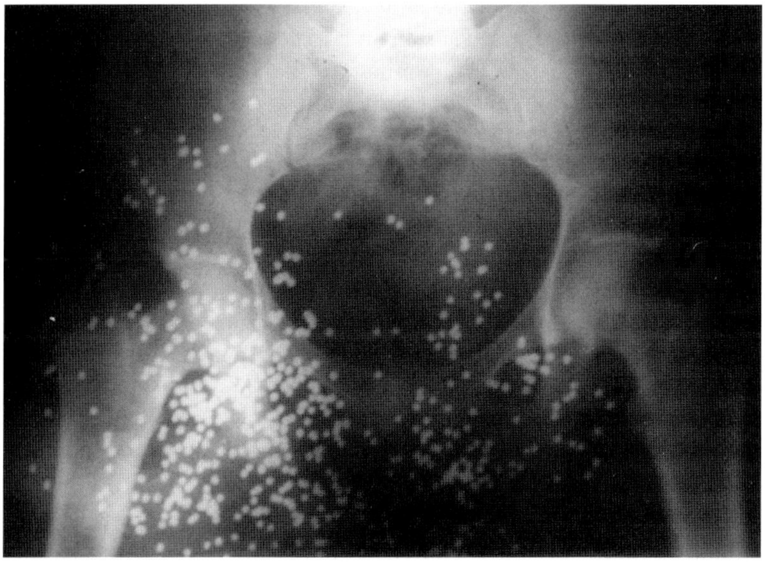

Fig. 17.1. Shotgun wounds

of length and direction so that the entire potential area of injury can be imaged.

17.2.4 Impalement

Impalement injuries are a special form of penetrating abdominal injury. With impalement, the penetrating object remains within the body and the patient may arrive at the hospital with the object in place. Such objects should not be removed in the field because they sometimes tamponade injuries to vascular structures and thus prevent exsanguination. Impalement objects should be removed in the controlled environment of the operating room. Imaging impalements can be very challenging. The radiologist should assure that imaging does not risk moving the impalement object. Creativity may be necessary to perform angiography, contrast enema, or other examinations. Depending upon the location of the impalement, imaging may require the prone or in decubitus position to prevent injury.

17.2.5 Iatrogenic Penetrations

Medical misadventures are the most common source of penetrating injuries not caused by violence. Instrumentation with endoscopes may result in penetration of bowel, bladder, ureter, and vasculature. Laparoscopic surgery has brought with it a set of injuries related to these techniques. A discussion of iatrogenic injuries is beyond the scope of this chapter.

17.2.6 Locations of Injuries

17.2.6.1 Rationale

For evaluation of penetrating abdominal trauma, it is important to divide the location of penetration into anatomical zones (Ferrada and Birolini 1999). Each zone has different structures at risk and the likelihood of injury to these structures depends upon the area of penetration. The imaging paradigm for penetrations of each zone is different. Localizing the penetration for imaging, however, must be a conscious effort by the traumatologist in concert with the radiologist. All entry and exit wounds should be identified. All clothing must be removed to allow complete inspection. Skin folds and creases should be assessed. The patient should be turned to assess the entire back. It is dangerous to assume that there is only one wound. In many situations, the wounding agent will pass through several zones of the abdomen. Sometimes it is impossible to assess the trajectory of wounding agents. Stab wounds, for example, may have only an entry wound. Bullets may extend superficially before entering the abdomen. Bullet holes in the skin may be tangential grazes that do not enter deep tissues. Nonetheless, for gunshot wounds, there should be an exit wound or a retained bullet associated with each entry wound. The location of penetrating abdominal wounds is important since the management of wounds to the anterior abdomen is different from those to the flank and/or back. Wounds to the anterior abdomen can be easily dissected locally to assess if the peritoneum has been penetrated. The flank and back cannot be easily explored locally since there are thick paraspinal muscles and there is a greater distance to the retroperitoneum. Moreover, the likelihood of organ injury is different in each area and the types of structures that must be evaluated differ as well. Penetration in each zone results in a different prevalence of injury.

17.2.6.2 Thoracoabdominal Zone

The thoracoabdominal region is the area extending from the nipples to the costal margin. It includes the lower thoracic cage the and inferior aspect of the mediastinum. Structures at risk include the lower lobes of the lungs as well as the diaphragms, heart, liver, and spleen and occasionally the colon. Wounds can be predominantly thoracic or abdominal or a combination of the two.

17.2.6.3 Anterior Abdominal Zone

The abdomen is the area bounded superiorly by the costal margin, laterally by the anterior axillary line, and inferiorly by the symphysis pubis and inguinal crease. The area includes all intraperitoneal organs. Physical assessment of this zone is facilitated by the development of peritonitis when structures within the peritoneum are injured. Of anterior abdominal gunshot wounds, 80% penetrate the peritoneum with up to 95% of these resulting in significant intraabdominal injuries (Henneman 1989). There are one or two visceral or vascular injuries in 60% of patients and three or more injuries in the remainder. The exact frequency of various organ injuries varies among different surgical series. The small bowel and colon tend to be the most frequently injured organs. Other commonly injured organs include the liver, vasculature, stomach, and kidneys. Compared with stab wounds, gunshot wounds have a 2.5 times greater likelihood of vascular injuries.

Approximately 66% of patients with anterior abdomen stab wounds have penetration of the peritoneum and roughly 50% of these patients present with overt peritoneal signs and hemodynamic instability requiring immediate laparotomy (Henneman 1989). Only 50%–60% of the other half of patients with peritoneal violation have significant intraabdominal injuries. On average, two visceral or vascular injuries are found at laparotomy (Feliciano and Rozycki 1995). The most commonly injured organs include small bowel, liver, colon, diaphragm, and stomach (Feliciano and Rozycki 1995).

17.2.6.4
Flank and Back Zone

The flanks are defined as the areas between the anterior axillary line and the posterior axillary line from the sixth intercostal space to the iliac crest. The back is the region between the right and left posterior axillary lines from the tip of the scapula to the iliac crest. The dense paraspinal muscles and vertebral structures provide a significant barrier which protects the retroperitoneal structures (Henneman 1989). Less than 25% of stab wounds to the back and/or flank cause visceral damage. The organs at risk are the diaphragm, the liver, and the spleen superiorly, the colon and small intestine, the kidney and ureters, the vasculature, and the spine and its contents. Because of the lower probability of injury in penetrations of the back and flank, imaging plays an important role in the assessment of hemodynamically stable patients with back and flank penetrations.

17.2.6.5
Pelvic Zone

The pelvis is defined as the area extending from the iliac crests to the bottom of the ischium. Anteriorly, it is also part of the abdomen; laterally and posteriorly it includes the gluteal region and the back. The clinical and diagnostic algorithms for penetrations of the anterior pelvis are similar to that for other anterior abdominal wounds, that is, minimal diagnostic workup because of the high likelihood of multiple organ injury and the fairly good clinical correlation. Surgical exploration for most injuries is mandatory.

However, there are some noteworthy differences from anterior abdominal penetrations. Posterior pelvic penetrations are often benign because of the ample surrounding musculature of the buttocks, as well as osseous protection from the pelvic bones and spine. Genitourinary injuries are common because of the large area occupied by the bladder. Vascular injuries are frequent because of the prominent place of the aortoiliac vessels in the pelvis.

17.3
Imaging

While CT has become established as the imaging study of choice for most abdominal injuries, a variety of other imaging modalities are also used in the workup of patients with penetrating trauma. They include plain films, contrast examinations, US, CT, and angiography. At the current time, the role of MRI in the management of these patients is unclear, but MR is not likely to play a great role in the emergency management of these patients. Bullets are composed of various metals whose response to the strong magnetic field cannot be predicted because the composition of missiles cannot be determined in the acute setting.

17.3.1
Radiography

17.3.1.1
Chest Radiography

Chest radiography plays an important role in the management of penetrating abdominal trauma, particularly those wounds in the thoracoabdominal zone. Thoracoabdominal injuries, which can extend from the chest into the abdomen or from the abdomen into the chest or mediastinum, can cause troubles and confusion for the traumatologist who must decide on priorities. Should the abdomen or the chest be explored and in what sequence? Is chest drainage necessary? Is hypotension or hypoxia during exploratory laparotomy secondary to occult tension pneumothorax or hemothorax ? Therefore, a single portable radiograph of the chest may be performed when clinical conditions allow. It remains contraindicated when abdominal penetration is associated with hemodynamic instability. In such circumstances, it is more prudent to proceed to abdominal exploration. A chest film can be performed in the operating room if stabilization can be accomplished before the laparotomy.

The chest film provides information about the location of bullets and allows estimations of the trajectory of the missile (Fig. 17.2). It can suggest diaphragmatic wounding in such cases. It is useful to place radio-opaque markers on entry and exit wounds so that trajectory can be inferred. It is important to determine whether the pleural space and lung have been violated. Hemothorax should be evacuated before exploration because it is more difficult after the abdomen has been exposed. Pneumothorax can be subtle or obvious, but in either case, tube thoracostomy is indicated prior to induction of anesthesia and positive pressure ventilation when even a small pneumothorax is identified. Determination that there has been mediastinal traverse by a missile is critical as these wounds risk injury to the heart, the great vessels, esophagus, and airway. Widening of the mediastinal shadow, indistinctness of the descending aorta, air in the mediastinum all suggest such injury. Cardiac injury and tamponade is a more difficult radiological assessment because cardiac penetration does not necessarily lead to a large amount of blood in the pericardial sac. Because of the acute nature of this accumulation, only small amounts of blood are required to cause hemodynamic effects. Therefore, a normal heart size on chest radiography cannot be used to infer the absence of cardiac injury.

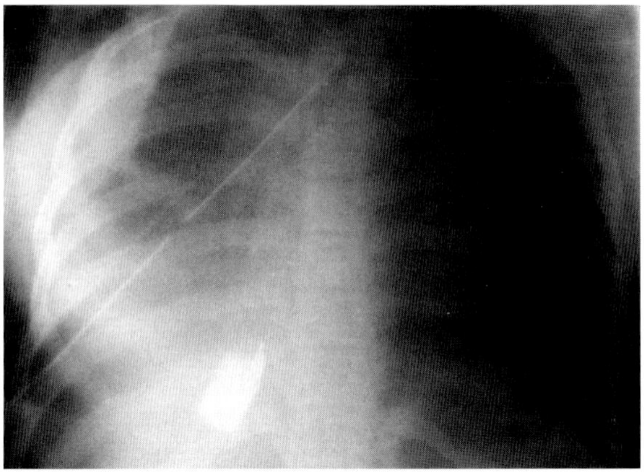

Fig. 17.2. Chest radiograph

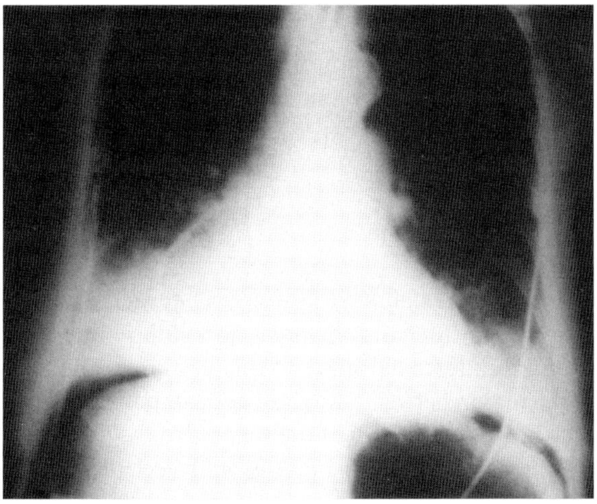

Fig. 17.3. Chest radiograph demonstrates pneumoperitoneum after gunshot wound of the abdomen. The portable chest radiograph is often performed in the supine position. It was fortuitous that this film was obtained with the patient sitting in the bed

In some circumstances chest radiography can identify pneumoperitoneum resulting from bowel perforation (Fig. 17.3). This is an important finding because it creates an immediate indication for exploratory surgery. Rapid identification and treatment of bowel perforations is the standard. However, free peritoneal air is more often not visible; it is absent in 50%–85% of patients with bowel perforations. Reasons for this may be technical, as only supine or semi-erect views are usually obtained. Moreover, most bowel injuries are localized to the small intestine and there may be only a small amount of air expelled through a small hole.

17.3.1.2 Abdominal Radiography

Abdominal radiographs have a limited role in the management of penetrating trauma. They have even less value in the assessment of abdominal stab wounds. The role of abdominal radiography is much more marginal than the chest radiograph. When there is obvious evidence of abdominal penetration with clinical signs of hemodynamic instability or peritonitis, abdominal radiography is contraindicated. The amount of useful information is very limited. Surgeons base their clinical decisions upon other clinical criteria and abdominal radiography does not contribute greatly in those decisions.

The utility of supine abdominal radiographs in the management of patients with abdominal gunshot wounds is controversial. Abdominal radiographs are potentially useful since they can detect bullet fragments, abnormal gas collections, and other radio-opaque foreign bodies such as dirt or cloth. Propo-

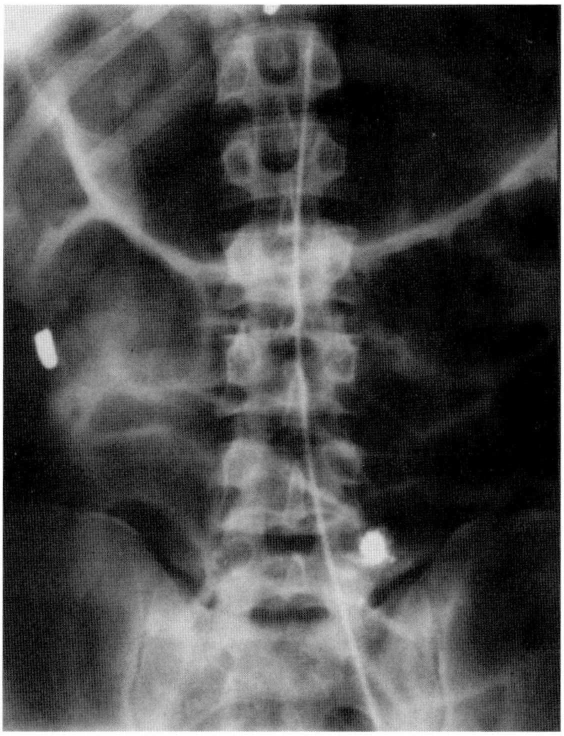

Fig. 17.4. Abdominal film

nents of preoperative supine abdominal radiographs in the hemodynamically unstable patient suggest that these findings may lead to surgical exploration in an area remote from the suspected bullet path (QUIGLEY and BRET 1995). In addition, a cluster of small bullet fragments is a strong indicator of tissue damage in that region (HOLLERMAN et al. 1990b). Most authors do not share this opinion.

There are a few valid indications for abdominal radiography. In stable patients with gunshot wounds or shrapnel wounds, radiography can identify bullets and other foreign bodies (Fig. 17.4). This can confirm the clinical determination that a bullet has entered the abdominal cavity. These images can sometimes help determine a gross estimation of the trajectory of the missile and provide the traumatologist with a list of potential organ injuries. Fractures of the ribs, spine, and pelvis can be identified. Bullet fragmentation can be seen.

Pneumoperitoneum is the most important finding. The presence of free intraperitoneal air is a very significant finding. Yet, it is often not recognized or visible. It is not seen in the majority of cases of bowel perforation. Perhaps the small bowel injuries do not leak much air. Most of these patients are imaged by portable techniques. Perhaps the helpful erect film was not performed. Other causes of pneumoperitoneum can be seen in trauma. Associated neck or mediastinal injury may track air into the peritoneum. This possibility is suggested by subcutaneous emphysema, pneumomediastinum, or tension pneumothorax on the chest radiograph.

Other air collections can also be seen (Fig. 17.5). These do not resemble bowel gas or pneumoperitoneum. Small pockets of streaks and bubbles may be seen with duodenal and retroperitoneal colonic injury. They can also be sucked in from the outside by the negative cavity formed as the bullet projects through the body. Migration of bullets on sequential radiographs may be identified (Fig. 17.6). This finding suggests that the bullet is located within a hollow structure, including the vasculature, the bowel, the urinary, or biliary drainage systems. Intravascular bullets may migrate to the heart and other arteries and veins. Bullets within the peritoneum or pleura can also migrate. Bullets can also move around within abscesses and other collections. Other foreign bodies can also be identified (Fig. 17.7).

However, the supine abdominal radiograph is unable to localize abnormalities in three dimensions. To be truly effective in assessing trajectory, it would be helpful to obtain a lateral view of the abdomen at the same time. This will help determine whether flank and back gunshot wounds have traversed into the peritoneal cavity or whether they are lodged in the back muscles or the anterior abdominal wall.

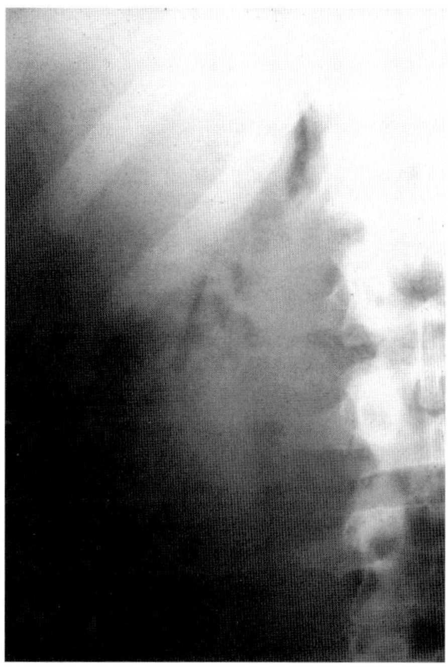

Fig. 17.5. Retroperitoneal air

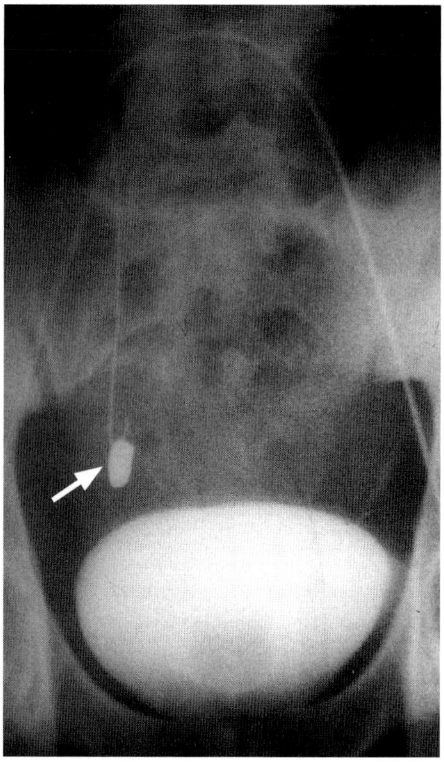

a

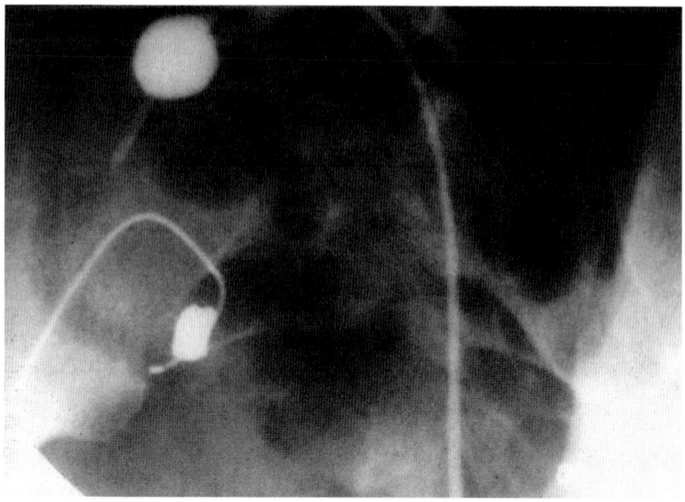

b

Fig. 17.6a, b. Migratory bullet. The patient sustained a gunshot wound to the upper portion of the right flank and the bullet was found in the pelvis (*arrow*). Peritoneal lavage failed to demonstrate any hemoperitoneum. Median sternotomy was performed and a perforation of the right ventricle was repaired. **a** Since the bullet was not found, a radiograph of the abdomen was performed. This showed the bullet to be in the pelvis, suggesting that inferior migration through the vena cava had occurred. **b** A balloon was placed in the lower inferior vena cava to prevent further migration of the bullet back toward the heart. A snare was used to retrieve this bullet

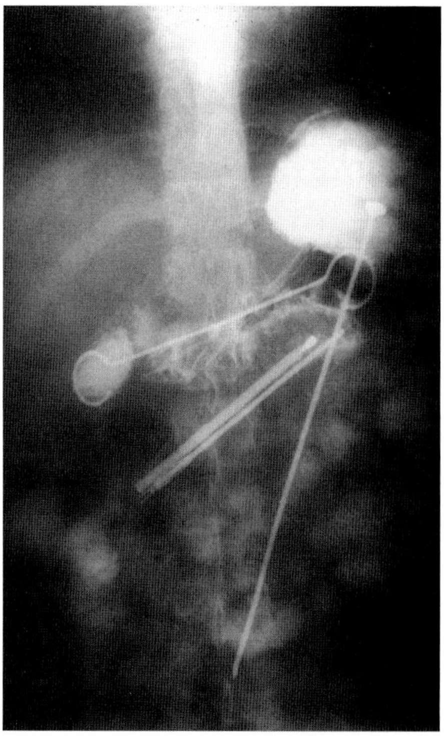

Fig. 17.7. Foreign body identification. This psychotic prison inmate swallowed metallic foreign bodies in attempts to remain out of prison. Visualized on this image are radio antennae and a spoon

The use of iodinated contrast medium prior to the abdominal radiography requires discussion. For many years, traumatologists have injected iodinated contrast medium 5–10 min prior to the abdominal radiograph (Fig. 17.8). The purpose of this was to identify the kidneys, to assure that there were two of them, and that they both excreted. The rationale was to assure that nephrectomy was not performed in a patient with a single kidney. Advocates also argued that it was also helpful to identify a kidney adjacent to a hematoma and to identify anomalously positioned kidneys. This practice is, for the most part, no longer utilized by traumatologists.

To summarize, while there are some interesting findings of abdominal radiography, I do not advocate imaging of hemodynamically unstable patients or of patients with clear clinical signs of abdominal penetration after abdominal gunshot wounds. I think that the likelihood of significant injury is high and that the delay to obtain them rarely is worth the extra time in hemorrhagic shock.

17.3.1.3 Contrast Radiography

Contrast studies were previously the primary methods of evaluating penetration injuries. Contrast stud-

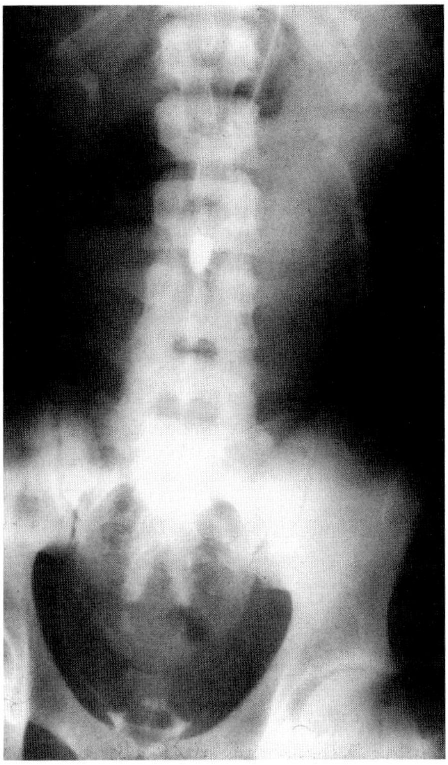

Fig. 17.8. One-shot urogram. A single portable film of the abdomen was performed prior to exploration of this patient with a gunshot wound of the abdomen. The image shows poor visualization of the left renal collecting system and urinary extravasation

ies of the gastrointestinal tract were, in the past, the procedures of choice for assessment of missed bowel perforations. Intravenous urography and cystography were frequently performed to assess retroperitoneal penetrations. However, the high-radiation dosage, the cost, the inaccuracy of these studies, and the development of CT have led to a marked reduction in these procedures. They continue to have some value in postoperative assessment of penetrating trauma, but this usually follows CT. Leaks following repair and strictures are still studied by these methods.

Intravenous Urography

The role of the "one-shot" intravenous pyelography (IVP) in patients with penetrating trauma is controversial. The primary indication for radiological evaluation to stage renal trauma from penetrating injuries is proximity of the injury to the genitourinary system (Carrol and McAninch 1989). A one-shot IVP has been used to evaluate those patients with suspected renal trauma who are too unstable to undergo a CT scan. The one-shot IVP is usually performed by administering 1.5 ml/kg of intravenous contrast followed by a portable radiograph approximately 5–10 min later. The purpose of the one-shot IVP is to detect renal injuries and to assess for the presence of contralateral renal function.

Recent studies have suggested that one-shot IVP has no significant value in the management of unstable patients with suspected renal trauma (Stevenson and Battistella 1994; Patel and Walker 1997). Patel reported a series of 40 patients with penetrating trauma and found the one-shot IVP had a sensitivity of 25%, a specificity of 76%, and a positive predictive value of 20%. The results of the one-shot IVP did not alter the decision for laparotomy in any of the patients who underwent exploratory laparotomy (Patel and Walker 1997). Stevenson reported a series of 239 patients with blunt or penetrating trauma and found the one-shot IVP had a sensitivity of 73%, a specificity of 92%, and a positive predictive value of 73%. In addition, Stevenson also found that only 1.3% of their patients had their surgical management altered by the IVP (Stevenson and Battistella 1994).

Multiple studies have also shown that excretory urography is limited in its ability to identify renal injuries (Scott et al. 1969; Wilson and Ziegler 1987). For example, Scott et al. and Wilson and Ziegler reported that IVPs were normal in 33% and 34%, respectively, of patients with known penetrating renal injuries. Some surgeons, in the minority, prefer to have an image of the abdomen to assess that there is an excreting kidney contralateral to an injured kidney. At Kings County Hospital, the authors abandoned this practice in 1985. Ureteric injury is often difficult to detect. Hematuria may be absent. Contusion of the ureter may result in no demonstrable injury on urography. However, contusion in the poorly vascularized ureter may deteriorate; the result is mural breakdown with leakage of urine into the surrounding tissue. Urography is still used by many to assess the ureter (Fig. 17.9). Urographic findings include proximal hydronephrosis, contrast extravasation and urinoma, and failure to visualize the distal ureter.

Cystography

The plans, protocols, and rationale for imaging the lower genitourinary tract in penetrating trauma is different from that of blunt trauma in several respects. Hematuria may be absent in many patients with penetrating urinary injuries. This is especially true for ureteric injuries. Bladder injuries are often both intra-

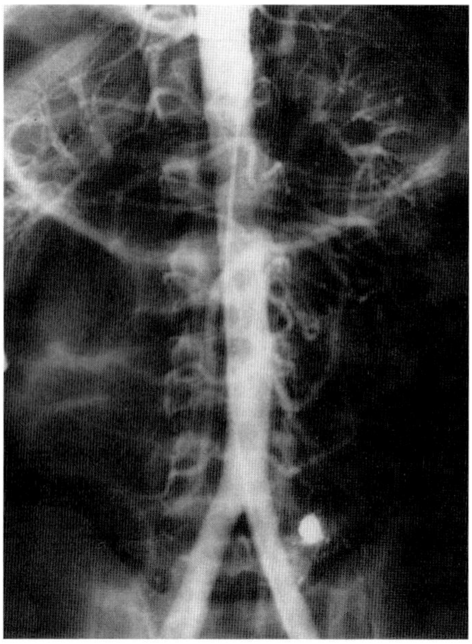

Fig. 17.9. Ureteric laceration

peritoneal and extraperitoneal because penetrations violate fascial barriers without distinction.

Therefore the workup of the lower urinary tract is different from that of blunt trauma. In blunt trauma, cystography precedes urography so that complete bladder emptying can be accomplished. This is helpful in the assessment of the bladder. The ureter is not a likely injury in blunt trauma. On the contrary, with penetrating pelvic trauma, ureteric injury may occur and must be excluded. Therefore, in penetration of the true pelvis, there must be good visualization of the ureters and we must tailor the examination to assure this. Because bladder injury may coexist with distal ureteric injury, extravasation from the bladder may obscure a leak from a ureter. So urography must precede cystography in these patients.

Cystography is performed in the same manner as for blunt trauma. Scout images in the frontal and lateral projections are followed by full distension and opacification of the bladder with at least 400 ml of a 30% concentration of iodinated contrast medium instilled in a retrograde fashion. Frontal and lateral radiographs are performed with the bladder filled and after evacuation. Injuries are diagnosed by identifying extravasation of contrast medium. Because penetrations do not discriminate fascial barriers, intraperitoneal and extraperitoneal may coexist. Moreover, fistulous connections between the bladder and neighboring structures can also occur (Fig. 17.10). Posterior urethral injuries may also be seen in association with the bladder injury (Fig. 17.11).

Gastrointestinal Studies

Contrast studies of the gastrointestinal tract were previously the primary diagnostic studies in trauma but, with the development of computed cross-sectional imaging modalities, these studies have markedly diminished in value and utilization. Contrast gastrointestinal series and enemas have been relegated to the assessment and evaluation of postoperative complications such as sepsis. The primary reasons

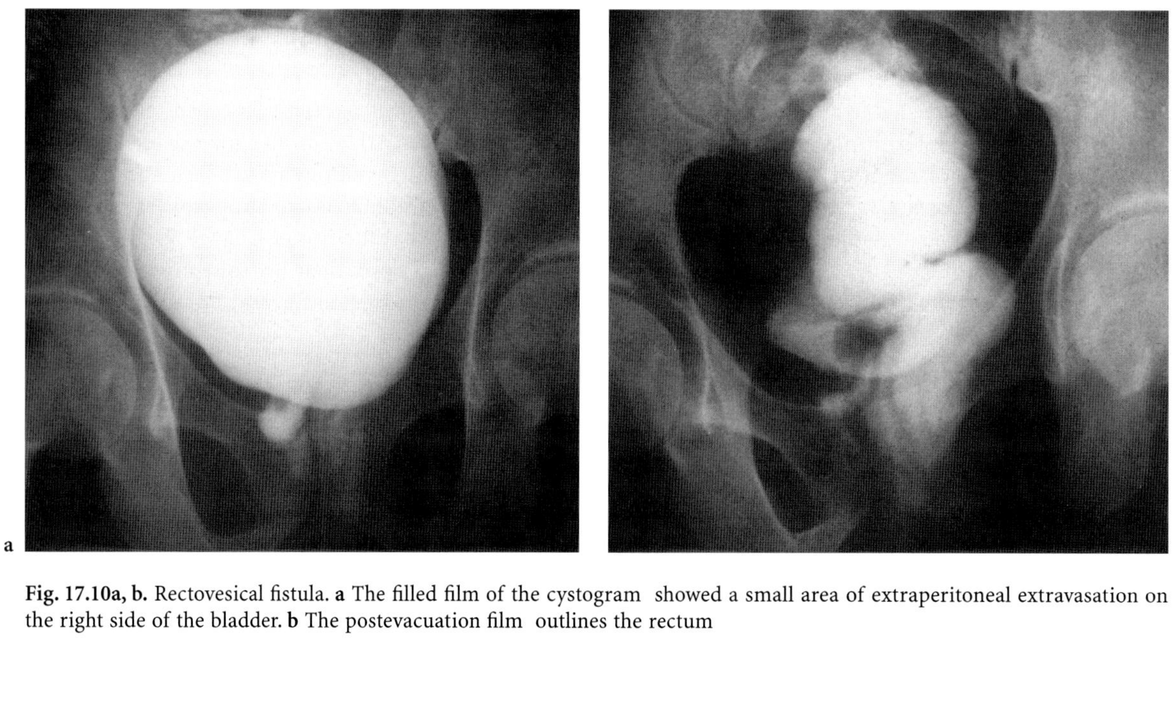

Fig. 17.10a, b. Rectovesical fistula. **a** The filled film of the cystogram showed a small area of extraperitoneal extravasation on the right side of the bladder. **b** The postevacuation film outlines the rectum

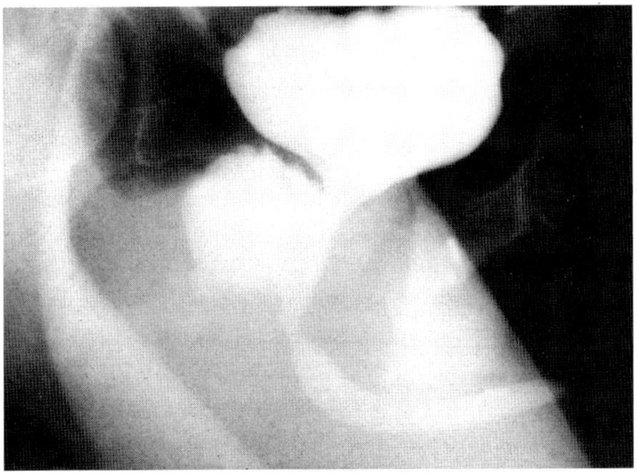

Fig. 17.11. Prostatic urethral injury. Perineal gunshot wound led to a urethrogram that showed a large cavitation of the prostate gland with contained extravasation from the prostatic urethra

for these studies include the detection of bowel anastomosis breakdown and evaluation of postoperative stricture and obstructions (Figs. 17.12 and 17.13).

Esophagography

Esophagography, however, remains essential for the assessment of the distal esophagus when there are thoracoabdominal penetrations with mediastinal traverse (Fig. 17.14). These injuries cannot be identified during laparotomy. Simultaneous operative exploration of the mediastinum is usually not warranted because of the morbidity of that procedure. Rather contrast studies

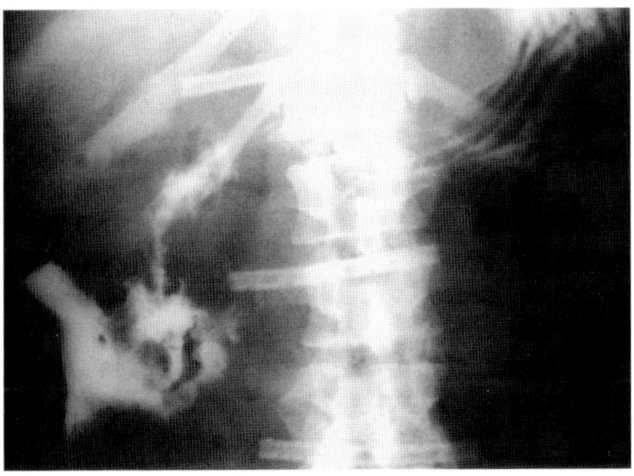

Fig. 17.12. Duodenal dehiscence. Postoperative drainage and sepsis lead to evaluation of the duodenal repair by water-soluble contrast study. This showed extravasation from the duodenal repair and accumulation in the space adjacent to the duodenal repair

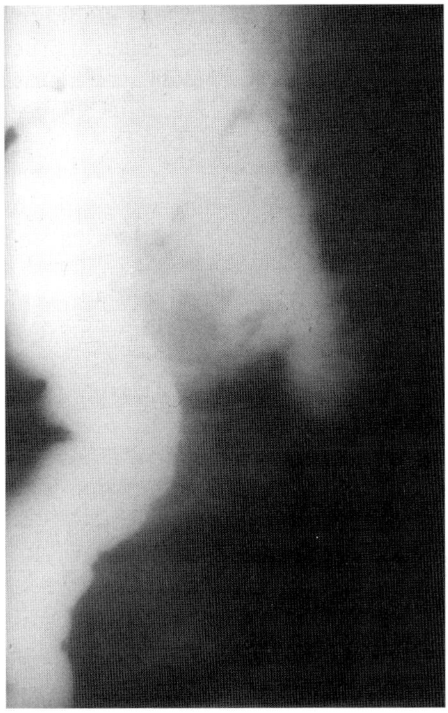

Fig. 17.13. Colonic injury. The patient sustained a stab wound of the back. Clinical observation was attempted because CT had not been established at that time. A water-soluble enema demonstrated extravasation from the colon

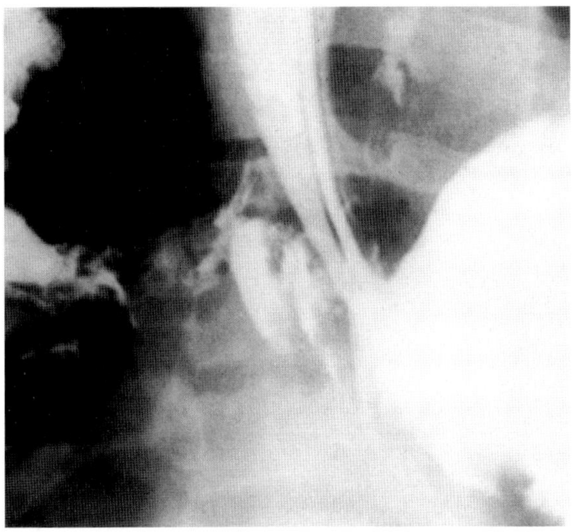

Fig. 17.14. Esophageal perforation. This patient sustained a thoracoabdominal gunshot wound with mediastinal traverse. A water-soluble contrast esophagogram was performed. It demonstrated through and through perforations of the distal esophagus just above the diaphragm. The majority of extravasated contrast medium was in the right chest but a small amount is seen in the left pleural space

are performed to diagnose and exclude esophageal injury. While these authors have little hesitation to use barium suspensions for suspected esophageal injuries above the level of the carina, there are compelling reasons to use a water-soluble contrast agent when there is a thoracoabdominal penetration. It is impossible to prevent the barium from traversing the esophagus into the bowel from which it would leak into the peritoneum if there were a concomitant peritoneal bowel perforation. Barium peritonitis is a difficult problem leading to intense inflammation, which is difficult to control and results in very serious adhesions. Since bowel perforations are the most common injury, we attempt to avoid this problem by using water-soluble material. However, since Gastrografin is so hypertonic, and because the risks of aspiration are not insignificant in these patients, iso-osmolar contrast agents are recommended.

The diagnostic accuracy of esophagography at our institution has been outstanding. Sensitivity and specificity greater than 98% have been obtained for the past 20 years. The diagnosis of esophageal perforation is straightforward. Contrast spillage into the mediastinum or pleural spaces, or both, defines the injury. It is important to specifically identify the site of injury as the surgical approach may differ.

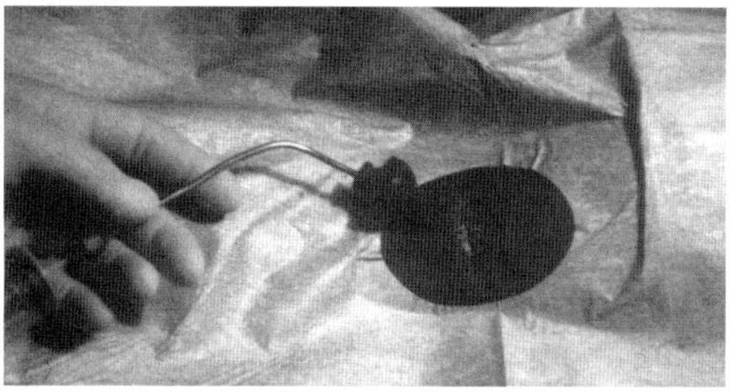
a

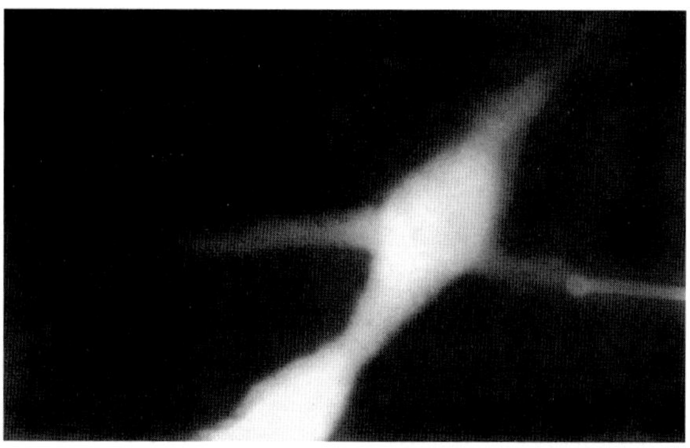
b

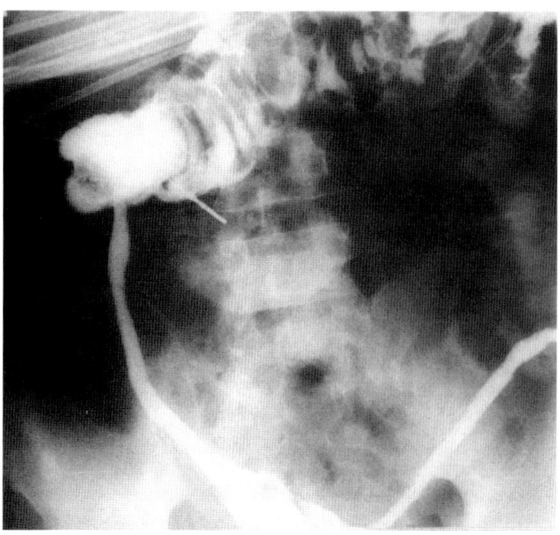
c

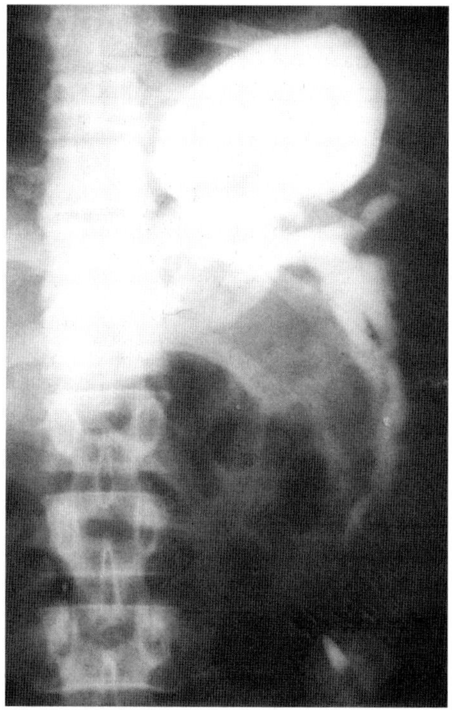
d

Fig. 17.15a–d. Evaluation of draining sinus tracts. **a** The triangular acorn-shaped device is ideally suited to occluding the drain tract and allowing visualization of the entire cavity. **b** The patient developed drainage from a left flank drain tract. The initial sinus tract study, performed by placing a urinary catheter into the tract, failed to demonstrate anything significant. The catheter went directly horizontal and failed to delineate the tract that extended downward toward the pelvis. **c** With use of the acorn it was possible to delineate the entire tract, which extended down into the pelvis and then extended cephalad to demonstrate a fistula from the right colon. **d** Gastrocutaneous fistula. Postoperative drainage after gunshot wound of the stomach, kidney, diaphragm, and pancreas was studied by a contrast gastrointestinal examination that did not identify the problem. Sinography shown here demonstrated quite clearly that there was fistula from a breakdown of the gastric repair

Sinography

Enteric leaks are a common complication of penetrating abdominal trauma (Fig. 17.15). Draining sinuses and abscess formation are frequent sequelae of penetrating bowel trauma. Leaks result from several causes, including undetected injury, progression of contusion, and serosal injury to full thickness disruptions, intestinal obstruction, and dehiscence of anastomotic sewn or stapled repairs. Caused by poor technique, local infection, ischemia, or progressive degeneration of microscopic contusion caused by high-velocity wounding agents, these complications are a major source of morbidity and late mortality after penetrating trauma. They may present as sepsis, leakage of fluid from drain tracts and incisions, abscesses, or wound infection.

The diagnosis of these leaks is sometimes cryptic and often time-consuming. Numerous diagnostic tests may be required to arrive at the correct diagnosis. Various contrast studies, including computed tomography, gastrointestinal series, contrast enemas, and enteroclysis have been used to detect the source of these leaks. However, the most direct method of identifying both enteric leaks and fistulas is sinography. Because penetrating trauma so frequently injures the hollow viscera, enteric fistulas and sinus tracts are common complications, often associated with abdominal abscesses. Contamination of the peritoneum and retroperitoneum from spillage of food and feces at the time of injury creates a poor environment for healing and breakdown of anastomoses should be considered when postoperative sepsis occurs. Because of the risks of leaks from bowel and other hollow viscera, surgeons frequently placed drains around injuries to allow egress of infected material. When these drains and drain tracts persist in leakage, the radiologist should consider evaluation of the drain or tract. Retrograde sinography is the best method of detecting enteric fistulas. Rather than rely upon leakage under lower pressure to opacify the tract and cavity when the contrast is administered within the gastrointestinal tract, sinography directly opacifies the tract and cavity under pressure. There is no ability to bypass the leaking area as is the case with GI opacification.

We treat these studies as infected drainage procedures. Antibiotics are administered intravenously as prophylaxis against bacteremia. The wound is cleaned with Betadine solution and covered with a sterile towel. Absorbent gauze is placed at the injection site to prevent artifacts caused by contrast leakage into the surrounding skin, sheets, etc. We place an "acorn" device into the sinus opening to completely occlude its orifice in attempts to prevent reflux. We do not put tubes into the tract, as this may result in the bypass of and failure to diagnose side tracts and short enteric connections. Sterile 30%–60% water-soluble contrast medium is injected under fluoroscopic control until all aspects of the cavity are seen and enteric communications have been excluded. Delay in imaging may result in further opacification of the normal GI tract and make it impossible to determine the site of the fistulous communication.

17.3.2 Ultrasonography

US has many features which make it well suited for the evaluation of patients with abdominal trauma: it is rapid, noninvasive, portable, and relatively inexpensive (Rozycki 1995; Rozycki et al. 1998a; Boulanger et al. 1999; Rozycki and Newman 1999). In addition, US can be performed serially to reassess the patient if his or her clinical status changes. US relies primarily upon the detection of intraperitoneal fluid, which is a secondary sign of abdominal trauma. Consequently, US may potentially miss significant injuries if they do not result in hemoperitoneum. US has been used in the evaluation of abdominal trauma since the early 1980s. Focused assessment with sonography for trauma (FAST), a directed ultrasound examination of the abdominal and pericardial cavities for free fluid, was first described by Tso et al. (1992). Since this report by Tso et al., there have been numerous studies assessing the utility and role of US in the evaluation of blunt abdominal trauma (Boulanger et al. 1995; McKenney et al. 1996; Rozycki et al. 1998b). FAST has been incorporated into trauma algorithms as a screening test for patients with blunt abdominal trauma, with selective use of CT or diagnostic peritoneal lavage (DPL), depending on FAST and clinical findings. These studies have shown US has a sensitivity ranging from 81% to 90% and a specificity ranging from 96% to 98%.

While there have been multiple studies of US in blunt abdominal trauma, there have been limited studies of US use in penetrating abdominal trauma. Rozycki et al. reported their experience of US in the evaluation of 74 patients with penetrating abdominal trauma (Rozycki et al. 1993). The sensitivity of US was 77% and the specificity was 86%. Injuries which resulted in false negative studies included small bowel perforation, colon perforation, ruptured hemidiaphragm, liver laceration, and splenic laceration. However, all of the patients in the false negative group had injuries requiring mandatory celiotomies, so US would not have altered their management. In 1995, Rozycki et al. reported their experience with US in an additional 76 patients with penetrating abdominal trauma (Rozycki et al. 1995). In this study, US had a sensitivity of 83.8% and a specificity of 97.4%. False negative studies were associated with the same types of injuries as their previous study. Also, as in their 1993 study, all patients in the false negative group had mandatory celiotomy based on the nature of their injuries.

For the patient with penetrating thoracoabdominal injuries, US has the potential to detect hemopericardium, traumatic pleural effusions, and diaphragmatic rupture (Rozycki et al. 1998a). Several studies have demonstrated that US can decrease the time to diagnosis of penetrating cardiac injury and improve both the survival rate and neurological outcome (Plummer et al. 1992; Rozycki et al. 1996; Rozycki et al. 1999). The mean performance time for pericardial examination has been reported to be 0.8 min, with a mean time from US to operation of approximately 12 min (Rozycki et al. 1996). US also is useful for detecting traumatic pleural effusions. Sisley et al. (1998) compared ultrasound and portable supine chest radiographs in 360 patients with blunt or penetrating torso injuries. This study showed that US is as accurate as portable chest radiographs for detecting traumatic effusion, but is significantly faster. US also has the potential to determine the presence of diaphragmatic injuries (Ammann et al. 1988). Ipsilateral hemoperitoneum and pleural effusion in patients with penetrating thoracoabdominal wounds increases the chances of a diaphragmatic injury. Another reported application of US in penetrating thoracoabdominal trauma is the examination of wound tracts to determine if violation of the peritoneum or pleura has occurred. Fry et al. reported a pilot study of 29 patients with penetrating trauma to the thorax or abdomen (Fry et al. 1995). Wound tracts were examined using a 7-MHz transducer and injuries were considered extraperitoneal or extrapleural if the entire tract was visualized and it was superficial to the deepest fascial structure. Positive and negative predictive accuracy was 100% in this study. This small study suggests that US has the potential to be a safe alternative to local wound exploration.

While the role of US in blunt abdominal trauma is clearly defined, its role in patients with penetrating thoracoabdominal trauma is still evolving. Potential roles of US in penetrating trauma that have been suggested include rapid screening of patients with multiple injuries, triage of multiple simultaneous trauma admissions, and detection of hemothorax and hemopericardium without a chest radiograph.

17.3.3 Computed Tomography

17.3.3.1 Indications

CT is the single best study to use in the assessment of abdominal penetration when clinical circumstances warrant and allow imaging. It is the only examination that can comprehensively assess all organs and all compartments of the abdomen. It can detect subtle evidence of pneumoperitoneum, quantify hemoperitoneum and retroperitoneal hemorrhage, and localize solid and hollow visceral injuries. It has high specificity and acceptable sensitivity. It replaces a battery of imaging examinations, including intravenous urography, upper and lower gastrointestinal injuries, thus lowering overall radiation exposure and cost. It is cost-effective because it eliminates the expense and time to perform several other alternative examinations, shortens time to diagnosis and exclusion, and results in cost savings by requiring less hospital time and fewer admissions.

The role of CT in penetrating abdominal trauma has evolved considerably as the surgical management has changed from mandatory exploratory laparotomy to a more conservative selective approach over the past 15 years. The management of penetrating trauma to the abdomen and the role of CT varies depending upon the exact location of the injury as well as the clinical status of the patient. In general, we manage patients with penetrating injuries to the anterior abdomen differently than patients who have sustained injuries involving the back and/or flank. Patients with evidence of hemodynamic instability, peritoneal signs, or organ evisceration undergo immediate exploratory laparotomy. Consequently, we use CT primarily for those patients with penetrating trauma who are hemodynamically stable. CT has many features that make it well suited for the evaluation of patients with penetrating trauma to the abdomen. CT is widely available and is a rapid diagnostic test. CT provides a complete anatomical assessment of the abdomen as well as the retroperitoneum.

Current approaches to the management of the hemodynamically stable patient with penetrating trauma to the back and/or flank include clinical observation, diagnostic peritoneal lavage (DPL) and CT (JACKSON and THAL 1979; PECK and BERNE 1981; PHILLIPS et al. 1986; HIMMELMAN et al. 1991; BOYLE et al. 1997). Retroperitoneal organs are well protected by the posterior musculature and fascia and are infrequently injured (HENNEMAN 1989). However, physical examination of this area is generally poor since signs of peritoneal irritation may not be initially apparent due to tamponading effects of retroperitoneal structures. For example, between 2% and 6% of significant occult injuries may be missed on serial physical examinations, even as late as 48 h after injury (FLETCHER et al. 1989). While DPL is a reliable predictor of intraperitoneal injury, it is a poor test to evaluate for possible retroperitoneal injuries. Because a missed injury may lead to significant morbidity, CT has been used in the management of hemodynamically stable patients to help detect occult intraperitoneal or retroperitoneal injuries. Overall, CT scanning with triple contrast in patients with penetrating trauma to the back and/or flank has an accuracy rate of 97%–100%. Sensitivity and specificity range from 87.5% to 100% and 98% to 100%, respectively. Negative predictive values have ranged from 97.9% to 100% (PHILLIPS et al. 1986; HAUSER et al. 1987; FLETCHER et al. 1989; REHM et al. 1989; HIMMELMAN et al. 1991; KIRTON et al. 1997; ALBRECHT et al. 1999).

CT has also been incorporated into the management algorithm of patients with penetrating injuries to the anterior abdomen (GROSSMAN et al. 1998; GINZBURG et al. 1998). Recent studies have suggested that carefully selected patients with gunshot wounds to the anterior abdomen can be managed nonoperatively (CHMIELEWSKI et al. 1995; DEMETRIADES et al. 1997). Triple-contrast CT scans have been used in these patients to assess the projectile trajectory and to help determine if there has been penetration of the peritoneum. CT criteria of peritoneal penetration include pneumoperitoneum, free intraperitoneal fluid, documented solid-organ injury, extravasation of contrast material, and obvious peritoneal penetration. In general, patients with peritoneal penetration undergo exploratory laparotomy while patients with negative studies are observed. Patients with equivocal findings may undergo laparoscopy or laparotomy. GINZBURG et al. (1998) reported a 54% specificity, a 100% negative predictive value, and 71% accuracy for CT in anterior abdominal penetrating injuries. Recent scientific presentations, as yet unpublished, have illustrated that CT is able to diagnose intraperitoneal penetrations. In some cases laparotomy can be avoided, when an isolated hepatic injury is discovered.

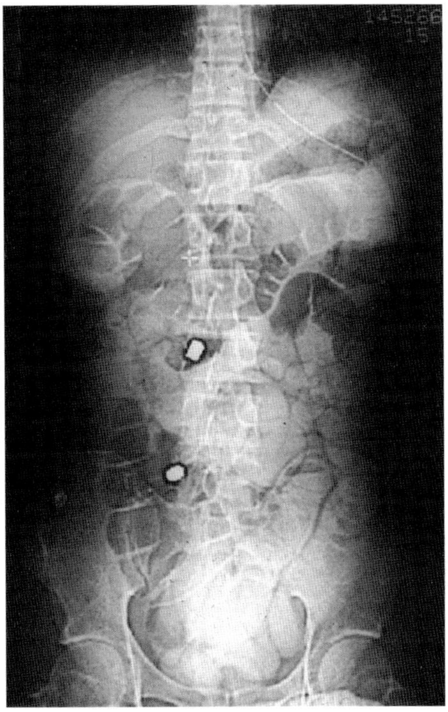

Fig. 17.16. CT scout view. A patient with gunshot wound of the back underwent CT examination. The scout view shows a bullet in the abdomen embedded in the spine. ECG lead pads were placed on the entry wound and clearly demonstrate the trajectory of the bullet

17.3.3.2 Technique

Scout View

The digital scout view has several uses (Fig. 17.16). It may identify and localize opaque bullets, thus allowing a crude assessment of their trajectory. This is made more accurate when opaque markers are placed at any entry and exit wounds prior to imaging. The scout view can determine by this technique whether there has been thoracoabdominal traverse and also facilitate assessment of the diaphragm. The scanogram provides a global view of the ribs, spine, pelvis, and hips and may identify fractures.

Contrast Administration for Penetrating Trauma

Proper technique for CT scans in patients with penetrating trauma to the back and/or flank is critical to avoid missing injuries. While several studies have used only oral and intravenous contrast, most studies suggest that triple-contrast – oral, rectal, and intravenous – CT should be performed (PHILLIPS et al. 1986;

Hauser et al. 1987; Fletcher et al. 1989; Rehm et al. 1989; Himmelman et al. 1991; Kirton et al. 1997; Albrecht et al. 1999). Colon injuries from penetrating trauma to the back and/or flank are infrequent, but missed colon injuries can cause serious infectious complications such as abdominal abscesses or retroperitoneal phlegmon. Moreover, delayed repair of missed colonic injuries is more difficult because of the inflammation from fecal soilage. The opportunity for simple repair may be lost and the more morbid colostomy may be required. Consequently, most studies suggest that rectal contrast is essential since it increases the ability to detect subtle alterations in the colon. A dilute contrast enema – 30 ml water-soluble contrast in 1 l of water – is administered on the scan table immediately before scanning. It is important that contrast adequately fills the colon, especially on the side of the injury. Placing the patient in right lateral decubitus may be necessary to adequately opacify the right colon and cecum.

Intravenous contrast (1.5–2 cc/kg) is administered intravenously. Oral contrast (300 cc 3% Gastrografin aliquots) is administered via the nasogastric tube 60 min, 15 min, and immediately prior to scanning.

17.3.3.3 Results

Identifying the Sites of Penetration

We place radio-opaque makers on all entry and exit wounds to help interpret the study. Detection of some injuries and exclusion of others can be difficult, as the findings may be subtle. A search of the entire abdomen without a zone of interest and focus can lead to errors. A variety of marking devices are available. Radio-opaque markers such as mammography localization beads and CT guidance devices are excellent methods for identifying wounds. However, we use the pads used for attaching electrodes from an electrocardiography unit. They do not create significant artifacts, are readily available and inexpensive, and remain attached to the site quite easily.

Interpretation

The primary role of CT in penetrating trauma to the back and/or flank is to triage patients into two groups, those who can be discharged after local wound care and those who may require intervention or further observation. Multiple studies have categorized CT findings of penetrating trauma slightly differently from blunt trauma, categorizing the diagnoses into several distinct groups (Phillips et al. 1986; Hauser et al. 1987; Fletcher et al. 1989; Rehm et al. 1989; Himmelman et al. 1991; Kirton et al. 1997; Albrecht et al. 1999). We use a six-tier method of description that leads to a variety of options for patient care. These include:

- Normal
  - An examination is considered normal if CT shows that the trajectory appears to be outside the abdominal compartments and does not violate the transversalis fascia (Fig. 17.17). There must be no intraperitoneal fluid and no evidence of pneumoperitoneum or retroperitoneal air. There are no hematomas. The bowel wall is thin without edema or intramural hematoma or air. There is no urinary or bowel contrast extravasation. A normal examination provides good justification to discharge the patient from the emergency department without further observation or admission, provided the scan correlates with the patient's condition.

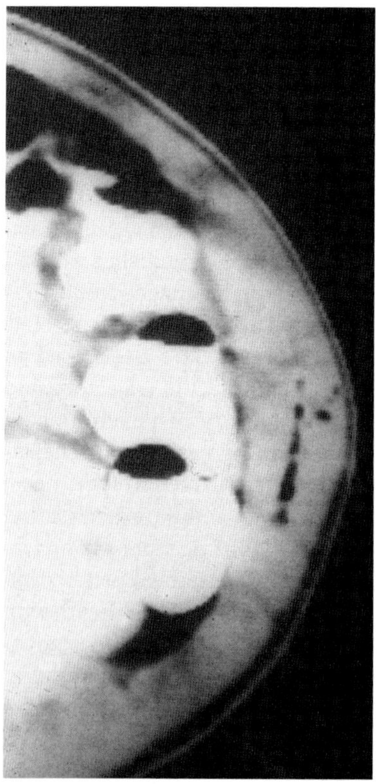

Fig. 17.17. Negative CT. Close-up of left flank shows a small amount of air between the internal oblique and the external oblique muscles. There was no hematoma. The colon showed no extravasation

- Low risk
  - A low-risk scan does not meet all of the above criteria (Figs. 17.18, 17.19). The trajectory of the penetration is either indeterminate or is located near abdominal viscera. There is no pneumoperitoneum or hemoperitoneum. There may be hematomas but they are located in the abdominal wall and do not infiltrate the wall of the bowel of the mesentery, nor do they extend into the retroperitoneum. Furthermore, there is no direct evidence of any solid visceral injuries. There is no gastrointestinal contrast extravasation. The decision to discharge the patient from the emergency department without admission is more clinical. Patients are often observed for several hours prior to discharge. Bowel wall contusion is more difficult to exclude.

- High risk
  - This interpretation means that while there is no direct evidence of visceral injury, the penetration is noted to be adjacent to abdominal organs or viscera (Figs. 17.20–17.23). Retroperitoneal hematomas or hematomas adjacent to organs are commonly seen. The hematomas may abut against the hollow viscera but they do not directly infiltrate or thicken the bowel wall. Emphysema may be seen within the retroperitoneum or abdominal wall, but no contrast extravasation is detected. Emphysema is nonspecific because air can be introduced during high-velocity missile wounding and one cannot assume that extraluminal air originated from bowel perforations.

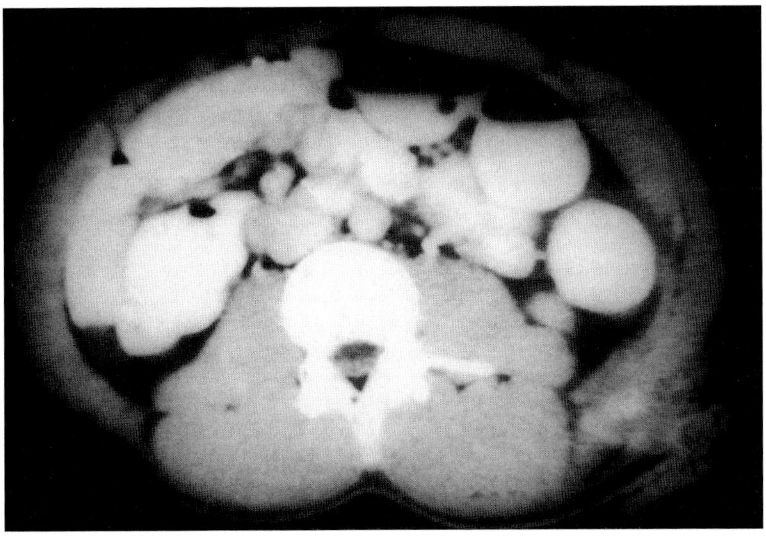

Fig. 17.18. Low-risk scan. There is a superficial hematoma in the left flank with active bleeding. The fat surrounding the colon is clean with no infiltration. The bowel wall is not thickened. This patient required no treatment

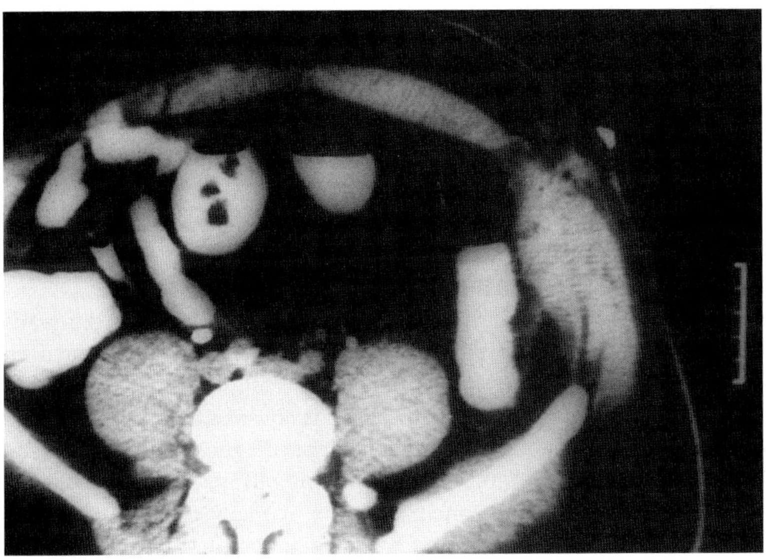

Fig. 17.19. Low-risk scan. the patient sustained a stab wound in the left flank. CT shows a hematoma in the internal oblique muscle but the subjacent colon has no evidence of edema or extravasation. The patient was observed for 24 h and discharged

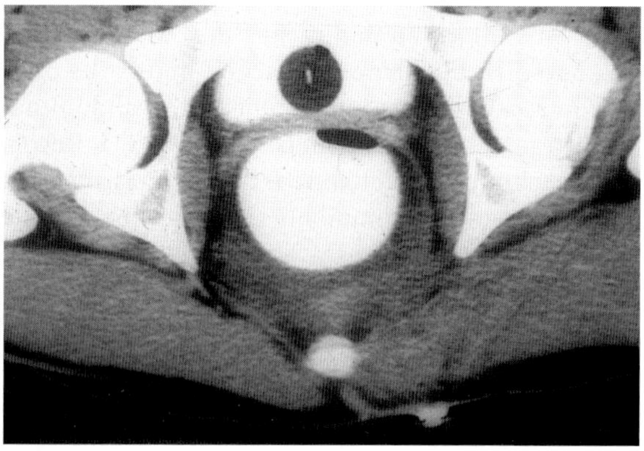

Fig. 17.20. High-risk scan. The patient sustained a stab wound to the buttock which is identified by the marker to the left of the sacrum. There is hematoma surrounding the rectum but there is no leak of air or contrast medium. Patient was managed by observation

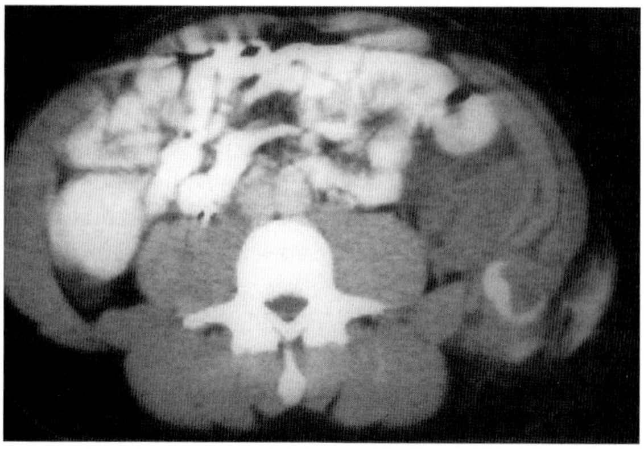

Fig. 17.21. High-risk scan. There is a large hematoma in the left retroperitoneum space that is displacing the colon anteriorly. The contrast extravasation in the hematoma does not extend to the colon. The colon wall is difficult to delineate. No extravasated air was present. This patient was observed for several days and then discharged

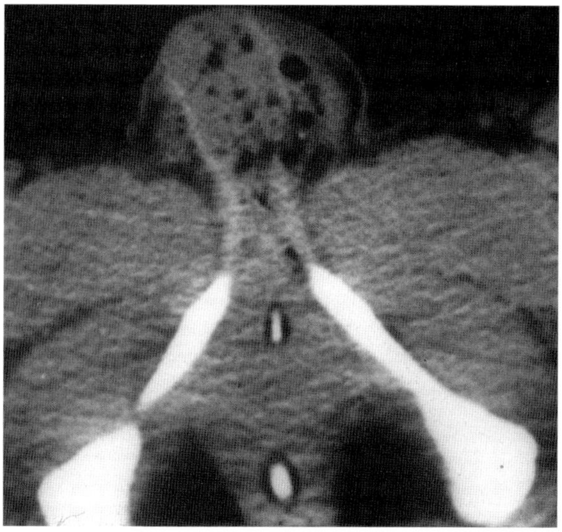

Fig. 17.22. Emphysema in the penis and scrotum secondary to gunshot wound of the pelvis. This patient sustained only the genitourinary injury. There was no bowel injury. Emphysema such as this is a nonspecific finding that is suspicious for bowel injury but not definitive. Patients with extensive emphysema should be observed carefully or explored

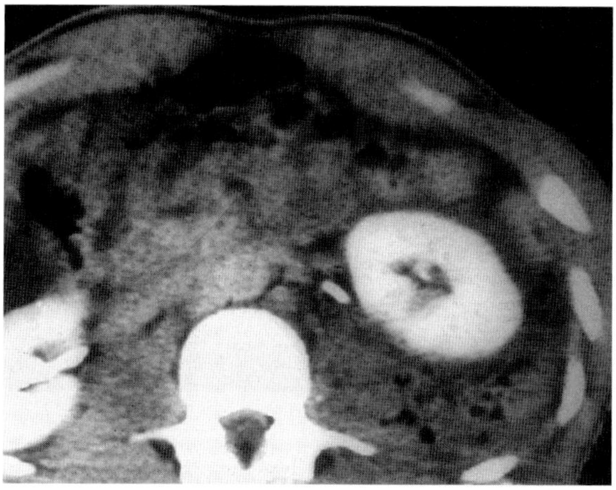

Fig. 17.23. Perinephric emphysema. This patient sustained a gunshot wound of the back. There was a perinephric hematoma that contained air. There was no bowel injury identified at exploration. Emphysema can enter the tissues through temporary cavitation

- Patients with such injuries are managed on clinical criteria. If there are signs of injury, then exploratory laparotomy is undertaken. Otherwise, these patients are usually observed for variable time as inpatients. They are discharged after their clinical presentation has improved. It is feasible to perform a repeat study in some of these patients to assess the progression of disease.

- Diagnostic of hollow visceral injury
  - The diagnosis of bowel injuries can be readily made if specific findings are identified (Figs. 17.24–17.33). While emphysema in hematomas or wounds is nonspecific, free intraperitoneal air is considered diagnostic of bowel injury, unless there are mitigating circumstances such as pneumothorax or mediastinal emphysema. However, even when pneumothorax is present,

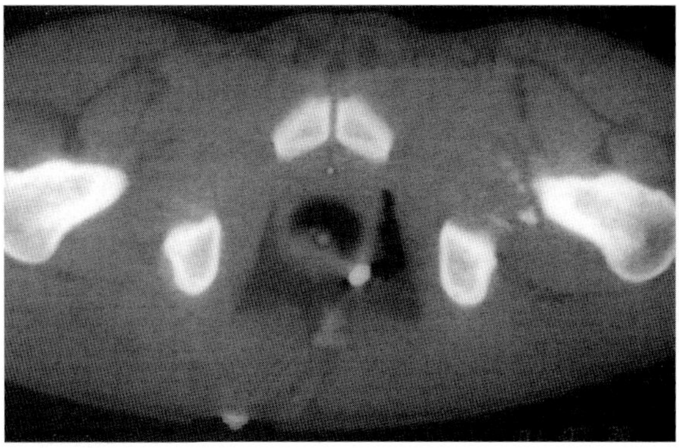

Fig. 17.24. Perirectal emphysema. The trajectory of this bullet can be inferred by the path from the marker on the right of the anus to the left of the rectum. The perirectal emphysema is probably from the bullet. Endoscopy failed to show an injury to the colon

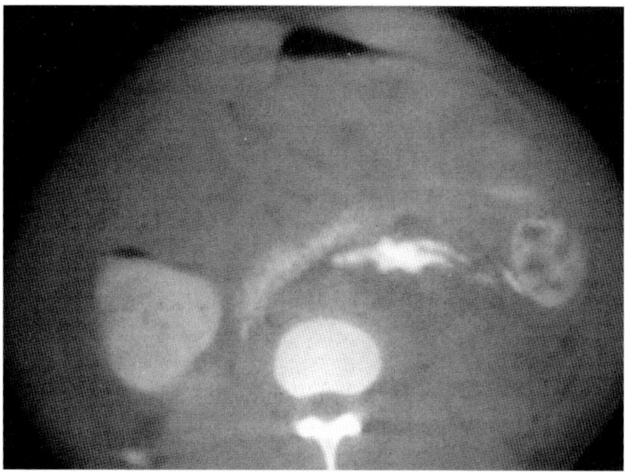

Fig. 17.25. Pneumoperitoneum after gunshot wound of the colon. A wide window image such as this is helpful in assessing pneumoperitoneum

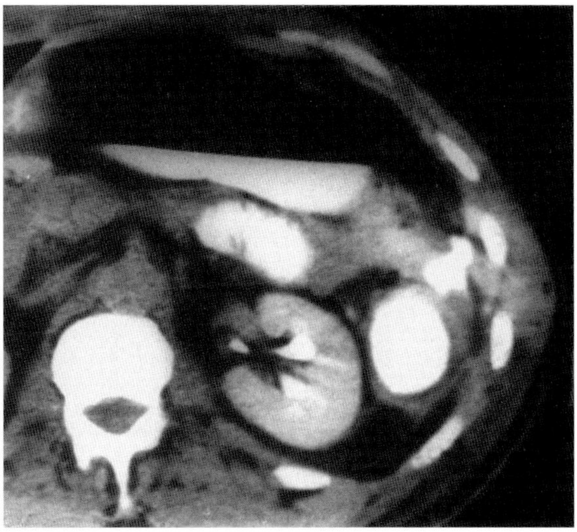

Fig. 17.26. Colon injury. There is thickening of the wall of the colon and extravasation anterior to the bowel

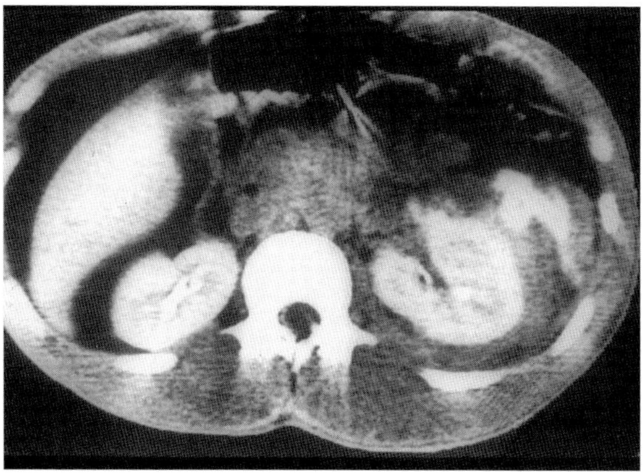

Fig. 17.27. Gunshot wounds of the left kidney and the descending colon. CT shows perinephric hematoma surrounding the left kidney. There is extravasation of contrast from the colon into the perinephric space. Since fascial boundaries are disrupted, the etiology of the extravasation can sometimes be quite difficult to prove

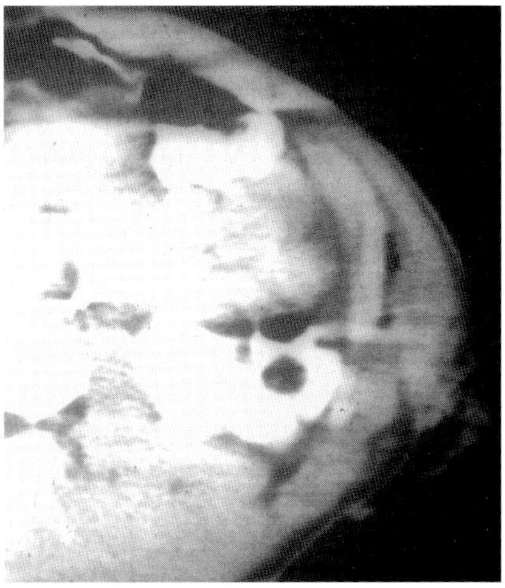

Fig. 17.28. Colonic laceration. This patient sustained a stab wound of the flank. The contrast extravasates out of the stab wound

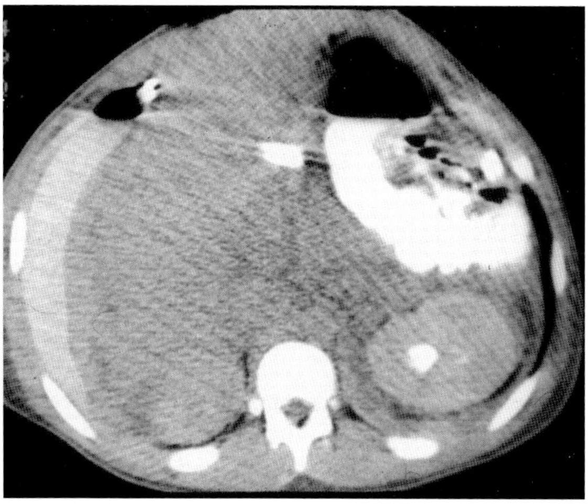

Fig. 17.29. Transverse colon perforation after gunshot wound. There is contrast and air in the right paracolic gutter

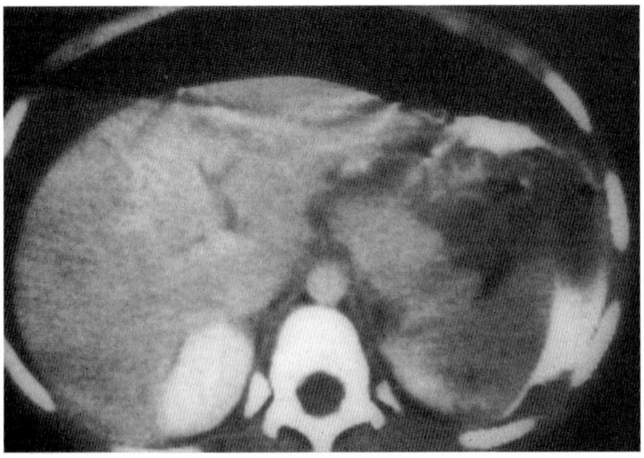

Fig. 17.30. Gastric penetration. This patient has a large amount of pneumoperitoneum. There is also contrast in the left paracolic gutter

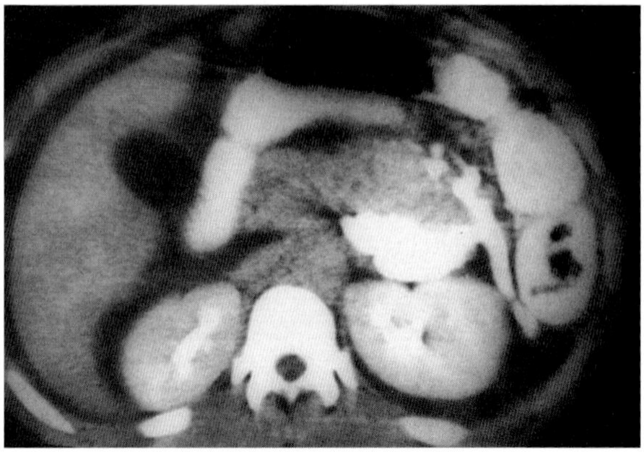

Fig. 17.31. Duodenal/jejunal laceration. This patient sustained a stab wound of the back. There is extravasation anterior to the kidney in the lesser sac

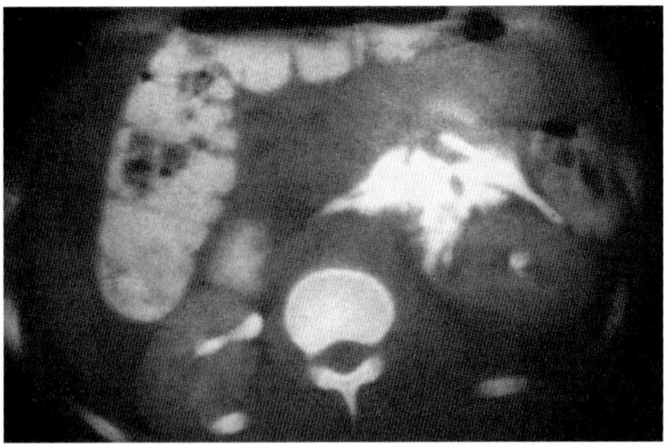

Fig. 17.32. Proximal ureteric transection. This CT shows extravasation in a similar location to Fig. 17.31. At wide window it is clear that the density of the extravasated contrast medium is much greater than the 3% solution used to opacify the colon. This represents contrast medium concentrated within the kidney

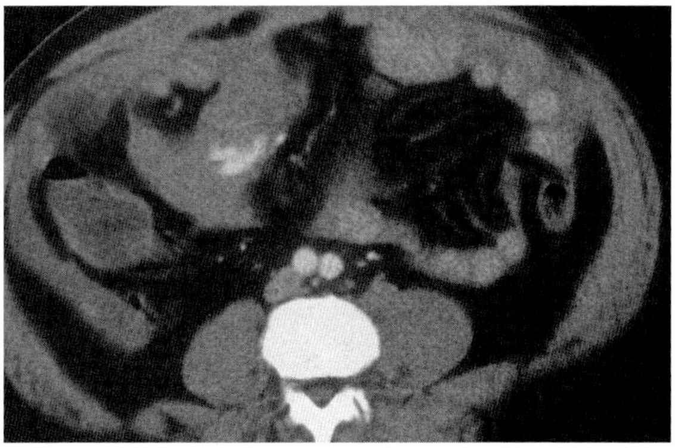

Fig. 17.33. Mesenteric hematoma. This patient sustained a gunshot wound of the abdomen that resulted in a hematoma in the mesentery of the ileum. Active bleeding was noted. At exploration, bleeding from the ileocolic artery was treated by ligation. Bowel integrity was confirmed. No infarction was detected

pneumoperitoneum is considered a serious observation, one that usually is an indication for exploratory laparotomy. The detection of free air is facilitated by looking at these images with a wide window setting, such as for bone or lung. The widened window allows better discrimination between intraluminal air and adjacent free air. The wide window helps in the assessment of the bowel wall as well.

Pneumoperitoneum is most likely to be present when there is injury to intraperitoneal hollow visceral injuries such as gastric or small-bowel perforations. Free peritoneal air may be caused by colonic injury as well, especially when there is injury to the transverse colon or the flexures. Pneumoperitoneum is less likely to be seen when there is retroperitoneal colonic injury, but extraluminal air may be present within the retroperitoneum. Another sign of colonic injury is the presence of bubbling of air and fluid out the entry or exit site during the enema. When this occurs, it is sufficient to direct the patient to the operating theater; no further imaging is necessary.

There are specific findings of bowel perforation. These include air within the wall of the bowel, especially when associated with intramural edema or hematoma in the bowel wall. Mesenteric hematoma is also considered a serious finding and exploration is usually warranted to assure that there is no bowel ischemia or infarction resulting from mesenteric arterial injury. The most reliable and specific finding of bowel perforation is extravasation of contrast medium from the bowel. This may appear as free contrast extravasation within the peritoneum. This classic observation of contrast medium outlining the outer wall of the bowel and opacifying the peritoneal spaces may be seen with enteric, gastric, and colonic injury. Contrast extravasation in the retroperitoneum is likely to be caused by colonic or duodenal injury. This appears as streaky localized collections of contrast medium.

Contrast extravasation may originate from bowel, urinary tract, or vasculature. Differentiating these may be difficult at conventional narrow soft tissue windows. Wide window images are useful in this situation. The contrast extravasating from the genitourinary tract is usually highly concentrated, far more than the 3% contrast administered within the bowel. It is usually readily differentiated from the 3% contrast medium administered in the bowel or the diluted contrast medium from vascular extravasation.

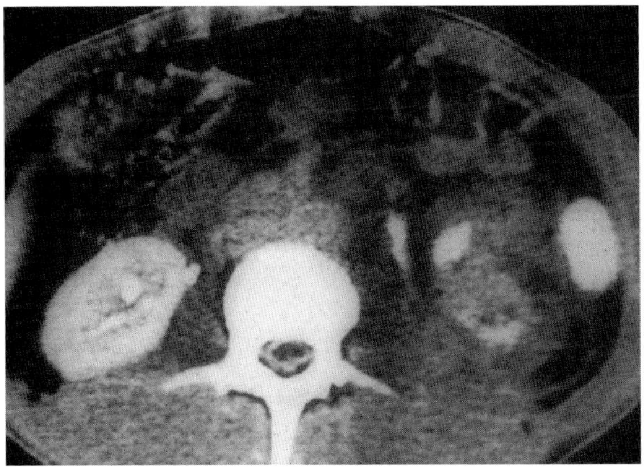

Fig. 17.34. Gunshot wound of the kidney. There is poor enhancement of the kidney associated with perinephric hematoma. Adjacent colon injury could not be excluded so laparotomy was performed. This confirmed the findings. Nephrectomy was performed

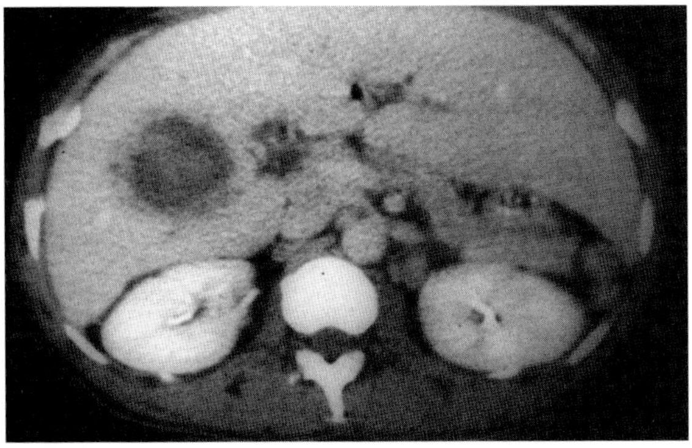

Fig. 17.35. Hepatic injury

- Diagnostic of Solid Visceral Injury
  - The diagnosis of solid visceral injuries is straightforward (Figs. 17.34, 17.35). The findings are similar to those seen with blunt trauma. These include nonenhancing soft tissue masses within or adjacent to the solid viscera, which represent intraparenchymal, subcapsular, or extrinsic hematomas. Segmental areas of nonenhancement suggest vascular disruptions. Active blush of contrast medium suggests active arterial hemorrhage.

There are a few noteworthy differences between blunt and penetrating injuries. Lacerations often have a linear appearance or expand along a linear path that represents the laceration. Gunshot wounds may leave bits of metal along the trajectory. Adjacent lacerations of multiple organs, unusual in blunt trauma, is more frequently seen after penetration. Because penetrations do not respect fascial planes, hematomas may spread in unusual ways. Hematomas adjacent to the organ are called sentinel hematomas because they point to the organ that sustained injury. When penetration disrupts normal fascial boundaries, hematomas spread beyond their expected confines. Therefore, perivisceral hematomas sometimes cannot be used to identify the organ of injury.

Similarly, extravasation of urinary contrast medium from penetration of the urinary collecting system may spread in nonanatomical ways. Extravasation may be seen into the pleural space, the spine, into the peritoneum, to name a few unusual locations.

Evaluation of the ureter is mandatory for penetrating abdominal trauma. While uncommon after blunt trauma, this structure must be scrutinized during the reading of CT after penetrating trauma. The findings may be subtle. Proximal hydronephrosis is usually present. Contrast extravasation may be focal and surround the ureter. Extravasation may also spread into multiple compartments. Differentiation of urinary and bowel contrast may be difficult but is possible by exploiting the differences in density between urinary and bowel contrast. Wide window images facilitate this differentiation.

- Suspicions for Vascular Injury
  - Some authors suggest that certain CT findings represent evidence of arterial injury and they consider such findings indications for angiography (Phillips et al. 1986) (Fig. 17.36). A large retroperitoneal hematoma adjacent to an organ suggests bleeding from that structure. The identification of a contrast blush is a compelling

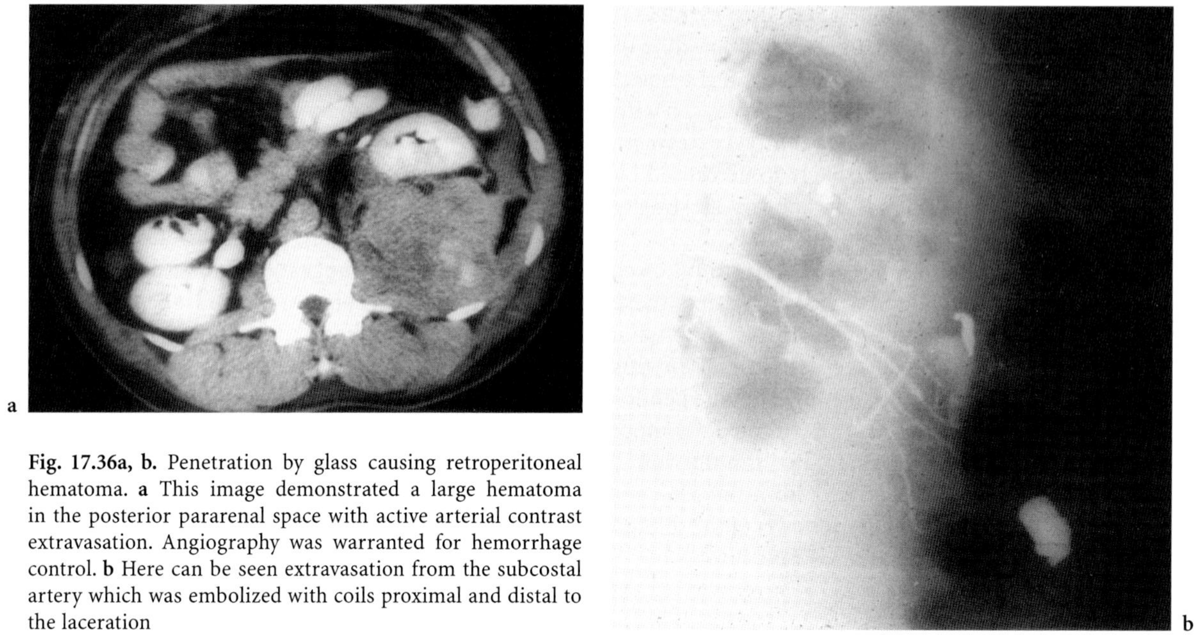

Fig. 17.36a, b. Penetration by glass causing retroperitoneal hematoma. a This image demonstrated a large hematoma in the posterior pararenal space with active arterial contrast extravasation. Angiography was warranted for hemorrhage control. b Here can be seen extravasation from the subcostal artery which was embolized with coils proximal and distal to the laceration

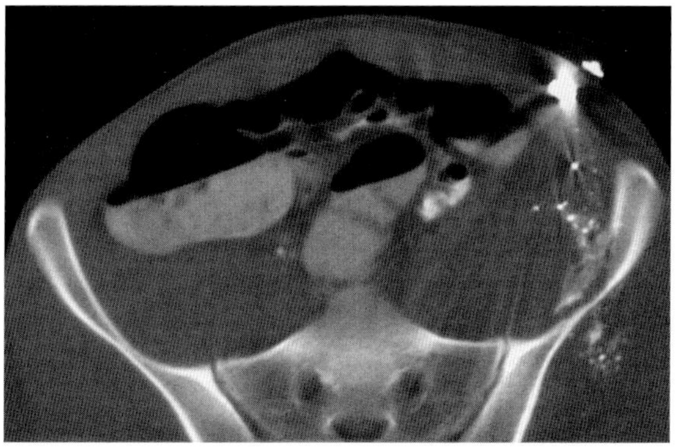

Fig. 17.37. Gunshot wound to the ilium extending lateral to the vessels and ureter

sign that there is active hemorrhage. When segments of organs do not perfuse, vascular injury should be suspected. Other CT findings that may be a potential indication for angiography include large perinephric hematomas, hepatic lacerations, and renal lacerations

- Other Findings
  - The evaluation of CT for penetrating trauma is not complete without evaluation of the adjacent nonabdominal structures (Figs. 17.37, 17.38). Spinal canal disruptions and fractures of the spine are highly morbid injuries that should be assessed. Intrathecal bullets and bony fragments should be assessed and described. Fluid collec-

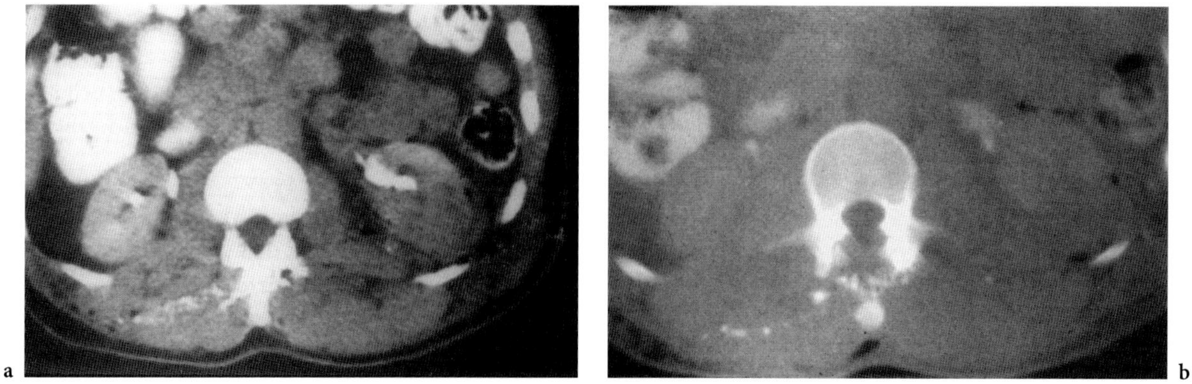

Fig. 17.38a, b. This patient sustained a gunshot wound to the lumbar vertebra. The bullet has extended from right to left through the paraspinal muscles, the posterior elements of L2, and into the left kidney

tions in the paraspinal regions may sometimes represent disruptions in the thecal sac. Fractures of the pelvis and ribs should also be identified. Pneumothorax, hemothorax, and hemopericardium must be assessed.

17.3.3.4
Economics of CT

In 1985 we reported the efficacy of CT for the evaluation of penetrations of the back and flank. We concluded that the test was cost-effective by expediting surgical exploration and reducing delays and complications, by avoiding unnecessary laparotomy, by decreasing admissions, and by lowering length of stay.

In addition to improving triage of patients with penetrating abdominal injuries, CT has the potential to decrease hospital stay and costs (Rehm et al. 1989; Kirton et al. 1997; Albrecht et al. 1999). CT scans are expensive, but may decrease overall costs if patients with low-risk scans are discharged directly from the emergency department or within 24 h. Albrecht et al. showed that length of stay was significantly less in patients with low-risk scans and no associated injuries as compared to all other treatment groups (Albrecht et al. 1999). While several studies have shown that CT can decrease length of hospital stay, none of these studies have proven that overall costs are decreased. In addition, a study by McAllister et al. (1994) suggested that CT scans were effective in detecting occult injuries but added considerable cost and rarely altered clinical management.

17.3.4
Angiography/Interventional Radiology

17.3.4.1
Development

Angiography and transcatheter embolization have become an essential component in the management of both penetrating and blunt trauma to the abdomen (Margolies et al. 1972; Matalon et al. 1979; Sclafani et al. 1982, 1995; Panetta et al. 1985; Sclafani and Sclafani 1996; Velhamos et al. 1999, 2000). The potential embolization for injuries was first illustrated in 1966 when Boijsen et al. (1966) suggested the use of transcatheter intraarterial epinephrine for hemostasis of hepatic arterial hemorrhage. In 1972, Margolies and colleagues described the use of embolization for hemorrhage associated with pelvic fractures (Sclafani et al. 1982). As experience with angiography and embolization grew, it became clear that this technique would be applicable to a variety of types and sites of traumatic injuries. Angiography and embolization have been reported most commonly for blunt trauma to the liver, spleen, retroperitoneum, and pelvis (Margolies et al. 1972; Matalon et al. 1979; Panetta et al. 1985; Sclafani et al. 1995; Velhamos et al. 1999, 2000). However, recent trends toward nonoperative management has helped to increase the role and utility of angiography and embolization in penetrating abdominal trauma (Velhamos et al. 1999, 2000).

Multiple studies have documented the safety and efficacy of angiography and embolization in penetrating abdominal trauma. In 1982, one of the authors reported the first large series of traumatized patients who underwent angiography and embolization for penetrating injuries (Sclafani et al. 1982). Embolization was successful in 83% of the cases with no complications. Velhamos et al. (2000) reported a 91% success rate in 40 patients with penetrating abdominal injuries with no major complications. Other series and case reports have shown that angiography and embolization can be used successfully to treat hemorrhage from penetrations of the liver, spleen, kidneys, mesentery, pelvis, and retroperitoneal vasculature (Sclafani et al. 1984; Uflacker et al. 1984; Fisher and Ben-Menachem 1985; Fisher et al. 1989; Eastham et al. 1992; Heyns and Van Vollenhoven 1992; Reilly et al. 1996).

17.3.4.2
Indications

Indications for angiography and percutaneous embolization in patients with penetrating trauma usually relate to problems that remain after urgent laparotomy has been performed. It is uncommon at this juncture to consider, other than incidental, nonoperative management of major vascular injuries caused by penetrating trauma. Most patients present with multiple injuries and blood loss, leading to urgent laparotomy.

Indications for angiography include:

- Persistent bleeding despite surgical intervention
- Bleeding from injuries managed nonoperatively, notably renal and hepatic penetrations
- Prior to an urgent operation to control bleeding sites that are difficult to access surgically such as deep intraparenchymal false aneurysms
- As a preventive measure in patients who are hemodynamically stable, but whose injuries are frequently associated with major bleeding

- As part of damage-control surgery
- From late vascular complications of vascular penetrations such as arteriovenous, arterioportal fistulas, and false aneurysms

17.3.4.3 Damage Control

Recently surgeons have used angiography as a component of damage-control surgery. In this approach, surgeons attempt to control obvious hemorrhage, then pack and close the abdomen so that resuscitation can be accomplished and hypothermia and coagulopathy have been corrected. The patient returns to the operating room for further management and definitive repair of non-life-threatening injuries only after resuscitation has been achieved.

Angiography is frequently used to assess for vascular injuries within the liver, kidney, and retroperitoneum prior to reexploration. By embolizing deep visceral vascular injuries before reexploration, surgeons can treat the hollow visceral injuries and provide necessary drainage under more controlled circumstances. The timing of angiography and embolization is important, but there is no definitive data to suggest what is the best time for intervention. Velhamos and colleagues (2000) compared four different times of angiography and embolization to determine if timing affected success rate of bleeding control.

The four groups included:

- Directly to the angiography suite from the ER
- To the angiography suite after a short period of resuscitation in the ICU
- To the angiography suite immediately after laparotomy
- To the angiography suite after a short time in the ICU following laparotomy

Velhamos found no significant difference in the outcomes of these four groups. The advantage of utilizing angiography and embolization early is that it may avoid potential complications from hemodynamic compromise such as extensive blood loss, hypothermia and a hypocoagulable state exacerbating blood loss, and multiple blood transfusions. Since there is no definitive data to support the timing of angiography and embolization, each case must be managed on an individual basis. Certain patients such as those with comorbidities and minimal reserve, the elderly, those with coagulopathy, or those who cannot receive blood transfusions such as Jehovah's witnesses may benefit from earlier intervention with angiography and embolization.

Technique

We recommend aortography of the abdomen or thoracoabdomen as the initial screening examination in most patients who need angiographic evaluation for penetrating injury. In many of these difficult situations, previously unidentified aortic injury must be excluded. Furthermore, injuries are often multiple and unsuspected intraperitoneal or retroperitoneal bleeding sites may be detected by aortography. In addition, aortography can identify anomalies and potential arterial displacements and surgical ligations. Selective catheterization and angiography is usually required for definitive diagnosis and therapy.

Angiographic Findings

The most common and reliable sign of arterial injury after penetration, similar to that for blunt trauma, is the presence of extraluminal contrast extravasation. Other signs of arterial injury include arterial occlusion, laceration, transection, false aneurysm, intimal flap, intraluminal thrombosis, and fistulas (Sclafani et al. 1986).

Because penetrating trauma may injure multiple continuous structures violating fascial separations without discrimination, the likelihood of arterial fistulas is higher. Communications between arteries and many other structures have been described. In most situations, these fistulas connect systemic arteries and veins. In the abdomen, however, connections between the systemic arteries and the adjacent portal venous system must also be considered and excluded. Systemic arterial communications to hollow structures such as the biliary tree, the urinary collecting system, the gastrointestinal tract, and the pleural space must also be considered.

Embolization

The details of embolization are beyond the scope of this chapter. Embolization is most commonly indicated if arterial extravasation of contrast is seen. Other indications for embolization include false aneurysms, arteriovenous fistula, transection, or laceration. Occlusions should also be treated, as occlusions may represent thrombosis or vasospasm. Preemptive embolization of occlusions may avoid complications that may occur when vasospasm resolves and leaves a disrupted vessel free to bleed. Surgical gelatin and steel coils are the most common embolic agents used in trauma since they are simple to use, inexpensive, and readily available, rapidly control hemorrhage, and limit tissue ischemia and infarction. Gelatin is the agent of choice to occlude small branches that are bleeding within the retroperitoneum or from solid viscera. Permanent agents such as polyvinyl alcohol are unnecessary. We recommend injection of 2- to 3-mm pledgets through a 1-ml syringe in 0.1- to 0.3-ml increments until there is stasis of contrast and no further extravasation. Steel coils are used primarily for large vessel occlusions, such as those required for arteriovenous fistula or large vessel lacerations. Steel coils are also used for proximal arterial occlusions to decrease arterial pressure without parenchymal arterial occlusion or thrombosis

17.3.4.4 Delayed Posttraumatic Complications

Drainage of Abscesses

Sepsis, exceeded only by hemorrhage and head injury, is the third deadly killer of the traumatized patient. It is responsible for many of the deaths that occur in the later phases of trauma care. It prolongs hospitalization and leads to many morbidities. The incidence of abscess formation after penetrating abdominal trauma varies from 2% to 10%. The reasons for this are multifactorial. The presence of multiple organ injuries, especially pancreaticoduodenal, colonic, splenic, and vascular injury increases the likelihood of infection. Fragmentation of injured organs may leave behind devitalized areas that undergo necrosis and secondary infection. Hollow visceral injuries lead to contamination with bile, urine, feces, food, and other enteric contents that form a nidus for infection. Removal of injured organs such as the spleen, kidney, and pancreas lead to anatomical dead spaces that can accumulate these fluids. Finally, trauma in itself diminishes cellular immunity.

Computed tomography is the method of choice for the diagnosis of posttraumatic abscesses, which should be suspected when signs of sepsis manifest more than 1 week after trauma and when there are no signs of pulmonary or urinary infection. Fluid collections present after 5–7 days in the presence of clinical signs of infection are suggestive of infection. However, in some circumstances, noninfected hematomas, seromas, and ascitic collections may give an appearance that resembles abscesses. Moreover, some fluid collections may be loculated bland fluid without infection. The only definitive way to make the diagnosis is sampling of these fluid collections. Percutaneous aspiration under CT guidance is the preferred method of doing this. While US is advocated by many as a good alternative, the likelihood of multiple collections, leaks, and other abnormalities that may not be detected by US make CT preferable in the trauma situation. The percutaneous techniques of drainage are beyond the scope of this chapter but fall into two methods: percutaneous needle aspiration and drainage or transsinus drainage. Since drains are placed in the abdomen for evacuation of many penetrating wounds, their formed tracts can be used for access to deep collections without the small risk of inadvertent puncture of some normal structure.

Urinary Leaks

Injuries to the urinary collecting system are much more common after penetrating trauma than after blunt trauma (Fig. 17.39). Blunt upper urinary collecting system injuries usually involve the calyceal system and are often confined within the kidney or within the perinephric space by the perirenal fascia. Penetration disrupts all anatomical barriers and the extent of leakage from the collecting system depends upon the trajectory of the offending object. Moreover, ureteral injury is exceedingly rare after blunt trauma as it is fixed and deep. With penetrating trauma, it is as likely to sustain injury as any other structure of similar size. Notably, with penetration, injury of

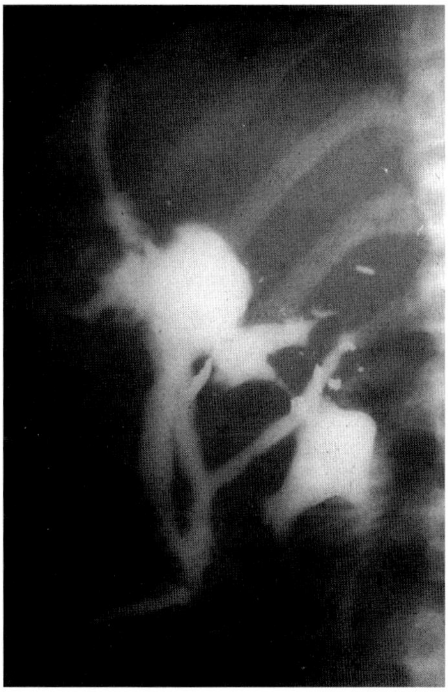

Fig. 17.39. Urinary leak

the ureter may be occult and may be unrecognized during operative intervention. When visualized in the operating theater, the ureter may be merely ecchymotic with no disruption or leakage apparent. These contusions may progress to more serious injuries. The blast effect to the ureter in combination with its poor blood supply render these contusions prone to delayed full thickness disruption postoperatively. For the same reasons, repaired ureteric injuries are also at risk of dehiscence. The leak of urine from these disruptions can develop into a discrete collection, a urinoma, that can be sterile but often becomes infected. Urine leaks can also be more diffuse and result in azotemia from reabsorption of urine from the peritoneum. Urinomas may cause increasing distal obstruction, which results in an increase in the urinary leakage.

The treatment of these ureteric disruptions is threefold. The urine must be diverted to eradicate the collection. This is most easily and most reliably performed by antegrade nephrostomy. Retrograde diversion has not been successful very often because of the distortion created by the urinoma and the inability of the urologist to manipulate the catheter across the dehiscence. Once the renal collecting system has been accessed, a stent should be placed across the injured area. This stent should be of ample size, 12 French or larger, because stenosis can be anticipated. Finally the urinoma should be percutaneously catheterized to externally drain residual urine. Cultures of the urinoma may enable proper antibiotic therapy.

Enteric Fistulas

Because the bowel is the organ most frequently injured by penetration, it is not surprising that complications of bowel injuries occur with some frequency. Dehiscence of repairs and missed injuries or breakdown of incomplete lacerations all can lead to abscesses and enteric fistulas.

Fistulas, not only to bowel but also to other hollow viscera, are best identified and characterized by sinography, the retrograde injection of contrast medium into a draining sinus. The treatment of these leaks is good drainage and eradication of the associated abscesses. Often catheters can be placed through the existing sinus tract for drainage. It is important to look for reasons that the enteric fistula has not closed spontaneously. In the trauma situation, these include foreign bodies, infections, and distal obstructions from either internal herniations, adhesions, or strictures. Enteric imaging such as enteroclysis should be considered when these fistulas do not close.

Biliary Leakage

Leakage of bile is a serious complication of hepatic and extrahepatic bile duct penetrations (Fig. 17.40). It may lead to jaundice, peritonitis, sepsis, and abscess formation. Fistulas to the skin, the pleura, and the vasculature can be very difficult to identify and to treat. Bilomas, the collection of bile in the liver, may become infected or expand, leading to rupture. The best test for diagnosing these fistulas is biliary scintigraphy because it provides, noninvasively, direct evidence of bile leakage. Isotope may accumulate inside the liver or extend out of the liver. Sinography is useful in assessing biliary cutaneous fistulas because it allows opacification under sufficient pressure to fill the biliary tree.

Biliary connections to the vasculature present with gastrointestinal hemorrhage, intermittent jaundice, and biliary colic. The vascular connections of greatest concern are those to the hepatic artery, although connections to the portal vein or hepatic veins may also occur. The treatment of these fistulas is embolization of the connecting artery.

Most bilomas are self-limiting and require no specific treatment. They result from laceration or transection of biliary ducts, usually within the liver. As the drainage through the injured duct is not continuous, bile collects in a cavitation as a biloma. With poor outflow, pressure builds within the cavity and bile segment, eventually resulting in biliary cirrhosis to that segment. The severed ends of the bile duct scar and are obliterated. Either the biloma stabilizes or involutes. In some situations, infection of the collection occurs, leading to sepsis. Such infected bilomas are abscesses and require percutaneous drainage. Larger ductal structures that are injured require further interventions in addition to drainage of bilomas. Stenting procedures may be useful in allowing biliary egress from the liver and healing of the biliary laceration.

17.4 Conclusion

The incidence of penetrating abdominal trauma increased dramatically between 1966 and 1996. By some estimates, it might become the most common cause of traumatic death in the United States by the year 2003. Diagnostic imaging has become increasingly important in the management of civilian penetrating abdominal trauma. CT appears to be the most widely utilized imaging modality for penetrating abdominal trauma and is used primarily to appropriately triage

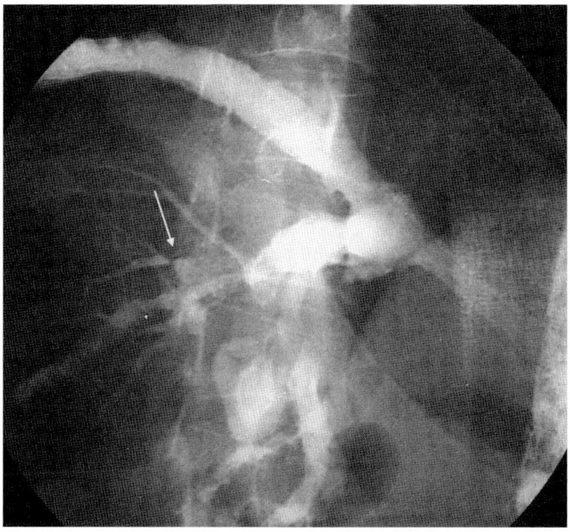
a

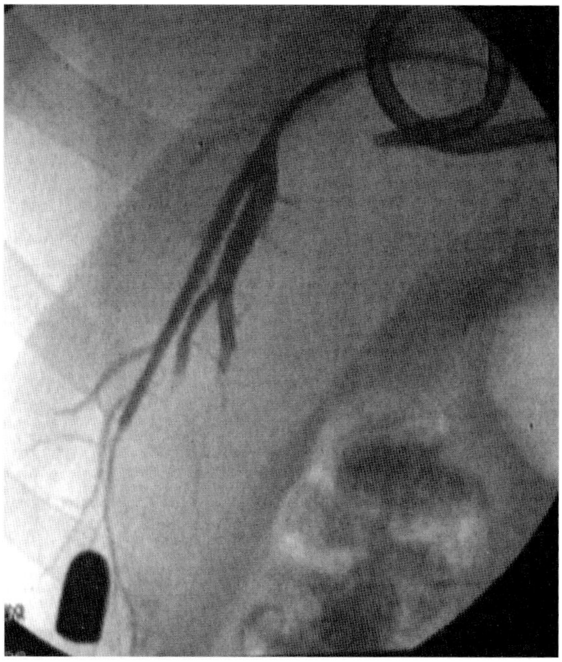
b

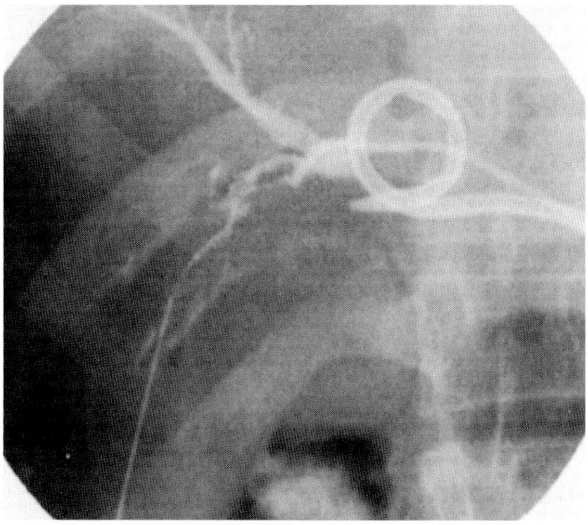
c

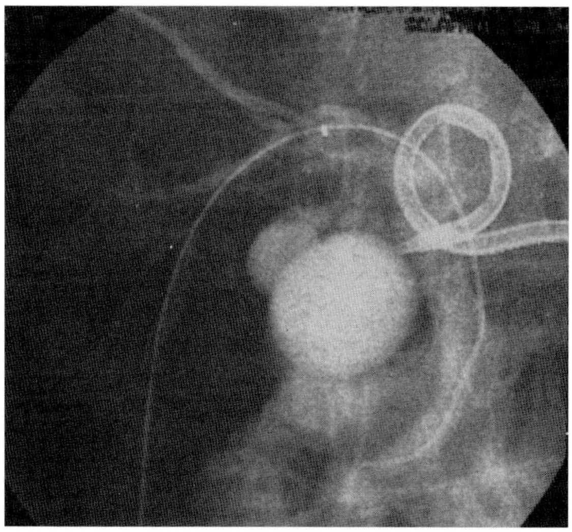
d

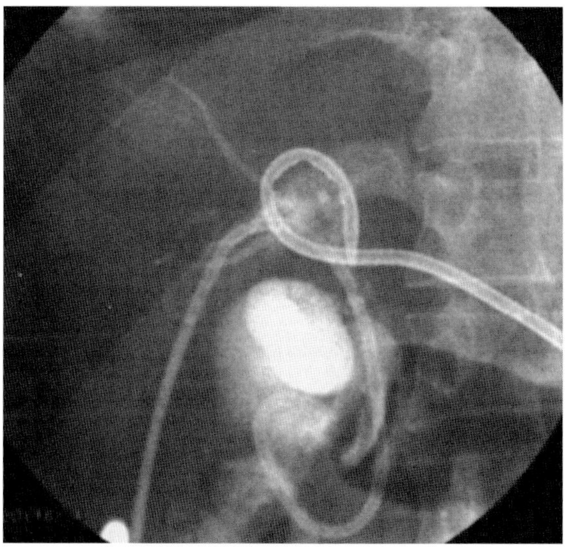
e

Fig. 17.40a–e. Radiological intervention for biliary trauma. **a** Sinus tract injection with biliary fistula. **b** Catheterization of the transected bile duct from the sinus tract. **c** Percutaneous needle puncture of the peripheral portion of the duct. **d** Micropuncture system advanced through the liver into the common bile duct. **e** Placement of a 12-French stent in the duodenum patients into two groups, those who can be discharged after local wound care and those who may require surgical intervention or further observation. While US has been used extensively in the evaluation of blunt abdominal trauma, its role in the evaluation of penetrating abdominal trauma is evolving. Recent trends toward nonoperative management have increased the role and utility of angiography and embolization in penetrating abdominal trauma. Angiography and embolization have been used in patients with penetrating trauma for persistent bleeding despite surgical intervention, bleeding from injuries managed nonoperatively, and bleeding later in posttraumatic course due to complication of vascular injuries.

References

Albrecht RM, Vigil A, Schermer CR et al (1999) Stab wounds to the back/flank in hemodynamically stable patients: evaluation using triple-contrast computed tomography. Am Surgeon 65:683–687

Ammann A, Brewer WH, Maull KI et al (1988) Traumatic rupture of the diaphragm; real-time sonographic diagnosis. AJR 140:915–919

Boijsen E, Judkins MP, Simay A (1966) Angiographic diagnosis of hepatic rupture. Radiology 86:66–72

Boulanger BR, Brenneman FD, McLellan BA et al (1995) A prospective study of emergent abdominal sonography after blunt trauma. J Trauma 39:325–330

Boulanger BR, Rozycki GS, Rodriquez A (1999) Sonographic assessment of traumatic injury: future developments. Surg Clin North Am 79:1297–1316

Boyle EM, Maier RV, Salzar JD et al (1997) Diagnosis of injuries after stab wounds to the back and flank. J Trauma 42: 260–265

Carroll PR, McAninch JW (1989) Staging of renal trauma. Urol Clin North Am 16:193–201

Chmielewski GW, Nicholas JM, Dulchavsky SA, Diebel LN (1995) Nonoperative management of gunshot wounds of the abdomen. Am Surg 61:665–668

Demetriades D, Velhamos G, Cornwell E et al (1997) Selective nonoperative management of gunshot wounds of the anterior abdomen. Arch Surg 132:178–183

Eastham JA, Wilson TG, Larsen DW, Ahlering TE (1992) Angiographic embolization of renal stab wounds. J Urol 148:268–270

Feliciano DV, Rozycki GS (1995) The management of penetrating abdominal trauma. Adv Surg 28:1–39

Ferrada R, Birolini D (1999) New concepts in the management of patients with penetrating abdominal wounds. Surg Clin North Am 79:1331–1356

Fisher RG, Ben-Menachem Y (1985) Embolization procedures in trauma: the abdomen-extraperitoneal. Semin Int Radiol 2:148–156

Fisher RG, Ben-Menachem Y, Whigham C (1989) Stab wounds of the renal artery branches: angiographic diagnosis and treatment by embolization. AJR 152:1231–1235

Fletcher TB, Setiawan H, Harrell RS, Redman HC (1989) Posterior abdominal stab wounds: role of CT evaluation. Radiology 173:621–625

Fry WR, Smith S, Schneider JJ, Organ CH (1995) Ultrasonographic examination of wound tracts. Arch Surg 130: 605–608

Ginzburg E, Carrillo EH, Kopleman T et al (1998) The role of computed tomography in selective management of gunshot wounds to the abdomen and flank. J Trauma 45: 1005–1009

Grossman MD, May AK, Schwab CW et al (1998) Determining anatomic injury with computed tomography in selected torso gunshot wounds. J Trauma 45:446–453

Hauser CJ, Huprich JE, Bosco P et al (1987) Triple-contrast computed tomography in the evaluation of penetrating posterior abdominal injuries. Arch Surg 122:1112–1115

Henneman PL (1989) Penetrating abdominal trauma. Emerg Clin North Am 7:647–666

Heyns CF, van Vollenhoven P (1992) Increasing role of angiography and segmental artery embolization in the management of renal stab wounds. J Urol 147:1231–1234

Himmelman RG, Martin M, Gilkey S, Barrett JA (1991) Triple-contrast CT scans in penetrating back and flank trauma. J Trauma 31:852–855

Hollerman JJ, Fackler ML, Coldwell DM, Ben-Menachem Y (1990a) Gunshot wounds: 1. Bullets, ballistics, and mechanisms of injury. AJR 155:685–690

Hollerman JJ, Fackler ML, Coldwell DM, Ben-Menachem Y (1990b) Gunshot wounds: 2. Radiology. AJR 155:691–702

Jackson GL, Thal ER (1979) Management of stab wounds of the back and flank. J Trauma 19:660–664

Kirton OC, Wint D, Thrasher B et al (1997) Stab wounds to the back and flank in the hemodynamically stable patient: a decision algorithm based on contrast-enhanced computed tomography with colonic opacification. Am J Surg 173: 189–193

Margolies MN, Ring EJ, Waltman AC et al (1972) Arteriography in the management of hemorrhage from pelvic fractures. N Engl J Med 287:317–321

Matalon TSA, Athanasoulis CA, Margolies MN et al (1979) Hemorrhage with pelvic fractures: efficacy of transcatheter embolization. AJR 113:859–864

McAllister E, Perez M, Albrink MH et al (1994) Is triple-contrast computed tomographic scanning in the selective management of stab wounds to the back? J Trauma 37:401–403

McKenney MG, Martin L, Lentz K et al (1996) 1000 consecutive ultrasounds for blunt abdominal trauma. J Trauma 40: 607–612

Panetta T, Scalfani SJ, Goldstein AS et al (1985) Percutaneous transcatheter embolization for massive bleeding from pelvic fractures. J Trauma 25:1021–1029

Patel VG, Walker MK (1997) The role of "one-shot" intravenous pyelogram in evaluation of penetrating abdominal trauma. Am Surg 63:350–353

Peck J, Berne T (1981) Posterior abdominal stab wounds. J Trauma 21:298–306

Phillips T, Sclafani SJA, Goldstein A et al (1986) Use of contrast-enhanced CT enema in the management of penetrating trauma to the flank and back. J Trauma 26:593–601

Plummer D, Brunette D, Asinger R, Ruiz E (1992) Emergency department echocardiography improves patient outcome in penetrating cardiac injury. Ann Emerg Med 21:709–712

Quigley MJ, Bret PM (1995) Occult pseudoaneursyms of the

abdominal aorta following gunshot wound: the importance of plain film findings. J Trauma 38:269–272
Rehm CG, Sherman R, Hinz TW (1989) The role of CT scan in evaluation for laparotomy in patients with stab wounds of the abdomen. J Trauma 29:446–450
Reilly KJ, Shapiro MB, Haskal ZJ (1996) Angiographic embolization of a penetrating traumatic renal arteriovenous fistula. J Trauma 41:763–765
Rozycki GS (1995) Abdominal US in trauma. Surg Clin North Am 75:175–191
Rozycki GS, Newman PG (1999) Surgeon-performed ultrasound for the assessment of abdominal injuries. Adv Surg 33:243–259
Rozycki GS, Ochsner MG, Jaffin JH, Champion HR (1993) Prospective evaluation of surgeon's use of ultrasound in the evaluation of trauma patients. J Trauma 34:515–527
Rozycki GS, Ochsner MG, Schmidt JA et al (1995) A prospective study of surgeon-performed ultrasound as the primary adjuvant modality for injured patient assessment. J Trauma Injury Inf Crit Care 39:492–500
Rozycki GS, Feliciano DV, Schmidt JA et al (1996) The role of surgeon-performed ultrasound in patients with possible cardiac wounds. Ann Surg 223:737–746
Rozycki GS, Feliciano DV, Davis TP (1998a) US as used in thoracoabdominal trauma. Surg Clin North Am 78:295–310
Rozycki GS, Ballard RB, Feliciano DV et al (1998b) Surgeon-performed ultrasound for the assessment of truncal injuries: lessons learned from 1540 patients. Ann Surg 228: 557–567
Rozycki GS, Feliciano DV, Ochsner G et al (1999) The role of ultrasound in patients with possible penetrating cardiac wounds: a prospective multicenter study. J Trauma 46:543–552
Sclafani AP, Sclafani SJA (1996) Angiography and transcatheter embolization of vascular injuries of the face and neck. Laryngoscope 106:168–173
Sclafani SJA, Shaftan GW, Mitchell WG et al (1982) Interventional radiology in trauma victims: analysis of 51 consecutive patients. J Trauma 22:353–360
Sclafani SJA, Shaftan GW, McAuley J et al (1984) Interventional radiology in the management of hepatic trauma. J Trauma 24:256–262
Sclafani SJA, Cooper R, Shaftan GW et al (1986) Arterial trauma: diagnostic and therapeutic angiography. Radiology 161:165–172
Sclafani SJA, Shaftan GW, Scalea TM et al (1995) Nonoperative salvage of computed tomography-diagnosed splenic injuries: utilization of angiography for triage and embolization for hemostasis. J Trauma 39:818–827
Scott R, Carlton CE, Goldman M (1969) Penetrating injuries of the kidney: analysis of 181 patients. J Urol 101:247–253
Sisley AC, Rozycki GS, Ballard RB et al (1998) Rapid detection of traumatic effusion using surgeon-performed ultrasonography. J Trauma 44:291–297
Stevenson J, Battistella FD (1994) The "one-shot" intravenous pyelogram: is it indicated in unstable trauma patient before celiotomy? J Trauma 36:828–834
Tso P, Rodriquez A, Cooper C et al (1992) Sonography in blunt abdominal trauma: a preliminary progress report. J Trauma 33:39–43
Uflacker R, Paolini RM, Lima S (1984) Management of traumatic hematuria by selective renal artery embolization. J Urol 132:662–667
Velhamos GC, Demetriades D, Chahwan S et al (1999) Angiographic embolization for arrest of bleeding after penetrating trauma to the abdomen. Am J Surg 178:367–373
Velhamos GC, Chahwan S, Falabella A et al (2000) Angiographic embolization for intraperitoneal and retroperitoneal injuries. World J Surg 24:539–545
Wilson RF, Ziegler DW (1987) Diagnostic and treatment problems in renal injuries. Am Surg 53:399–402

18 Imaging of Abdominal Injuries in the Pediatric Age Group

W. A. Bhatti and H. Carty

CONTENTS

- The imaging features of abdominal trauma in adults and children are similar
- This chapter aims to deal with the difference between the two groups, including the mechanism of injury, optimal imaging modalities, salient imaging features, and potential pitfalls in the evaluation of pediatric abdominal trauma
- Diagnostic imaging of abdominal trauma should be aggressive and management should be conservative

W. A. Bhatti, MD
Professor of Paediatric Radiology, Alder Hey Children's Hospital, Eaton Road, Liverpool L12 2AP, UK
H. Carty, MD
Professor of Paediatric Radiology, Alder Hey Children's Hospital, Eaton Road, Liverpool L12 2AP, UK

18.1 Introduction

This chapter deals with the salient features and potential pitfalls of imaging in abdominal trauma in childhood. Most injuries described have similar typical imaging appearance to those in adults. The purpose of this chapter is to concentrate on the differences between the two groups. It will not address iatrogenic trauma. In recent years, noninvasive imaging has become the cornerstone in the investigation of abdominal trauma, with every attempt made to manage the child conservatively. The hemodynamically unstable child with significant abdominal trauma, increasing abdominal girth, and peritonism will require an exploratory laparotomy. The stable child with no significant abdominal signs will be managed conservatively. The role of imaging is to determine the extent of trauma, thus guiding management decisions.

18.2 Incidence

Motor vehicle accidents account for the majority of blunt abdominal trauma. Bicycle handlebar and injury related to restraining devices such as seatbelts are also a significant cause of abdominal injury. Data collected prospectively from the National Trauma Registry in United States from 1985 to 1991 showed that 86% of the abdominal injuries were secondary to blunt abdominal trauma (Cooper et al. 1994). The incidence of blunt abdominal trauma is higher in Western Europe than in the United States, where gunshot wounds and knife injuries are slightly more common.

The mortality rate associated with blunt abdominal trauma was 9% in the above-mentioned study. Liver, spleen, and renal injuries occurred in approximately 30% of injuries and gastrointestinal injuries in 15%.

18.3 Mechanism

The abdominal organs in smaller children are more susceptible to injury for a number of reasons. The solid abdominal organs lie more anteriorly and lower in children, due to the horizontal position of the diaphragm. The skin is thin, the abdominal musculature poorly developed, and cartilaginous ribs provide little protection for these organs.

There are two different mechanisms that may result in injury following blunt abdominal trauma. Firstly, compressive forces: these may result in compression of a solid organ or viscus against a fixed structure such as the spine. This may be experienced from a direct blow or external compression as with a handlebar injury. This type of injury may result in contusion or subcapsular hematoma of the liver or spleen or perforation if a hollow viscus is involved. Secondly, deceleration forces such as are experienced in road traffic accidents and seatbelt injuries. Following such events, stretching and/or linear shearing forces may result in laceration or injury to mesenteric and renal vessels. The Chance-type transverse fracture through the lumbar vertebra is usually the result of such deceleration injuries. In reality a combination of the two types of injury may exist, as described in "lap belt complex," where a constellation of injuries including flexion-distraction injury to the lumbar spine such as Chance fracture, ecchymosis of the abdominal wall, and injury to the small intestine may occur (Newman et al. 1990) (Fig. 18.1).

Penetrating injuries, including stabbing and shooting injuries, produce a different pattern of injury. The peritoneal cavity may be breached and any organ lying in the path of the penetrating instrument may be injured. The management of such injuries differs from that of blunt abdominal trauma and is managed more aggressively, particularly if there is suspicion that the peritoneum has been breached.

18.4 Clinical Presentation

The clinical presentation and mechanism of abdominal trauma may vary with the age of the

a
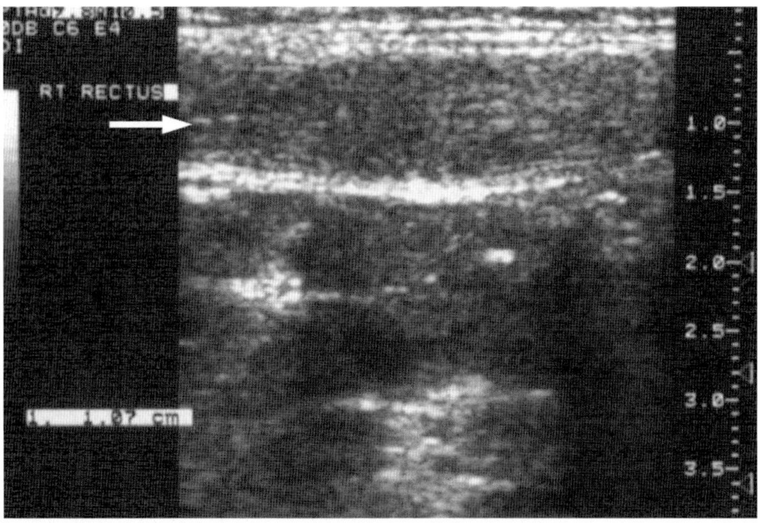

b
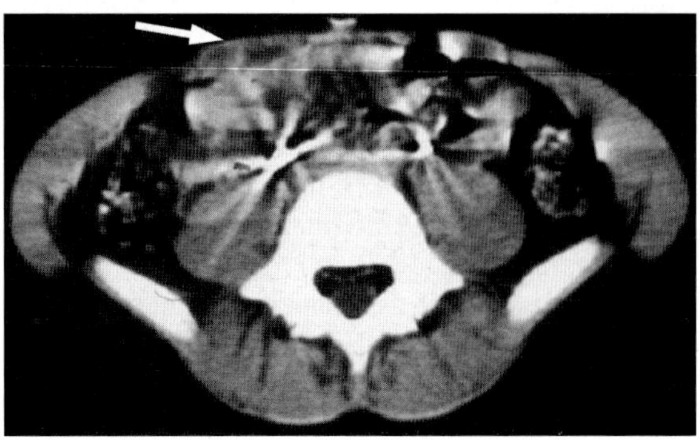

Fig. 18.1a,b. Rectus sheath hematoma. **a** Ultrasound scan showing thickening of the rectus sheath following blunt abdominal trauma(*arrow*). **b** CT confirmed these finding of right rectus sheath hematoma (*arrow*)

child. In an infant or toddler, in the absence of a history of motor vehicle accident, nonaccidental injury must be considered and an accurate account of events leading to the injury with careful correlation with clinical and imaging finding is mandatory. Such children subjected to physical abuse are often more severely ill than those presenting with accidental trauma as there is frequently a delay in seeking medical attention. Careful superficial examination looking for signs of neglect, unexplained bruising, finger marks, or petechiae might alert the attendant medical personnel. A child admitted with significant abdominal trauma may present in shock secondary to hypovolemia. Physical examination may be unreliable in up to 30% of children, particularly when the child has a reduced level of consciousness (DUPRIEST et al. 1982). The abdomen should be inspected for bruising, laceration, increasing abdominal girth, and seatbelt marks. A skilled, gentle, and patient doctor with continued consultation with the parents should examine the child. The child should be carefully assessed as per the Advanced Trauma Life Support (ATLS) guidelines looking for other associated life-threatening injuries, including tension pneumothorax, pelvic, and lumbar fractures. Visual inspection of the external genitalia looking particularly for blood at the meatus in a boy with suspected pelvic fractures is essential. Examination per rectum or per vagina should be limited to where it may affect the overall management of the patient, having obtained parental consent. Blood is obtained once i.v. access has been gained and sent for a full blood count, urea and electrolytes, serum amylase, transaminases, blood grouping and cross-matching.

Monitoring vital signs is important to gauge cardiovascular status, particularly tachycardia. Children are able to maintain a normal blood pressure despite significant blood loss, owing to their considerable physiological reserve (STEIN et al. 1994). Children have an efficient compensatory mechanism and their blood pressure falls only when 40% of their blood volume is lost (RANCE et al. 2000).The inferior vena cava (IVC) itself can be a useful gauge to assess the state of hydration, particularly in children, who can maintain a nearly normal blood pressure and pulse even when severely volume depleted. The IVC on CT normally appears oval or plump in well-hydrated subjects. In the fluid-depleted it will appear thin and flat on several of the axial slices. Imaging in severe abdominal trauma is as per departmental policy, which may include plain radiographs, ultrasound, or CT examinations.

18.5 Imaging

An accurate account of events leading to the trauma is important to optimize imaging investigations, where possible. Good clinical evaluation will direct the clinician to the site of injury and possible injured structures. There is often a combination of different structures, which may be involved depending on the site of trauma. A knowledge of the type of combination injuries may help in identifying the spectrum of injuries sustained. The combination injuries to the upper abdomen may be categorized into three main groups, based on the site of abdominal injury. Injury to the right side of the abdomen includes visceral injury of the liver, right kidney, right adrenal gland, and right hemidiaphragm combined with right lung contusion, rib fractures, and hemo- or pneumothorax. On the left similarly, injury may include the same organs substituting splenic for liver injuries. A central blow to the abdomen as experienced during a playground fight or steering wheel injury may result in the third group midline injuries. The spectrum of injury encountered may include injury to the left lobe of the liver, the pancreas, duodenum, transverse colon, small bowel, small bowel mesentery, aorta, and the IVC. The sternum and lower ribs and cardiac injury may also occur.

Plain radiographs, US, and CT are the imaging modalities used as first-line in the investigation of abdominal trauma.

18.5.1 Plain Radiographs

Plain abdominal radiographs are often requested in the acute trauma setting, but a normal abdominal radiograph does not exclude abdominal injury. The supine abdominal radiograph may often be normal or show nondiagnostic abnormalities. Free intraperitoneal air (as little as 1–2 ml) may be detected on the supine film. Large amounts of free air may appear as a large central lucent region resembling a football. Free air may outline the falciform or umbilical ligaments and can be seen on both sides of the bowel wall. Rarely, free air is seen in the scrotum of toddlers. The sensitivity for detecting free air can be increased by performing an erect chest or lateral decubitus abdominal X-ray with the right side up. Failing this, in smaller children, a shoot-through lateral radiograph can be performed. Acute gastric dilatation on plain radiographs is commonly seen in children who have

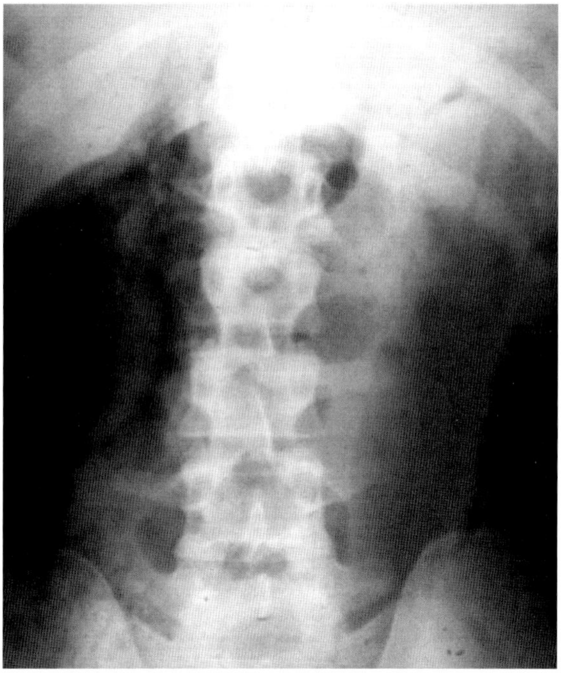

Fig. 18.2. Nonaccidental injury. Hyperlucency in the right side of the abdomen, outlining the inferior margin of the right lobe of the liver, consistent with free intraperitoneal air

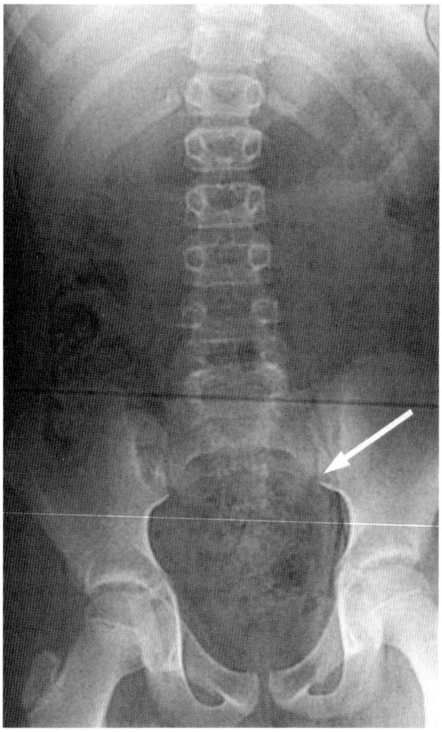

Fig. 18.3. Retroperitoneal air is shown outlining the left psoas muscle (*arrow*)

sustained blunt abdominal trauma. Skeletal injury fractures of the spine or pelvis are best detected on radiographs, but may need CT to further assess them. Retroperitoneal air occurs from penetrating injury or from severe soft tissue injury, allowing air to dissect upwards (Figs. 18.2, 18.3).

18.5.2 Ultrasound

The properties of ultrasound (US), including its portability, speed, and lack of ionizing radiation, should be ideally suited in the investigation of pediatric abdominal trauma. There are several drawbacks: it can be uncomfortable for the patient, bowel gas may obscure the organs, bony or thoracic injuries cannot be identified, and it is operator-dependent. US is a good screening examination in the following patients with possible abdominal injury (McKenny 1999):

- Suspected intraabdominal injury in a multiple trauma patient with altered sensorium, i.e., secondary to drug, alcohol, or head trauma, or with spinal cord injury
- Unexplained hypotension in trauma patients
- Multiple trauma patients undergoing general anesthesia for orthopedic, neurosurgical, or other injuries

In the acute setting, focused abdominal sonogram in trauma (FAST) scans may be used to assess free intraperitoneal fluid, an indication of hemoperitoneum or rupture of the intestine (Thourani et al. 1998). An abdominal US should examine all organs as well as identify free fluid (Fig. 18.4). If any part of

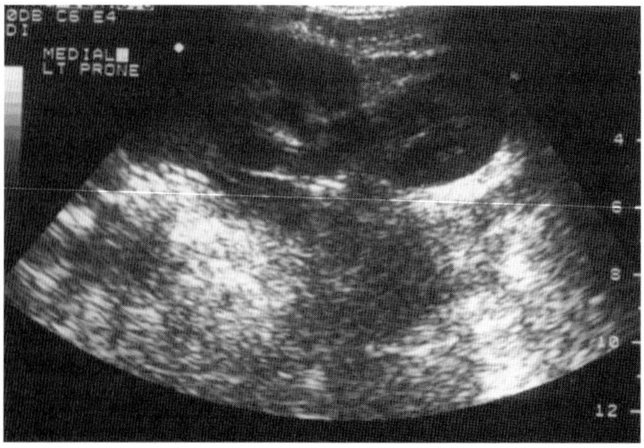

Fig. 18.4. Ultrasound of a fractured left kidney

the abdomen has not been examined owing to bowel gas or overlying subcutaneous emphysema, then further evaluation by CT is needed. Unstable patients with a positive ultrasound are taken to operating room, stable patients with a positive ultrasound are examined by CT (McKenney 1999).

18.5.3 Computed Tomography

CT has become the gold standard for the assessment of abdominal trauma particularly solid parenchymal injuries. CT is the investigation of choice in children with severe abdominal trauma, particularly when associated chest or bony injuries are suspected (Richardson et al. 1997). It has several advantages over ultrasound in that it allows a complete abdominal assessment, including the bowel and mesentery, detection of free air and bone injuries.

US examination of the abdomen is preferred in the non-trauma setting but in trauma CT is indicated in the following circumstances (Carty 1999):

- Hemodynamically stable but potentially significant intraabdominal injury by history
- Significant initial fluid resuscitation requirements without an obvious source of blood loss
- Multiple system injury, especially with head injury
- Inability to perform an adequate abdominal examination
- Hemoglobin below 10 g/dl that is not explained by an obvious source of blood loss
- Hematuria associated with signs of abdominal injury

In multiple trauma patients with suspected head trauma, a non-contrast-enhanced CT examination of the brain is performed prior to other contrast enhanced studies. For abdominal CT in the acute trauma setting, 2 ml/kg of intravenous contrast is recommended with a 50-s delay prior to scanning to achieve optimal solid organ enhancement. Oral contrast is not routinely used and the benefits are limited, as most sick children fail to drink the contrast (Shankar et al. 1999). Water can be used in the place of standard oral contrast (Fig. 18.5). Depending on the size of the child, either a 5-mm or 10-mm slice thickness is used with coverage from above the diaphragm down to include the pelvis. The images obtained are viewed on soft tissue as well as lung settings to assess for the presence of free intraperitoneal air. Images are viewed on soft tissue and bony windows (Fig. 18.6).

18.5.4 Magnetic Resonance Imaging

MRI has little role in the acute trauma setting apart from suspected spinal cord trauma.

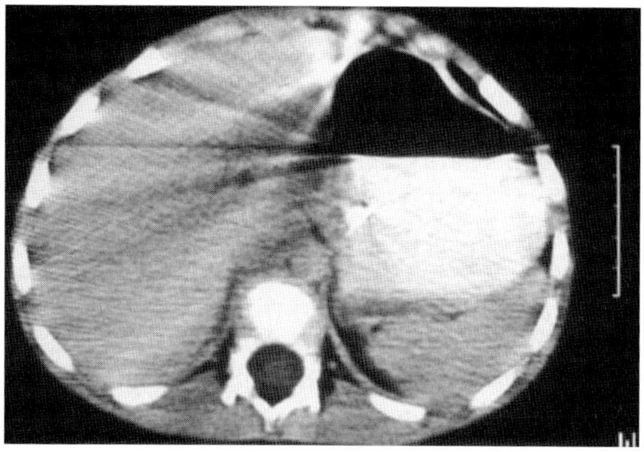

Fig. 18.5. Streak artifact showing a pitfall associated with the use of oral contrast

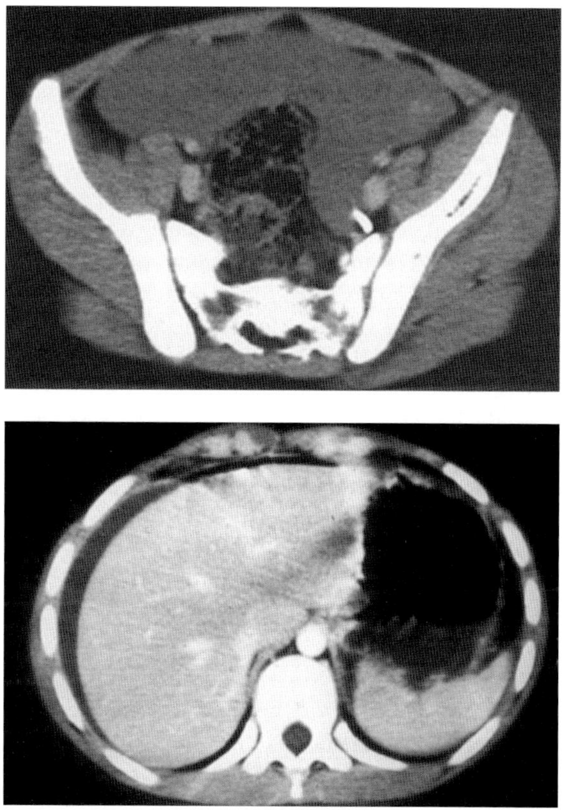

a

b

Fig. 18.6. a CT pelvis showing free intraperitoneal fluid. b CT abdomen, showing free fluid and intraperitoneal air outlining the liver

18.6 Imaging Features of Pediatric Abdominal Trauma

18.6.1 Hemoperitoneum/Hemopericardium

Diagnostic peritoneal lavage has now been abandoned in children. It is an invasive procedure associated with major complications, including injury to the bladder, bowel, and vascular injuries in 2% of patients (Fischer et al. 1978). It may require sedation and there are diagnostic problems, where lavage may be misinterpreted as free fluid on US and CT examinations. Diagnostic peritoneal lavage has been criticized for being unable to quantify free fluid and its lack of specificity.

US examination of the abdomen can readily assess for the presence of free intraperitoneal fluid. The FAST technique assesses the presence of fluid in the right upper quadrant, Morison's pouch, the perisplenic and subphrenic spaces, and the pelvis (Chiu et al. 1997). Hemopericardium can be detected if present by scanning in the subxiphoid region. Free fluid on US appears as an echo-poor area. It cannot be distinguished from blood. On CT it may have greater attenuation than fluid in the urinary or gall bladder, but may have the same attenuation. Interrogation of the attenuation values of the free fluid may help differentiate hemoperitoneum, which has a value of 30 HU from ascites, urine, bile, or intestinal contents that may measure between 0 and 10 HU. Hemoperitoneum may vary depending on whether it is fresh blood (unclotted), which measures 30–45 HU, or clotted blood, which may measure 40–60 HU. Higher-density sentinel clots surrounded by lower-density fluid may be observed around sites of active bleeding. The finding of active extravasation of contrast during CT is an indication for emergency surgery. The density of extravasated contrast may range from 85 to 370 HU.

18.6.2 Liver Trauma

The inferior margin of the liver lies exposed and unprotected by ribs and a direct punch can result in a laceration or fracture. The left lobe of the liver is more commonly injured by a direct blow, as it is compressed against the spine, and this is more common in abuse. In comparison, the larger right lobe, particularly the posterior segment, is more often injured in accidental trauma, owing to its proximity to the rib cage and spinal column (Stalker et al. 1986). Optimal image enhancement of the liver can be achieved by administering 2 ml/kg of intravenous contrast with a 50-s delay, which highlights the contrast between normal and abnormal liver and surrounding collections. The imaging features of liver injury are similar to those in adults: subcapsular hematoma, parenchymal contusions, and lacerations are the commonest. A rise in the serum transaminase is a good indicator of liver injury. Subcapsular hematomas typically appear as low-density areas on CT and hypoechoic lesion on ultrasound examination. In fresh hematomas, there may be a central high-density clotted blood surrounded by low-density unclotted blood or sentinel clot. Contusions appear as low-density areas within the liver parenchyma and lacerations as branching irregular low-density areas traversing the liver parenchyma (Fig. 18.7).

Ascites in children in the presence of liver trauma is suggestive of severe hepatic trauma. Special attention should be paid to lacerations involving the bare area of the liver, where injury can result in a retroperitoneal hemorrhage. Periportal areas of low attenuation have been described in the setting of abdominal trauma and nontraumatic conditions such as hepatitis or liver transplantation and are found in 80% of children with hepatic injury. The periportal tracking in liver trauma is frequently focal and associated with adjacent liver laceration or hemorrhage. It has little prognostic significance in the pediatric setting and is thought to represent periportal lymphoedema subsequent to rapid rehydration with i.v. fluids (Fig. 18.8). Complications following hepatic trauma include a biloma, disrup-

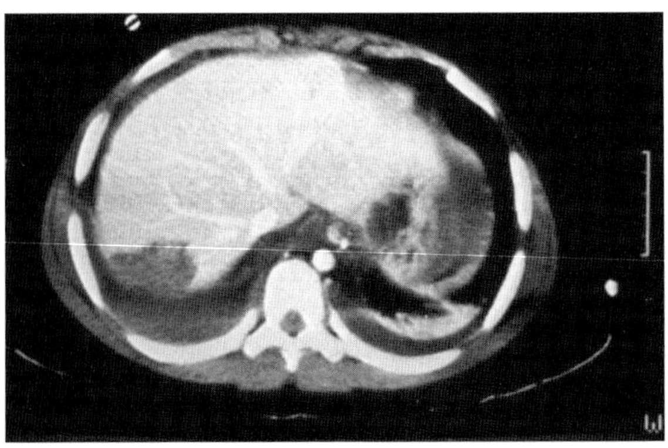

Fig. 18.7. Hepatic trauma. Laceration involving the posterior segment of the right lobe of the liver with associated intraperitoneal hematoma and pleural effusions. This is a difficult region to visualize on ultrasound

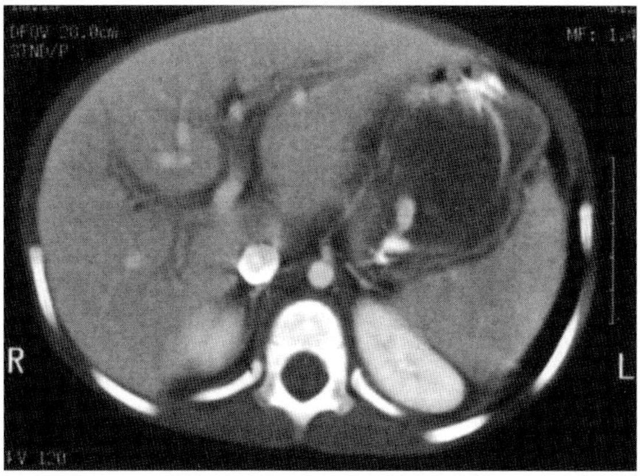

Fig. 18.8. Periportal tracking. Zones of low attenuation shown in the liver tracking the course of the portal vein and its branches, following blunt abdominal trauma. In the pediatric setting this has little prognostic value

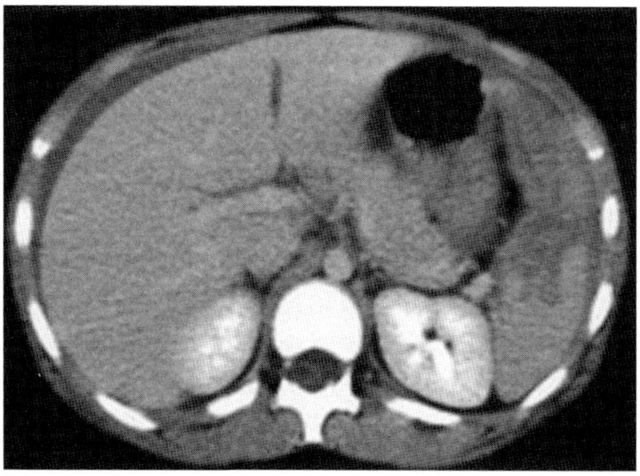

Fig. 18.9. Splenic hematomas. Multiple splenic hematomas with free intraperitoneal hematoma. Beware the appearance of inhomogeneous enhancement of the spleen during the arterial phase

tion of hepatic or bile duct, hepaticobiliary fistula, or even portal vein thrombosis. Most of these can be determined by follow-up ultrasound scanning, but may require further CT scans, endoscopic retrograde cholangiopancreatography (ERCP) or even angiography for diagnosis. Occasionally, hepatic trauma may be associated with diaphragmatic injury that is not manifest on initial imaging or lacks physical signs. Awareness of the association will increase pickup for the potentially catastrophic complication. In child abuse, the most common injuries are subcapsular hematomas, parenchymal contusions, and lacerations, usually as a result of a direct blow (Carty 1991; Ruess et al. 1995). The size and extent of the liver injury do not correlate with the need for surgery, as many lesions resolve spontaneously.

18.6.3 Splenic Trauma

Blunt abdominal trauma accounts for the vast majority of all splenic injuries. Although motor vehicle accidents account for the greatest number of cases, sporting injuries, karate, cricket ball, and even hockey stick injuries are becoming increasingly more common. Trauma to the spleen results from a blow to the left lower chest or left upper quadrant of the abdomen. The presentation is dependent on the extent of blood loss and injury, but may include vague left-sided thoracic chest pain, which may radiate to the left shoulder (Kehr's sign), abdominal pain, and in cases of severe hemorrhage, collapse (Fig. 18.9). The spleen may be pathologically enlarged by a preexisting cyst, lymphoma, leukemia, and infectious mononucleosis and prone to injury following minor trauma. Splenic enlargement detected after minor trauma is rarely due to the acute injury but is secondary to preexisting pathology. Similarly, in certain parts of Africa and Asia where malaria or kala azar are endemic, the spleen is particularly at risk. The initial abdominal radiographs are often normal but may reveal splenomegaly. In the presence of a large splenic hematoma, there may be displacement of the gastric air bubble or transverse colon. There may be radiographically visible left lower-rib fractures, pneumothorax, or elevated hemidiaphragm, but the absence of left lower-rib fractures does not rule out splenic injury. There may be associated injuries as per left-sided combination injuries of the renal and adrenal glands. CT is important in the accurate diagnosis and quantifying splenic trauma in the pediatric population where splenic conservation is all important. CT performed with i.v. contrast will readily identify the spectrum of splenic injuries, including subcapsular hematoma, laceration, contusion, fragmentation, and rarely splenic hilar vessel injuries. The appearances are similar to those in the adult.

Potential diagnostic pitfalls include imaging too soon after the bolus such that there is inhomogeneous enhancement of the spleen, splenic lobulation, or clefts, which may simulate lacerations. Contrast-enhanced CT examination reveals the normal enhancing splenic parenchyma from the lower-density hematoma or contusions. It is important to distinguish perisplenic from intrasplenic fluid in that perisplenic blood does not indent the spleen but subcapsular hematomas do.

Injury to the splenic vascular pedicle following a severe road traffic accident where shearing forces are experienced should be readily identifiable and requires immediate attention, either angiographic embolization in an attempt to conserve the spleen or operative removal. The fear of overwhelming postsplenectomy infection (OPSI) has altered the management from splenectomy to splenic conservation where possible. Children have a better outlook than adults in this respect, partly explained by the thicker splenic capsule and more responsive splenic vessel, which contracts more markedly in response to a hemodynamic insult in children than in adults. Postsplenectomy patients are prone to pneumococcal infection and thus must be vaccinated against this. Parents should be informed and receive adequate advice about sepsis prophylaxis. Delayed rupture may occur several days after injury and initial clinical and radiological assessment and careful monitoring is required for patients managed conservatively. True delayed rupture following an initial intact splenic capsule is rare, but carries a worse prognosis. US monitoring is required for patients managed conservatively. Long-term surveillance is required to monitor resolution and to detect complications such as splenic cysts, pseudoaneurysms, or arteriovenous fistulae. Occasionally the spleen may heal with a resultant large splenic cyst, which is vulnerable and prone to injury, especially during contact sports. Suitable advice should be given and the decision to operate will depend on the child's health style.

18.6.4 Pancreatic Trauma

Traumatic pancreatitis in children is rare and is usually the result of accidental abdominal trauma. In trauma, as the pancreas crosses the vertebral column, compression of the pancreas against the vertebral column may occur from a direct punch, a handlebar injury, or injury by a sporting implement such as a hockey stick or cricket ball. In adolescent "joyriders" who fail to use safety seatbelts, blunt pancreatic injury may result from impaction against a steering wheel. Penetrating injuries such as stab wounds may also cause pancreatic injury (Fig. 18.10). In a small but significant number of patients, traumatic pancreatitis may result from nonaccidental injury from repeated kicks or blows to the abdomen. The pancreas is more prone to injury in children than in adults. This is in part related to the thicker envelope of retroperitoneal fatty tissue in adults, which surrounds and cushions the pancreas, and the more developed abdominal musculature in adults. Clinically, the patient may present with shock, vomiting, and abdominal pain but the signs are nonspecific. In cases of abuse, the presentation may be delayed. The presenting child may have suffered significant weight loss, diarrhea, and chronic abdominal pain and may have a palpable mass due to a pseudocyst. The serum amylase is not always raised in the acute phase and may be delayed and peak 24 h after the initial insult.

The scope of injuries to the pancreas includes contusions, laceration, and transection. Thin-section CT is the imaging modality of choice. The appearance of pancreatitis may range from a normal appearing gland to diffuse enlargement. CT may be normal if performed within 24 h of injury, before the development of radiological change (Smith et al. 1988). The CT features indicative of pancreatitis include fluid in the lesser sac, anterior para-renal space, and fascial thickening. The pancreas may show normal enhancement or in severe trauma, heterogeneous enhancement. Complications include pancreatic necrosis or phlegmon and pseudocyst formation, which appears as a well-defined water density collection related to the pancreas. This may be single or loculated and when large enough, indents the stomach and causes gastric outlet obstruction. Pancreatic laceration and fractures appear as low attenuation interruptions in the pancreatic parenchyma, but caution must be exercised as the pancreas in children can return to its normal contour immediately after injury. In cases of suspected damage to the pancreatic duct, ERCP or MRCP can be performed to assess the integrity of the duct, as instrumentation may exacerbate pancreatitis (Fig. 18.11). US has a limited role in pancreatic

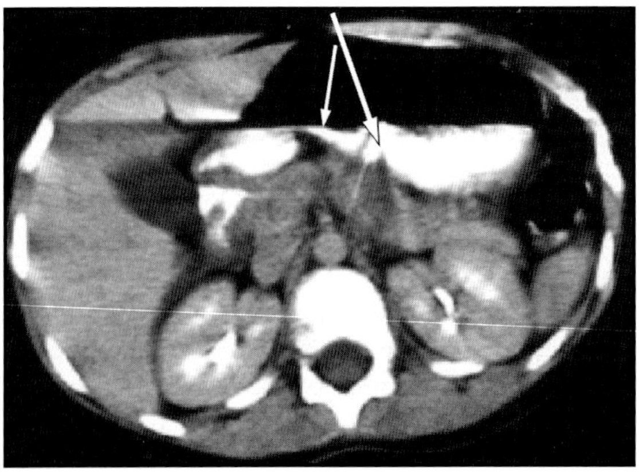

Fig. 18.10. CT pancreatic laceration. This patient suffered a blow to the anterior abdomen resulting in the pancreatic lacerations (*arrows*). Note the small amount of hematoma in the left anterior pararenal space

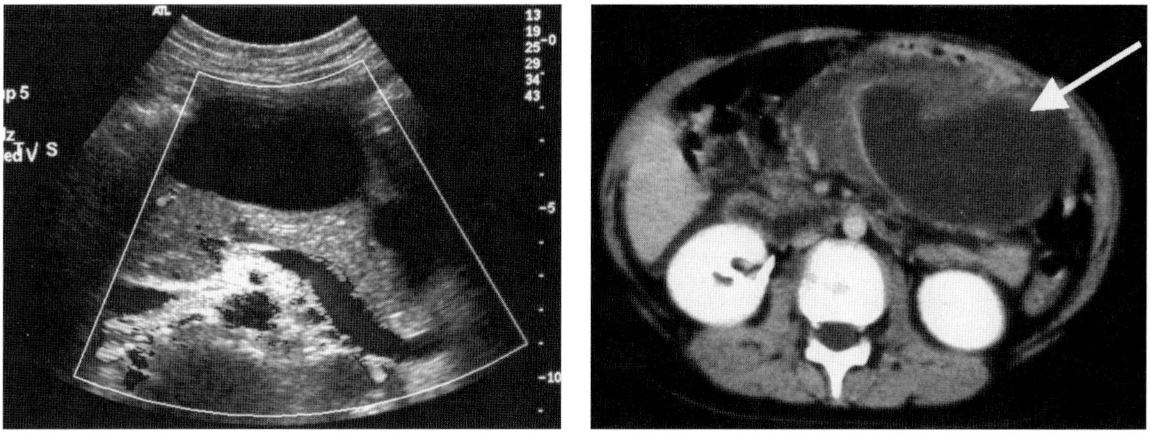

a b

Fig. 18.11a, b. Pancreatic pseudocyst. **a** US and **b** CT of the abdomen. Pancreatic pseudocyst (*arrow*) as a complication following traumatic pancreatitis

trauma in the acute setting: it is uncomfortable, the tail is poorly assessed, and bowel gas may obscure adequate visualization. Serial US examination can be performed for follow-up in patients who have experienced a pancreatic injury to assess resolution or detect complications. A typical but rare finding on an abdominal radiograph is the presence of a sentinel loop of isolated dilated bowel loop in the upper abdomen. Long-term complications are seen once the acute injury has resolved.

18.6.5 Urinary Tract Trauma

18.6.5.1 Renal Injuries

Injuries to the kidneys following blunt abdominal trauma are more common in children than in adults for a number of reasons. The abdominal musculature and perinephric fat is thinner and the kidneys are larger in proportion to the body size. Preexisting anomalies such as hydronephrosis, horseshoe, or pelvic kidneys also make them susceptible to injury owing to the size or location. Dependent on the history, individuals with suspected renal injury and microhematuria following blunt injury can be monitored by serial ultrasound (Mayor et al. 1995). Normal function in the contralateral kidney must be demonstrated before any form of surgery can be contemplated. In practice this is achieved by contrast-enhanced CT. Renal trauma is common and the imaging features are similar to those in adults. The spectrum of injuries includes renal contusion, renal cortical laceration, fractured kidney, shattered kidney, subcapsular hematoma, traumatic renal artery occlusion, or renal vein thrombosis. An imaging classification considering four grades has been widely adopted.

US has potential advantages over other imaging features in evaluation of the kidneys. It is mobile and can rapidly provide valuable information about the renal morphology and perfusion using Doppler. Doppler examination will reveal acute renal arterial occlusion whene there has been no time for development of collaterals. It is also good at demonstrating perfusion defects in which intrarenal arteries have been damaged and in the assessment of late complications such as arteriovenous fistula, where high systolic velocities in the artery supplying the fistula are demonstrated and may be transmitted into the venous waveform. Doppler examination is operator-dependent and good results can be achieved by a skilled operator. In the severely injured patient, high-quality images may not be obtained for a number of reasons and thus contrast-enhanced CT is the modality of choice in these individuals (Fig. 18.12).

On CT, lacerations appear as irregular linear low-attenuation areas that may extend from the periphery of the renal parenchyma to the intrarenal collecting ducts. They may be associated with contrast extravasation into the perirenal space or the renal collecting system. The leakage of contrast following a major laceration should be distinguished from active arterial bleeding, which appears earlier on the CT scan (Fig. 18.13). Rarely but not infrequently, trauma to the abdomen may reveal an underlying renal abnormality such as polycystic disease, a Wilms tumor, hydronephrosis, or large renal cysts. The preexisting renal

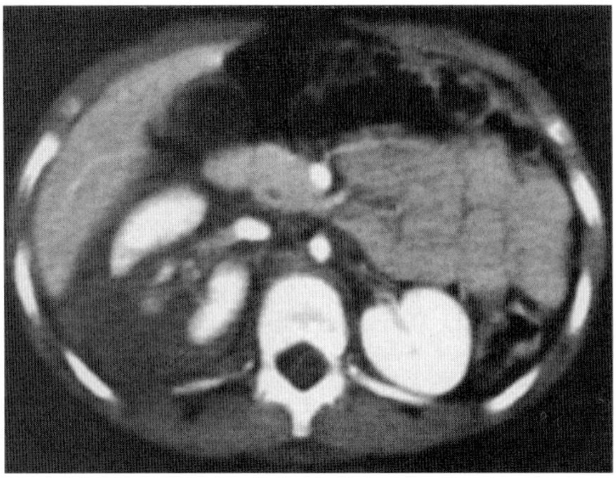

Fig. 18.12. Category II injury. Laceration of the right kidney communicating with the pelvicalyceal system. Hemorrhage is seen in the right perirenal space and peritoneal cavity

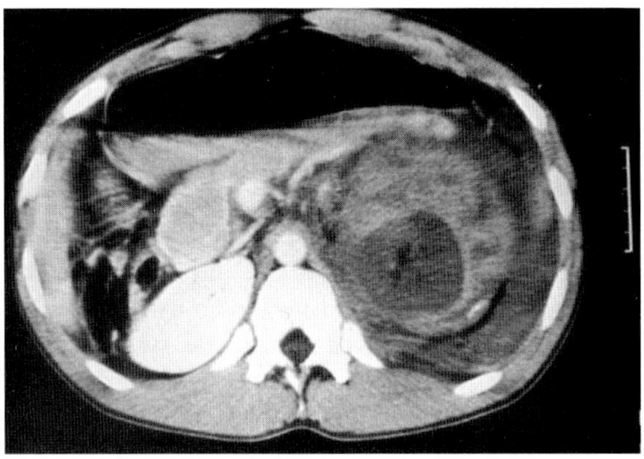

Fig. 18.13. Category III renal injury. Left renal pedicle injury with associated perirenal hematoma. Notice the left kidney is devascularized, with no contrast uptake. Note the gastric dilatation and left-sided retroperitoneal air related to the left perirenal hematoma, thought to relate to a tear in the fourth part of the duodenum

abnormality predisposes the kidney to increased risk of injury after blunt abdominal trauma. Category I injuries are managed conservatively but category III and IV require surgery. Category II may require further imaging and may need surgery (Fig 18.14).

Long-term follow-up by radionuclide imaging is required to assess residual function and monitor long-term complications such as hypertension and renal atrophy (Figs. 18.15 and 18.16).

18.6.5.2 Ureteric Injuries

Injuries to the ureter are rare, but may result from direct forces that may compress it against the ribs or the upper lumbar vertebrae, resulting in transection or more commonly partial rupture. Most injuries are sited within the proximal ureter and around the pyeloureteral junction (PUJ). The diagnosis may be made on CT but delayed images may be required or an intravenous urogram (IVU) (Siegle and Balfe 1989). Perinephric, perihilar, or retroperitoneal extravasation of contrast may be shown. There may be PUJ obstruction. This type of injury is managed by insertion of ureter stents to bridge the partial rupture or open anastomosis in complete transection. There is a long-term risk of ureteric stricture formation.

18.6.5.3 Bladder Injuries

The bladder in a small child, when full, lies quite exposed in an intraabdominal position and is susceptible to injury. Bladder rupture should be suspected in children with gross macrohematuria or anuria following blunt abdominal trauma. There are two types of bladder injury which may result: intraperitoneal rupture and extraperitoneal rupture. On clinical examination, blood may be visible at the urethral meatus and thus an indirect urethrogram should be performed to assess the integrity of the urethra. On the abdominal radiograph, there may be fractures involving the pelvic bones and pubic rami. Ultrasound examination may reveal free intraperitoneal fluid in the case of

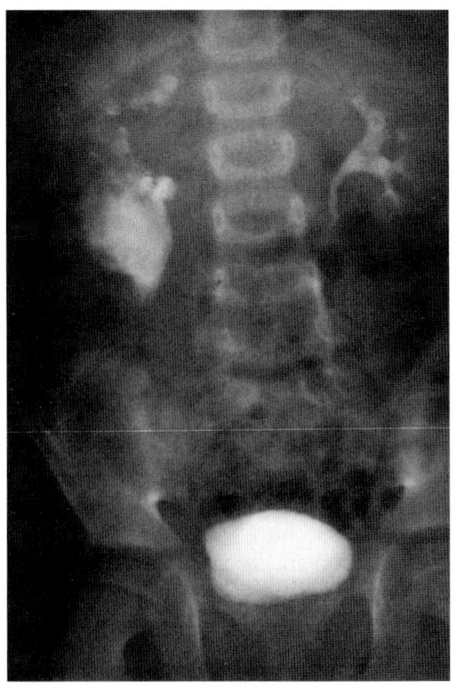

Fig. 18.14. Posttraumatic right-sided urinoma

intraperitoneal rupture. The definitive diagnosis and site of rupture is determined by performing a cystogram. Contrast-enhanced CT may miss the diagnosis, particularly when there is little contrast in the ureter or bladder, but a delayed CT examination following administration of intravenous contrast improves the sensitivity (Sivit et al. 1995). In all abdominal CT, the bladder catheter should be clamped before starting.

Extraperitoneal bladder rupture is more common and is diagnosed on cystography when there is perivesical extravasation of contrast. The contrast may track superiorly and anteriorly to the umbilicus into the prevesical space. Secondary signs including perivesical hematoma or fluid may be seen on ultrasound or CT.

Intraperitoneal bladder rupture will result in peritonitis. On CT there may be free fluid of similar attenuation to water and a small bladder. Cystography will reveal extravasation of contrast into the paracolic gutters and outlining the bowel loops, which allows differentiation between intra- and extraperitoneal rupture.

Most cases are managed conservatively, with either suprapubic or transurethral catheterization without any adverse long-term affects (Figs. 18.17 and 18.18).

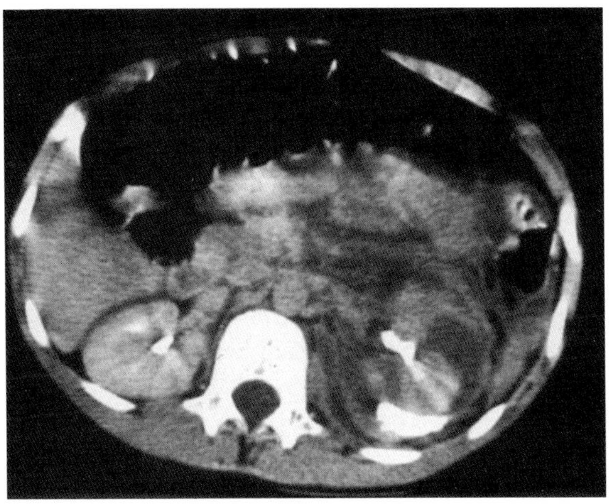

Fig. 18.15. Left-sided injury: laceration through the midpole to the pelvicalyceal system with leakage of excreted contrast into the perirenal space

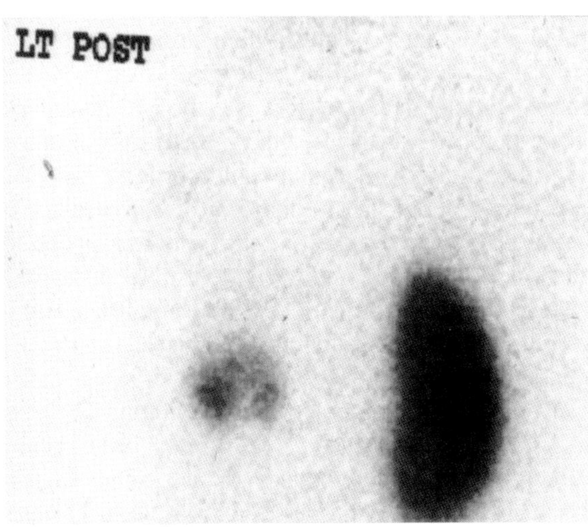

Fig. 18.16. Posttraumatic renal atrophy. Follow-up radioisotope scan shows atrophy of the affected left kidney

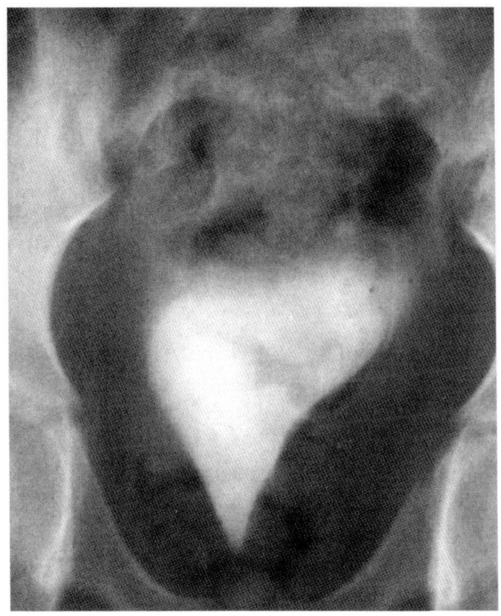

Fig. 18.17. Intraperitoneal bladder rupture. Intraperitoneal rupture occurs when the bladder is full at the time of lower abdominal trauma. Usually, as in this case, the dome is involved, with contrast extending up the paracolic gutters

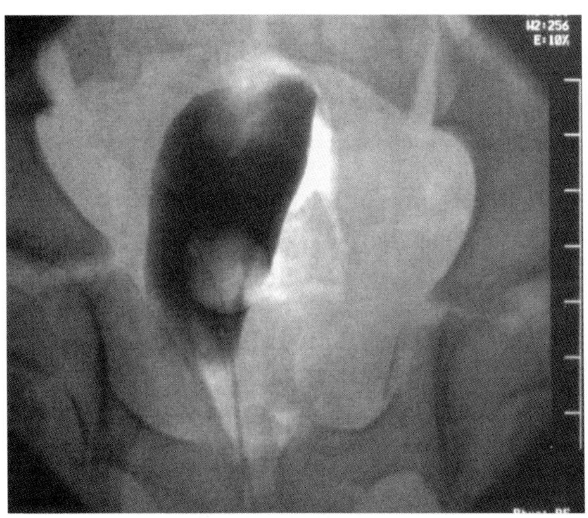

Fig. 18.18. Extraperitoneal bladder rupture. The bladder appears pear-shaped and there is loss of obturator fat planes. Note the pelvic fracture involving the left ischium

18.6.5.4 Urethral Injuries

Hematuria is a poor predictor of the severity of injury and may be present without overt renal or bladder injury being secondary to urethral injury. This is more common in boys, where the urethra is fixed, compared to a more mobile urethra in girls. Presentation with blood at the urethral meatus is common, difficulty in voiding, and even urinary retention. There may be associated pelvic fractures. Urethral injuries are investigated by retrograde urethrography in boys prior to urethral catheterization to prevent inadvertently converting a partial tear to a full thickness tear. Posterior urethral injuries are associated with pelvic fractures and occur solely in boys, where the bladder base is fixed to the urogenital diaphragm. Anterior urethral injuries are not associated with pelvic fractures and are seen in straddle injuries or occasionally in abused children. Owing to the close proximity of the vagina to the urethra in girls, injuries are usually concurrent and may require primary repair. Long-term sequelae include urethral strictures, which are managed by urethral dilatation or urethroplasty (Fig. 18.19).

18.6.5.5 Adrenal Injuries

Injury to the adrenal glands is rare and an incidence of 0.03% is reported after blunt abdominal trauma (Burks et al. 1992). The adrenal glands are well protected owing to their deep location and surrounding fat and thus injury is often associated with injury to other surrounding organs including the kidney, spleen, or pancreatic tail.

When identified, it is usually an incidental finding on CT performed for blunt abdominal trauma, when one adrenal gland is affected, but may become clinically apparent in bilateral adrenal injuries where there is adrenocortical insufficiency. Bilateral adrenal hemorrhage secondary to blunt abdominal trauma is the subject of occasional case reports (Rammelt et al. 2000). Clinically, in bilateral adrenal trauma, there may be vague abdominal pain, pyrexia, and hypotension. Trauma to the adrenal glands resulting in adrenal hemorrhage is well recognized in neonates and seen in child abuse, as well as in blunt and penetrating abdominal trauma (Nimkin et al. 1994). On CT there is an oval area within the gland of predominantly low attenuation, thickening of the ipsilateral diaphragmatic crus, infiltration of the surrounding fat with hemorrhage, and the presence of intraperitoneal free fluid. MRI yields little additional information and its use may be limited to cases of adrenal hemorrhage within adrenal neoplasm, whereby in- and out-of-phase imaging may be utilized. Neonatal adrenal hemorrhage is monitored by ultrasound.

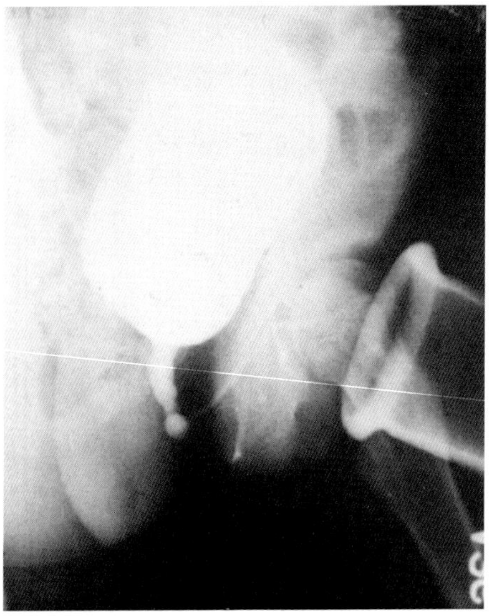

Fig. 18.19. Posttraumatic urethral stricture. Micturating cystogram showing a urethral stricture following a straddle injury

18.6.6 Hollow Viscus Injury

Hollow viscus injuries can result from motor vehicle accidents, child abuse and neglect, or rarely following ingestion of sharp foreign bodies. This can result in mesenteric injuries, bowel hematoma, perforation or transection. The mesenteric side of the bowel is more prone to vascular tears and the antimesenteric side to perforation. These injuries are more common in the jejunum than the duodenum or large bowel in accidental injury. The mechanism of bowel injury is secondary to external compressive forces applied to the bowel against the spine, for example, in seatbelt injuries or from a direct blow to the abdomen. High-resolution CT scans allow the clinician to accurately and expeditiously assess the presence of injury to the solid abdominal viscera, but a continuing problem facing the trauma surgeon is the unrecognized hollow viscus injury. The incidence of associated hollow viscus injury and multiple solid organ injury ranges from 0.7% to 26.5% in the overall pediatric trauma population (Nance et al. 1997). Delayed presentation of bowel injury may occur and present as intestinal obstruction. This is secondary to an ischemic stricture or the herniation of a loop of small bowel through a traumatic mesenteric defect (Fig. 18.20).

18.6.7 Seatbelt Injuries/Lap Belt Complex

Road traffic accident injuries may result in a lap seat belt complex-type injury in children wearing a lap belt or a three-point restraint in the rear seat of a vehicle where the shoulder belt component has been lifted and placed behind or under the shoulders (Newman et al. 1990). Infants and toddlers are more susceptible to this type of injury on sudden deceleration due to their reduced anteroposterior diameter, thin abdominal wall, and higher center of gravity. Owing to the poorly developed iliac spines, there is a tendency for the lap belt to rise cephalad and this is demonstrated in studies that show the location of the ecchymosis secondary to the seat belt is in an elevated position.

CT may reveal pneumoperitoneum, hemoperitoneum, bowel wall thickening, duodenal hematoma, mesenteric hematoma, bowel wall enhancement, and even extravasation of oral contrast.

Extravasation of intravascular contrast is an urgent indication for surgery and may be seen in sudden deceleration injuries resulting in mesenteric vessel injury. Injury to the colon is rare, as the pelvis and its peripheral abdominal location protect it. The transverse colon as it traverses the vertebral column may undergo similar injuries to those described in the duodenum.

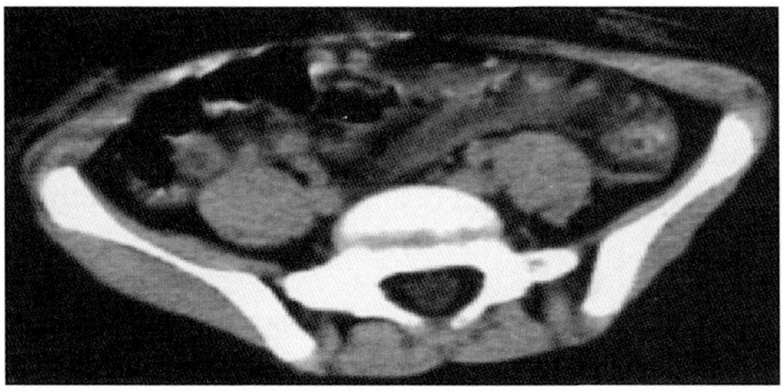

Fig. 18.20. Traumatic herniation of a bowel loop. This child remained unwell after an initial CT, which was reported as normal. Review of the CT showed a trapped loop of bowel herniating through a tear in the mesentery

18.6.8 Lumbar Spine Injuries: Chance Fractures

Lumbar spine injuries may result following a road traffic accident and although rare, should not be missed as delay in diagnosis and treatment can result in long-term morbidity. Typically, the subject is restrained by a lap seatbelt which is designed such that the hip joints and the pelvis, through rotation, absorb the energy on sudden deceleration. On impact, small children with immature iliac spines submarine below the seatbelt, and, owing to the large size of their head relative to the body, sustain a hyperflexion type injury to the lumbar spine, as well as significant abdominal trauma. The L1 and L2 are the vertebra commonly involved in this form of injury, which is usually a transverse fracture or a Chance fracture (Reid et al. 1990). There has been an increase in the number of these fractures with the increasing use of seatbelts. This may be visible on the plain AP and lateral radiograph of the spine, but thin-section CT is requested for accurate assessment. Injury to the conus or filum may result in neurological damage (Fig. 18.21).

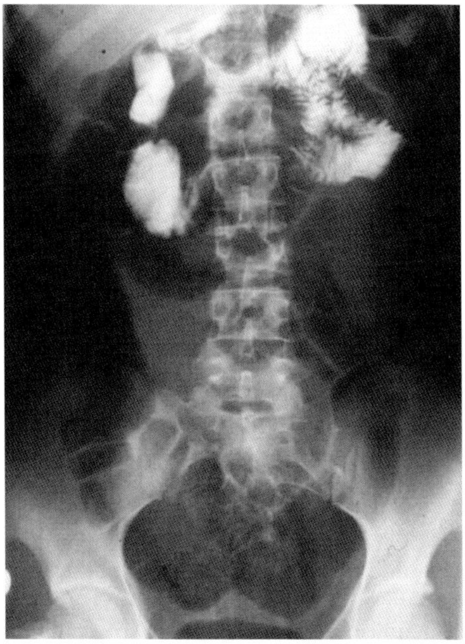

Fig. 18.21. Bowel/mesenteric injury and Chance fracture. This patient sustained an anterior abdominal injury in a road traffic accident. Note the Chance type fracture through the L3 and associated duodenal/mesenteric hematoma affecting the third part of the duodenum on this contrast study

18.6.9 Nonaccidental Injuries

18.6.9.1 The Battered Child

Major blunt abdominal trauma due to child abuse is rare, but has a high associated morbidity and mortality. Typically the preschool child, the infant and toddlers are the most affected. The child may present with bilious vomiting, unexplained shock or anemia. The histories are often inaccurate and presentation is often delayed. The history is the key point to the diagnosis, as there is discrepancy between the clinical state of the child and the history described. Most injuries result from acute compression against the vertebral column of the hollow viscus or solid organ, as may have resulted from a direct blow or kick to the abdomen. This may result in submucosal or subserosal bleeding leading to partial or complete obstruction of the affected bowel.

The duodenum and jejunum are the most frequent gastrointestinal injuries sustained in abuse and are typically located in the second and third parts (Kirks 1983; Kleinman 1990). There may be associated biliary or pancreatic injury in approximately 25% of cases. The plain abdominal X-ray may reveal proximal small-bowel obstruction. Upper GI contrast examination may reveal the extent of the intramural hematoma with thickening of the proximal mucosal folds, giving a coiled spring appearance in the acute phase. The thickened folds may persist during resolution of the hematoma and thus nonaccidental injury must be considered if these are identified. The hematoma may be visualized on ultrasound or CT and there may be associated proximal duodenal dilatation. Most cases are managed conservatively (Fig. 18.22). Small bowel perforation may occur at sites of fixation, including the second and third part of the duodenum, just distal to the ligament of Treitz and the ileocecal junction. Free air may be seen on the supine abdominal radiograph as previously described (see plain radiographs). Physicians must be wary, particularly in patients who are ventilated, those with pneumomediastinum from trauma, and those who may have had a diagnostic peritoneal lavage, who may show extraluminal gas on their abdominal films; differentiation from these causes and bowel perforation is paramount in order to avoid unnecessary laparotomies. The pitfall for the unwary is the presence of intraperitoneal gas due to tracking of air into the peritoneum from a pneumomediastinum or following peritoneal lavage.

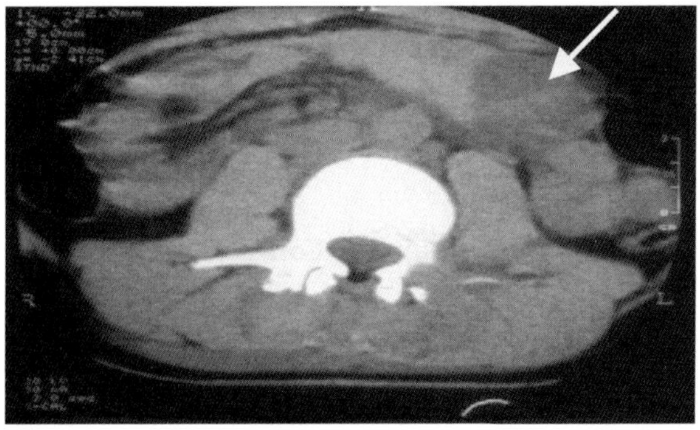

Fig. 18.22. Duodenal and jejunal hematoma (*arrow*) in a patient with a Chance-type lumbar fracture. Note the loss of the left postvertebral fat planes secondary to postvertebral hematoma

18.6.9.2 Sexual Abuse and Genital Trauma

In cases of severe lower abdominal trauma in which a pelvic fracture is suspected, the integrity of the bladder, urethra, or colon may be compromised and contrast examinations including cystogram and urethrogram may be warranted. Straddle injuries associated with cycling or perineal injuries related to jumping fences may result in laceration or hematomas affecting the vulva or scrotum that rarely require imaging. Imaging is rarely required in cases of suspected genital trauma, a significant proportion of which are secondary to sexual abuse. Presentation is often delayed, in which case the child may present with pelvic sepsis or penetrating vaginal tears that may be associated with significant retroperitoneal hematoma. A radiological survey may be warranted to identify fractures. Similarly, anal and rectal injuries may be seen in association with sexual abuse and present with perineal and pelvic abscesses. Rarely, a child may present in shock with peritonitis secondary to rectal tears as a result of forceful penetration.

18.6.10 Diaphragmatic Trauma

Diaphragmatic ruptures occur in 0.8–8% of blunt abdominal injuries, being more frequent on the left than the right owing to the protection provided by the liver. Diagnosis is often difficult, can be delayed, and carries a significant mortality risk. Tears frequently involve the posterior and lateral peripheral muscular portions of the diaphragm. Diagnosis may be delayed in intubated patients, where the positive intrathoracic pressure prevents herniation of abdominal contents into the thorax, and are only manifest after extubation. The diagnosis is often difficult to make on plain films, where there may be nonspecific findings, including pleural effusions, atelectasis, lung contusions, and altered, sometimes raised, diaphragmatic contour. Specific findings include the stomach within the thorax or herniation of solid viscera such as the liver, spleen, or even kidneys (Fig. 18.23). Fluoroscopy may reveal paradoxical movement in diaphragmatic paralysis. Fluoroscopy with oral contrast may reveal herniated intrathoracic bowel content. Ultrasound may demonstrate diaphragmatic hernia if there is associated herniation of a solid organ, but computed tomography with coronal and sagittal reconstructions is the technique of choice and allows direct visualization of tears and intrathoracic organ herniation. Although MRI provides superb images, it has a limited role in the acute setting, but may be utilized in cases of delayed presentation or equivocal cases where nonionizing, multiplanar MRI would be preferred, using a T1-weighted sequence the diaphragm appears as a hypointense homogeneous band. Contrast studies with follow-through images are definitive.

a

b

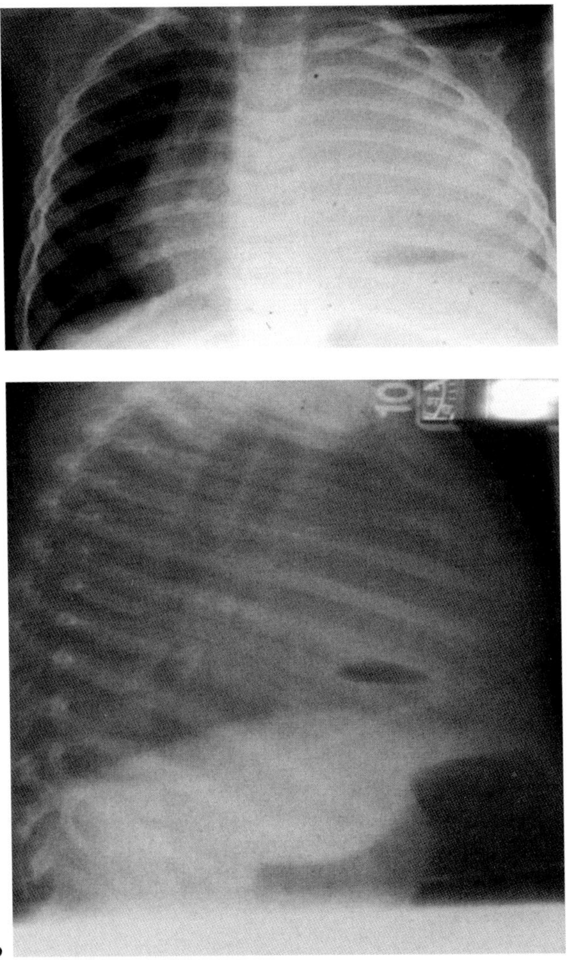

Fig. 18.23a,b. Traumatic diaphragmatic hernia. **a** Note the complete opacification of the left hemithorax secondary to contusions and effusion and an air-filled viscus above the left hemidiaphragm. **b** This is clearly seen on the lateral chest radiograph

18.7 Conclusion

The use of computed tomography, particularly helical CT, has improved the diagnostic accuracy of pediatric blunt abdominal trauma with most patients being managed conservatively. Plain films and ultrasound are important tools with a defined role but CT, with its multiformat reconstruction, speed, and windowing to assess soft tissues and bone and detect free gas, is the now the investigation of choice. Radionuclide imaging may be required in the follow-up monitoring of renal injury.

References

Burks DW, Mirvis SE, Shanmuganathan K (1992) Acute adrenal injury after blunt abdominal trauma: CT finding. AJR 58: 503–507

Carty H (1991) The nonskeletal injuries of child abuse, part 2. The body. Yearbook Paediatric Radiol 3

Carty H (1999) Emergency pediatric radiology. (Medical radiology, Diagnostic imaging and radiation oncology) Springer, Berlin Heidelberg New York, p 364

Chiu WC, Cushing BM, Rodriguez A et al (1997) Abdominal injuries without hemoperitoneum: a potential limitation of focused abdominal sonography for trauma (FAST). J Trauma 42:617–623

Cooper A, Barlow B, Discala C, String D (1994) Mortality and truncal injury. The pediatric perspective. J Pediatr Surg 29: 33–38

Dupriest RW, Rodriguez A, Shatney CH (1982) Peritoneal lavage in children and adolescents with blunt abdominal trauma. Am Surg 48:460–462

Fischer RP, Beverlin BL, Engrave LH (1978) Diagnostic peritoneal lavage: fourteen years and 2,586 patients later. Am J Surg 136:701–706

Kirks DR (1983) Radiological evaluation of visceral injury in the battered child syndrome. Paediatr Ann 12:888–891

Kleinman PK (1990) Diagnostic imaging in child abuse. AJR 155:703–707

Mayor B, Gudinchet F, Wicky S, Reinberg O, Schnyder P (1995) Imaging evaluation of blunt renal trauma in children:

diagnostic accuracy of intravenous pyelography and ultrasonography. Pediatr Radiol 25:214–218

McKenney KL (1999) Ultrasound of blunt abdominal trauma. Advances in emergency radiology II. Radiol Clin North Am 37:879–893

Nance ML, Peden GW, Shapiro MB et al (1997) Solid viscus injury predicts major hollow viscus injury in blunt abdominal trauma. J Trauma 43:618–623

Newman K, Bowman LM, Eichelberger MR et al (1990) The lap belt complex: intestinal and lumbar spine injury in children. J Trauma 30:1133–1140

Nimkin K, Teeger S, Wallach MT, Duvally JC, Spevak MR, Kleinman PK (1994) Adrenal haemorrhage in abused children: imaging and post-mortem findings. AJR 162:661–663

Rammelt S, Mucha D, Amlang M, Zwipp H (2000) Bilateral adrenal haemorrhage in blunt abdominal trauma. J Trauma 48:332–335

Rance CH, Singh SJ, Kimble R (2000) Blunt abdominal trauma in children. J Paediatr Child Health 36:2–6

Reid AB, Letts RM, Black GB (1990) Pediatric Chance fractures: association with intra-abdominal injuries and seatbelt use. J Trauma 30:384–391

Richardson MC, Hollman AS, Dacis CF (1997) Comparison of computed tomography and ultrasonographic imaging in the assessment of blunt abdominal trauma in children. Br J Surg 84:1144–1146

Ruess L, Sivit CJ, Eichelberger MR et al (1995) Blunt hepatic and splenic trauma in children; correlation of a CT severity scale with clinical outcome. Paediatr Radiol 25:321–325

Shankar KR, Lloyd DA, Kitteringham L, Carty H (1999) Oral contrast with computed tomography in the evaluation of blunt abdominal trauma in children. Br J Surg 86: 1073–1077

Siegle MJ, Balfe DM (1989) Blunt renal and ureteral trauma in childhood: CT patterns of fluid collections. AJR 152: 1043–1047

Sivit CJ, Cutting JP, Eichelberger MR (1995) CT diagnosis and localization of rupture of the bladder in children with blunt abdominal trauma: significance of contrast material extravasation in the pelvis. AJR 164:1243–1246

Smith SD, Nakayama DK, Gantt N, Lloyd D, Rowe MI (1988) Pancreatic injuries in childhood due to blunt trauma. J Pediatr Surg 23:610–614

Stalker HP, Kaufman RA, Towbin RB (1986) Patterns of liver injury in childhood: CT analysis. AJR 147:1199–1203

Stein JP, Freeman JA, Kaji DM (1994) Blunt renal trauma in the paediatric population: indications for radiographic evaluation. Urology 44:406–410

Thourani HV, Pettitt BJ, Schmidt JA, Cooper WA, Rozycki GS (1998) Validation of surgeon-performed emergency abdominal ultrasonography in pediatric trauma patients. J Pediatr Surg 33:322–328

19 Post-traumatic Venothromboembolic Disease: Diagnosis and Prevention

B. Ghaye

CONTENTS

B. Ghaye
Department of Medical Imaging, University Hospital Sart Tilman, Domaine Universitaire du Sart Tilman B35, 4000 Liège, Belgium

- The association between trauma and venous thromboembolism has been known for more than 50 years. Trauma is considered as one of the main causes of fatal pulmonary embolism.
- Although the risk factors that predispose to deep venous thrombosis in trauma patients have been well described, embolic events are unpredictable.
- Thromboprophylaxis is indicated in high-risk trauma patients, and inferior vena cava filters may have a role in the prevention of pulmonary embolism. Preventive caval filter placement should be considered early after admission.
- The diagnosis of pulmonary embolism is particularly difficult in trauma patients. Spiral CT angiography of pulmonary arteries should be a well-suited technique in this setting.
- Trauma patients are susceptible to uncommon sites of venous thrombosis in the abdomen and to uncommon causes of pulmonary embolism, including embolism of fat, liver tissue, bile, air and foreign bodies.

19.1 Introduction

Deep venous thrombosis (DVT) is a common but elusive disease that can result in suffering and death, if not recognized and treated effectively. DVT occurs in about 2 million patients in the US each year. DVT and pulmonary embolism (PE) are the two aspects of the same disease process, termed venous thromboembolism (VTE). It is estimated that in the US, 600,000 patients develop PE and 60,000 die of this complication each year (Hirsh and Hoak 1996). The prevalence of PE detected at autopsy among hospitalized patients is 14%–26% (Lindblad et al. 1991;

Stein and Henry 1995; Patriquin et al. 1998). One-third of PE episodes caused or contributed to death of the patients, 70% of which were not suspected clinically (Stein and Henry 1995). These results have not changed over the 3 last decades, despite progress in medicine and prophylaxis (Lindblad et al. 1991). Silent PE is most commonly detected in a high-risk population, including trauma patients. Approximately 10% of patients with PE do not survive the initial embolic event. When untreated, PE is fatal in up to 30% of patients, which can be reduced to 2%–10% if diagnosed and treated promptly with anticoagulation (Dalen and Alpert 1975; Moser 1990; Matsumoto and Tegtmeyer 1995; Carson et al. 1992). Such therapy, however, is not without risk, with an estimated 10%–30% complication rate (Urokinase Pulmonary Embolism Trial 1973; Gervin 1975; Kashtan et al. 1980; Cheely et al. 1981; Fihn et al. 1993; Landefeld and Beyth 1993).

Although sepsis and multiorgan failure remain the primary cause of the late mortality in trauma patients, increasing evidence suggests that VTE is now the third most common cause of death in patients who survive the first 24 h (Sevitt and Gallagher 1961; Fitts et al. 1964; Coon 1976; Shackford and Moser 1988; Geerts et al. 1996). One of the most dramatic aspects of PE is that one-quarter to one-half of the patients, who suddenly died from PE during their convalescence, would otherwise be expected to survive their devastating injuries and be able to return to normal life (Green et al. 1990; Rosenthal et al. 1994; Rodriguez et al. 1996; Owings et al. 1997). Since improved trauma care has reduced the early mortality rate, a large population of severely injured patients survives for prolonged periods of time in the ICU, leaving more patients at risk for late death. Immobilized by multiple fractures, spinal cord or head injuries, or life support systems, the trauma patients are at increased risk for VTE (Shackford and Moser 1988; Kudsk et al. 1989).

VTE is a major posttraumatic complication, manifesting few specific symptoms and thus rendering the clinical diagnosis insensitive and unreliable (Goldhaber et al. 1982; Hull and Pineo 1996; Stein 1996). Untreated DVT has been associated with a 50% or higher rate of PE over a 3-month period and a 10%–30% fatality rate, making early detection and treatment essential (Hillner et al. 1992). Reliance on the diagnosis and treatment of established VTE may expose susceptible patients to unacceptable risks as the first manifestation of the disease may be fatal PE (Clagett et al. 1998). Two-thirds of patients who will eventually die from PE survive less than 30 min, too quickly for any treatment to be effective (Donaldson et al. 1963).

Complications of VTE are costly, accounting for 9% of hospital re-admission following trauma (Battistella et al. 1997). In addition to being the primary source of PE, DVT may result in up to 50% of the patients in a postphlebitic syndrome, which manifests with painful edema, and in some circumstances skin ulceration and impaired mobility, months to years after the initial event, resulting in high cost associated with treatment, hospitalization and time loss from being out of work (Strandness et al. 1983; Patton et al. 1996; Prandoni et al. 1996, 1997, 1998; Bermudez et al. 1997; Meissner 1998; Erstad 1998). Much less commonly, venous occlusion may be complete, resulting in phlegmasia cerulea dolens and possible limb loss, due to venous gangrene, because of secondary arterial insufficiency and resulting compartment syndrome (Hirschmann 1987; Weaver et al. 1988).

Therefore, maximal thromboprophylaxis is essential in trauma patients, particularly in the severely injured. Multiple methods have been used for prophylaxis of VTE: the most commonly used are low-dose heparin, mechanical prophylaxis, low-molecular-weight heparin, and vena cava filter placement (Pasquale et al. 1998; Velmahos et al. 2000). Published results of these prophylaxis methods are usually inconsistent in the trauma population, as the conclusions are usually extrapolated from other populations, including elective surgical, orthopedic or medical patients.

19.2 History

As early as 1856, Virchow identified, the classic triad of risk factors leading to the development of venous thrombosis: changes in blood flow, vessel injury, and changes in the blood (Virchow 1856). The first relationship between VTE and trauma was initially demonstrated by McCartney in 1934, who first reported an increased incidence of fatal PE (3.8%) among over 1600 patients dying after trauma, with a significantly higher incidence in the elderly, in women and in patients with lower extremity fractures. Trauma accounted for 20% of all cases of fatal PE found at postmortem (McCartney 1934, 1935). Fifty percent of deaths occurred more than 2 weeks and 25% more than 4 weeks after injury, compared with nontrauma postoperative patients, in whom PE occurred earlier in the hospital course. Bauer was one of the first to recommend routine use of thromboprophylaxis in trauma patients (Bauer 1944). Autopsies of over 1000 World War II fatalities disclosed DVT in 62% and PE in 6.2% (Hamilton and Angevine 1946). The importance of the relationship between VTE and trauma was first demonstrated in the clinicopathological study of Sevitt and Gallagher in 1961, who reported 65% of DVT in 125 patients without embolism who died after trauma or burning, and 20.3% of PE in 468 autopsies after injury. In the vast majority, VTE was considered to cause or seriously contribute to death (Sevitt and Gallagher 1961). These authors had also described efficacy of anticoagulant therapy, as prophylaxis of DVT and/or PE in injured patients (Sevitt and Gallagher 1959). Postmortem findings stimulated the assessment of trauma patients by serial venography. A 35.5% rate of DVT was demonstrated in 124 patients 3 weeks after the accident, although thrombus formation was observed as early as 24 h after injury (Freeark et al. 1967). Nevertheless, DVT was difficult to diagnose in trauma patients, as most of the cases of DVT were asymptomatic or patients were too sick to be moved to the radiology suite for venography. Consequently, many patients were left undiagnosed and untreated, developing PE and a postphlebitic syndrome.

Over the next 15 years, other studies were published that first identified groups of patients with specific injuries who had a high risk of DVT and fatal PE in the general population. Conclusive evidence showing the benefit of DVT prophylaxis in the general surgical patient group appeared in the 1970s. Combined data on more than 12,000 patients included in randomized trials during the 1970s and the 1980s, showed that low-dose heparin reduced the incidence of DVT by 68% and PE by 49% (National Institutes of Health Consensus Conference 1986). This conference recognized the high risk of DVT in young multitrauma patients. Patients with head or spinal cord injuries had at least a 40% risk of developing DVT and 1%–4% risk of fatal PE. The conference called for randomized prospective studies and recommended the use of prophylactic measures aimed at decreasing DVT, especially in victims considered to be at high risk.

An incidence of 63% of DVT was found on venograms in 38 patients who were immobilized for more than 10 days following trauma. Almost all DVTs were clinically silent and the need for surveillance in these high-risk patients became obvious (Kudsk et al. 1989). The first study identifying risk factors of DVT in trauma patients was performed in 1990 (Shackford et al. 1990). Shackford and colleagues studied 719 patients admitted to the trauma center; 177 had at least one risk factor of DVT. The 10 risk factors defined were: age >45 years, bed rest >3 days, prior history of DVT, spine fracture, paraplegia, coma, lower extremity or pelvic fractures, major venous injury, or a complex wound of a lower extremity. No patient without at least one of the identified risk factors developed VTE, while 7% with at least one risk factor had complications of VTE (4 PEs, 8 DVTs), despite prophylaxis with low-dose heparin or mechanical prophylaxis when applicable.

19.3 Incidence

It is well documented that only one-third of fatal PEs are diagnosed before death (Goldhaber et al. 1982). It is difficult to establish the true incidence of VTE after trauma, as most episodes of DVT or PE are clinically silent, especially in patients with multiple neurological or extremity injuries (Myllynen et al. 1985; Knudson et al. 1992, 1994; Meyer et al. 1995). The incidence of DVT or PE in any population depends on the diligence with which it is sought, the sensitivity of the screening test and how frequently they are performed, the nature and the complexity of the injuries and the age of the population. These considerations have led to discrepancies in the incidence of VTE among different reports, particularly in trauma patients (Meissner 1998). Because most thrombi are asymptomatic, studies employing strictly clinical criteria for the diagnosis obviously underestimate the incidence of VTE. It is not surprising that studies based on autopsy findings or venography show the highest rate of DVT (Hamilton and Angevine 1946; Sevitt and Gallagher 1961; Freeark et al. 1967; Kudsk et al. 1989; Geerts et al. 1994). In a review of eight studies (one on autopsy findings and seven using venography), the reported incidence of DVT in trauma patients without thromboprophylaxis varied between 18% and 90% (average 42%), whereas the associated incidence of PE has been estimated between 4% and 22% (average 10%) (Shackford and Moser 1988). These observations clearly placed trauma patients among the highest risk group for VTE (Geerts et al. 2001). A relationship could be found between survival period or duration of bed rest and the incidence of DVT. In patients dying within 4 days of injury, 19% had DVT. Then, the frequency raised rapidly to 47% if death occurred between day 4–7 after injury. From day 8 on, the incidence of thrombosis seems to plateau, ranging between 75% in patients dying during the 3rd week, and 90% in patients dying during the next few weeks (SEVITT and GALLAGHER 1961). In a large venographic study on trauma patients who underwent no thromboprophylaxis, a rate of 57.6% of DVT was reported. The incidence varied according to the type of injuries: face, chest or abdominal injuries, 50%; major head injuries, 54%; spinal cord injuries, 62%; and lower extremity injuries, 69%. Only 1.5% of DVTs were symptomatic and 18% were located at or above the popliteal level (GEERTS et al. 1994). VTE has been reported in 41%–100% of patients who have complete paralysis after spinal cord injury (TODD et al. 1976; MYLLYNEN et al. 1985; GREEN et al. 1990; YELNIK et al. 1991). Four percent of fatal PE with no clinical signs of DVT have been reported, despite thromboprophylaxis (YELNIK et al. 1991). Of trauma patients requiring ventilatory support for more than 7 days, 21 of 109 (19.2%) suffered a confirmed PE (O'MALLEY and ROSS 1990). The clinical significance of calf thrombi in this population is unknown, but such thrombi cannot be ignored. Since many trauma patients do not become fully mobile for weeks to months, these thrombi have the potential to extend and cause delayed proximal DVT and PE. Patients with penetrating trauma not involving major veins have a lower risk of thrombosis than patients who sustained blunt injury (DENNIS et al. 1993; HOYT et al. 1993; FREZZA et al. 1996).

A meta-analysis of 73 studies including patients with different types of prophylaxis reported a mean rate of DVT of 11.8% (95%, confidence interval, 10.4–13.1) and a mean rate of PE of 1.5% (95% confidence interval, 1.1–1.8; VELMAHOS et al. 2000). Although the overall incidence of PE in trauma patients is low, PE remains a significant cause of late death (5% in patients surviving more than 1 week; WINCHELL et al. 1994). The mortality rate for trauma patients with PE is ten times the mortality rate for patients who did not sustain PE (TUTTLE-NEWHALL et al. 1997). Nevertheless, despite various types of prophylaxis, an evidence of 43% of DVT was still reported recently (GREENFIELD et al. 1997).

19.4 Pathogenesis

Virchow's classic triad of DVT risk factors is currently interpreted as comprising stasis, endothelial damage and hypercoagulability (KNUDSON et al. 1994). Trauma patients often present with all three risk factors at admission, and with clinical DVT and/or PE manifesting within 72 h. The relative importance of each component in an individual patient remains poorly defined (MEISSNER 1998).

- Stasis in trauma patients can result from immobilization due to critical illness, skeletal injuries or paralysis (MAMMEN 1992). Furthermore, spinal cord injuries produce loss of the muscular pump and of sympathetic tone of the lower extremity vessels, increasing venous stasis (MYLLYNEN et al. 1985). Compression of the inferior vena cava (IVC) by an intra-abdominal hematoma, or in-adequate resuscitation (ERSTAD 1998) and a high level of PEEP (VELMAHOS et al. 1998) may further increase the venous stasis.

- Endothelial damage can be produced by direct lesions in penetrating trauma, fractures, or following insertion of a venous catheter. Direct pressure on the endothelium due to immobilization can increase the endothelial damage (MAMMEN 1992; WILSON et al. 1994).

- Hypercoagulability in trauma patients has been known for more than 50 years. Multiple transfusions, sepsis, surgery, dehydration (RUIZ et al. 1991), transient bacteremia (WILSON et al. 1994), shock and poor perfusion (BRATHWAITE et al. 1993) will exacerbate the hypercoagulability. Endothelial cells have pro- and anticoagulant activity; the disruption of this delicate balance after major trauma may explain both early bleeding and late clotting (PALOMBO et al. 1991; KNUDSON et al. 1996; DRIES 1996). Trauma produces a critically important response of the hemostatic system on the coagulation and the fibrinolytic aspect, which are both necessary to control life-threatening hemorrhage and secondarily promote perfusion to healing tissue through vascular recanalization. The inability to down-regulate the cascade of coagulation, once hemostasis has been obtained, can lead to pathological thrombosis (SCHMIDT et al. 1992; OWINGS et al. 1996; MAMMEN 1992; ENGELMAN et al. 1996). Consequently, severe trauma patients first have coagulopathy followed by a hypercoagulable state occurring soon after injury (HARRIGAN et al. 1985; ENDERSON et al. 1991; SCHMIDT et al. 1992; GANDO et al. 1992; KNUDSON et al. 1996).

19.5 Risk Factors for Venous Thromboembolism in Trauma Patients

Patients can be classified as being at low, moderate, high or highest risk on the basis of well-defined clinical criteria. The choice of prophylaxis should be tailored to the patient's risk (HIRSH and HOAK 1996). Table 19.1 demonstrates the risk of VTE in surgical and trauma patients. Patients with major trauma or spinal cord injuries have been considered to be at the highest risk for VTE, requiring maximal prophylaxis.

Early investigators identified advanced age, immobilization and lower-extremity fractures as risk- factors for DVT in trauma patients (MCCARTNEY 1934, HAMILTON and ANGEVINE 1946; SEVITT and GALLAGHER 1961). More recently, the identification of high-risk subgroups has been important in defining those patients who might benefit from appropriate use of prophylaxis or serial screening studies. In many patients, multiple risk factors may be present and the risks are cumulative. Although the incidence of VTE varies widely in different papers, depending upon the population studied and the method used for detection of DVT, common risk factors were identified.

- VTE is more likely to complicate blunt than penetrating trauma (KNUDSON et al. 1994).
- Age is the most important risk factor, and as the average age of the Europe and United States population increases, VTE may become more frequent (KUDSK et al. 1989; SHACKFORD et al. 1990; O'MALLEY and ROSS 1990; RUIZ et al. 1991; KNUDSON et al. 1992, 1994; BURNS et al. 1993; DENNIS et al. 1993; ROGERS et al. 1993; GEERTS et al. 1994; NAPOLITANO et al. 1995; UPCHURCH et al. 1995; ABELSETH et al. 1996; HAENTJENS et al. 1996; PIOTROWSKI et al. 1996; GREENFIELD et al. 1997; HEADRICK et al. 1997; TUTTLE-NEWHALL et al. 1997; GEERTS et al. 1999; WOJCIK et al. 2000).
- The Injury Severity Score (ISS) (O'MALLEY and ROSS 1990; RUIZ et al. 1991; BUERGER et al. 1993; BURNS et al. 1993; HOYT et al. 1993; GEERTS et al. 1994; HILL et al. 1994; WINCHELL et al. 1994; NAPOLITANO et al. 1995; TUTTLE-NEWHALL et al. 1997; KELLER et al. 2000).
- Prolonged immobilization (FREEARK et al. 1967; SHACKFORD et al. 1990; RUIZ et al. 1991; KNUDSON et al. 1992, 1994; DENNIS et al. 1993; NAPOLITANO et al. 1995; GEERTS et al. 1999).
- Coma (DENNIS et al. 1993; ROGERS et al. 1993; WINCHELL et al. 1994; NAPOLITANO et al. 1995).

Table 19.1. Levels of thromboembolic risk in surgical patients without prophylaxis [Modified from GALLUS et al. (1994), NICOLAIDES et al. (1997), HIRSH and HOAK (1996), GEERTS et al. (2001)]

Level of risk	Calf DVT %	Proximal DVT %	Clinical PE %	Fatal PE %	Successful prevention strategies
Low risk Minor surgery in patients <40 years with no additional risk factors	2	0.4	0.2	0.002	No specific measure Aggressive mobilization
Moderate risk Minor surgery in patients with additional risk factors; nonmajor surgery in patients aged 40–60 years with no additional risk factors; major surgery in patients <40 years with no additional risk factors	10–20	2–4	1–2	0.1–0.4	LDH, LMWH, ES or PCD
High risk Nonmajor surgery in patients >60 years or with additional risk factors; major surgery in patients >40 years or with additional risk factors	20–40	4–8	2–4	0.4–1.0	LDH, LMWH, or PCD
Highest risk Major surgery in patients >40 years plus prior VTE, cancer, or hypercoagulable state; hip or knee arthroplasty, hip fracture surgery; major trauma; spinal cord injury	40–80	10–20	4–10	0.2–5	LMWH, oral anticoagulants, PCD/ES+LDH/LMWH, or adjusted-dose heparin

LDH, low-dose heparin; *LMWH*, low-molecular-weight heparin; *ES*, elastic stockings; *PCD*, pneumatic compressive device; *VTE*, venous thrombo-embolism

- Spinal cord injury (Todd et al. 1976; Myllynen et al. 1985; Shackford and Moser 1988; Dennis et al. 1993; Rogers et al. 1993; Geerts et al. 1994; Winchell et al. 1994; Meyer et al. 1995; Napolitano et al. 1995; Piotrowski et al. 1996).
- Pelvic bone fracture (O'Malley and Ross 1990; White et al. 1990; Buerger et al. 1993; Hoyt et al. 1993; Rogers et al. 1993; Knudson et al. 1994; Winchell et al. 1994; Tuttle-Newhall et al. 1997).
- Lower extremity bone fracture (Freeark et al. 1967; Maliska et al. 1985; Shackford and Moser 1988; Ruiz et al. 1991; Hoyt et al. 1993; Rogers et al. 1993; Knudson et al. 1994; Geerts et al. 1994; Hill et al. 1994; Winchell et al. 1994; Haentjens et al. 1996; Headrick et al. 1997; Tuttle-Newhall et al. 1997).
- Iatrogenic factors such as central venous catheters appear to be a risk for upper extremity thrombi in trauma patients. The increased risk can be related to trauma of venous endothelium, intravascular foreign body impeding blood flow or administration of potentially caustic factors. Central venous catheters should be removed as soon as possible after resuscitation and/or operative procedure (O'Malley and Ross 1990; Burns et al. 1993; Meredith et al. 1993; Hammers et al. 1996).
- Other iatrogenic factors include: blood transfusion (Knudson et al. 1992; Geerts et al. 1994; Gearhart et al. 2000), repair or ligation of major venous injury (Cargile et al. 1992; Dennis et al. 1993; Sue et al. 1995), and longer operating time or time from injury to orthopedic operation since early operative fixation of fractures of lower extremity decreases the rate of DVT (Webb et al. 1992; Abelseth et al. 1996).
- Underlying pre-existing conditions also increase the risk (Webb et al. 1992; Knudson et al. 1992; Weinmann and Salzman 1994; Spain et al. 1997). An increased incidence of DVT has been noted among trauma patients with coagulopathy at admission (Knudson et al. 1992; Spain et al. 1997).

A risk assessment profile was proposed to define the level of VTE risk (Table 19.2). This profile takes into account underlying conditions, iatrogenic factors and injury-related factors. Each risk factor was weighed. A risk assessment profile for thromboembolism (RAPT) score of 5 or more, which required a minimum of two factors, was assessed to define the high-risk population (Greenfield et al. 1997). Such a VTE risk factor assessment can be used to adapt prophylaxis of trauma patients (Diagram 19.1). The elimination of DVT screening with US and pharmacological and mechanical prophylaxis therapy in the low-risk group has been reported to be safe and to reduce hospital costs (Cafferata et al. 1998; Gearhart et al. 2000).

Table 19.2. Assessment of venous thromboembolic risk factors in adult trauma patients (age ≥15 years) [Modified from Greenfield et al. (1997), with permission]

Factor	Weight
Underlying conditions	
Obesity (>120% metropolitan life table)	2
Malignancy	2
Abnormal coagulation factors at admission	2
Pregnancy (including 8 weeks postpartum)	2
History of thromboembolism	3
Iatrogenic factors	
Central femoral line >24 h	2
Four or more transfusions during 1st 24 h	2
Surgical procedures >2 h	2
Repair or ligation of major venous injury	3
Injury-related factors	
AIS ≥ 3 for chest	2
AIS ≥3 for abdomen	2
Spinal fractures	2
Coma (GCS <8 for >4 h)	3
Immobility (excluding pelvic fractures) requiring bedrest >5 days	3
Complex lower extremity fracture	4
Pelvic fracture requiring bedrest >5 days or operative fixation	4
Spinal cord injury (complete or incomplete) with para- or quadriplegia	4
Age	
40–59 years	2
60–74 years	3
≥75 years	4

AIS, abbreviated injury score; *GCS*, Glasgow Coma Scale

19.6 Time to Diagnosis

A procoagulant condition is present directly after injury, which explains why DVT and PE can occur during the first 24 h of hospitalization after trauma (Ruiz et al. 1991; Rogers et al. 1993; Hill et al. 1994; Hammers et al. 1996; Owings et al. 1997; Erstad 1998). A venographic study reported DVT in 20% of patients on the 1st day after trauma (Freeark et al. 1967). In one case, PE was reported as early as 2 h after accident (Rogers et al. 2000). This may be one of the reasons of the apparent failure of prophylaxis of VTE

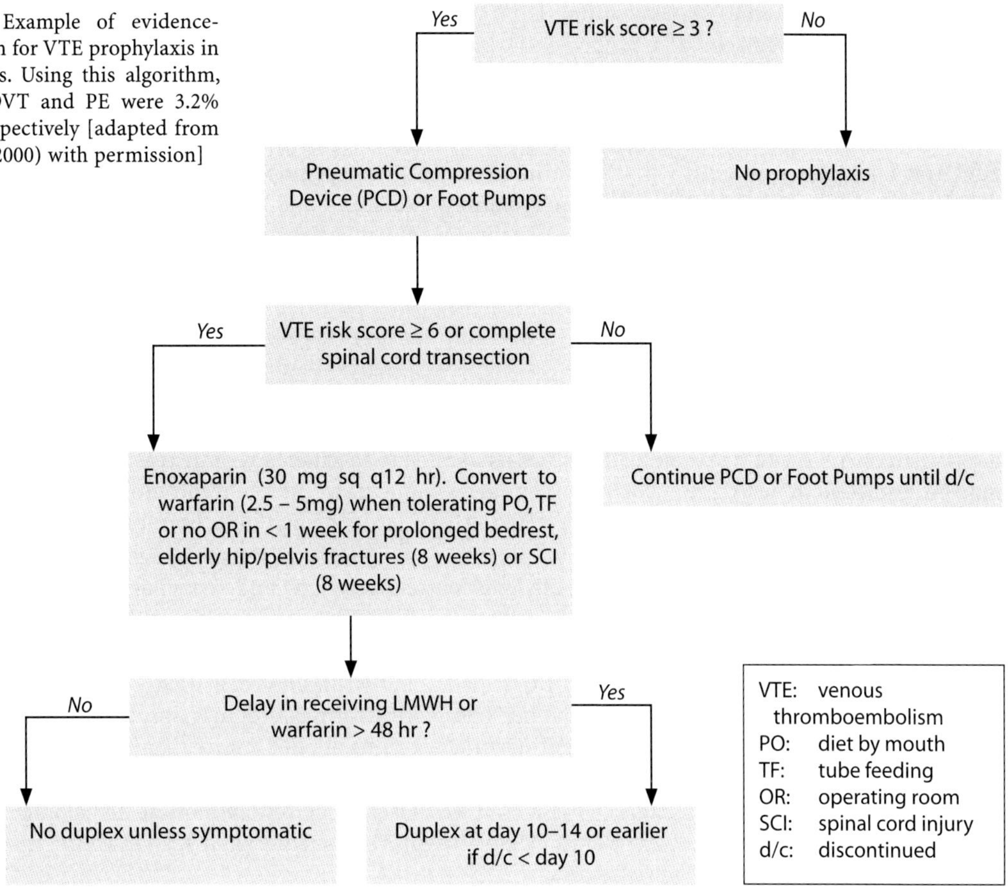

Diagram 19.1. Example of evidence-based algorithm for VTE prophylaxis in trauma patients. Using this algorithm, incidence of DVT and PE were 3.2% and 0.033% respectively [adapted from Wojcik et al. (2000) with permission]

at large in many published series and emphasizes the need for starting treatment early. Some series report 40%–70% of PE occurring during the 1st week after trauma (O'Malley and Ross 1990; Shackford et al. 1990; Rogers et al. 1993; Rodriguez et al. 1996; Hammers et al. 1996). As VTE manifests few specific symptoms and the clinical assessment is insensitive, the correct diagnosis is frequently delayed. The mean time from trauma to diagnosis of PE varies from 7 to 21 days in clinical studies (O'Malley and Ross 1990; Shackford et al. 1990; Ruiz et al. 1991; Rogers et al. 1993; Burns et al. 1993; Dennis et al. 1993; Knudson et al. 1994, 1996; Hill et al. 1994; Piotrowski et al. 1996; Hammers et al. 1996; Rodriguez et al. 1996; Wojcik et al. 2000).

19.7 Prophylaxis

Given the substantial risk of VTE, routine prophylaxis has become the standard of care for trauma patients. There are three major methods of preventing DVT and/or subsequent PE. The first involves pharmacological steering of coagulation, the second attempts to decrease stasis by increasing venous return from lower extremities, and the third concerns vena cava filter placement.

19.7.1 Low-Dose Heparin

The subcutaneous administration of low-dose heparin (LDH) two or three times a day at a dose of 5000 U is used for prophylaxis against DVT and PE. Until recently, LDH was the most widely accepted means of prophylaxis in the general surgical, orthopedic and urological patients (Clagett and Reisch 1988). In the general surgical population, LDH is given subcutaneously 2 h before operation and after surgery and is continued until the patients are fully ambulatory or discharged. Despite the fact that subcutaneous LDH is clearly effective in these patients, it is probably inappropriate as an isolated measure in high-risk trauma patients. Trauma patients differ from the general surgical patients in that prophylactic LDH cannot be given prior to the accident, thus much of its benefit may be lost (Ruiz et al. 1991; Meissner 1998). Once an intravascular clot has formed, LDH has no effect on fibrinolysis. In addition, trauma has been demonstrated to cause activation of the coagulation system, which may be more profound than in general surgery, rendering LDH insufficient (Ruiz et al. 1991; Knudson et al. 1994; Upchurch et al. 1995). Only a few studies have specifically looked at the use of LDH in trauma patients (Table 19.3). Most are nonrandomized or uncontrolled small studies, and most of the results were nonsignificant. Furthermore, LDH is associated with bleeding complications and its use may be precluded in head trauma or visceral injuries treated with expectant observation (Spain et al. 1997; Meissner 1998). A meta-analysis of 1102 patients revealed no benefit of heparin in VTE prophylaxis in trauma patients (9.9% with heparin; 7.2% without; P=0.77). Furthermore, the use of heparin provided no reduction in the occurrence of clinically detected PE (1.3% PE with heparin, 2.2% PE without heparin; P=0.16) (Upchurch et al. 1995). Recent trauma guidelines have concluded that there is enough accumulated data to warrant not using LDH in a trial in high-risk trauma patients (Pasquale et al. 1998).

19.7.2 Compression Devices

External pneumatic compression devices (PCDs) are an established form of prophylaxis for prevention of DVT in postoperative patients (Turpie et al. 1977, 1989; Clagett and Reisch 1988; Woolson and Watt 1991; Comerota et al. 1992; Fisher et al. 1995; Ramos et al. 1996). Single or multiple bladder systems can be used (Salzman et al. 1987). The sequential compression devices consist of a pair of sleeves containing multiple chambers, which are sequentially inflated from the ankle to the knee or mid-thigh (Fisher et al. 1995). Such devices theoretically act trough the complementary mechanisms of increasing blood velocities, reducing stasis and concentration of coagulation material, increasing plasmatic fibrinolytic activity by stimulating the release of bioactive agents from the blood vessel endothelium and reducing endothelial damage from venodilatation (Tarnay et al. 1980; Salzman et al. 1987; Summaria et al. 1988; Comerota et al. 1992; Fisher et al. 1995; Jacobs et al. 1996). PCDs would seem to be an ideal form of prophylaxis for the trauma patient, as they can be applied earlier than anticoagulation in patients with neurological injuries, major surgery or extensive visceral or retroperitoneal hematoma (Dennis et al. 1993; Spain et al. 1997; Velmahos et al. 1998). The

Table 19.3. Prophylactic use of low-dose heparin in trauma patients

Reference	Study design	Population	No. of patients		VTE incidence (%)		Results
			LDH	No LDH	LDH	No LDH	
Shackford et al. (1990)	Prospective nonrandomized	177 (719 admitted) high-risk (defined) patients receiving LDH, PCD or no prophylaxis	18	25	6	4	NS
Ruiz et al. (1991)	Prospective nonrandomized	100 consecutive severely injured (ISS ≥10) patients receiving LDH or no prophylaxis	50	50	28	2	P<0.0001
Dennis et al. (1993)	Prospective semirandomized	395 (ISS >9) patients receiving LDH, PCD or no prophylaxis	92	114	3	9	P<0.05
Knudson et al. (1994)	Prospective semirandomized	251 high-risk (defined) patients receiving LDH, PCD or no prophylaxis	63	91	3	4	NS
Napolitano et al. (1995)	Prospective nonrandomized	458 (5170 admitted) high-risk (defined) patients receiving LDH and/or PCD or no prophylaxis, screened by US	128	42	9	12	NS
Headrick et al. (1997)	Prospective nonrandomized	228 (1566 admitted) high-risk (defined) patients	20	24	25	25	NS

LDH, Low-dose heparin; *PCD*, pneumatic compression devices; *ISS*, Injury Severity Score; *NS*, nonsignificant; *US*, Ultrasound; *VTE*, venous thromboembolism.

Table 19.4. Prophylactic use of pneumatic compressive devices in trauma patients

Reference	Study design	Population	No. of patients		VTE incidence (%)		Results
			PCD	No PCD	PCD	No PCD	
SHACKFORD et al. (1990)	Prospective nonrandomized	177 (719 admitted) high-risk (defined) patients receiving LDH, PCD or no prophylaxis	81	25	6	4	NS
DENNIS et al. (1993)	Prospective semirandomized	395 patients (ISS >9) receiving LDH, PCD or no prophylaxis	189	114	3	9	P<0.05 especially for neurological trauma
GERSIN et al. (1994)	Prospective nonrandomized	32 trauma patients with GCS ≤8	14	18	28	22	NS
KNUDSON et al. (1994)	Prospective semirandomized	251 high-risk (defined) patients receiving LDH, PCD or no prophylaxis	58	103	7	7	P=0.057 for neurological trauma
NAPOLITANO et al. (1995)	Prospective nonrandomized	458 (5170 admitted) high-risk (defined) patients receiving LDH and/or PCD or no prophylaxis, screened by US	129	42	12	12	NS
FISHER et al. (1995)	Prospective randomized	304 patients with hip and pelvic fracture	145	159	6	18	P=0.03 for patients with hip fracture
HEADRICK et al. (1997)	Prospective nonrandomized	228 (1566 admitted) high-risk (defined) trauma patients	130	24	14	25	NS

LDH, low-dose heparin; *PCD*, pneumatic compression devices; *ISS*, Injury Severity Score; *NS*, nonsignificant.

results of different studies comparing the use of PCDs to no prophylaxis in trauma patients are shown in Table 19.4. With the exception of hip fracture, results were nonsignificant, although a tendency of decreasing DVT can be seen in patients with neurotrauma. PCDs cannot be applied in up to 35% of patients for various reasons: presence of cast or plaster, external fixation or traction devices, severe lower extremity wounds and potential lower extremity ischemia (SHACKFORD et al. 1990). Some teams have applied PCDs to the arms, which are known to have a high level of fibrinolytic activity, and demonstrated a reduction in DVT (KNIGHT and DAWSON 1976). PCDs have no effect in preventing clot formation in the pelvic veins (FISHER et al. 1995). Rare cases of complications are reported and include pressure necrosis (PARRA et al. 1989), peroneal palsy and compartment syndrome (PITTMAN 1989; LACHMAN et al. 1992), superficial skin changes (2%) (KNUDSON et al. 1996) or PE (SIDDIQUI et al. 2000).

Finally, a meta-analysis of studies conducted in over 1100 patients revealed no difference in the prophylaxis in trauma patients treated with LDH and PCD (11.8% VTE), LDH alone (9.3%), PCDs alone (7.3%), or no prophylaxis (7.1%) (KNUDSON et al. 1992, 1994; DENNIS et al. 1993; UPCHURCH et al. 1995; HEADRICK et al. 1997). Trauma guidelines currently recommend the use of PCDs in high-risk trauma patients, especially in patients with contraindications to anticoagulation, despite the lack of strong data to support their use (KELSEY et al. 2000).

19.7.3 Foot Pumps

Foot pumps (FPs) or arteriovenous impulse (AVI) compression systems, which require only access to the foot, have been suggested as an alternative when PCDs cannot be applied (ANGLEN et al. 1998; ELLIOTT et al. 1999). These devices work on the principle of the physiological foot pump, that is, normally accomplished by walking (COMEROTA et al. 1992; SPAIN et al. 1998). They can also be placed inside a cast if necessary. The results of FPs in trauma patients remain controversial. Two studies have demonstrated similar effectiveness of FPs compared to PCDs (PURTILL et al. 1997; SPAIN et al. 1998), while two others showed better results with PCDs (KNUDSON et al. 1996; ELLIOTT et al. 1999). Another study using FPs in trauma patients evidenced 57% of DVT at venography with 11% of proximal DVT and 2%

of PE, which is similar to trauma patients who do not receive prophylaxis (Geerts et al. 1999). FPs can thus be used as a substitute for sequential compression devices (PCDs) in high-risk trauma patients who cannot wear PCDs (Pasquale et al. 1998; Elliott et al. 1999).

19.7.4 Low-Molecular-Weight Heparin

Low-molecular-weight heparin (LMWH) contains the unique pentasaccharide required for specific binding to antithrombin III. Compared to unfractionated heparin, the advantages of LMWH in low doses include a higher and more predictable bioavailability (85% vs 10%), a longer biological half-life (one injection daily), less heparin-induced thrombocytopenia and theoretically fewer bleeding complications for equivalent antithrombotic doses (Hull et al. 1992; Warkentin et al. 1995; Leizorovicz 1996). LMWH rapidly achieves a peak level within 3–5 h after administration. Because hemostasis is not established in most patients until 12–24 h after operation, delaying the administration to 12–24 h ensures that wounds have been stabilized (Colwell et al. 1999).

Since 1984, numerous clinical trials with LMWH have been undertaken in patients undergoing major surgical procedures. Four large meta-analyses demonstrated a lower incidence of DVT using LMWH compared to unfractionated heparin in orthopedic surgery and a similar incidence in general surgery. There was no difference in the risk of major bleeding, although a tendency of a higher bleeding rate with LMWH in general surgery was suggested. No difference was found for PE. Minor bleeding was significantly reduced in the LMWH group, whereas no difference was found for major bleeding complications (Nurmohamed et al. 1992; Leizorovicz et al. 1992; Palmer et al. 1997a, b).

The number of available studies evaluating LMWH prophylaxis is limited for trauma patients (Table 19.5):

In the largest series comparing LMWH vs LDH, LMWH was more effective in prevention of DVT after major trauma (Geerts et al. 1996). The rates of DVT and proximal vein thrombosis were reduced by 43% and 65%, respectively, compared to 19% and 12% with LDH. The bleeding rate (2.9%) was not

Table 19.5. Prophylactic use of low-molecular-weight heparin in trauma patients

Reference	Study design	Population	No. of patients				VTE incidence (%)				Results	Diagnostic methods of DVT
			LMWH	PCD	FP	LDH	LMWH	PCD	FP	LDH		
Green et al. (1990)	Prospective randomized	41 from 87 patients with complete spinal cord injury	20	0	0	21	0	0	0	5 (24%)	*P*<0.02	IPG, US, serial Venography
Knudson et al. (1996)	Prospective randomized	202 from 372 high-risk (defined) patients	120	61	21	0	1 (1%)	1 (1.6%)	1 (5%)	0	NS (~historical control: 9.1% rate of DVT; *P*=0.037)	US
Geerts et al. (1996)	Prospective randomized	265 (1076 admitted) (ISS≥9) patients	129	0	0	136	Global: 40 (31%), Proximal: 8 (6.2%)	0	0	Global: 60 (44.1%), Proximal: 20 (14.7%)	Global: *P*=0.01, Proximal: *P*=0.01	Venography
Greenfield et al. (1997)	Prospective semi-randomized	53 high-risk (defined) patients	11	20	15	7	27%	40%	40%	56%	Pilot study → no conclusion	US
Cohn et al. (1999)	Prospective randomized	66 from 104 moderate-to high-risk (defined) patients	34	32	0	0	0	2 (6.2%)	0	0	NS, 5 bleeding complications in each group	Serial US
Norwood et al. (2001)	Prospective	118 from 439 (ISS≥9) patients	118	0	0	0	2 (1.7%)	0	0	0	0	US

LDH, low-dose heparin; *PCD*, pneumatic compression devices; *FP*, foot pumps; *NS*, Nonsignificant; *LMWH*, low-molecular-weight heparin; *US*, ultrasound.

significantly different from LDH (0.8%), although patients with intracranial bleeding were excluded from the trial. The authors suggested that from the perspective of the risks of VTE and its prevention, a major trauma should be considered analogous to orthopedic surgery of the lower extremity rather than to general surgery. The exact effect of LMWH on bleeding complications in trauma patients remains unclear (SPAIN et al. 1998). A 5% rate of bleeding complications possibly related to the use of LMWH was reported despite defined contraindications, which were severe neurological injury (GCS ≤8 or spinal cord injury), liver or spleen injuries managed conservatively, evidence of continued bleeding after 24 h, neck hematoma at admission and platelet count below 50,000 at 24 h after injury (KNUDSON et al. 1996).

LMWH can be safely started within 36 h of injury and there is generally no need for withdrawal in the event of a subsequent surgical procedure (GEERTS et al. 1996). LMWH or oral anticoagulation should be continued for several weeks after the injury in patients who remain at high risk for VTE. Refinements in contraindication to early initiation of LMWH include intracranial bleeding, incomplete spinal cord injury with perispinal hematoma, ongoing uncontrolled bleeding, and uncorrected coagulopathy (GEERTS et al. 2001).

These conditions may account to 25% of patients with major trauma at admission. Head injuries without frank hemorrhage, complete spinal cord injuries, laceration or contusion to the lung, liver, spleen or kidney, or the presence of retroperitoneal hematoma do not contraindicate the use of LMWH prophylaxis when no active bleeding is evidenced (GEERTS et al. 2001; NORWOOD et al. 2001). Cost-effectiveness is demonstrated by an estimated $2300 cost per additional life-year saved (DEVLIN et al. 1998). The current trauma guidelines recommend the use of LMWH in pelvic or complex lower extremity fractures, requiring operative fixation or bedrest longer than 5 days, and spinal cord injury with complete or incomplete motor paralysis (KELSEY et al. 2000).

19.7.5 Inferior Vena Cava Filter

19.7.5.1 General Use of Inferior Vena Cava Filters

The concept of ligating a vein in the management of VTE was first performed by John Hunter in 1784 on a femoral vein and by Bottini in 1893 at the level of the IVC (cited in REEKERS et al. 1999). Surgical ligation, plication and clipping of the IVC were the methods of choice until the early 1970s. A high associated morbidity and mortality of up to 21%–41% have been reported, although this rate probably reflects the underlying status more than the process itself (CRANE 1964; NABSETH and MORAN 1965). In 1969, an intracaval umbrella-type filter was introduced in clinical practice (MOBIN-UDDIN et al. 1969). The first model was associated with a high rate of caval occlusion (60%–70%). In 1973, a new filter, capturing emboli without impeding blood flow, was introduced (GREENFIELD et al. 1973). These filters, having a large caliber of 22–24 F, must be inserted by means of venotomy.

The next step in the development of inferior vena cava filter (IVCF) was the percutaneous insertion of the device, thanks to the progressive reduction in filter size (Fig. 19.1). In 1977, a Nitinol filter composed of a memory shape alloy, was inserted through a 9-F delivery system via an antecubital vein (SIMON et al. 1977). The lower external diameter of the introducer carried a lower rate of venous thrombosis at the insertion site. Complications of IVCF have been markedly reduced over the years by modifications in the filter design (Fig. 19.2). New filters are made of biocompatible metals, which are not thrombogenic and are magnetic resonance-compatible. The easy access to caval interruption partly explains the increase in indications coming in the 1980s and the 1990s, with great differences among European countries (ALEXANDER et al. 1994). Large series or meta-analyses have reported the effectiveness and the complications of IVCF in patients with VTE. The overall frequency of recurrent PE is between 2% and 5.6%, with approximately 0.7%–3.8% of fatal recurrent PE (BECKER et al. 1992; FERRIS et al. 1993; GREENFIELD and PROCTOR 1995; BALLEW et al. 1995; REEKERS et al. 1999; GIRARD et al. 2000; ATHANASOULIS et al. 2000). Death from PE, despite IVCF, can be explained by the fact that small clots can pass through the filter, especially when nonautomatically centered filters are placed in an eccentric oblique position, through collateral circulation or by the formation of clots in or above the filter (KATSAMOURIS et al. 1988; TARDY et al. 1996; GIRARD et al. 2000).

Complications can be listed as follows:

- Fatal complications of IVC are rare, only four cases have been reported in a large review of the literature (BALLEW et al. 1995).

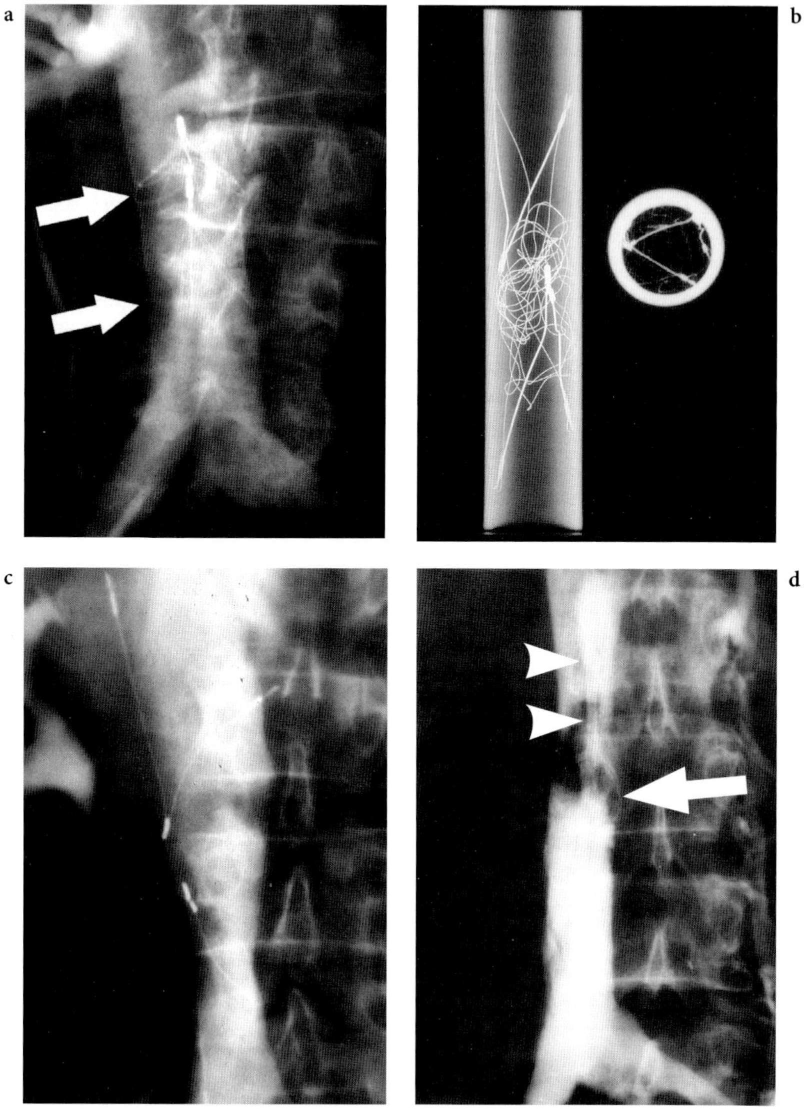

Fig. 19.1a–d. Types of inferior vena cava filters. **a** Simon Nitinol filter. The filter (*arrows*) is anchored to the caval wall by the caudal prongs only. **b** Bird's nest filter: in vitro deployment shows coiling of the filament within a tube in a longitudinal and axial view. **c** Bird's nest filter: the filter adapts to a large diameter of the inferior vena cava. The anchoring prongs are highly radio-opaque, but not the filaments. **d** Protect infusion catheter filter. The temporary filter was introduced via a jugular vein access. The arrowheads point at the catheter. A thrombus is entrapped at the level of the filter (*arrow*) with cranial extension, resulting either from venous embolism or local thrombosis

- Complications during insertion are reported in 4%–11% (mean, 5%): hematoma at insertion site, air embolism, wound infection, pneumothorax, vocal cord paralysis or hoarseness, retroperitoneal pain, stroke, deployment problems, and misplacement of IVCF (tilting, asymmetry of filter struts, anatomical variants or embolization to the heart or pulmonary arteries).
- DVT at the insertion site. The reported incidence varied from 0% to 41%. The femoral route for insertion should be preferred as, in opposition to insertion via the jugular vein, IVCF will protect against lung embolization of a potential DVT at the insertion site.
- Caval obstruction. The reported frequency varies from 3.2% to 30%, depending on the type of filter. Occlusion usually results from entrapment of a major embolus by the filter, rather than thrombus formation in loco. Caval occlusion most frequently occurs in patients with neoplasms.
- Subsequent new DVT and venous insufficiency. The influence of IVCF on a new DVT is difficult to estimate, as venous insufficiency can also be encountered in patients treated only with anticoagulation. The reported incidence is 0%–59%.
- Caval wall penetration by the filter has been reported in 0%–29% of patients, and rarely has clinical symptoms from vascular or GI tract perforation.
- Filter migration. Late migration occurs most frequently caudally, and rarely to the cardiac cavities. The reported incidence is 0.1%–69%.
- Filter fracture can be seen in 0.2%–2.2%, depending on the type of filter.

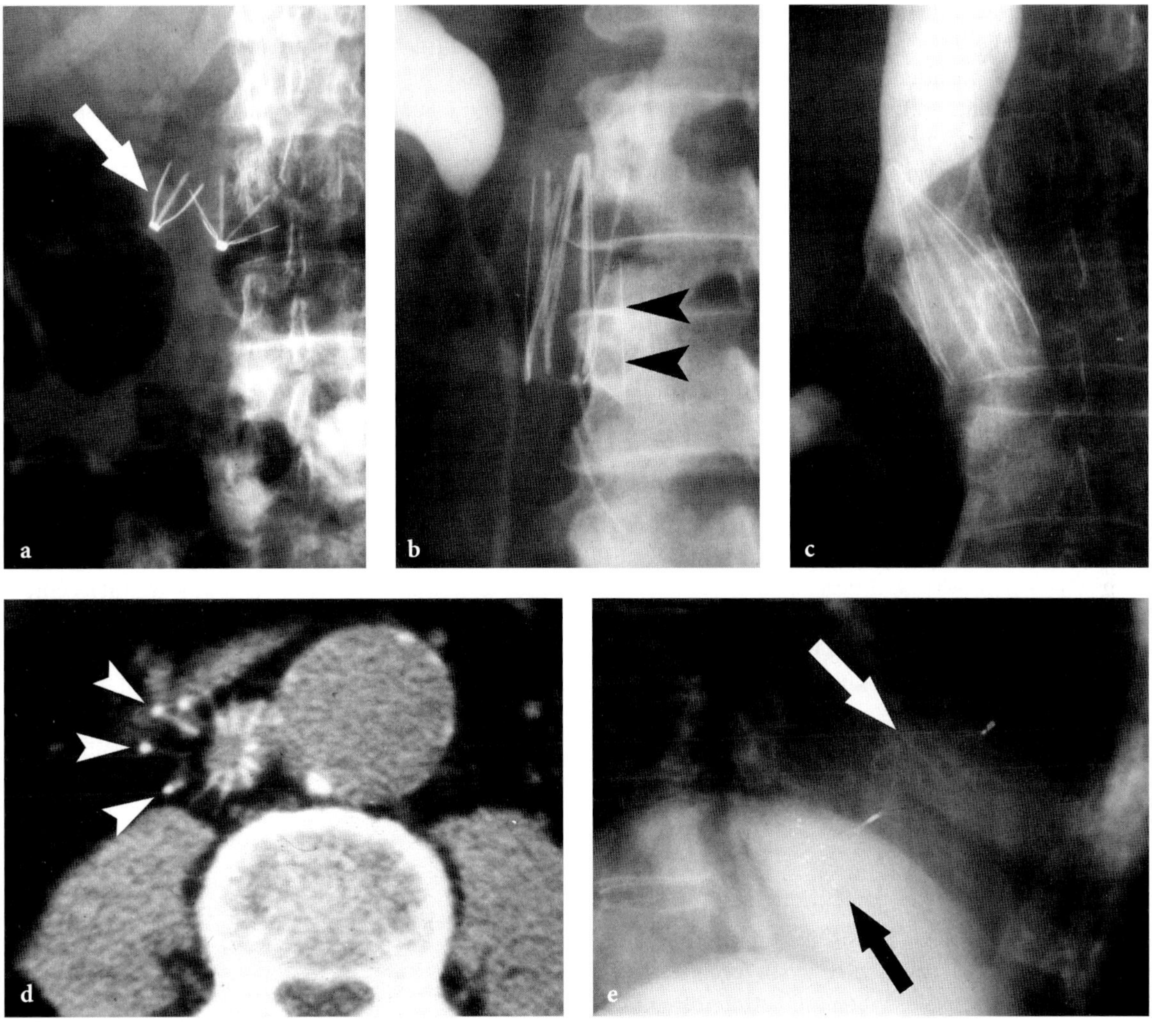

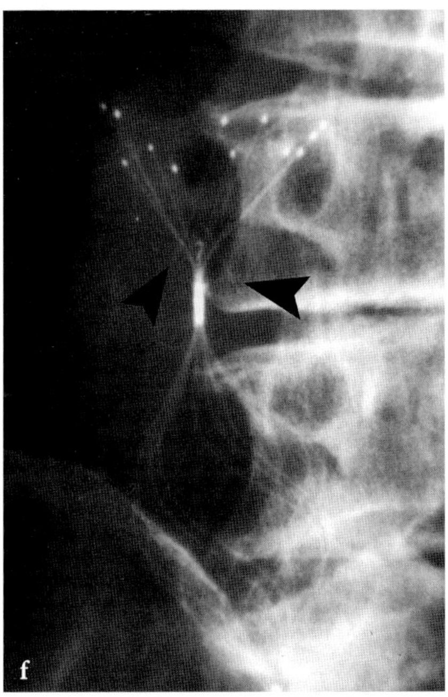

Fig. 19.2a–f. Complications of inferior vena cava filter. **a** Mobin-Udin umbrella. The stiff insertion device of this filter was occasionally responsible for misplacement of the filter, as in this case, in the right renal vein (*arrow*). Another filter was correctly placed in the IVC. **b** Fracture of a strut in a LGM filter (*arrowheads*). **c** Cone-shaped filters adopt a position parallel to the IVC at the level of placement. Filtering capability is decreased, in case of angulation of the IVC adjacent to the filter. **d** Perforation of the wall of IVC. When local chronic retraction of the IVC has occurred at the level of filter placement, the prongs of some filter designs (here a Gunther basket filter) may perforate the caval wall (*arrowheads*), usually without consequences. **e** Migration of Gunther basket filter to the right heart. This Gunther basket filter had been introduced the wrong way through the femoral vein and was immediately washed to the right heart (*arrows*). Percutaneous retrieval was successful. **f** Fracture of struts in a Gunther basket filter (*arrowheads*)

The ideal filter does not exist. As the hundreds of published papers reporting immediate and long-term outcome of patients with IVCF are difficult to compare, the relative efficacy and safety of the available devices is difficult to assess (Greenfield et al. 1999). Furthermore, cost is variable from country to country: in the US an IVCF costs approximately US $5000, whereas average cost is US $800 in Europe (Girard et al. 2000). To date, only one multicenter randomized trial has evaluated the benefits and risks of IVCF and anticoagulation versus anticoagulation alone in 400 patients with proximal DVT. This study demonstrated a short-term benefit of IVCF, with a significant lower rate of recurrent PE (1.1 vs 4.8%) at day 12, whereas the difference was no longer significant at 2 years follow-up (3.4% vs 6.3%). These results were opposed by a significant increase of recurrent DVT and possibly postphlebitic syndrome (20.8% vs 11.6%). There was no difference concerning both short- and long-term mortality, and bleeding complications between both groups (Decousus et al. 1998). These results may suggest a theoretical argument in favor of temporary filters.

19.7.5.2 Prophylactic Inferior Vena Cava Filter in Trauma Patients

Prophylactic inferior vena cava filter (PIVCF) is a form of PE prophylaxis that is used more frequently in trauma patients, especially when even a minor amount of bleeding as a complication of anticoagulation cannot be tolerated (Pasquale et al. 1998). When thromboprophylaxis fails, anticoagulation with heparin followed by oral anticoagulation remains the method of choice for prevention of progression or recurrence of VTE. Bleeding complications are certainly the most significant risk in trauma patients. A 36% rate of severe bleeding has been reported, even in low-risk trauma patients, necessitating termination of therapy. Complications included recurrent PE, subdural hematoma, hemothorax, hemopericardium, heparin-induced thrombocytopenia, retroperitoneal hematoma and a drop in blood pressure or hemoglobin level. Age over 55 years was associated with an increased risk and was an indication for IVC filter placement (Brathwaite et al. 1993).

Two major indications for IVCF have to be considered in trauma patients: therapeutic, when VTE has been proved by diagnostic methods, and prophylactic, in patients at high risk of PE. Thromboprophylaxis with LDH or compression devices reduces the rate of VTE to 10%, which remains higher than the reported rate of 5%–7% in general surgical patients, even though trauma patients are usually younger and have no previous history of venous disease (Khansarinia et al. 1995). Furthermore, 14% of the high-risk group could not receive prophylaxis because of a contraindication to anticoagulation, and up to 35% cannot effectively tolerate compression devices (Shackford et al. 1990). The risk factors are present within the first hours following injury. Delaying anticoagulation prophylaxis until the patient has had an operation or waiting for a decrease in bleeding risk, may result in increased morbidity or mortality (Greenfield et al. 2000). Ideally, IVCF should be inserted immediately after admission to a trauma center for a maximal protection against PE (Khansarinia et al. 1995). This has led to an increasing use of prophylactic IVCF in high-risk trauma patients over the past 10 years in an attempt to decrease the incidence of PE and has even become standard practice in many trauma centers (Britt et al. 1996; McMurtry et al. 1999). The indications for IVCF in trauma patients can be derived from nontrauma patients (Pasquale et al. 1998) and are listed in Table 19.6.

Table 19.6. Indications of inferior vena cava filter placement

Absolute indications:
Recurrent PE despite full anticoagulation
DVT and contraindication to full anticoagulation
DVT and major bleeding while on full anticoagulation
Progression of DVT (iliofemoral) despite anticoagulation
Extended or Debated indications:
After massive PE, when recurrent PE may prove fatal
Free-floating DVT in pelvic veins or IVC
During or after surgical embolectomy
Prophylactic indications:
Severe closed head injury (GCS <8)
Spinal cord injury
Complex pelvic fracture
Multiple long-bone fractures
Major eye injury

Table 19.7 is extracted from the clinical studies published so far on the use of prophylactic IVCF in trauma patients with no previous episode of VTE. Most studies are nonprospective, nonrandomized and uncontrolled trials, comparing results with historical controls and using variable outcomes and periods of follow-up, rendering any comparison difficult (Velmahos et al. 2000; Wojcik et al. 2000). Nevertheless, it is obvious that although early placement of prophylactic IVCF does not prevent DVT, it prevents the occurrence of PE in high-risk patients, with a success rate of 97%–100%, although the pos-

sibility of PE originating from upper extremity vein thrombosis is not eliminated. The overall mortality rate of PE is significantly reduced in some series (KHANSARINIA et al. 1995), but not significantly in others (RODRIGUEZ et al. 1996). One report suggests inserting IVCF, once DVT has been diagnosed by serial US (HEADRICK et al. 1997). Since there is no question that prophylactic IVCF reduces the rate of PE, the real issue is how to define the high-risk population that can benefit from IVCF, the short-term and long-term complications and the cost-effectiveness of prophylactic IVCF.

19.7.5.3
High-Risk Population

The more predictable high-risk population that can benefit from IVCF prophylaxis remains undetermined. Only 9%–30% of patients will present DVT after IVCF insertion, suggesting that 70%–91% are unnecessary. One study found four groups of trauma patients that accounted for 92% of PE:

- Age over 55 years with isolated long bone fracture
- Severe head injury with coma
- Multiple long bone fractures and pelvic fracture
- Spinal cord injury with paraplegia or quadriplegia

The authors estimated that the risk of PE in these groups ranged from 2.1% (head injuries) to 5.4% (spinal cord injuries), a relative risk that is 21–54 times that of the global trauma population (0.1%) of the same study. The three latter categories were considered candidates for prophylactic IVCF and represented less than 5% of trauma patients. The overall incidence of PE dropped from 1% in historical controls to 0.25% when using IVCF (ROGERS et al. 1993).

Another trauma center defines four high-risk groups for PE despite prophylaxis by LDH, PCD or both when not contraindicated:

- Head and spinal cord injuries
- Head injury and long bone fracture
- Severe pelvis and long bone fracture
- Multiple long bone fractures

They estimated that routine prophylactic placement of IVCF in those patients (particularly the three latter categories, representing 2% of their trauma population) should significantly decrease the incidence of PE (WINCHELL et al. 1994).

Both studies concluded that patients with an estimated risk of PE despite prophylaxis of greater that 2%–5% are reasonable candidates for IVCF prophylaxis, especially if conventional measures cannot be used.

Patients with para- or quadriplegia remain at risk for PE long after termination of acute care (75% of PE occur after acute care discharge), at a time when standard prophylaxis is often discontinued (WILSON et al. 1994). Spinal cord injuries may be one of the best indications for prophylactic IVCF, as they represent 4% of all trauma admissions, but account for 31% of all post-traumatic PE, with 0.3–20% being lethal.

Patients with penetrating iliofemoral venous injury are also a high-risk group, with VTE occurring in 43%–75% of patients (DENNIS et al. 1993; SUE et al. 1995). Nevertheless, the best indication remains high-risk patients who are not candidates for pharmacological or mechanical prophylaxis.

19.7.5.4
Short- and Long-Term Complications

There is much controversy about the relatively low incidence of fatal PE, the perceived risk of filter insertion, the filter's permanence and its potential for late complications (QUIRKE et al. 1997). Inserting a prophylactic IVCF in a young trauma patient without pre-existing VTE is not a benign intervention and requires a basic understanding of the risk-benefit ratio (WOJCIK et al. 2000). Local venous thrombosis at the insertion site is a rare event. Half of DVTs are contralateral to the insertion site (LANGAN et al. 1999). The short-term IVC patency varied between 90% and 100%. Some authors think that the mere presence of IVCF does not contribute to significant morbidity and the underlying process, post-traumatic VTE, is the cause of caval thrombosis, as the filter traps potential emboli usually early in the clinical course (RODRIGUEZ et al. 1996). Considering the alternative of allowing the embolus to proceed to the lung, it seems appropriate to accept the risk of early obstruction, particularly because many will ultimately recanalize (GREENFIELD et al. 1994; PATTON et al. 1996). A case of phlegmasia cerulea dolens following insertion of a Greenfield filter has been reported (WEBB et al. 1992).

The long-term follow-up is presented in Table 19.8. Whether insertion of prophylactic IVCF renders patients more prone to subsequent DVT and postphlebitic syndrome is controversial (PATTON et al. 1996; RODRIGUEZ et al. 1996). Nevertheless, the 24.6% incidence of DVT after IVCF placement highlights the importance of providing DVT prophylaxis whenever possible. There seems to be no propensity towards an increased prevalence of DVT or caval

Table 19.7. Prophylactic inferior vena cava filter in trauma patients

Reference	Type of study	Patient population	Method of diagnosis for PE and DVT	PIVCF group							Control groups						Results
											No PIVCF group			Historical			
				(*n*)	PE (%)	DVT (%)	Insertion compli-cations (%)	Delay between trauma & insertion	IVC patency (%)	Associated treatment	(n)	PE (%)	DVT (%)	(*n*)	PE (%)	DVT (%)	
Webb et al. (1992)	Nonrandomized prospective	24 HR (defined) trauma pts from 51 undergoing surgery for acetabular fractures	Clinical	24	0	1 (4.12)	0	During surgery	-	LDH and PCD	27	2 (7.4) 1 fatal	1 (3.7)	-	-	-	PIVCF is efficacious for preventing fatal PE in this HR group
Matous et al. (1993)	Nonrandomized retrospective	52 HR (defined) from 5280 admitted trauma pts (1%)	-	52	0	-	-	-	-	-	-	-	-	-	-	-	-
Rogers et al. (1993)	Nonrandomized prospective	34 HR (defined) pts with CI to AC, from 792 admitted trauma pts (4.3%)	PE: clinical DVT: IPG weekly	34	0	6 (17.6)	0	<3 d	89	PCD	758	2 (0.26)	-	2525	25 (1) 7 fatal	-	Less PE in the study group vs historical control (0.25% vs 1%) (*P*<0.05)
Leach et al. (1994)	Nonrandomized retrospective	200 HR (defined) from 10948 admitted trauma pts (1.8%)	-	200	0	-	8 (4)	-	100	-	10748	4 fatal (0.04)	-	1257	11 (0.9)	-	Less fatal PE during the study period compared to historical control
Rosenthal et al. (1994)	Nonrandomized retrospective	67 trauma pts including 29 having CI to AC or PCD from 161 admitted trauma pts with ISS >16	Clinical	29	0	-	1 (3)	-	100	-	38	1 (2.6)	9 (23.6)	94	22 (23.4) 5 fatal	19 (20)	Less PE in the study group vs historical control (1.5% vs 23.4%)
Wilson et al. (1994)	Nonrandomized prospective	15 consecutive pts with traumatic spinal cord injury	PE: clinical DVT: IPG weekly	15	0	0	0	-	82	LDH or PCD	-	-	-	111	7 (6.3) 3 fatal	-	PIVCF is effective for preventing PE in this condition
Khansarinia et al. (1995)	Nonrandomized prospective	108 HR (defined) from 6558 admitted trauma pts (1.6%)	PE: clinical DVT: US screening weekly	108	0	10 (9)	2 (1.85)	11.9 d	-	LDH or PCD if not CI	6448	2 fatal (0.03)	-	216	13 (6) 9 fatal	-	Less PE in the PIVCF group vs historical control, *P*<0.009 Less PE-related death, *P*<0.03
Rogers et al. (1995)	Nonrandomized prospective	63 HR (defined) pts having CI to AC, from 3151 admitted trauma pts (2%)	PE: clinical DVT: IPG weekly	63	1 (1.6) 1 fatal	19 (30)	2 (3.1)	4.3 d	96	PCD	3088	6 (0.2)	-	2525	25 (1) 7 fatal	-	Less PE in the study group vs historical control (0.2% vs 1%) (*P*<0.001)

Zolfaghari et al. (1995)	Nonrandomized retrospective	29 trauma pts with extended indications for PIVCF among 3005 admitted trauma pts (1 %)	Clinical	29	0	–	0	11.4 d	–	LDH or PCD	2976	– (<1)	–	–	–	–	Aggressive use of PIVCF decreased the incidence of PE
Patton et al. (1996)	Nonrandomized retrospective	110 HR (defined) from 15526 admitted trauma pts (0.7%)	Clinical	110	0	7 (6.4)	6 (5.4)	10.4 d	99	LDH and PCD if not CI							–
Rodriguez et al. (1996)	Nonrandomized prospective	40 HR (defined) trauma pts	Clinical	40	1 (2.5)	6 (15)	0	3 d	90	LDH or PCD	–	–	–	80	14 (17.5) 8 fatal	15 (19)	Less PE in the IVCF group vs control, P=0.02 No significant difference for PE-related mortality DVT: DTV: IVCF group vs control, NS
Gosin et al. (1997)	Nonrandomized retrospective	250 HR (defined) trauma pts	PE: clinical	99	0	–	0	1 week	–	–	1531 151 HR	15 (1) 4 (2.6)	–	249	12 (4.8)	–	Less PE in the study group vs historical control, P=0.045 Less PE in the IVCF group vs historical control, P<0.02
Rogers et al. (1997)	Nonrandomized prospective	35 HR (defined) pts from 940 admitted orthopedic trauma pts (3.7%)	PE: clinical DVT: IPG weekly	35	1 (2.8)	–	2 (5.7)	<3 d	94	PCD	905	1 (0.1)	–	1150	11 (1) 4 fatal	–	Less PE in the study group vs historical control (0.2% vs 1%) (P<0.04)
Rogers et al. (1998)	Nonrandomized prospective	132 HR (defined) trauma pts having CI to AC, from 5280 admitted trauma pts (2.5%)	PE: clinical DVT: IGP or US weekly	132	3 (2.3) 1 fatal	16 (12)	4 (3)	<3 d	97	PCD	–	–	–	–	–	–	–
Langan et al. (1999)	Nonrandomized retrospective	187 HR (defined) from 7333 admitted trauma pts (2.5%)	Clinical US at FU	187	1 (0.5)	24 (12.8)	3 (1.6)	–	100	LDH or PCD if not CI	3788	5 (0.13)	61 (1.6)	–	–	–	PE: IVCF group vs control: NS More DVT in the IVCF group vs control, P=0.001
McMurtry et al. (1999)	Non randomized retrospective	248 HR (defined) from 28227 admitted trauma pts (0.9 %)	Clinical	248	4 (1.6)	6 (2.4)	7 (2.8)	5 d	99	PCD or LDH if not CI	27979	108 (0.4)	–	–	–	–	Increased use of PIVCF failed to reduce the rate of PE

AC, anticoagulation; CI, contraindication; d, days; DVT, deep vein thrombosis; FU, follow-up; HR, high risk; IPG, impedance plethysmography; ISS, injury severity score; LDH, low-dose heparin; NS, nonsignificant; n, number; PCD pneumatic compression device; PE, pulmonary embolism; PIVCF, prophylactic inferior vena cava filter; pts, patients; US, ultrasound.

Table 19.8. Long-term follow-up of prophylactic inferior vena cava filter

Reference	No.	No. of pts for follow-up	PE (%)	New DVT (%)	Leg swelling (%)	IVC occlusion (%)	Mean follow-up (months)
Rosenthal et al. (1994)	29	25	0	0	0	0	32.8
Patton et al. (1996)	110	45	0	14	11	0	19
Rodriguez et al. (1996)	40	38	1	6	4	4	12
Rogers et al. (1998)	132	47	3	10	–	1	20
Langan et al. (1999)	187	75	1	24	27	0	19.4
Greenfield et al. (2000)	249	197	3	39	38	5	29
Wojcik et al. (2000)	191[a]	64[b]	0	28	3	0	28.9
TOTAL	938	491 (52.3)	8 (1.6)	121 (24.6)	83 (16.9)	10 (2)	26.1

[a] Include both prophylactic and therapeutic inferior vena cava filter.
[b] Only patients with prophylactic IVCF are considered.

thrombosis over time (Greenfield et al. 1994; Patton et al. 1996). Long-term follow-up shows high caval patency (98%) and a low rate of PE (1.6%). The incidence of PE is higher in patients who had a severe strut malposition or filter tilting (Rogers et al. 1998). In a study comparing the long-term outcomes of prophylactic and therapeutic IVCF over a 9-year period, the prophylaxis group had less lower extremity edema, was anticoagulated less often, used support stocking less often, but had a comparable incidence of venous ulceration (Greenfield et al. 2000). Early or late entrapment of IVCF by blind manipulation of a guidewire or catheter, frequently used in trauma patients, can usually be avoided with careful technique. In any case of doubt or problem, imaging modalities should be obtained (Streib and Wagner 2000; Barraco and Scalea 2000).

19.7.5.5 Cost-Effectiveness

Need and risk of IVCF in trauma patients should be assessed by clinical judgment (Gosin et al. 1997). More focused risk stratification is needed to select the 25% of the trauma patients who are at risk of VTE, to decrease the number of IVCF and improve cost-effectiveness (Langan et al. 1999; Greenfield et al. 2000).

19.7.5.6 Bedside Insertion of IVCF

Most patients with massive injuries, who require an IVCF, can be safely transported to the interventional radiological suite for placement. In some trauma patients with relative contraindications to transportation out of the ICU, IVCF can be placed at the patient's bedside, with fluoroscopy guidance (Sing et al. 1998, 2001; Tola et al. 1999), portable duplex US (Nunn et al. 1997; Neuzil et al. 1998; Benjamin et al. 1999; Sato et al. 1999), or a combined fluoroscopy-US technique (Rose et al. 1997). Fluoroscopy has the advantage of allowing cavography, used to localize the renal veins. Iodinated contrast-medium injection is required, although bedside carbon dioxide vena cavagrams have been recently described (Dewald et al. 2000; Sing et al. 2000, 2001). Recently, US has been used to guide the bedside insertion of IVCF. US makes it possible to visualize the optimal site of filter placement and the size of the vena cava; deployment and position of the filter are immediately apparent. An adequate visualization of the anatomical landmarks is achieved in 85%–93%. Main causes of failure of insertion under US guidance are obesity, bowel gas or subcutaneous emphysema, or massive abdominal injuries. A dilated IVC may require insertion of a Bird's nest filter, which is, however, best achieved under fluoroscopic guidance. Introduction of IVCF at the patient's bedside under US guidance is more operator-dependent, as demonstrated by the learning curves (Nunn et al. 1997; Sato et al. 1999). The use of intravascular US as an imaging guidance has also been recently described (Bonn et al. 1999; Matsumura and Morasch 2000; Ebaugh et al. 2001). The early results of beside insertion of IVCF suggest a complication rate similar to those described with the standard fluoroscopic guidance. Cost is decreased, compared to the use of a radiological suite or operating room, although cost savings can vary from country to country.

19.7.5.7 Temporary Filter

In contrast to patients with nontrauma-related DVT, who have a lifelong increased risk of recurrent DVT, most trauma patients do not have a decreased life expectancy and have reversible risk factors for VTE, which means that their theoretical risk will return to baseline (McMurtry et al. 1999). Most trauma patients require a short period of protection with a filter before prophylactic anticoagulation can be initiated. This consideration has been suggested as a potential indication for temporary or retrievable IVCF (Quirke et al. 1997).

As most complications of IVCF are delayed, it is assumed that early retrieval of the filter would reduce the rate of complications. The potential clinical indications of temporary or retrievable IVCF are reported in Table 19.9.

Table 19.9. Potential indications of temporary or retrievable IVCF (Modified from Millward [1998] and Zwaan et al. [1998])

- Prophylaxis in trauma patients
- Protection during thrombolytic therapy for lower extremity DVT
- Patients presenting with VTE and a short term contraindication to anticoagulation (i.e., neurosurgery)
- Prophylactic placement after PE or DVT in patients with poor cardiopulmonary reserve or with contraindication to anticoagulation
- Protection during abdominal surgery in patients with known pelvic DVT
- DVT during pregnancy
- Free-floating iliac vein or IVC clot
- Orthopedic surgery

There are two types of nonpermanent IVCF.

- The temporary IVCF is a filter attached to a catheter or a guidewire with a proximal extremity that protrudes from the insertion site or is buried in the soft tissue adjacent to the puncture site. Compared to retrievable IVCF, temporary IVCFs have a higher risk of infection, which limits the duration for which the device may be kept in place. Furthermore, the risk of air embolism, skin infection and hematoma is higher. They must be removed despite ongoing contraindications to anticoagulation, requiring in some cases placement of a permanent filter. If contraindication to anticoagulation is anticipated to be longer than 10 days, a permanent IVCF should be directly inserted (Millward 1998).
- The retrievable IVCF is a permanent filter that can be removed by snaring a hook on the filter. Such IVCFs have a relatively complex and higher-cost removal technique compared to the temporary filter (Millward 1998). Experimental work in vitro has demonstrated that the clot-trapping ability of temporary IVCF devices is superior to that of permanent IVCFs, especially for small and multiple clots (Stoneham et al. 1995).

Numerous temporary and retrievable filters are currently under evaluation. At the moment, there is, however, insufficient evidence for promoting routine clinical use. Some of the nonpermanent IVCFs are modified versions of existing permanent filters. Design of these filters evolves rapidly. Some have a short half-life and others are withdrawn from the market due to lethal complications. The temporary IVCFs include the Günther Temporary Filter (Millward et al. 1994; Vos et al. 1997; Zwaan et al. 1998), the Protect Infusion Catheter (Millward 1998; Hughes et al. 1999), the Bird's Nest Filter (Cope et al. 1996), the Nitinol Retrievable Filter (Nakagawa et al. 1994), the Tempofilter (Bovyn et al. 1997) (withdrawn from the market), the Antheor Filter (Zwaan et al. 1998; Millward 1998), the Prothia Filter (Thery et al. 1990), the Filcard and the Lysofilter (Pieri et al. 1993) and others including the DIL filter, the FCP-2002 Filter and the Angiocor Filter (Zwaan et al. 1998, Millward 1998). The retrievable filters include the Amplatz Filter (Epstein et al. 1989), the Günther Tulip Filter (Neuerburg et al. 1993, 1997; Khong and John 1997; Millward et al. 2000), and the Irie Filter (Irie et al. 1995; Vesely et al. 1996).

The complications reported include vein thrombosis at the insertion site, IVC thrombosis, recurrent PE after filter retrieval, infection of the device, hematoma at the insertion site, requirement of replacement by a permanent filter, air embolism, filter rupture, migration, tilting and cardiac perforation (Thery et al. 1992; Vos et al. 1997; Bovyn et al. 1997; Neuerburg et al. 1997; Zwaan et al. 1998; Millward et al. 1998, 2000). The rate of complication varied between the different types of temporary or retrievable IVCFs and even between different teams using the same device. For example, Vos and Zwaan had a low rate of complications using the Günther Temporary Filter, whereas Millward abandoned the use of this type of filter due to a 47% rate of complications. This may be partly explained by the variable patient selection in preliminary studies (Millward et al. 1994; Millward 1998; Vos et al. 1997; Zwaan et al. 1998).

Five papers reported the use of temporary or retrievable filters in trauma patients (Millward 1998; Millward et al. 1994, 2000; Bovyn et al. 1997; Hughes et al. 1999). The filter is left in place until the contraindication to anticoagulation has vanished. For temporary filters, the jugular route is preferred, as the direction to the IVC is straighter, it has fewer restrictions on patient mobility, and a lower risk of infection. This route, however, can be problematic when a permanent filter has to be inserted before retrieval of a temporary filter, and more risky when retrieval is required due to heart catheterization. A preretrieval inferior vena cavagram, intravascular ultrasound or abdominal CT should always be performed before the procedure, as a large amount of clots can be trapped in the device (Fig. 19.1D). Local thrombolysis can be given in such cases, the thrombolytic agent being perfused through the lumen of the catheter of retrievable filters. Otherwise, a permanent IVCF can be inserted above the temporary filter. Small clots are allowed to embolize to the lungs. Most of the clots adherent to the filter can be retrieved along with the device. Up to 40% of filters have trapped thrombi without IVC thrombosis at the time of removal (Thery et al. 1990; Millward 1998). The learning curve for retrieval of the device is short; the procedure takes a mean of 5.3 min (2–13 min) of fluoroscopy (Millward et al. 2000). The maximum duration of implantation time shows a considerable variation between devices, varying from 12 to 55 days (Bovyn et al. 1997). The Günther Tulip Filter should be retrieved by 13 days, but one series reported successful retrieval after a mean of 23 days (Abbott 1999).

Overall, the risk-benefit ratio is favorable in trauma patients (Pasquale et al. 1998). Some authors consider placement of prophylactic IVCF only when no other option is available (McMurtry et al. 1999), while others advocate their use together with DVT prophylaxis whenever possible, until a proven better method of PE protection is found (Langan et al. 1999).

Prophylaxis should be continued after hospital discharge in some high-risk patients and those requiring prolonged bedrest or rehabilitation until they achieve normal ambulatory status, as many as 40% of VTE episodes can occur after discharge (Schwarcz et al. 2001).

In summary, providing thromboprophylaxis to patients who have sustained multiple post-traumatic injuries remains a significant challenge (Greenfield et al. 2000). A recent meta-analysis of trauma series showed no clear advantage of one method of prophylaxis over another and over no prophylaxis at all, probably related to many factors, including a nonuniform population and a small sample size (Velmahos et al. 2000). A large prospective and randomized multicenter trial based on the design published by Greenfield is ongoing. It is comparing results of prophylaxis using LDH, PCD, FPs and LMWH as well as the use of the IVC filter. The following conclusions are based on the 6th ACCP consensus conference on antithrombotic therapy (Geerts et al. 2001). Thromboprophylaxis must be discussed on a per patient basis, according to his or her VTE risk, bleeding risk, trauma condition and prognosis. The appropriate prophylaxis has to be started as soon as possible and should be continued until discharge. LMWH seems to be the simplest, most efficient and cost-effective thromboprophylactic method that is currently available for high-risk trauma patients when not contraindicated (Goldhaber 1998; Wade and Chisholm 2000). More effective and safer new indirect thrombin inhibitors and direct thrombin inhibitors are currently under investigation (Pini 1999). PCDs may be useful in patients with intracranial bleeding and possibly as the initial prophylaxis for patients at high risk of bleeding until anticoagulation can be started. The potential benefit and cost-effectiveness of the combination of mechanical and pharmacological prophylaxis remain to be demonstrated. IVCF insertion is primarily indicated for patients with documented threatening DVT and contraindication to full anticoagulation. The prophylactic insertion of IVCF remains controversial.

19.8 Screening of Venous Thromboembolism

The limited effectiveness of most prophylactic methods has led to the concept of a systematic screening for nonsymptomatic DVT in high-risk trauma patients. The availability of a sensitive and specific noninvasive diagnostic technique for DVT would be useful both for daily clinical practice and for clinical trials on the prevention of DVT (Agnelli et al. 1995). Serial surveillance using duplex US, impedance plethysmography or ^{125}I-fibrinogen leg scanning has been used. Although attractive, this approach is expensive and can be applied only to a limited number of patients at risk (Clagett et al. 1998; Geerts et al. 2001). More promising is the use of biological markers of thrombosis.

19.8.1 D-dimers

A simple, noninvasive and cost-effective screening blood test that could help determine, with a high negative predictive value (NPV), which patients are at risk for VTE, would be useful to prevent fatal PE. There is currently no reliable such test for trauma patients.

Most recent studies focused on D-dimers, which are a specific cleavage product of the degradation of cross-linked fibrin strands by fibrinolytic proteins (Enderson et al. 1991; Schmidt et al. 1992; Bounameaux and Perrier 1996; Owings et al. 1996, 2000, 2001). There are different D-dimer assay methods currently available. The ELISA and SimpliRED tests have a higher NPV (93%–100%) than the latex test (±80%) (Owings et al. 2000). The SimpliRED, which can be performed on whole blood samples, is easier, quicker and less expensive than the ELISA test, allowing for repetitive tests. The SimpliRED assay is semiquantitative, compared to the quantitative ELISA test (Egermayer et al. 1998; Chen et al. 1999; Owings et al. 2000). New rapid immunoturbidimetric techniques such as the Liatest assay have also been developed (Indik and Alpert 2000). D-dimers have a low specificity, as they may be elevated in other situations that occur in trauma patients such as surgery, infections, sepsis, large hematomas, intravascular coagulation or adult respiratory distress syndrome (ARDS) (Schmidt et al. 1992). As all trauma patients have vascular damage, all will have positive tests with high levels of D-dimers immediately after injury, responsible for the low positive predictive value (PPV) of the test (Engelman et al. 1996). D-dimers begin to decay by 24 h, and by 48–72 h, they decrease towards a normal or a near-normal level even in severely injured patients (Enderson et al. 1991; Schmidt et al. 1992; Chen et al. 1999; Owings et al. 2000). It is postulated that a second rise would detect VTE in patients without recent surgery, ARDS or sepsis. SimpliRED assay results with a sensitivity of 100%, specificity of 43%, PPV of 35% and NPV of 100% have been reported in trauma or surgical patients (Owings et al. 2000). Nevertheless, recent results from an emergency department reported a sensitivity of only 65% and NPV of 81% using the SimpliRED technique (Farrell et al. 2000). Other problems exist with the use of D-dimers for screening in trauma patients (Owings et al. 2001): first, VTE is known to occur early after injury, with a rate of 85% false-positive D-dimers at that time, and second, D-dimers are frequently increased in patients at a higher risk for VTE (advanced age, high ISS), which makes the PPV too low to be valuable. It was recently concluded that D-dimer tests should best serve to exclude VTE in less severely injured patients, and with a suspicion of VTE more than 48 h after trauma. Unstable and severely injured patients should undergo more aggressive work-up and treatment (Owings et al. 2000, 2001). A recent uncontrolled study suggested adapting the dose of LMWH prophylaxis in relation to daily monitoring of D-dimer level in trauma surgery (Peetz et al. 2000). Recent preliminary studies suggested a benefit by combining D-dimer measurements with spirometric or volumetric capnogram measurements (Anderson et al. 1999; Kline et al. 2001; Rodger et al. 2001).

19.8.2 Duplex Ultrasonography

19.8.2.1 US in the Nontrauma Population

The accuracy of duplex US in the detection of acute DVT of the lower extremities depends on a number of variables, most notably whether the patients have symptoms suggestive of venous congestion and how the US examination was performed (Cornuz et al. 1999). Patients presenting with symptoms of acute DVT are likely to have much more extensive, proximal and occlusive DVT that frequently involves the femoropopliteal venous segments where DVT is readily detected. Two large meta-analyses have demonstrated that, in symptomatic patients, the technique was highly accurate for detecting DVT in the femoropopliteal segments (mean sensitivity, 95%; specificity, 95%; PPV, 95%; NPV, 95%). The sensitivity for calf DVT was lower (84%) than that for above-knee DVT (Comerota et al. 1993; Rose 1998).

Asymptomatic high-risk patients in a surveillance program are likely to have smaller, more often nonocclusive thrombi, which are frequently isolated in the difficult-to-visualize calf veins (Rose et al. 1994). A review in asymptomatic high-risk patients showed that the sensitivity of US dropped to 76% for above-knee DVT and 30% for calf veins (Comerota et al. 1993; Rose 1998). The overall results of the most recent studies were better, probably due to the improved instrumentation and operator experience. Considering only level-one studies, the following results were obtained: a sensitivity of 62%, a specificity of 97% and a PPV of 66% for proximal DVT; a sensitivity of 48% and a PPV of 93% at the calf level (Wells et al. 1995).

19.8.2.2
Ultrasound in the Trauma Population

A clinical suspicion of DVT should always be confirmed by other tests, because patients with minimal leg symptoms may have extensive venous thrombosis, whereas the classic symptoms and signs such as pain, tenderness and swelling of the leg, can be caused by nonthrombotic disorders, especially in patients with trauma of the lower limbs. Venous thrombi will produce symptoms if they obstruct the venous outflow, cause inflammation of the vein wall and perivascular tissue, or embolize into the pulmonary circulation (Hirsh and Hoak 1996). Many of these patients are mechanically ventilated, with or without sedation, or comatose and therefore unable to communicate their symptoms, or respond appropriately to attempts to elicit tenderness. They also often have other pathological processes that can provide adequate explanations for the nonspecific signs associated with PE (O'Malley and Ross 1990; Geerts et al. 1994; Velmahos et al. 1998). The practice of routine surveillance US in high-risk trauma patients may reduce the occurrence of major PE and lead to earlier diagnosis and treatment of lower extremity DVT before PE supervenes (Ruiz et al. 1991; Napolitano et al. 1995; Headrick et al. 1997; van den Berg et al. 1999).

19.8.2.3
Advantages and Disadvantages

Although not infallible, venography is recognized as the gold standard for detecting DVT (Rogoff and DeWeese 1960; Weinmann and Salzman 1994). Venography would be difficult to implement for DVT screening in trauma patients. It requires mobilization and transport of the patients to the radiological suite, cooperation of the patients, and is expensive and moderately invasive. Furthermore, venous puncture may be impossible in up to 20% of patients with leg injury (Geerts et al. 1994; Meissner 1998). Venography may be nondiagnostic in up to 19% of the patients (Geerts et al. 1996).

The advantages of US as a screening technique, compared to venography, are the following: it is safe, noninvasive, repeatable, no contrast medium is used and the procedure can be performed at the patient's bedside. Compared to hemodynamic tests, it is more accurate, less patient-dependent, more rapid, and allows a precise location of the site of DVT. Furthermore, it may allow evaluation of the age of the thrombus or other pathologies (hematoma, Baker's cyst, etc.), provide anatomical/functional information, and is widely available.

The disadvantages of US are operator- and patient-dependence, limitation by open wounds, edema, obesity, calcified arterial disease, bandages, and orthopedic hardware (casts, cervical spine collar, external fixators or traction devices, blind areas such as the adductor canal and abdomen or pelvis (bowel gas; Comerota et al. 1993; Hammers et al. 1996; Meissner 1998).

19.8.2.4
Results

There are several studies available, using US as a serial screening method for DVT in high-risk trauma patients (Table 19.10). These studies are subject to methodological criticism, as venography was not used to confirm the diagnosis in doubtful cases or in patients presenting with PE and negative US, leading to the speculation that US screening may have missed clinically significant DVT (Winchell et al. 1994; Pasquale et al. 1998). US detected 2.4%–43% of DVT despite prophylaxis. 50%–75% of DVT were partly occlusive. More than 80% of DVT detected by US were nonsymptomatic. Four studies screened both lower and upper extremities (Burns et al. 1993; Knudson et al. 1994, 1996; Hammers et al. 1996). As many as 30% of DVTs were found in the upper extremities (seven patients after central line placement and one after direct trauma; Hammers et al. 1996). A 28% prevalence of subclavian vein thrombosis due to catheter placement and subsequent 12% documented embolism to the lungs have been reported (Horattas et al. 1988). It has also been reported that 15%–25% of patients had incomplete US studies (Knudson et al. 1992; Burns et al. 1993; Dennis et al. 1993; Greenfield et al. 1997; Gearhart et al. 2000). Iliac veins were analyzable in 10%–59%, femoral veins in 81%–95%, popliteal veins in 73%–77%, calf veins in 67%–75%, IVC in 65%, internal jugular veins in 71% and axillary and subclavian veins in 83% (Hammers et al. 1996; Greenfield et al. 1997). US screening may miss DVT distal to the popliteal level, or proximal to the iliac veins, DVT that occurs and resolves within screening intervals and DVT that is present but not detected because of inherent limitations to US. Despite prophylaxis and venous screening, fatal PE still occurred without warning in 25% of patients presenting PE. The results of serial US screening are not significantly different from other studies that only performed US based on the presence of signs and symptoms of possible DVT or PE

(Meyer et al. 1995; Spain et al. 1997). Those studies also confirmed a high incidence of DVT among critically injured patients, despite an aggressive strategy for prophylaxis.

One of the main limitations of US screening is that it gives poor results for calf vein thrombosis. There are few data regarding the importance of these thrombi in high-risk patients. While some authors do not consider calf DVT as significant (Moser and LeMoine 1981; Gottlieb and Widjaja 1999; Gottlieb et al. 1999), others found a 20%–30% risk of proximal extension or chronic venous insufficiency if left untreated (Kakkar et al. 1969; Lagerstedt et al. 1985; Philbrick and Becker 1988; Comerota et al. 1993; Lohr et al. 1991, 1995). Furthermore, minimal calf DVT can be associated with 20%–30% PE, usually small, which may be insignificant in young patients, but may be clinically relevant in patients with limited cardiopulmonary reserve (Browse and Thomas 1974; Havig 1977; Passman et al. 1997; Meissner 1998; Ohgi et al. 1998).

19.8.2.5
Cost-Effectiveness

The cost per test varies from US $250 to $420, resulting in US $4200–18,000 per DVT diagnosed (Burns et al. 1993; Napolitano et al. 1995; Hammers et al. 1996; Piotrowski et al. 1996; Spain et al. 1997; Satiani et al. 1997; Gearhart et al. 2000). In non-trauma patients with an initial negative US, the cost of US follow-up has been estimated at US $390,000 per additional life saved, and US $3,500,000 per life saved for a second follow-up study (Hillner et al. 1992).

Routine US screening was more cost-effective in patients with an anticipated length of hospital stay of less than 2 weeks (Brasel et al. 1997). However, as many as 50% of DVTs may occur up to 3 weeks or longer after injury (Napolitano et al. 1995), it is not cost-effective to serially screen all trauma patients for DVT (Satiani et al. 1997). Therefore, high-risk trauma patients who are prone to develop DVT need to be identified (Pasquale et al. 1998). Routine screening may have a role among very high-risk patients, particularly those who are not candidates for either pharmacological or mechanical prophylaxis (Meissner 1998). One report recommended the use of US screening only in patients with spinal cord injuries (Meyer et al. 1995). Routine screening has not been demonstrated to reduce the frequency of clinically significant outcomes, such as nonsymptomatic VTE or fatal PE. Broad applications of effective methods of prophylaxis have been more cost-effective and are probably safer than selective intensive surveillance.

19.8.3
Impedance Plethysmography

Impedance plethysmography (IPG) has a high sensitivity and specificity for patients who present with signs and symptoms of DVT. A review of the literature showed a sensitivity of 90% and a specificity of 94% for proximal DVT (Wheeler et al. 1994). Concerning screening in nonsymptomatic patients, sensitivity was 12%–37% and specificity 90%–99% (Agnelli et al. 1995). Many limiting factors such as inadequate patient's relaxation, reduced arterial inflow and extravascular compressing lesions (hematoma, edema), can produce false-positive results (Rogers et al. 1993; Weinmann and Salzman 1994). Complete serial IPG cannot be performed in 50% of the trauma patients, due to the lack of cooperation in head-injured patients, or lower extremities orthopedic injuries interfering with placement of the device (Norcross et al. 1991). Furthermore, IPG is reliable for above-knee thrombosis if thrombi are less than 5 days old (Shackford and Moser 1988). The reported low sensitivity of IPG in detecting DVT precludes its use for screening of asymptomatic trauma patients at high risk for DVT (Shackford et al. 1990; Rogers et al. 1993; Geerts et al. 1994).

19.8.4
Bedside Leg Scanning

^{125}I-fibrinogen leg scanning (IFLS) is also known as fibrinogen uptake test (FUT). A review of 15 studies on screening for postoperative DVT showed that IFLS had a sensitivity of 45%–82% and a specificity of 79% for proximal and distal DVT and a sensitivity of 55%–88% and a specificity of 92% for isolated calf thrombosis, when compared to venography (Lensing and Hirsh 1993). These results were barely improved when IPG and IFLS were combined (sensitivity 50%, specificity 93%; Cruickshank et al. 1989). The technique is difficult to perform and its sensitivity can be excessive; hematoma, for example, can be a source of false-positive results. On the other hand, an organized thrombus may not be detected (Shackford and Moser 1988; Yelnik et al. 1991). The potential role of Tc-99m apcitide thromboscintigraphy, which allows differentiation between acute and chronic thrombosis, has yet to be evaluated in the trauma patient population (Blum and Handmaker 2000).

Table 19.10. Ultrasound Screening of Post-traumatic DVT

Reference	Patient population	Type of study	Screening technique	Level of screening	Gold standard	Prophylaxis	Results
Knudson et al. (1992)	113 trauma patients (defined)	Prospective semirandomized	Doppler + B-mode US Within 24 h of admission, then every 5 days for 3 weeks	Proximal	No	LDH (33%) or PCD and stockings (67%)	8 DVT detected (7%) despite prophylaxis 7 PE (6%), 4 with negative US 15% of patients with incomplete US studies 5 DVT and 1 PE asymptomatic
Burns et al. (1993)	57 HR (defined) from 400 admitted trauma patients (14%)	Prospective nonrandomized	Color duplex US twice weekly	Proximal and distal Upper extremities	No	LDH, PCD or PIVCF in 85%	12 DVT detected (21%), all asymptomatic despite prophylaxis in 9 33% were located in the pelvis or in upper extremities 2 PE (3.5%) with negative US 23% of patients with incomplete US study
Dennis et al. (1993)	395 trauma patients with ISS⩾9	Prospective semirandomized	Duplex US: 30% Doppler US: 70% Within 48 h of admission, Then every 5 days	Proximal	No	LDH or PDC in 71% Control in 29%	18 DVT detected (4.6%) (prophylaxis in 8) 4 PE (1%), 3 fatal with negative US 20% of patients with incomplete US studies
Hill et al. (1994)	100 consecutive trauma patients with ISS ≥10	Prospective nonrandomized	Duplex US on days 1, 3, 6, 10 and 21 or until discharge	–	No	LDH (50%)	15 DVT detected (15%) despite prophylaxis in 14 No PE
Knudson et al. (1994)	251 trauma patients with defined risk	Prospective semirandomized	Duplex US within 24 h of admission, then every 5–7 days	Proximal and distal Some upper extremities	No	LDH, PCD or control	15 DVT detected (6%) 12 DVT were asymptomatic 2 PE (0.8%) with negative US (1 fatal)
Napolitano et al. (1995)	458 trauma patients from 5170 admitted requiring admission to surgical ICU and immobilization in bed (9%)	Prospective nonrandomized	Duplex US twice weekly	Proximal	No	LDH and/or single-chamber PCD (92%)	45 proximal DVT detected (10%) despite prophylaxis (30 on the first US) 1 clinical PE (0.2%)
Hammers et al. (1996)	136 HR (defined) from 937 admitted trauma patients (14.5%)	Prospective nonrandomized	Color duplex US within 2 days of admission, then weekly	Proximal Upper extremities	No	LDH and/or PCD IVCF if CI to LDH and PCD (20 patients)	19 asymptomatic DVT detected (14%) despite prophylaxis (70% in lower limbs, 30% in upper extremities) 3 clinical PE (2.2%)

Knudson et al. (1996)	372 HR (defined) trauma patients	Prospective semirandomized	Duplex US within 24 h of admission, then every 5–7 days	Proximal and distal Upper extremities	No	LMWH, FP or PCD and stockings	9 DVT detected (2.4%) despite prophylaxis 8 DVT were asymptomatic 1 clinical PE (0.3%) with positive US
Piotrowski et al. (1996)	343 HR (defined) from 3154 admitted trauma patients (10.9%)	Prospective nonrandomized	Color duplex US within 2 days of admission, weekly for 3 weeks, biweekly for 3 weeks, then monthly	Proximal	No	LDH, stockings and/or PCD (96%)	20 DVT detected (5.8%) despite prophylaxis 17 DVT were asymptomatic 3 clinical PE (0.9%), 2 fatal with negative US
Greenfield et al. (1997)	53 HR (defined) trauma patients	Prospective semirandomized	Color duplex within 24 h of admission, then days 3 & 6, then weekly for 4 weeks	Proximal and distal	No	LDH, LMWH, PCD or FP PIVCF in 50%	23 DVT detected (43%) despite prophylaxis (17 proximal) No PE
Headrick et al. (1997)	228 HR (defined) from 1566 admitted trauma patients (14.5%)	Prospective nonrandomized	Color duplex US within 3 days of admission, then weekly	Proximal and distal	No	LDH and/or PCD (90%) IVCF when proximal DVT detected	39 DVT detected (17%) despite any type or combination of prophylaxis (97% proximal DVT) 32 DVT were asymptomatic 1 fatal PE (0.4%) in the non-IVCF group, despite anticoagulation Significant difference in comparison to a historical control (6 PE) $P<0.05$
Velmahos et al. (1998)	200 HR (defined) trauma patients	Prospective nonrandomized	Duplex US weekly	Proximal	No	LDH (46%) and/or PCD (97.5%) IVCF in 17%	26 DVT detected (13%) despite any type or combination of prophylaxis 4 clinical PE (2%), all with negative US
Gearhart et al. (2000)	102 HR (defined) trauma patients	Prospective nonrandomized	Duplex US weekly	Proximal and distal	No	LDH or LMWH and PCD or FP	11 DVT detected (10.8%) despite prophylaxis 7 DVT were asymptomatic 1 clinical PE (1%) with negative US 25% of patients with incomplete US
Schwarcz et al. (2001)	241 HR (defined) trauma patients	Retrospective nonrandomized	Duplex US within 72 h, then weekly	Proximal and distal	No	LMWH	13 DVT detected (5.4%) despite prophylaxis (8 on the first US); 12 DVT were asymptomatic 2 clinical PE (0.8%) with negative US

LDH, low-dose heparin; *DVT*, deep venous thrombosis; *US*, ultrasound; *PE*, pulmonary embolism; *PCD*, pneumatic compression device; *PIVCF*, prophylactic inferior vena cava filter; *IVCF*, inferior vena cava filter; *ISS*, Injury Severity Scale; *ICU*, intensive care unit; *CI*, contra-indication; *LMWH*, low-molecular-weight heparin; *HR*, high-risk; *FP*, foot pumps.

19.8.5 Bedside Lung Scanning

In the 1960s, perfusion lung scanning at the patient's bedside was reported (Shibata et al. 1966). The test was manually performed with a portable scintillation probe, along the anterior and lateral aspect of the thorax, and sometimes a posterior view was obtained. Good correlation was achieved compared to conventional scintiscanogram, to detect massive or lobar PE. Currently, some ICU units are equipped with mobile gamma camera, allowing perfusion or ventilation/perfusion lung scanning to be performed at the patient's bedside, even in intubated patients. Some projections, such as the posterior view, cannot be performed at the bedside, potentially leading to undiagnosed PE. Nevertheless, results reported are similar to those obtained in the nuclear medicine units (refer to Chap. 19.9.2; Jolliet et al. 1995).

19.8.6 Bedside Pulmonary Angiography

Bedside pulmonary angiography (PA) has been performed by injection of contrast medium through a catheter, placed in the right ventricle or the main pulmonary artery, allowing detection of massive PE (Calinog et al. 1972; Trujillo et al. 1976) or through a Swan-Ganz catheter (Loop et al. 1975; Dougherty et al. 1980; Le Page and Gracia 1982). A flow-directed Swan-Ganz catheter allows for multiple limited segmental angiograms. The technique is simple, safe, reliable and can be repeated at frequent intervals when necessary. Unfortunately, a very low sensitivity (<50%) and a specificity of only 60% was reported when compared to conventional PA (Le Page and Gracia 1982). In emergency conditions, some still perform bedside pulmonary angiography through a Swan-Ganz catheter, allowing thrombolytic therapy to be started immediately (Tanaka et al. 1995).

19.9 Diagnosis

So far, there are no specific studies on investigation of PE in trauma patients. The following chapters will thus review the different imaging modalities for PE, applied to the general hospital patient population. Chest X-ray, ventilation/perfusion (V/Q) lung scan and pulmonary angiography (PA) were classically used before the 1990S. Each modality has advantages and disadvantages with varying sensitivities and specificities. However, no single modality has been shown to be appropriate in every patient. The V/Q lung scan together with chest X-ray have been the first-line tests for more than 30 years, but 60%–70% of V/Q scans are nondiagnostic (PIOPED Investigators 1990). If results were inconclusive, imaging of the veins of the lower limbs (by US or impedance plethysmography) was performed. If the diagnosis was still unclear, the patient went on to PA. This diagnostic algorithm, however, was generally underused. At the beginning of the 1990s, it was emphasized that there is a clear need for a technique to demonstrate PE that should be accurate, safe, noninvasive, easily and rapidly performed, widely accepted and cost-effective (Gurney 1993; Gefter et al. 1995; Goodman and Lipchik 1996). Spiral CT angiography (SCTA) of the pulmonary arteries has the potential to fulfill these requirements.

19.9.1 Chest X-ray

Before the 1960s, chest X-ray was the only imaging modality when PE was suggested clinically. The chest X-ray is still frequently performed in patients suspected of PE as it is fast, low cost and easy to perform. The radiological signs of PE on chest X-ray have been described for more than 60 years (Westermark 1938; Hampton and Castleman 1940; Fleischner et al. 1941; Fleischner and Udis 1952; Fleischner 1962; Figley et al. 1967; Bynum and Wilson 1978). The classic signs include:

- Hemidiaphragmatic elevation (Even et al. 1979)
- Pleural-based truncated cone (Hampton's hump) representing pulmonary infarct or hemorrhage (Hampton and Castleman 1940; Dalen et al. 1977; Wilson et al. 1986)
- Gradual decrease in size over weeks to months of infarct (melting sign; Woesner et al. 1971)
- Plate-like atelectasis (Fleischner's lines; Fleischner et al. 1941)
- Pleural effusion (Bynum and Wilson 1978)
- Focal area of local pulmonary oligemia (Westermark's sign) (Westermark 1938)
- Proximal dilation of pulmonary arteries (sausage sign; Palla et al. 1983; Stein et al. 1992b)
- Abrupt distal tapering of the occluded vessel (knuckle sign; Williams and Wilcox 1963)
- Enlargement of the right heart cavities (Stein et al. 1992b)

- Azygos vein and/or superior vena cava (SVC) dilatation (FLEISCHNER and UDIS 1952)
- Pulmonary edema (FLEISCHNER 1962)

The nature and the extent of the abnormalities vary considerably among different studies and are also influenced by multiple factors: the population studied, the magnitude of arterial obstruction, diagnostic delay, coexistence of cardiopulmonary disease and probably the experience of the reader. Table 19.11 shows results in published series since 1973. Sensitivity of chest X-ray is limited, as no abnormality is demonstrated in up to 40%–50% of cases. A normal chest X-ray is found most commonly in younger patients (STEIN et al. 1991; GREEN et al. 1992). Specificity is also controversial since the publication of two studies. The first study demonstrated a large interobserver variation among nine readers, with a sensitivity varying from 8% to 52% (mean 33%), and a specificity from 31% to 80% (mean 59%). There was no correlation between level of training or experience and interobserver performance (GREENSPAN et al. 1982). In the second study, the positive predictive value of each sign varied from 14% to 27% and the negative predictive value from 73% to 75% (WORSLEY et al. 1993). These studies concluded that chest X-ray does not provide adequate information to accurately establish or exclude the diagnosis of PE. Nevertheless, these studies suffered from the absence of serial chest X-rays, which are necessary to appreciate subtle signs, such as changes in the size of the pulmonary arteries or of an area of oligemia. Despite these limitations, chest X-ray has a pivotal role in the evaluation of PE patients, as it may provide an alternative diagnosis to explain the patient's symptoms (pneumonia, pulmonary edema, pneumothorax, rib fracture) and it is essential for proper evaluation of the V/Q scan (KELLEY and ELLIOTT 1974; BUCKNER et al. 1989). Opacities appearing 4 h to 5 days (mean 1.8 days) in areas of abnormal perfusion scan strongly suggest the diagnosis of PE (VIX1983). The combination of serial chest X-rays with clinical symptoms and signs, blood gases and EKG will suggest the need for further examination.

19.9.2 Pulmonary Scintigraphy

The perfusion (Q) lung scan is obtained by injecting a radiotracer, which is trapped in the capillary and arteriolar bed of the lung, and reflects the relative distribution of perfusion of the lungs. A ventilation (V) lung scan was introduced to increase the specificity of the Q scan on the premise that the V scan is preserved in areas of reduced perfusion due to PE (V/Q mismatch). Conversely, in parenchymal lung disease, it was anticipated that reduced regional ventilation resulting in a reduced perfusion would be detected by V scan (V/Q match) (DENARDO et al. 1970). Subsequent studies

Table 19.11. Chest X-ray in the diagnosis of PE

Reference	No. of patients	Normal (%)	Infiltration (infarct/hemorrhage) (%)	Condensation Atelectasis (%)	Pleural effusion (%)	Hemidiaphragm elevated (%)	Focal oligemia (%)	Dilatation of proximal pulmonary artery (%)	Right heart enlargement (%)
BYNUM and WILSON (1978)	155	19 (12)	70 (45)	25 (16)	79 (51)	–	–	–	–
MOSES et al. (1974)	41	3 (7)	22 (54)	11 (27)	21 (51)	7 (17)	1 (2)	2 (5)	7 (17)
GREEN et al. (1992)	77	26 (34)	19 (25)	19 (25)	24 (31)	–	–	1 (1)	2 (3)
STEIN et al. (1991)	260	20 (8)	98 (38)	179 (69)	127 (49)	67 (26)	55 (21)	55 (21)	46 (18)
DAUTZENBERG et al. (1982)	91	4 (4)	8 (9)	35 (38)	56 (61)	69 (76)	–	67 (73)	–
MANGANELLI et al. (1995)	118	–	38 (32)	28 (24)	67 (57)	87 (74)	15 (13)	91 (77)	62 (52)
UPET[a] (1973)	128	–	53 (41)	26 (20)	36 (28)	52 (41)	19 (15)	30 (23)	9 (7)
TOTAL	870	72 (11)	308 (35)	322 (37)	408 (47)	282 (44)	90 (14)	246 (34)	126 (20)

[a] *UPET*, Urokinase Pulmonary Embolism Trial.

demonstrated that a V/Q match cannot be used to rule out PE, as it can occur early in the course of PE. Similarly, only 68% of PEs are evidenced in case of V/Q mismatch (Hull et al. 1985). Furthermore, V/Q scan provides only indirect evidence for PE rather than direct visualization of clots and has a poor spatial resolution. Thirty years of experience, improved technology and multiple criteria revision have not altered this fact (Goodman et al. 1997). Nevertheless, until recently, the V/Q lung scan has been the initial noninvasive procedure of choice for the assessment of patients with suspected PE. The V/Q scan can only offer a level of probability for PE, based on the size and the number of perfusion defects, which are not specific for emboli. In the 1980s, a large multi-institutional study was conducted (PIOPED), designed to evaluate the efficacy of various conventional methods for the diagnosis of PE. The PIOPED data set has been extremely useful, as it contains precise description on a very large number of patients suspected of PE undergoing V/Q scan, chest X-ray and PA, as well as extensive clinical data. The V/Q scans were grouped into four categories according to the probability that the findings were related to acute PE: normal/near normal, low-, intermediate- and high-probability (PIOPED Investigators 1990). Results are reported in Table 19.12.

Improvement of the results was achieved by combining the results of V/Q scan with the clinical likelihood of PE a priori. The clinical likelihood of PE was high in 10%, and low in 26%, and was in agreement with the final diagnosis in 68% and 91%, respectively, demonstrating that clinical assessment was more often correct in excluding PE. Results were intermediate in the majority of the patients (64%).

One of the major contributions of the PIOPED study was to estimate the sensitivity and specificity of V/Q scans, demonstrating a high sensitivity and limited specificity, as confirmed thereafter in another large study (Hull and Raskob 1991). The sensitivity of a high-probability V/Q scan was 41%–57% and specificity was 90%–97%. When high and intermediate-probability were combined into a single diagnostic category, sensibility increased to 69%–82% while specificity decreased to 52%–75%. When the low-probability category was also included, sensitivity reached 98% while specificity decreased to 10%–51%. These results underscore the need for further workup in patients with a low- or intermediate-probability V/Q scan.

19.9.2.1 High-probability V/Q Scan

A high-probability V/Q scan was found in 13% of patients. It lacked sensitivity since it failed to identify 59% of patients with PE. Usually, a high-probability V/Q scan indicates PE when associated with a high clinical probability a priori (PPV=96%). Unfortunately, the PPV is reduced to 74%, when patients had a history of previous VTE. Results also decreased to 56% when associated with low clinical suspicion (PIOPED Investigators 1990; Table 19.12).

19.9.2.2 Normal or Near-Normal Probability V/Q Scan

Normal findings on a Q scan exclude the presence of clinically important PE (NPV of up to 98%) with reliability similar to PA (Kipper et al. 1982; Hull et al. 1990, 1994; Van Beek et al. 1995; Worsley and Alavi 1995). Nevertheless, the sensitivity of the Q scan is less than 100% for single emboli. Experimentally in dogs, 83% of obstructing clots (90% in vessels larger than 1 mm and 33% in vessels smaller than 1 mm) and 26% of partially occluding clots are detected (Alderson et al. 1978). This has also been reported in clinical practice, particularly in the case of large central nonobstructive PE (Remy-Jardin et al. 1996; Schoepf et al. 2000). PE can also be demonstrated at PA in 10% of lobes with a normal V/Q scan (Arborelius et al. 1985). Thus in clinical settings, the high sensitivity of the perfusion scan is due to the occur-

Table 19.12. Results of the PIOPED study [Modified from PIOPED Investigators (1990), with permission]

V/Q	Frequency	PE +	Clinical likelihood of PE		
Probability	(%)	Global (%)	High (%)	Intermediate (%)	Low (%)
High	13	87	96	88	56
Intermediate	39	30	66	28	16
Low	34	14	40	16	4
Normal/near normal	14	4	0	6	2

V/Q, ventilation/perfusion lung scan; *PE*, pulmonary embolism.

rence of multiple emboli, at least one of which causes a perceptible perfusion defect (GURNEY 1993).

19.9.2.3
Intermediate-Probability Lung Scan

The intermediate-probability lung scan is not helpful and is also called indeterminate-probability. In this category, 24%–33% of patients have PE (PIOPED INVESTIGATORS 1990; FERRETTI et al. 1997; GARG et al. 1998).

19.9.2.4
Low-Probability V/Q Scan

A low-probability V/Q scan with a strong clinical suspicion that there is no PE is generally accurate in ascertaining the absence of PE (NPV=96%). When the clinical assessment and V/Q results are discordant, the probability of PE ranges from 16% to 88%, which is not sufficiently accurate to be used as a basis for patient care (Table 19.12). While retrospective studies have suggested that patients with a low-probability V/Q scan have a favorable prognosis, despite the absence of anticoagulation or additional testing, others have suggested that as many as 25% of patients with a low-probability scan have angiographic evidence of PE (HULL and RASKOB 1991). Therefore, V/Q findings should be reported only as being normal, high-probability or nondiagnostic (MOSER 1990; HULL et al. 1995). In the PIOPED study, interobserver agreement was excellent for high-probability (95%), very low-probability (92%) and normal probability (94%), whereas it was only 75% for intermediate-probability and 70% for low-probability, which compounds the diagnostic difficulties. Approximately 70% of the patients had nondiagnostic V/Q scan (low- or indeterminate-probability) and required further diagnostic evaluation to confirm or exclude VTE definitely (PIOPED INVESTIGATORS 1990).

The addition of screening for DVT would decrease the number of patients who require PA from 72% to 33% (STEIN et al. 1993). Such an approach is nevertheless uncommonly followed in routine practice (ROSEN et al. 1995). In patients with adequate cardiopulmonary reserve and a nondiagnostic V/Q scan, thrombotic extension from submassive PE is not an important cause of morbidity and in most patients, recurrent embolism originates from proximal DVT, which means that the use of serial testing for DVT is an effective strategy. In patients with negative results, the follow-up demonstrated a recurrence of 1.9% VTE, of which 8% were fatal (HULL et al. 1994). On the contrary, in patients with inadequate cardiopulmonary reserve, which may be encountered in trauma patients with respiratory involvement, and nondiagnostic V/Q scan, there is a serious risk of death from the emboli already present. Considering the low-probability cohort, the frequency of VTE on follow-up was 11.7%, two-thirds of which were fatal within days of entry, with autopsy-proven PE. This contrasts strikingly with the good prognosis in patients with adequate cardiopulmonary reserve (0.14% death), and emphasizes that the term "low-probability V/Q scan" should be abandoned (HULL et al. 1995). With COPD, the V/Q scan was reported as normal in 5%, high-probability in 5% and nondiagnostic in 90%. Patients with previous cardiac or pulmonary disease also showed a nondiagnostic V/Q scan in 78% of the cases (LESSER et al. 1992). In patients who are chronically ill, hospitalized, or who have an abnormal chest X-ray, the likelihood of a false-positive V/Q scan is very high, and of a true negative is low (ROBIN 1977). When a thoracic injury is present in trauma patients, the diagnostic difficulties of V/Q scan can be further increased (SHACKFORD and MOSER 1988). In the PIOPED study, patients with a history of immobilization, trauma to the lower extremities, recent surgery or central venous instrumentation within 3 months prior to symptoms, were more likely to have a false-negative (low or very low-probability) lung scan interpretation (Table 19.13). For the low-probability V/Q scan, the prevalence of PE was 21% in patients with two of the above-mentioned risk factors, whereas others have a 4% prevalence of PE (WORSLEY et al. 1994; WORSLEY and ALAVI 1995).

In summary, the present role of the V/Q lung scan is controversial. By using several revisions of the original PIOPED criteria, it should be possible to decrease the number of indeterminate and low V/Q scans (and read them as low-probability or very low-probability scans, respectively) and provide a more accurate assessment (GOTTSCHALK et al. 1993; GOTT-

Table 19.13. V/Q lung scan in trauma patients (% of pulmonary embolism) [Modified from WORSLEY and ALAVY (1995), with permission]

V/Q interpretation	Risk factors		
	0	1	2
High	82	84	97
Intermediate	25	37	45
Low/very low	4	12	21
Normal	0	0	0

SCHALK 2000; SOSTMAN et al. 1994; STEIN and GOTTSCHALK 2000). Serial testing for DVT in patients with a nondiagnostic V/Q scan makes it possible to detect more patients requiring anticoagulation but delays final diagnosis, adds to the cost and may be difficult to implement (GOODMAN and LIPCHIK 1996). A recent Italian study combined a different interpretation of the Q scan (based on the shape of perfusion defect rather than on their size or number) without a V scan, combined with chest X-ray, electrocardiographic and clinical symptoms. They were able to reduce the need for PA in about 25% of the patients with abnormal scans (THE PISA-PED INVESTIGATORS 1995; MINIATI et al. 1996, 1999). For others, V/Q scans have been reported as "essential, but often not helpful" (SOSTMAN et al. 1982). Although the role of the V/Q scan for accurately diagnosed PE has undergone numerous refinements, the application of scintigraphy for diagnosing acute PE remains a challenge that can confound rather than clarify diagnosis (BIELLO et al. 1979; HULL et al. 1985; PIOPED INVESTIGATORS 1990; RUBIN 1997; STEIN 1997).

19.9.3 Pulmonary Angiography

Since its introduction in 1938 (ROBB and STEINBERG 1938), pulmonary angiography (PA) has been considered the gold standard for demonstration of PE, because a correctly performed normal PA excludes the diagnosis of PE, and demonstration of an intraluminal filling defect in a pulmonary artery establishes the diagnosis (HIRSH and HOAK 1996).

19.9.3.1 Underuse of Pulmonary Angiography and Consequences

In clinical practice, despite excellent sensitivity and specificity, PA has not gained widespread acceptance. The reasons for the underuse of PA are multiple. PA is invasive, expensive, requires technical expertise or may not be readily available in some clinical settings or hospitals. Some clinicians do not refer to PA, relying on the low incidence of recurrent PE if examinations of the lower limb veins are negative. But the main reason for underuse of PA remains its invasiveness (KHORASANI et al. 1997). Nevertheless, PA has been demonstrated to have a low mortality rate (<0.5%) and morbidity rate (0%–5%), which are in fact lower than the complication rate of an empirical anticoagulation (5%–30%) (DALEN et al. 1971; MILLS et al. 1980; CHEELY et al. 1981; PERLMUTT et al. 1987; STEIN et al. 1992a; VAN BEEK et al. 1996a; VAN ROOIJ et al. 1995; ZUCKERMAN et al. 1996; NILSSON et al. 1998). Most of the complications were observed in patients who were in critical condition when undergoing PA. The severity of the underlying condition renders the patient vulnerable to the procedure, whereas the most accurate diagnosis is needed in these patients (STEIN et al. 1992a). Although rare, since the use of pigtail catheters, most of the complications (cardiac arrhythmia, cardiac perforation, endocardial and myocardial injury) are related to heart catheterization and not to contrast-medium injection (PIOPED INVESTIGATORS 1990; NILSSON et al. 1998). Pulmonary hypertension has been discussed as being an additional cause of morbidity (DALEN et al. 1971; MILLS et al. 1980; PERLMUTT et al. 1987; ZUCKERMAN et al. 1996) or not (STEIN et al. 1992a; VAN ROOIJ et al. 1995; NILSSON et al. 1998). Despite its place as a cornerstone in multiple published diagnostic algorithms, clinicians underused PA, unwilling to expose patients with unstable cardiovascular conditions to a potentially risky procedure (SOSTMAN et al. 1982; SCHLUGER et al. 1994; HENSCHKE et al. 1995; KHORASANI et al. 1997; PATRIQUIN et al. 1998). Finally, the treatment decision for patients with a nondiagnostic V/Q scan seems to be based on the best clinical guess, which is known to be unreliable, or even worse, as a result of misinterpretation by the clinician of a low or indeterminate V/Q scan report (BONE 1993; GRAY et al. 1993; KEMBER et al. 1997). Consequently, a significant number of patients with PE may not have been diagnosed or treated and, on the other hand, a significant number who did not have PE have nonetheless been anticoagulated.

19.9.3.2 Results

The emergence of SCTA has highlighted the problems of comparing a new diagnostic technique with an established but fallible test (HANSELL 1997; QANADLI et al. 2000). Although PA has long been considered to be the most accurate technique available for detecting PE, its diagnostic accuracy has not been tested against an independent gold standard. Such a study was performed on pigs and showed that for emboli that are equivalent in size to human subsegmental pulmonary vessels, PA had a sensitivity of 87% and a predictive positive value of 88% (BAILE et al. 2000). Inter-reader agreement is variable and is clearly related to the quality of examination. Reader agreement is good from the main pulmonary artery to the segmental level (83%–100%), but is poor to moderate at the subsegmental level (13%–66%) (QUINN et al. 1987; STEIN et al. 1992a, 1999; DIFFIN et al. 1998; NILSSON et al. 1999). In clinical practice, the rate of false-negative examinations has been estimated between 1% and 9%, primarily because of the difficulty of visualizing small subsegmental clots, suggesting that PA is reliable only for larger emboli in the main to segmental pulmonary arteries (WELLMAN 1986). The intraobserver agreement of PA is good (K=0.74) (STEIN et al. 1999). Special techniques can be used to improve visualization of PE in small arteries: cineangiography (MEISTER et al. 1972; NILSSON et al. 1999), balloon-occlusion angiography (WILSON and BYNUM 1976; FERRIS et al. 1984; VAN ROOIJ et al. 1995), superselective angiography (BOOKSTEIN 1969) or wedge angiography (STEIN 1971). Clots can be demonstrated in arteries less than 1 mm in diameter, using superselective injections (BOOKSTEIN 1969). Nevertheless, the patient's outcome, the ultimate test of the usefulness of a study, has demonstrated that a negative PA has few adverse outcomes for the patient, suggesting that small peripheral PE may have little consequence. The recurrence rate at follow-up studies varied from 0% to 4.2%, including exceptional fatal issues (NOVELLINE et al. 1978; CHEELY et al. 1981; STEIN et al. 1992a; VAN ROOIJ et al. 1995; HENRY et al. 1995; VAN BEEK et al. 1996a,b; NILSSON et al. 1999). The rate of nondiagnostic PA is usually below 3%. Nevertheless, larger nondiagnostic or uncertain results (11% and 17%) were also reported (DALEN et al. 1971; THE PISA-PED INVESTIGATORS 1995).

19.9.3.3 Digital Subtraction Pulmonary Angiography

Currently, the digital subtraction technique is applied, although it requires good breath-holding capabilities. Pulmonary digital subtraction angiography (DSA) is a methodological step backward as, compared to conventional PA, it has lower spatial resolution and is more prone to respiratory and cardiac artifacts. Nevertheless, digital images allow a wide latitude of postprocessing, transforming DSA into advantages: images can be viewed subtracted or not, may be enhanced, magnified or visualized in cine mode (DARCY 1998). The first studies were performed with peripheral intravenous injection of contrast medium. Results were variable with adequate imaging varying from 76% to 94%, a sensitivity of 81%–100% and a specificity of 64%–96% compared to conventional PA, when injection was performed in a peripheral vein or centrally in the SVC or right atrium, respectively (POND et al. 1983; MUSSET et al. 1988). These DSA images had sufficient resolution to confirm central emboli, but were insufficient to rule out small PE. Advantages were a smaller amount of contrast medium injected, lower cost and lower risk due to the absence of transcardiac catheterization, as well as faster imaging and decreased procedural time. Insufficient results led investigators to use the subtraction technique with direct injection of contrast medium in the pulmonary arteries, to allow more accurate assessment of the peripheral pulmonary arteries. Recent studies compared the results of conventional and subtraction techniques. The sensitivity, accuracy and interobserver agreement were equivalent or even better using DSA compared to conventional PA (VAN ROOIJ et al. 1995; VAN BEEK et al. 1996b; JOHNSON et al. 1998; HAGSPIEL et al. 1998).

19.9.4 Computed Tomography

19.9.4.1 Introduction

In 1978, SINNER initially described the diagnosis of PE with CT (SINNER 1978). In 1980, GODWIN reported for the first time the direct demonstration of endovascular clots in central PE using sequential CT (GODWIN et al. 1980). In 1984, Breatnach reported the first CT case of a segmental embolus (BREATNACH and STANLEY 1984). During the 1980s, incremental contrast-enhanced CT was occasionally performed, when the risk of complication of PA was high, for the follow-up of central PE and for preoperative delineation of organized central thrombus. Nevertheless, the potential advantage of CT for the diagnosis of PE remained doubtful, until the technical development of helical CT, which allowed the acquisition of a volume data set in a single breath-hold, at the peak of contrast enhancement using only a moderate amount of IV contrast (VOCK et al. 1990). The first prospective study comparing spiral CT angiography (SCTA) of pulmonary arteries with PA in 42 patients was published in 1992 (REMY-JARDIN et al. 1992). The next year, Teigen reported his experience on the use of electron beam computed tomography (EBCT) for the diagnosis of central PE in 86 patients (TEIGEN et al. 1993). Since these preliminary studies, SCTA dramatically improved the evaluation of pulmonary arteries down to 2–3 mm in diameter in routine clinical practice.

19.9.4.2 Advantages of Spiral CT Angiography

Direct Visualization of Pulmonary Emboli

SCTA can demonstrate endoluminal clots, whereas PA and V/Q lung scan show most commonly indirect signs of PE such as regional perfusion defect or abrupt cut-off of the pulmonary arteries (Remy-Jardin et al. 1992). Furthermore, central PEs are often more apparent on SCTA because on PA, the emboli are usually seen end-on (Teigen et al. 1993; Enzweiler et al. 2002). The vascular signs of acute PE on SCTA include the following (Remy-Jardin et al. 1992; Kuzo and Goodman 1997; Hansell 1997; Chartrand-Lefevre et al. 1999; Figs. 19.3–19.6):

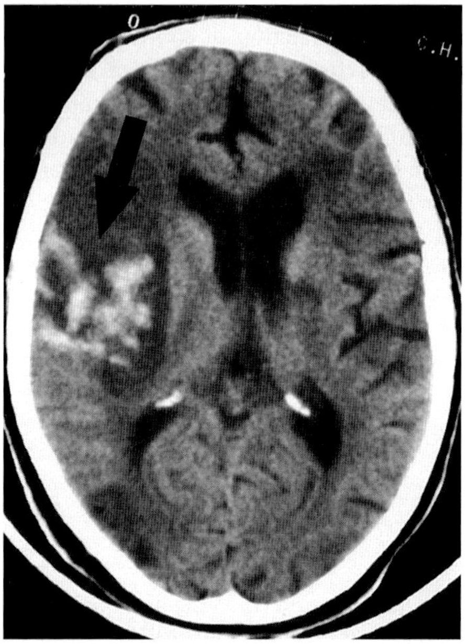

a

Fig. 19.3a–e. Massive pulmonary embolism in a 75-year-old woman. A post-traumatic femoral fracture was treated surgically 2 weeks earlier and a splenic contusion was treated conservatively. The patient was discharged on day 10 under prophylactic dose of low-molecular-weight heparin. She was readmitted on day 13 with a left hemiparesis. **a** Cerebral CT showed a large hemorrhagic right frontal infarct. **b, c, d** Due to refractory hypoxemia, 2-mm-thick contrast-enhanced spiral CT scan of pulmonary arteries was obtained, showing massive PE in lobar and segmental arteries (*arrowheads*). The patient eventually died on day 14 from myocardial infarct, due to paradoxical embolism that was confirmed at autopsy. **e** 10-mm-thick contrast-enhanced spiral CT scan shows a linear intrasplenic hypodensity compatible with a post-traumatic laceration (*arrow*)

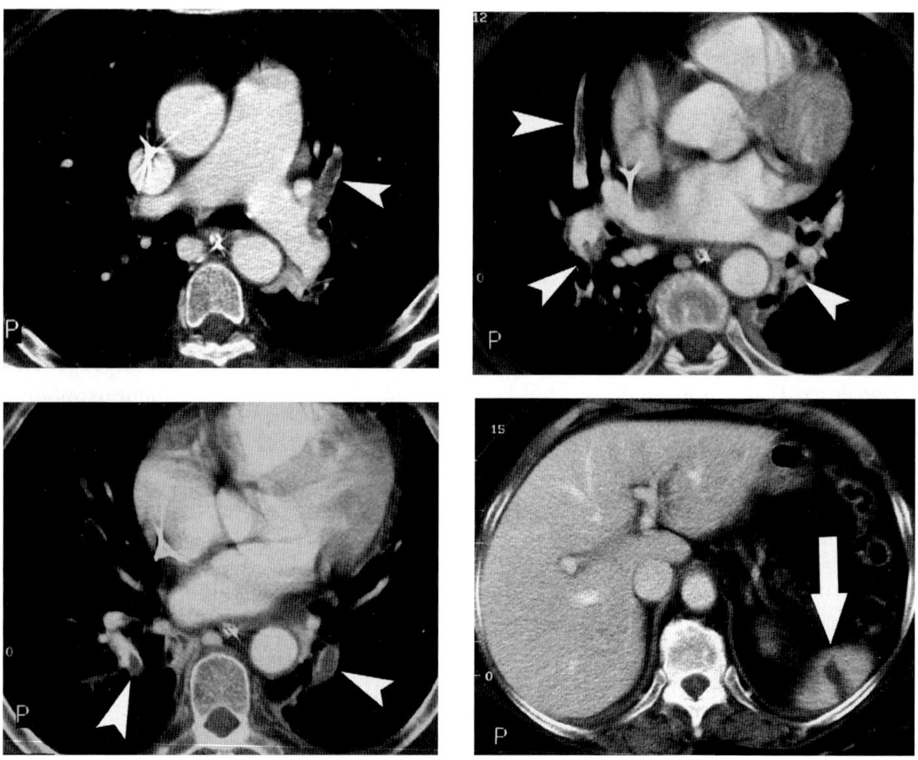

b c d e

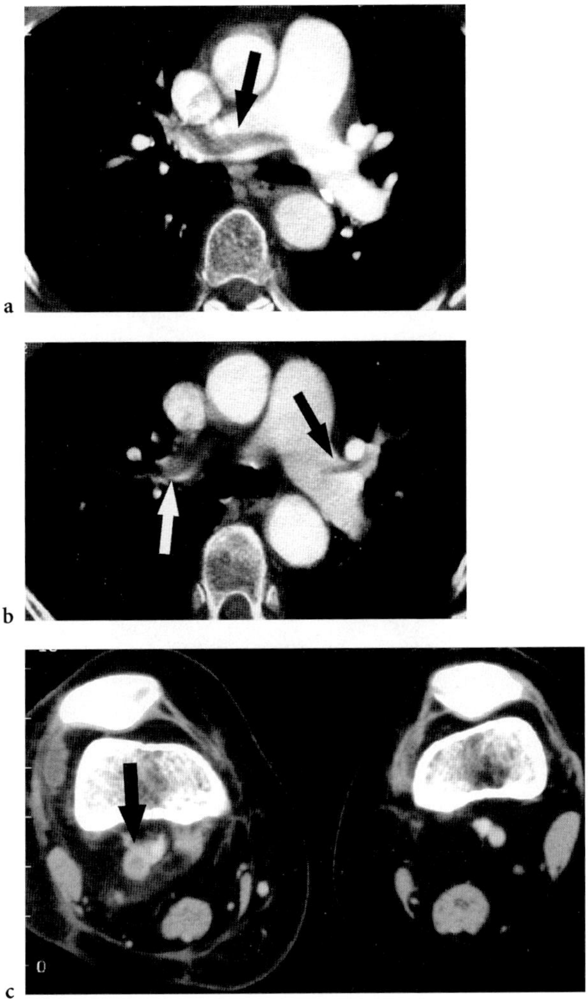

Fig. 19.4a–c. Massive PE in a patient with lower limb trauma. A 75-year-old woman presented with a traumatic fracture of the right hip that was treated by osteosynthesis. She was discharged at day 11. At day 13, she presented with atrial fibrillation to the emergency department. (**a, b**): 2-mm-thick contrast-enhanced spiral CT shows clots in the central pulmonary arteries (*arrows*). **c** 5-mm-thick axial CT venography shows DVT at the level of the right popliteal vein (*arrow*)

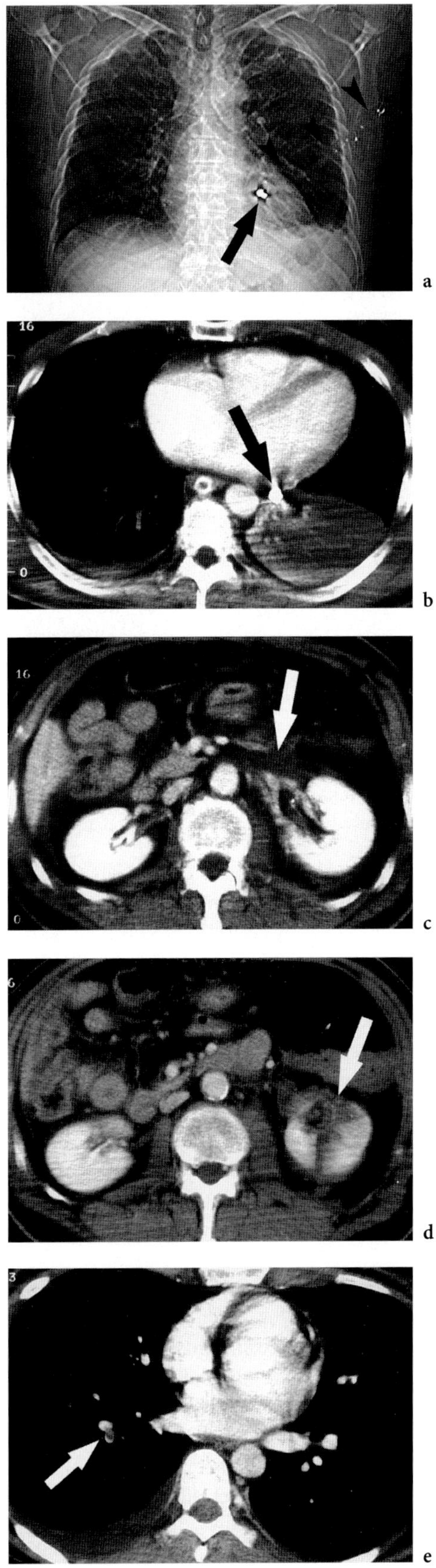

Fig. 19.5a–e. Asymptomatic PE in a patient with penetrating trauma. A 56-year-old male was shot. Two bullets penetrated the left flank and the left hemithorax. **a** Digital chest X-ray demonstrates a bullet (*arrow*) projecting over the left heart. Fragments of the bullet are shown in the left axilla and left lung along the missile path (*arrowheads*). **b** Spiral CT of the thorax performed at admission showed a small left pneumothorax (not shown), left lower lobe atelectasis and a bullet located behind the left ventricle (*arrow*). A left chest tube was inserted (not shown). **c, d** Spiral CT of the abdomen performed at admission showed pneumoperitoneum (not shown), hematoma of the left kidney at the renal hilum and laceration of lower pole (*arrows*). The bullet was shown in front of the sacrum (not shown). Laparotomy was performed for left renal hemostasis, and suture of the perforated gastric wall. **e** Spiral CT of the thorax performed before discharge with 5-mm-thick slices revealed asymptomatic PE in the segmental arteries of the right lower lobe (*arrow*)

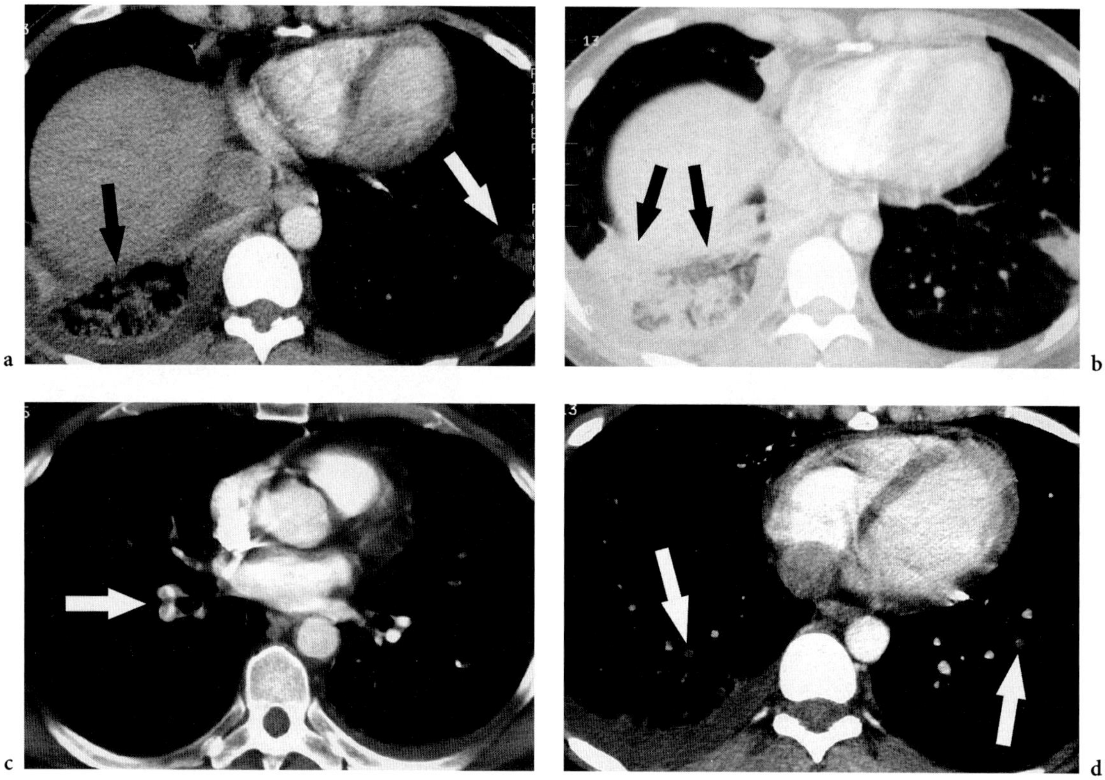

Fig. 19.6a–d. Pulmonary embolism following a fall in a staircase. A 33-year-old woman presented with right chest pain. She had a history of minor chest and lower limb trauma 5 days earlier. **a, b** 2-mm-thick contrast-enhanced spiral CT shows typical pulmonary infarct in both lower lobe (*arrows*). Note a right pleural effusion. **c, d** 2-mm-thick contrast-enhanced spiral CT shows segmental and subsegmental PE in the lower lobes (*arrows*)

- Central partial intravascular filling defect surrounded by contrast medium (CM) presenting the polo mint sign, when perpendicular to the long axis of the vessels, or the railway sign when parallel to the long axis.
- Eccentric partial filling defect or mural defect surrounded by CM presenting an acute angle with the vessel wall.
- Complete filling defect not surrounded by CM and occupying the entire arterial vessel section. The corresponding artery is frequently dilated compared to the opposite side.

Indirect Findings of Pulmonary Embolism

- The most commonly observed ancillary finding is the wedge-shaped pleural-based consolidation corresponding to the Hampton hump (Figs. 19.6, 19.7). Its frequency in patients with PE varied from 25% to 62% (Chintapalli et al. 1988; Coche et al. 1998; Shah et al. 1999; Johnson et al. 1999). In more than 50% of pulmonary infarction, low attenuation areas may be seen within the lesion and represent preserved, uninfarcted secondary pulmonary lobules (Balakrishnan et al. 1989). Wedge-shaped consolidation is also nonspecific as it may be seen in pneumonia, tumor, hemorrhage, edema, atelectasis and fibrosis (Ren et al. 1990). On the other hand, infarcts are not always wedge-shaped or subpleural on CT (Sinner 1978; Balakrishnan et al. 1989; Johnson et al. 1999).
- The vascular sign is a thickened vessel leading to the apex of the consolidation, increasing the specificity for infarction, but is infrequent or difficult to recognize (Balakrishnan et al. 1989; Ren et al. 1990).
- Others. Atelectasis and pleural effusion are frequent but nonspecific findings (Coche et al. 1998; Shah et al. 1999; Johnson et al. 1999). Dilatation of the right main pulmonary artery and the left interlobar pulmonary artery and linear bands have been found most commonly in patients with PE in one study (Coche et al. 1998). Areas of oligemia are considered to be of limited utility for the diagnosis of acute PE (Coche et al. 1998; Johnson et al. 1999).

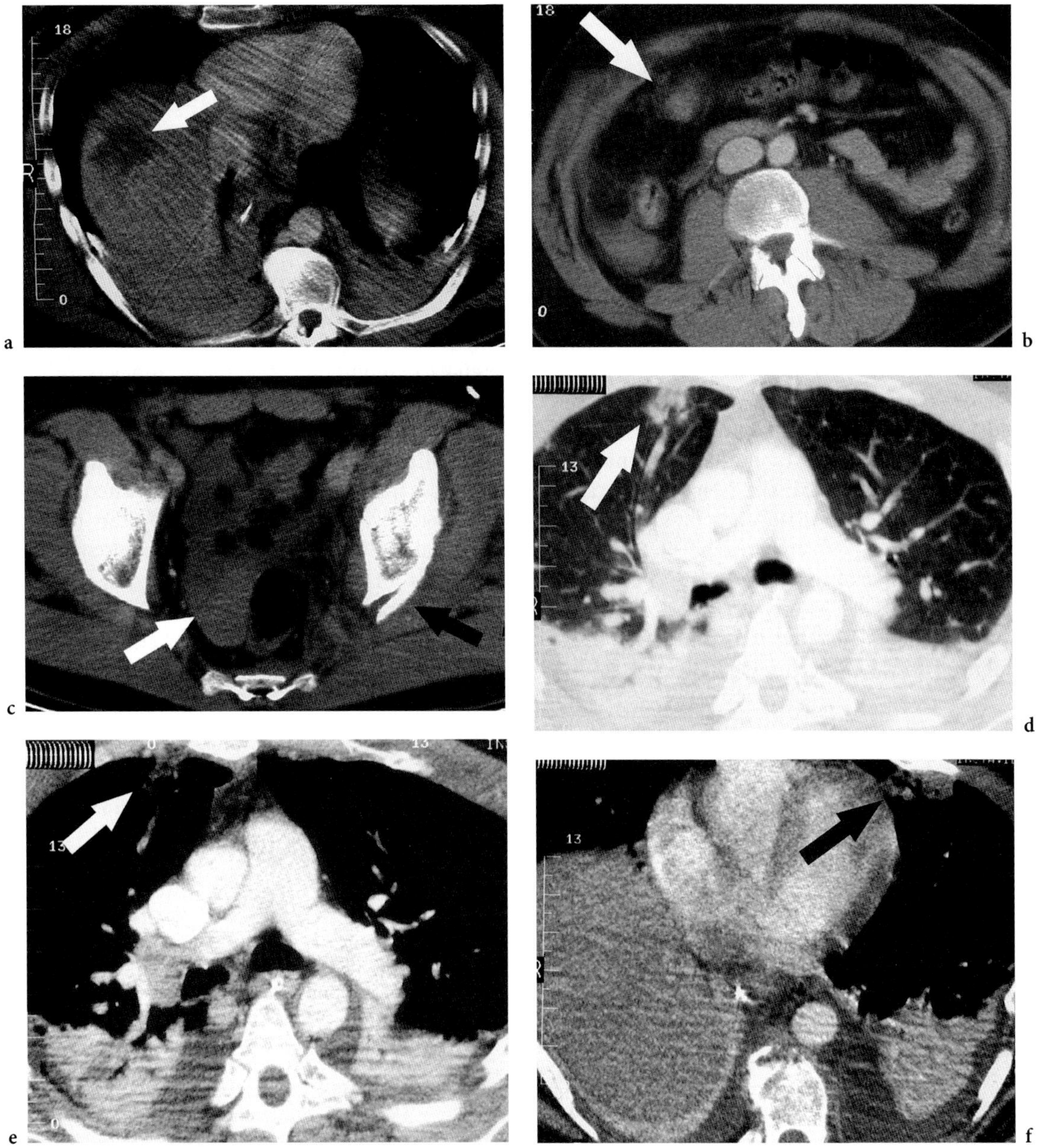

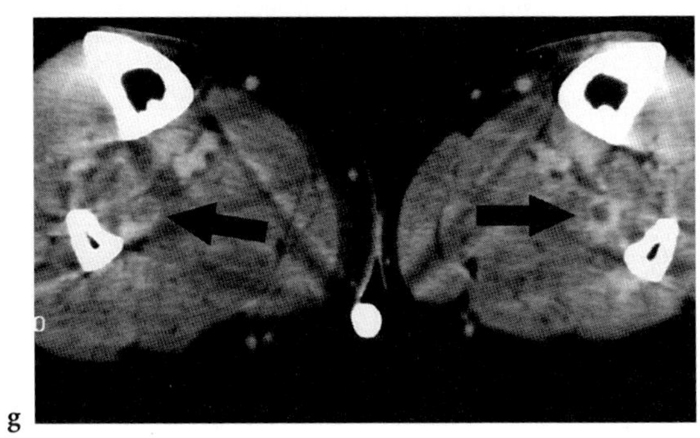

Fig. 19.7a–g. Deep venous thrombosis and pulmonary embolism following a car accident. A 37-year-old male was involved in a severe car accident, and presented with abdominal and chest injuries and multiple long-bone fractures. Anticoagulation prophylaxis was started with delay on day 13, due to hemothorax, thoracic flap and multiple orthopedic surgical procedures. On day 17, the patient presented with dyspnea and temperature while still intubated. **a–c** Spiral CT of the abdomen performed at admission showed liver contusion (**a**), peri-intestinal (*arrow*) and dependent hemoperitoneum (**b**) and hemoperitoneum in the perivesical compartment (**c**) (*arrow*) that were conservatively managed. **d–f** 2-mm-thick contrast-enhanced spiral CT shows multiple nonenhancing wedge-shaped bilateral peripheral pulmonary infiltrates (*arrows*), compatible with pulmonary infarcts. **g** 5-mm-thick axial CT venography shows clots in peroneal veins bilaterally (*arrows*)

Estimation of the Age of the Embolic Event

Differences in morphology of clots and arteries can be used to estimate the age of the thromboembolic event (Table 19.14) (Kauczor et al. 1999). SCTA is superior to V/Q scan in this setting. In the PIOPED study, 74% of patients with a history of PE, and in whom a high-probability V/Q scan was obtained, actually had PE, whereas 91% of patients without a history of PE, had PE (PIOPED Investigators 1990).

High Sensitivity and Specificity

By comparing experimentally SCTA (1 mm collimation) and PA with a true gold standard (cast in a pig model), both techniques were found to be comparable for detecting subsegmental-sized emboli (Baile et al. 2000). Nevertheless, some clinicians are not totally persuaded of the effectiveness of SCTA as a result of the wide range of sensitivities and specificities (Rathbun et al. 2000; Mullins et al. 2000). The most important factor affecting the results was the improvement of spiral CT technology (Ghaye et al. 2002b). For a 5-mm collimation, results varied from 53% to 100% (sensitivity) and from 78% to 100% (specificity); for 3-mm collimation, results varied from 67% to 92% and from 91% to 100%, respectively; and for 2-mm collimation results varied from 94% to 95% and from 94% to 97% (Table 19.15). In studies including patients with nondiagnostic V/Q scan, SCTA demonstrated 14%–44% positive results for PE (Remy-Jardin et al. 1996; Van Rossum et al. 1996a; Garg et al. 1998; Ferretti et al. 1997), which is similar to results (22%) obtained using pulmonary angiography (PIOPED Investigators 1990). Correlative studies have demonstrated that the accuracy of SCTA is greater than for the V/Q lung scan (Table 19.16). Another study comparing SCTA and V/Q scans as the initial investigation for acute PE, found a significantly higher proportion of confident diagnosis when SCTA was used (90%) compared to the V/Q scan (54%) (Cross et al. 1998). A review study, comparing a meta-analysis of seven single-slice SCTA studies with the V/Q scanning results in the PIOPED study, showed that overall accuracy of SCTA was better than the V/Q lung scan (Cueto et al. 2001).

Table 19.14. Criteria for spiral CT angiography diagnosis and estimation of age of pulmonary embolism [Modified from Kauczor et al. (1999), with permission]

Criteria	Acute PE	Subacute PE	Chronic PE
Filling defect	Central, eccentric, intraluminal Lack of opacification	Wall adherent (acute angle), convex Lack of opacification	Wall adherent (obtuse angle), concave Intraluminal webs Signs of thrombus recanalization Calcification
Vascular wall			Irregular wall thickening
Intra-pulmonary vessels	Dilated or normal	Dilated or normal	Smaller than normal Abnormal proximal to distal tapering Variation in size of segmental vessels Complete retraction of segmental vessels (cut-off)
Parenchyma	Infiltration (hemorrhage) Round or wedge-shaped pleural-based consolidation	Pleural-based wedge-shaped consolidation	Translobular lines Plate-like atelectasis Mosaic perfusion Bronchial dilatation in abnormal areas
Pleura	Pleural effusion	Pleural effusion	Pleural effusion
Pulmonary hypertension	Right heart enlargement with normal wall thickness (<5 mm)	Right heart enlargement, interventricular septal shift Dilation of central pulmonary arteries	Right heart enlargement with thickening of the wall (>5 mm) Negative axis of interventricular septum Dilation of central pulmonary arteries Dilation and tortuosity of bronchial arteries Pericardial effusion, ascites

Table 19.15. Published studies for the diagnosis of pulmonary embolism using spiral CT angiography

Reference	No. of patients	Indications	Prevalence of PE (%)	Colli-mation (mm)	Lowest anatomical level of interpretation	Sensitivity (%)	Specificity (%)
Remy-Jardin et al. (1992)	42	Clinical suspicion of PE or unexplained abnormal chest X-ray	18 (43)	5	Segmental	18/18 (100)	23/24 (96)
Blum et al. (1994)	10	Clinical suspicion of massive PE	7 (70)	5	Segmental	7/7 (100)	3/3 (100)
Steiner et al. (1994)	38	Clinical suspicion of PE	30 (79)	5	Segmental	30/30 (100)	8/8 (100)
Goodman et al. (1995)	20	Nondiagnostic V/Q, negative US	11 (55)	5	Segmental Subsegmental	6/7 (86) 7/11 (64)	12/13 (92) 8/9 (89)
Remy-Jardin et al. (1996)	75	Patients referred for PA with clinical suspicion of PE	43 (57)	3–5	Segmental	39/43 (91)	25/32 (78)
Sostman et al. (1996)	28 [53]	Clinical suspicion of PE	20 (38)	5	Subsegmental	5 readers: 62%–92% (75)	73%–100% (89)
Van Rossum et al. (1996a)	77	Abnormal V/Q with clinical suspicion of PE	40 (52)	5	Segmental	38/40 (95)	36/37 (97)
Van Rossum et al. (1996b)	149	Clinical suspicion of PE	68 (46)	5	Segmental	Observer 1: 64/68 (94) Observer 2: 56/68 (82)	78/81 (96) 75/81 (93)
Christiansen (1997)	70	High clinical suspicion of PE	22 (31)	5	Segmental Subsegmental	17/19 (89) 19/22 (86)	49/51 (96) 44/48 (92)
Mayo et al. (1997)	139	Clinical suspicion of PE	46 (33)	3	Segmental	40/46 (87)	88/93 (95)
Pruszczyk et al. (1997)	49	Suspicion of PE at transthoracic echo-cardiography	40 (82)	5	Subsegmental	39/40 (97)	(90)
Drucker et al. (1998)	47	Patients with clinical suspicion of PE referred for PA	15 (32)	5	Segmental	Group A: 9/15 (60) Group B: 8/15 (53)	26/32 (81) 31/32 (97)
Garg et al. (1998)	54	Nondiagnostic V/Q, negative US or discordant V/Q and clinical probability	14 (26)	3	Subsegmental	4/6 (67)	18/18 (100)
Herold et al. (1999)	391	Clinical suspicion of PE	–	3 (2–5)	Subsegmental	Local reading: (95) Expert reading: (87)	(97) (90)
Kim et al. (1999)	110	Clinical suspicion of PE	25 (23)	3	(Sub)segmental	23/25 (92)	82/85 (96)
Van Strijen et al. (1999)	238	Clinical suspicion of PE	– (51)	5	Segmental Subsegmental	(86) (69)	NA (86)
Blachere et al. (2000)	179	Clinical suspicion of PE	68 (38)	2–3	Subsegmental	Observer 1: 64/68 (94) Observer 2: (94)	104/111 (94) (95)
Qanadli et al. (2000)	158	Clinical suspicion of PE	62 (39)	2.5	Subsegmental	56/62 (90)	89/95 (94)
Perrier et al. (2001)	299	Clinical suspicion of PE in outpatients	118 (39)	3	Subsegmental	(70)	(91)

Table 19.16. Comparison of spiral CT angiography and ventilation/perfusion lung scan

Reference method	Diagnostic	Results				Conclusion
	Sensitivity (%)	Specificity (%)	PPV (%)	NPV (%)		
Mayo et al. (1997)	SCTA	87	95	95	95	SCTA is more correct (P<0.01)
	V/Q	65	94	83	84	
Van Rossum et al. (1998a)	SCTA	75	90	93	90	SCTA is more accurate (P<0.01)
	V/Q	49	74	96	85	
Kim et al. (1999)	SCTA	92	96	88	97	-
	V/Q	72	94	78	92	
Blachere et al. (2000)	SCTA	1st observer: 94	94	95	96	SCTA performs better (P<0.05)
		2nd observer: 94	95	95	97	
	V/Q	1st observer: 81	74	82	76	
		2nd observer: 76	80	78	82	

SCTA, spiral CT angiography; *PPV*, positive predictive value; *NPV*, negative predictive value.

Alternative Diagnosis

One of the main advantages of SCTA is that it provides an alternative diagnosis explaining the symptoms of the patient, which are not suggested by other diagnostic imaging techniques such as the V/Q scan, PA or US. SCTA demonstrated pleural or parenchymal abnormalities that could explain a defect seen at V/Q scanning with low or indeterminate-probability in 57% of patients (Van Rossum et al. 1996a). The rate of alternative diagnoses varied from 11% to 85% (Ferretti et al. 1997; Cross et al. 1998; Garg et al. 1998; Van Rossum et al. 1998a; Kim et al. 1999; Garg et al. 1999; Lorut et al. 2000; Montgomery et al. 2000; Remy-Jardin et al. 2000a). Alternative diagnoses are provided more frequently and with more precision than on PA (Van Beek and Reekers 1999). The most common diagnoses in patients without PE included pneumonia, atelectasis, pneumothorax, pneumomediastinum, pericardiac or pleural effusion, aortic dissection, cardiovascular disease, interstitial lung disease, post-traumatic or postoperative changes, abscess, esophagitis, mucous plugging, bronchial infection, chronic obstructive pulmonary disease (COPD), bronchopleural fistula, mediastinitis, pulmonary hypertension, aspiration pneumonia, septic emboli, diaphragmatic hernia, esophageal rupture and malignancies, most of which can also be seen following trauma.

Interobserver Variability

Good to excellent interobserver variability was demonstrated and compared favorably with agreement for PA and V/Q scan (Table 19.17).

The interobserver agreement is significantly dependent on the technical quality of the examination for SCTA and PA, and independent for V/Q (Herold et al. 1998). The interobserver variation was good to very good until the segmental level (K=0.72–0.88) (Mayo et al. 1997; Chartrand-Lefebvre et al. 1999; Domingo et al. 2000) and until the subsegmental level (K=0.72–0.97) (Van Rossum et al. 1996b; Herold et al. 1998; Blachere et al. 2000; Qanadli et al. 2000; Remy-Jardin et al. 2000a; Perrier et al. 2001). Although some authors found a considerable learning curve for interpreting SCTA, especially for the detection of small emboli (Garg et al. 1999; Ost et al. 2001), excellent interobserver agreement was found for six observers with different levels of experience (K=0.85) (Chartrand-Lefebvre et al. 1999), between senior and junior CT radiologists without prior experience with SCTA (K=0.90) (Van Rossum et al. 1998b) and between a senior and junior chest radiologist (K=0.97) (Remy-Jardin et al. 2000a). In this last study, using thin collimation (2 or 3 mm), the agreement was excellent for the different levels of interpretations: lobar level (K=0.99), segmental level (K=0.98), subsegmental level (K=0.97). For the latter level, significantly better results were achieved using 2-mm compared to 3-mm collimation. The intraobserver variation is also excellent (K=0.87) (Chartrand-Lefebvre et al. 1999). The interob-

Table 19.17. Interobserver agreement for spiral CT angiography, ventilation/perfusion lung scan and pulmonary angiography

Reference	SCTA	V/Q	PA
Mayo et al. (1997)	K=0.85	K=0.61	88%
Herold et al. (1998)	K=0.72	K=0.39	K=0.46
Blachere et al. (2000)	K=0.72	K=0.22	K=0.83
Qanadli et al. (2000)	K=0.86		K=0.78

SCTA, spiral CT angiography; *V/Q*, ventilation/perfusion; *PA*, pulmonary angiography.

server agreement should be further increased with multidetector CT, using thinner collimation as most causes of disagreement concerned partial volume effect, small sized arteries, motion artifact and technically suboptimal examination.

Severity Assessment of Pulmonary Embolism

Preliminary studies have been performed to attempt to quantify the degree of obstruction of the pulmonary bed similar to the Miller score (Miller et al. 1971), the Walsh score (Walsh et al. 1973), or the Simon score (Simon et al. 1984) at PA. One study used modified Miller and Walsh scores (Bankier et al. 1997). Refinements tried to differentiate partial versus complete obstruction of each artery by weighting on a two-point scale (Qanadli et al. 2001) or on a five-point scale, to provide additional information on the residual perfusion distal to the embolus (Mastora et al. 2001). Similar to MR imaging, EBCT can provide morphological, volumetric and functional information on the effect of thromboembolism at a microvascular level on lung perfusion. Such objective measurements may provide additional information that is more important for treatment than the direct visualization of emboli at SCTA alone (Schoepf et al. 2000). Other studies used cardiac morphological criteria (Sobotka et al. 1999; Reid and Murchison 1998). In one study, minor acute PE was associated with a short axis ratio (right ventricle/left ventricle) below 1.1/1. In all cases of severe acute PE, the ratio was over 1.5/1. Straightening or shifting to the left of the interventricular septum and reflux of contrast medium into the IVC can also be seen, but are more difficult to quantify (Reid and Murchison 1998). The acute dilatation of the right ventricle can thus be a useful sign to assess the severity of the pathophysiological effect of PE, in addition to the mechanical obstruction by intravascular clots, as the release of vasoactive agents can further increase the pulmonary vascular resistance by a reflex pulmonary vasoconstriction (Lualdi and Goldhaber 1995).

Wide Availability

SCTA is a routine 24-h-a-day technique. During the night, a CT scan is more easily accessible than a nuclear medicine study. This is one of the main reasons that makes SCTA the first choice for diagnosis of PE in many institutions.

Rapidity

The average time for SCTA is 10–15 min and for V/Q scan 45 min. Therefore the time spent outside the ICU unit is far less for patients undergoing SCTA rather than V/Q scan, a difference that can be extremely important in critically ill patients requiring monitoring and special nursing care (Pesola and Pesola 2000; Montgomery et al. 2000).

Minimally Invasive

SCTA obviates the complications encountered by heart catheterization at PA in high-risk patients.

Cost-Effectiveness

SCTA is less expensive than V/Q (1.4 times less) and pulmonary angiography (2–8 times less) although it can vary among institutions and countries (Goodman et al. 1997; Van Erkel et al. 1999). Using a study model, the cost-effectiveness of various algorithms for PE diagnosis was evaluated, including V/Q scan, D-dimer assay, pulmonary angiography, lower limb vein US and SCTA. They analyzed the probability of PE and DVT, the accuracy and complications of the different modalities, the prognosis in treated and untreated patients, and the cost of diagnosis and treatment. The five strategies with the lowest mortality rate at 3 months and the lowest associated cost per life saved included SCTA, usually in combination with US examination of the lower limbs (Van Erkel et al. 1996). Further refinements of this model concluded that the most cost-effective approach was US of the lower limbs followed by SCTA if the US findings were negative (Van Erkel and Pattynama 1998). A slightly different study model found that the use of SCTA ± US of lower limbs as a first-line test was associated with the highest expected survival but at a higher cost compared to other diagnostic strategies

(Paterson and Schwartzman 2001). Difficulties in such model studies are large variations in the cost of different tests (i.e., the V/Q lung scan) and in the current performance of improving test (i.e., SCTA). The ability of SCTA to provide an alternative diagnosis was not considered. As patient survival is primarily influenced by the sensitivity of SCTA, even better results can be expected with multislice CT.

Follow-up

SCTA is useful for evaluating the resolution and recanalization of emboli (Godwin et al. 1980; Remy-Jardin et al. 1992, 1997c; Van Rossum et al. 1998c). Although perfusion lung scans are commonly used for this purpose, the changing pattern of perfusion may be confusing or misleading in some patients with central clots; the dissolution and fragmentation of central emboli with a peripheral migration can lead to an apparent worsening of perfusion defects, with chest pain and a misleading diagnosis of recurrent PE (Moser et al. 1973; Urokinase Pulmonary Embolism Trial 1973).

Volume of Contrast Medium

SCTA used less iodinated contrast medium than PA: the mean dose (33.7 g) of iodine injected during SCTA was significantly lower than that injected at selective digital PA (51.3 g) (Qanadli et al. 2000). The dose is expected to be further reduced when using multislice CT (MSCT).

19.9.4.3 Limitations of SCTA

Contraindications to Iodinated Contrast Medium Injection

Renal failure, hypersensitivity to iodinated contrast medium, and severe heart failure may account for contraindications in 2.4%–12% of patients (Ferretti et al. 1997; Remy-Jardin et al. 2000b). Perhaps in the future, the use of gadolinium as a contrast medium agent will be effective with MSCT.

Moderate Amount of Irradiation

SCTA of pulmonary arteries is responsible for a higher effective dose of irradiation than the V/Q lung scan (Robinson 1996). SCTA nevertheless provides a lower radiation dose to the fetus compared to lung perfusion scanning (Winer-Muram et al. 1999). Reducing the collimation may be associated by a substantial increase in the radiation dose delivered to the patient, even with the use of multislice CT (Schoepf et al. 2002). Studies dealing with so-called low-dose CT angiograms are needed.

Inconclusive Examinations

The range of failed or indeterminate SCTA is reported between 2% and 13% (Van Rossum et al. 1996a,b; Remy-Jardin et al. 1996; Mayo et al. 1997; Chartrand-Lefebvre et al. 1999; Garg et al. 1999; Kim et al. 1999; Lomis et al. 1999; Blachere et al. 2000; Qanadli et al. 2000; Remy-Jardin et al. 2000a; Ost et al. 2001; Gottsäter et al. 2001; Perrier et al. 2001). This is in contrast with the nondiagnostic V/Q scan rate, which varies considerably (within the range of 30% to 80%) and in the same range of nondiagnostic PA, which varies from 0% to 17% (Dalen et al. 1971; Hull et al. 1983; PIOPED Investigators 1990; Van Rooij et al. 1995; Van Beek et al. 1996a; Nilsson et al. 1998, 1999). Technical problems are encountered in less than 3% of patients (Remy-Jardin et al. 2000a). Inconclusive examinations are usually related to breathing artifacts (very dyspneic patients are allowed to breath quietly during acquisition), a poor signal-to-noise ratio and insufficient opacification of pulmonary arteries, which may occur in 1%–10% (Remy-Jardin et al. 1996; Van Rossum et al. 1996a,b; Kuzo and Goodman 1997; Kim et al. 1999).

Learning Curve and Pitfalls in Interpretation

The correct interpretation of a SCTA examination of the pulmonary arteries requires a certain level of experience and knowledge of interpretative pitfalls. Interpretative pitfalls may be technically, anatomically or patient-related, resulting in pseudo-filling defects (Teigen et al. 1993; Remy-Jardin et al. 1997a; Kuzo and Goodman 1997; Hansell 1997). Technically related pitfalls include inadequate selection of injection parameters or improper selection of the duration of the apnea according to the patient's respiratory condition. A compromise has to be chosen between high longitudinal spatial resolution and short duration of apnea. Breathing artifacts can result in inhomogeneous opacification of pulmonary arteries in addition to hypodense doubling or blurring of vessels. Soft tissue reconstruction algorithms are mandatory as the high-spatial-frequency reconstruction algorithm frequently used for imaging the thorax shows a high attenuation rim around vertically oriented vessels. Image noise can degrade image quality, especially in heavy patients or in patients with a large pleural effusion. Beam hardening artifacts from contrast in the superior vena cava may create pseudo-filling defects in the arteries of the right upper lobe. Such artifacts may be reduced using a saline push immediately after contrast-medium injection, which produces a washout of the contrast medium in the superior vena cava (Vogel et al. 2001).

Anatomical landmarks and variants need to be known for accurate interpretation. Knowledge of the size and location of intersegmental lymph nodes is important (Remy-Jardin et al. 1995a). Bronchovascular anatomy is also an important prerequisite, as veins may exhibit a pseudo-filling defect due to slow flow. Finally, physiological or pathological factors may influence the SCTA technique or result in examinations that are difficult to interpret: superior vena cava obstruction, cardiomyopathy, focal or globally increased pulmonary resistance and cardiac or pulmonary shunts may require longer scan delays, whereas circumferential perivascular edema, the peribronchovascular course of dilated bronchial arteries or mucous plugging of small bronchi may simulate PE.

Subsegmental PE

The level beyond the segmental level is more difficult to interpret due to small vessel diameter, limited spatial resolution, insufficient enhancement and spatial orientation of vessels and thrombi (Kauczor et al. 1999). SCTA has been criticized for its inability to detect subsegmental PE. However, this limitation also seems to be inherent to both PA and V/Q scanning (Diffin et al. 1998; Stein et al. 1999; Gottsäter et al. 2001). It is well known from balloon-occlusion angiography studies that peripheral PEs are missed during conventional angiography (Bynum et al. 1979; Ferris et al. 1984). In the PIOPED study, all but one of the patients with subsegmental PE as the largest clot had low or intermediate results (nondiagnostic) (Stein and Henry 1997). In a recent study, SCTA detected more subsegmental PE than PA (92 vs 56) and 75% of isolated PE seen at PA. In this setting, SCTA performed obviously better than PA (Qanadli et al. 2000).

Analyzability of Pulmonary Vessels

One of the main advantages of cross-sectional imaging is the absence of overlapping structure in opposition to PA. Initially performed with a 5-mm collimation, 78% of segmental arteries could be correctly analyzed (Ferretti et al. 1997). Subsegmental arteries were considered beyond the scope of SCTA (Goodman et al. 1995). The reduction of the collimation to 3 mm enables correct depiction of 85% of segmental arteries and 37%–43% of subsegmental arteries. Further reduction to 2 mm improves the analyzability of subsegmental arteries to 61%–65% (Remy-Jardin et al. 1997b, 2000b). The recent introduction of MSCT offers a further improvement in performance, in particular the ability to scan larger anatomical volumes with high spatial resolution. A recent anatomical study demonstrated that when using a 4×1-mm collimation and a reconstruction slice thickness of 1.25 mm, 94% of subsegmental arteries and 74% of subsubsegmental arteries were correctly analyzed (Ghaye et al. 2001).

Frequency of Isolated Subsegmental Pulmonary Embolus

The correct diagnosis of acute PE with SCTA is improved by the presence of multiple emboli, while only one is necessary to be confidently recognized for the diagnosis. When a clot breaks off the deep veins of the leg and migrates to the lungs, it fragments in the right heart, showering the lung with emboli that vary in size (Gurney 1993). Thus PE splits into an average of 4–11 fragments with one or more large enough to be detected by CT (Urokinase Pulmonary Embolism Trial 1973; Remy-Jardin et al. 1992; Teigen et al. 1993; Oser et al. 1996; Ferretti et al. 1997; Shah et al. 1999; Blachere et al. 2000; Qanadli et al. 2000). There is a wide range of reported isolated subsegmental emboli both on PA and on SCTA. The true incidence of isolated subsegmental PE is unknown, even in studies using PA, as the interobserver agreement at the subsegmental level varies from 13% to 66% (Quinn et al. 1987; Stein et al. 1992a, 1999). It seems that in a broad selection of patients, less than 10% will have isolated subsegmental PE (PIOPED Investigators 1990; Remy-Jardin et al. 1996, 2000a; Stein and Henry 1997; Nilsson et al. 1999; Blachere et al. 2000; Qanadli et al. 2000), whereas in a highly selected population, limited clinical series or retrospective evaluation, higher frequencies were reported (Goodman et al. 1995; Oser et al. 1996; Goodman and Lipchik 1996; Van Rossum et al. 1996b). Nevertheless, two large studies reported a frequency of 4%–5.9% of all patients and 17%–22.3% of patients with acute positive findings (Diffin et al. 1998; De Monye et al. 2000).

Clinical Significance of Subsegmental Pulmonary Embolism

The clinical importance of subsegmental PE is controversial. Small emboli are frequent and a healthy lung acts as a filter to protect the systemic circulation

(Gurney 1993). Its dual blood supply helps to preserve the integrity of the embolized segment. Small subsegmental PE has been untreated in angiographic studies with less than 1.6% of patients presenting with symptomatic PE in 6–12 months of follow-up (Henry et al. 1995). In the PIOPED population, among patients with only segmental arteries or smaller branches showing PE on PA, fatal and nonfatal events were nonsignificantly different between untreated and treated patients (Stein et al. 1995). Nevertheless, small emboli can be of clinical importance for patients with limited cardiopulmonary reserve (Hull et al. 1995; Remy-Jardin et al. 1996) and are an important indicator for current DVT, which potentially heralds more severe embolic events, in a sense, the tip of the iceberg (Oser et al. 1996). Lower limb vein investigation for DVT can be used as an alternative method in some patients with adequate cardiopulmonary reserve or a low or moderate clinical suspicion of PE (Hull et al. 1994; Wells et al. 1998). However, in trauma patients, half of PE supervenes despite US screening. As long as the controversy on the importance of isolated subsegmental PE is not resolved (will it be one day?), all PE must be considered important (Goodman et al. 1995).

Multislice CT

Three recent studies evaluated the benefit of multislice CT on the detection of subsegmental PE (Fig. 19.8). The first compared single-slice CT (3-mm collimation) and multislice CT (2.5-mm collimation) and found that the latter technique improved the conspicuity of peripheral arteries and identified significantly more peripheral filling defects. Improvements were attributed to the thinner collimation, faster scanning and more homogeneous contrast enhancement possible using multislice CT (Raptopoulos and Boiselle 2001). The second study assessed the influence of reconstructed slice thickness on the detection of subsegmental PE, using multislice CT. Following acquisition with a 4×1-mm collimation, 1-mm-thick reconstructed sections allowed detection of 14% and 40% more of subsegmental PE compared to 2-mm- and 3-mm-thick reconstructed sections, respectively. The benefit was more substantial for vessels with an oblique course to the scanning plane, i.e., middle lobe and lingula. Diagnostic confidence, interobserver agreement and reproducibility of findings were increased and the number of indeterminate results was decreased (Schoepf et al. 2002). The third study evaluated the impact of multislice CT on image quality and diagnostic value for PE compared to single-slice CT. The overall quality of SCTA was significantly higher using multislice CT, particularly for subsegmental arteries. This was related to a higher spatial resolution along the longitudinal axis of the patient and to a decrease in respiratory and cardiac motion artifacts. Interestingly, accurate interpretation of subsegmental vessels was particularly improved in patients with underlying pulmonary disease, a patient population in which the diagnosis of PE is known to be difficult (Remy-Jardin et al. 2002).

Negative Predictive Value of Spiral CT Angiography

One solution to determine the fate of small missed clots is to evaluate the outcome of patients with negative SCTA, namely to determine the rate of subsequent PE (negative predictive value). Although most clinicians readily accept a SCTA-based positive diagnosis of PE, many are hesitant to accept a negative SCTA as a definite exclusion of PE (Goodman et al. 2000). The majority of subsequent PEs occur within the first weeks after treatment for PE or exclusion of PE: 50% of PE recurrence and 90% of PE-related death in treated patients occurred within 1–2 weeks (Carson et al. 1992; Hirsh 1998). Therefore, the mean follow-up of 3 months is acceptable to differentiate missed VTE and a new episode of VTE in a high-risk patient. Nevertheless, the rate of subsequent VTE remains an indirect indicator of the false-negative rate of a test, as in patients with high-risk factors, a new episode of PE does not necessarily mean that the first test was wrongly negative. The results of ten series published in the literature are reported in Table 19.18. This table demonstrates that a negative SCTA may be able to exclude clinically significant VTE with the same level of confidence as negative PA (0%–4.2%) (Novelline et al. 1978; Cheely et al. 1981; Hull et al. 1983; Henry et al. 1995; Van Rooij et al. 1995; Van Beek et al. 1996a,b; Nilsson et al. 1999) or even approaching a normal lung scintigraphy (0%–0.7%) (Hull et al. 1994; Van Beek et al. 1995; Garg et al. 1999; Goodman et al. 2000; Van Beek et al. 2001). Fatal PE varied from 0% to 0.9%. These results require confirmation in further studies, as validity of most of published material is hampered by the small number of autopsies obtained and the high percentage of patients lost for follow-up.

Fig. 19.8a–f. Pulmonary embolism in a patient with chest trauma. A 36-year-old male was involved in a car accident. No traumatic lesion was disclosed at admission. Brain CT was unremarkable. Body CT was not obtained. On the fourth day of hospitalisation, he presented with chest pain and moderate dyspnea. Multidetector spiral CT of the thorax (collimation 3 mm) showed a traumatic dissection and rupture of the aortic isthmus (*arrows*) and multiple central and peripheral pulmonary emboli (*arrowheads*) on axial view and multiplanar reformatting. Couresy of Jean-Paul Maréchal, MD, Clinique André Renard, Herstal Belgium

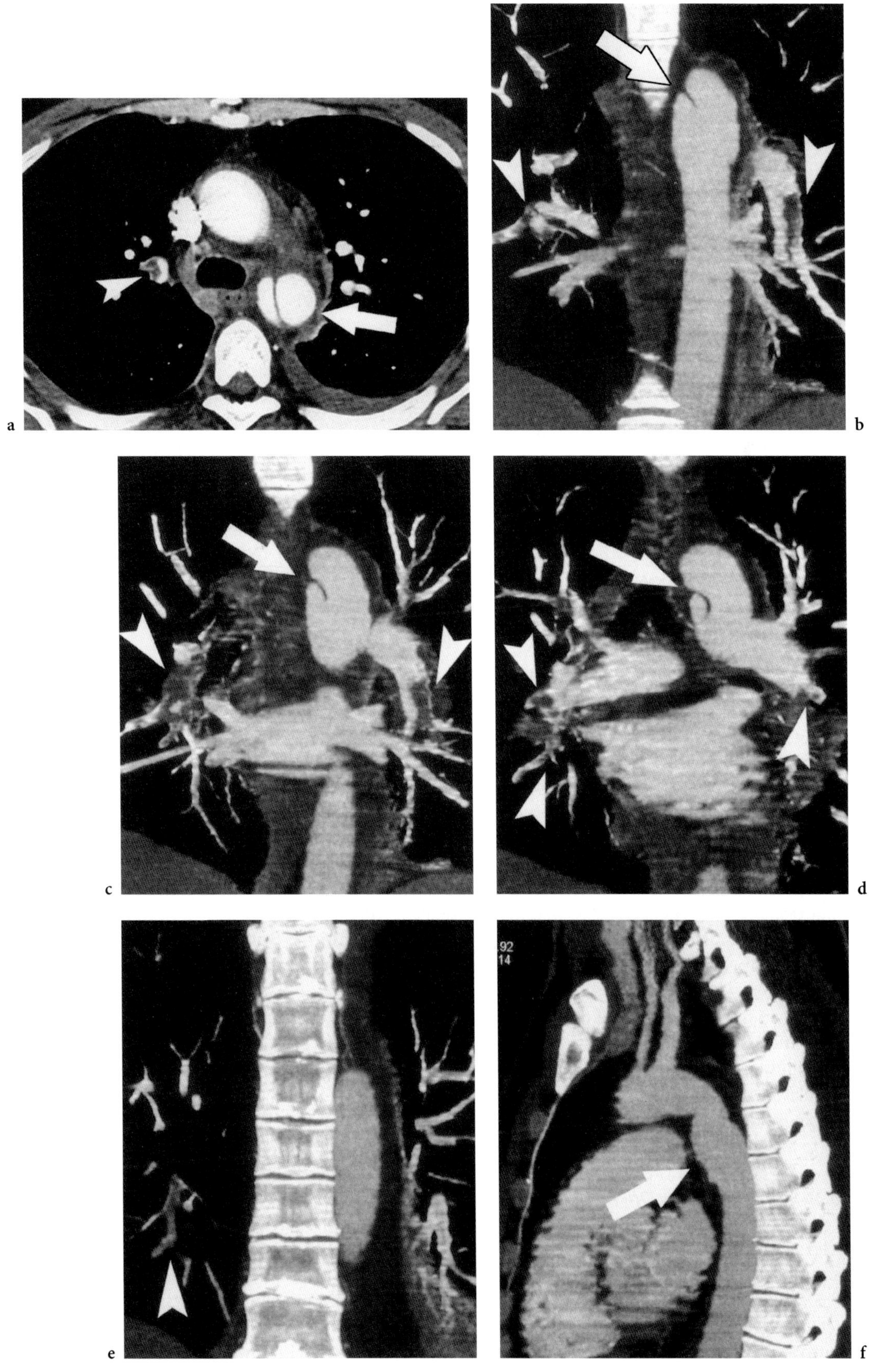

Table 19.18. Follow-up of patients with negative spiral CT angiography

Reference	Entry criteria	No. of patients	SCTA (negative or indeterminate)	Patients with follow-up	Length of follow-up (months)	NPV (%)
Ferretti et al. (1997)	Nondiagnostic V/Q US normal	164	125	109	3	94.6
Krestan et al. (1998)	Clinical suspicion of PE	485	325	155	>3	99.5
Garg et al. (1999)	Nondiagnostic V/Q US normal	126	82	78	6	98.7
Lomis et al. (1999)	Clinical suspicion of PE	143	113	100	6	100
Goodman et al. (2000)	Clinical suspicion of PE, abnormal chest X-ray	393	285	198	3	99
Remy-Jardin et al. (2000a)	Clinical suspicion of PE	370	217 39[a]	59 12	3	100 83.3[a]
Gottsäter et al. (2001)	Clinical suspicion of PE	305	244	215	3	98.6
Ost et al. (2001)	Nondiagnostic V/Q, high clinical suspicion of PE	103	71	71	6	93–96
Swensen et al. (2002)	Clinical suspicion of PE	1512	1010	993	3	99.5
Remy-Jardin et al. (2002)	Clinical suspicion of PE	125[b] 134[c]	98 110	62 91	3	100 99

NPV, negative predictive value.
[a] Indeterminate results. [b] Single-slice CT. [c] Multislice CT.

Large Number of Images

The total number of images from SCTA is in the range of 100–200 using single detector CT (SDCT) and 500–1000 using multislice CT (MSCT). The use of monitor reading has become essential for the analysis of pulmonary arteries, using cine-mode viewing, which results in an increased PE detection rate (Gosselin et al. 1998; Goodman et al. 2000). Monitors are also helpful for multiplanar reconstruction (MPR) in different orientations to differentiate intra- and extravascular structures and to improve diagnostic confidence (Remy-Jardin et al. 1995b). Double-screen monitors presenting the acquisition in mediastinal and parenchymal windows simultaneously can provide more accurate diagnosis, impeding false-positive results, due to respiratory or vascular artifacts. Window settings should also be adapted to the degree of vascular enhancement in order not to miss small emboli (Brink et al. 1997).

Small Size or Obliquely Oriented Arteries

Arteries from the lingula remain the most difficult to interpret due to their small caliber, their oblique or horizontal course, or susceptibility to cardiac artifact. MSCT with the adjunct of cardiac gating should improve analysis of the vessels.

In summary, SCTA should be considered as the initial imaging modality of choice, particularly in patient subgroups, which are known to be associated with a high rate of nondiagnostic V/Q scans, such as in-patients (including trauma patients) and patients with a history of cardiopulmonary disease or abnormalities on chest X-ray.

19.9.5 Combined Spiral CT Angiography–CT Venography

While clots in the lung clearly influence the cardiopulmonary status of the patient, the major risk of death is from recurrent PE, as supported by the data of the PIOPED study, in which 90% of patients dying from PE actually died from a recurrent embolic event (Carson et al. 1992). Completing nondiagnostic V/Q scan or negative PA or SCTA by imaging of the lower extremity veins (usually serial) in patients with suspected PE has already been advocated in the past (Hull et al. 1983, 1985; Stein et al. 1993; Goodman and Lipchik 1996; Sostman 1997; Lomis et al. 1999). Nevertheless, serial US or impedance plethysmography may be difficult to implement and delay the final diagnosis (Goodman and Lipchik 1996). The combination of SCTA of pulmonary arteries and CT venography (CTV) of lower limbs and abdominal veins in one session was first reported in 1998 (Loud et al. 1998). CTV is performed immediately after SCTA acquisition without additional injection of contrast medium or separate venipuncture, adding negligible time to the study. The acquisition of CTV should be obtained after a delay of 3–3.5 min after starting contrast medium injection (Yankelevitz et al. 2000; Szapiro et al. 2001; Bruce et al. 2001). The combined SCTA-CTV provides a comprehensive evaluation of patients suspected of PE: it is a simple diagnostic (one-stop shop) algorithm: if one is positive, the patient is treated; if both are negative, no treatment is indicated. Criteria for the diagnosis of DVT with CTV include (Figs. 19.4, 19.7):

- Filling defect in an opacified vein
- High-contrast rim of the venous wall
- Venous dilatation as compared with the normal contralateral side
- Obliteration of perivenous fat, suggestive of edema
- Opacification of collateral veins (Zerhouni et al. 1980; Baldt et al. 1996; Loud et al. 1998)

CTV can be performed using either the sequential technique (Ghaye et al. 2000; Loud et al. 2000, 2001; Katz et al. 2000; Garg et al. 2000; Garg and Mao 2001), spiral technique (El Hajjam et al. 1999; Cham et al. 2000; Duwe et al. 2000; Muller et al. 2001; Wildberger et al. 2002) or mixed sequential and spiral technique (Coche et al. 2001; Nicolas et al. 2001). By comparing the results of CTV to US, results had an 89%–100% sensitivity and a 94%–100% specificity (Loud et al. 2000, 2001; Coche et al. 2001; Duwe et al. 2000; Garg et al. 2000). General intertechnique agreement varied from 0.84 to 1.0 (El Hajjam et al. 1999; Ghaye et al. 2000). CTV also demonstrated the extension of DVT more precisely, which may be important information before an intervention such as insertion of an inferior vena cava filter. CTV also demonstrated DVT in pelvic or abdominal veins that are not assessed by US, as well as additional findings that may explain the patient's symptoms (GI tract perforation, subdiaphragmatic abscess or abdominal hematoma; Ghaye et al. 2002a). CTV increases the percentage of positive cases by 11%–36% compared to SCTA alone (Cham et al. 2000; Katz et al. 2000; Garg et al. 2000; Coche et al. 2001; Loud et al. 2001; Nicolas et al. 2001). This technique is particularly useful in the ICU and in trauma patients, who are often intubated and in whom one cannot assess leg symptoms. Furthermore, the quality of SCTA may be limited by breathing artifacts in these patients. The presence of dressings, casts, trophic skin changes and the lack of mobility in trauma patients make US difficult to perform whereas they do not represent a problem for CTV (Ghaye et al. 2000; Ghaye and Dondelinger 2002).

19.9.6 Magnetic Resonance Imaging

To date, magnetic resonance angiography (MRA) does not have a widespread use in emergency medicine and in critically ill patients, mainly because of long examination time, difficulties in patient monitoring, higher cost and the limited availability or access of MR in most centers. Nevertheless, MRA is evolving as a promising alternative technique in the direct and noninvasive evaluation of VTE disease (Gefter et al. 1995; Kauczor 1998; Hoffmann et al. 1999). The main advantages over CT are the absence of nephrotoxic iodinated contrast medium and ionizing radiation (Woodard et al. 1995). Unfortunately, trauma patients may frequently present contraindications for MR examination, especially those with orthopedic hardware, although improvements are continuously made in the MR compatibility of most materials.

The limitations of the first 2D time-of-flight (TOF) technique used in the early 1990s, which allowed visualization of central vessels only, have been overcome by advances in MR software and hardware, with strong gradients and the use of 3D-gradient echo sequences. Small studies have compared the value of MRA with PA in the diagnosis of PE (Table 19.19).

Early studies were performed without injection of contrast medium and showed sensitivities from 55% to 100% and specificities from 60% to 78%. Subsequent studies with contrast-medium injection showed sensitivities of 46%–100% and specificities from 90%–100%, including analysis of peripheral PE. The interobserver agreement varied from 0.38 to 0.83, demonstrating that a certain level of experience is required for correct interpretation (Grist et al. 1993; Sostman et al. 1996; Meaney et al. 1997; Gupta et al. 1999). Like the combined use of SCTA and CTV, MR of the pulmonary arteries can be completed by MR venography of the lower limbs and pelvis (Grist et al. 1993; Sostman et al. 1993), which have results similar to conventional venography (Evans et al. 1993; Carpenter et al. 1993; Ruehm et al. 2000). The advent of blood-pooled agents should further increase the accuracy of the technique (Ahlström et al. 1999). Another approach is the direct and selective visualization of clots in lower limb DVT and in pulmonary emboli due to the predictable T1 changes in clots (Moody et al. 1997, 1998). Recent experimental stud-

Table 19.19. Magnetic resonance in the diagnosis of acute pulmonary embolism

Reference	No. of patients	Gold standard (No.)	Sequence	Anatomical level of interpretation	Sensitivity (%)	Specificity (%)	K
Grist et al. (1993)	20	PA (14) Others (6)	2D TOF Fast GRE	Segmental	92–100	62	0.38
Holland et al. (1993)	16	PA (12) Others (4)	-	Central	79	100	-
Schiebler et al. (1993)	18	PA (8) Others (16)	2D TOF, SE, Cine SPAMM	Main Lobar	86 55	78 60	-
Erdman et al. (1994)	34	PA (34)	SE, multiphasic SE, GRE	Segmental	90	77	-
Loubeyre et al. (1994)	23	PA (23)	Fast GRE turboFLASH + gadolinium	Central	70	100	-
Laissy et al. (1995)	28	PA (28)	2D TOF 2D TurboFLASH + gadolinium	Segmental	50	100	-
Sostman et al. (1996)	25 [53]	PA (-) VQ (-)	2D GRASS	Subsegmental	5 readers: 14–86 (46)	67–100 (90)	
Meaney et al. (1997)	30	PA (30)	Fast GRE + gadolinium	Segmental	75–100	95–100	0.57–0.83
Gupta et al. (1999)	36	PA (36) + gadolinium	Fast GRE	Subsegmental	85	96	0.54

PA, pulmonary angiography; *TOF*, time-of-flight; *GRE*, gradient-recalled echo; *SE*, spin-echo; *SPAMM*, spatial modulation of magnetization; *FLASH*, fast low-angle shot; *GRASS*, gradient-recalled acquisition in steady state.

ies showed that pulmonary arteries are visible down to the subsegmental level (Goyen et al. 2001) and MR was equivalent to SCTA for demonstration of small PE (Reittner et al. 2001). MRI is a promising method for complete morphological and functional work-up in patients with VTE, including imaging of PE and DVT, perfusion imaging of the pulmonary microcirculation, ventilation imaging and assessment of the right ventricle function and flow in the pulmonary arteries, all findings that may be necessary for adequate treatment of patients (Kauczor 1998; Meaney et al. 1999).

MR can be more specific than CT for the characterization of pulmonary infarction, as methemoglobin contained in pulmonary infarction will produce a high signal on T1-weighted images (Kessler et al. 1991).

19.9.7 Echocardiography

Echocardiography (ECG) is usually performed using a transthoracic (TTE) or a transesophageal (TEE) approach. The use of intravascular ultrasound remains within the field of research (Porter et al. 1994; Tapson et al. 1994). ECG can be used as a first-line method at the bedside in unstable trauma patients, as it allows the diagnosis of acute right heart failure, visualizes clots in the right heart or in some locations of the central pulmonary arteries, depending on TTE or TEE use (Vignon et al. 1994; Pruszczyk et al. 2001). When positive, immediate treatment can be started, but in case of doubt, SCTA should be performed before initiating treatment (Kasper et al. 1997b; Krivec et al. 1997; Karavidas et al. 2000). ECG can provide alternative diagnoses such as aortic dissection, pericardial tamponade or myocardial infarction. ECG can be helpful in assessing right heart dysfunction by demonstrating right ventricle (RV) dilatation and hypokinesis, straightening, leftward bowing or paradoxical motion of the interventricular septum, decreased left ventricular volume, loss of inspiratory collapse of the IVC, tricuspid regurgitation and dilatation of pulmonary artery (Kasper et al. 1986; Jardin et al. 1997). The McConnell sign, a distinct echocardiographic pattern of regional RV dysfunction in which the apex is spared, appears to be specific for acute PE (McConnell et al. 1996). The presence of RV hypertrophy (wall thickness >5–6 mm) help to differentiate between acute and subacute or chronic massive PE (Prakash and Matsukubo 1983; Kasper et al. 1993). ECG can assess the prognosis of acute PE, an acute RV afterload stress being associated with a high rate of complications and mortality (Kasper et al. 1997a,b; Pruszczyk et al. 1997).

With respect to the diagnosis of PE, TEE performs better than TTE (Steiner et al. 1996; Antakly-Hanon et al. 1998; Miniati et al. 2001). Nevertheless, the combination of TTE, US of lower limb veins and a clinical score has a sensitivity of 89% (97% when PE is massive) and a specificity of 74% (Grifoni et al. 1998). TEE suffers from operator dependency, topographical limitation due to pulmonary air and central airways, and technical limitations, which may impede using TEE in up to 40% of patients (very dyspneic or mechanically ventilated patients, nondiet rest, etc.) (Antakly-Hanon et al. 1998). The results of four studies comparing ECG with SCTA demonstrated higher accuracy for SCTA. TEE showed an 80%–85% sensitivity and an 86%–100% specificity for central PE. Concerning peripheral PE, results are 55%–59% and 77%, respectively, which are insufficient to warrant this test in a routine clinical setting (Steiner et al. 1996; Pruszczyk et al. 1997, 2001; Antakly-Hanon et al. 1998). Comparison of imaging modalities for the diagnosis of pulmonary embolism are presented in Table 19.20.

19.10 Post-traumatic Venous Thrombosis in the Abdomen

Patients with major abdominal venous injuries have a mortality rate approaching 50%, usually resulting from exsanguinating hemorrhage (Cohen et al. 1980). A less well-known entity concerns post-traumatic intra-abdominal venous thrombosis.

19.10.1 Thrombosis of the Inferior Vena Cava

Trauma of the inferior vena cava (IVC) is a relatively rare event occurring in 0.4%–5.4% of penetrating trauma and in about 0.9% of blunt trauma abdominal injuries (Leppäniemi et al. 1994). Injury to the IVC is serious, as more than one-third of patients die before reaching the hospital and another third die during the course of treatment. High mortality is determined by associated organ injury and pericaval containment in case of transmural laceration of the IVC (Grmoljez et al. 1976; Ombrellaro et al. 1997). Thrombosis of the IVC is a rare disease. A review of the literature since 1987 has demonstrated that thrombosis has been associated with a large number of diseases (Peck et al. 1998; Table 19.21). Despite the high incidence of lower limb DVT, post-traumatic thrombosis of the IVC has been rarely reported (Henne-Bruns and Kremer 1992; Geerts et al. 1994), although Sevitt

Table 19.20. Comparison of imaging modalities for pulmonary embolism [Modified from Goodman et al. (1997), with permission]

	V/Q scan	US	PA	SCTA	MR	TEE
Sensitivity	>96%	<50%[a]	>95%	>90%[b]	>80%	>80%[d]
Specificity	>20%	NA	>95%	>95%[b]	>90%	>90%
Morbidity	0	0	~ 2%	0.04%[c]	0.0003–0.7%	~0.5%
Mortality	0	0	<1%	<0.00005%[c]	~0	<0.05%
Availability	+++	++++	++	++++	++	+++
Alternative Dx	<+	NA	<+	+++	+++	+
Cost (US$)[e]	1.3 ×[e]	0.3 ×[e]	2.3 ×[e]	1 ×[e]	1.5–7.5 ×	0.5–1 ×
Bedside	+	++++	<+	–	–	++++

V/Q, ventilation/perfusion lung scan; *US*, ultrasound; *PA*, pulmonary angiography; *SCTA*, spiral CT angiography; *MR*, magnetic resonance; *TEE*, transesophageal echography; *NA*, not available.
[a] Percentage of patients with proven pulmonary embolism who have positive Doppler studies of lower extremity veins.
[b] Results of single detector CT.
[c] Mortality, morbidity from nonionic contrast.
[d] For central PE.
[e] Mean cost in five European and one US hospitals (Van Erkel et al. 1999).

Table 19.21. Causes of inferior vena cava thrombosis [Modified from PECK et al. (1998), with permission]

IVC filters
Femoral vein catheterization
Venous prosthetic devices
Budd-Chiari syndrome
Congenital abnormalities of the IVC
IVC aneurysm
Abdominal aortic aneurysm
Retroperitoneal fibrosis
Retroperitoneal hematoma
Behçet's syndrome
Primary tumor of the IVC
Compression or invasion by tumors (liver, kidney, lymphoma, pancreas, adrenal, lymphadenopathies, etc.)
Hepatic abscess
Chronic pancreatitis
Pancreatic cysts
Blunt abdominal trauma
Postoperative sequelae of laparoscopy
Postpartum ovarian vein thrombosis
Liver transplantation
Systemic amyloidosis
Septic thrombophlebitis
Acute staphylococcal osteomyelitis
Burns
Antiphospholipid syndrome
Membranous lupus nephritis
Coagulation abnormalities
Ulcerative colitis
Strenuous athletics
Others

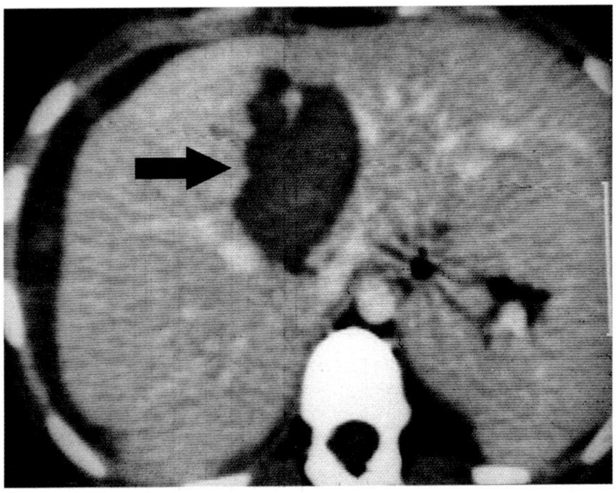

a

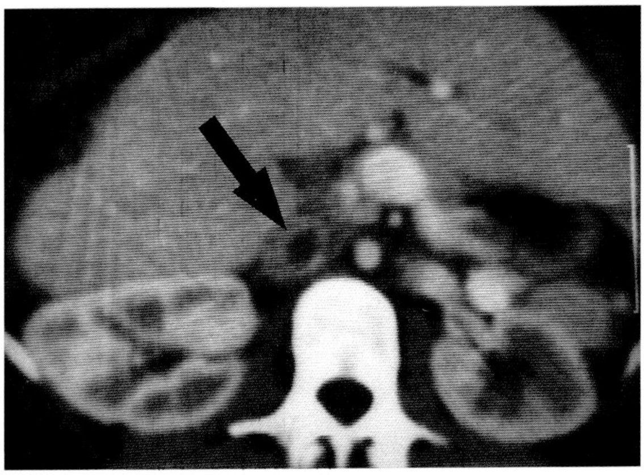

b

Fig. 19.9a, b. Post-traumatic IVC thrombosis. **a** Contrast-enhanced abdominal CT performed 4 days after trauma showed a 6-cm intrahepatic hematoma (*arrow*), with mixed densities, and perihepatic hemoperitoneum with fresh clots. **b** A nonocclusive segmental thrombus was seen in the infrarenal IVC. No significant PE occurred. Conservative management of liver injury

and GALLAGHER have noticed extension of lower limb DVT into the IVC in 5% of patients (SEVITT and GALLAGHER 1961). To the best of our knowledge, only 24 post-traumatic IVC thromboses have been reported in the English, French, German and Japanese literature (Table 19.22). All reported cases resulted from blunt trauma. The clinical features usually remain vague and nonspecific and the diagnosis is usually made by chance (Fig. 19.9). Symptoms include nonspecific abdominal pain (36%), low back pain (14%), or renal disease (23%). Nine patients (41%) presented with Budd-Chiari syndrome. Associated lower limb DVT is reported in 23% of cases only and lower limb swelling in 41%, indicating that lack of these symptoms cannot rule out the presence of IVC thrombosis. Sometimes patients remain nonsymptomatic, particularly when thrombus is not occlusive. Seven patients (32%) experienced PE before diagnosis, two proved to be fatal. No recurrence or new episode of PE was mentioned after the diagnosis.

US can fail to demonstrate IVC thrombosis, especially in the infrarenal segment, due to frequent bowel gas distension in trauma patients (TAKEUCHI et al. 1995). In case of suspicion, abdominal CT could solve the problem (CAMPBELL et al. 1981; NAGY and DUARTE 1990; KUKI et al. 1995; PATEL et al. 1996; KIMOTO et al. 1998; CELLARIER et al. 1999).

Different mechanisms have been proposed for traumatic IVC thrombosis (CAMPBELL et al. 1981; TAKEUCHI et al. 1995):

- An endothelial injury of the venous wall resulting from compression or shearing forces that directly lead to caval mural thrombosis which progressed to occlusion

- Caval stasis secondary to compression of the IVC by pericaval or retroperitoneal hematoma
- Traumatic hepatic or renal vein thrombosis extending into the IVC
- The presence of a central IVC catheter

It is noteworthy that prolonged immobility, which is one of the most important predisposing factors of post-traumatic DVT, was usually not present (Takeuchi et al. 1995).

A prothrombotic condition was present in less than half of patients, particularly in patients with membranous obstruction of the IVC (Balian et al. 1998). Nearly half of the patients presented with Budd-Chiari syndrome. Budd-Chiari syndrome results from hepatic venous outflow obstruction with hepatomegaly, ascites, abdominal pain and deterioration of liver function, eventually progressing to liver failure or portal hypertension. The anatomical location of the traumatic obstruction can be the major hepatic veins (Brink and Botha 1955) or the IVC above the hepatic veins (Little and Montgomery 1952; Hales and Scatliff 1966; Deutsch et al. 1972; Grmoljez et al. 1976; Kuki et al. 1995; Coue et al. 1996; Patel et al. 1996; Balian et al. 1998). It is now admitted that membranous obstruction of the IVC results from localized thrombosis and trauma has been suggested as one of the main factors involved in the development of thrombosis (Balian et al. 1998). The other causes listed in the literature are congenital, post-thrombotic and postinfectious (Coue et al. 1996). The development of membranous stenosis occurs as a result of laceration of the IVC during the initial injury. Then the inflammatory endothelial proliferation during the healing process leads to stenosis and secondary thrombosis extends in the hepatic venous outflow and the IVC. The IVC adjacent to the point of diaphragmatic fixation seems to be particularly vulnerable to compression or shearing injury (Patel et al. 1996). Budd-Chiari syndrome is often fatal in its acute form, which makes prompt diagnosis and immediate treatment necessary (Kuki et al. 1995).

The overall delay between injury and symptomatic presentation of IVC thrombosis ranged from 2 days to 7 years. In patients without associated chronic signs of IVC thrombosis (membranous obstruction), the delay ranged from 13 days to 3 months, most appearing in the first 6 weeks. This delay is almost the same as for post-traumatic lower limb DVT. The delay in patients presenting with Budd-Chiari syndrome or a membranous obstruction of the IVC ranged from 2 days to 7 years, most of them appearing some months or years after trauma, which means that post-traumatic Budd-Chiari syndrome is usually delayed rather than acute.

Different treatment modalities have been proposed for the management of IVC thrombosis. Anticoagulation remains essential if not contraindicated. As for lower limb DVT, IVC filters, temporary or definite, may be indicated as IVC thrombosis can progress under anticoagulation (Girard et al. 1989; Cellarier et al. 1999). In case of extensive IVC thrombosis, associated with renal or liver failure, or contraindication to anticoagulation, surgical thrombectomy, membranectomy and/or angioplasty should be performed. Treatment using percutaneous mechanical thrombectomy, PTA and fibrinolysis have also been described for post-traumatic Budd-Chiari syndrome (Patel et al. 1996; Balian et al. 1998).

19.10.2 Other Thromboses

19.10.2.1 Renal Veins

Traumatic renal vein thrombosis usually occurs in combination with arterial and/or parenchymal injury and follows severe abdominal trauma. Isolated renal vein thrombosis is extremely rare and has been described after localized abdominal trauma (Laakso et al. 1982; Sapir et al. 1982; Fanney et al. 1990; Nau et al. 1992; Berkovich et al. 2001). According to Berkovich, among the eight case reports in the literature, this author described the only convincing traumatic isolated vein thrombosis without arterial injury, renal disease or evidence of a medical disorder that could be responsible for thrombus formation (Berkovich et al. 2001). Though nephrotic syndrome is now considered the cause rather the consequence of renal vein thrombosis, Laakso reported the case of unilateral renal vein thrombosis following a horse kick associated with traumatic proliferative glomerulonephritis and nephrotic syndrome (Laakso et al. 1982). Based on the degree of obstruction and collaterality, the clinical presentation varies from an absence of symptoms to back pain or hematuria. In rare cases, PE, sometimes fatal, may be the presenting sign of traumatic renal vein thrombosis (Nau et al. 1992). CT is the modality of choice for diagnosis, showing clots in a dilated renal vein, usually associated with renal enlargement, delayed or absent collecting system enhancement, prolonged corticomedullary differentiation, infiltration of perinephric fat and thickening of renal fascia (Berkovich et al. 2001). Treatment options include anticoagulation, local thrombolysis or in some conditions surgery.

Table 19.22. Post-traumatic thrombosis of the inferior vena cava

Reference	Age/sex	Mechanism of injury	Type of vascular injury	Clinical presentation: Signs associated with IVC thrombosis	Lower limb edema	Lower limb thrombosis	Associated abdominal injuries	Location of IVC thrombosis	Other abdominal thrombosis	Delay between injury and clinical presentation	PE	Treatment	Outcome
Little and Montgomery (1952)	57/M	Road accident (hit by a truck)	IVC stenosis at the level of diaphragm (endothelial injury?)	Lower limb edema, abdominal pain, Budd-Chiari syndrome	+	–	–	Supra- and infrarenal IVC	Renal vein, hepatic veins	3 months	–	Antibiotic therapy	Death at d 45 after admission (9 months after trauma)
Hales and Scatliff (1966)	28/M	Sport accident (baseball bat)	–	Budd-Chiari syndrome, hematemesis	–	–	–	Supra- and infrarenal IVC	Renal veins, hepatic veins, portal vein	7 years	–	Surgical by-pass	Death 22 years after trauma
Pasquier et al. (1969)	27/M	Crush trauma of both thighs	Lower limb DVT extending to iliac veins and IVC, compression by retroperitoneal hematoma	Back pain, altered general condition, fever	+	+	–	Infrarenal IVC	–	6 weeks	–	Thrombectomy + AC	–
Deutsch et al. (1972)	–	–	–	Budd-Chiari syndrome	–	–	–	Suprarenal IVC	Hepatic vein →IVC→ right heart	–	+	–	Death 2 weeks later
	–	–	–	Budd-Chiari syndrome	–	–	–	Suprarenal IVC	–	–	–	–	–
Grmoljez et al. (1976)	57/M	Crush injury to thorax and abdomen	Transmural laceration of IVC (pericaval hematoma)	Back pain, DVT (bilateral), circulatory collapse, progressive hematuria, Budd-Chiari syndrome under AC	+	+	–	Mediastinal + supra- and infrarenal IVC	Renal veins	6 weeks	+	AC + thrombectomy + surgical repair of IVC laceration	OK
Kittredge et al. (1979)	30/M	–	–	–	–	–	–	Suprarenal IVC	–	7 years	–	–	OK
Campbell et al. (1981)	21/M	Car accident	Endothelial injury	Abdominal pain, fatigue	–	–	Minor liver laceration	Retrohepatic + infrarenal IVC	–	13 days	+	AC	OK
Bauer et al. (1983)	25/M	Abdominal contusion	Endothelial injury	Abdominal wall edema	+	+	–	Supra- and infrarenal IVC	–	–	–	AC	OK
Nagy and Duarte (1990)	55/M	Car accident	Endothelial injury	Abdominal and back pain	–	–	–	Infrarenal IVC	–	18 days	–	PIVCF + AC	OK
Knudson et al. (1992)	33/F	Car accident	Endothelial injury	–	–	–	Splenic/liver laceration	–	–	21 days	+	AC	–

Mayzlik et al. (1992)	49/M	Lumbar impact «squash»	–	Nephrotic syndrome	+	+	–	Suprarenal IVC	–	2 months	–	Surgery (thrombectomy)	OK
Nau et al. (1992)	30/M	Slight sport trauma	Endothelial injury	PE	–	–	–	IVC at the level of left renal vein	Left renal vein	6 weeks	+	AC, Fibrinolysis	Death 4 h after fibrinolysis (from PE)
Burks et al. (1992)	46/M	Car accident	Compression by adrenal hematoma	NA	NA	NA	Adrenal hematoma	Infrarenal IVC	–	4 weeks	NA	PIVCF	NA
Kuki et al. (1995)	20/M	Car accident	Endothelial laceration	Budd-Chiari syndrome, acute renal failure	+	–	Liver necrosis	Suprarenal IVC	Hepatic veins, renal veins	3 weeks	–	Surgery (thrombectomy and angioplasty)	OK
Takeuchi et al. (1995)	21/M	Car accident	Compression by retroperitoneal hematoma, central IVC catheter	Abdominal pain, hematuria	–	–	Pelvic fracture, retroperitoneal hematoma, hemoperitoneum	Infrarenal IVC	–	14 days	+	–	Death (acute PE)
Coue et al. (1996)	29/M	Motorcycle accident	Membranous obstruction	Lower limb pain, abdominal pain, Budd-Chiari syndrome	–	–	Renal contusion, dissection of renal artery	No acute thrombosis	–	3 years	–	PTA × 2	Relapse at 11 month surgical angioplasty
Patel et al. (1996)	36/F	Car accident	Endothelial injury	Abdominal pain, Budd-Chiari syndrome, fever, oliguria	+	+	Small liver laceration, perforation of small intestine	Infra and suprarenal IVC	Renal veins, right hepatic vein	5 weeks	–	Urokinase + PTA, AC, percutaneous mechanical thrombectomy	OK
Balian et al. (1998)	31/M	Road accident	Membranous obstruction	Fatigue, abnormal liver tests	–	–	Right kidney injury	No acute thrombus	–	3 years	–	AC + PTA	Relapse of membranous obstruction→ surgical angioplasty
	17/M	Motorcycle accident	Membranous obstruction	Abdominal pain, Budd-Chiari syndrome	+	–	Spleen hematoma	Infrarenal IVC →right atrium	Hepatic veins, renal veins	2 days	–	AC, angioplasty, stenting of IVC	Relapse at 1 year→ surgery
Kimoto et al. (1998)	35/M	Fall (3 m)	Endothelial injury	Abdominal pain, fever	–	–	Liver laceration	Infrarenal IVC	–	35 days	–	Surgery (thrombectomy)	OK
Cellarier et al. (1999)	50/M	Car accident	Endothelial injury	PE	+	–	Pelvic fracture, abdominal contusion	Infrarenal IVC	–	3 months	+	Temporary IVCF + surgery + AC	OK

AC, anticoagulation; *DVT*, deep venous thrombosis; *F*, female; *IVC*, inferior vena cava; *M*, male; *PE*, pulmonary embolism; *PIVCF*, prophylactic inferior vena cava filter; *PTA*, percutaneous transluminal angioplasty.
Two more cases of the Japanese literature are reported by Takeuchi et al. (1995).

19.10.2.2 Hepatic Veins

Traumatic Budd-Chiari syndrome may be encountered without thrombosis or membranous obstruction of the IVC. Usually, it results from compression of the hepatic veins by a large liver hematoma (Nicoloff et al. 1964) or intrathoracic liver hernia following rupture of the diaphragm (Fernandez-Gonzalez et al. 1994). Two cases of isolated hepatic vein thrombosis presenting clinically as Budd-Chiari syndrome 3 months after major trauma have been reported (Brink and Botha 1955; Izard et al. 1995). The deceleration probably caused torsion of the hepatic veins without rupture, producing severe endothelial injury.

19.10.2.3 Portal Venous System

Portal Vein

Abdominal blunt trauma is an exceptional cause of portal vein thrombosis. To the best of our knowledge, ten case reports have been published in the literature (Duvoux et al. 1994 including a review of seven cases in literature; Beaufort et al. 1996; Prignet et al. 1996). In adults, portal vein thrombosis is usually associated with liver cirrhosis, hepatocellular carcinoma or other intra-abdominal tumor, abdominal inflammatory of infectious disease, myeloproliferative disease and hemostasis abnormalities. Clinical signs of portal vein thrombosis are usually poor and nonspecific: abdominal pain, vomiting, diarrhea a few days or a few weeks after trauma or late hepatocellular insufficiency (Beaufort et al. 1996; Prignet et al. 1996), or gastrointestinal bleeding due to portal hypertension associated with formation of portal cavernoma and esophageal varices (Beaufort et al. 1996). Rare reports used anticoagulation successfully as the only treatment modality, and surgery was advocated in some cases (Duvoux et al. 1994).

Mesenteric and Splenic Veins

Post-traumatic portal vein thrombosis can extend to the superior mesenteric and splenic vein (Beaufort et al. 1996). Isolated post-traumatic superior mesenteric vein thrombosis has been rarely reported. Avulsion producing massive hemorrhage is the most frequent (McCune et al. 1952; Courcy et al. 1984; Claikens et al. 1998). Post-traumatic intestinal infarction of venous origin manifests in the first 24 h or is delayed from 2 days to 1 month. The rapidity and severity of symptoms are related to the proximal or distal location of the thrombus and the capability of formation of collaterals (Jekic 1980). Anticoagulation is mandatory, with a usually large surgical resection of infarcted bowel and venous disobstruction (Courcy et al. 1984). Splenic vein thrombosis is a rare complication of splenectomy or arterial splenic embolization. It may sometimes extend to the portal and/or mesenteric vein, usually in patients with hematological disorders (Petit et al. 1994).

Hepatic Arteriovenous Fistula

Without communication with the caval system, thrombosis of the portal system cannot produce pulmonary embolism. Two cases of blunt and penetrating abdominal trauma producing a large communication between the hepatic artery and the hepatic veins through a large liver hematoma have been reported. Both produced massive fatal PE (Huguet et al. 1975; Lagache et al. 1980).

19.11 Uncommon Causes of Pulmonary Embolism

The microvascular pulmonary bed has the property to filter any substance of approximately 10 μm or greater that gains access to the venous circulation (King and Harmon 1994). This can result in obstruction to blood flow, injury to the lung parenchyma and impairment of gas exchanges. In addition to cruor embolism, numerous disorders may be conceptualized as embolic disease to the lung (Table 19.23).

Many of these so-called emboli can be produced at the time of trauma or during the recovery period. Other types of emboli can be found in blunt abdominal trauma patients and do not involve the pulmonary circulation:

- Nucleus pulposus embolism, arterial or venous, causing spinal cord ischemia (Toro et al. 1994)
- Atheromatous embolization in the visceral or peripheral arterial bed (Hertzer 1977; Kiechle et al. 1983).

19.11.1 Fat Embolism

Fat embolism syndrome (FES) is extensively debated in the literature in terms of its etiology, risk, patho-

Table 19.23. Uncommon causes of pulmonary embolism

- Tumor
  - Solid tumor (renal cell carcinoma, right atrium myxoma or lymphoma, pulmonary artery sarcoma, endocardial metastases, etc.)
  - Endovascular lymphoma
- Hematopoietic cell
  - Tumoral (acute or chronic myeloblastic leukemia)
  - Sickle cell disease
  - Leukostasis
- Septic emboli
  - Infected thrombophlebitis
  - Lemierre syndrome
  - Infected indwelling catheter
  - Osteomyelitis
  - Hydatid
- IV drug addict
  - Septic emboli
  - Talc
  - Cellulosis
  - Cotton
  - Starch
- Air
- Fat
- Amniotic fluid
- Bone marrow
- Skin, hair
- Osseous or cartilaginous fragments
- Parasite (schistosomiasis)
- Parenchyma (liver, brain)
- Extraneous material:
  - Missile
  - Indwelling catheters
- Cardiac vegetations
- Others
  - Mercury
  - Barium sulfate
  - Iodinated oil
  - Sclerotherapy material
  - Methylmethacrylate cement (percutaneous vertebroplasty, orthopedic surgery)
  - Vegetable

physiology, diagnosis and treatment, which makes FES one of the least clearly understood complications of trauma. Since the first clinical diagnosis of FES following trauma (Von Bergmann 1873), blunt trauma has been recognized as a primary cause of FES. The causes of FES are multiple and include traumatic, surgical, and nontraumatic origin (Table 19.24).

FES and fat embolism are not synonymous: FES is a phenomenon secondary to fat embolism (Lindeque et al. 1987; Johnson and Lucas 1996; Bulger et al. 1997).

19.11.1.1 Pathophysiology and Clinical Manifestations

The classic triad of FES consists of respiratory distress, cerebral dysfunction and a petechial rash (Table 19.25).

Table 19.24. Causes of fat embolism (Modified from Fabian [1993]; King and Harmon [1994]; Johnson and Lucas [1996])

Bone fracture
(especially shaft of long-bone and pelvic fractures)
Orthopedic procedures
Adipose tissue injuries
Burns
External cardiac massage
Liver trauma
Liposuction
Osteomyelitis
Diabetes mellitus
Pancreatitis
Sickle cell disease
Liver steatosis
Bone marrow harvesting and transplant
Bone tumor lysis
Decompression sickness
High-altitude flights
Renal transplantation
Epilepsy
Severe infection
Extracorporeal circulation
Cardiopulmonary by-pass
Steroid therapy
Chemotherapy
Parenteral infusion of lipids

The clinical recognition of FES may be difficult, as most signs are also commonly found in severe trauma patients without FES. Furthermore, there is no standard definition of FES and Gurd's criteria are criticized (Gurd and Wilson 1974; Lindeque et al. 1987).

The first step of fat embolism is a traumatic mechanical release due to local high pressure of fat globule from bone marrow (or adipose tissue) in small veins, which eventually embolized into the lungs and in systemic small arteries via cardiac or intrapulmonary shunts.

Sudden Death

All patients with fractures have fat in their blood and subclinical fat embolism occurs in 47%–100% of trauma patients (Ten Duis et al. 1988; Hulman 1995; Johnson and Lucas 1996; Mudd et al. 2000). An initial mechanical effect that is severe enough can lead to right heart strain or failure, secondary to pulmonary hypertension (Heine et al. 1998). No correlation is found between the presence and the amount of fat and the severity of the clinical manifestations, which means that obstruction is probably not the only mechanism, but may compound other thoracic problems. However, multiple reports of macroscopic fat embolus large enough to obstruct large

Table 19.25. Clinical diagnostic criteria of fat embolism syndrome (Adapted from GURD and WILSON [1974] and TAKAHASHI et al. [1999])

Major (at least 1)	
	Respiratory symptoms with positive radiographic changes
	Cerebral signs unrelated to head injury or any other condition
	Petechial rash
Minor (at least four)	
	Tachycardia
	Pyrexia
	Retinal changes (fat or petechiae)
	Jaundice
	Urinary changes (anuria, oliguria, fat globules)
Laboratory data (at least one)	
	Sudden drop in hemoglobin level
	High erythrocyte sedimentation rate
	Fat macroglobulinemia
	Sudden thrombocytopenia

pulmonary arteries and resulting in sudden death have been reported (MAYRON et al. 1985; BRANDT et al. 1998; SHEAFOR et al. 1998; RAVENEL et al. 2002). Others have noted that there may be a local activation of the coagulation at the fracture site by the association of intravascular bone marrow, venous stasis and vascular damage which may initiate the formation of mixed fatty and cruor macroemboli up to 3 cm in size (SIKORSKI 1983; HOFMAN et al. 1998). They also postulate that this mechanism is responsible for postsurgical or post-traumatic DVT, which explains the poor efficacy of postprocedure or post-trauma prophylactic anticoagulation.

Respiratory Insufficiency

Pulmonary findings are usually the earliest symptoms. Eighty percent of circulating fat globules are trapped in the pulmonary vascular bed while a minority will enter the systemic circulation and are responsible for systemic symptoms. Hypoxemia, dyspnea and tachypnea are the most frequent findings due to vascular obstruction. The neutral fat of the fat globule is not toxic. Degradation by an endothelial lipase produces free fatty acids, which are toxic for the vascular endothelium and the lung parenchyma, with variable degrees of respiratory distress, which may lead to adult respiratory distress syndrome (ARDS) (RISEBOROUGH and HERNBORN 1976; KING and HARMON 1994). Symptoms typically occur within 24–96 h after trauma. Delayed presentation, up to 2 weeks, can occur. The V/Q scan frequently demonstrates a typical mottled appearance with numerous subsegmental perfusion defects, even when chest X-ray is normal (MILSTEIN et al. 1974; PARK et al. 1986). The V/Q scan may also exhibit a pattern that is interpreted as low-probability for PE. Chest X-ray classically shows snowstorm infiltration. Chest CT demonstrates nonspecific findings of permeability lung edema, with bilateral areas of consolidation, often in a predominant dependent position. Early findings of small ill-defined, predominantly centrolobular micronodules have been reported that may represent small foci of alveolar edema caused by ARDS or hemorrhage secondary to a transient coagulopathy. Micronodules and areas of ground glass attenuation may predominate in the upper zones (HEYNEMAN and MÜLLER 2000; ARAKAWA et al. 2000; CHOI et al. 2002) (Fig. 19.10). Demonstration on CT of a macroscopic fat embolus in the pulmonary arteries has been recently reported (RAVENEL et al. 2002).

Neurological Impairment

Patients often present with confusion, sometimes progressing to delirium or even coma. Focal neurological deficits may be encountered (JACOBSON et al. 1986). Neurological symptoms are usually self-limited. CT may be normal, or may show multiple low-density areas in the white matter (infarction), abnormal gyral enhancement, cerebral edema or areas of hemorrhage (SAKAMOTO et al. 1983; JACOBSON et al. 1986; BEERS et al. 1988). MR better evidences ischemic lesions as early as 4 h after onset of symptoms and which are not demonstrated on CT (KAWANO et al. 1991). These lesions are reversible after 2 weeks in patients with favorable outcome and definite in patients with poor outcome (TAKAHASHI et al. 1999).

Petechial Rash

Petechiae, which are nearly pathognomonic of FES, are seen in only 50% of patients, and usually after the onset of respiratory and neurological symptoms. They are usually located in the nondependent areas of the head, neck and chest.

Pyrexia

Mild pyrexia within 24 h combined with fractures may have a predictive value (TEN DUIS et al. 1988).

Others

Other findings include ocular manifestations (fat in the conjunctivae, ischemic or Purtscher's retinopathy), which occur in 50%–60% (BUCKLEY and JAMES

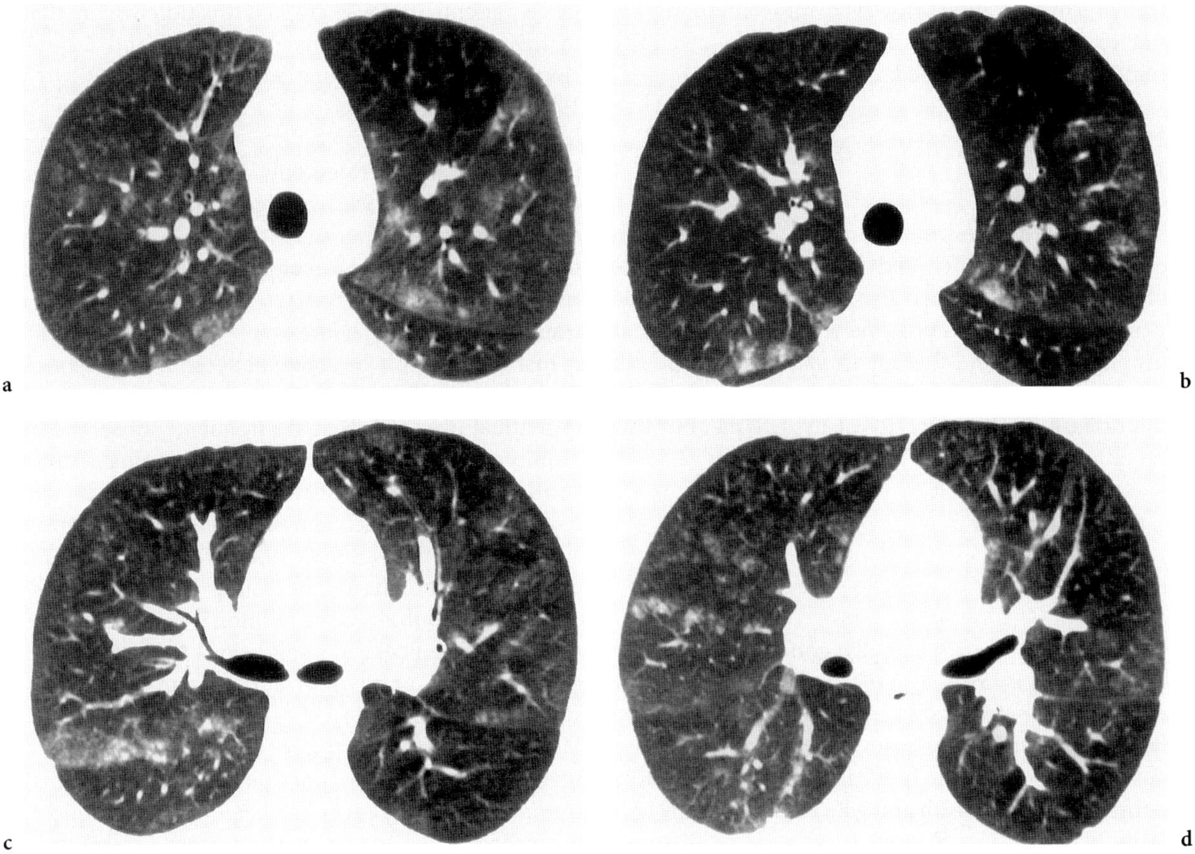

Fig. 19.10a–d. Post-traumatic fat embolism. A 68-year-old man was admitted after a car accident. A fracture of the right femoral shaft was repaired by internal fixation. He presented on day 2 with somnolence, petechiae on the anterior part of the thorax and hypoxemia at 60 mmHg despite assisted ventilation. **a–d** High-resolution CT shows multiple areas of ground glass attenuation and lung consolidation in dependent position, and small ill-defined centrolobular micronodules predominantly distributed in nondependent zones. Findings are compatible with fat embolism. Recovery was uneventful

1996), lipiduria without clinical renal impairment, jaundice and multiple coagulation abnormalities.

19.11.1.2
Incidence

The reported incidence of FES varies from 1% to 29% (Riska and Myllynen 1982; Lindeque et al. 1987; Ten Duis et al. 1988; King and Harmon 1994; Johnson and Lucas 1996; Bulger et al. 1997). An incidence from 0.5% to 3.5% is reported with isolated long-bone fracture and from 5% to 10% with multiple skeletal trauma (Johnson and Lucas 1996). The incidence is decreased in open fracture or closed fracture treated operatively within 24 h. The decompression of the fracture results in less mobilization of fat in the circulation (Riska and Myllynen 1982; Ten Duis et al. 1988).

19.11.1.3
Laboratory Tests

No laboratory test for fat offers specific diagnostic certainty. Stainable fat in the blood probably occurs at some point after nearly every fracture but may no longer be detectable once the syndrome has clinically developed. Stainable fat in the sputum, urine and cerebrospinal fluid has a similar lack of sensitivity and specificity (King and Harmon 1994).

Recently several authors have evaluated the usefulness of bronchoalveolar lavage fluid analysis (Chastre et al. 1990; Vedrinne et al. 1992; Mimoz et al. 1995) and microvascular cytology from a Swan-Ganz catheter (Masson and Ruggieri 1985; Castella et al. 1992; Qingshan et al. 1996), suggesting that these could be used to directly visualize the fat globules from recovered fluid. However, these methods are not yet widely accepted clinically and their validity remains to be determined.

19.11.1.4 Treatment

Treatment is first respiratory support and prevention of hypovolemic shock and restoration of adequate blood volume. Fracture decompression should be performed as soon as possible. It was postulated that prophylactic steroid therapy in patients at high risk for developing FES tends to reduce the incidence of the disease and the severity of hypoxemia, but this remains highly controversial (LINDEQUE et al. 1987; KALLENBACH et al. 1987).

19.11.1.5 Prognosis

Clinical outcome is generally good. Mortality for clinical FES is 5%–20% (FABIAN 1993; JOHNSON and LUCAS 1996; BULGER et al. 1997). Nevertheless, fat emboli, originating from subcutaneous adipose tissue, were reported to be a cause of death in 60% of patients beaten to death and who expired within 12 h (HISS et al. 1996).

19.11.2 Embolism of Liver Tissue

Pulmonary embolism of hepatic tissue is considered to be exceptional. We found 42 reported cases, usually in the forensic literature. A review of the literature in 1959 reported 11 cases (JOHNSTON 1959) and another one 9 additional cases in 1971 (NUNES 1971). One of the possible consequences of abdominal trauma is the release of organ tissue in the venous circulation and eventually embolization in the pulmonary arteries (GREENBERG 1986; WALZ and WALZ 1992). Blunt or penetrating trauma can result to some degree in disarrangement of liver structure and laceration of the walls of small vessels and inferior vena cava. The first reports were made by JUERGENS and VON RECKLINGHAUSEN in 1886. In a review of 1310 autopsies of trauma in the Armed Forces Institute of Pathology (AFIP), 287 had mild to severe liver injury. Only six had microscopic fragments of liver tissue in the pulmonary arteries (JOHNSTON 1959). Another study on 50 autopsies with severe liver laceration demonstrated the presence of 13 liver emboli in the lung. Ten patients presented only one embolus and three patients up to 13 emboli. It is noteworthy that in this study, 25 bone marrow emboli and 2 bone spicules were also observed in the lung (NUNES 1971). Another autopsy study of 104 patients with injury of the liver, including 40 with severe liver laceration, demonstrated only one microscopic liver embolus (STRAUS 1942). In opposition to pulmonary embolism of tumoral, necrotic or infected hepatic tissue, the presence of normally structured hepatic tissue in the pulmonary arteries always results from trauma (STRAUS 1942; JOHNSTON 1959; NUNES 1971). A distinction must be made between a fragment of liver tissue in the pulmonary arterial bed and small individual liver cells that are frequently observed in pulmonary capillaries unrelated to trauma (JOHNSTON 1959). The fate of such liver emboli is unknown. Experimental work showed resolution within 1 month but one clinical case presented with an organized thrombus at day 49 after injury. The presence of liver emboli in the pulmonary embolism has essentially medicolegal applications to determine if trauma is ante- or postmortem, as it can be used as a sign of vital reaction (JOHNSTON 1959; NUNES 1971; MOAR 1984). All described case reports followed severe blunt and sometimes penetrating abdominal trauma. One case report has been described following external cardiac massage for terminal respiratory arrest, which can call forensic interest into question (CHO and ANTHONY 1976). The obstruction of a major blood vessel by massive liver fragments is extremely rare. Table 19.26 presents cases in which liver embolism was responsible or contributed significantly to the death of the patient.

19.11.3 Foreign Body or Missile Embolism

Missile embolism is a rare complication of penetrating trauma. However, a rapid increase in the number of cases has been observed in the last few years due to the rise in urban civilian gunshot wounds. A first description was given by DAVIS in 1834 (PATEL et al. 1989). When a low velocity missile (e.g., an air-rifle) enters a blood vessel, most of its kinetic energy may have already been lost. Therefore, the force of the blood stream can sweep the missile away, resulting in embolization to a site that may be at a considerable distance from the entry site. The diagnosis of a missile embolus should be suspected if the missile is not found in the expected area, if there is no exit wound or if it is demonstrated radiographically in a location distant from the site of injury (MATTOX et al.

Table 19.26. Fatal pulmonary embolism of liver tissue

Reference	Age/sex	Mechanism of injury	Associated injuries	Symptoms	Delay between trauma and death	Pathology	
						Liver	Pulmonary arteries
Lippincott and Breck (1943)	M	Crush	Fracture of two right ribs	–	45 min	Rupture of liver Tear of IVC	Macerated hepatic tissue in right auricle and PA that was completely occluded over 5 cm
Greenberg (1986)	20/M	Fall	Right kidney laceration, pulmonary contusions, hemoperitoneum	Ventricular fibrillation, cardiac arrest	After admission	"Pulpified" liver	0.5 cm liver fragment occluding the right PA
Voitk and Munkittrick (1986)	21/M	Snowmobile accident	Hemoperitoneum, laceration of right adrenal	Cardiopulmonary arrest	Several hours	Severe laceration of the liver Tear of IVC	Large fragment (2 cm) in the right PA + multiple small fragments
Takatsu et al. (1988)	4/M	Hit by a truck	Fracture of ribs, contusions and laceration of lungs, spleen and right kidney, massive retroperitoneal hematoma and hemoperitoneum	–	Dead on arrival	Laceration of liver Tear of IVC	Occlusion of IVC through the rent → Right atrial cavity (liver herniation) No microscopic emboli
Michalodimitrakis and Tsatsakis (1998)	17/M	Crush	–	–	–	Multiple lacerations of liver Tear in IVC	Complete occlusion of the right PA

PA, pulmonary arteries; *IVC*, inferior vena cava.

1979; Patel et al. 1989). The majority (around 80%) of missiles involve the arterial system. In a review of literature in 1987, 126 cases of venous missile embolism were described since 1900 (Shannon et al. 1987). The clinical manifestations are related to the site of penetration, associated visceral injury and the site of embolization. Most of venous emboli (65%) are asymptomatic and the diagnosis is frequently delayed. Chest pain, dyspnea, hemoptysis or dysrhythmia can be observed in some patients (Nagy et al. 1994). The factors affecting the destination of an embolus include the site of injury, the size of the missile, vascular anatomy, flow dynamics, the action of adjacent muscle groups and the body position of the patient during and subsequent to wounding. In the literature review of venous missile embolism by Shannon et al. (1987), the entry point was supradiaphragmatic in 33%, including head veins (4%), neck veins (5%), thoracic veins (13%), or right heart (10%). The entry point was infradiaphragmatic in 67%, including femoral vein (10%), iliac vein (18%), IVC (33%) or visceral vein (5%). The site of embolization was the pulmonary arteries (37%), the right heart (atrium, 3% and ventricle, 47%), IVC (8%), peripheral vein (4%) and paradoxical or systemic embolism (4%) (Shannon et al. 1987). Bizarre embolization sites and, for example, retrograde migration from the heart to the IVC or paradoxical arterial embolization are described in less than 5% of the patients (Mattox et al. 1979; Wascher and Gwinn 1995).

Management of these missile emboli remains controversial and includes thoracotomy, arteriotomy, lobectomy, percutaneous catheter extraction or simple observation (Rich et al. 1978; Shannon et al. 1987; Kortbeek et al. 1992; Nagy et al. 1994; Ezberci and Kargi 1999). However, when comparing results of early missile extraction versus simple observation or retrieval when symptomatic, the rate of complication is 2% versus 25% and mortality 2% versus 6%, respectively (Shannon et al. 1987).

Complications occurring during observation include neurosis, thrombosis, gangrene, sepsis, bronchial erosion, hemorrhage and pulmonary infarction. Experience indicates that the risk of complication is greater than current morbidity of early removal. Therefore the indication of removal is based on technical feasibility rather than on physiological rationale. The feasibility and safety of missile extraction is enhanced by increasing experience with the percutaneous technique of foreign body retrieval. On the other hand, there is global agreement for embolectomy when pulmonary complications occur. The need for delayed removal (>6 weeks) is influenced by size, shape, location and potential bacterial contamination (GI tract perforation): a missile that is large (>5 mm), irregular, located near a major vascular bifurcation, embedded in the heart chambers or having penetrated the GI tract should be removed (Shannon et al. 1987). Other authors considered that small, smooth, uncontaminated and firmly lodged missiles in the right heart producing no arrhythmia or valvular dysfunction can be safely observed (Nagy et al. 1994).

19.11.4 Bile Embolism

Bile is one of the most uncommon embolisms to the lung. The first case was reported by Brown in 1952 (Brown and Walsh 1952). Until 1993, only 14 cases had been reported. They followed trauma in 11 patients, producing communication between the bile ducts and the hepatic veins (Kihira et al. 1993). Nine were iatrogenic (biopsy, percutaneous cholangiography or drainage, surgery). Only two followed blunt trauma with rupture of the liver (Doerig 1972) or gunshot wound with secondary liver abscess (Doyle and Gray 1968). Bile embolism was the cause or significantly contributed to death in eight cases and sepsis in four. Usually, bile embolism produces no major emboli, but diffuse small emboli in small arteries, arterioles and capillaries occasionally surrounded by fibrin. Associated small infarctions have also been described (Doyle and Gray 1968). Thirteen of the 14 patients had cholestasis at the time of bile embolism. Cholestasis results in a higher pressure within the bile ducts than in the hepatic veins. Associated trauma can thus facilitate the entry of pressured bile in the systemic circulation. The association of a cholestasis is believed to be an important component in the mechanism of bile embolism. Usually, bilirubin is dissolved when entering the bloodstream. In the event of cholestasis, the bile may remain insoluble due to prolonged inspissation, dehydration or inflammation (Mehta and Rubenstone 1967; Doyle and Gray 1968). There may also be a direct pulmonotoxic effect as experimental work after liver trauma showed edema, hemorrhage and destruction of capillary endothelium (McCurdy et al. 1970). It is nevertheless probable that subclinical bile embolism may occur more frequently. A review of literature reported 50 cases of bilhemia, fatal in 25. It followed blunt trauma in 23 patients and was iatrogenic in 14 patients (Sandblom et al. 2000). Clinically, there is no way to differentiate bile embolism from other types of PE, which makes the combination of cholestasis with trauma essential. The low amount of fibrin associated with bile emboli would imply that anticoagulation or thrombolytic therapy would probably be ineffective (Peven and Yokoo 1983; Balogh 1984).

Treatment options of the source of bilhemia include biliary sphincterotomy, percutaneous transhepatic or nasobiliary drainage, occlusion of the fistula with biliary covered stent via endoscopy or angiographic procedure and surgical resection (Struyven et al. 1982; Gable et al. 1997; Sandblom et al. 2000).

19.11.5 Venous Air Embolism

Venous air embolism (VAE) is an uncommon problem that can lead to substantial morbidity and mortality. The causes of VAE are multiple (O'Quin and Lakshminarayan 1982; Orebaugh 1992; King and Harmon 1994). VAE can be directly associated with head, neck, thoracic or abdominal trauma or surgery (Estrera et al. 1990; Orebaugh 1992). In head and neck trauma, air enters the venous system due to frequent subatmospheric pressure in veins located above the heart. Pneumothorax, pneumomediastinum or bronchopulmonary venous fistula can favor ingress of air in the systemic or pulmonary veins. The presence or insufflation of air or gas in the peritoneum or retroperitoneum can lead to VAE in the systemic or portal system. Nevertheless, the most common cause of VAE remains central venous catheterization. Administration of air can occur in situations that decrease the intravenous pressure below ambient air pressure, such as strained respiration. The majority of VAE occurs however during manipulation of the catheter.

Signs and symptoms vary from nonexistent to cardiovascular collapse, depending on the amount and rate of air entry and the position of the body (Orebaugh 1992). With a bolus administration, VAE is obstructing the right ventricular ejection, causing decreased pulmonary and systemic arterial pressure. With infusion, the obstruction is located at the level of the pulmonary arterioles causing pulmonary hypertension and systemic hypotension (O'Quin and Lakshminarayan 1982). In humans, the fatal volume is estimated to be between 100 and 500 ml of air at 100 ml/s, but lower volumes may be fatal in severely injured patients with compromised hemodynamics. It is possible for 100 ml of air per second to flow through 14-gauge catheters with a 5-cm H_2O drop across it (Flanagan et al. 1969). Signs of paradoxical emboli (heart, central nervous system) may be encountered in some patients by passage of air through a patent foramen ovale or across the pulmonary capillaries or arteriovenous pulmonary shunts (Gottdiener et al. 1988; Black et al. 1991). Chest X-ray is usually normal or shows pulmonary infiltrates reflecting pulmonary edema. Sometimes an air/fluid level can be seen in the right heart chambers (Peters 1988; O'Quin and Lakshminarayan 1982), which may also be demonstrated on echocardiography (Gottdiener et al. 1988; Marcus et al. 1991). Treatment includes immediate patient positioning in a left lateral decubitus and a Trendelenburg position, closed-chest cardiac massage or removal of air through central venous catheter, administration of 100% oxygen and/or hyperbaric oxygen therapy. Most patients recover with supportive care. Since many cases are undiagnosed and untreated, the actual rate of severe complications and mortality remains unknown. Arterial air embolism is rarer than VAE among iatrogenic problems (Schneider et al. 2000). Two cases of arterial or venous air embolism have been recently reported, occurring during initial CT work-up of trauma patients with pulmonary contusions. In order to obtain images in strict inspiratory apnea, the sedated patients were curarized and lungs were manually inflated by a balloon. The patients presented immediate cardiopulmonary arrest due to massive air embolism. The probable mechanism involved is bronchiolopulmonary vein fistula located in a lung contusion area (Segura et al. 1998; Schneider et al. 2000).

We found 18 cases of VAE following abdominal trauma in the literature, usually resulting in hepatoportal venous gas (Shuck et al. 1974; Traverso 1981; Vauthey and Matthews 1988; Friedman et al. 1991; Ho and Hu 1995; Dill-Macky 1997; Kelly et al. 1997; Gurland et al. 1998; Torriero et al. 1998; Muscari et al. 1999; Wu et al. 2000; Kingsley et al. 2000; Scaglione et al. 2001). Only one series has been published and reports that intravascular gas was detected in less than 1% of patients (5/730), with abdominal blunt trauma systematically screened on US at admission. All VAEs were considered to be benign, involving portal vein, IVC and hepatic veins (Brown et al. 1999). Six other case reports were considered to be benign (Vauthey and Matthews 1988; Kelly et al. 1997; Dill-Macky 1997; Gurland et al. 1998; Muscari et al. 1999; Scaglione et al. 2001). The postulated mechanisms are a disruption of the bowel mucosa or a sudden increase in intra-abdominal pressure, caused by the impact that forced intraluminal gas into the bowel wall, where it is absorbed by the portal circulation. Once in the portal system, the gas may pass into the hepatic veins via the sinusoids. Gas in the inferior vena cava may arise from a site of portosystemic communication. Nevertheless, other case reports reflected vascular injury and bowel necrosis. Pneumatosis intestinalis was often associated. Immediate laparotomy or laparoscopy was advocated in such conditions, as mortality ranged from 75% to 90% (Traverso 1981; Friedman et al. 1991; Ho and Hu 1995; Hong et al. 1997; Kingsley et al. 2000).

19.11.6 Amniotic Fluid Embolism

Etiologies of amniotic fluid embolism are multiple, including usually iatrogenic trauma. It has been extremely rarely reported following blunt abdominal trauma resulting in membrane and uterine vein rupture (Olcott et al. 1973; Judich et al. 1998). The result is embolization of large amounts of amniotic fluid debris within the pulmonary circulation. The clinical presentation is variable and pathophysiology is debated. The delay between trauma and clinical symptoms may varies from 0 to 48 h. The cardinal signs associate cyanosis, cardiovascular collapse, sudden onset of respiratory distress, major coagulation disorder in 40% of the patients and signs of central nervous system irritability in 20% (Clark 1991; King and Harmon 1994). The presence of massive pulmonary embolism on angiography due to amniotic embolism has also been reported (Bauer et al. 1995). Maternal mortality is very high, 80%–100%, of which 25%–50% die within 1 h of onset of symptoms. Diagnosis is usually performed by blood aspiration of amniotic fluid debris from the pulmonary circulation. The presence of fetal matter in the pulmonary circulation can nevertheless be found in asymptomatic women, which suggests the presence of subclinical amniotic fluid embolism (McDougall and Duke 1995).

19.11.7 Cerebral Tissue Embolism

Post-traumatic pulmonary embolism of cerebral tissue is a rare event reported at autopsy following massive head trauma (Ogilvy et al. 1988) and birth trauma or forceps deliveries (Hauck et al. 1990; Baergen et al. 1997). The persistence of cerebral tissue in the lung is a direct and continuous source of tissue thromboplastin and may render treatment of coagulopathy difficult in their survival time (Ogilvy et al. 1988; Rosendale et al. 1992; Collins and Davis 1994; Simonetti et al. 1998). Autopsy review of patients with severe head trauma reported a incidence varying from 2% to 10% when using immunohistochemical staining (Collins and Davis 1994). Massive embolism of cerebral tissue with emboli up to 1 cm in diameter has been reported (Wacks and Bird 1970; Legier and Rinaldi 1973; Hatfield and Challa 1980; Ogilvy et al. 1988; Kunz et al. 1990; Davis et al. 1991; Miyaishi et al. 1994). To the best of our knowledge, 48 cases have been reported so far in the literature (Staats et al. 1965; Nishiyama 1966; Simpson and Blumbergs 1991; Rosendale et al. 1992; Collins and Davis 1994; Miyaishi et al. 1994; Simonetti et al. 1998). One of the clinical interests of pulmonary embolism of cerebral tissue is that recipients of transplanted lung from donors who suffered severe head trauma have been reported to have early severe and lethal graft dysfunction due to multiple thrombi, diffuse alveolar damage and alveolar hemorrhage (Rosendale et al. 1992). A recent case report of cerebral tissue embolism in a transplanted lung with massive pulmonary arterial thrombosis was treated successfully with long-term anticoagulation (Simonetti et al. 1998).

19.11.8 Bone and Bone Marrow Embolism

In opposition to bone marrow embolism (which can produce fat embolism syndrome), embolism of bone spicule is a very rare event. Some are described following trauma (normal or weakened bone), orthopedic surgery and bone marrow transplantation (Nunes 1971; Jenny-Möbius et al. 1999).

19.12 Conclusion

Venous thromboembolism is the third most common cause of death, after sepsis and multiorgan failure, in trauma patients who survive the first 24 h. The clinical diagnosis is unreliable, which makes optimal thromboprophylaxis essential, particularly in severely injured patients. Thromboprophylaxis must be discussed on a per patient basis, according to the patient's VTE risk, bleeding risk, trauma condition and prognosis. In patients suspected of having VTE, the combination of pulmonary artery SCTA and CTV of lower limb and abdominal veins allows a complete one-session evaluation.

References

Abbott GT (1999) Prophylactic use of temporary IVC filters for prevention of pulmonary thromboembolization in a district general hospital (abstract). J Vasc Interv Radiol 10: 288–289

Abelseth G, Buckley RE, Pineo GE, Hull R, Rose MS (1996) Incidence of deep-vein thrombosis in patients with fractures of the lower extremity distal to the hip. J Orthop Trauma 10:230–235

Agnelli G, Radicchia S, Nenci GG (1995) Diagnosis of deep vein thrombosis in asymptomatic high-risk patients. Haemostasis 25:40–48

Ahlström KH, Johansson LO, Rodenburg JB, Ragnarsson AS, Akeson P, Börseth A (1999) Pulmonary MR angiography with ultrasmall superparamagnetic iron oxide particles as a blood pool agent and a navigator echo for respiratory gating: pilot study. Radiology 211:865–869

Alderson PO, Doppman JL, Diamond SS, Mendenhall KG, Barron El-Girton M (1978) Ventilation-perfusion lung imaging and selective pulmonary angiography in dogs with experimental pulmonary embolism. J Nucl Med 19: 164–171

Alexander JJ, Yuhas JP, Piotrowski JJ (1994) Is the increasing use of prophylactic percutaneous IVC filters justified? Am J Surg 168:102–106

Anderson JT, Owings JT, Goodnight JE (1999) Bedside noninvasive detection of acute pulmonary embolism in critically ill surgical patients. Arch Surg 134:869–875

Anglen JO, Goss K, Edwards J, Huckfeldt RE (1998) Foot pump prophylaxis for deep venous thrombosis: the rate of effective usage in trauma patients. Am J Orthop 27:580–582

Antakly-Hanon Y, Vieillard-Baron A, Qanadli SD et al (1998) Transoesophageal echocardiography in the diagnosis of pulmonary embolism with acute cor pulmonale. Arch Malad Cœur Vaiss 91:843–848

Arakawa H, Kurihara Y, Nakajima Y (2000) Pulmonary fat embolism syndrome: CT findings in six patients. J Comput Assist Tomogr 24:24–29

Arborelius MJ, Fredin H, Nyman U, Hellekant C (1985) Angiographic evaluation of scintigraphic abnormalities in screening for pulmonary embolism after total hip replacement. Acta Radiol 26:511–518

Athanasoulis CA, Kaufman JA, Halpern EF, Waltman AC, Geller SC, Fan CM (2000) Inferior vena cava filters: review of a 26-year single-center clinical experience. Radiology 216:54–66

Baergen RN, Castillo MM, Mario-Singh B, Stehly AJ, Benirschke K (1997) Embolism of fetal brain tissue to the lungs and the placenta. Pediatr Pathol Lab Med 17:159–167

Baile EM, King GG, Muller NL et al (2000) Spiral computed tomography is comparable to angiography for the diagnosis of pulmonary embolism. Am J Respir Crit Care Med 161:1010–1015

Balakrishnan J, Meziane MA, Siegelman SS, Fishman EK (1989) Pulmonary infarction: CT appearance with pathologic correlation. J Comput Assist Tomogr 13:941–945

Baldt MM, Zontsich T, Stümpflen A et al (1996) Deep venous thrombosis of the lower extremity: efficacy of spiral CT venography compared with conventional venography in diagnosis. Radiology 200:423–428

Balian A, Valla D, Naveau S et al (1998) Post-traumatic membranous obstruction of the inferior vena cava associated with a hypercoagulable state. J Hepatol 28:723–726

Ballew KA, Philbrick JT, Becker DM (1995) Vena cava filter devices. Clin Chest Med 16:295–305

Balogh K (1984) Pulmonary bile emboli. Arch Pathol Lab Med 108:814–816

Bankier AA, Janata K, Fleischmann D et al (1997) Severity assessment of acute pulmonary embolism with spiral CT: evaluation of two modified angiographic scores and comparison with clinical data. J Thor Imaging 12:150–158

Barraco RD, Scalea TM (2000) Dislodgment of inferior vena cava filters during central line placement: case report. J Trauma 48:140–142

Battistella FD, Torabian SZ, Siadatan KM (1997) Hospital readmission after trauma: an analysis of outpatient complications. J Trauma 42:1012–1016

Bauer FE, Janisch HD, Banzer D, Hampel KE (1983) Traumatic caused thrombosis of the vena cava inferior. Dtsch Z Verdau Stoffwechselkr 43:267–271

Bauer G (1944) Thrombosis following leg injuries. Acta Chir Scand 90:229–248

Bauer P, Lelarge P, Hennequin L, Lambert H, Larcan A (1995) Thrombo-embolism during amniotic fluid embolism. Intensive Care Med 21:384

Beaufort P, Perney P, Coste F, Masbou J, Le Bricquir Y, Blanc F (1996) Post-traumatic thrombosis of the portal vein. Presse Med 25:247–248

Becker DM, Philbrick JT, Selby JB (1992) Inferior vena cava filters. Indications, safety, effectiveness. Arch Intern Med 152:1985–1994

Beers GJ, Nichols GR, Willing SJ (1988) CT demonstration of fat-embolism-associated hemorrhage in the anterior commissure. AJNR Am J Neuroradiol 9:212–213

Benjamin ME, Sandager GP, Cohn EJ Jr et al (1999) Duplex ultrasound insertion of inferior vena cava filters in multitrauma patients. Am J Surg 178:92–97

Berkovich GY, Ramchandani P, Preate DL, Rovner ES, Shapiro MB, Banner MP (2001) Renal vein thrombosis after martial arts trauma. J Trauma 50:144–146

Bermudez KM, Knudson MM, Nelken NA, Shackleford S, Dean CL (1997) Long-term results of lower-extremity venous injuries. Arch Surg 132:963–968

Biello DR, Mattar AG, Osei-Wusu A et al (1979) Interpretation of indeterminate lung scintigrams. Radiology 133:189–194

Blachere H, Latrabe V, Montaudon M et al (2000) Pulmonary embolism revealed on helical CT angiography: comparison with ventilation-perfusion radionuclide lung scanning. Am J Roentgenol 174:1041–1047

Black M, Calvin J, Chan KL, Walley WM (1991) Paradoxic air embolism in the absence of an intracardiac defect. Chest 99:754–755

Blum AG, Delfau F, Grignon B et al (1994) Spiral-computed tomography versus pulmonary angiography in the diagnosis of acute massive pulmonary embolism. Am J Cardiol 74:96–98

Blum JE, Handmaker H (2000) Role of small-peptide radiopharmaceuticals in the evaluation of deep venous thrombosis. Radiographics 20:1187–1193

Bone RC (1993) The low-probability lung scan. A potentially lethal reading. Arch Intern Med 153:2621–2622

Bonn J, Liu JB, Eschelman DJ, Sullivan KL, Pinheiro LW, Gardiner GA Jr (1999) Intravascular ultrasound as an alternative to positive-contrast vena cavography prior to filter placement. J Vasc Interv Radiol 10:843–849

Bookstein JJ (1969) Segmental arteriography in pulmonary embolism. Radiology 93:1007–1012

Bounameaux H, Perrier A (1996) Role of D-dimer in the exclusion of pulmonary embolism. Semin Respir Crit Care Med 17:31–37

Bovyn G, Gory P, Reynaud P, Ricco JB (1997) The Tempofilter®: a multicenter study of a new temporary caval filter implantable for up to six weeks. Ann Vasc Surg 11:520–528

Brandt SE, Zeegers WS, Ceelen TL (1998) Fatal pulmonary fat embolism after dorsal spinal fusion. Eur Spine J 7:426–428

Brasel KJ, Borgstrom DC, Weigelt JA (1997) Cost-effective prevention of pulmonary embolus in high-risk trauma patients. J Trauma 42:456–462

Brathwaite CEM, Mure AJ, O'Malley KF, Spence RK, Ross SE (1993) Complications of anticoagulation for pulmonary embolism in low-risk trauma patients. Chest 104:718–720

Breatnach E, Stanley RJ (1984) CT diagnosis of segmental pulmonary artery embolus. J Comput Assist Tomogr 8: 762–764

Brink AJ, Botha D (1955) Budd-Chiari syndrome: diagnosis by hepatic venography. Br J Radiol 28:330–331

Brink J, Woodard P, Horesh L et al (1997) Depiction of pulmonary emboli with spiral CT: optimization of display window settings in a porcine model. Radiology 204:703–708

Britt LD, Zolfaghari D, Kennedy E, Pagel KJ, Minghini A (1996) Incidence and prophylaxis of deep vein thrombosis in a high-risk trauma population. Am J Surg 172:13–14

Brown CY, Walsh GC (1952) Fatal bile embolism following liver biopsy. Ann Intern Med 36:1529–1533

Brown MA, Hauschildt JP, Casola G, Gosink BB, Hoyt DB (1999) Intravascular gas as an incidental finding at US after blunt abdominal trauma. Radiology 210:405–408

Browse NL, Thomas ML (1974) Source of non-lethal pulmonary emboli. Lancet 16:258–259

Bruce D, Loud PA, Klippenstein DL, Grossman ZD, Katz DS (2001) Combined CT venography and pulmonary angiography: how much venous enhancement is routinely obtained? Am J Roentgenol 176:1281–1285

Buckley SA, James B (1996) Purtscher's retinopathy. Postgrad Med J 72:409–412

Buckner CB, Walker CW, Purnell GL (1989) Pulmonary embolism: chest radiographic abnormalities. J Thorac Imaging 4:23–27

Buerger PM, Peoples JB, Lemmon GW, McCarthy MC (1993) Risk of pulmonary emboli in patients with pelvic fractures. Am Surg 59:505–508

Bulger EM, Smith DG, Maier RV, Jurkovich GJ (1997) Fat embolism syndrome: a 10-year review. Arch Surg 132:435–439

Burks DW, Mirvis SE, Shanmuganathan K (1992) Acute adrenal injury after blunt abdominal trauma: CT findings. AJR Am J Roentgenol 158:503–507
Burns GA, Cohn SM, Frumento RJ, Degutis LC, Hammers L (1993) Prospective ultrasound evaluation of venous thrombosis in high-risk trauma patients. J Trauma 35:405–408
Bynum LJ, Wilson JE (1978) Radiographic features of pleural effusions in pulmonary embolism. Am Rev Respir Dis 117: 829–834
Bynum LJ, Wilson JE, Christensen EE, Sorensen C (1979) Radiographic techniques for balloon-occlusion pulmonary angiography. Radiology 133:518–520
Cafferata HT, Morrison S, Duer C, Depalma RG (1998) Venous thromboembolism in trauma patients: standardized risk factors. J Vasc Surg 28:250–259
Calinog TA, Magovern GJ, Fisher DL, McGinnis G, Salvoza M (1972) Newer approaches in the bedside diagnosis of massive pulmonary embolism. Preliminary report. J Thorac Cardiovasc Surg 63:300–304
Campbell DN, Liechty RD, Rutherford RB (1981) Traumatic thrombosis of the inferior vena cava. J Trauma 21:413–415
Cargile JS, Hunt JL, Purdue GF (1992) Acute trauma of the femoral artery and vein. J Trauma 32:364–370
Carpenter JP, Holland GA, Baum RA, Owen RS, Carpenter JT, Cope C (1993) Magnetic resonance venography for the detection of deep venous thrombosis: comparison with contrast venography and duplex Doppler ultrasonography. J Vasc Surg 18:734–741
Carson JL, Kelley MA, Duff A et al (1992) The clinical course of pulmonary embolism. N Engl J Med 326:1240–1245
Castella X, Valles J, Cabezuelo MA, Fernandez R, Artigas A (1992) Fat embolism syndrome and pulmonary microvascular cytology. Chest 101:1710–1711
Cellarier G, Carli P, Laurent P, Bonal J, Thouard H, Dussarat GV (1999) Post-traumatic caval thrombosis: a case report and a review of the literature. Presse Med 28:1575–1578
Cham MD, Yankelevitz DF, Shaham D et al (2000) Deep venous thrombosis: detection by using indirect CT venography. Radiology 216:744–751
Chartrand-Lefebvre C, Howarth N, Lucidarme O et al (1999) Contrast-enhanced helical CT for pulmonary embolism detection: inter- and intraobserver agreement among radiologists with variable experience. Am J Roentgenol 172:107–112
Chastre J, Fagon JY, Soler P et al (1990) Bronchoalveolar lavage for rapid diagnosis of the fat embolism syndrome in trauma patients. Ann Intern Med 113:583–588
Cheely R, McCartney WH, Perry JR et al (1981) The role of noninvasive tests versus pulmonary angiography in the diagnosis of pulmonary embolism. Am J Med 70:17–22
Chen JP, Rowe DW, Enderson BL (1999) Contrasting post-traumatic serial changes for D-dimer and PAI-1 in critically injured patients. Thromb Res 94:175–185
Chintapalli K, Thorsen K, Olson DL, Goodman LR, Gurney J (1988) Computed tomography of pulmonary thromboembolism and infarction. J Comput Assist Tomogr 12: 553–559
Cho SY, Anthony C (1976) Pulmonary embolism by hepatic tissue after external cardiac massage (letter to the editor). JAMA 236:140–141
Choi JA, Oh YW, Kim HK, Kang KH, Choi YH, Kang EY (2002) Nontraumatic pulmonary fat embolism syndrome: radiologic and pathologic correlations. J Thor Imaging 17:167–169
Christiansen F (1997) Diagnostic imaging of acute pulmonary embolism. Acta Radiol 38:1–33
Clagett GP, Reisch JS (1988) Prevention of venous thromboembolism in general surgical patients. Ann Surg 227–240
Clagett GP, Anderson FA, Geerts W et al (1998) Prevention of venous thromboembolism. Chest 114:531S–560S
Claikens B, Brugman E, Verbrugghe J (1998) Post-traumatic thrombosis of a segmental branch of the inferior mesenteric vein. J Belge Radiol 81:286–287
Clark SL (1991) Amniotic fluid embolism. Crit Care Clin 7: 877–882
Coche EE, Müller NL, Kim KI, Wiggs BR, Mayo JR (1998) Acute pulmonary embolism: ancillary findings at spiral CT. Radiology 207:753–758
Coche EE, Hamoir XL, Hammer FD, Hainaut P, Goffette PP (2001) Using dual-detector helical CT angiography to detect deep venous thrombosis in patients with suspicion of pulmonary embolism: diagnostic value and additional findings. Am J Roentgenol 176:1035–1039
Cohen D, Johansen K, Cottingham K, Clayson K, Simonowitz D (1980) Trauma to major visceral veins: an underemphasized cause of accident mortality. J Trauma 20:928–932
Cohn SM, Moller BA, Feinsteiin AJ, Burns GA, Ginzburg E, Hammers LW (1999) Prospective trial of low-molecular-weight heparin versus unfractionated heparin in moderately injured patients. Vasc Surg 33:219–223
Collins KA, Davis GJ (1994) A retrospective and prospective study of cerebral tissue pulmonary embolism in severe head trauma. J Forensic Sci 39:624–628
Colwell CW Jr, Collis DK, Paulson R et al (1999) Comparison of Enoxaparin and warfarin for the prevention of venous thromboembolic disease after total hip arthroplasty: evaluation during hospitalization and three months after discharge. J Bone Joint Surg Am 81:932–940
Comerota AJ, Katz ML, White JV (1992) Why does prophylaxis with external pneumatic compression for deep vein thrombosis fail? Am J Surg 164:265–268
Comerota AJ, Katz ML, Hashemi HA (1993) Venous duplex imaging for the diagnosis of acute deep venous thrombosis. Haemostasis 23:61–71
Coon WW (1976) Risk factors in pulmonary embolism. Surg Gynecol Obstet 143:385–390
Cope C, Baum RA, Duszak RA Jr (1996) Temporary use of a Bird's nest filter during iliocaval thrombolysis. Radiology 198:765–767
Cornuz J, Pearson SD, Polak JF (1999) Deep venous thrombosis: complete lower extremity venous US evaluation in patients without known risk factors – outcome study. Radiology 211:637–641
Coue O, Fornes P, Paraf F, Couetil JP, Bruneval P (1996) Budd-Chiari syndrome secondary to traumatic stenosis of the inferior vena cava. Gastroenterol Clin Biol 20:196–199
Courcy PA, Brotman S, Oster-Granite ML, Soderstrom CA, Siegel JH, Cowley RA (1984) Superior mesenteric artery and vein injuries from blunt abdominal trauma. J Trauma 24:843–845
Crane C (1964) Femoral vs caval interruption for venous thromboembolism. N Engl J Med 278:819
Cross JJ, Kemp PM, Walsh CG, Flower CD, Dixon AK (1998) A randomized trial of spiral CT and ventilation perfusion scintigraphy for the diagnosis of pulmonary embolism. Clin Radiol 53:177–182
Cruickshank MK, Levine MN, Hirsh J et al (1989) An evaluation of impedance plethysmography and ^{125}I-fibrinogen

leg scanning in patients following hip surgery. Thromb Haemost 62:830–834
Cueto SM, Cavanaugh SH, Benenson RS, Redclift MS (2001) Computed tomography scan versus ventilation-perfusion lung scan in the detection of pulmonary embolism. J Emerg Med 21:155–164
Dalen JE, Alpert JS (1975) Natural history of pulmonary embolism. Prog Cardiovasc Dis 17:259–270
Dalen JE, Brooks HL, Johnson LW, Meister SG, Szucs MM, Dexter L (1971) Pulmonary angiography in acute pulmonary embolism: indications, techniques, and results in 367 patients. Am Heart J 81:175–185
Dalen JE, Haffajee CI, Alpert JS, Howe JP, Ockene IS, Paraskos JA (1977) Pulmonary embolism, pulmonary hemorrhage and pulmonary infarction. N Engl J Med 296:1431–1435
Darcy MD (1998) Pulmonary digital subtraction angiography: ready for prime time. Radiology 207:11–12
Dautzenberg B, Silva A, Chaumier P, Sors C (1982) La radiographie standard dans l'embolie pulmonaire. Rev Fr Mal Resp 10:468–469
Davis GJ, McCloud LC, Nichols GR, Martin AW (1991) Cerebral tissue pulmonary embolization due to head trauma: a case report with immunohistochemical confirmation. J Forensic Sci 36:921–925
De Monye W, van Strijen MJL, Huisman MV et al (2000) Suspected pulmonary embolism: prevalence and anatomic distribution in 487 consecutive patients. Radiology 215: 184–188
Decousus H, Leizorovicz A, Parent F et al (1998) A clinical trial of vena caval filters in the prevention of pulmonary embolism in patients with proximal deep-vein thrombosis. N Engl J Med 338:409–415
Denardo G, Goodwin DA, Ravasini R, Dietrich PA (1970) The ventilatory lung scan in the diagnosis of pulmonary embolism. N Engl J Med 282:1334–1336
Dennis JW, Menawat S, von Thron J et al (1993) Efficacy of deep venous thrombosis prophylaxis in trauma patients and identification of high-risk groups. J Trauma 35:132–139
Deutsch V, Rosenthal T, Adar R, Mozes M (1972) Budd-Chiari syndrome: study of angiographic findings and remarks on etiology. Am J Roentgenol 116:430–439
Devlin JW, Petitta A, Shepard AD, Obeid FN (1998) Cost-effectiveness of enoxaparin versus low-dose heparin for prophylaxis against venous thrombosis after major trauma. Pharmacotherapy 18:1335–1342
Dewald CL, Jensen CC, Park YH et al (2000) Vena cavography with CO_2 versus with iodinated contrast material for inferior vena cava filter placement: a prospective evaluation. Radiology 216:752–757
Diffin DC, Leyendecker JR, Johnson SP, Zucker RJ, Grebe PJ (1998) Effect of anatomic distribution of pulmonary emboli on interobserver agreement in the interpretation of pulmonary angiography. Am J Roentgenol 171:1085–1089
Dill-Macky MJ (1997) Benign hepatic portal venous gas following blunt abdominal trauma. Aust Radiol 41:166–168
Doerig M (1972) Gallenembolie nach posttraumatischem Budd-Chiari-Syndrom. Helv Chir Acta 39:191–194
Domingo ML, Marti-Bonmati L, Dosda R, Pallardo Y (2000) Interobserver agreement in the diagnosis of pulmonary embolism with helical CT. Eur J Radiol 34:136–140
Donaldson GA, Williams C, Scannell JG et al (1963) A reappraisal of the application of the Trendelenburg operation to massive fatal embolism: report of a successful pulmonary-artery thrombectomy using a cardiopulmonary bypass. N Engl J Med 268:171–174
Dougherty JE, Lasala AF, Fieldman A (1980) Bedside pulmonary angiography utilizing an existing Swan-Ganz catheter. Chest 77:43–46
Doyle WF, Gray JM (1968) Bile embolization following hepatic trauma. Arch Path 85:559–561
Dries DJ (1996) Activation of the clotting system and complement after trauma. New Horiz 4:276–288
Drucker EA, Rivitz SM, Shepard JA et al (1998) Acute pulmonary embolism: assessment of helical CT for diagnosis. Radiology 209:235–241
Duvoux C, Radier C, Gouault-Heilmann M, Texier JP, Le Cudonnec B, Dhumeaux D (1994) A rare cause of portal vein thrombosis: the abdominal blunt trauma. Gastroenterol Clin Biol 18:165–167
Duwe KM, Shiau M, Budorick NE, Austin JHM, Berkmen YM (2000) Evaluation of the lower extremity veins in patients with suspected pulmonary embolism: a retrospective comparison of helical CT venography and sonography. Am J Roentgenol 175:1525–1531
Ebaugh JL, Chiou AC, Morasch MD, Matsumura JS, Pearce WH (2001) Bedside vena cava filter placement guided with intravascular ultrasound. J Vasc Surg 34:21–26
Egermayer P, Town GI, Turner JG, Heaton DC, Mee AL, Beard MEJ (1998) Usefulness of D-dimer, blood gas, and respiratory rate measurements for excluding pulmonary embolism. Thorax 53:830–834
El Hajjam M, Qanadli SD, Mignon F, Sissakian J, Chagnon S, Lacombe P (1999) Combined double helical CT phlebography of the lower extremities and CT pulmonary angiography: new approach for thromboembolic disease diagnosis (abstract). Radiology 213:126
Elliott CG, Dudney TM, Egger M et al (1999) Calf-thigh sequential pneumatic compression compared with plantar venous pneumatic compression to prevent deep-vein thrombosis after non-lower extremity trauma. J Trauma 47:25–32
Enderson BL, Chen JP, Robinson R, Maull KI (1991) Fibrinolysis in multisystem trauma patients. J Trauma 31:1240–1246
Engelman DT, Gabram SGA, Allen L, Ens GE, Jacobs LM (1996) Hypercoagulability following multiple trauma. World J Surg 20:5–10
Enzweiler CN, Wiese TH, Lembcke AE et al (2002) Electron beam tomography of interpulmonary saddle embolism: extent and vascular distribution. J Comput Assist Tomogr 26:26–32
Epstein DH, Darcy MD, Hunter DW et al (1989) Experience with the Amplatz retrievable vena cava filter. Radiology 172:105–110
Erdman WA, Peshock RM, Redman HC et al (1994) Pulmonary embolism: comparison of MR images with radionuclide and angiographic studies. Radiology 190:499–508
Erstad BL (1998) Venous thromboembolism in multiple trauma patients. Pharmacotherapy 18:1011–1023
Estrera AS, Pass LJ, Platt MR (1990) Systemic arterial air embolism in penetrating lung injury. Ann Thorac Surg 50:257–261
Evans AJ, Sostman HD, Knelson MH et al (1993) Detection of deep venous thrombosis: prospective comparison of MR imaging with contrast venography. Am J Roentgenol 161: 131–139
Even P, Sors H, Reynaud P, Safran D, Duroux P; Ruff F (1979) Regional alveolar hypoventilation induced by alveolar hypocapnia. Bull Eur Physiopath Resp 15:145–166

Ezberci F, Kargi H (1999) Surgical management of a pulmonary artery missile embolism after an air rifle wound to the liver. South Med J 92:1207–1209
Fabian TC (1993) Unraveling the fat embolism syndrome. N Engl J Med 329:961–963
Fanney DR, Casillas J, Murphy BJ (1990) CT in the diagnosis of renal trauma. Radiographics 10:29–40
Farrell S, Hayes T, Shaw M (2000) A negative simpliRED D-dimer assay result does not exclude the diagnosis of deep vein thrombosis or pulmonary embolus in emergency department patients. Ann Emerg Med 35:121–125
Fernandez-Gonzalez AL, Llorens R, Herreros JM, Cato J, Lecumberri F, Longo J (1994) Blunt traumatic rupture of the right hemidiaphragm and Budd-Chiari syndrome. Ann Thorac Surg 58:559–561
Ferretti GR, Bosson JL, Buffaz PD et al (1997) Acute pulmonary embolism: role of helical CT in 164 patients with intermediate-probability at ventilation-perfusion scintigraphy and normal results at duplex US of the legs. Radiology 205:453–458
Ferris EJ, Holder JC, Lim WN et al (1984) Angiography of pulmonary emboli: digital studies and balloon-occlusion cineangiography. Am J Roentgenol 142:369–373
Ferris EJ, McCowan TC, Carver DK, McFarland DR (1993) Percutaneous inferior vena cava filters: follow-up of seven designs in 320 patients. Radiology 188:851–856
Figley MM, Gerdes AJ, Ricketts HJ (1967) Radiographic aspects of pulmonary embolism. Semin Roentgenol 2:389–405
Fihn SD, McDonnell M, Martin D et al (1993) Risk factors for complications of chronic anticoagulation. A multicenter study. Ann Intern Med 118:511–520
Fisher CG, Blachut PA, Salvian AJ, Meek RN, O'Brien PJ (1995) Effectiveness of pneumatic leg compression devices for the prevention of thromboembolic disease in orthopaedic trauma patients: a prospective, randomized study of compression alone versus no prophylaxis. J Orthop Trauma 9: 1–7
Fitts WT, Lehr H, Bitner RL et al (1964) An analysis of 950 fatal injuries. Surgery 56:663–668
Flanagan J, Gradishar I, Gross R et al (1969) Air embolism: a lethal complication of subclavian venipuncture. N Engl J Med 281:488–489
Fleischner FG (1962) Pulmonary embolism. Clin Radiol 13: 169–182
Fleischner FG, Udis SW (1952) Dilatation of the azygos vein. A roentgen sign of venous engorgement. Am J Roentgenol 67:569–575
Fleischner F, Hampton AO, Castleman B (1941) Linear shadows in the lung (interlobar pleuritis, atelectasis and healed infarction). Am J Roentgenol 46:610–618
Freeark RJ, Boswick J, Fardin R (1967) Post-traumatic venous thrombosis. Arch Surg 95:567–573
Frezza EE, Siram SM, van Thiel DH, Mezghebe MH (1996) Venous thromboembolism after penetrating chest trauma is not a cause of early death. J Cardiovasc Surg 37:521–524
Friedman D, Flancbaum L, Ritter E, Trooskin SZ (1991) Hepatic portal venous gas identified by computed tomography in a patient with blunt abdominal trauma: a case report. J Trauma 31:290–292
Gable DR, Allen JW, Harrel DJ, Carrillo EH (1997) Endoscopic treatment of post-traumatic "bilhemia": case report. J Trauma 43:534–536
Gallus AS, Salzman EW, Hirsh J (1994) Prevention of VTE. In: Colman RW, Hirsh J, Marder VJ et al (eds) Hemostasis and thrombosis: basic principles and clinical practice, 3rd edn. Lippincott, Philadelphia, pp 1331–1345
Gando S, Tedo I, Kubota M (1992) Posttrauma coagulation and fibrinolysis. Crit Care Med 20:594–600
Garg K, Mao J (2001) Deep venous thrombosis: spectrum of findings and pitfalls in interpretation on CT venography. AJR Am J Roentgenol 177:319–323
Garg K, Welsh CH, Feyerabend AJ et al (1998) Pulmonary embolism: diagnosis with spiral CT and ventilation-perfusion scanning – correlation with pulmonary angiographic results or clinical outcome. Radiology 208:201–208
Garg K, Sieler H, Welsh CH, Johnston RJ, Russ PD (1999) Clinical validity of helical CT being interpreted as negative for pulmonary embolism: implications for patient treatment. Am J Roentgenol 172:1627–1631
Garg K, Kemp JL, Wojcik D et al (2000) Thromboembolic disease: comparison of combined CT pulmonary angiography and venography with bilateral leg sonography in 70 patients. Am J Roentgenol 175:997–1001
Gearhart MM, Luchette FA, Proctor MC et al (2000) The risk assessment profile score identifies trauma patients at risk for deep vein thrombosis. Surgery 128:631–640
Geerts WH, Code KI, Jay RM, Chen E, Szalai JP (1994) A prospective study of venous thromboembolism after major trauma. N Engl J Med 331:1601–1606
Geerts WH, Jay RM, Code KI et al (1996) A comparison of low-dose heparin with low-molecular-weight heparin as prophylaxis against venous thromboembolism after major trauma. N Engl J Med 335:701–707
Geerts W, Jay R, Code K et al (1999) Venous foot pump as thromboprophylaxis in major trauma. Thromb Haemost 82 [Suppl]:650–651
Geerts WH, Heit JA, Clagett GP et al (2001) Prevention of venous thromboembolism. Chest 119:132S–175S
Gefter WB, Hatabu H, Holland GA, Gupta KB, Henschke CI, Palevsky HI (1995) Pulmonary thromboembolism: recent developments in diagnosis with CT and MR imaging. Radiology 197:561–574
Gersin K, Grindlinger GA, Lee V, Dennis RC, Wedel SK, Cachecho R (1994) The efficacy of sequential compression devices in multiple trauma patients with severe head injury. J Trauma 37:205–208
Gervin AS (1975) Complications of heparin therapy. Surg Gynecol Obstet 140:789–796
Ghaye B, Dondelinger RF (2002) Non-traumatic thoracic emergencies: CT venography in an integrated diagnostic strategy of acute pulmonary embolism and venous thrombosis. Eur Radiol 12:1906–1921
Ghaye B, Szapiro D, Willems V, Dondelinger RF (2000) Combined CT venography of the lower limbs and spiral CT angiography of pulmonary arteries in acute pulmonary embolism: preliminary results of a prospective study. JBR-BTR 83:271–278
Ghaye B, Szapiro D, Mastora I et al (2001) Peripheral pulmonary arteries: how far in the lung does multi-detector row spiral CT allow analysis? Radiology 219:629–636
Ghaye B, Szapiro D, Willems V, Dondelinger RF (2002a) Pitfalls in CT venography of the lower limbs and abdominal veins. Am J Roentgenol 178:1465–1471
Ghaye B, Remy J, Remy-Jardin M (2002b) Non-traumatic thoracic emergencies: CT diagnosis of acute pulmonary embolism: the first 10 years. Eur Radiol 12:1886–1905
Girard P, Hauuy MP, Musset D, Simonneau G, Petitpretz P

(1989) Acute inferior vena cava thrombosis: early results of heparin therapy. Chest 95:284–291
Girard P, Tardy B, Decousus H (2000) Inferior vena cava interruption: how and when? Annu Rev Med 51:1–15
Godwin JD, Webb WR, Gamsu G, Ovenfors CO (1980) Computed tomography of pulmonary embolism. Am J Roentgenol 135:691–695
Goldhaber SZ, Hennekens CH, Evans DA, Newton EC, Godleski JJ (1982) Factors associated with correct antemortem diagnosis of major pulmonary embolism. Am J Med 73: 822–826
Goldhaber SZ (1998) Pulmonary embolism. N Engl J Med 339: 93–104
Goodman LR, Lipchik RJ (1996) Diagnosis of acute pulmonary embolism: time for a new approach. Radiology 199:25–27
Goodman LR, Curtin JJ, Mewissen MW et al (1995) Detection of pulmonary embolism in patients with unresolved clinical and scintigraphic diagnosis: helical CT versus angiography. Am J Roentgenol 164:1369–1374
Goodman LR, Lipchik RJ, Kuzo RS (1997) Acute pulmonary embolism: the role of computed tomography imaging. J Thor Imag 12:83–86
Goodman LR, Lipchik RJ, Kuzo RS, Liu Y, McAuliffe TL, O'Brien DJ (2000) Subsequent pulmonary embolism: risk after a negative helical CT pulmonary angiogram – prospective comparison with scintigraphy. Radiology 215:535–542
Gosin JS, Graham AM, Ciocca RG, Hammond JS (1997) Efficacy of prophylactic vena cava filters in high-risk trauma patients. Ann Vasc Surg 11:100–105
Gosselin MV, Rubin GD, Leung AN, Huang J, Rizk NW (1998) Unsuspected pulmonary embolism: prospective detection on routine helical CT scans. Radiology 208:209–215
Gottdiener JS, Papademetriou V, Notargiacomo A, Park WY, Cutler J (1988) Incidence and cardiac effects of systemic venous air embolism. Arch Intern Med 148:795–800
Gottlieb RH, Widjaja J (1999) Clinical outcomes of untreated symptomatic patients with negative findings on sonography of the thigh for deep vein thrombosis: our experience and a review of the literature. Am J Roentgenol 172: 1601–1604
Gottlieb RH, Widjaja J, Mehra S, Robinette WB (1999) Clinically important pulmonary emboli: does calf vein US after outcomes? Radiology 211:25–29
Gottsäter A, Berg A, Centergard J, Frennby B, Nirhov N, Nyman U (2001) Clinically suspected pulmonary embolism: is it safe to withhold anticoagulation after a negative spiral CT? Eur Radiol 11:65–72
Gottschalk A (2000) New criteria for ventilation-perfusion lung scan interpretation: a basis for optimal interaction with helical CT angiography. Radiographics 20:1206–1210
Gottschalk A, Sostman HD, Coleman RE et al (1993) Ventilation-perfusion scintigraphy in the PIOPED study, part II. Evaluation of the scintigraphic criteria and interpretations. J Nucl Med 34:1119–1126
Goyen M, Laub G, Ladd ME et al (2001) Dynamic 3D MR angiography of the pulmonary arteries in under four seconds. J Magn Reson Imaging 13:372–377
Gray HW, McKillop JH, Bessent RG (1993) Lung scan reporting language: what does it mean? Nucl Med Commun 14: 1084–1087
Green D, Lee MY, Lim AC et al (1990) Prevention of thromboembolism after spinal cord injury using low-molecular-weight heparin. Ann Intern Med 113:571–574
Green RM, Meyer TJ, Dunn M, Galssroth J (1992) Pulmonary embolism in younger adults. Chest 101:1507–1511
Greenberg MJ (1986) Pulmonary artery embolism with liver tissue (letter to the editor). Ann Emerg Med 15:1119–1120
Greenfield LJ, Proctor MC (1995) Twenty-year clinical experience with the Greenfield filter. Cardiovasc Surg 3:199–205
Greenfield LJ, McCurdy JR, Brown PP, Elkins RC (1973) A new intracaval filter permitting continued flow and resolution of emboli. Surgery 73:599–606
Greenfield LJ, Proctor MC, Cho KJ et al (1994) Extended evaluation of the titanium Greenfield vena caval filter. J Vasc Surg 20:458–464
Greenfield LJ, Proctor MC, Rodriguez JL, Luchette FA, Cipolle MD, Cho J (1997) Posttrauma thromboembolism prophylaxis. J Trauma 42:100–103
Greenfield LJ, Rutherford RB and the Participants in the Vena Caval Filter Consensus Conference (1999) Recommended reporting standards for vena caval filter placement and patient follow-up. J Vasc Interv Radiol 10:1013–1019
Greenfield LJ, Proctor MC, Michaels AJ, Taheri PA (2000) Prophylactic vena caval filters in trauma: the rest of the story. J Vasc Surg 32:490–497
Greenspan RH, Ravin CE, Polansky SM, McLoud TC (1982) Accuracy of the chest radiograph in diagnosis of pulmonary embolism. Invest Radiol 17:539–543
Grifoni S, Olivotto I, Cecchini P et al (1998) Utility of an integrated clinical, echocardiographic, and venous ultrasonographic approach for triage of patients with suspected pulmonary embolism. Am J Cardiol 82:1230–1235
Grist TM, Sostman HD, McFall JR et al (1993) Pulmonary angiography with MR imaging: preliminary clinical experience. Radiology 189:523–530
Grmoljez PF, Donovan JF, Willman VL (1976) Traumatic inferior vena caval obstruction. J Trauma 16:746–748
Gupta A, Frazer CK, Ferguson JM et al (1999) Acute pulmonary embolism: diagnosis with MR angiography. Radiology 210: 353–359
Gurd AR, Wilson RI (1974) The fat embolism syndrome. J Bone Joint Surg 56B:408–416
Gurland B, Dolgin SE, Shlasko E, Kim U (1998) Pneumatosis intestinalis and portal vein gas after blunt abdominal trauma. J Pediatr Surg 33:1309–1311
Gurney JW (1993) No fooling around: direct visualization of pulmonary embolism. Radiology 188:618–619
Haentjens P and The Belgian Fraxiparine Study Group (1996) Thromboembolic prophylaxis in orthopaedic trauma patients: a comparison between a fixed dose and an individually adjusted dose of a low molecular weight heparin (nadroparin calcium). Injury 27:385–390
Hagspiel KD, Polak JF, Grassi CJ, Faitelson BB, Kandarpa K, Meyerovitz MF (1998) Pulmonary embolism: comparison of cut-film and digital pulmonary angiography. Radiology 207:139–145
Hales MR, Scatliff JH (1966) Thrombosis of the inferior vena cava and hepatic veins (Budd-Chiari Syndrome). Ann Intern Med 65:768–781
Hamilton T, Angevine D (1946) Fatal pulmonary embolism in 100 battle casualties. Milit Surg 99:450–458
Hammers LW, Cohn SM, Brown JM et al (1996) Doppler color flow imaging surveillance of deep vein thrombosis in high-risk trauma patients. J Ultrasound Med 15:19–24
Hampton AO, Castleman B (1940) Correlation of postmortem chest teleroentgenograms with autopsy findings with spe-

cial reference to pulmonary embolism and infarction. Am J Roentgenol 43:305–326
Hansell DM (1997) Spiral computed tomography and pulmonary embolism: current state. Clin Radiol 52:575–581
Harrigan C, Lucas CE, Ledgerwood AM, Walz DA, Mammen EF (1985) Serial changes in primary hemostasis after massive transfusion. Surgery 98:836–844
Hatfield S, Challa VR (1980) Embolism of cerebral tissue to lungs following gunshot wound to head. J Trauma 20:353–355
Hauck AJ, Bambara JF, Edwards WD (1990) Embolism of brain tissue to the lung in a neonate. Arch Pathol Lab Med 114: 217–218
Havig O (1977) Deep vein thrombosis and pulmonary embolism: an autopsy study with multiple regression analysis of possible risk factors. Acta Chir Scand 479:1–93
Headrick JR, Barker DE, Pate LM, Horne K, Russell WL, Burns RP (1997) The role of ultrasonography and inferior vena cava filter placement in high-risk trauma patients. Am Surg 63:1–8
Heine TA, Halambeck BL, Mark JB (1998) Fatal pulmonary fat embolism in the early postoperative period. Anesthesiology 89:1589–1591
Henne-Bruns D, Kremer B (1992) Injuries of the portal vein and vena cava due to blunt abdominal trauma. Zentralbl Chir 117:343–347
Henry JW, Relyea B, Stein PD (1995) Continuing risk of thromboemboli among patients with normal pulmonary angiograms. Chest 107:1375–1378
Henschke CI, Mateescu I, Yankelevitz DF (1995) Changing practice patterns in the workup of pulmonary embolism. Chest 107:940–945
Herold CJ, Remy-Jardin MJ, Grenier PA et al (1998) Prospective evaluation of pulmonary embolism: initial results of the European multicenter trial (ESTIPEP) (abstract). Radiology 209:299
Herold CJ, Hahne J, Ghaye B et al (1999) Prospective evaluation of pulmonary embolism: diagnostic performance of spiral CT angiography in the ESTIPEP trial (abstract). Radiology 213:126–127
Hertzer NR (1977) Peripheral atheromatous embolization following blunt abdominal trauma. Surgery 82:244–247
Heyneman LE, Müller NL (2000) Pulmonary nodules in early fat embolism syndrome: a case report. J Thorac Imaging 15:71–74
Hill SL, Berry RE, Ruiz AJ (1994) Deep venous thrombosis in the trauma patient. Am Surg 60:405–408
Hillner BE, Philbrick JT, Becker DM (1992) Optimal management of suspected lower-extremity deep venous thrombosis: an evaluation with cost assessment of 24 management strategies. Arch Intern Med 152:165–175
Hirschmann JV (1987) Ischemic forms of acute venous thrombosis. Arch Dermatol 123:933–936
Hirsh J (1998) Low-molecular-weight heparin: a review of the results of recent studies of the treatment of venous thromboembolism and unstable angina. Circulation 98: 1575–1582
Hirsh J, Hoak J (1996) Management of deep vein thrombosis and pulmonary embolism. Circulation 93:2212–2245
Hiss J, Kahana T, Kugel C (1996) Beaten to death: why do they die? J Trauma 40:27–30
Ho MC, Hu RH (1995) Hepatic portal vein gas following blunt colon injury: report of a case. J Formos Med Assoc 94: 578–580
Hoffmann U, Schima W, Herold C (1999) Pulmonary magnetic resonance angiography. Eur Radiol 9:1745–1754
Hofmann S, Huemer G, Salzer M (1998) Pathophysiology and management of the fat embolism syndrome. Anaesthesia 53:35–37
Holland GA, Gefter WB, Baum RA, Gupta KB, Cope C, Kressel HY (1993) Prospective comparison of pulmonary MR angiography and ultrafast CT for diagnosis of pulmonary thromboembolic disease (abstract). Radiology 189:234
Hong JJ, Gadaleta D, Rossi P, Esquivel J, Davis JM (1997) Portal vein gas, a changing clinical entity. Report of 7 patients and review of the literature. Arch Surg 132:1071–1075
Horattas MC, Wright DJ, Fenton AH et al (1988) Changing concepts of deep venous thrombosis of the upper-extremity: report of a series and review of the literature. Surgery 104:561–567
Hoyt DB, Simons RK, Winchell RJ et al (1993) A risk analysis of pulmonary complications following major trauma. J Trauma 35:524–531
Hughes GC, Smith TP, Eachempati SR, Vaslef SN, Reed RL II (1999) The use of a temporary vena caval interruption device in high-risk trauma patients unable to receive standard venous thromboembolism prophylaxis. J Trauma 46: 246–249
Huguet C, Gallot D, Charles JF, Coloigner M, Marre P, Tiengou L (1975) Pulmonary embolism, the unrecognized risk of post-traumatic arterio-venous fistulas of the hepatic veins. J Chir 110:341–348
Hull RD, Pineo GF (1996) Clinical features of deep venous thrombosis. In: Hull RD, Raskob GE, Pineo FG (eds) Venous Thromboembolism: An Evidence-Based Atlas. Futura, Armonk, pp 87–91
Hull RD, Raskob GE (1991) Low-probability lung scan findings: a need for change. Ann Intern Med 114:142–143
Hull RD, Hirsh J, Carter CJ et al (1983) Pulmonary angiography, ventilation lung scanning, and venography for clinically suspected pulmonary embolism with abnormal perfusion lung scan. Ann Intern Med 98:891–899
Hull RD, Hirsh J, Carter CJ et al (1985) Diagnostic value of ventilation-perfusion lung scanning in patients with suspected pulmonary embolism. Chest 88:819–827
Hull RD, Raskob GE, Coates G, Panju AA (1990) Clinical validity of a normal perfusion lung scan in patients with suspected pulmonary embolism. Chest 97:23–26
Hull RD, Raskob GE, Pineo GF et al (1992) Subcutaneous low-molecular-weight heparin compared with continuous intravenous heparin in the treatment of proximal-vein thrombosis. N Engl J Med 326:975–982
Hull RD, Raskob GE, Ginsberg JS et al (1994) A noninvasive strategy for the treatment of patients with suspected pulmonary embolism. Arch Intern Med 154:289–297
Hull RD, Raskob GE, Pineo GF, Brant RF (1995) The low-probability lung scan. A need for change in nomenclature. Arch Intern Med 155:1845–1851
Hulman G (1995) The pathogenesis of fat embolism. J Pathol 176:3–9
Indik JH, Alpert JS (2000) Detection of pulmonary embolism by D-dimer assay, spiral computed tomography, and magnetic resonance imaging. Prog Cardiovasc Dis 42:261–272
Irie T, Yamauchi T, Makita K, Kusano S (1995) Retrievable IVC filter: preliminary in vitro and in vivo evaluation. J Vasc Intervent Radiol 6:449–454
Izard G, Houri R, Randrianasolo S, Gailleton R (1995) Acute

trauma-induced Budd-Chiari syndrome. Presse Med 24: 1209–1210
Jacobs DG, Piotrowski JJ, Hoppensteadt DA, Salvator AE, Fareed J (1996) Hemodynamic and fibrinolytic consequences of intermittent pneumatic compression: preliminary results. J Trauma 40:710–717
Jacobson D, Terrence C, Reinmurth O (1986) The neurologic manifestations of fat embolism. Neurology 36:847–851
Jardin F, Dubourg O, Bourdarias JP (1997) Echocardiographic pattern of acute cor pulmonale. Chest 111:209–217
Jekic M (1980) L'infarctus intestinal traumatique. Helv Chir Acta 47:631–633
Jenny-Möbius U, Bruder E, Stallmach T (1999) Recognition and significance of pulmonary bone embolism. Int J Legal Med 112:195–197
Johnson MJ, Lucas GL (1996) Fat embolism syndrome. Orthopedics 19:41–47
Johnson MS, Stine SB, Shah H, Harris VJ, Ambrosius WT, Trerotola SO (1998) Possible pulmonary embolus: evaluation with digital subtraction versus cut-film angiography – prospective study in 80 patients. Radiology 207:131–138
Johnson PT, Wechsler RJ, Salazar AM, Fisher AM, Nazarian LN, Steinter RM (1999) Spiral CT of acute pulmonary thromboembolism: evaluation of pleuroparenchymal abnormalities. J Comput Assist Tomogr 23:369–373
Johnston EH (1959) Liver embolism to the lung as a complication of trauma. US Armed Forces Med J 10:1143–1151
Jolliet P, Slosman DO, Ricou B, Suter PM, Chevrolet JC (1995) Pulmonary scintigraphy at the bedside in intensive care patients with suspected pulmonary embolism. Intensive Care Med 21:723–728
Judich A, Kuriansky J, Engelberg I, Haik J, Shabtai M, Czerniak A (1998) Amniotic fluid embolism following blunt abdominal trauma in pregnancy. Injury 29:475–477
Kakkar VV, Howe CT, Flanc C, Clarke MB (1969) Natural history of postoperative deep-vein thrombosis. Lancet 2: 230–232
Kallenbach J, Lewis M, Zaltzman M, Feldman C, Orford A, Zwi S (1987) "Low-dose" corticosteroid prophylaxis against fat embolism. J Trauma 27:1173–1176
Karavidas A, Matsakas E, Lazaros G, Panou F, Foukarakis M, Zacharoulis A (2000) Emergency bedside echocardiography as a tool for early detection and clinical decision making in cases of suspected pulmonary embolism. A case report. Angiology 51:1021–1025
Kashtan J, Conti S, Blaisdell FW (1980) Heparin therapy for deep venous thrombosis. Am J Surg 140:836–840
Kasper W, Meinertz T, Henkel B et al (1986) Echocardiographic findings in patients with proved pulmonary embolism. Am Heart J 112:1284–1290
Kasper W, Geibel A, Tiede N et al (1993) Distinguishing between acute and subacute massive pulmonary embolism by conventional and Doppler echocardiography. Br Heart J 70:352–356
Kasper W, Konstantinides S, Geibel A, Tiede N, Krause T, Just H (1997a) Prognostic significance of right ventricular afterload stress detected by echocardiography in patients with clinically suspected pulmonary embolism. Heart 77: 346–349
Kasper W, Konstantinides S, Geibel A et al (1997b) Management strategies and determinants of outcome in acute major pulmonary embolism: results of a multicenter registry. J Am Coll Cardiol 30:1165–1171
Katsamouris AA, Waltman AC, Delichatsios MA, Athanasoulis CA (1988) Inferior vena cava filters: in vitro comparison of clot trapping and flow dynamics. Radiology 166:361–366
Katz DS, Loud PA, Klippenstein DL, Shah RA, Grossman ZD (2000) Extra-thoracic findings on the venous phase of combined computed tomographic venography and pulmonary angiography. Clin Radiol 55:177–181
Kauczor HU (1998) Contrast-enhanced magnetic resonance angiography of the pulmonary vasculature. A review. Invest Radiol 33:606–617
Kauczor HU, Heussel CP, Thelen M (1999) Update on diagnostic strategies of pulmonary embolism. Eur Radiol 9:262–275
Kawano Y, Ochi M, Hayashi K, Morikawa M, Kimura S (1991) Magnetic resonance imaging of cerebral fat embolism. Neuroradiology 33:72–74
Keller ME, Metzler MH, Phillips JO, Huckfeldt RE, Spadone DP (2000) Evaluation of a disease management plan for prevention and diagnosis of thromboembolic disease in major trauma patients. Curr Surg 57:456–459
Kelley MJ, Elliott LP (1974) The radiological evaluation of the patient with suspected pulmonary thromboembolic disease. Med Clin North Am 59:3–36
Kelly BS, Meyers P, Choe KA, Hurst J, Luchette FA (1997) Traumatic pneumatosis cystoides intestinalis with portal venous air embolism. J Trauma 42:112–114
Kelsey LJ, Fry DM, Vanderkolk WE (2000) Thrombosis risk in the trauma patient. Prevention and treatment. Hematol Oncol Clin North Am 14:417–430
Kember PG, Euinton HA, Morcos SK (1997) Clinicians' interpretation of the indeterminate ventilation-perfusion scan report. Br J Radiol 70:1109–1111
Kessler R, Fraisse P, Krause D, Veilon F, Vandevenne A (1991) Magnetic resonance imaging in the diagnosis of pulmonary infarction. Chest 99:298–300
Khansarinia S, Dennis JW, Veldenz HC, Butcher JL, Hartland L (1995) Prophylactic Greenfield filter placement in selected high-risk trauma patients. J Vasc Surg 22:231–236
Khong PL, John PR (1997) Technical aspects of insertion and removal of an inferior vena cava IVC filter for prophylactic treatment of pulmonary embolus. Pediatr Radiol 27: 239–241
Khorasani R, Gudas TF, Nikpoor N, Polak JF (1997) Treatment of patients with suspected pulmonary embolism and intermediate-probability lung scans: is diagnostic imaging underused? Am J Roentgenol 169:1355–1357
Kiechle FL, McLaughlin JH, Yang SS, Bernstein J (1983) Atheromatous embolization. Am J Emerg Med 3:299–301
Kihira T, Konishi T, Shiraishi T, Yatani R, Nakano T (1993) Fatal bile pulmonary embolism following percutaneous transhepatic cholangiodrainage: case report and literature review. Angiology 44:725–730
Kim K, Müller NL, Mayo JR (1999) Clinically suspected pulmonary embolism: utility of spiral CT. Radiology 210:693–697
Kimoto T, Kohno H, Uchida M et al (1998) Inferior vena caval thrombosis after traumatic liver injury. HPB Surg 11:111–116
King MB, Harmon KR (1994) Unusual forms of pulmonary embolism. Clin Chest Med 15:561–580
Kingsley DD, Albrecht RM, Vogt DM (2000) Gastric pneumatosis and hepatoportal venous gas in blunt trauma: clinical significance in a case report. J Trauma 49:951–953
Kipper MS, Kortman KE, Ashbur WL et al (1982) Long-term follow-up of patients with suspected pulmonary embolism and a normal lung scan. Chest 82:411–415

Kittredge RD, Gordon DH, Mitty HA, Sprayregen S (1979) Systemic venous blood return via the portal vein. Radiology 131:37–41
Kline JA, Israel EG, Michelson EA, O'Neil BJ, Plewa MC, Portelli DC (2001) Diagnostic accuracy of a bedside D-dimer assay and alveolar dead-space measurement for rapid exclusion of pulmonary embolism: a multicenter study. JAMA 285: 761–768
Knight MTN, Dawson R (1976) Effect of intermittent compression of the arms on deep venous thrombosis in the legs. Lancet 11:1265–1267
Knudson MM, Collins JA, Goodman SB, McCrory DW (1992) Thromboembolism following multiple trauma. J Trauma 32:2–11
Knudson MM, Lewis FR, Clinton A, Atkinson K, Megerman J (1994) Prevention of venous thromboembolism in trauma patients. J Trauma 37:480–487
Knudson MM, Morabito D, Paiement GD, Shackleford S (1996) Use of low-molecular-weight heparin in preventing thromboembolism in trauma patients. J Trauma 41:446–459
Kortbeek JB, Clark JA, Carraway RC (1992) Conservative management of a pulmonary artery bullet embolism: case report and review of the literature. J Trauma 33:906–908
Krestan CR, Klein N, Kreuser S, Minar E, Janeta J, Herold CJ (1998) Value of a negative spiral-CT angiography in patients with suspected acute PE: retrospective analysis of PE recurrence and outcome. Presented at the 6th annual meeting of the European Society of Thoracic Imaging in Bologna, June 1998
Krivec B, Voga G, Zuran I et al (1997) Diagnosis and treatment of shock due to massive pulmonary embolism. Approach with transesophageal echocardiography and intrapulmonary thrombolysis. Chest 112:1310–1316
Kudsk KA, Fabian TC, Baum S, Gold RE, Mangiante E, Voeller G (1989) Silent deep vein thrombosis in immobilized multiple trauma patients. Am J Surg 158:515–519
Kuki S, Taketani S, Matsumura R et al (1995) Acute Budd-Chiari syndrome due to inferior vena cava occlusion following blunt trauma. Thorac Cardiovasc Surg 43:227–229
Kunz G, Pedal I, Schmidt G (1990) Massive pulmonary brain tissue embolism. Beitr Gerichtl Med 48:317–323
Kuzo RS, Goodman LR (1997) CT evaluation of pulmonary embolism: technique and interpretation. Am J Roentgenol 169:959–965
Laakso M, Pentikäinen PJ, Lampainen E, Romppanen T, Naukkarinen A, Collan Y (1982) Trauma, renal vein thrombosis and subsequent nephrotic syndrome. Ann Clin Res 14:140–144
Lachmann EA, Rook JL, Tunkel R, Nagler W (1992) Complications associated with intermittent pneumatic compression. Arch Phys Med Rehab 73:482–485
Lagache G, Soots G, Guiset J, Cecat P (1980) Massive pulmonary embolism due to post-traumatic pseudo-aneurysm due to rupture of the left hepatic artery, revealed by dissecting aneurysm below the capsule of the right lobe of the liver. J Chir 117:27–30
Lagerstedt CI, Olsson CG, Fagher BO, Öqvist BW, Albrechtsson U (1985) Need for long-term anticoagulant treatment in symptomatic calf-vein thrombosis. Lancet 7:515–518
Laissy JP, Bancal C, Sekkal S et al (1995) Pulmonary MR angiography at 1.0 T: early results with k-space segmented and post-contrast TurboFLASH two-dimensional time-of-flight sequences. Eur J Radiol 20:9–15
Landefeld CS, Beyth RJ (1993) Anticoagulant-related bleeding: clinical epidemiology, prediction and prevention. Am J Med 95:315–328
Langan EM, Miller RS, Casey WJ, Carsten CG, Graham RM, Taylor SM (1999) Prophylactic inferior vena cava filters in trauma patients at high risk: follow-up examination and risk/benefit assessment. J Vasc Surg 30:484–490
Leach TA, Pastena JA, Swan KG, Tikellis JL, Blackwood JM, Odom JW (1994) Surgical prophylaxis for pulmonary embolism. Am Surg 60:292–295
Legier J, Rinarldi I (1973) Gross pulmonary embolization with cerebral tissue following head trauma. J Neurosurg 39:109–113
Leizorovicz A (1996) Comparison of the efficacy and safety of low-molecular-weight heparins and unfractionated heparin in the initial treatment of deep venous thrombosis. Drugs 52:30–37
Leizorovicz A, Haugh MC, Chapuis F-R, Samama MM, Boissel J-P (1992) Low molecular weight heparin in prevention of perioperative thrombosis. BMJ 305:913–920
Lensing AWA, Hirsh J (1993) ^{125}I-fibrinogen leg scanning: Reassessment of its role for the diagnosis of venous thrombosis in post-operative patients. Thromb Haemost 69:2–7
Le Page JR, Gracia RM (1982) The value of bedside wedge pulmonary angiography in the detection of pulmonary emboli: a predictive and prospective evaluation. Radiology 144:67–73
Leppäniemi AK, Savolainen HO, Salo JA (1994) Traumatic inferior vena caval injuries. Scand J Thorac Cardiovasc Surg 28:103–108
Lesser BA, Leeper KV, Stein PD et al (1992) The diagnosis of acute pulmonary embolism in patients with chronic obstructive pulmonary disease. Chest 102:17–22
Lindblad B, Sternby NH, Bergqvist D (1991) Incidence of venous thromboembolism verified by necropsy over 30 years. BMJ 302:709–711
Lindeque BGP, Schoeman HS, Dommisse GF, Boeyens MC, Vlok AL (1987) Fat embolism and the fat embolism syndrome. A double-blind therapeutic study. J Bone Joint Surg 69-B:128–131
Lippincott SW, Breck MR (1943) Embolism from liver tissue in pulmonary artery. Arch Path 36:423
Little RD, Montgomery POB (1952) Case report of stenosis of the vena cava with vena caval and hepatic vein thrombosis related to trauma. Ann Intern Med 37:197–203
Lohr JM, Kerr TM, Lutter KS, Cranley RD, Spirtoff K, Cranley JJ (1991) Lower extremity calf thrombosis: to treat or not to treat? J Vasc Surg 14:618–623
Lohr JM, James KV, Deshmukh RM, Hasselfeld KA (1995) Calf vein thrombi are not a benign finding. Am J Surg 170: 86–90
Lomis NN, Yoon HC, Moran AG, Miller FJ (1999) Clinical outcomes of patients after a negative spiral CT pulmonary arteriogram in the evaluation of acute pulmonary embolism. J Vasc Intervent Radiol 10:707–712
Loop JW, Archer G, Northrop CH (1975) Bedside pulmonary arteriography. Radiology 114:469–471
Lorut C, Ghossains M, Horellou MH, Achkar A, Fretault J, Laaban JP (2000) A noninvasive diagnostic strategy including spiral computed tomography in patients with suspected pulmonary embolism. Am J Respir Crit Care Med 162: 1413–1418
Loubeyre P, Revel D, Douek P et al (1994) Dynamic contrast-enhanced MR angiography of pulmonary embolism: com-

parison with pulmonary angiography. Am J Roentgenol 162:1035–1039
Loud PA, Grossman ZD, Klippenstein DL, Ray CE (1998) Combined CT venography and pulmonary angiography: a new diagnostic technique for suspected thromboembolic disease. Am J Roentgenol 170:951–954
Loud PA, Katz DS, Klippenstein DL, Shah RD, Grossman ZD (2000) Combined CT venography and pulmonary angiography in suspected thromboembolic disease: diagnostic accuracy for deep venous evaluation. Am J Roentgenol 174: 61–65
Loud PA, Katz DS, Bruce DA, Klippenstein DL, Grossman ZD (2001) Deep venous thrombosis with suspected pulmonary embolism: detection with combined CT venography and pulmonary angiography. Radiology 219:498–502
Lualdi JC, Goldhaber SZ (1995) Right ventricular dysfunction after acute pulmonary embolism: pathophysiologic factors, detection, and therapeutic indications. Am Heart J 130: 1276–1282
Maliska P, Tiercelin G, Vallée C, Baer M, Pasteyer J (1985) Routine preoperative venography for patients undergoing delayed surgery for limb trauma. Ann Fr Anesth Reanim 4:23–26
Mammen EF (1992) Pathogenesis of venous thrombosis. Chest 102:640S–644S
Manganelli D, Palla A, Donnamaria V, Giuntini C (1995) Clinical features of pulmonary embolism. Doubts and certainties. Chest 107:25S–32S
Marcus RH, Weinert L, Neumann A, Borow KM, Lang R (1991) Venous air embolism. Chest 99:784–785
Masson RG, Ruggieri J (1985) Pulmonary microvascular cytology. A new diagnostic application of the pulmonary artery catheter. Chest 88:908–914
Mastora I, Masson P, Galland E et al (2001) Severity of acute pulmonary embolism: evaluation of a new spiral CT angiographic score in correlation with echocardiographic data (abstract). Eur Radiol 11:137
Matous SK, Castle JM, Puyana JC (1993) The use of inferior vena cava filters in the trauma patient. J Trauma 36:159
Matsumoto AH, Tegtmeyer CJ (1995) Contemporary diagnostic approaches to acute pulmonary emboli. Radiol Clin North Am 33:167–183
Matsumura JS, Morasch MD (2000) Filter placement by ultrasound technique at the bedside. Semin Vasc Surg 13: 199–203
Mattox KL, Beall AC Jr, Ennix CL, Debakey ME (1979) Intravascular migratory bullets. Am J Surg 137:192–195
Mayo JR, Remy-Jardin M, Müller NL et al (1997) Pulmonary embolism: prospective comparison of spiral CT with ventilation-perfusion scintigraphy. Radiology 205:447–452
Mayron R, Ruiz E, Mestitz ST, Omlie WR (1985) Tissue-fat pulmonary embolism occurring in a patient with a severe pelvic fracture. J Emerg Med 2:251–256
Mayzlik J, Prochazka V, Michalsky R, Docekal B (1992) Surgical treatment of post-traumatic thrombosis of the inferior vena cava. Rozhl Chir 71:43–46
McCartney JS (1934) Pulmonary embolism following trauma. Am J Pathol 10:709–710
McCartney JS (1935) Pulmonary embolism following trauma. Surg Gynecol Obstet 61:369–379
McConnell MV, Solomon SD, Rayan ME, Come PC, Goldhaber SZ, Lee RT (1996) Regional right ventricular dysfunction detected by echocardiography in acute pulmonary embolism. Am J Cardiol 78:469–473
McCune WS, Keshishian JM, Blades BB (1952) Mesenteric thrombosis following blunt abdominal trauma. Ann Surg 135:606–614
McCurdy WC, Hawley WD, Coalson JJ, Greenfield LZ (1970) Pulmonary complications following liver trauma. J Trauma 10:690–698
McDougall RJ, Duke GJ (1995) Amniotic fluid embolism syndrome: case report and review. Anaesth Intens Care 23: 735–740
McMurtry AL, Owings JT, Anderson JT, Battistella FD, Gosselin R (1999) Increased use of prophylactic vena cava filters in trauma patients failed to decrease overall incidence of pulmonary embolism. J Am Coll Surg 189:314–320
Meaney JFM, Weg JG, Chenevert TL, Stafford-Johnson D, Hamilton BH, Prince MR (1997) Diagnosis of pulmonary embolism with magnetic resonance angiography. N Engl J Med 336:1422–1427
Meaney JFM, Johansson LOM, Ahlstrom H, Prince MR (1999) Pulmonary magnetic resonance angiography. J Magn Reson Imaging 10:326–338
Mehta S, Rubenstone AI (1967) Pulmonary bile thromboemboli. A report of two cases. Am J Clin Pathol 47:490–496
Meissner MH (1998) Deep venous thrombosis in the trauma patient. Sem Vasc Surg 11:274–282
Meister SG, Brooks HL, Szucs MM, Banas JS Jr, Dexter L, Dalen JE (1972) Pulmonary cineangiography in acute pulmonary embolism. Am Heart J 84:33–37
Meredith JW, Young JS, O'Neil EA, Snow DC, Hansen KJ (1993) Femoral catheters and deep venous thrombosis: a prospective evaluation with venous duplex sonography. J Trauma 35:187–191
Meyer CS, Blebea J, Davis K Jr, Fowl RJ, Kempczinski RF (1995) Surveillance venous scans for deep venous thrombosis in multiple trauma patients. Ann Vasc Surg 9:109–114
Michalodimitrakis M, Tsatsakis A (1998) Massive pulmonary embolism by liver tissue. Med Sci Law 38:85–87
Miller GA, Sutton GC, Kerr IH, Gibson RV, Honey M (1971) Comparison of streptokinase and heparin in treatment of isolated acute massive pulmonary embolism. Br Med J 2:681–684
Mills SR, Jackson DC, Older RA, Heaston DK, Moore AV (1980) The incidence, etiologies, and avoidance of complications of pulmonary angiography in a large series. Radiology 136: 295–299
Millward SF (1998) Temporary and retrievable inferior vena cava filters: current status. J Vasc Interv Radiol 9:381–387
Millward SF, Bormanis J, Burbridge BE, Markman SJ, Peterson RA (1994) Preliminary clinical experience with the Gunther temporary inferior vena cava filter. J Vasc Interv Radiol 5: 863–868
Millward SF, Bhargava A, Aquino J Jr et al (2000) Günther tulip filter: preliminary clinical experience with retrieval. J Vasc Interv Radiol 11:75–82
Milstein D, Nusynowitz ML, Lull RJ (1974) Radionuclide diagnosis in chest disease resulting from trauma. Semin Nucl Med 4:339
Mimoz O, Edouard A, Beydon L et al (1995) Contribution of bronchoalveolar lavage to the diagnosis of post-traumatic pulmonary fat embolism. Intensive Care Med 21:973–980
Miniati M, Pistolesi M, Marini C et al (1996) Value of perfusion lung scan in the diagnosis of pulmonary embolism: results of the prospective investigative study of acute pulmonary embolism diagnosis (PISA-PED). Am J Respir Crit Care Med 154:1387–1393

Miniati M, Prediletto R, Formichi B et al (1999) Accuracy of clinical assessment in the diagnosis of pulmonary embolism. Am J Respir Crit Care Med 159:864–871

Miniati M, Monti S, Pratali L et al (2001) Value of transthoracic echocardiography in the diagnosis of pulmonary embolism: results of a prospective study in unselected patients. Am J Med 110:528–535

Miyaishi S, Moriya F, Yamamoto Y, Ishizu H (1994) Massive pulmonary embolization with cerebral tissue due to gunshot wound to the head. Brain Inj 8:559–564

Moar JJ (1984) Pulmonary embolism due to hepatic tissue – a forensic vital sign? S Afr Med J 66:699–700

Mobin-Uddin K, McLean R, Jude JR (1969) A new catheter technique of interruption of inferior vena cava for prevention of pulmonary embolism. Am Surg 35:889–894

Montgomery AB, Gilkeson RC, Glauser J, Applegate KE (2000) The role of spiral CT using the pulmonary embolus protocol: a comparison of emergency department and hospitalized populations. Emerg Radiol 7:25–30

Moody AR, Liddicoat A, Krarup K (1997) Magnetic resonance pulmonary angiography and direct imaging of embolus for the detection of pulmonary emboli. Invest Radiol 32: 431–440

Moody AR, Pollock JG, O'Connor AR, Bagnall M (1998) Lower-limb deep venous thrombosis: direct MR imaging of the thrombus. Radiology 209:349–355

Moser KM (1990) Venous thromboembolism. Am Rev Respir Dis 141:235–249

Moser KM, LeMoine JR (1981) Is embolic risk conditioned by location of deep venous thrombosis? Ann Intern Med 94: 439–444

Moser KM, Longo AM, Ashburn WL, Guisan M (1973) Spurious scintiphotographic recurrence of pulmonary emboli. Am J Med 55:434–443

Moses DC, Silver TM, Bookstein JJ (1974) The complementary roles of chest radiography, lung scanning, and selective pulmonary angiography in the diagnosis of pulmonary embolism. Circulation 49:179–188

Mudd KL, Hunt A, Matherly RC et al (2000) Analysis of pulmonary fat embolism in blunt force fatalities. J Trauma 48: 711–715

Muller C, Kopka L, Funke M, Funke C, Grabbe E (2001) Diagnosis of lung embolism and underlying venous thrombosis in multi-slice spiral CT. Rofo Fortschr Geb Rontgenstr Neuen Bildgeb Verfahr 173:528–535

Mullins MD, Becker DM, Hagspiel KD, Philbrick JT (2000) The role of spiral volumetric computed tomography in the diagnosis of pulmonary embolism. Arch Intern Med 160: 293–298

Muscari F, Suc B, Lagarrigue J (1999) Hepatic portal venous gas: is it always a sign of severity and surgical emergency? Chirurgie 124:69–72

Musset D, Rosso J, Petitpretz P et al (1988) Acute pulmonary embolism: diagnostic value of digital subtraction angiography. Radiology 166:455–459

Myllynen P, Kammonen M, Rokkanen P, Böstman O, Lalla M, Laasonen E (1985) Deep venous thrombosis and pulmonary embolism in patients with acute spinal cord injury: a comparison with nonparalyzed patients immobilized due to spinal fractures. J Trauma 25:541–543

Nabseth DC, Moran JM (1965) Reassessment of the role of inferior-vena-cava ligation in venous thromboembolism. N Engl J Med 273:1250–1253

Nagy KK, Duarte B (1990) Post-traumatic inferior vena caval thrombosis: case report. J Trauma 30:218–221

Nagy KK, Massad M, Fildes J, Reyes H (1994) Missile embolization revisited: a rationale for selective management. Am Surg 60:975–979

Nakagawa N, Cragg AH, Smith TP, Castaneda F, Barnhart WH, Dejong SC (1994) A retrievable Nitinol vena cava filter: experimental and initial clinical results. J Vasc Interv Radiol 5:507–512

Napolitano LM, Garlapati VS, Heard SO et al (1995) Asymptomatic deep venous thrombosis in the trauma patient: is an aggressive screening protocol justified? J Trauma 39:651–659

National Institutes of Health Consensus Conference (1986) Prevention of venous thrombosis and pulmonary embolism. JAMA 256:744–749

Nau T, Heinze W, Hayduk K (1992) Fatal pulmonary embolism after thrombolysis in post-traumatic renal-vein thrombosis. Dtsch Med Wochenschr 117:1318–1320

Neuerburg J, Günther RW, Rassmussen E et al (1993) New retrievable percutaneous vena cava filter: experimental in vitro and in vivo evaluation. Cardiovasc Intervent Radiol 16:224–229

Neuerburg JM, Günther RW, Vorwerk D et al (1997) Results of a multicenter study of the retrievable tulip vena cava filter: early clinical experience. Cardiovasc Intervent Radiol 20: 10–16

Neuzil DF, Garrard CL, Berkman RA, Pierce R, Naslund TC (1998) Duplex-directed vena caval filter placement: report of initial experience. Surgery 123:470–474

Nicolaides AN, Bergqvist D, Hull R et al (1997) Prevention of VTE: International consensus statement (guidelines according to scientific evidence). Int Angiol 16:3–38

Nicolas M, Debelle L, Laurent V et al (2001) Incremental lower extremity CT venography, a simplified approach for the diagnosis of deep venous thrombosis in patients with pulmonary embolism. J Radiol 82:251–256

Nicoloff DM, Fortuny IE, Dewall RA (1964) Acute Budd-Chiari secondary to intrahepatic hematoma following blunt abdominal trauma: treatment by open intracardiac surgery. J Thorac Cardiovasc Surg 47:225–229

Nilsson T, Carlsson A, Mare K (1998) Pulmonary angiography: a safe procedure with modern contrast media and technique. Eur Radiol 8:86–89

Nilsson T, Turen J, Billström A, Mare K, Carlsson A, Nyman U (1999) Validity of pulmonary cine arteriography for the diagnosis of pulmonary embolism. Eur Radiol 9:276–280

Nishiyama RH (1966) Cerebral tissue emboli in the lungs: a finding in severe head trauma. Mil Med 131:1309–1310

Norcross ED, Alexander JB, O'Malley KF, Spence RK, Ross SE (1991) The failure of serial pneumatic cuff venous occlusion plethysmography to predict patients at risk for pulmonary emboli after trauma. Am Surg 57:169–170

Norwood SH, McAuley CE, Berne JD et al (2001) A potentially expanded role for enoxaparin in preventing venous thromboembolism in high risk blunt trauma patients. J Am Coll Surg 192:161–167

Novelline RA, Baltarowich OH, Athanasoulis CA, Waltman AC, Greenfield AJ, McKusick KA (1978) The clinical course of patients with suspected pulmonary embolism and a negative pulmonary arteriogram. Radiology 126:561–567

Nunes MA (1971) Pulmonary embolism by hepatic tissue. J Forensic Sci 16:57–67

Nunn CR, Neuzil D, Naslund T et al (1997) Cost-effective

method for bedside insertion of vena caval filters in trauma patients. J Trauma 43:752–758
Nurmohamed MT, Rosendaal FR, Büller HR et al (1992) Low-molecular-weight heparin versus standard heparin in general and orthopaedic surgery: a meta-analysis. Lancet 340:152–156
Ogilvy CS, McKee AC, Newman NJ, Donnelly SM, Kiwak KJ (1988) Embolism of cerebral tissue to lungs: report of two cases and review of the literature. Neurosurgery 23:511–516
Ohgi S, Tachibana M, Ikebuchi M, Kanaoka Y, Maeda T, Mori T (1998) Pulmonary embolism in patients with isolated soleal vein thrombosis. Angiology 49:759–764
Olcott C IV, Robinson AJ, Maxwell TM, Griffin HA (1973) Amniotic fluid embolism and disseminated intravascular coagulation after blunt abdominal trauma. J Trauma 13: 737–740
O'Malley KF, Ross SE (1990) Pulmonary embolism in major trauma patients. J Trauma 30:748–750
Ombrellaro MP, Freeman MB, Stevens SL, Diamond DL, Goldman MH (1997) Predictors of survival after inferior vena cava injuries. Am Surg 63:178–183
O'Quin RJ, Lakshminarayan S (1982) Venous air embolism. Arch Intern Med 142:2173–2176
Orebaugh SL (1992) Venous air embolism: clinical and experimental considerations. Crit Care Med 20:1169–1177
Oser RF, Zuckerman DA, Gutierrez FR, Brink JA (1996) Anatomic distribution of pulmonary emboli at pulmonary angiography: implications for cross-sectional imaging. Radiology 199:31–35
Ost D, Rozenshtein A, Saffran L, Snider A (2001) The negative predictive value of spiral computed tomography for the diagnosis of pulmonary embolism in patients with nondiagnostic ventilation-perfusion scans. Am J Med 110:16–21
Owings JT, Bagley M, Gosselin R, Romac D, Disbrow E (1996) Effect of critical injury on plasma antithrombin activity: low antithrombin levels are associated with thromboembolic complications. J Trauma 41:396–406
Owings JT, Kraut E, Battistella F, Cornelius JT, O'Malley R (1997) Timing of the occurrence of pulmonary embolism in trauma patients. Arch Surg 132:862–867
Owings JT, Gosselin RC, Battistella FD, Anderson JT, Petrich M, Larkin EC (2000) Whole blood D-dimer assay: an effective noninvasive method to rule out pulmonary embolism. J Trauma 48:795–800
Owings JT, Gosselin RC, Anderson JT, Battistella FD, Bagley M, Larkin EC (2001) Practical utility of the D-dimer assay for excluding thromboembolism in severely injured trauma patients. J Trauma 51:425–430
Palla A, Donnamaria V, Petruzzelli S, Rossi G, Riccetti G, Giuntini C (1983) Enlargement of the right descending pulmonary artery in pulmonary embolism. Am J Roentgenol 141:513–517
Palmer AJ, Koppenhagen K, Kirchhof B, Weber U, Bergemann R (1997a) Efficacy and safety of low-molecular-weight heparin, unfractionated heparin and warfarin for thrombo-embolism prophylaxis in orthopaedic surgery: a meta-analysis of randomised clinical trials. Haemostasis 27:75–84
Palmer AJ, Schramm W, Kirchhof B, Bergemann R (1997b) Low-molecular-weight heparin and unfractionated heparin for prevention of thrombo-embolism in general surgery: a meta-analysis of randomised clinical trials. Haemostasis 27:65–74
Palombo JD, Blackburn GL, Forse RA (1991) Endothelial cell factors and response to injury. Surg Gynecol Obstet 173: 505–515
Park HM, Ducret RP, Brindley DC (1986) Pulmonary imaging in fat embolism syndrome. Clin Nucl Med 11:521–522
Parra RO, Farber R, Feigl A (1989) Pressure necrosis from intermittent pneumatic compression stockings. N Engl J Med 321:1615
Pasquale M, Fabian TC and the EAST Ad Hoc Committee on Practice management Guideline Development (1998) Practice management guidelines for trauma from the eastern association for the surgery of trauma. J Trauma 44:941–957
Pasquier J, Alex R, Descos L, Duquesnel J, Croisille M, Tran Minh V (1969) A propos d'un cas de thrombose extensive à la veine cave inférieure, d'origine traumatique probable. J Radiol Electrol Med Nucl 50:849
Passman MA, Moneta GL, Taylor LM et al (1997) Pulmonary embolism is associated with the combination of isolated calf vein thrombosis and respiratory symptoms. J Vasc Surg 25:39–45
Patel KR, Cortes LE, Semel L, Sharma PVP, Clauss RH (1989) Bullet embolism. J Cardiovasc Surg 30:584–590
Patel NH, Bradshaw B, Meissner MH, Townsend MF (1996) Post-traumatic Budd-Chiari syndrome treated with thrombolytic therapy and angioplasty. J Trauma 40:294–298
Paterson DI, Schwartzman K (2001) Strategies incorporating spiral CT for the diagnosis of acute pulmonary embolism: a cost-effectiveness analysis. Chest 119:1791–1800
Patriquin L, Khorasani R, Polak JF (1998) Correlation of diagnostic imaging and subsequent autopsy findings in patients with pulmonary embolism. Am J Roentgenol 171:347–349
Patton JH, Fabian TC, Croce MA, Minard G, Pritchard E, Kudsk KA (1996) Prophylactic Greenfield filters: acute complications and long-term follow-up. J Trauma 41:231–237
Peck KE, Bonoan JT, Cunha BA (1998) Postlaparoscopic traumatic inferior vena caval thrombosis. Heart Lung 27: 279–282
Peetz D, Hafner G, Hansen M et al (2000) Dose-adjusted thrombosis prophylaxis in trauma surgery according to levels of D-dimer. Thromb Res 98:473–483
Perlmutt LM, Braun SD, Newman GE, Oke EJ, Dunnick NR (1987) Pulmonary arteriography in the high-risk patient. Radiology 162:187–189
Perrier A, Howarth N, Didier D et al (2001) Performance of helical computed tomography in unselected outpatients with suspected pulmonary embolism. Ann Intern Med 135: 88–97
Pesola GR, Pesola HR (2000) Spiral CT diagnosis of pulmonary embolus. Am J Emerg Med 18:441–443
Peters SG (1988) Mediastinal air-fluid level and respiratory failure. Chest 94:1063–1064
Petit P, Bret PM, Atri M, Hreno A, Casola G, Gianfelice D (1994) Splenic vein thrombosis after splenectomy: frequency and role of imaging. Radiology 190:65–68
Peven DR, Yokoo H (1983) Bile pulmonary embolism: report of a case and a review of the literature. Am J Gastroenterol 78:830–834
Philbrick JT, Becker DM (1988) Calf deep venous thrombosis. A wolf in sheep's clothing? Arch Intern Med 148:2131–2138
Pieri A, Santoro G, Duranti A, Mori F, Vannuzzi A, Benelli L (1993) Temporary caval filters. Our experience. Preliminary analysis of 24 cases. Phlébologie 46:457–466
Pini M (1999) Future prospects of prophylaxis for deep vein thrombosis. Blood Coagul Fibrinolysis 10:S19–S27

PIOPED Investigators (1990) Value of the ventilation/perfusion scan in acute pulmonary embolism. Results of the Prospective Investigation of Pulmonary Embolism Diagnosis (PIOPED). JAMA 263:2753–2759
Piotrowski JJ, Alexander JJ, Brandt CP, McHenry CR, Yuhas JP, Jacobs D (1996) Is deep vein thrombosis surveillance warranted in high-risk trauma patients? Am J Surg 172: 210–213
Pittman GR (1989) Peroneal nerve palsy following sequential pneumatic compression. JAMA 261:2201–2202
Pond GD, Ovitt TW, Capp MP (1983) Comparison of conventional pulmonary angiography with intravenous digital subtraction angiography for pulmonary embolic disease. Radiology 147:345–350
Porter TR, Mohanty PK, Pandian NG (1994) Intravascular ultrasound imaging of pulmonary arteries. Methodology, clinical applications, and future potential. Chest 106:1551–1557
Prakash R, Matsukubo H (1983) Usefulness of echocardiographic right ventricular measurements in estimating right ventricular hypertrophy and right ventricular systolic pressure. Am J Cardiol 51:1036–1040
Prandoni P, Lensing AW, Cogo A et al (1996) The long-term clinical course of acute deep venous thrombosis. Ann Intern Med 25:1–7
Prandoni P, Villalta S, Bagatella P et al (1997) The clinical course of deep-vein thrombosis. Prospective long-term follow-up of 528 symptomatic patients. Haematologica 82: 423–428
Prandoni P, Lensing AWA, Prins MR (1998) Long-term outcomes after deep venous thrombosis of the lower extremities. Vasc Med 3:57–60
Prignet JM, Duval JL, Raynard B et al (1996) Portal vein thrombosis and esophageal rupture secondary to blast injury. Gastroenterol Clin Biol 20:103–105
Pruszczyk P, Torbicki A, Pacho R et al (1997) Noninvasive diagnosis of suspected severe pulmonary embolism. Chest 112:722–728
Pruszczyk P, Torbicki A, Kuch-Wocial A, Szulc M, Pacho R (2001) Diagnostic value of transoesophageal echocardiography in suspected haemodynamically significant pulmonary embolism. Heart 85:628–634
Purtill L, Gens DR, Joseph LA, Sandager GP, Flinn W (1997) Randomized prospective comparison of foot pumps versus calf pumps for deep venous thrombosis prophylaxis in trauma patients (abstact). J Trauma 43:197
Qanadli SD, El Hajjam M, Mesurolle B et al (2000) Pulmonary embolism detection: prospective evaluation of dual-section helical CT versus selective pulmonary arteriography in 157 patients. Radiology 217:447–455
Qanadli SD, El Hajjam M, Vieillard-Baron A et al (2001) New CT index to quantify arterial obstruction in pulmonary embolism: comparison with angiographic index and echocardiography. Am J Roentgenol 176:1415–1420
Qingshan T, Boxun Z, Chengxuan M, Xinhua Z (1996) A new method of early diagnosis of fat embolism syndrome. An experimental study of the pulmonary microvascular cytology. Chin Med J 109:173–175
Quinn MF, Lundell CJ, Klotz TA et al (1987) Reliability of selective pulmonary arteriography in the diagnosis of pulmonary embolism. Am J Roentgenol 149:469–471
Quirke TE, Ritota PC, Swan KG (1997) Inferior vena caval filter use in U.S. trauma centers: a practitioner survey. J Trauma 43:333–337
Ramos R, Salem BI, de Pawlikowski MP, Coordes C, Eisenberg S, Leidenfrost R (1996) The efficacy of pneumatic compression stockings in the prevention of pulmonary embolism after cardiac surgery. Chest 109:82–85
Raptopoulos V, Boiselle PM (2001) Multi-detector row spiral CT pulmonary angiography: comparison with single-detector row spiral CT. Radiology 221:606–613
Rathbun SW, Raskob GE, Whitsett TL (2000) Sensitivity and specificity of helical computed tomography in the diagnosis of pulmonary embolism: a systematic review. Ann Intern Med 132:227–232
Ravenel JG, Heyneman LE, McAdams HP (2002) Computed tomography diagnosis of macroscopic pulmonary fat embolism. J Thor Imag 17:154–156
Reekers JA, Harmsen H, Hoogeveen YL, Günther RW (1999) Vena cava filter devices – types, effectiveness, indications, complications in pulmonary embolism. In: Oudkerk M, van Beek E Jr, ten Cate YW (eds) Pulmonary Embolism. Blackwell Science, London, pp 332–351
Reid JH, Murchison JT (1998) Acute right ventricular dilatation: a new helical CT sign of massive pulmonary embolism. Clin Radiol 53:694–698
Reittner P, Coxson HO, Nakano Y et al (2001) Pulmonary embolism: comparison of gadolinium-enhanced MR angiography with contrast-enhanced spiral CT in a porcine model. Acad Radiol 8:343–350
Remy-Jardin M, Remy J, Wattinne L, Giraud F (1992) Central pulmonary thromboembolism: diagnosis with spiral volumetric CT with the single-breath-hold technique – comparison with pulmonary angiography. Radiology 185:381–387
Remy-Jardin M, Duyck P, Remy J et al (1995a) Hilar lymph nodes: identification with spiral CT and histological correlations. Radiology 196:387–394
Remy-Jardin M, Remy J, Cauvain O, Petyt L, Wannebroucq J, Beregi JP (1995b) Diagnosis of central pulmonary embolism with helical CT: role of two-dimensional multiplanar reformations. Am J Roentgenol 165:1131–1138
Remy-Jardin M, Remy J, Deschildre F (1996) Diagnosis of pulmonary embolism with spiral CT: comparison with pulmonary angiography and scintigraphy. Radiology 200: 699–706
Remy-Jardin M, Remy J, Artaud D, Deschildre F, Fribourg M, Beregi JP (1997a) Spiral CT of pulmonary embolism: technical considerations and interpretive pitfalls. J Thor Imag 12:103–117
Remy-Jardin M, Remy J, Artaud D, Deschildre F, Duhamel A (1997b) Peripheral pulmonary arteries: optimization of the spiral CT acquisition protocol. Radiology 204:157–163
Remy-Jardin M, Louvegny S, Remy J et al (1997c) Acute central thromboembolic disease: posttherapeutic follow-up with spiral CT angiography. Radiology 203:173–180
Remy-Jardin M, Remy J, Baghaie F, Fribourg M, Artaud D, Duhamel A (2000a) Clinical value of thin collimation in the diagnostic workup of pulmonary embolism. Am J Roentgenol 175:407–411
Remy-Jardin M, Baghaie F, Bonnel F, Masson P, Duhamel A, Remy J (2000b) Thoracic helical CT: influence of subsecond scan time and thin collimation on evaluation of peripheral pulmonary arteries. Eur Radiol 10:1297–1303
Remy-Jardin M, Tillie-Leblond I, Szapiro D et al (2002) CT angiography of pulmonary embolism in patients with underlying respiratory disease: impact of multislice CT (MSCT) on image quality and diagnostic accuracy. Eur Radiol 12:1971–1978

Ren H, Kuhlman JE, Hruban RH, Fishman EK, Wheeler PS, Hutchins GM (1990) CT of inflation-fixed lungs: wedge-shaped density and vascular sign in the diagnosis of infarction. J Comput Assist Tomogr 14:82–86
Rich NM, Collins KA, Davis GJ, Andersen CA, McDonald PT, Kozloff L, Ricotta JJ (1978) Missile emboli. J Trauma 18: 236–239
Riseborough EJ, Herndon JH (1976) Alterations in pulmonary function, coagulation and fat embolism in patients with fractures of the lower limbs. Clin Orthop 115:248–267
Riska EB, Myllynen P (1982) Fat embolism in patients with multiple injuries. J Trauma 22:891–894
Robb GP, Steinberg I (1938) A practical method of visualization of the chambers of the heart, the pulmonary circulation and the great vessels in man. J Clin Invest 17:507–510
Robin ED (1977) Overdiagnosis and overtreatment of pulmonary embolism: the emporor may have no clothes. Ann Intern Med:775–781
Robinson PJ (1996) Ventilation-perfusion lung scanning and spiral computed tomography of the lungs: competing or complementary modalities? Eur J Nucl Med 23:1547–1553
Rodger MA, Jones G, Rasuli P et al (2001) Steady-state end-tidal alveolar dead space fraction and D-dimer: bedside tests to exclude pulmonary embolism. Chest 120:115–119
Rodriguez JL, Lopez JM, Proctor MC et al (1996) Early placement of prophylactic vena caval filters in injured patients at high risk for pulmonary embolism. J Trauma 40:797–804
Rogers FB, Shackford SR, Wilson J, Ricci MA, Morris CS (1993) Prophylactic vena cava filter insertion in severely injured trauma patients: indications and preliminary results. J Trauma 35:637–642
Rogers FB, Shackford SR, Ricci MA, Wilson JT, Parsons S (1995) Routine prophylactic vena cava filter insertion in severely injured trauma patients decreases the incidence of pulmonary embolism. J Am Coll Surg 180:641–647. Comment: J Am Coll Surg 180:725--726
Rogers FB, Shackford SR, Ricci MA, Huber BM, Atkins T (1997) Prophylactic vena cava filter insertion in selected high-risk orthopaedic trauma patients. J Orthop Trauma 11:267–272
Rogers FB, Strindberg G, Shackford SR et al (1998) Five-year follow-up of prophylactic vena cava filters in high-risk trauma patients. Arch Surg 133:406–411
Rogers FB, Osler TM, Shackford SR (2000) Immediate pulmonary embolism after trauma: case report. J Trauma 48: 146–148
Rogoff SM, DeWeese JA (1960) Phlebography of the lower extremity. JAMA 172:1599–1606
Rose SC (1998) Venous duplex US. In: 1998 Syllabus: RSNA categorical course in Diagnostic Radiology: Vascular Imaging. Ferris EJ, Waltman AC, Fishman EK, Polak JF, Potchen EJ (eds) Oak Book, IL pp 139–156
Rose SC, Zwiebel WJ, Miller FJ (1994) Distribution of acute lower extremity deep venous thrombosis in symptomatic and asymptomatic patients: imaging implications. J Ultrasound Med 13:243–250
Rose SC, Kinney TB, Valji K, Winchell RJ (1997) Placement of inferior vena caval filters in the intensive care unit. J Vasc Interv Radiol 8:61–64
Rosen MP, Weintraub J, Donohoe K, Porter DH, Kim D, McArdle C (1995) Role of lower extremity US in patients with clinically suspected pulmonary embolism. J Vasc Interv Radiol 6:439–441
Rosendale BE, Keenan RJ, Duncan SR et al (1992) Donor cerebral emboli as a cause of acute graft dysfunction in lung transplantation. J Heart Lung Transplant 11:72–76
Rosenthal D, McKinsey JF, Levy AM, Lamis PA, Clark MD (1994) Use of Greenfield filter in patients with major trauma. Cardiovasc Surg 2:52–55
Rubin GD (1997) Helical CT for the detection of acute pulmonary embolism: experts debate. J Thoracic Imaging 12:81–102
Ruehm SG, Wiesner W, Debatin JF (2000) Pelvic and lower extremity veins: contrast-enhanced three-dimensional MR venography with a dedicated vascular coil – initial experience. Radiology 215:421–427
Ruiz AJ, Hill SL, Berry RE (1991) Heparin, deep venous thrombosis, and trauma patients. Am J Surg 162:159–162
Sakamoto T, Sawada Y, Yukioka T, Yoshioka T, Sugimoto T, Taneda M (1983) Computed tomography for diagnosis and assessment of cerebral fat embolism. Neuroradiology 24:283–285
Salzman EW, McManama GP, Shapiro AH et al (1987) Effect of optimization of hemodynamics on fibrinolytic activity and antithrombotic efficacy of external pneumatic calf compression. Ann Surg 206:636–641
Sandblom P, Jackobsson B, Lindgren H, Lunderquist A (2000) Fatal bilhemia. Surgery 127:354–357
Sapir DG, Moulsdale JE, Zimmerman JM (1982) Unilateral renal vein thrombosis without proteinuria. Am J Med Sci 283:89–93
Satiani B, Falcone R, Shook L, Price J (1997) Screening for major deep vein thrombosis in seriously injured patients: a prospective study. Ann Vasc Surg 11:626–629
Sato DT, Robinson KD, Gregory RT et al (1999) Duplex directed caval filter insertion in multi-trauma and critically ill patients. Ann Vasc Surg 13:365–371
Scaglione M, Lassandro F, Pinto E et al (2001) Gastric pneumatosis and portal vein gas: incidental findings at helical CT after blunt abdominal trauma. Emerg Radiol 8:162–164
Schiebler ML, Holland GA, Hatabu H et al (1993) Suspected pulmonary embolism: prospective evaluation with pulmonary MR angiography. Radiology 189:125–131
Schluger N, Henschke C, King T et al (1994) Diagnosis of pulmonary embolism at a large teaching hospital. J Thor Imaging 9:180–184
Schmidt U, Enderson BL, Chen JP, Maull KI (1992) D-dimer levels correlate with pathologic thrombosis in trauma patients. J Trauma 33:312–320
Schneider F, Lutun P, Zollner G, Gaudias J, Pinto L, Tempe JD (2000) Favorable outcome in a large left heart air embolism: lessons from an unusual complication of a noninvasive chest scan. Crit Care Med 28:1217–1219
Schoepf UJ, Bruening R, Konschitzky H et al (2000) Pulmonary embolism: comprehensive diagnosis by using electron-beam CT for detection of emboli and assessment of pulmonary blood flow. Radiology 217:693–700
Schoepf UJ, Holzknecht N, Helmberger TK et al (2002) Subsegmental pulmonary emboli: improved detection with thin-collimation multi-detector row spiral CT. Radiology 222:483–490
Schwarcz TH, Quick RC, Minion DJ, Kearney PA, Kwolek CJ, Endean ED (2001) Enoxaparin treatment in high-risk trauma patients limits the utility of surveillance venous duplex scanning. J Vasc Surg 34:447–452
Segura P, Kleinhans E, Schmitt A, Dosch JC, Tulasne PA (1998) Massive gas embolism following lung inflation for thoracic CT scan in a multiple trauma patient with lung contusions. Ann Fr Anesth Reanim 17:728–734

Sevitt S, Gallagher NG (1959) Prevention of venous thrombosis and pulmonary embolism in injured patients. Lancet 2: 981–989

Sevitt S, Gallagher NG (1961) Venous thrombosis and pulmonary embolism. A clinico-pathological study in injured and burned patients. Br J Surg 48:475–489

Shackford SR, Moser KM (1988) Deep venous thrombosis and pulmonary embolism in trauma patients. J Intensive Care Med 3:87–98

Shackford SR, Davis JW, Hollingsworth-Fridlund P, Brewer NS, Hoyt DB, Mackersie RC (1990) Venous thromboembolism in patients with major trauma. Am J Surg 159:365–369

Shah AA, Davis SD, Gamsu G, Intriere L (1999) Parenchymal and pleural findings in patients with and patients without acute pulmonary embolism detected at spiral CT. Radiology 211:147–153

Shannon FL, McCroskey BL, Moore EE, Moore FA (1987) Venous bullet embolism: rationale for mandatory extraction. J Trauma 27:1118–1122

Sheafor DH, Foti TM, Vaslef SN, Nelson RC (1998) Fat in the inferior vena cava associated with caval injury. Am J Roentgenol 171:181–182

Shibata HR, Ross W, Stephens-Newsham L, McLean LD (1966) Bedside diagnosis of massive pulmonary embolism. Arch Surg 93:250–257

Shuck JM, Malan LJ, Hammar MD (1974) Pneumatosis cystoides intestinals due to blunt abdominal trauma. J Trauma 14:435–440

Siddiqui AU, Buchman TG, Hotchkiss RS (2000) Pulmonary embolism as a consequence of applying sequential compression device on legs in a patient asymptomatic of deep vein thrombosis. Anesthesiology 92:880–882

Sikorski JM (1983) Venous thrombosis produced by the local injection of fat. J Bone Joint Surg 65B:340–345

Simon M, Kaplow R, Saltzman E, Freiman D (1977) A vena cava filter using thermal shape memory alloy: experimental aspects. Radiology 125:85–94

Simon M, Sharma GV, Sasahara AA (1984) An angiographic method for quantitating the severity of pulmonary embolism and the effects of therapy. Int Angiol 3:389–392

Simonetti VA, Basha MA, Allenspach L, Klosterman KG, Nakhleh R, Higgins RSD (1998) Donor cerebral tissue pulmonary emboli in a functioning transplanted lung. Clin Genet 12:504–507

Simpson DA, Blumbergs PC (1991) Embolism of cerebral tissue: a cause of coagulopathy and cerebral infarction? Surg Neurol 35:159–162

Sing RF, Smith CH, Miles WS, Messick WJ (1998) Preliminary results of bedside inferior vena cava filter placement. Safe and cost-effective. Chest 114:315–316

Sing RF, Cicci CK, Lequire MH, Stackhouse DJ (2000) Bedside carbon dioxide cavagrams for inferior vena cava filters: peliminary results. J Vasc Surg 32:144–147

Sing RF, Jacobs DG, Heniford BT (2001) Bedside insertion of inferior vena cava filters in the intensive care unit. J Am Coll Surg 192:570–576

Sinner WN (1978) Computed tomographic patterns of pulmonary thromboembolism and infarction. J Comput Assist Tomogr 2:395–399

Sobotka A, Khalil A, Parrot A et al (1999) Acute pulmonary embolism: quantitative, easy and non-invasive assessment of severity with spiral CT angiography (abstract). Eur Radiol 9:227

Sostman HD (1997) Opinion response to acute pulmonary embolism: the role of computed tomographic imaging. J Thorac Imag 12:89–92

Sostman HD, Ravin CE, Sullivan DC, Mills SR, Glickman MG, Dorfman GS (1982) Use of pulmonary angiography for suspected pulmonary embolism: influence of scintigraphic diagnosis. Am J Roentgenol 139:673–677

Sostman HD, Debatin JF, Spritzer CE, Coleman RE, Grist TM, McFall JR (1993) MRI in venous thromboembolic disease. Eur Radiol 3:53–61

Sostman HD, Coleman RE, de Long DM, Newman GE, Paine S (1994) Evaluation of revised criteria for ventilation-perfusion scintigraphy in patients with suspected pulmonary embolism. Radiology 193:103–107

Sostman HD, Layish DT, Tapson FV et al (1996) Prospective comparison of helical CT and MR imaging in clinically suspected acute pulmonary embolism. J Magn Reson Imaging 6:275–281

Spain DA, Richardson JD, Polk HC, Bergamini TM, Wilson MA, Miller FB (1997) Venous thromboembolism in the high-risk trauma patient: do risks justify aggressive screening and prophylaxis? J Trauma 42:463–469

Spain DA, Bergamini TM, Hoffmann JF, Carrillo EH, Richardson JD (1998) Comparison of sequential compression devices and foot pumps for prophylaxis of deep venous thrombosis in high-risk trauma patients. Am Surg 64: 522–525

Staats OJ, Ceballos R, Miller RE (1965) Brain tissue embolization secondary to cerebral trauma. Ala J Med Sci 2:394–396

Stein PD (1971) Wedge arteriography for the identification of pulmonary emboli in small vessels. Am Heart J 82:618–623

Stein PD (1996) The clinical diagnosis of acute pulmonary embolism. In: Hull RD, Raskob GE, Pineo FG (eds) Venous Thromboembolism: An Evicence-Based Atlas. Futura, Armonk, pp 161–167

Stein PD (1997) Opinion response to acute pulmonary embolism: the role of computed tomographic imaging. J Thoracic Imaging 12:86–89

Stein PD, Gottschalk A (2000) Review of criteria appropriate for a very low-probability of pulmonary embolism on ventilation-perfusion lung scans: a position paper. Radiographics 20:99–105

Stein PD, Henry JW (1995) Prevalence of acute pulmonary embolism among patients in a general hospital and at autopsy. Chest 108:978–981

Stein PD, Henry JW (1997) Prevalence of acute pulmonary embolism in central and subsegmental pulmonary arteries and relation to probability interpretation of ventilation/perfusion lung scans. Chest 111:1246–1248

Stein PD, Gottschalk A, Saltzman HE, Terrin ML (1991) Diagnosis of acute pulmonary embolism in the elderly. J Am Coll Cardiol 18:1452–1457

Stein PD, Athanasoulis C, Alavi A et al (1992a) Complications and validity of pulmonary angiography in acute pulmonary embolism. Circulation 85:462–468

Stein PD, Athanasoulis C, Greenspan RH, Henry JW (1992b) Relation of plain chest radiographic findings to pulmonary arterial pressure and arterial blood oxygen levels in patients with acute pulmonary embolism. Am J Cardiol 69: 394–396

Stein PD, Hull RD, Saltzman HA, Pineo G (1993) Strategy for diagnosis of patients with suspected acute pulmonary embolism. Chest 103:1553–1559

Stein PD, Henry JW, Relyea B (1995) Untreated patients with pulmonary embolism. Outcome, clinical, and laboratory assessment. Chest 107:931–935

Stein PD, Henry JW, Gottschalk A (1999) Reassessment of pulmonary angiography for the diagnosis of pulmonary embolism: relation of interpreter agreement to the order of the involved pulmonary arterial branch. Radiology 210: 689–691

Steiner P, Phillips F, Wesner D, Lund GK, Kreymann G, Nicolas V, Crone-Munzebrock W (1994) Primary diagnosis and follow-up in acute pulmonary embolism: comparison of digital subtraction angiography and spiral CT. Rofo Fortschr Geb Rontgenstr Neuen Bildgeb Verfahr 161:285–291

Steiner P, Lund GK, Debatin JF et al (1996) Acute pulmonary embolism: value of transthoracic and transesophageal echocardiography in comparison with helical CT. Am J Roentgenol 167:931–936

Stoneham GW, Burbridge BE, Millward SF (1995) A temporary inferior vena cava filters: in vitro comparison with permanent IVC filters. J Vasc Interv Radiol 6:731–736

Strandness DE Jr, Langlois Y, Cramer M, Randlett A, Thiele BL (1983) Long-term sequelae of acute venous thrombosis. JAMA 250:1289–1292

Straus R (1942) Pulmonary embolism caused by liver tissue. Arch Path 33:69–71

Streib EW, Wagner JW (2000) Complications of vascular access procedures in patients with vena cava filters. J Trauma 49: 553–558

Struyven J, Cremer M, Pirson P, Jeanty P, Jeanmart J (1982) Post-traumatic bilhemia: diagnosis and catheter therapy. AJR 138:746–747

Sue LP, Davis JW, Parks SN (1995) Iliofemoral venous injuries: an indication for prophylactic caval filter placement. J Trauma 39:693–695

Summaria L, Caprini JA, McMillan R et al (1988) Relationship between postsurgical fibrinolytic parameters and deep vein thrombosis in surgical patients treated with compression devices. Am Surgeon 3:156–160

Swensen SJ, Sheedy PF Jr, Ryu JH et al (2002) Outcomes after withholding anticoagulation from patients with suspected acute pulmonary embolism and negative computed tomographic findings: a cohort study. Mayo Clin Proc 77: 130–138

Szapiro D, Ghaye B, Willems V, Zhang L, Albert A, Dondelinger RF (2001) Evaluation of CT time-density curves of lower-limb veins. Invest Radiol 36:164–169

Takahashi M, Suzuki R, Osakabe Y et al (1999) Magnetic resonance imaging findings in cerebral fat embolism: correlation with clinical manifestations. J Trauma 46:324–327

Takatsu A, Shigeta A, Abe M, Kitune K, Kawai T (1988) Embolism of massive hepatic tissue in inferior vena cava and right atrium after closed liver injury. Am J Forensic Med Pathol 9:233–235

Takeuchi M, Maruyama K, Nakamura M et al (1995) Post-traumatic inferior vena caval thrombosis: case report and review of the literature. J Trauma 39:605–608

Tanaka H, Hiraoka N, Baba M et al (1995) Two cases of acute massive pulmonary embolism diagnosed by pulmonary angiography with Swan-Ganz catheter. Japan J Thor Dis 33:312–317

Tapson VF, Davidson CJ, Kisslo KB, Stack RS (1994) Rapid visualization of massive pulmonary emboli utilizing intravascular ultrasound. Chest 105:888–890

Tardy B, Mismetti P, Page Y et al (1996) Symptomatic inferior vena cava filter thrombosis: clinical study of 30 consecutive cases. Eur Respir J 9:2012–2016

Tarnay TJ, Rohr PR, Davidson AG, Stevenson MM, Byars EF, Hopkins GR (1980) Pneumatic calf compression, fibrinolysis, and the prevention of deep vein thrombosis. Surgery 88:489–496

Teigen CL, Maus TP, Sheedy PF, Johnson CM, Stanson AW, Welch TJ (1993) Pulmonary embolism: diagnosis with electron-beam CT. Radiology 188:839–845

Ten Duis HJ, Nijsten MWN, Klasen HJ, Binnendijk B (1988) Fat embolism in patients with an isolated fracture of the femoral shaft. J Trauma 28:383–390

The Pisa-Ped Investigators (1995) Invasive and noninvasive diagnosis of pulmonary embolism. Preliminary results of the prospective investigative study of acute pulmonary embolism diagnosis (PISA-PED). Chest 107:33–38S

Thery C, Asseman P, Amrouni N et al (1990) Use of new removable vena cava filter in order to prevent pulmonary embolism in patients submitted to thrombolysis. Eur Heart J 11:334–341

Thery C, Bauchart JJ, Lesenne M et al (1992) Predictive factors of effectiveness of streptokinase in deep venous thrombosis. Am J Cardiol 69:117–122

Todd JW, Frisbie JH, Rossier AB et al (1976) Deep venous thrombosis in acute spinal cord injury: a comparison of ^{125}I fibrinogen leg scanning, impedance plethysmography and venography. Paraplegia 14:50–57

Tola JC, Holtzman R, Lotttenberg L (1999) Bedside placement of inferior vena cava filters in the intensive care unit. Am Surg 65:833–838

Toro G, Roman GC, Navarro-Roman L, Cantillo J, Serrano B, Vergara I (1994) Natural history of spinal cord infarction caused by nucleus pulposus embolism. Spine 19:360–366

Torriero F, Macori F, Misiti A, Iacari V, Anaveri G (1998) A case of gas occurrence in the venous hepato-portal area after blunt trauma of the abdomen. Radiol Med 96:118–120

Traverso LW (1981) Is hepatic portal venous gas an indication for exploratory laparotomy? Arch Surg 116:936–938

Trujillo MH, Castillo A, Esparna J (1976) Bedside pulmonary angiography in the critically ill patient. Crit Care Med 43: 151–152

Turpie AGG, Gallus AS, Beattie WS, Hirsh J (1977) Prevention of venous thrombosis in patients with intracranial disease by intermittent pneumatic compression of the calf. Neurology 27:435–438

Turpie AGG, Hirsh J, Gent M, Julian D, Johnson J (1989) Prevention of deep vein thrombosis in potential neurosurgical patients. A randomized trial comparing graduated compression stockings alone or graduated compression stockings plus intermittent pneumatic compression with control. Arch Intern Med 149:679–681

Tuttle-Newhall JE, Rutledge R, Hultman CS, Fakhry SM (1997) Statewide, population-based, time-series analysis of the frequency and outcome of pulmonary embolus in 318,554 trauma patients. J Trauma 42:90–99

Upchurch GR, Demling RH, Davies J, Gates JD, Knox JB (1995) Efficacy of subcutaneous heparin in prevention of venous thromboembolic events in trauma patients. Am Surg 61: 749–755

Urokinase Pulmonary Embolism Trial (1973) A national cooperative study. Circulation 47 [Suppl 2]:1–108

Van Beek EJR, Reekers JA (1999) The value of pulmonary

angiography for the differential diagnosis of pulmonary embolism. Eur Radiol 9:1310–1316
Van Beek EJ, Kuyer PM, Schenk BE, Brandjes DP, Ten Cate JW, Buller HR (1995) A normal perfusion lung scan in patients with clinically suspected pulmonary embolism. Frequency and clinical validity. Chest 108:170–173
Van Beek EJR, Reekers JA, Batchelor DA, Brandjes DP, Büller HR (1996a) Feasibility, safety and clinical utility of angiography in patients with suspected pulmonary embolism. Eur Radiol 6:415–419
Van Beek EJR, Bakker AJ, Reekers JA (1996b) Pulmonary embolism: interobserver agreement in the interpretation of conventional angiographic and DSA images in patients with nondiagnostic lung scan results. Radiology 198:721–724
Van Beek EJR, Brouwers EM, Song B, Bongaerts AH, Oudkerk M (2001) Lung scintigraphy and helical computed tomography for the diagnosis of pulmonary embolism: a meta-analysis. Clin Appl Thromb Hemost 7:87–92
Van den Berge E, Bathgate B, Panagakos E et al (1999) Duplex screening as a method of quality assurance of perioperative thromboembolism prophylaxis. Int Angiol 18:210–219
Van Erkel AR, Pattynama PM (1998) Cost-effective diagnostic algorithms in pulmonary embolism: an updated analysis. Acad Radiol 5 [Suppl 2]: 321–327
Van Erkel AR, van Rossum AB, Bloem JL, Kievit J, Pattynama PM (1996) Spiral CT angiography for suspected pulmonary embolism: a cost-effectiveness analysis. Radiology 201: 29–36
Van Erkel AR, van den Hout WB, Pattynama PM (1999) International differences in health care costs in Europe and the United States: do these affect the cost-effectiveness of diagnostic strategies for pulmonary embolism? Eur Radiol 9:1926–1931
Van Rooij WJ, Den Heeten GJ, Sluzewski M (1995) Pulmonary embolism: diagnosis in 211 patients with use of selective pulmonary digital subtraction angiography with a flow-directed catheter. Radiology 195:793–797
Van Rossum AB, Treurniet FE, Kieft GJ, Smith SJ, Schepers-Bok R (1996a) Role of spiral volumetric computed tomographic scanning in the assessment of patients with clinical suspicion of pulmonary embolism and an abnormal ventilation/ perfusion lung scan. Thorax 51:23–28
Van Rossum AB, Pattynama PM, Tjin A, Ton ER et al (1996b) Pulmonary embolism: validation of spiral CT angiography in 149 patients. Radiology 201:467–470
Van Rossum AB, Pattynama PM, Mallens WM, Hermans J, Heijerman HG (1998a) Can helical CT replace scintigraphy in the diagnostic process in suspected pulmonary embolism? A retrolective-prolective cohort study focusing on total diagnostic yield. Eur Radiol 8:90–96
Van Rossum AB, van Erkel AR, van Persijn van Meerten EL, Ton ER, Rebergen SA, Pattynama PM (1998b) Accuracy of helical CT for acute pulmonary embolism: ROC analysis of observer performance related to clinical experience. Eur Radiol 8:1160–1164
Van Rossum AB, Pattynama PM, Tjin A, Ton E, Kieft GJ (1998c) Spiral CT appearance of resolving clots at 6-week follow-up after acute pulmonary embolism. J Comput Assist Tomogr 22:413–417
Van Strijen MJ, de Monye W, Kieft GJ, Bloem JL (1999) Diagnosis of pulmonary embolism with spiral CT: a prospective cohort study in 617 consecutive patients (abstract). Radiology 213 [Suppl]:128
Vauthey JN, Matthews CC (1988) Portal vein air embolization after blunt abdominal trauma. Am Surg 54:586–588
Vedrinne JM, Guillaume C, Gagnieu MC, Gratadour P, Fleuret C, Motin J (1992) Bronchoalveolar lavage in trauma patients for diagnosis of fat embolism syndrome. Chest 102:1323–1327
Velmahos GC, Nigro J, Tatevossian R et al (1998) Inability of an aggressive policy of thromboprophylaxis to prevent deep venous thrombosis (DVT) in critically injured patients: are current methods of DVT prophylaxis insufficient? J Am Coll Surg 187:529–533
Velmahos GC, Kern J, Chan LS, Oder D, Murray JA, Shekelle P (2000a) Prevention of venous thromboembolism after injury: an evidence-based report, part I. Analysis of risk factors and evaluation of the role of vena caval filters. J Trauma 49:132–139
Velmahos GC, Kern J, Chan LS, Oder D, Murray JA, Shekelle P (2000b) Prevention of venous thromboembolism after injury: an evidence-based report, part II. Analysis of risk factors and evaluation of the role of vena caval filters. J Trauma 49:140–144
Vesely TM, Krysl J, Smith SR, Killion D, Hicks ME (1996) Preliminary investigation of the Irie inferior vena caval filter. J Vasc Interv Radiol 7:529–535
Vignon P, Mentec H, Terre S, Gastinne H, Gueret P, Lemaire F (1994) Diagnostic accuracy and therapeutic impact of transthoracic and transesophageal echocardiography in mechanically ventilated patients in the ICU. Chest 106: 1829–1834
Virchow R (1856) Ein Vortrag über die Thrombose vom Jahre 1845. In: Virchow R (ed) Gesammelte Abhandlungen zur wissenschaftlichen Medizin. Meidinger, Frankfurt, pp 478–486
Vix VA (1983) The usefulness of chest radiographs obtained after a demonstrated perfusion scan defect in the diagnosis of pulmonary emboli. Clin Nucl Med 8:497–500
Vock P, Soucek M, Daepp M, Kalender WA (1990) Lung: spiral volumetric CT with single-breath-hold technique. Radiology 176:864–867
Vogel N, Kauczor HU, Heussel CP, Ries BG, Thelen M (2001) Artifact reduction in bolus-enhanced spiral CT of pulmonary arteries using a saline bolus. Rofo Fortschr Geb Rontgenstr Neuen Bildgeb Verfahr 173:460–465
Voitk AJ, Munkittrick RC (1986) A fatal pulmonary embolus composed of gross liver tissue. Can J Surg 29:218–219
Von Bergmann E (1873) Ein Fall tödlicher Fettembolie. Berl Med Wochenschr 10:385
Vos LD, Tielbeek AV, Bom EP, Gooszen HC, Vroegindeweij D (1997) The Günther temporary inferior vena cava filter for short-term protection against pulmonary embolism. Cardiovasc Intervent Radiol 20:91–97
Wacks MR, Bird HA (1970) Massive gross pulmonary embolism of cerebral tissue following severe head trauma. J Trauma 10:344–348
Wade WE, Chisholm MA (2000) Deep venous thrombosis prophylaxis in trauma: cost analysis. Blood Coag Fibrinol 11:101–106
Walsh PN, Greenspan RH, Simon M et al (1973) An angiographic severity index for pulmonary embolism. Circulation 47/48 [Suppl]:101–108
Walz MV, Walz MK (1992) Pulmonary embolism caused by liver tissue. Aktuel Traumatol 22:102–103
Warkentin TE, Levine MN, Hirsh J et al (1995) Heparin-induced thrombocytopenia in patients treated with low-

molecular-weight heparin or unfractionated heparin. N Engl J Med 332:1330–1335

Wascher RA, Gwinn BC Jr (1995) Air rifle pellet injury to the heart with retrograde caval migration. J Trauma 38: 379–381

Weaver FA, Meacham PW, Adkins RB, Dean RH (1988) Phlegmasia cerulea dolens: therapeutic considerations. South Med J 81:306–312

Webb LX, Rush PT, Fuller SB, Meredith JW (1992) Greenfield filter prophylaxis of pulmonary embolism in patients undergoing surgery for acetabular fracture. J Orthop Trauma 6:139–145

Weinmann EE, Salzman EW (1994) Deep-vein thrombosis. N Engl J Med 331:1630–1641

Wellman HN (1986) Pulmonary thromboembolism: current status report on the role of nuclear medicine. Semin Nucl Med 16:236–274

Wells PS, Lensing AWA, Davidson BL, Prins MH, Hirsh J (1995) Accuracy of ultrasound for the diagnosis of deep venous thrombosis in asymptomatic patients after orthopedic surgery. Ann Intern Med 122:47–53

Wells PS, Ginsberg JS, Anderson DR et al (1998) Use of a clinical model for safe management of patients with suspected pulmonary embolism. Ann Intern Med 129:997–1005

Westermark N (1938) On the roentgen diagnosis of lung embolism. Acta Radiol 19:357–372

Wheeler HB, Hirsh J, Wells P, Anderson FA Jr (1994) Diagnostic tests for deep vein thrombosis. Clinical usefulness depends on probability of disease. Arch Intern Med 154:1921–1928

White RH, Goulet JA, Bray TJ, Daschbach MM, McGahan JP, Hartling RP (1990) Deep-vein thrombosis after fracture of the pelvis: assessment with serial duplex-ultrasound screening. J Bone Joint Surg 72A:495–500

Wildberger JE, Mahnken AH, Sinha AM, Haage P, Schaller S, Gunther RW (2002) A differentiated approach to pulmonary embolism and deep venous thrombosis using multislice CT (abstract). Eur Radiol 12 [Suppl]:262

Wilson JE III, Bynum LJ (1976) An improved pulmonary angiographic technique using a balloon-tipped catheter. Am Rev Respir Dis 114:1137–1144

Wilson AG, Joseph AEA, Butland RJA (1986) The radiology of aseptic cavitation in pulmonary infarction. Clin Radiol 37: 327–333

Wilson JT, Rogers FB, Wald SL, Shackford SR, Ricci MA (1994) Prophylactic vena cava filter insertion in patients with traumatic spinal cord injury: preliminary results. Neurosurgery 35:234–239

Winchell RJ, Hoyt DB, Walsh JC, Simons RK, Eastman AB (1994) Risk factors associated with pulmonary embolism despite routine prophylaxis: implications for improved protection. J Trauma 37:600–606

Winer-Muram HT, Boone JM, Tankiwale A, Lombardo GL, Russi TJ, Muram D (1999) Helical CT for pregnant patients with suspected pulmonary embolism: is it safe? (abstract) Radiology 213 [Suppl]:128

Woesner ME, Sanders I, White GW (1971) The melting sign in resolving transient pulmonary infarction. Am J Roentgenol 111:782–790

Wojcik R, Cipolle MD, Fearen I, Jaffe J, Newcomb J, Pasquale MD (2000) Long-term follow-up of trauma patients with a vena caval filter. J Trauma 49:839–843

Woodard PK, Sostman HD, MacFall JR et al (1995) Detection of pulmonary embolism: comparison of contrast-enhanced spiral CT and time-of-flight MR techniques. J Thor Imaging 10:59–72

Woolson ST, Watt JM (1991) Intermittent pneumatic compression to prevent proximal deep venous thrombosis during and after total hip replacement. A prospective, randomized study of compression alone, compression and aspirin, and compression and low-dose warfarin. J Bone Joint Surg 73A:507–512

Worsley DF, Alavi A (1995) Comprehensive analysis of the results of the PIOPED study. J Nucl Med 36:2380–2387

Worsley DF, Alavi A, Aronchick JM, Chen JTT, Greenspan RH, Ravin CE (1993) Chest radiographic findings in patients with acute pulmonary embolism: observations from the PIOPED study. Radiology 189:133–136

Worsley DF, Palevsky HI, Alavi A (1994) A detailed evaluation of patients with acute pulmonary embolism and low- or very-low-probability lung scan interpretations. Arch Intern Med 154:2737–2741

Wu JW, Chen MY, Auringer ST (2000) Portal venous gas: an unusual finding in child abuse. J Emerg Med 18:105–107

Yankelevitz DF, Gamsu G, Shah A et al (2000) Optimization of combined CT pulmonary angiography with lower extremity CT venography. Am J Roentgenol 174:67–69

Yelnik A, Dizien O, Bussel B et al (1991) Systematic lower limb phlebography in acute spinal cord injury in 147 patients. Paraplegia 29:253–260

Zerhouni EA, Barth KH, Siegelman SS (1980) Demonstration of venous thrombosis by computed tomography. Am J Roentgenol 134:753–758

Zolfaghari D, Johnson B, Weireter LJ, Britt LD (1995) Expanded use of inferior vena cava filters in the trauma population. Surg Annu 27:99–105

Zuckerman DA, Sterling KM, Oser RF (1996) Safety of pulmonary angiography in the 1990s. J Vasc Interv Radiol 7:199–205

Zwaan M, Lorch H, Kulke C et al (1998) Clinical experience with temporary vena cava filters. J Vasc Interv Radiol 9:594–601

20 Systematic CT Examination of Thoracoabdominal Polytrauma Victims at Admission

R. F. Dondelinger, P. Deleuse, G. Ponghis, V. Willems

CONTENTS

R. F. Dondelinger, MD
Professor and Chairman, Department of Medical Imaging, University Hospital Sart Tilman, Domaine Universitaire du Sart Tilman B35, 4000 Liège, Belgium
P. Deleuse, MD
Department of Medical Imaging, University Hospital Sart Tilman, Domaine du Sart Tilman B35, 4000 Liège, Belgium
G. Ponghis, MD
Resident, Department of Medical Imaging, University Hospital Sart Tilman, Domaine du Sart Tilman B35, 4000 Liège, Belgium
V. Willems, MD
Department of Medical Imaging, University Hospital Sart Tilman, Domaine du Sart Tilman B35, 4000 Liège, Belgium

- CT may be the best single imaging modality for evaluating blunt polytrauma patients, provided the equipment is accessible in the resuscitation environment.
- Interpretation of a CT examination of a trauma patient on a viewing console gave similar results to film reading.
- Trivial hemoperitoneum without intraperitoneal injury or with only retroperitoneal or pelvic injury was seen on CT at admission in 8% and 15% respectively (1.2% and 2.8% of all trauma patients).
- Significant hepatosplenic injury without peritoneal fluid detected on CT at admission was seen in 8% of the cases.
- Contrast medium extravasation was seen on CT in 7% of the cases and 2% of all trauma victims were treated by hemostatic arterial embolization.

20.1 Patient Population

In the USA, annually more years of life are lost by trauma than by cardiovascular disease and cancer together, as predominantly young victims are involved in traffic accidents, or labor and sports injuries. In Germany, about 50,000 annual deaths are due to trauma, 1,500,000 individuals are injured and a large number remain temporarily or permanently disabled (Klotter et al. 1993).

Trauma victims with obvious or suspected head and face, spinal, thoracic, or abdominal injury were studied in our department with CT at admission, after initial resuscitation. Records from 469 consecutive patients were reviewed for the time period from June 1994 to October 1999. Patients with isolated brain, facial, or cervical spine injury were not considered in this study. Patients who were investigated with US alone or were taken immediately to the operating room were excluded. There were 355 males and 114 females (ratio 3:1) included in the study. Age varied from 2 to 98 years with a mean of 35.9. Four hundred fifty-seven (97.5%) patients had sustained blunt trauma. The largely predominant cause was a traffic accident, involving the car driver, one or several passengers, bicycle or motorcycle drivers, or pedestrians. Other infrequent causes were falls, or labor or sports accidents. Twelve (2.5%) victims were wounded by penetrating injury, 8 by gunshot and 4 by a stab wound. A total number of 562 CT studies were obtained, i.e., 1.2 examinations per patient during hospitalization. We obtained 396 (84.4%) CT examinations, either immediately at admission or after resuscitation. After the first 24 h of admission, (18.4%) CT examinations were obtained and are not considered in the study. Thirty-two patients had 43 CT examinations that were repeated during hospitalization and are excluded from the study.

This retrospective study was based on the 396 CT studies obtained immediately at admission. Distribution of patients per year during the study period was as follows: 11 (3%) patients in 1994, 44 (11%) in 1995, 71 (18%) in 1996, 107 (27%) in 1997, 80 (20%) in 1998 and 83 (21%) in 1999. Cumulative distribution of patients per month for the study period is indicated in Fig. 20.1.

We examined 889 (48%) patients between 8 A.M. and 6 P.M., 116 (29%) patients between 6 P.M. and midnight, and 91 (23%) between midnight and 8 A.M.

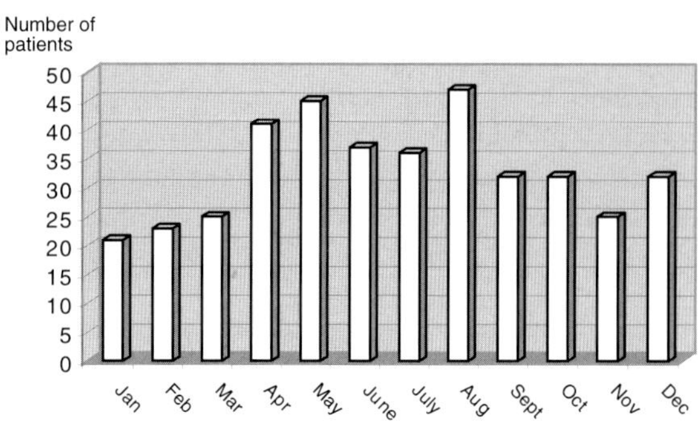

Fig. 20.1. Mean number of CT examinations per month obtained immediately at admission (from June 1994 to October 1999)

20.2 Technique

All patients were examined on the same CT equipment (PQ 2000, Picker, Cleveland, Ohio, USA) with helical acquisition capability, that was upgraded in 1998 to a PQ 5000. This equipment is located adjacent to the Emergency Department. The 40 m^2 room also contains an angiography unit (Omnicon, Picker) linked with the CT through a rotating patient support. This patient support has a radiolucent carbon table top that can be operated as a free floating support, with a manual handle, when in the angiographic position. Rotation from the angiographic to the CT position or vice versa is activated manually and takes a few seconds. A contrast medium injector dedicated to CT and another power injector for angiographic studies is available in the suite. Mural outlets for anesthesiology are available for patient monitoring in both positions, for CT and angiography. Two angiography monitors are ceiling mounted and a CT slave monitor is positioned in the examination room on a mobile chart, together with the fluoro-CT monitor (Capasso et al. 1996; Kos et al. 1999).

Among the total number of 396 examinations obtained at admission, 75 (19%) covered the abdomen and the pelvis including the base of the thorax, 315 (79%) covered the entire abdomen and thorax, and 6 examinations (1%) covered only the thorax. In 2 of 390 abdominal (0.5%) examinations, oral contrast was given. Hemodynamically stable, stabilized, and marginally stable patients were included. Patient resuscitation and monitoring was continued in the CT room. CT examinations including the abdomen were conducted before and after i.v. contrast medium injection, thoracic examinations were performed only after i.v. contrast enhancement. For abdominal and thoracic examinations, a caudocranial acquisition was obtained, followed by a craniocaudal spiral, covering also the pelvis. Additional acquisitions were obtained when necessary. In 390 of 396 patients (98.5%) a nonionic contrast agent was given intravenously.

20.3 Study Protocol

The main objective of the study was to review the accuracy of CT in the initial assessment of trauma patients and to compare the results obtained by film interpretation with reviewing the examination on a console. It has been suggested that the CT images obtained on trauma patients should be read immediately on the console, as it will become standard with the widespread use of multislice CT (Wechsler et al. 1996). Diagnostic findings were correlated with the medical records of the patients.

For this retrospective survey, initial radiological reports, obtained from film reading and formulated by senior radiologists, were compared with a second reading done by another senior radiologist, on a viewing station (Voxel Q, Picker) without taking films. For this reading, done by the same observer, 38 types of injuries were considered, which are listed in Table 20.1.

Table 20.1. Type of injuries considered for reviewing CT examinations at admission

Pneumothorax
Pneumomediastinum
Pneumopericardium
Pleural effusion
Lung contusion
Phrenic rupture
Thoracic cage fracture
Hemopericardium
Hemomediastinum
Aortic injury
Esophageal injury
Thoracic spine fracture
Lumbar spine fracture
Kidney
Bladder
Adrenal
Spleen
Liver
Pancreas
Gallbladder
Hemoperitoneum
Pneumoperitoneum
GI tract injury
Muscular hematoma
Contrast medium extravasation
Pelvic bone fracture
Retroperitoneal hematoma

Pneumothorax, pleural effusion, lung contusion, and renal and adrenal injury were considered separately for both sides. Thoracic cage fractures included fractures of the sternum, ribs, clavicle and scapula. The following scores were used to evaluate severity of injury:

- Pneumothorax. Minor: less than 1 cm thickness; large: total lung collapse; moderate: between 1 cm and total lung collapse.
- Pleural effusion. Small: 1 cm; moderate: 1–5 cm; large: >5 cm.
- Lung contusion. Involvement of 1, 2, or 3 lobes was considered. Minimal contusion: <10% of lobe volume; moderate: 10–50%; large: >50%.
- Hemomediastinum. Minimal: limited obliteration of mediastinal fat; large: displacement of mediastinal vessels or pleura; moderate: between the two.
- Hemopericardium. Small: <5 mm; moderate: 5–10 mm; large:>10 mm.

Hepatic and splenic injuries were classified according to the scores given by Mirvis et al. (1989a, b). Renal injuries were classified according to Federle et al. (1981). Pancreatic injuries were classified approximately according to the surgical classification by Jurkovich and Carrico (1990). Hemoperitoneum was searched for in the following five compartments: right subphrenic space, left subphrenic space, Morison's pouch, inframesocolic and right or left paracolic gutter, and the perivesical space. The volume of hemoperitoneum was estimated as minor when less than 1 cm, moderate when 1–5 cm, and large when greater than 5 cm.

20.4 Abdominal Injury

Among 396 CT examinations obtained at admission, 390 (98%) covered the abdomen and pelvis. Table 20.2 lists abdominal and pelvic injuries found in these 390 examinations.

20.4.1 Hemoperitoneum

A peritoneal effusion was observed in 82 of 390 (21%) patients.

20.4.1.1 Distribution and Amount

We examined these patients in detail, to learn more about the relevance of hemoperitoneum seen on CT at admission and for patient management. For 72 of 82 patients, full medical records were available. We considered the five of the peritoneal compartments listed above for retrospective evaluation of hemoperitoneum volume. Hemoperitoneum was almost equal-

Table 20.2. CT findings in abdominal injury at admission, (n=390)

Hemoperitoneum	82 (21.0%)
Spleen	43 (11.0%)
Liver	40 (10.2%)
Gastrointestinal tract or mesentery	7 (1.8%)
Pneumoperitoneum	5 (1.2%)
Pancreas	4 (1.0%)
Gallbladder	4 (1.0%)
Pelvic or abdominal wall hematoma	88 (22.6%)
Pelvic fracture	79 (20.2%)
Retroperitoneal hematoma	49 (12.6%)
Lumbar spine fracture	35 (9.0%)
Renal	26 (6.7%)
Adrenal	18 (4.6%)
Urinary bladder	1 (0.2%)

ly distributed in all five compartments (15–23%). At admission, CT showed no predominance, either for subphrenic spaces or for the perivesical compartments. When hemoperitoneum was observed in one compartment only, it was of minimal volume in 53% of the cases; when present in all five compartments, it occupied a large volume in at least one compartment (perivesical) in 50% of the cases.

20.4.1.2
Hemoperitoneum Associated with Visceral Injury

Fifty-five out of 72 victims (76%) had at least one visceral injury associated with hemoperitoneum. When hemoperitoneum was limited to one compartment, which occurred in 17out of 72 (23%) of the cases, a visceral injury was present in 8 (47%) cases. When hemoperitoneum was observed in 2, 3, or 4 peritoneal compartments, a visceral injury was seen in 11 of 14 (79%), 11 of 14 (79%), and 10 of 11 (91%) cases, respectively. When hemoperitoneum was seen in all five peritoneal compartments, a visceral injury was present in 15 of 16 (94%) of the patients. Table 20.3 shows the type of visceral abdominal injuries that were associated with hemoperitoneum.

The grade of splenic injury seemed to be related to the amount of hemoperitoneum, but without statistical significance. Grades I and II splenic injuries showed hemoperitoneum limited to 1–3 compartments in 11 out of 15 (73%) cases, whereas grades III and IV splenic contusion was associated with hemoperitoneum in 4–5 compartments in 8 out of 13 (61%). No correlation was found between severity of hepatic contusion and distribution of hemoperitoneum.

Table 20.3. Visceral injuries associated with hemoperitoneum in 72 patients

Spleen	28 (39%)
Liver	25 (35%) including 1 false negative CT (grade I)
Gastrointestinal tract and mesos	3 (4%)
Pancreas	2 (3%)
Urinary bladder	1 (1%) false negative CT

Twenty surgical interventions were performed in 18 of 72 patients (25%) for repair of visceral injuries (Table 20.4).

One splenectomy was done in emergency before CT. One perforation of the gastrointestinal tract and the rupture of the urinary bladder were missed on CT. Only one celiotomy done at day 0 was nontherapeutic. The risk of requiring a laparotomy increased with the number of peritoneal compartments filled with hemoperitoneum: 12% of patients with hemoperitoneum in one compartment were operated on, as well as 21%, 36%, and 56% of patients with hemoperitoneum present in 3, 4, and 5 compartments, respectively.

20.4.1.3
Hemoperitoneum Without Visceral Injury

Isolated hemoperitoneum without evidence of visceral injury on CT was said to be secondary to significant injury to the gastrointestinal tract or mesos in the vast majority of patients. Recent reports have shown that hemoperitoneum can be the sole indicator of an abdominal visceral trauma (Chiu et al. 1997; Shanmuganathan et al. 1999).

In our study, in 17 of 72 (23%) patients with peritoneal fluid, no intraperitoneal organ injury was seen on CT at admission. Unilateral periadnexal fluid in young women, fluid limited to the gallbladder fossa, and images with questionable artifacts were excluded.

Table 20.4. Type and timing of abdominal interventions done for visceral injuries associated with hemoperitoneum

Type of surgery	No. of patients (%)	Time of intervention
Splenectomy	9 (32%)	6 at day 0 3 at day 1
Hepatic packing	2 (8.5%)	2 at day 0
Gastrointestinal repair	3 (100%)	2 at day 0 1 at day 1
Urinary bladder repair	1 (100%)	1 at day 5
Partial pancreatectomy	2 (100%)	1 at day 1 1 at day 2
Exploratory laparotomy	3 (4%)	1 at day 0 1 at day 6 1 at day 9

Densities measured on hemoperitoneum were not considered, as they can be extremely variable, from 60 to 100 HU for recent clot to 0 HU for supernatant serum in a nondependent position (FEDERLE and JEFFREY 1983; LEVINE et al. 1996). Among these 17 patients, CT was negative for any intraperitoneal injury in 6 cases. Hemoperitoneum of minimal or moderate volume was present in only one compartment in four of them, and in two other patients, a minimal hemoperitoneum was present in three compartments. In the 11 remaining patients, CT was positive for pelvic or retroperitoneal injury. Peritoneal effusion was seen in one or two compartments in 5 of 11 (45%) and 3 of 11 (27%) trauma victims, respectively. In victims with pelvic or retroperitoneal injury, the parietal peritoneal leaflet had probably ruptured, allowing extraperitoneal blood to spread into the peritoneal cavity. In these patients, diagnostic peritoneal lavage would have shown a false positive result. In none of these 17 patients was a significant intraperitoneal injury missed, as no patient with isolated hemoperitoneum required surgical repair of an intraperitoneal injury. This observation is in contradiction with other reports, claiming that in patients with isolated hemoperitoneum, exploratory laparotomy was therapeutic in 94% of patients for repair of bowel and mesenteric injury (CUNNINGHAM et al. 1998). In another report, a distinction is made between mesenteric and nonmesenteric fluid. Small amounts of hemoperitoneum as the sole indicator of trauma may be treated conservatively, except for mesenteric fluid, which raises a strong suspicion of gastrointestinal rupture (LEVINE et al. 1995).

20.4.1.4
Visceral Injury Without Hemoperitoneum

Recent reports have shown that 11% of hepatic injuries and 12% of splenic injuries have no free peritoneal fluid on CT (OCHSNER et al. 2000). In this study, we observed 25 significant abdominal injuries in 14 of 308 patients (5%), without hemoperitoneum seen on CT at admission, which are detailed in Table 20.5. In 10 other patients (3%), combined intra- and retroperitoneal injuries without hemoperitoneum were found.

20.4.2
Splenic Injury

Splenic injury predominated slightly over hepatic injury, as found in other surgical series (COX 1984). Forty-three of 390 (11%) patients had splenic injury; 18 (42%) had grade I, 9 (21%) had grade II, 8 (18.5%) had grade III, and 8 (18.5%) had grade IV. Associated abdominal and thoracic injuries are listed in Table 20.6.

Twenty-seven (63%) patients had benign splenic injury (grade I or II) and 16 (37%) had severe (grade III or IV) splenic contusion. Among associated abdominal injuries, pelvic fractures and renal contusion were seen predominantly in 33% and 23%, respectively. The left kidney was injured together with the spleen in 60% of all associated renal injuries. An associated left adrenal contusion was seen in one case. Hepatic contusion was associated in four (9%)

Table 20.5. Visceral abdominal injuries seen in 14/308 patients without hemoperitoneum

Type and grade of injury	No. of patients
Spleen	9
Grade I: 7	
Grade II: 2	
Liver	10
Grade I: 6	
Grade II: 1	
Grade III: 3	
Pancreas	1
Grade II: 1	
Pneumoperitoneum	3
Gastrointestinal tract or mesos	2 (surgery in 2)

Table 20.6. Splenic contusion and associated abdominal and thoracic injuries

Splenic injury	Type of associated injuries	No. of patients
Grade I: 7 Grade II: 1 Grade III: 2 Grade IV: 4	Pelvic fracture	14
Grade I: 2 Grade III: 1 Grade IV: 1	Liver injury Grade III: 2 Grade II: 1 Grade II: 1	4
	Kidney (right 4, left 6)	10
	Adrenal (right 3, left 1)	4
	Pancreas (grade II, III)	2
	GI tract (caecum, intestine)	2
	Lumbar spine fracture	4
	Pneumothorax (left 12, right 3, bilateral 5)	20
	Pleural effusion (left 10, right 2, bilateral 9)	21
	Thoracic cage fracture (left 13, right 4, bilateral 2, sternal fracture 1)	20
	Pulmonary contusion (left 4, right 2, bilateral 20)	26
	Thoracic aorta rupture	2

cases. Injury was located in the right lobe in three patients, and in the right and left lobe in one patient. Lumbar spine fractures were seen in four (9%) cases. No thoracic spine fracture was found in association with splenic injury. Pancreatic, gastrointestinal tract injury, and thoracic aorta rupture were associated with an equal frequency of 5%. Thoracic cage fractures predominated on the left side (35% vs 14% for the right side). About half of the patients with splenic injury show left lower rib fractures (McCort 1964). Pulmonary or pleural injury was associated in 60% and 49% of the cases.

20.4.3 Hepatic Injury

Hepatic injury was observed in 40 of 390 patients (10%) with a similar frequency to splenic trauma. Grade I injury was present in 12 patients (30%), grade II in 9 (23%), grade III in 18 (45%,) and grade IV in 1 (2%). Benign hepatic injury (grade I or II) was present in 53% and severe injury (grade III or IV) in 47% of the cases. Table 20.7 lists associated abdominal and thoracic injuries.

Pelvic fractures were observed in 11 (27%) patients with hepatic injury and lumbar spine fractures occurred in 4 (10%). Two patients had a combined pelvic and lumbar spine fracture. Splenic injury was associated in four (10%) cases. Adrenal injury was common and seen in nine (23%) cases, all located on the right side. Right renal contusion was seen in six (15%) of the cases. Pleural and pulmonary injury was seen in 47% and 65% of the cases, with a significant predominance of the right side for pleural effusion and pneumothorax. Thoracic cage fractures predominated on the right side (40% vs 10% for the left side). About 50% of patients with hepatic injury have right lower rib fractures (McCort 1964).

Table 20.7. Hepatic contusion and associated abdominal and thoracic injuries

Hepatic injury	Type of associated injuries	No. of patients
	Pelvic fracture	11
Grade I: 4 Grade II: 2 Grade III: 5		
	Lumbar spine fracture	4
Grade I: 1 Grade III: 3		
	Spleen	4
Grade II: 2	grade III or IV: 2	
Grade III: 2	grade I: 2	
	Adrenal (all right-sided)	9
	Kidney (all right-sided)	6
	Pulmonary contusion (right 5, left 2, bilateral 19)	26
	Pleural effusion (right 8, left 1, bilateral 10)	19
	Thoracic cage fracture (right 13, left 1, bilateral 3)	17
	Pneumothorax (right 7, left 2, bilateral 3)	12

20.4.4 Renal Injury

Renal injury was observed in 26of 390 (7%) cases. Right renal injury was present in 18 (69%), left renal injury in 7 (27%), and bilateral renal injury in 1 case (4%). Eleven patients (42%) had renal injury without associated splenic or hepatic injury. A grade I renal injury was present in 14 (52%), a grade II in 4 (15%), and a grade III in 9 (33%) cases. Table 20.8 lists associated abdominal and thoracic injuries.

Splenic injury coexisted with renal injury in 10 of 26 patients (38%), followed by adrenal injury, which occurred in 7 of 26 patients (27%). Adrenal injury was homolateral to renal injury in all cases. Hepatic injury was associated with renal injury in six cases (23%); the right kidney was involved in all cases. The right kidney and the right adrenal were involved together with hepatic contusion in four cases (15%). Among all cases of renal injury, hemoperitoneum was found in 18 of 26 cases (69%). Isolated hemoperitoneum without intraperitoneal injury was found in three cases with renal injury (12%). The right kidney was more often associated with lumbar spine fracture (6 vs 2). Pulmonary contusion was seen in 65% and pleural effusion in 23% of the cases.

20.4.5 Adrenal Injury

Contusion of the adrenal gland may give an intraglandular or periglandular hematoma, obscuring the margins of the gland. Hematoma shows as an enlarged gland and blurs the periglandular fat. Hematoma can extend caudally, preferentially on the left side, where the adrenal is less confined than on the right side. Glandular or periglandular hematoma was seen in 18 (5%) of the cases, and may give a pseudo-enlargement of the right diaphragmatic crus. The right adrenal gland was involved in 17 out of 18 (94%) of the cases, the left adrenal in 1 case (6%). Four (9%) splenic injuries were associated with adrenal contusion: three

Table 20.8. Renal contusion and associated abdominal and thoracic injuries

Renal injury	Type of associated injuries	No. of patient
Grade I: 5 Grade III: 2	Adrenal (right 6, left 1)	7 (27%)
Grade III (left)	Pancreas (grade II)	1 (4%)
Right 5, bilateral 1 Grade I: 4 Grade II: 1 Grade III: 2	Lumbar spine	6 (23%)
Right 6, left 1 Grade I: 6 Grade II: 1	Pelvic fracture	7 (27%)
Right 3 Grade I: 2 Grade III: 1	Hemoperitoneum without intraperitoneal visceral injury	3 (12%)
Right 12, left 4, bilateral 1 Grade I: 12 Grade II: 1 Grade III: 5	Retroperitoneal hematoma	17 (65%)
	Pulmonary contusion (right 12, left 4, bilateral 1)	17 (65%)
	Thoracic cage fracture (right 5, left 5)	10 (38%)
	Pneumothorax (right 4, left 3)	7 (27%)
	Pleural effusion (right 8, left 4)	12 (23%)

right adrenals and one left were involved. Splenic injury was grade III in one and grade IV in three cases. Nine hepatic injuries (22.5%) were associated with adrenal contusion, all located on the right side. Seven renal injuries (27%) were associated with adrenal injury, all homolateral. No adrenal contusion was observed as an isolated finding. The predominance of unilateral, right adrenal injury and the association with homolateral intraabdominal visceral injury was confirmed in children (Sivit et al. 1992).

20.4.6 Lumbar Spine and Pelvic Fractures

Lumbar spine fractures occurred in 35 of 390 (9%) patients in this series. Figures of 10% of concomitant lumbar spine fractures and abdominal injuries were reported in the literature (Rabinovici et al. 1999). In our study, 11% of lumbar spine fractures were associated with splenic or hepatic injury, 17% were concomitant to renal injury. Pelvic fractures were noted in 79 of 390 (20%) patients. Eighteen percent of pelvic fractures were associated with splenic injury, and 33% of all splenic contusion were associated with pelvic fractures. Fourteen percent of all pelvic fractures were concomitant to hepatic injury, and 28% of all hepatic injuries were associated with pelvic fractures. For renal injuries, figures were 9% and 27%, respectively. The association of hepatosplenic injuries combined with pelvic fractures was emphasized in other reports (Miltner et al. 1992). In one recent report, splenic, hepatic, or renal injuries were found concomitant to pelvic fractures in 59% (Siegmeth et al. 2000).

20.4.7 Other Injuries

Gastrointestinal tract or mesenteric contusion was seen in seven (1.8%) cases. In surgical series, gastroduodenal and pancreatic injury, resulting from blunt trauma and requiring celiotomy accounted for 0.4% (Cox 1984). In our series, pneumoperitoneum was observed in five (1%) cases and was associated with hemoperitoneum in three cases.

Pancreatic contusion was seen in four (1.0%) cases: two were grade II and two were grade III. One pancreatic contusion had no associated abdominal injury. In another case, only hemoperitoneum was found associated with pancreatic injury. In a third case, splenic and left renal injury was seen, and in a fourth case, splenic injury was associated. Three cases were associated with hemoperitoneum. Two more pancreatic injuries, missed at admission, were diagnosed on delayed scans.

Gallbladder injury was observed in four case (1%) at admission and one other case was confirmed on repeated CT.

One (0.2%) urinary bladder, with extraperitoneal rupture and associated with pelvic and lumbar spine fractures, was missed on CT at admission.

20.5 Thoracic Injury

20.5.1 Pneumothorax

Pneumothorax was detected in 87 of 321 (27%) patients, who underwent either a complete thoracic and abdominal CT examination or only a complete thoracic examination. The total number of pneumothoraces was 106. Twenty-nine (27%) pneumothoraces were located on the right side, 39 (37%) on the left side, and in 19 patients, pneumothorax was bilateral (36%). Forty-nine of 106 (46%) pneumothoraces were minimal, 54 (51%) were moderate, and 3 (3%) were large, with total lung collapse.

20.5.2 Pulmonary Contusion

Pulmonary contusion was present in 171of 321 patients (53%). In 32 (19%) patients, contusion was located in the right lung; 21 (12%) patients had contusion in the left lung. Bilateral pulmonary contusion was noted in 118 (69%) patients.

20.5.3 Pleural Effusion

We noted 222 pleural effusions in 135 out of 321 patients (42%) cases. Twenty-three (10%) pleural effusions were right-sided; 25 (11%) were left-sided. Of these, 174 effusions were bilateral (78%). In 110 of 222 (50%) right-sided pleural effusions, 77 (70%) were of minimal volume and 33 (30%) were of moderate amount. In 112 left-sided pleural effusions, 78 (70%) were of minimal amount, 30 (27%) of moderate and 4 (4%) of large amount.

20.5.4 Thoracic Cage Fractures

Thoracic cage fractures occurred in 119 of 321 patients (40%). Right or left rib fractures were seen in 54 (17%) and 61 (19%) patients, respectively; in 2 of these cases (4%), costal fractures were bilateral. Right clavicular fractures were seen in nine (3%) patients and left-sided fractures in nine (3%) patients. A fracture of the right scapula was seen in seven patients (2%) and a left scapular fracture in six (2%) patients. A sternal fracture was observed in nine (3%) cases. A combination of costal, clavicular, scapular, or sternal fractures was seen in 31 out of 119 (26%) the cases. Pulmonary contusion was associated with homolateral rib fractures in 39 out of 54 cases (72%) on the right side and 49 out of 61 (80%) on the left side.

20.5.5 Hemomediastinum

Hemomediastinum was seen in 47 of 321 (15%) cases and was classified as minor in 12 (26%), moderate in 11 (23%), and large or displacing the pleura in 24 (51%) cases. Isolated hemomediastinum without other thoracic injury occurred in 26 of 47 (55%) cases. In 21 of 47 (45%) cases of patients with hemomediastinum, the injury that was responsible for the hemomediastinum was evidenced: thoracic aortic injury in 5 patients, thoracic spine fracture in 8, fracture of the lumbar spine in 4, and fracture of the thoracic and lumbar spine in 5. Hemomediastinum caused by isthmic thoracic aortic injury or spinal fracture predominates in a posterior location. Isolated hemomediastinum, caused by rupture of small mediastinal veins, is predominantly located in the anterior mediastinum.

20.6 Contrast Extravasation

Twenty-nine sites of contrast medium extravasation were observed in 26 of 396 (7%) trauma victims on CT examination at admission. Sites of extravasation are listed in Table 20.9.

In three patients, hemorrhage was observed in two different sites: retroperitoneal space and pelvis in two patients, spleen and pelvis in one patient. The spleen showed extravasation more frequently than the liver, but no grade I or II splenic or hepatic injury showed active extravasation. Interestingly, it was shown that even low-grade splenic injury in adults may show delayed rebleeding, whereas low-grade injury has a more consistent response to conservative management (Mirvis et al. 1989b).

Demonstration of an active bleeding site enables "focused arteriography and embolization" or "focused surgery" for immediate hemostasis, without exploration of the entire abdominal cavity or unnecessary selective arteriographic catheterization (Di Giacomo et al. 1996). In this series, eight (2% of all trauma victims) hemostatic arterial embolization procedures were performed immediately after completion of the CT examination, in four splenic, two hepatic, and two renal injuries,

Table 20.9. Sites of extravasation of contrast medium seen in 26/396 (7%) patients on CT at admission

Site of extravasation	No. of extravasation sites
Spleen	8
Retroperitoneal space	7
Liver	4
Kidney	3
Pelvis	3
Thoracic aorta	2
Mesentery	1
Portal vein	1

using the combined CT-angiography unit. Patients were hemodynamically marginally stable or unstable (Kos et al. 1999). In the past, 2.3% of abdominal trauma victims underwent diagnostic angiography; today almost all arteriographies performed are therapeutic (Strauch 1973).

20.7 Free Air

Free air, which is not subcutaneous emphysema, pneumoperitoneum, retropneumoperitoneum, or air extending from a pneumomediastinum to the abdomen, may be seen on CT following blunt injury. Free gas bubbles are seen close to joints, such as in front of the sacroiliac joints, or in the vertebral canal, and result from a sudden stretching or elongation of joints or a vacuum phenomenon.

20.8 Results

20.8.1 Incidence of Abnormal CT Examinations

Patient selection for CT investigation has changed over the last years. In 1994, when CT examination of trauma patients was not systematic at admission in our department, patients with trivial injury were not included, which accounted for a higher percentage of examinations showing significant posttraumatic injuries. Actually, the number of examinations showing either thoracic or abdominal significant injuries lies between 69% and 91%. Table 20.10 lists results obtained during the last 6 years. Although it is estimated that abdominal trauma accounts only for 10–20% of admissions, the possibility of exploring head, face, spine, thorax, and abdominal injuries with one examination justifies systematic CT.

20.8.2 Diagnostic Errors

Significant and obvious injuries were omitted in the initial reports and others were also omitted during reviewing. During review, CT of all examinations obtained at admission by the same experienced radiologist, 44 diagnoses that were reported in the original report were missed.

Table 20.10. CT examinations at admission showing significant thoracic or abdominal injuries

Year	Total no. of CT	No. (%) of CT examinations positive for injury at admission
1994	11	8 (73)
1995	44	40 (91)
1996	71	59 (84)
1997	107	81 (76)
1998	80	59 (74)
1999	83	57 (69)

Table 20.11 lists the false negative diagnoses that were not described during review of the cases on the console. Most missed findings were minimal injuries. Among these diagnostic errors, pneumoperitoneum, renal contrast extravasation, aortic injury, pneumothorax, and intercostal hemorrhage may have had pejorative consequences on patient management. All errors of interpretation were attributed to fatigue of the reader, who reviewed a series of cases at the end of a working day, without having clinical information, except the gender and age of the patient. Two false positive diagnoses were formulated: one hepatic contusion, grade I, and one minimal pleural effusion. Diagnostic errors formulated on the initial reports were similar in nature than those committed by the secondary reader and are not listed here. Misdiagnosis could be related to inadequate examination technique concerning contrast enhancement, slice thickness, anatomical variants, wrong perception of pathophysiology of trauma, perception errors,

Table 20.11. False negative diagnoses missed during case review on the console

Small bone fracture	17
Compartmental hemoperitoneum	6
Hepatic contusion (grade I)	3
Splenic contusion (grade I)	2
Pneumothorax	2
Pneumomediastinum	2
Pneumoperitoneum	1
Renal contusion (grade I)	1
Renal contrast extravasation	1
Pancreatic contusion	1
Esophageal contusion	1
Abdominal periaortic contusion	1
Aortic pseudoaneurysm	1
Lung contusion	1
Pleural effusion	1
Muscle contusion	1
Pleural contrast extravasation	1
Psoas muscle contrast extravasation	1

or rare injury. Comparative results obtained by film reading and case review on the console are given in Table 20.12.

Forty-five (11%) of 396 patients examined by CT died during a 1-year follow-up. Forty (89%) deaths were related to injury, five patients (11%) died due to a non-posttraumatic cause. Four of 396 (1%) patients were lost to follow-up. None of the 40 deaths could retrospectively be attributed to misdiagnosis of significant injury on CT at admission.

Table 20.12. Comparison between the original reports obtained on film reading and second reading on a viewing station (expressed in percentage)

	Film reading (%)	Review on viewing station (%)
Sensitivity	80.9	96.8 ($P<0.05$)
Specificity	99.7	99.9
Positive predictive value	97.7	99.8
Negative predictive value	98.2	99.5

20.9 Conclusion

Isolated blunt abdominal injuries are rare. Trauma victims with obvious or suspected abdominal injuries should also undergo thoracic, pelvic, and lumbar spine CT. Certain patterns of association of abdominal injuries or abdominal and bone injuries can be identified according to the type of trauma or direction of impact. Benign hemoperitoneum may be isolated and significant visceral injuries may be present without hemoperitoneum. Reviewing CT examinations on a console gives equivalent results to film reading. Sensitivity and specificity of CT are high and mismanagement caused by misreading CT at admission is rare.

References

Capasso P, Trotteur G, Flandroy P, Dondelinger RF (1996) A combined CT and angiography suite with a pivoting table. Radiology 199:561–563

Chiu WC, Cushing BM, Rodriguez A et al (1997) Abdominal injuries without hemoperitoneum: a potential limitation of focused abdominal sonography for trauma (FAST). J Trauma 42:617–623

Cox EF (1984) Blunt abdominal trauma. A 5-year analysis of 870 patients requiring celiotomy. Ann Surg 199:467–474

Cunningham MA, Tyroch AH, Kaups KL, Davis JW (1998) Does free fluid on abdominal computed tomographic scan after blunt trauma require laparotomy? J Trauma 44:599–602

Di Giacomo JC, McGonigal MD, Haskal ZJ et al (1996) Arterial bleeding diagnosed by CT in hemodynamically stable victims of blunt trauma. J Trauma 40:249–252

Federle MP, Jeffrey RB (1983) Hemoperitoneum studied by CT. Radiology 148:187–192

Federle MP, Kaiser JA, McAninch JW, Jeffrey RB, Mall JC (1981) The role of computed tomography in renal trauma. Radiology 141:455–460

Jurkovich G, Carrico C (1990) Pancreatic trauma. Surg Clin North Am 70:575–593

Klotter HJ, Nies C, Zielke A, Sitter H, Rothmund M (1993) Choice of diagnostic modalities in blunt abdominal trauma. Chirurg 64:841–848

Kos X, Fanchamps JM, Trotteur G, Dondelinger RF (1999) Radiologic damage control: evaluation of a combined CT and angiography suite with a pivoting table. Cardiovasc Intervent Radiol 22:124–129

Levine CD, Patel UJ, Wachsberg RH, Simmons MZ, Baker SR, Cho KC (1995) CT in patients with blunt abdominal trauma: clinical significance of intraperitoneal fluid detected on a scan with otherwise normal findings. AJR 164:1381–1385

Levine CD, Patel UJ, Silverman PM, Wachsberg RH (1996) Low attenuation of acute traumatic hemoperitoneum on CT scans. AJR 166:1089–1093

McCort JJ (1964) Radiographic examination in blunt abdominal trauma. Radiol Clin North Am 2:121–143

Miltner E, Wiedmann HP, Leutwein B et al (1992) Liver and spleen ruptures in authentic car-to-car side collisions with main impact at front door or B-pillar. Am J Forensic Med Pathol 13:2–6

Mirvis SE, Withley NO, Wainwright JR, Gends DR (1989a) Blunt hepatic trauma in adults: CT-based classification and correlation with prognosis and treatment. Radiology 172:27–32

Mirvis SE, Withley NO, Gends DR (1989b) Blunt splenic trauma in adult: CT-based classification and correlation with prognosis and treatment. Radiology 171:33–39

Ochsner MG, Knudson MM, Pachter HL et al (2000) Significance of minimal or no intraperitoneal fluid visible on CT scan associated with blunt liver and splenic injuries: a multicenter analysis. J Trauma 49:505–510

Rabinovici R, Ovadia P, Mathiak G, Abdullah F (1999) Abdominal injuries associated with lumbar spine fractures in blunt trauma. Injury 30:471–474

Shanmuganathan K, Mirvis SE, Sherbourne CD, Chiu WC, Rodriguez A (1999) Hemoperitoneum as the sole indicator of abdominal visceral injuries: potential limitations of screening abdominal US for trauma. Radiology 212:423–430

Siegmeth A, Mullner T, Kukla C, Vecsei V (2000) Associated injuries in severe pelvic trauma. Unfallchirurg 103: 572–581

Sivit CJ, Ingram JD, Taylor GA, Bulas DI, Kushner DC, Eichelberger MR (1992) Posttraumatic adrenal hemorrhage in children: CT findings in 34 patients. AJR 158:1299–1302

Strauch GO (1973) Major abdominal trauma in 1971: a study of Connecticut by the Connecticut Society of American Board Surgeons and the Yale Trauma Program. Am J Surg 125:413–418

Wechsler RJ, Spettell CM, Kurtz AB et al (1996) Effects of training and experience in interpretation of emergency body CT. Radiology 199:171–72

21 Respective Merit of Imaging and Other Diagnostic Modalities in Abdominal Injuries

R. F. DONDELINGER

CONTENTS

- Diagnostic investigation of trauma should be intense and when necessary aggressive, but management should be conservative.
- A traumatized patient may have several significant or life-threatening injuries; the most important one is not necessarily the most obvious (JURKOVICH and CARRICO 1992).
- Laparotomy should not be delayed by time-consuming studies in the unstable patient (JONES et al. 1983).
- A negative laparotomy is preferable to an undiagnosed critical injury, but it is optimal to avoid both (PETERSEN and SHELDON 1979).

R. F. DONDELINGER, MD
Professor and Chairman, Department of Medical Imaging, University Hospital Sart Tilman, Domaine Universitaire du Sart Tilman B35, 4000 Liège, Belgium

21.1 Introduction

In this chapter, the clinical symptoms and findings, the different imaging modalities and other tests obtained in the acute abdominal trauma victim are reviewed and their respective merits in the diagnosis of abdominal injuries are discussed. Results concerning specific abdominal organ injuries are not considered, as they are discussed in detail in the previous chapters. The implication of imaging in decisions on management and the therapeutic potential of angiography is also discussed in the previous chapters.

21.2 History of Trauma

In many cases, no reliable history of trauma can be established at admission of the victim, either because the patient is unconscious or because he or she is confused after the shock and is not able to remember the exact circumstances of an accident or an assault. The mental status of a conscious trauma victim may also be altered by brain injury, drugs, or medication. Other victims may remain stoic and deny any complaints or injury. Finally, the patient may be comatose with no proof of identification and it is possible that no-one witnessed the accident.

However, to sense the severity of potential internal injuries, the mechanism of trauma should be established by the description given by the victim or other witnesses. The need to extract a victim, or ejection from a car, indicates severe trauma. A traffic accident in which one or several persons have died alerts one to potentially severe injuries in survivors. Car passengers restrained by the seatbelt sustain the same deceleration forces as the car; unrestrained victims experience additional forces, responsible for injuries from the inside of the car. Restrained passengers experience more abdominal hollow viscus injuries than those who are unrestrained, due to the sudden increase in intraluminal pressure. Inflated airbags may also be responsible for additional injuries. Stretching forces and shear forces are exerted on different fixed points within the abdomen, depending on the trauma mechanism, and consequently direction of impact exposes different organs to injury:

- Lateral impacts create more severe injuries than frontal ones.
- The orientation of a fracture line in the liver can be anticipated according to the impact.
- Crushing forces of the mid-abdomen are likely to fracture the left lobe of the liver, the pancreas, or the bile ducts that are bent over the lumbar spine.
- In the contrecoup mechanism, the organ injury lies on the opposite site from the impact.
- Organs that are located in the same area and are exposed to the same impact forces are often injured together. Thus, sets of lesions that are frequently associated can be defined: for instance, spleen, tail of pancreas, left kidney, left colon or liver, right adrenal, right kidney are classic associations.
- The pancreas, the bile ducts and the adrenals, particularly on the left, are rarely injured alone, due to their protected location; associated injuries have to be searched for systematically.
- Pelvic bone and lumbar spine fractures must also always lead to imaging of the abdomen and pelvis, as visceral injuries are frequently associated.
- The impact of a bicycle handlebar, a ski pole or a hockey stick produces localized "almost penetrating" injuries of abdominal organs without a wound; the organs directly underlying the impact site must be scrutinized with particular attention.

Finally, intensive resuscitation with vigorous cardiac massage at the site of accident may have created additional hepatic or splenic iatrogenic injury.

In practice, history taking after trauma most often gives only little information on the number and type of expected abdominal injuries. Careful history taking is more important in a nonacute setting, when acute clinical symptoms are delayed manifestations of an ignored or occult trauma. Contusion to some abdominal organs may remain occult for a long time. A history of an apparently minor trauma may be found in cases of delayed splenic rupture, while posttraumatic symptomatic pancreatic pseudocyst or some intraparenchymal vascular lesions may be incidentally discovered.

History taking should bring to light any previous surgery, organomegaly, congenital or acquired diseases, renal insufficiency, respiratory diseases, diabetes mellitus, catabolic drug therapy (steroids), coagulopathies, anticoagulant drug treatment, and bone fragility, which might be responsible for more severe injuries despite minor trauma. Preexisting lesions inside a contused organ may produce major clinical symptoms despite negligible trauma (see Chap. 13): for instance, Crohn's colitis may perforate after a minor blow to the abdomen, the liver may bleed after a moderate contusion to a large subcapsular hemangioma or a pedunculated adenoma, or to any other highly vascularized hepatic lesion. Simple acts such as vomiting, defecation, or coitus might rupture a weakened spleen or liver.

Child abuse is a special and delicate problem. Its frequency is generally underestimated in civilized countries, despite horrific numbers of cases being published in annual statistics. Isolated pancreatic injury in a child without a clear history of midabdominal trauma, for instance, should raise the suspicion of an intentional sharp blow. In the case of child abuse, adults report contradicting history, give an evasive description, or invent an injury mechanism that does not explain the pathophysiology of the injuries observed.

21.3 Clinical Abdominal Examination

In blunt abdominal trauma, clinical symptoms are generally present, but localized or specific complaints are rare. In adults, brain and facial injuries, thoracic cage fractures, pelvic or spine fractures, or limb injuries are usually more visible – to the victim, rescuers, and witnesses – than abdominal injuries. Thoracic injuries are usually more electively symptomatic and painful and distract the attention from less critical abdominal pain.

However, abdominal pain is a frequent complaint following blunt trauma, and was found in more than 90% of patients with an abdominal injury. Pain is either vague and diffuse over the entire abdomen, or more or less localized in a quadrant or flank. Abdominal pain is sensitive for the presence of abdominal injury, but not specific. Half of patients with abdominal pain have no significant abdominal injury (Ruf et al. 1985). Lack of specificity is caused by overlap of thoracic and upper abdominal symptoms or of symptoms caused by lumbar spine or pelvic fractures and associated visceral injuries. Injury to the posterior area of the liver or spleen, close to the diaphragm, can cause difficulty in breathing, singultus, or pain in the right or left shoulder that is not related to a scapular trauma; this is referred to as Kehr's sign (LOWENFELS 1966). In adults, associated rib fractures, rather than an underlying hepatic or splenic injury, are often responsible for pain felt in the right or left upper abdominal quadrant, but should alert one to an underlying visceral contusion. Blood extending to the paracolic gutters may induce flank pain and is often associated with liver or spleen laceration.

Apart from abdominal pain, externalized blood (vomiting or coughing blood, hematuria, urethral or rectal bleeding) yields valuable information on the site of injury, even when reported as a single episode after the trauma.

At inspection, the abdomen may be globally distended by hemoperitoneum. Local deformity may be seen, due to a subcutaneous or muscular wall hematoma or pelvic bone fracture. Ecchymoses on the abdominal wall give an indication on the site of maximum impact and to the possible location of an underlying abdominal injury. Ecchymoses from seatbelt injury raise the suspicion of gallbladder, duodenopancreatic, or intestinal rupture. The Cullen sign is the observation of periumbilical discoloration, secondary to blood in the peritoneal cavity. Inspection of a swollen scrotum indicates scrotal hematoma with possible testicular injury or, in some pediatric cases, the presence of hemoperitoneum through a persistent communication between the peritoneal cavity and scrotum.

Physical examination of the abdomen in a blunt trauma victim is often superficial and shortened, because it is considered to give poor results compared to cross section imaging, which can be rapidly obtained. However, palpation and auscultation of the abdomen is crucial and offers suggestive signs of injury, particularly to intraperitoneal viscera. A continuous increase in abdominal distension in a hypotensive patient indicates an increase in hemoperitoneum. The Ballance sign consists of dullness by percussion of the flank and indicates blood in the paracolic gutter. The absence of bowel sounds, generalized direct tenderness, rebound tenderness, muscular guarding, spasm or rigidity, or bruising, point to significant abdominal injury in penetrating and in blunt trauma. Peritoneal irritation, when observed at admission, should always raise the suspicion of gastrointestinal rupture (SHAFTAN 1969; CUSHING et al. 1997).

The retroperitoneal space is less accessible to palpation, but a massive retroperitoneal hematoma may also be palpable in the flank. Hematoma in the abdominal muscular wall can be seen and palpated, but limits deep abdominal palpation and may wrongly suggest intraabdominal hematoma. Palpation of a deep mass or hematoma carries an increased probability of intraabdominal visceral injury (ALLEN et al. 1998). Introducing a nasogastric tube may show return of blood, suggestive of either gastrointestinal injury, hemobilia or pancreatic hemorrhage externalized through the papilla. Bleeding from the urethra during catheter insertion suggests perineal and urethral injury. Blood at rectal digital examination indicates rectal or intestinal injury or posttraumatic intestinal ischemia. A displaced prostate can be palpated in pelvic injury or massive hemoperitoneum in the Douglas pouch.

Overall, clinical abdominal examination is sensitive in 45%–92% and specific in 45%–56% in abdominal contusion, and misleading in almost half of the patients (OLSEN and HILDRETH 1971; RODRIGUEZ et al. 1982; RUF et al. 1985; FABIAN et al. 1986; GRUESSNER et al. 1989; ROTHLIN et al. 1992; KLOTTER et al. 1992, 1993; SCHURINK et al. 1997). Clinical examination reveals association of multiple abdominal injuries in only 26% of the cases (LANG 1990) and is the least reliable for the detection of injury to retroperitoneal or deep abdominal organs such as the pancreas, bile ducts, bowel, mesentery, large vessels, etc. Patients with paraplegia or assisted ventilation generally have an equivocal abdominal examination.

It was claimed in the past that "no diagnostic test beats a good history and careful examination" in evaluating trauma patients, and that "radiologic studies should be done to confirm a clinical suspicion, not just for the sake of completeness" (KURTZMAN 1977). Today, clinical orientation may draw the attention to a pelvic abdominal quadrant or provide an incentive to look for a particular type of injury, but overall, no clinical examination can surpass the completeness of a well-conducted CT examination that covers brain, thorax, abdomen, spine, and pelvis in a polytrauma patient.

However, the hemodynamic condition of the patient and the gross clinical findings always take precedence in the sequence of management, including imaging, of the trauma patient. In critical patients, imaging will be limited or abbreviated, so that urgent surgery can be performed. Fundamental advise to radiologists is well formulated in Ben Menachem's laws:

- The number of imaging examinations in the emergency room should be inversely proportional to the number and severity of injuries present or suspected. Do not diagnose the patient to death!

- Obvious and superficial injuries are not necessarily the most life-threatening and should not distract the attention from a systematic search for a nonvisible bleeding source.

21.4 Laboratory Findings

Laboratory evaluation of the acute trauma victim at admission is limited to hemoglobin, hematocrit, white blood cell, type and cross-matching (Strauch 1973).

Hematocrit and hemoglobin do not immediately reflect the amount of posttraumatic blood loss and therefore are not reliable indicators of internal abdominal bleeding in the acute phase. Hemodilution and major body fluid shifts are also responsible for variations in hematocrit values. Furthermore, serial hematocrit evaluation is superseded by rapidly obtained imaging at admission, which gives direct assessment of the amount of hemoperitoneum or the volume of a collected hematoma. A falling hematocrit value may be secondary to other causes such as orthopedic intervention and does not necessarily mean visceral rebleeding.

Leukocytosis is neither a reliable indicator of specific abdominal injury nor related to severity of injury (Berman et al. 1958; Perry 1965). An elevated leukocyte count may be found in gastrointestinal rupture and also in abdominal intra- or retroperitoneal parenchymal injury and may be seen in the absence of abdominal injury.

Serum amylase was suggested as a specific indicator of pancreatic injury (Elman et al. 1929). The value of determining serum amylase has been discussed in the chapter on pancreatic injuries (see Chap. 7). Suffice it to mention the main reasons for lack of predictive value of serum amylase: false-negative results may be caused by blood sampling carried out too early, within the first 3 h of trauma, a limited penetrating pancreatic injury, or injury limited to the tail of the pancreas. False-positive elevation is seen with a great variety of injuries to other organs or other pathological conditions such as gastrointestinal rupture or arterial mesenteric occlusion. The increase in serum amylase on serial tests is the most valuable indicator of pancreatic injury and prompts intensive imaging (Cleveland et al. 1963; Adams et al. 1968; Bach and Frey 1971; White and Benfield 1972; Olsen 1973; Takishima et al. 1997). When properly used, the positive and negative predictive value of serum amylase for pancreatic or gastrointestinal injury was 1.5% and 3%, respectively, in a large study (Boulanger et al. 1993).

Significantly increased liver enzymes (serum glutamic-oxaloacetic transaminase, SGOT and serum glutamic-pyruvic transaminase, SGPT) are frequently observed together with hepatic injury, even in the absence of clinical complaints, but elevation may also occur in shock condition or in drug addicts (Oldham et al. 1984; Sahdev et al. 1991; Coant et al. 1992; Lam et al. 1999). Alkaline phosphatase is a less useful predictor of hepatic injury.

A rapid increase in serum bilirubin indicates posttraumatic bilhemia, secondary to an intrahepatic bile-venous fistula. Delayed raised bilirubin levels, by peritoneal resorption, is suggestive of intraperitoneal bile leakage, and a late increase in bilirubin is indicative of a posttraumatic biliary stricture.

Urinalysis evidences microscopic hematuria, which does not correlate well with severity of renal injury (Peterson 1978). Avulsion of a vascular renal pedicle can occur without hematuria.

21.5 Diagnostic Peritoneal Lavage

Diagnostic abdominal paracentesis was introduced at the beginning of the last century to evaluate abdominal trauma (Saloman 1906). The four-quadrant needle aspiration method was not found reliable and was abandoned in favor of diagnostic peritoneal lavage (DPL) (Brittain 1963; Canizaro et al. 1964; Root et al. 1965). DPL detected lesser quantities of intraperitoneal blood than aspiration, and a negative lavage constitutes a reliable indicator of absence of intraperitoneal bleeding. Lavage is positive, when gross, nonclotting blood returns or more than 100,000 red blood cells/mm^3 or more than 500 leukocysts/mm^3 are observed. Elevated amylase, presence of bile, leukocytes, or bacteria, food elements in the fluid, or draining of the lavage fluid from other thoracic or abdominal tubes are other positive signs of abdominal injury involving the peritoneal cavity, particularly the bile ducts or the gastrointestinal tract.

In the past, DPL was found to be more accurate than physical findings for deciding on early intervention. Indications were liberal: DPL was used in unconscious patients suffering from multiple trauma or in shock, patients for whom a history could not be taken, those with unreliable clinical findings, pelvic or spinal fractures, and in all trauma patients with an unreliable or equivocal abdominal examination. There are no absolute contraindications for DPL. Relative contraindications are preterm pregnancy, extensive postoperative abdominal scarring, and distended bowel loops.

Today, DPL has been largely superseded by CT in the assessment of hemoperitoneum (FEDERLE and JEFFREY 1983). Although it has high sensitivities and specificities of 95%–99%, it takes the same time or longer than a multislice CT examination, and results are technique-dependent (GILL et al. 1975; BROTMAN et al. 1981; PACHTER and HOFSTETTER 1981; SCHEELE and WAGNER 1981; SCHRIEFERS and GEROMETTA 1981; KLAUE 1983; GOMEZ et al. 1987; HANNA et al. 1987; HAWKINS et al. 1988; MEYER et al. 1989; REED et al. 1992; COLUCCIELLO 1993; CROCE et al. 1995; SINGH et al. 1997; NAGY et al. 2000).

Open DPL may have a sensitivity of 100%, but a specificity of 80% (NAGY et al. 2000). In some surgical series of blunt abdominal trauma patients treated with celiotomy, DPL was responsible for a negative celiotomy in up to 10.2% of cases, and laparotomy based on findings of DPL was shown to be nontherapeutic in a large number of cases (19%–39%) (GILL et al. 1975; COX 1984; HENNEMAN et al. 1990; DROST et al 1991; FRYER et al. 1991). Management of trauma victims with an indeterminate or weak positive DPL (20,000–100,000 red blood cell count/mm^3) was a source of controversy. In these patients, around 4%, repetition of DPL was advocated, but the majority of repeated DPL either produced an indeterminate result again or became negative, and laparotomy, carried out in this group, was therapeutic in a few cases only. When CT was obtained after DPL, it showed a high number of low-grade intraabdominal injuries that could be treated conservatively (DE MARIA 1991). In the past, before the era of CT, in order to reduce unnecessary or delayed surgery following indeterminate results of DPL, radionuclide imaging was advocated as the initial screening modality, followed by DPL depending on results obtained from imaging (DANZL and BERG 1977). In our experience, 1.5% of all adult blunt abdominal trauma victims had peritoneal effusion without any significant abdominal injury on CT at admission, and 4.3% of patients had no detectable intraperitoneal injury. In case of isolated hemoperitoneum or hemoperitoneum associated with trivial visceral injury or retroperitoneal injury, a positive DPL would lead to unnecessary laparotomy (COLUCIELLO 1993). In the literature, 11% of children with abdominal trauma were reported to have unexplained isolated peritoneal fluid (TAYLOR and SIVIT 1995). Rupture of the posterior parietal peritoneal leaflet may occur together with pelvic or retroperitoneal hematoma and result in a positive DPL, which leads to unnecessary or risky laparotomy (FREEMAN and FISCHER 1976; HUBBARD et al. 1979). On the other hand, in our experience, 20%–25% of adults who had significant injuries to the spleen or liver had no peritoneal effusion at all on CT. In other studies, 34% of adults and 37% of children with abdominal injuries or 11% of liver injuries and 12% of splenic injuries had no free fluid seen on CT and could be missed by DPL (TAYLOR and SIVIT 1995; SHANMUGANATHAN et al. 1999; OCHSNER et al. 2000). In a few patients, we have even observed pneumoperitoneum on CT, without peritoneal fluid. When US was used as a reference, 7% of abdominal injuries were without hemoperitoneum (LUCCIARINI et al. 1993; ROZYCKI et al. 1993; MCKENNEY et al. 1994). Anecdotally, an injured spleen, in an intrathoracic location through a diaphragmatic rupture was without intraperitoneal bleeding (BEN-MENACHEM et al. 1981). The improvement of patient rescue and transport by load and go means that many trauma patients are investigated less than 1 h after trauma, before significant hemoperitoneum is seen.

A leukocyte count of over 300/mm^3 from DPL indicates immediate laparotomy. The ratio between white and red cell count in the lavage fluid from DPL divided by the ratio of the same parameters in the circulating blood was shown to improve the early diagnosis of bowel perforation. A cell count ratio greater than 1 predicts hollow viscus perforation with a sensitivity and specificity of 100% and 97%, respectively, indicating laparotomy (FANG et al. 1998).

Finally, DPL is not totally innocuous and may provoke a limited number of complications. Reported complication rates varied from 0% to 3%. In a randomized study, a 5.7% rate of complications was noted with closed lavage and 0% with open lavage (PACHTER and HOFSTETTER 1981). Another large study noted no difference between open and closed DPL (NAGY et al. 2000). Complications are usually benign and include puncture of the gastrointestinal tract, urinary bladder, ovary, or a large vessel, mesenteric laceration, or erroneous extraperitoneal or subcutaneous infusion of lavage fluid.

DPL was compared with CT and US in the literature (FABIAN et al. 1986; MEYER et al. 1989; HOFFMANN et al. 1992; GOLETTI et al. 1994). Sensitivities of both diagnostic methods varied from 75% to 94%, but there were almost no false positives. US and CT showed similar results in comparison with DPL, which was found to be less operator-dependent than imaging and less expensive than CT. Today, it may be concluded that the debate about DPL versus CT is closed.

CT has largely superseded DPL in the evaluation of blunt abdominal trauma in the vast majority of trauma centers in Europe and in the United States. The sequence of DPL, followed by CT in patients with a positive DPL, which was suggested in the past, has also been abandoned (Baron et al. 1993). In patients with multiple injuries who are marginally stable, DPL can still be obtained if the CT examination is not readily available or requires patient transport to a location other than the resuscitation environment.

21.6 Laparotomy

Laparotomy was the gold standard for diagnosis of traumatic abdominal injuries before the advent of reliable cross section imaging. Now, diagnostic laparotomy in blunt abdominal trauma of low or moderate severity has lost most of its past importance (Feussner et al. 1999). Imaging is the primary investigation and should be carried out promptly and efficaciously by expert trauma radiologists. However, laparotomy should not be delayed by time-consuming studies in the unstable patient (Jones et al. 1983). A lifesaving crash or damage control laparotomy is indicated in patients in shock, who are brought to the emergency operating room immediately, without imaging. A necessary laparotomy should be carried out without delay to stop hemorrhage, but unnecessary laparotomy should be avoided. A negative exploratory laparotomy may be seen in up to 16% of trauma victims, depending on patient selection (Sayers et al. 1992). In the majority of patients who have sustained blunt abdominal contusion, their hemodynamic status allows cross section imaging first. As a consequence of the generally adopted conservative treatment in abdominal visceral injuries, laparotomy may become delayed in some patients who would urgently need it. General causes of delay are an obscured history of trauma, admission to an inadequate hospital or department, and particularly unreliable or misinterpreted diagnostic imaging. However, a small percentage of abdominal injuries may also be missed at laparotomy. Delay time of diagnosis of an injury missed at laparotomy may vary from hours to months. Causes of missing an injury intraoperatively include inexperience of the surgeon, a hostile abdomen, insufficient organ mobilization, or insufficient retroperitoneal exploration. Injuries missed during surgery carry significantly higher complication and mortality rates than diagnosed injuries: 83% and 17% versus 39% and 6%, respectively (Sung and Kim 1996).

Retroperitoneal hemorrhage should not be primarily explored by a laparotomy, but should be investigated angiographically, combined with hemostatic embolization for active bleeding. Pelvic hemorrhage associated with pelvic bone fractures is primarily treated by external fixation and if necessary by arterial embolization. Surgical dissection of a retroperitoneal or pelvic hematoma might create catastrophic bleeding before the surgeon is able to localize the bleeding source and stop the hemorrhage.

21.7 Laparoscopy

Laparoscopy or coelioscopy is not a completely safe investigation of abdominal trauma (Leppaniemi and Elliot 1996; Memon and Fitzgibbons 1997). Although it might indicate open surgery with confidence, precious time may be lost and several abdominal compartments or organs are not adequately visualized (Townsend et al. 1993; Elliott et al. 1998). Significant injuries to the liver, pancreas, gastrointestinal tract (small intestine), and urinary bladder can be missed in up to 16% or 19% of victims with blunt or penetrating trauma (Klotter et al. 1993; Rossi et al. 1993; Elliott et al. 1998). Even active hemorrhage may be overlooked (Livingston et al. 1992). However, in pediatric abdominal trauma, laparoscopy or minimal access surgery was advocated as a valuable method of investigation (Chen et al. 1995). It is reasonable to include laparoscopy in a protocol, if nonsurgical management of penetrating trauma is elected and CT is questionable for peritoneal penetration (Ginzburg et al 1998).

21.8 Imaging

Abdominal cross section imaging is now the standard initial evaluation of the majority blunt trauma victims. It should provide complete information on all injuries present at admission. A rapid, complete and reliable diagnostic work-up contributes to orientate correct treatment, to prevent complications and sequelae and to avoid unnecessary procedures and reduce hospitalization time. A significant shift in imaging techniques has occurred in the past 20 years. Angiography has been abandoned as a diagnostic modality, the use of nuclear imaging is limited to a few specific situations, and CT has superseded US in most centers (Kurtzman 1977).

21.8.1 Abdominal Radiographs

Plain films of the abdomen covering the abdomen from diaphragm to perineum were crucial in the investigation of trauma patients before the advent of cross section imaging. Anterior-posterior supine, erect, and left lateral decubitus films with horizontal X-ray beam were necessary for a complete evaluation and particularly to assess pneumoperitoneum (Freeark 1982). Plain films of the abdomen may be obtained quickly on a radiographic table with digital films, which can be immediately reviewed on the screen. Signs suggesting abdominal injury are listed in Table 21.1.

Abdominal radiographs were claimed to be accurate in the assessment of abdominal injury in 11% and suggestive of injury in 34%–40% of cases (Cantor 1970; Williams and Zollinger 1959). Normal abdominal films do not rule out significant abdominal and pelvic injury and positive findings for abdominal fluid are not specific to recognize location, severity, and extent of injury. Free intraperitoneal air may warrant immediate surgery, but extraperitoneal or subcutaneous emphysema may be confusing and perforation of the digestive tract can be missed in a high number of cases (Sperling and Rigler 1937; Jacobson and Carter 1951; Elkin and Cohen 1962; Gould and Thorworth 1963; Berk 1970; Ting and Renter 1973; Love 1975; Mindelzun and McCort 1984; Espinoza and Rodriguez 1997; Frick et al. 1999; Neugebauer et al. 1999). False positive plain films of the abdomen may lead to unnecessary laparotomy in about 20% of cases; false negative films are responsible for a delayed laparotomy with a possible lethal outcome in 17% of cases (Kern and Klaue 1975; Bivins et al. 1978).

At present, and in the light of CT, the merit of plain abdominal films is low in blunt trauma. Even foreign bodies (e.g., bullets) that are easily recognized are more precisely localized and their trajectory or penetration to the depth of a knife wound are better assessed with CT.

Table 21.1. Suggestive signs of abdominal trauma on plain films

Slight lumbar spine scoliosis in a young patient
Right or left lower rib fractures
Lumbar spine or transverse process fractures
Pelvic bone fractures
Free intraperitoneal air
Retroperitoneal or exoperitoneal loculated air
Intraportal air (intrahepatic)
Air in bile ducts or gallbladder
Displaced air (stomach, colon, rectum)
Abnormal course of nasogastric tube
Dilated stomach
Increase in serration of the greater curvature of the stomac
Air in the duodenal loop
Duodenal fold widening or coiled spring or stack of coins sign
Paralytic ileus
Spasm of bowel segment
Irregular distensibility of a bowel segment
Localized intramural bowel mass
Thumbprinting in bowel wall
Diffuse thickening of bowel wall
Colon cut-off sign
Airless abdomen
Abdominal "ground glass" appearance
Medial positioning of small bowel loops
Perivesical spaces "dog ear sign"
Obscured paracolic gutters
Loss of definition of hepatic and splenic colon flexure
Enlarged organ (lower pole of spleen or right lobe of liver)
Soft tissue mass, displacing or not digestive air
Displaced organ contour (kidney)
Blurred psoas muscle limit or no psoas shadow
Asymmetrical loss of normal concavity or bulging of soft tissue of the flank
High position of a hemidiaphragm or signs of visceral trans-diaphragmatic hernia (particularly on the left side)

Although plain films give poor results in abdominal visceral injury, it is worthwhile to consider the likelihood of visceral abdominal injuries that might be associated with bone fractures, which are seen on plain films:

- Of adult patients with hepatic or splenic injury, 30%–50% have associated right or left lower rib fractures (McCort 1964, 1973).
- There is a high association between lumbar spine, pelvic fracture, and renal injury.
- Pelvic fractures are frequently associated with bladder and urethral injury.
- A Chance fracture of the lumbar spine is likely to be associated with bowel perforation.

21.8.2 Radiographic Contrast Studies

Selective radiographic contrast studies are only rarely obtained as a primary investigation at admission.

21.8.2.1 Intravenous Urography

Intravenous urography or pyelography (IVP) is not sensitive for renal parenchymal injuries that do not involve the pyelocaliceal system, but a normal IVP has a reliable negative predictive value for significant renal injury. IVP is specific for massive urine extravasation, but misses minor or moderate leaks, does not accurately assess the severity of renal trauma, and gives no information on associated injuries (Federle et al. 1981; Federle 1983). IVP is no longer obtained as a primary investigation in abdominal or retroperitoneal trauma. Radiographic films may be taken after contrast-enhanced CT in renal injuries with major laceration of the excretory system.

21.8.2.2 Retrograde Urethrocystography

Retrograde urethrography is necessary to demonstrate urethral rupture precisely. Retrograde urethrocystography is more accurate in evidencing urinary bladder rupture than CT with delayed imaging after opacification of the bladder. However, CT cystography obtained with retrograde contrast injection is better able to show limited extravasation of contrast than conventional CT or conventional retrograde cystography. CT cystography should be routine when pelvic visceral injury, gross hematuria, and pelvic fractures are suspected (Peng et al. 1999; Fishman and Horton 2000).

21.8.2.3 Digestive Tract Contrast Radiography

Contrast opacifications of the gastrointestinal tract are rarely obtained in the acute trauma victim. Oral administration of hydrosoluble iodinated contrast material carries the risk of vomiting and aspiration pneumonia and is therefore not used in routine CT in acute trauma cases at admission. Upper gastrointestinal tract contrast opacification can demonstrate esophageal, gastric, or duodenal rupture, but gives no information on associated injuries. Colon enema is unrealistic in a polytrauma patient. Overall, intestinal or colon contusion, mural hematoma, or mesenteric hemorrhage are not assessed with sufficient confidence by contrast opacification (Glazer et al. 1981; Karnaze et al. 1981).

21.8.2.4 Endoscopic Retrograde Cholangiopancreatography

Endoscopic retrograde cholangiopancreatography is indicated in a selected group of patients when biliary or pancreatic duct laceration is suspected and no urgent intervention is required. Accuracy of evidencing ductal rupture is almost 100% and the technique is often effective for treatment of biliary or pancreatic duct fistulas, by catheter drainage or temporary stenting (Deviere 1987; Sugimoto et al. 1993; Harrell et al. 1998; Griffen et al. 2000).

21.8.2.5 Sinograms

Sinograms or fistulographs obtained by injection of contrast medium into the tract of a stab wound were advocated in the past to evaluate peritoneal penetration, but a high false-negative rate and limited information compared to CT has contributed to the abandonment of this type of examination (Aragon and Eiseman 1976; Demetriades and Rabinowitz 1987). Triple contrast helical CT was recently shown in a prospective study to accurately predict peritoneal violation and the need of laparotomy in these patients (Shanmuganathan et al. 2001).

Sinograms can be obtained in the late posttraumatic phase, when a cutaneous fistula has occurred and communicates with the bile or pancreatic ducts, the urinary excretory system, or the gastrointestinal tract. Many external fistulas can be treated by a controlled percutaneous catheter diversion.

21.8.3 Ultrasound

Ultrasonography (US) has been in clinical use for the evaluation of abdominal trauma since the 1970s (Kristensen et al. 1971). US is mobile, rapid, and cheap and can be immediately obtained at admission, irrespective of the hemodynamic condition of the patient, without interruption of resuscitation maneuvers such as tracheal intubation, placement of IV lines etc. (Schlager et al. 1994; Goletti et al. 1994). In contrast to CT, it does not require sedation in children and could therefore replace CT with equivalent results in 76% of pediatric patients (Katz et al. 1996).

US is credited with a sensitivity of 78%–99% and a specificity of 93%–99% in the detection of intraperitoneal fluid (GRUESSNER et al. 1989; KIMURA and OTSUKA 1991; HOFFMANN et al. 1992; LIU et al. 1993; ROTHLIN et al. 1993; ROZYCKI et al. 1993; GLASER et al. 1994; GOLETTI et al. 1994; MCKENNEY M et al. 1994, MCKENNEY KL et al. 1998; BOULANGER et al. 1996). When searching for free intraperitoneal blood, all supra- and inframesocolic compartments have to be screened. In our experience, we have found no predilection at admission for blood to accumulate in a particular peritoneal compartment. On delayed control examinations, blood preferentially sedimentates in the perivesical spaces. Others have found no correlation between fluid location and site of injury (MCKENNEY 1999).

General radiologists, trauma-dedicated radiologists, and intensive care physicians and surgeons claim similar results in abdominal evaluation of trauma patients with US. Focused assessment with sonography for trauma (FAST) or a standardized six-point trauma US examination was introduced as a surgical means for rapid evaluation of the abdomen in the shock room. The examination is limited to detection of intraperitoneal fluid and major parenchymal injuries (CHIU et al. 1997; ROZYCKI et al. 1998a,b; SCALEA et al. 1999; NUNES et al. 2001). Surgeons claim, that the method is easy to learn for this purpose, as no sophisticated findings are searched for, particularly in the hemodynamically unstable patient (FÖRSTER et al. 1993; TSO et al. 1992; MCKENNEY MG et al. 1996, 1998, SMITH et al. 1998). In fact, US has the potential to show the presence of intraperitoneal fluid in less than 1 min of scanning. Subxiphoid scanning of the base of the pericardiac sac also rapidly confirms tamponade of the heart by a pericardiac effusion. This preliminary information is sufficient to decide on the site of immediate intervention in patients in shock (LENTZ et al. 1996; WHERETT et al. 1996). However, in hemodynamically stable children, FAST was shown in a comparison with CT to be an unreliable screening test of abdominal injury: sensitivity was only 30% and specificity 100% (MUTABAGANI et al. 1999). During a quick abdominal survey with US, a significant false-negative rate of 20%–30% might be expected in the surgical or emergency medicine literature, (JEHLE et al. 1993; MA et al. 1995; ROZYCKI et al. 1995; BOULANGER et al. 1995, 1996; LENTZ et al. 1996; WHERETT et al. 1996; THOMAS et al. 1997). Surgeons and radiologists using FAST reported up to 17%–29% of abdominal injuries without hemoperitoneum (CHIU et al. 1997; SHANMUGANATHAN et al. 1999). Indeed, immediately after trauma, fresh clotted blood in the peritoneal cavity or subcapsular or intraparenchymal hematoma show a high echogenicity, similar to that of a plain parenchyma, making the diagnosis of collected blood versus a solid parenchyma difficult (WICKS et al. 1978; SIGEL et al. 1981, 1982; COELMO et al. 1982; VAN SONNENBERG et al. 1983; HASHIMOTO et al. 1984). Echogenicity of collected blood then decreases progressively with time and appears anechoic and easy to see after 4–5 days, due to hemolysis. One of the most frequent causes of false-positive US is nontrauma-related free intraperitoneal fluid, particularly physiological free pelvic fluid in women of reproductive age (BROWN et al. 2001).

There is a general agreement that organ specific injuries are more difficult to detect than intraperitoneal fluid with US. Results depend on many factors, such as organ size, organ location, penetrating wound dressing and pain. Meteorism, ileus, subcutaneous emphysema or massive pneumoperitoneum are specific limitation to abdominal US (AMICI et al. 1982; AUFSCHNAITER and KOFLER 1983; ROTHLIN et al. 1992). Sensitivity for individual abdominal organ injuries is lower than that for detection of hemoperitoneum and varies from 36% to 100%, and specificity varies from 88% to 100% in mostly retrospective studies. The variable individual organ-injury sensitivities have been discussed in the literature. Liver, spleen, and kidney injuries are detected with 92.4%, 90.0%, and 92.2% sensitivity rates, respectively. In splenic and in hepatic injuries, the frequently associated lower rib fractures limit the applicability of the ultrasound probe for a complete examination, due to pain. Relying on splenomegaly, as suggested in initial reports, is not specific for splenic injury. Differentiation of fresh subcapsular and perisplenic blood may be difficult; clefts and lacerations may pose problems (ASHER et al. 1976). Similar limitations apply to hepatic injury, where US may be sufficient to assess benign injury accurately, located at the periphery (HANEY et al 1982; KULIGOSWKA et al. 1984). Duodenopancreatic injuries are picked up with a sensitivity of 71.4% and gastrointestinal trauma with 34.7% only (YOSHII et al. 1998). Small pneumoperitoneum, devascularized intestine, or localized mural gastrointestinal thickening easily escape US (FOLEY and TEELE 1979; O'MALLEY and SALEM 1979; FON et al. 1980). In a prospective study, significant differences in results were obtained versus experience of the operator: sensitivity and specificity of 45% and 99%, respectively, by the experienced surgeon and 30% and 100%, respectively, by the beginner (ROTHLIN et al. 1992).

In the combined evaluation of hemoperitoneum and visceral injuries by US, overall sensitivities, specificities, and accuracy of 84%–95%, 88%–95%, and 86%–95%, respectively, were found (Hauenstein et al. 1982; Kuhn et al. 1983; Gruessner et al. 1989; Tso et al. 1992; Rothlin et al. 1992, 1993; Bode et al. 1993; Boulanger et al. 1993; McElveen and Collin 1997; Akgur et al. 1997; Singh et al. 1997; Bain et al. 1998; McKenney KL et al. 1998; Smith et al. 1998; Abu-Zidan et al. 1999; Shih et al. 1999).

Other valuable information, besides hemoperitoneum and parenchymal contusion, cannot be obtained accurately with US: active bleeding, degree of perfusion of abdominal organs, free retroperitoneal air, specific demonstration of extravasation of urine, etc.

Finally, the hemodynamic status of the patient influences results: in hypotensive patients, the sensitivity of US increased from 76% to 100% compared with normotensive patients for indication of laparotomy (Rozycki et al. 1998a,b; Brown et al. 2001).

21.8.4 Computed Tomography

Computed tomography (CT) was rapidly recognized as a valuable tool in the evaluation of trauma patients. Unlike US, agitated adults and children under the age of 6 require adequate sedation for CT (Druy and Rubin 1979; Mall and Kaiser 1980; Berger and Kuhn 1981; Mahboubi 1985).

In the literature, CT examination technique varied between Europe and the United States, due to different patient selection criteria and differences in radiological culture. In many centers in the US, exclusively hemodynamically stable patients were investigated, but more recently, marginally stable patients have also been included, as is the case in Europe (Raptopoulos 1994). CT equipment is now installed in the emergency environment, allowing for CT evaluation, including marginally stable patients without time loss and without patient transport (Hauser and Bohndorf 1999). Resuscitation is continued during CT examination, while imaging is completed. In marginally stable patients, there is no time to administer oral contrast. Furthermore, oral contrast, when extravasated through a gastrointestinal perforation, may be impossible to distinguish from extravasated vascular contrast medium, indicating active hemorrhage. Only in stable patients is there time enough for oral administration of dilute (2%–5%) water soluble contrast material, either given through a nasogastric tube or orally for 20–40 min before the CT examination (Shuman 1997). However, neither oral nor rectal contrast is essential for the diagnosis of abdominal injury. Upper GI opacification may increase the sensitivity for injuries of the pancreas, duodenum, and intestine, but without a proven effect on management. On the other hand, examination time is lengthened and increases the risk of vomiting and aspiration (Kinnunen et al. 1994; Tsang et al. 1997).

The use of standardized examination protocols, as described in Chap. 3, is indispensable for helical single and multislice scanning. A completely negative CT in a patient with blunt injury is of great value, as it allows discharge of the patient after a short observation period of several hours, without formal hospitalization. CT in that respect is much more reliable than US, due to its simultaneous applicability to brain, lung, viscera, and bone (Fried et al. 1992; Brasel et al. 1996). A second opinion can be obtained by electronic transmission of the entire CT image set to an expert on call. Teleradiology is more problematic with other imaging tests (Feussner and Siewert 1996).

Early reports on the first 200 to 500 investigated patients had shown that there were only a few false positive or false negative interpretations of abdominal CT in trauma (Federle et al. 1982; Federle 1983). The great value of CT was established thereafter by numerous publications in the radiological and surgical literature (Marincek 1993; Clancy et al. 1993; Mirvis and Shanmuganathan 1994; Raptopoulos 1994; Sherck et al. 1994; Udekwu et al. 1996; Breen et al. 1997; Williams et al. 1997; Federle et al. 1998). Most published papers credit CT with overall sensitivities, constantly higher than 90%, and specificities which are close to 100% in the diagnosis of abdominal injuries in adults and in the pediatric age group (Roche et al. 1992). The advantage of CT is that it is less operator-dependent than US and overall less organ-specific, except for tubular structures (bile ducts, pancreatic ducts, ureter). However, several papers report differentiated results of CT in trauma. In a retrospective study on 256 victims who were explored with abdominal CT, sensitivity, specificity, and accuracy were 92.4%, 99.5%, and 97.6%, respectively; 24.2% of examinations were positive for visceral injury in this study. Injury-specific and sensitivities were lowest in the pancreas (0%), intestinal tract (41.6%) and urinary bladder (50%), accounting for a global 1.9% rate of false-negative diagnoses. No death or major complication was attributable to a delay in diagnosis caused by a false-negative CT (Udekwu et al. 1996). Sensitivities of 85%, 84%, and 67% were reported in another paper, for renal, hepatic and splenic injury, respectively (Lang 1990). In another paper, false positive findings were noticed in about one-third of the patients and 7% were false negative results (MATSUBARA et al. 1990). Overall, false-positive diagnoses obtained with CT are rare and mainly caused by perception errors by the observer. False-negative diagnoses, however, are caused by the nature of injury and the inability of CT to investigate some types of abdominal injuries correctly. Classic potential false-negative CT results are listed in Table 21.2.

CT identifies hemoperitoneum with similar or greater ease than US and distinguishes hemoperitoneum from retroperitoneal hematoma. Pneumoperitoneum, subcutaneous emphysema, wound dressing, and paralytic ileus do not limit a CT examination. CT has definitely replaced diagnostic peritoneal lavage (DPL) and is quicker. If DPL is still practiced, CT should be obtained before, as residual peritoneal fluid may be mistaken for hemoperitoneum (FEDERLE et al. 1982).

In a small prospective and randomized study, CT was shown to be more cost-effective than US and DPL (NAVARRETE-NAVARRO et al. 1996).

Measurement of densities does not separate peritoneal blood from ascites, urine, bile, bowel content, a ruptured cyst, or a mixture of these fluids. The blood density depends on hematocrit, physical state of blood, previous injection of contrast medium, free extravasation of contrast, and window width (ROBERTS et al. 1993).

The observation of an isolated hemoperitoneum, without associated visceral injury seen on CT, raises the question of whether laparotomy is indicated or not. In our experience, a CT negative for visceral injury and a nonsuspicious clinical examination allow for conservative, expectant observation (see Chap. 20). Other reports claim that laparotomy is indicated, as gastrointestinal injury needing repair is frequently present, despite a negative CT (CUNNINGHAM et al. 1998).

As CT is able to detect minimal density gradients, it was expected to diagnose small amounts of extravasated contrast medium and give superior results to angiography in abdominal hemorrhage (JEFFREY et al. 1991). There is no prospective comparative study of CT and angiography in the detection of active abdominal posttraumatic bleeding. In our personal experience, more than 90% of angiographies were indicated by a positive CT for contrast extravasation and 90% of angiographies were therapeutic by hemostatic embolization. The observation of active extravasation is a determining factor for proper patient management. In the spleen, for instance, it has a high predictive value for surgery or embolization, even in minor- or moderate-grade splenic injury (GAVANT et al. 1997; FEDERLE et al. 1998). Significant differences in CT attenuation values were found between active bleeding (25–370 HU, mean 132) and clotted blood (40–70 HU, mean 51) ($P<0.001$) (SHANMUGANATHAN et al. 1993). Progressive dilution of contrast medium in peritoneal fluid from the site of parenchymal capsular tear is an unequivocal sign of active hemorrhage and correctly localizes the site of bleeding. When hepatic and splenic trauma coexist, higher densities of clot are seen around the organ with most significant hemorrhage. However, neither the amount of hemoperitoneum, nor the volume of a hematoma close to a solid viscus sentinel clot sign are predictive of active hemorrhage, but the likelihood of laparotomy increases with the amount of hemoperitoneum observed on CT in our experience and in other studies (CROCE et al. 1995; PACHTER et al. 1996).

Table 21.2. Common false-negative diagnoses of CT in blunt abdominal trauma

Pancreatic duct rupture
Ureteral contusion
Urinary bladder (without CT cystography) or urethral rupture
Bile duct rupture
Mesenteric tear
Diaphragmatic rupture
Intestinal contusion or rupture without pneumoperitoneum
Small vascular injury (pseudoaneurysm) without contrast extravasation
Any low-grade parenchymal injury
Testicular injury

As trauma is a dynamic process, it has been argued that repetition of CT at regular time intervals is mandatory to evidence injuries that might have escaped the initial CT at admission or to disclose changes that might indicate rebleeding (increase in hematoma, high-density values appearing in a hematoma, pseudoaneurysm). Detection of pancreatic injury, perforation of the extrahepatic bile ducts, gallbladder, urinary bladder, or diaphragmatic rupture may benefit from a repeated CT. Traumatic injuries to the liver, spleen, kidney, and adrenal are usually all picked up at the initial CT. However, delayed bleeding may benefit from repeated CT, particularly in the spleen, known for its propensity to rebleed late (BUNTAIN et al. 1988; JEFFREY 1989). The question of missed concomitant gastrointestinal tract rupture is constantly raised as an argument against conservative treatment of hepatic or splenic contusion (FISCHER et al. 1988). In our experience, it is unlikely that significant gastrointestinal injury goes unnoticed, and in no patient with isolated hemoperitoneum did we notice a missed gastrointestinal injury that required surgical repair (see Chap. 20). However, small perforations of the gastrointestinal tract, the rectum for instance, may become visible only on repeated CT examinations, showing a fluid collection adjacent to the tear, which increases in size.

CT has largely replaced diagnostic peritoneal lavage, US, scintigraphy, and angiography. The main effects of CT on management of trauma lie in the decreased incidence of exploratory laparotomy, a more reliable and more systematic follow-up during hospitalization and follow-up, probably a shorter stay in the intensive care unit, with close observation and more targeted treatment (FEDERLE 1981).

21.8.5 Angiography

Angiography was introduced as a diagnostic modality of visceral injury in 1957 and was used in the 1960s and 1970s in the evaluation of abdominal trauma (NORELL 1957). Angiographic signs of visceral injury are not specific (Table 21.3) (VOGLER and BERGMANN 1963; BAUM et al. 1965; BOYSEN et al. 1966; LOVE et al. 1968; FREEARK et al. 1968; WENZ 1972; HAERTEL 1975).

Arteriography is no longer used as a primary tool in demonstrating abdominal injury. In the past, renal injury was best demonstrated by arteriography (LANG 1971, 1975, 1976). In splenic injury, arteriography was found to correlate poorly with the pathological findings and to be a poor predictor on management decision (FISHER et al. 1981). Only half of the splenic injuries seen on pathological examination were detected on splenic arteriography and a negative splenic angiogram was not reliable in 24% of the patients (FISHER et al. 1981). A high incidence of false positives was also noted, due to splenic lobulations, clefts, accessory spleen, or other anatomical or arterial variants or splenic infarcts (GOLD and REDMAN 1972). In hepatic injuries, arteriography gives similar results to those obtained with the spleen. Arterioportal flow may be seen in the contused liver in the absence of an arterioportal fistula (L'HERMINE et al. 1977). Hepatic vein injury is only rarely demonstrated angiographically (SCLAFANI et al. 1983). Posttraumatic vascular injuries in the gastrointestinal tract have been occasionally demonstrated. Arterial thrombosis, stretching, venous thrombus by compression of a hematoma were more frequently seen than active bleeding from a mesenteric or gastric artery. In the pancreas, severe life-threatening hemorrhage may occur after blunt or penetrating pancreatic injury. Pseudoaneurysm may develop later during the course of posttraumatic pancreatitis and is sometimes incorporated into the wall of a pseudocyst. Arteriography localizes the vascular injury precisely on an intra- or peripancreatic artery as in other parenchymas and allows for subsequent embolization (MARTY 1975). After abdominal surgery, systematic arteriography was used in determining the extent and prognosis of posttraumatic injuries, but has a limited role in asymptomatic patients (SCHORN and COLN 1977). However, the demonstration of a persistent pseudoaneurysm or arteriovenous fistula prompts endovascular occlusion, despite the patient being asymptomatic, to avoid later complications.

Table 21.3. Angiographic signs of abdominal injury

Arterial cut-off
Mural irregularities or flap
Laceration
Thrombosis
Dissection
Free-flow contrast extravasation
Stagnant intraparenchymal accumulation of contrast
Parenchymal blush
Stagnant arterial or venous flow
Diffuse vasoconstriction
Pseudoaneurysm
Arteriovenous fistula
Vessel displacement
Intraparenchymal avascular zones
Disruption of visceral contour
Displaced organ

Angiography, as a diagnostic modality of abdominal injury, has restrictions similar to radionuclide studies: it is time-consuming, not readily available in all hospitals admitting trauma patients and gives selective information depending on catheterization. Angiographic findings, except contrast-medium extravasation, are generally not specific for injury. The high diagnostic sensitivity with which angiography was credited was certainly overestimated when compared with the subtle injuries that can be shown by CT.

In our experience, most arteriographies in trauma patients are therapeutic. Active hemorrhage is seen as contrast extravasation and angiography visualizes the bleeding artery precisely, allowing in many cases for tissue-sparing hemostatic embolization in intraparenchymal arteries (SCLAFANI et al. 1995; HAGIWARA et al. 1996). Extravasation of contrast is most often seen as a localized blush within a parenchyma or around a vascular tear, with formation of a contained pseudoaneurysm or arteriovenous fistula either immediately or later. Overall, arteriography confirms arterial bleeding in 87% of cases, but results are affected by false negatives, caused by intermittent vasospasm, a decrease in blood pressure, spontaneous thrombus formation, venous bleeding, or inability to catheterize, and a few false positives such as normal adrenal parenchymal blush or collapsed intestine or vessels are seen end-on and simulate extravasation. Before the advent of CT as a systematic approach to trauma victims, abdominal arteriography was indicated in the marginally stable patient, who would probably require surgery and in whom a primary vascular lesion of the retroperitoneal space or pelvis was suspected (Class II). Patients in class I, who were unstable and in critical condition, were directed to surgery; patients who were stable were classified as class III and underwent CT (Ben Menachem 1981).

Today, patients in classes II and III undergo CT, when logistics allow doing so and arteriography is indicated, on the basis on the results of CT. In liver injuries, arteriography is indicated for selective catheter-directed embolization of pseudoaneurysm, arteriovenous fistula, or other complex arterioportal, arteriovenous hepatic or biliary fistula that are suspect on cross section imaging, provided they are sufficiently large.

21.8.6 Nuclear Medicine Studies

Nuclear medicine studies are not frequently used in Europe in the assessment of acute abdominal trauma, even though they are noninvasive, safe, and easy to perform. The main reasons for low acceptance are that nuclear medicine is not an integrated part of the Department of Medical Imaging, in many European countries the equipment is not available in the emergency environment, and nuclear medicine physicians are not available around the clock. The examination is time-consuming, the investigation is organ-specific and limited by at least 10% of equivocal or low-confidence results.

Contusion, laceration, and hematoma of the liver or spleen show as an intraparenchymal defect or a less defined zone of absent uptake or contour deformity. Multiple views are necessary when spleen and liver overlap, which might reduce errors in interpretation. Combined liver–lung or spleen–lung scans using technetium 99mm sulfur colloid were used in the past to investigate the dome of the liver, right diaphragm, and the base of the thorax (Delany and Jason 1981). Dynamic renal scans were used to elucidate injuries to the vascular pedicle or collecting system (Berger 1974). Uptake defects may be anatomical variants of a solid organ, a perfusion abnormality, or other preexisting anomalies that are not related to trauma; hemoperitoneum, pneumoperitoneum, and low-grade visceral injuries are not depicted (Little et al. 1967; Evans et al. 1972; Diamond et al. 1973; Gilday and Alderson 1974; Lutzker et al. 1974; Nebesar et al. 1974).

The Tc-99m-acetanilide iminodiacetic acid (Tc-99m-IDA) radiopharmaceuticals are useful to demonstrate biliary fistulae and intra- or extrahepatic accumulation of bile (Wiener and Vyas 1974; Henderson et al. 1978; Kuni et al. 1980; Christensen et al. 1981; Caride and Gibson 1982; Sty et al. 1982; Weissmann et al. 1982, 1983; Makhija and Schultz 1983; Gelfand 1984). The significance of visualization or nonvisualization of the gallbladder in trauma patients is the most reliable (Coletti et al. 1983).

Isotope angiography was suggested evidencing significant vascular injury by rapid, early sequential scanning. Tc-99m-human serum albumin or Tc-99m-labeled erythrocytes are positive by showing accumulation at the site of bleeding or in a pseudoaneurysm (Ruskin and Saenger 1963; Miskowiak et al. 1979). Lack of spatial resolution, vascular anatomy, and the necessity of repeating angiography for hemostatic embolization have limited the clinical application of the technique (Rosenthal 1974).

Studies in the past have claimed a 98% sensitivity in splenic and hepatic injury with a false-positive rate of 7%–10% (Federle 1983). In one study of 1833 cases, 106 true positive and 1727 true negative liver scans were reported, with no false-positive or false-negative results. Danzel and Berg found 207 splenic scans were positive for injury, 1621 were true negative, and 5 false positive were observed (Danzl and Berg 1977). Several studies established a comparison between scintigraphy and CT or scintigraphy and US (Froelich et al. 1982; Uthoff et al. 1983). Both methods showed erroneous results either with a similar rate or slightly higher rate with nuclear medicine. US had a detection rate of splenic injury that was inferior to that of scintigraphy.

21.8.7 Magnetic Resonance Imaging

The role of MRI in trauma is not defined. Experimental comparative studies have shown that 3D MRI in an animal model has a sensitivity and specificity of 100% versus 90% and 94% for CT in showing hepatic and renal injury and hemoperitoneum (Weishaupt et al. 2000). Serial postcontrast imaging with MRI is able to demonstrate active urine extravasation in acute renal trauma by increased signal intensity in communication with the collecting system, like CT (Marcos et al. 1998). Actually, acute trauma victims are not systematically evaluated with MRI for obvious logistical reasons and the length of the examination. MRI cannot compete with multislice CT (MSCT) in trauma imaging. In the nonacute setting, features such as magnetic resonance angiography (MRA) and magnetic resonance cholangiopancreatography (MRCP) can give valuable information on bile and pancreatic duct anatomy. Rapid multiplanar imaging is also offered now by multislice CT, which makes diagnoses such as diaphragmatic rupture and transphrenic herniation equally effective with both techniques (Mirvis et al. 1988; Daum-Kowalski et al. 1991; Boulanger et al. 1992; Dosios et al. 1993; Wataya et al. 1997; Shirasawa et al. 2001). A clinical comparative study between MRI and CT in the subacute posttraumatic phase (3-day interval between both examinations) concluded that MRI offered no significant advantage over CT for routine evaluation of acute abdominal trauma (McGehee et al. 1993).

21.9 Conclusion

Knowledge of the circumstances of trauma, the mechanism of injuries, and the fate of other involved victims helps to sense the severity of trauma. Clinical examination of the trauma victim is essential to decide on urgent management, despite powerful diagnostic imaging that is readily available in the emergency environment. CT has evolved as the optimal screening modality of polytrauma victims; US has a role in the shock room in unstable patients. Angiography is not used as a diagnostic modality, but exclusively for primary or secondary hemostasis.

Other imaging tests are used for solving specific problems in patients after initial trauma management.

References

Abu-Zidan FM, Sheikh M, Jadallah F, Windsor JA (1999) Blunt abdominal trauma: comparison of ultrasonography and computed tomography in a district general hospital. Australas Radiol 43:440–443

Adams JT, Libertino JA, Schwartz SI (1968) Significance of an elevated serum amylase. Surgery 63:877–884

Akgur FM, Aktug T, Olguner M, KovanlikaYA A, Hakguder G (1997) Prospective study investigating routine usage of ultrasonography as the initial diagnostic modality for the evaluation of children sustaining blunt abdominal trauma. J Trauma 42:626–628

Allen GS, Moore FA, Cox CS Jr, Wilson JT, Cohn JM, Duke JH (1998) Hollow visceral injury and blunt trauma. J Trauma 45:69–75

Amici F, Busilacchi P, De Nigris E et al (1982) Closed abdominal injuries: the diagnostic reliability of ultrasound. Radiol Med (Torino) 68:5–10

Aragon GE, Eiseman B (1976) Abdominal stab wounds: evaluation of sinography. J Trauma. 16:792–797

Asher WM, Parvin S, Virgilio RW et al (1976) Echographic evaluation of splenic injury after blunt trauma. Radiology 118:411–415

Aufschnaiter M, Kofler H (1983) Sonographic acute diagnosis in polytrauma. Aktuelle Traumatol 13:55–57

Bach RD, Frey CF (1971) Diagnosis and treatment of pancreatic trauma. Am J Surg 121:20–25

Bain IM, Kirby RM, Tiwari P et al (1998) Survey of abdominal ultrasound and diagnostic peritoneal lavage for suspected intra-abdominal injury following blunt trauma. Injury 29: 65–71

Baron BJ, Scalea TM, Sclafani SJ et al (1993) Nonoperative management of blunt abdominal trauma: the role of sequential diagnostic peritoneal lavage, computed tomography, and angiography. Ann Emerg Med 22:1556–1562

Baum S, Roy R, Finkelstein AK, Blakemore WS (1965) Clinical application of selective celiac and superior mesenteric arteriography. Radiology 84:279–294

Ben-Menachem Y, Fisher RG, Ward RE (1981) Are “occult” intra-abdominal and extraperitoneal injuries really occult. Radiol Clin North Am 19:125–140

Berger BC (1974) Radionuclide studies after urinary tract injury. Semin Nucl Med 4:371–393

Berger PE, Kuhn JP (1981) CT of blunt abdominal trauma in childhood. AJR 136:105–110

Berk RN (1970) Changing concepts in the plain film diagnosis of ruptured spleen. J Can Assoc Radiol 21:67–70

Berman JK, Habegger ED, Fields DC, Kilner WL (1958) Blood studies as an aid in differential diagnosis of abdominal trauma. JAMA 165:1537–1541

Bivins BA, Sachatello CR, Daugherty ME, Ernst CB, Griffin WO (1978) Diagnostic peritoneal lavage is superior to clinical evaluation in blunt abdominal trauma. Am J Surg 44:637–641

Bode PJ, Niezen RA, Van Vugt AB, Schipper J (1993) Abdominal ultrasound as a reliable indicator for conclusive laparotomy in blunt abdominal trauma. J Trauma 34:27–31

Boysen E, Judkins MP, Simay A (1966) Angiographic diagnosis of hepatic rupture. Radiology 86:66–72

Boulanger BR, Mirvis SE, Rodriguez A (1992) Magnetic resonance imaging in traumatic diaphragmatic rupture: case reports. J Trauma 32:89–93

Boulanger BR, Milzman DP, Rosati C, Rodriguez A (1993) The clinical significance of acute hyperamylasemia after blunt trauma. Can J Surg 36:63–69

Boulanger BR, Brennemann FD, McLellan BA et al (1995) A prospective study of emergent abdominal sonography after blunt trauma. J Trauma 39:325–330

Boulanger BR, McLellan BA, Brennemann FD et al (1996) Emergent abdominal ultrasound as a screening test in a

new diagnostic algorithm for blunt trauma. J Trauma 40: 867–874
Brasel KJ, Borgstrom DC, Kolewe KA, Weigelt JA (1996) Abdominal computed tomography scan as a screening tool in blunt trauma. Surgery 120:780–784
Breen DJ, Janzen DL, Zwirewich CV, Nagy AG (1997) Blunt bowel and mesenteric injury: diagnostic performance of CT signs. J Comput Assist Tomogr 21:706–712
Brittain RS (1963) Liver trauma. Surg Clin North Am 43:433–444
Brotman S, Shatney CH, Cowley RA (1981) False negative peritoneal lavage. Am Surg 47:309–310
Brown MA, Casola G, Sirlin CB, Patel NY, Hoyt DB (2001) Blunt abdominal trauma: screening US in 2693 patients. Radiology 218:352–358
Buntain WL, Gould HR, Maull KI (1988) Predictability of splenic lavage by computed tomography. J Trauma 28:24–34
Canizaro PD, Fitts CT, Swayer RB (1964) Diagnostic abdominal paracentesis: a proposed adjunctive measure. US Army Surgical Research Unit. Annual Report
Cantor MO (1970) Abdominal trauma. Thomas, Springfield, Illinois
Caride VJ, Gibson DW (1982) Noninvasive evaluation of bile leakage. Surg Gynecol Obstet 154:517–520
Chen MK, Schropp KP, Lobe TE (1995) The use of minimal access surgery in pediatric trauma: a preliminary report. J Laparoendosc Surg 5:295–301
Chiu WC, Cushing BM, Rodriguez A et al (1997) Abdominal injuries without hemoperitoneum: a potential limitation of focused abdominal sonography for trauma (FAST). J Trauma 42:817–822
Christensen PB, Oester-Joergensen E, Schoubye et al (1981) Scintigraphy with 99mTc-(2,6-diethylacetanilide)-iminodiacetic acid as a diagnostic test in traumatic lesions of the liver and biliary tract. Gastrointest Radiol 15:43–46
Clancy TV, Ragozzino MW, Ramshaw D, Churchill MP, Covington DL, Maxwell JG (1993) Oral contrast is not necessary in the evaluation of blunt abdominal trauma by computed tomography. Am J Surg 166:680–684
Cleveland HC, ReinschmidtT JD, Waddel WR (1963) Traumatic pancreatitis: an increasing problem. Surg Clin North Am 43:402–411
Coant PN, Kornberg AE, Brody AS, Edwards-Holmes K (1992) Markers for occult liver injury of physical abuse in children. Pediatrics 80:274–278
Coelmo JCU, Sigel B, Ryva JC et al (1982) B-mode sonography of blood clots. J Clin Ultrasound 10:323–327
Colletti PM, Barakos JA, Ralls PW, Siegel ME, Halls JM (1983) Hepatobiliary scintigraphy and scintiangiography in trauma. Clin Nucl Med 12:901–909
Colucciello SA (1993) Blunt abdominal trauma. Emerg Med Clin North Am 11:107–123
Cox EF (1984) Blunt abdominal trauma. A 5-year analysis of 870 patients requiring celiotomy. Ann Surg 199:467–474
Croce MA, Fabian TC, Menke PG et al (1995) Nonoperative management of blunt hepatic trauma is the treatment of choice for hemodynamically stable patients. Ann Surg 221: 744–745
Cunningham MA, Tyroch AH, Kaups KL, Davis JW (1998) Does free fluid on abdominal computed tomographic scan after blunt trauma require laparotomy? J Trauma 44:599–602
Cushing BM, Clark DE, Cobean R, Schenarts PJ, Rutstein LA (1997) Blunt and penetrating trauma – has anything changed? Surg Clin North Am 77:1321–1332
Danzl DF, Berg BC Jr (1977) Peritoneal lavage and scintigraphic evaluation of blunt abdominal trauma. JACEP 6:397–404
Daum-Kowalski R, Shanley DJ, Murphy T (1991) MRI diagnosis of delayed presentation of traumatic diaphragmatic hernia. Gastrointest Radiol 16:298–300
Delany HM, Jason RS (1981) Abdominal trauma. Surgical and radiological diagnosis. Springer, New York, pp 93–105
Demaria EJ (1991) Management of patients with indeterminate diagnostic peritoneal lavage results following blunt trauma. J Trauma 31:1627–1631
Demetriades D, Rabinowitz B (1987) Indications for operation in abdominal stab wounds. A prospective study of 651 patients. Ann Surg 205:129–132
Deviere J, Van Gansbeke D, Ansay J, De Toeuf J, Cremer M (1987) Endoscopic management of a posttraumatic biliary fistula. Endoscopy 19:136–139
Diamond AB, Meng CH, Woolanske AC et al (1973) Radionuclide demonstration of traumatic arterial injury. Radiology 109:623–628
Dosios T, Papachristos IC, Chrysicopoulos H (1993) Magnetic resonance imaging of blunt traumatic rupture of the right hemidiaphragm. Eur J Cardiothorac Surg 7:553–554
Drost TF, Rosemurgy AS, Kearny RE et al (1991) Diagnostic peritoneal lavage: limited indications due to evolving concepts in trauma case. Am Surg 57:126–130
Druy EM, Rubin BE (1979) Computed tomography in the evaluation of abdominal trauma. J Comput Assist Tomogr 3:40–44
Elkin M, Cohen G (1962) Diagnostic value of psoas shadow. Clin Radiol 13:210–217
Elliott DC, Rodriguez A, Moncure M et al (1998) The accuracy of diagnostic laparoscopy in trauma patients: a prospective, controlled study. Int Surg 83:294–298
Elman R, Arneson N, Graham EA (1929) Value of blood amylase estimations in the diagnosis of pancreatic disease. Arch Surg 19:943–967
Espinoza R, Rodriguez A (1997) Traumatic and nontraumatic perforation of hollow viscera. Surg Clin North Am 77: 1291–1304
Evans GW, Antin FG, McCarty HF et al (1972) Scintigraphy in traumatic lesions of liver and spleen. JAMA 222:665–668
Fabian TC, Mangiante EC, White TJ, Patterson CR, Boldreghini S, Britt LG (1986) A prospective study of 91 patients undergoing both computed tomography and peritoneal lavage following blunt abdominal trauma. J Trauma 26:602–608
Fang JF, Chen RJ, Lin BC (1998) Cell count ratio: new criterion of diagnostic peritoneal lavage for detection of hollow organ perforation. J Trauma 45:540–544
Federle MP (1981) Abdominal trauma: the role and impact of computed tomography. Invest Radiol 16:260–268
Federle MP (1983) Computed tomography of blunt abdominal trauma. Radiol Clin North Am 21:461–475
Federle MP, Jeffrey RB (1983) Hemoperitoneum studied by computed tomography. Radiology 148:187–192
Federle MP, Kaiser JA, McAninch JW et al (1981) The role of computed tomography in renal trauma. Radiology 141: 455–460
Federle MP, Crass RA, Jeffrey RB, Trunkey DD (1982) Computed tomography in blunt abdominal trauma. Arch Surg 117:645–650
Federle MP, Courcoulas AP, Powell M, Ferris JV, Peitzman AB (1998) Blunt splenic injury in adults: clinical and CT criteria for management, with emphasis on active extravasation. Radiology 206:137–142

Feussner H, Siewert JR (1996) Telemedicine – technical possibilities and practical applications. Chirurg 67:984–988
Feussner H, Papaziogas W, Siewert JR (1999) Modern diagnostic workup of blunt abdominal trauma. Chirurg 70:1246–1254
Fisher RG, Foucar K, Estrada B, Ben-Menchem Y (1981) Splenic rupture in blunt trauma – correlation of angiographic and pathological records. Radiol Clin North Am 19:141–146
Fischer RP, Miller-Crotschett RN, Reed RL II (1988) Gastrointestinal disruption: the hazard of nonoperative management in adults with blunt abdominal trauma. J Trauma 28:1445–1449
Fishman EK, Horton KM (2000) CT evaluation of bladder trauma: a critical look. Acad Radiol 7:309–310
Foley CL, Teele RL (1979) Ultrasound of epigastric injuries after blunt trauma. AJR 132:593–598
Fon GT, Hutner TB, Haber K (1980) Utility of ultrasound for diagnosis of mesenteric hematoma. AJR 134:381–384
Förster R, Pillasch J, Zielke A, Malewski U, Rothmund M (1993) Ultrasonography in blunt abdominal trauma: influence of the investigators' experience. J Trauma 34:264–269
Freeark R (1982) The abdomen in the patient with multiple injuries. Can J Surg 25:178–180
Freeark RJ, Love L, Baker RJ (1968) The role of aortography in the management of blunt abdominal trauma. J Trauma 8:557–571
Freeman T, Fischer RP (1976) The inadequacy of peritoneal lavage in diagnosing acute diaphragmatic rupture. J Trauma 16:538–540
Frick EJ Jr, Pasquale MD, Cipolle MD (1999) Small-bowel and mesentery injuries in blunt trauma. J Trauma 46:920–926
Fried AM, Humphries R, Schofield CN (1992) Abdominal CT scans in patients with blunt trauma: low yield in the absence of clinical findings. J Comput Assist Tomogr 16: 717–721
Froelich JW, Simeone JF, McKusick KA, Winzelberg GG, Strauss HW (1982) Radionuclide imaging and ultrasound in liver/ spleen trauma: a prospective comparison. Radiology 145: 457–461
Fryer JP, Graham TL, Fong HMT et al (1991) Diagnostic peritoneal lavage as an indicator for therapeutic surgery. Canad J Surg 34:471–476
Gavant ML, Schurr M, Frick PA et al (1997) Predicting clinical outcome of nonsurgical management of blunt splenic injury: using CT to reveal abnormalities of splenic vasculature. AJR 168:207–211
Gelfand MJ (1984) Scintigraphy in upper abdominal trauma. Semin Roentgenol 19:296–307
Gilday DL, Alderson PO (1974) Scintigraphic evaluation of liver and spleen injury. Semin Nucl Med 4:357–370
Gill W, Champion HR, Long WB, Jamaris J, Cowley RA (1975) Abdominal lavage in blunt trauma. Br J Surg 62:124–128
Ginzburg E, Carrillo EH, Kopelman T et al (1998) The role of computed tomography in selective management of gunshot wounds to the abdomen and flank. J Trauma 45:1005–1009
Glaser K, Tschemelitsch J, Klinger P, Wetscher G, Borden E (1994) Ultrasonography in the management of blunt abdominal and thoracic trauma. Arch Surg 129:743–747
Glazer GM, Buy JN, Moss AA et al (1981) CT in the detection of duodenal perforation. AJR 137:333–336
Gold RE, Redman HC (1972) Splenic trauma: assessment of problems in diagnosis. AJR 116:413–418
Goletti O, Ghiselli G, Lippolis PV et al. (1994) The role of ultrasonography in blunt abdominal trauma: results in 250 consecutive cases. J Trauma 36:178–181
Gomez GA, Alvarez R, Plasencia G et al (1987) Diagnostic peritoneal lavage in the management of blunt abdominal trauma: a reassessment. J Trauma 27:1–5
Gould JR, Thorworth WT (1963) Retroperitoneal rupture of duodenum due to blunt, nonpenetrating abdominal trauma. Radiology 80:743–747
Griffen M, Ochoa J, Boulanger BR (2000) A minimally invasive approach to bile peritonitis after blunt liver injury. Am Surg 66:309–312
Gruessner R, Mentges B, Duber C, Rückert K, Rothmund M (1989) Sonography versus peritoneal lavage in blunt abdominal trauma. J Trauma 29:242–246
Haertel M (1975) Röntgendiagnostik viszeraler Verletzungen nach stumpfem Abdominaltrauma. Thieme, Stuttgart
Hagiwara A, Yukioka T, Ohta S, Nitatori T, Matsuda H, Shimazaki S (1996) Nonsurgical management of patients with blunt splenic injury: efficacy of transcatheter arterial embolization. AJR 167:159–166
Haney PJ, Whitley NO, Brotman S et al (1982) Liver injury and complications in the postoperative trauma patient: CT evaluation. AJR 139:271–275
Hanna SS, Gorman PR, Harrison AW, Taylor G, Miller HA, Pagliarello G (1987) Blunt liver trauma at Sunnybrook Medical Center. J Trauma 27:965–969
Harrel DJ, Vitale GC, Larson GM (1998) Selective role for endoscopic retrograde cholangiopancreatography in abdominal trauma. Surg Endosc 12:400–404
Hashimoto BE, Laing FC, Jeffrey RB Jr et al (1984) Hemorrhagic pancreatic fluid collections examined by ultrasound. Radiology 150:803–808
Hauenstein KH, Wimmer B, Billmann P, Noldge G, Zavisic D (1982) Sonography of blunt abdominal trauma. Radiologe 22:106–111
Häuser H, Bohndorf K (1999) Radiological emergency management of multiple trauma patient. Emerg Radiol 6:61–69
Hawkins ML, Scofield WM, Carraway RP, Laws HL (1988) Diagnostic peritoneal lavage in blunt trauma. South Med J 81:293–296
Henderson RW, Lee YC, Telfer N (1978) Demonstration of traumatic hepato-pleural-cutaneous defect by 131I-rose bengal. Clin Nucl Med. 3:432–433
Henneman PL, Marx JA, Moore EE et al (1990) Accuracy on predicting necessary laparotomy following blunt and penetrating trauma. J Trauma 30:1345–1350
Hoffmann R, Nerlich M, Muggia-Sullam M et al (1992) Blunt abdominal trauma in cases of multiple trauma evaluated by ultrasonography: a prospective analysis of 291 patients. J Trauma 32:452–458
Hubbard SG, Bivins BA, Sachatello CR, Griffen WO Jr (1979) Diagnostic errors with peritoneal lavage in patients with pelvic fractures. Arch Surg 114:844–846
Jacobson G, Carter R (1951) Small intestinal rupture due to non-penetrating abdominal injury: roentgenological study. AJR 66:52–64
Jeffrey RB Jr (1989) CT diagnosis of blunt hepatic and splenic injuries: a look to the future. Radiology 171:17–18
Jeffrey RB Jr, Cardoza JD, Olcott EW (1991) Detection of active intra-abdominal arterial hemorrhage: value of dynamic contrast-enhanced CT. AJR 156:725–729
Jehle D, Guarino J, Karamanoukian H (1993) Emergency department ultrasound in the evaluation of blunt abdominal trauma. Am J Emerg Med 11:342–346
Jones TK, Walsh JW, Maull KI (1983) Diagnostic imaging in

blunt trauma of the abdomen. Surg Gynecol Obstet 157: 389–398
Jurkovich GJ, Carrico CJ (1992) Trauma: management of acute injuries. In: Sabiston DC Jr, Lyerly HK (eds) Textbook of surgery. Saunders, Philadelphia, pp 121–139
Karnaze GC, Sheedy PF, Stephens DH et al (1981) Computed tomography in duodenal rupture due to blunt abdominal trauma. J Comput Assist Tomogr 5:267–269
Katz S, Lazar L, Rathaus V, Erez I (1996) Can ultrasonography replace computed tomography in the initial assessment of children with blunt abdominal trauma? J Pediatr Surg 31: 649–651
Kern E, Klaue P (1975) Diagnose und Operationsindikation beim stumpfen Bauchtrauma. Dtsch Med Wochenschr 100: 660–664
Kimura A, Otsuka T (1991) Emergency center ultrasonography in the evaluation of hemoperitoneum: a prospective study. J Trauma 31:20–25
Kinnunen J, Kivioja A, Poussa K, Laasonen EM (1994) Emergency CT in blunt abdominal trauma of multiple injury patients. Acta Radiol 35:319–322
Klaue P (1983) Die Bedeutung der Lavage nach Beckenverletzungen. Langenbecks Arch Chir 361:85–89
Klotter HJ, Zielke A, Nies C, Sitter H, Rothmund M (1992) Sonographie beim akuten abdominellen Notfall. Chirurg 63:597–605
Klotter HJ, Nies C, Zielke A, Sitter H, Rothmund M (1993) Choice of diagnostic modalities in blunt abdominal trauma. Chirurg 64:841–848
Kristensen JK, Buemann B, Kuehl E (1971) Ultrasonic scanning in the diagnosis of splenic haematomas. Acta Chir Scand 137:653–657
Kuhn FP, Schreyer T, Schild H, Klose K, Gunther R (1983) Sonography in blunt abdominal trauma. ROFO Fortschr Geb Rontgenstr Nuklearmed 139:310–313
Kuligowska E, Mueller PR, Simeone JF, Fine C (1984) Ultrasound in upper abdominal trauma. Seminars Roentgenol 19:281–295
Kuni CC, Klingensmith WC 3rd, Koep LJ et al (1980) Communication of intrahepatic cavities with bile ducts: demonstration with Tc-99m-diethyl-IDA imaging. Clin Nucl Med 5:349–351
Kurtzman RS (1977) Radiology of blunt abdominal trauma. Surg Clin North Am 57:211–216
Lam EC, Janzen RM, Meloche RM, Trepanier PJ, Yoshida EM (1999) Acute pseudohepatitis in a chronic substance abuse secondary to occult seat belt injury. Can J Gastroenterol 13: 155–158
Lang EK (1971) Renal arteriography in the assessment of renal trauma. Radiology 98:103–107
Lang EK (1975) Arteriography in the assessment of renal trauma. J Trauma 15:553–559
Lang EK (1976) The role of arteriography in trauma. Radiol Clin N Am 14:353–370
Lang EK (1990) Intra-abdominal and retroperitoneal organ injuries diagnosed on computed tomograms obtained for assessment of renal trauma. J Trauma 30:1161–1168
Lentz KA, McKenney MG, Nunez DB, Martin L (1996) Evaluating blunt abdominal trauma: role for ultrasonography. J Ultrasound Med 15:447–451
Leppaniemi AK, Elliott DC (1996) The role of laparoscopy in blunt abdominal trauma. Ann Med 28:483–489
L'Hermine C, Grand M, Remond A, Van Kemmel M, Quandalle P (1977) Inversion of intrahepatic portal flow in contusions of the liver: a new concept of traumatic arterioportal fistulas (author's transl). J Radiol Electrol Med Nucl 58:609–619
Little JM, McRae J, Smitananda N, Morris JG (1967) Radioisotope scanning of liver and spleen in upper abdominal trauma. Surg Gynecol Obstet 125:725–729
Liu M, Lee CH, P'eng FK (1993) Prospective comparison of diagnostic peritoneal lavage, computed tomographic scanning, and ultrasonography for the diagnosis of blunt abdominal trauma. J Trauma 35:267–270
Livingston DH, Bartholomew JT, Blackwood J, Machiedo GW, Rush BF Jr (1992) The role of laparoscopy in abdominal trauma. J Trauma 33:471–475
Love L (1975) Radiology of abdominal trauma. JAMA 231: 1377–1380
Love L, Greenfield GB, Braun TW, Moncada R, Freeark RJ, Baker RJ (1968) Arteriography of splenic trauma. Radiology 91:96–102
Lowenfels AB (1966) Kehr's sign – a neglected aid in ruptures of the spleen. N Engl J Med 274:1019
Lucciarini P, Ofner D, Weber F, Lugenschmid D (1993) Ultrasonography in the initial evaluation and follow-up of blunt abdominal injury. Surgery 114:506–512
Lutzeker L, Koeningsberg M, Meng HF et al (1974) The role of radionuclide imaging in spleen trauma. Radiology 110: 419–423
Ma OJ, Mateer JR, Ogata M et al (1995) Prospective analysis of a rapid trauma ultrasound examination performed by emergency physicians. J Trauma 38:879–885
Mahboubi S (1985) Abdominal trauma in children: role of computed tomography. Pediatr Emerg Care 1:37–39
Makhija MC, Schultz S (1983) Bone scan that saved a laparotomy. Clin Nucl Med 8:555–556
Mall JC, Kaiser JA (1980) CT diagnosis of splenic laceration. AJR 134:265–269
Marcos HB, Noone TC, Semelka RC (1998) MRI evaluation of acute renal trauma. J Magn Reson Imaging 8:988–990
Marincek B (1993) Imaging in blunt abdominal trauma. Schweiz Med Wochenschr 123:473–479
Marty F (1975) Angiographic findings in pancreatic injury – 4 cases. In: Efficiency and limits of radiologic examination of the pancreas. Thieme, Stuttgart, pp 181–184
Matsubara TK, Fong HMT, Burns CM (1990) Computed tomography of the abdomen (CTA) in the management of blunt abdominal trauma. J Trauma 30:410–414
McCort JJ (1964) Radiographic examinations in blunt abdominal trauma. Radiol Clin North Am 2:121–143
McCort JJ (1973) Abdominal trauma. In: Margulis AR, Burhenne JH (eds) Alimentary tract roentgenology, vol 1. Mosby, St Louis, pp 228–270
McElveen TS, Collin GR (1997) The role of ultrasonography in blunt abdominal trauma: a prospective study. Am Surg 63:184–188
McGehee M, Kier R, Cohn SM, McCarthy SM (1993) Comparison of MRI with postcontrast CT for the evaluation of acute abdominal trauma. J Comput Assist Tomogr 17:410–413
McKenney KL (1999) Ultrasound of blunt abdominal trauma. Radiol Clin North Am 37:879–893
McKenney KL, Nunez DB, McKenney MG et al (1998) Sonography as the primary screening technique for blunt abdominal trauma: experience with 899 patients. AJR 170:979–1000
McKenney M, Lentz M, Nunez D et al (1994) Can ultrasound replace diagnostic peritoneal lavage in the assessment of blunt trauma? J Trauma 37:439–441

McKenney MG, Martin L, Lentz KA et al (1996) 1000 consecutive ultrasounds for blunt abdominal trauma. J Trauma 40: 607–609
McKenney MG, McKenney KL, Compton RP et al (1998) Can surgeons evaluate emergency ultrasound scans for blunt abdominal trauma? J Trauma 44:649–653
Memon MA, Fitztgibbons RJ (1997) The role of minimal access surgery in the acute abdomen. Surg Clin North Am 77:1333–1353
Meyer DM, Thal ER, Weigelt JA, Redman HC (1989) Evaluation of computed tomography and diagnostic peritoneal lavage in blunt abdominal trauma. J Trauma 29:1168–1171
Mindelzun RE, McCort JJ (1984) Upper abdominal trauma: conventional radiology. Semin Roentgenol 19:259–268
Mirvis SE, Shanmuganathan K (1994) Trauma radiology: part I. Computerized tomographic imaging of abdominal trauma. J Intensive Care Med 9:151–163
Mirvis SE, Keramati B, Buckman R, Rodriguez A (1988) MR imaging of traumatic diaphragmatic rupture. J Comput Assist Tomogr 12:147–149
Miskowiak J, Nielsen SL, Munck O, Burcharth F, Blichert-Toft M, Nadel MS (1979) Acute gastrointestinal bleeding detected with abdominal scintigraphy using technetium-99m-labeled albumin. Scand J Gastroenterol 14:389–394
Mutabagani KH, Coley BD, Zumberge N et al (1999) Preliminary experience with focused abdominal sonography for trauma (FAST) in children: is it useful? J Pediatr Surg 34: 48–52
Nagy KK, Roberts RR, Hoseph KT et al (2000) Experience with over 2500 diagnostic peritoneal lavages. Injury 31:479–482
Navarrete-Navarro P, Vazquez G, Bosch JM, Fernandez E, Rivera R, Carazo E (1996) Computed tomography vs clinical and multidisciplinary procedures for early evaluation of severe abdomen and chest trauma – a cost analysis approach. Inten Care Med 22:208–212
Nebesar RA, Rabinov KR, Potsaid MS (1974) Radionuclide imaging of the spleen in suspected splenic injury. Radiology 110:609–613
Neugebauer H, Wallenboeck E, Hungerford M (1999) Seventy cases of injuries of the small intestine caused by blunt abdominal trauma: a retrospective study from 1970 to 1994. J Trauma 46:116–121
Norell HG (1957) Traumatic rupture of the spleen diagnosed by abdominal aortography. Acta Radiol 48:449–452
Nunes LW, Simmons S, Kozar R, Kinback R, Hallowell MJ, Mulhern C Jr (2001) Feasibility and profitability of a radiology department providing trauma. US as a part of a trauma alert team. Acad Radiol 8:88–95
Ochsner MG, Knudson MM, Pachter HL et al (2000) Significance of minimal or no intraperitoneal fluid visible on CT scan associated with blunt liver and splenic injuries: a multicenter analysis. J Trauma 49:505–510
Oldham KT, Guice KS, Kaufman RA et al (1984) Blunt hepatic injury and elevated hepatic enzymes: a clinical correlation in children. J Pediatr Surg 19:457–461
Olsen WR (1973) The serum amylase in blunt abdominal trauma. J Trauma 13:200–204
Olsen WR, Hildreth DH (1971) Abdominal paracentesis and peritoneal lavage in blunt abdominal trauma. J Trauma 11: 824–829
O'Malley BP, Salem S (1979) Abdominal hematomas in unusual locations – contribution of ultrasound. J Can Assoc Radiol 30:182–183
Pachter HL, Hofstetter SR (1981) Open and percutaneous paracentesis and lavage for abdominal trauma: a randomized prospective study. Arch Surg 116:318–319
Pachter HL, Knudson MM, Esrig B et al (1996) Status of nonoperative management of blunt hepatic injuries in 1995: a multicenter experience with 404 patients. J Trauma 40: 31–38
Peng MY, Parisky YR, Cornwell EE III, Radin R, Bragin S (1999) CT cystography versus conventional cystography in evaluation of bladder injury. AJR 173:1269–1272
Perry JF (1965) A five-year survey of 152 acute abdominal injuries. J Trauma 5:53–61
Petersen SR, Sheldon GF (1979) Morbidity of a negative finding at laparotomy in abdominal trauma. Surg Gynecol Obstet 148:23–26
Peterson N (1978) The significance of delayed post-traumatic renal hemorrhage. J Urol 119:563–565
Raptopoulos V (1994) Abdominal trauma. Emphasis on computed tomography. Radiol Clin North Am 32:969–987
Reed RL, Merrel C, Meyers WC, Fischer RP (1992) Continuing evolution in the approach to severe liver trauma. Ann Surg 216:524–538
Roberts JL, Dalen K, Bosanko CM, Jafir SZ (1993) CT in abdominal and pelvic trauma. Radiographics 13:735–752
Roche BG, Bugmann P, Lecoultre C (1992) Blunt injuries to liver, spleen, kidney and pancreas in pediatric patients. Eur J Pediatr Surg 2:154–156
Rodriguez A, Dupriest RW Jr, Shatney CH (1982) Recognition of intra-abdominal injury in blunt trauma victims. A prospective study comparing physical examination with peritoneal lavage. Am Surg 48:457–459
Root HD, Hauser CW, McKinley CR et al (1965) Diagnostic peritoneal lavage. Surgery 57:663–667
Rosenthal L (1974) Intravenous radionuclide angiography in the diagnosis of trauma. Semin Nucl Med 4:395–409
Rossi P, Mullins D, Thal E (1993) Role of laparoscopy in the evaluation of abdominal trauma. Am J Surg 166:707–710
Rothlin M, Naf R, Amgwerd M, Candinas D, Trentz O (1992) How much experience is required for ultrasound diagnosis of blunt abdominal trauma? Langenbecks Arch Chir 377: 211–215
Rothlin MA, Remo N, Amgwerd M, Candinas D, Trentz O et al (1993) Ultrasound in blunt abdominal and thoracic trauma. J Trauma 34:488–495
Rozycki GS, Ochsner MG, Jaffin JH, Champion HR (1993) Prospective evaluation of surgeon's use of ultrasound in the evaluation of trauma patients. J Trauma 34:516–527
Rozycki GS, Ochsner MG, Schmidt JA et al (1995) A prospective study of surgeon performed ultrasound as the primary adjuvant modality for injured patient assessment. J Trauma 39:492–500
Rozycki GS, Ballard RB, Feliciano DV, Schmidt JA, Pennington SD (1998a) Surgeon-performed ultrasound for the assessment of truncal injuries: lessons learned from 1540 patients. Ann Surg 228:557–567
Rozycki GS, Ochsner MG, Feliciano DV et al (1998b) Early detection of hemoperitoneum by ultrasound examination of the right upper quadrant: a multicenter study. J Trauma 45:878–883
Ruf W, Mischkowsky T, Friedl W (1985) Diagnostic procedure in blunt abdominal trauma. Chirurg 56:673–679
Ruskin R, Saenger EL (1963) Liver scanning in the diagnosis of hemobilia. Radiology 81:980–983

Sahdev P, Garramone RR, Schwartz RJ, Steelman SR, Jacobs LM (1991) Evaluation of liver function tests in screening for intra-abdominal injuries. Ann Emerg Med 20:838–841
Saloman H (1906) Die diagnostische Punktion des Bauches. Berl Klin Wochenschr 43:45–46
Sayers RD, Bewes PC, Porter KM (1992) Emergency laparotomy for abdominal trauma. Injury 23:537–541
Scalea TM, Rodriguez A, Chiu WC et al (1999) Focused Assessment with Sonography for Trauma (FAST): results from an international consensus conference. J Trauma 46:466–472
Scheele J, Wagner W (1981) Importance of peritoneal lavage in the diagnosis of blunt abdominal trauma. MMW Munch Med Wochenschr 123:876–882
Schlager D, Lazzareschi G, Whitten D, Sanders AB (1994) A prospective study of ultrasonography in the ED by emergency physicians. Am J Emerg Med 12:185–189
Schorn L, Coln D (1977) Hepatic angiographic changes after trauma. Am J Surg 134:754–757
Schriefers KH, Gerometta P (1981) Stumpfe und offene Bauchveletzungen. Langenbecks Arch Chir 355:353–358
Schurink GW, Bode PJ, Van Luijt PA, Van Vugt AB (1997) The value of physical examination in the diagnosis of patients with blunt abdominal trauma: a retrospective study. Injury 28:261–265
Sclafani SJ, Gordon DH, Mitchell W (1983) Laceration of the inferior vena cava of angiographic demonstration. Cardiovasc Intervent Radiol 6:164–166
Sclafani SJ, Shaftan GW, Scalea TM et al (1995) Nonoperative salvage of computed tomography-diagnosed splenic injuries: utilization of angiography for triage and embolization for hemostasis. J Trauma 39:818–825
Shaftan GW (1969) Indications for operation in abdominal trauma. Am J Surg 99:657–664
Shanmuganathan K, Mirvis SE, Sover ER (1993) Value of contrast-enhanced CT in detecting active hemorrhage in patients with blunt abdominal or pelvic trauma. AJR 161: 65–69
Shanmuganathan K, Mirvis SE, Sherbourne CD, Chiu WC, Rodriguez A (1999) Hemoperitoneum as the sole indicator of abdominal visceral injuries: a potential limitation of screening abdominal US for trauma. Radiology 212: 423–430
Shanmuganathan K, Mirvis SE, Chiu WC, Killeen KL, Scalea TM (2001) Triple-contrast helical CT in penetrating torso trauma: a prospective study to determine peritoneal violation and the need for laparotomy. AJR 177:1247–1256
Sherck J, Shatney C, Sensaki K, Selivanov V (1994) The accuracy of computed tomography in the diagnosis of blunt small-bowel perforation. Am J Surg 168:670–675
Shih HC, Wen YS, Ko TJ, Wu JK, Su CH, Lee CH (1999) Noninvasive evaluation of blunt abdominal trauma: prospective study using diagnostic algorithms to minimize nontherapeutic laparotomy. World J Surg 23:265–269
Shirasawa B, Furukawa S, Tsushimi T et al (2001) Delayed traumatic diaphragmatic hernia diagnosed by MRI and direct coronal CT: report of a case. Kyobu Geka 54:885–887
Shuman WP (1997) CT of blunt abdominal trauma in adults. Radiology 205:297–306
Sigel B, Coelmo JCU, Spigos DG et al (1981) Ultrasonography of blood stasis and coagulation. Invest Radiol 16:71–76
Sigel B, Coelmo JCU, Schade SG et al (1982) Effect of plasma proteins and temperature on echogenicity of blood. Invest Radiol 17:29–33
Singh G, Arya N, Safaya R, Bose SM, Das KM, Khanna SK (1997) Role of ultrasonography in blunt abdominal trauma. Injury 28:667–670
Smith RS, Kern SJ, Fry WR, Helmer SD (1998) Institutional learning curve of surgeon-performed trauma ultrasound. Arch Surg 133:530–535
Sperling L, Rigler LG (1937) Traumatic retroperitoneal rupture of duodenum. Radiology 29:521–524
Strauch GO (1973) Major abdominal trauma in 1971: a study of Connecticut by the Connecticut Society of American Board Surgeons and the Yale Trauma Program. Am J Surg 125:413–418
Sty JR, Starshak RJ, Hubbard AM (1982) Radionuclide hepatobiliary imaging in the detection of traumatic biliary tract disease in children. Pediatr Radiol 12:115–118
Sugimoto K, Asari Y, Sakaguchi T, Owada T, Makawa K (1993) Endoscopic retrograde cholangiography in the nonsurgical management of blunt liver injury. J Trauma 35:192–199
Sung CK, Kim KH (1996) Missed injuries in abdominal trauma. J Trauma 41:276–282
Takishima T, Sugimoto K, Hirata M, Asari Y, Ohwada T, Kakita A (1997) Serum amylase level on admission in the diagnosis of blunt injury to the pancreas: its significance and limitations. Ann Surg. 226:70–76
Taylor GA, Sivit CJ (1995) Posttraumatic peritoneal fluid: is it a reliable indicator of intraabdominal injury in children? J Pediatr Surg 30:1644–1648
Thomas B, Falcone RE, Vasquez D et al (1997) Ultrasound evaluation of blunt abdominal trauma: program implementation, initial experience and learning curve. J Trauma 42:384–390
Ting YM, Renter SR (1973) Hollow viscus injury in blunt abdominal trauma. AJR 119:408–413
Townsend MC, Flancbaum L, Choban PS, Cloutier CT (1993) Diagnostic laparoscopy as an adjunct to selective conservative management of solid organ injuries after blunt abdominal trauma. J Trauma 35:647–651
Tsang BD, Panacek EA, Brant WE, Wisner DH (1997) Effect of oral contrast administration for abdominal computed tomography in the evaluation of acute blunt trauma. Ann Emerg Med 30:7–13
Tso P, Rodriguez A, Cooper C et al (1992) Sonography in blunt abdominal trauma: a preliminary progress report. J Trauma 33:39–44
Udekwu PO, Gurkin B, Oller DW (1996) The use of computed tomography in blunt abdominal injuries. Am Surg 62: 56–59
Uthoff LB, Wyffels PL, Adams CS, Zwicky GF Jr, Berg BC (1983) A prospective study comparing nuclear scintigraphy and computerized axial tomography in the initial evaluation of the trauma patient. Ann Surg 198:611–616
Van Sonnenberg E, Simeone JF, Mueller PR et al (1983) Sonographic appearance of hematoma in liver, spleen and kidney: a clinical, pathologic and animal study. Radiology 147:507–510
Vogler E, Bergmann M (1963) Angiography in blunt kidney trauma. ROFO 98:675–685
Wataya H, Tsuruta N, Takayama K, Mitsudomi T, Nakanishi Y, Hara N (1997) Delayed traumatic hernia diagnosed with magnetic resonance imaging. Nihon Kyobu Shikkan Gakkai Zasshi 35:124–128
Weishaupt D, Hetzer FH, Ruemm SG, Patak MA, Schmidt M, Debatin JF (2000) Three-dimensional contrast-enhanced

MRI using an intravascular contrast agent for detection of traumatic intra-abdominal hemorrhage and abdominal parenchymal injuries: an experimental study. Eur Radiol 10:1958–1964

Weissmann HS, Sugarman LA, Freeman LM (1982) Atlas of Tc-99m iminodiacetic acid (IDA) cholescintigraphy. Clin Nucl Med 7:231–239

Weissmann HS, Byun KJ, Freeman LM (1983) Role of Tc-99m IDA scintigraphy in the evaluation of hepatobiliary trauma. Semin Nucl Med 13:199–222

Wenz W (1972) Abdominale Angiographie. Springer, Berlin Heidelberg New York

Wherett LJ, Boulanger BR, McLellan BA et al (1996) Hypotension after blunt abdominal trauma: the role of emergent abdominal sonography in surgical triage. J Trauma 41:815–820

White PH, Benfield JR (1972) Amylase in the management of pancreatic trauma. Arch Surg 105:158–163

Wicks JD, Silver TM, Bree RL (1978) Gray scale features of hematomas: an ultrasonic spectrum. AJR 131:977–980

Wiener SN, Vyas M (1974) The scintigraphic demonstration of bile leakage utilizing 131I-rose bengal. J Nucl Med 15: 1044–1046

Williams RA, Black JJ, Sinow RM, Wilson SE (1997) Computed tomography-assisted management of splenic trauma. Am J Surg 174:276–279

Williams RD, Zollinger RM (1959) Diagnostic and prognostic factors in abdominal trauma. Am J Surg 97:575–581

Yoshii H, Sato M, Yamamoto S et al (1998) Usefulness and limitations of ultrasonography in the initial evaluation of blunt abdominal trauma. J Trauma 45:45–50

22 Hemostatic Arterial Embolization in Blunt Trauma Victims at Admission

R. F. DONDELINGER and G. TROTTEUR

CONTENTS

- Head injury should not be accepted as an explanation of shock, unless visceral hemorrhage is ruled out (WALT 1969).
- Marginally stable or unstable patients with retroperitoneal bleeding, evidenced on CT, should be directed to angiography and hemostatic embolization.
- Hemorrhage related to unstable pelvic fractures is preferably treated by external orthopedic fixation; persistent bleeding is treated by arterial embolization.
- Principles of hemostatic arterial embolization are different from tumor devascularization.

22.1 Introduction

For more than 20 years, suicide and trauma have been the leading causes of death in the male population under 25 and 40 years of age, respectively, and are responsible of the loss of more years of life than cancer and cardiovascular diseases together (TRUNKEY 1983). Traumatic injuries of the central nervous system, heart, and great vessels are responsible for the deaths that occur at the site of accident, whereas internal hemorrhage is the principal cause of mortality during the first 4 h following trauma; the vast majority of visceral nonbleeding injuries are compatible with survival. Therefore, urgent patient admission, rapid resuscitation, and hemodynamic stabilization are the prerequisites for setting management priorities, followed, when applicable, by aggressive and reliable investigation of all posttraumatic injuries for the selection of appropriate treatment. Urgent intervention is the cornerstone of posttraumatic hemostasis. It has

R. F. DONDELINGER, MD
Professor and Chairman, Department of Medical Imaging, University Hospital Sart Tilman, Domaine Universitaire du Sart Tilman B35, 4000 Liège, Belgium
G. TROTTEUR, MD
Department of Medical Imaging, University Hospital Sart Tilman, Domaine Universitaire du Sart Tilman B35, 4000 Liège, Belgium

been suggested for several decades that arteriographic embolization could be a useful adjunct in the treatment of persistent or recurrent postoperative bleeding, and a reasonable primary alternative to surgery in retroperitoneal or pelvic bleeding or in other selected patients with abdominal visceral hemorrhage. This chapter will be focused on blunt abdominal trauma.

22.2 Classification of Trauma Patients

History taking of the mechanism of trauma is helpful to anticipate the presence of potential posttraumatic injuries, to predict possible injury associations, and sense their severity. Despite the availability of powerful imaging, the gross clinical findings always take precedence in the sequence of management and imaging. Trauma victims may be classified into three categories for management orientation:

- Patients in class I, who remain hemodynamically unstable despite resuscitation, are directed to the operating room. Focused Assessment with Sonography for Trauma (FAST) or a standardized six-point trauma ultrasonography (US) examination was introduced as a means of rapid evaluation of the abdomen (and pericardium) in the shock room, and has replaced diagnostic peritoneal lavage, to decide on immediate laparotomy or thoracotomy, without additional imaging (Chiu et al. 1997; Rozycki et al. 1998; Scalea et al. 1999; Nunez et al. 2001).
- Patients in class II are marginally stable and will probably require surgery. However, when ongoing retroperitoneal hemorrhage is suspected, these patients should undergo angiography (Ben Menachem et al. 1981). Patients with pelvic bone fractures primarily undergo external orthopedic fixation, followed by angiographic evaluation, in the small group of patients in whom pelvic bleeding persists. Today, many of the marginally stable patients benefit from computed tomography (CT) to assess associated thoracoabdominal injuries, if the local logistics allow the examination to be done without delay in the resuscitation environment.
- Patients in class III are hemodynamically stable and are systematically evaluated with CT. Some patients with clinical suspicion of minimal single-organ injury or patients with no suspicion of internal injury do not need formal hospital admission.

According to this classification, based on the hemodynamic status, number, type, and severity of associated injuries, patients either undergo immediate surgery or hemostatic angiography, either alone or in combination with surgery, or they are included in a trial of expectant conservative management.

22.3 Trauma Patient Triage with Computed Tomography

Computed tomography largely contributes to management orientation of trauma victims. Spiral CT has been recognized as the modality of choice for investigation of blunt trauma, allowing for a rapid screening of injuries of the brain, face, thorax, abdomen, spine, and pelvis.

22.3.1 Significance of Hemoperitoneum for Patient Triage

CT and US are able to detect hemoperitoneum with confidence and have largely superseded diagnostic peritoneal lavage. However, the observation of hemoperitoneum is relatively irrelevant for management of stable patients. Peritoneal fluid confirms visceral bleeding but is not a reliable indicator of a need for hemostasis. In our experience, 1% of all adult patients with blunt abdominal trauma have hemoperitoneum without detectable abdominal organ injury and 4.3% have hemoperitoneum without intraperitoneal, but retroperitoneal injury. Small amounts of hemoperitoneum should be distinguished from fluid of other origin: ruptured adnexal cysts or follicle, biloma, urinoma, and others. In children, 11% were reported to have unexplained isolated peritoneal fluid (Taylor and Sivit 1995). In these patients, hemoperitoneum may be caused either by mesenteric vessel bleeding or by extension of retroperitoneal hematoma into the peritoneal cavity through a ruptured parietal peritoneal leaflet (Freeman and Fischer 1976; Hubbard et al. 1979). On the other hand, we and others have observed parenchymal hepatosplenic injuries of moderate severity grade and without hemoperitoneum in 11–25% of the cases, when CT was performed within one hour following trauma (Ochsner et al 2000).

22.3.2 Significance of Organ Injury Demonstration and Injury Severity Grading

There is general agreement that cross-section imaging evidences hemoperitoneum more easily than specific abdominal organ injury. A significant false negative rate of 20%–30% might be expected in the diagnosis of parenchymal injuries when using FAST. In hemodynamically stable patients, FAST was shown to be unreliable in comparison with CT, with a sensitivity of only 30% (Mutabagani et al. 1999). Furthermore, in polytrauma patients, US is not applicable to brain, lung and bone injury.

Early CT reports on the first 200 to 500 patients that were investigated for abdominal or pelvic trauma, had shown that there were only a few false positive or false negative interpretations of abdominal examinations (Federle et al. 1982; Federle 1983). Most papers published thereafter credited CT with overall sensitivities higher than 90% and specificities close to 100% in the diagnosis of abdominal parenchymal injuries in adults and in the pediatric age group. More differentiated injury-specific sensitivities were published for the pancreas (0%), gastrointestinal tract (42%), and urinary bladder (50%) (Udekwu et al. 1996). Some publications also reported lower sensitivities, of 85%, 84%, and 67% for renal, hepatic, and splenic injuries, respectively (Lang 1990). However, the accepted statement is that only a few percent of errors are observed in thoracoabdominal CT, and most missed injuries are generally not responsible for posttraumatic death; nor do they carry a life-threatening posttraumatic complication (Udekwu et al. 1996).

The amount of hemoperitoneum correlates with the need for laparotomy and with the severity of splenic injury, but not with the severity of hepatic injury, in our experience. High-grade (III–IV) splenic and hepatic injury may require hemostatic intervention more often than low-grade injury, but low-grade liver trauma (grades I and II) responds to expectant nonoperative treatment more consistently than splenic injury.

22.3.3 Demonstration of Ongoing Hemorrhage

It is well established that overall 50%–70% of all liver and splenic injuries have stopped bleeding at time of operation and can be treated conservatively, without surgery (Sclafani et al. 1984, 1995; Moore 1984; Anderson et al. 1986; Beal 1990). Therefore, imaging should be able to disclose active bleeding, which is expected to serve best as a triage of patients for urgent hemostatic intervention or expectant conservative treatment.

As CT is able to detect minimal density gradients, it was hypothesized that small amounts of extravasated contrast medium could be recognized and that CT could give equivalent or superior results to angiography in the diagnosis of active hemorrhage. In fact, ongoing bleeding (25–370 HU, mean, 132 HU) can be differentiated from clotted blood (40–70 HU) by measurement of CT attenuation values ($p<0.001$) (Shanmuganathan et al. 1993).

In the abdomen, contrast extravasation may be shown by spiral CT in 29% of the cases, depending on patient selection for CT, but it is uncertain if all extravasation seen on CT requires hemostatic embolization (Catalano et al. 1999). Extravasation of contrast medium was shown in the spleen to have a high predictive value for surgery, even in injuries of minor or moderate grade (Gavant et al. 1997; Federle et al. 1998). However, there is no prospective study on a large basis comparing CT and angiography in the detection of posttraumatic bleeding. In hemodynamically stable patients, correlation seemed good (Jeffrey et al. 1991). In our personal experience, more than 90% of these angiographies are indicated by a positive CT for contrast extravasation and 90% of angiographies are therapeutic by hemostatic embolization (Kurdziel et al. 1987; Dondelinger and Kurdziel 1991).

CT may show an intraparenchymal capillary blush, a pseudoaneurysm, an arteriovenous fistula, or contrast accumulation outside the organ capsule, dilution of contrast medium in peritoneal fluid, or sedimenting within a hematoma. Contrast diluting or sedimenting in peritoneal fluid, increasing size of a hematoma on serial CT examinations, or accumulation of contrast in interstitial tissue is a definite sign of ongoing bleeding. On the other hand, contrast observed in a hematoma that does not increase in size, a small parenchymal or muscular blush, a pseudoaneurysm, or an arteriovenous fistula do not necessarily indicate per se persisting bleeding. It is quite common to observe blushes of contrast in pelvic or retroperitoneal muscles that have a benign prognosis, compared with similar images seen in a plain parenchyma (Fig. 22.1). Although rare, some retroperitoneal bleeds of traumatic origin may involve ruptured veins and resemble nontraumatic spontaneous bleeding on

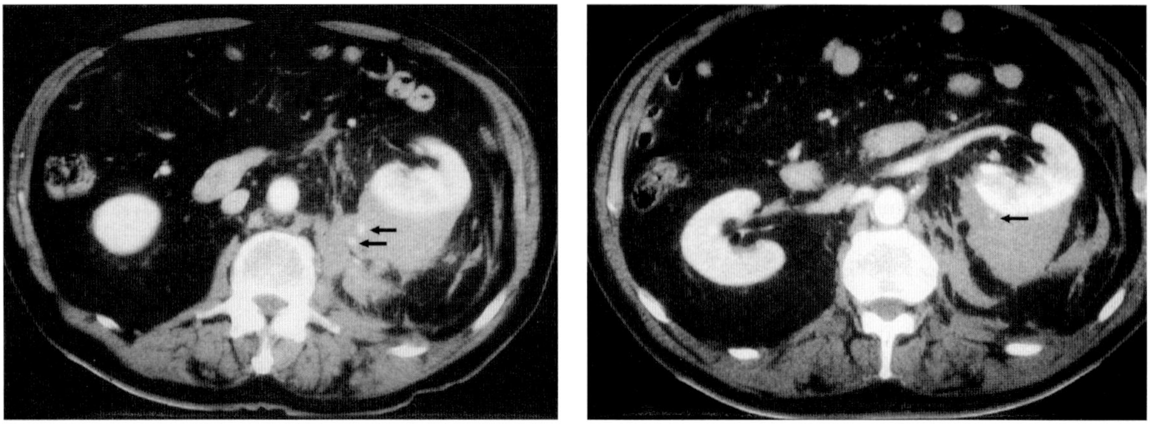

a b

Fig. 22.1a, b. This patient remained hemodynamically stable after a blunt trauma to the left flank. **a** CT at admission showed a moderate left posterior peri- and pararenal hematoma without renal injury, and two small foci of contrast extravasation (*arrows*) within the hematoma. CT suggests venous rather than arterial hemorrhage. **b** CT was repeated 24 h later and still showed a small spot of extravasated contrast material (*arrow*), with no increase in volume of the hematoma. No angiography was performed

imaging. In one study, the need of splenic intervention did not correlate with a contrast blush on CT, but correlated with injury grade, hypotension, and age (Omert et al. 2001). Some posttraumatic vascular lesions called immature pseudoaneurysms, particularly those of small size, may sometimes thrombose spontaneously and completely regress without intervention.

Therefore, the hemodynamic status of the patient, the number of blood transfusions, his or her ability to coagulate, metabolic parameters, and the overall assessment of severity of injury and type and number of associated lesions should be considered before indicating arteriography for hemostasis. Among CT findings, contrast extravasation is the most reliable sign for deciding on angiographic intervention or surgery, and is more important than description of the injury or assessment by grading systems. CT was found 90% sensitive and 98.6% specific in identifying patients with pelvic fractures requiring embolization (Pereira et al. 2000).

22.4 Diagnostic Arteriography

Angiography was introduced as a diagnostic modality of visceral injury in the mid-1950s and was used extensively during the 1960s and 1970s and less thereafter in the evaluation of visceral or large-vessel trauma (Norell 1957; Vogler and Bergmann 1963; Baum et al. 1965; Boijsen et al. 1966; Freeark et al. 1968; Love et al. 1968; Rose and Moore 1987). Angiographic signs of vascular or parenchymal injury are listed in Table 22.1. Some are not specific for a traumatic origin when taken as an isolated finding.

Overall, angiography confirms posttraumatic arterial bleeding in about 80%–98% of cases. In one study, no clinical factor predicted the likelihood to have a positive angiogram (Rose and Moore 1987; Velmahos et al. 2000 a, b). Results are mainly affected by false negatives, caused by intermittent vasospasm, spontaneous vaso-occlusion of a bleeding artery by thrombus formation, coexistence of several bleeding sites, venous or capillary bleeding that is not shown by

Table 22.1. Arteriographic signs of vascular or parenchymal injury

Arterial cut-off or transection	Stagnant arterial or venous flow
Mural irregularities or flap	Diffuse vasoconstriction
Laceration	Pseudoaneurysm
Thrombosis	Arteriovenous fistula
Dissection	Vessel displacement
Free-flow contrast extravasation	Intraparenchymal avascular zones
Stagnant intraparenchymal accumulation of contrast	Disruption of visceral contour
Parenchymal blush	Displaced organ

arteriography, technical inability to selectively catheterize the bleeding artery, insufficient concentration of iodine, or DSA technique related artifacts. False positives are a result of erroneous film interpretation: an adrenal blush, gastric or intestinal wall, a vessel seen end-on or overlying vessels, stagnant capillary flow or venous stasis should not be taken for contrast extravasation or a posttraumatic vascular lesion.

The arteriographic pathognomonic sign of extraluminal contrast extravasation is not 100% prognostic for ongoing hemorrhage: a limited extravasation within a parenchyma or within a hematoma may evolve in a self-contained manner into a pseudoaneurysm or an arteriovenous fistula that may persist or thrombose and regress or enlarge and rupture later. In our experience, there was an excellent overall correlation between CT and arteriography in demonstrating active bleeding, and the combination of the two modalities enhances diagnostic capabilities (Kurdziel et al. 1987; Kos et al. 1999).

22.5 Therapeutic Arteriography

22.5.1 Indications

As trauma victims are triaged by clinical assessment and CT for conservative management or intervention, arteriography is no longer used as a primary tool in demonstrating thoracoabdominal injury. In the pre-CT era, arteriography was first shown to be accurate in demonstrating renal injury (Lang 1976), but correlation was poor with the pathological findings in splenic injury and arteriography was found to be an unreliable predictor of management decision. A false-negative angiogram was observed in 24% of patients with splenic injury (Fisher et al. 1981). Similar criticism could be extrapolated to other parenchymal or extraparenchymal injuries studied angiographically. Over the past 20 years, with the advent of US and CT, the role of arteriography in trauma changed from a diagnostic to a therapeutic modality.

Although hemostatic embolization was recognized as an efficient means of treatment, arteriography is often not considered at the early posttraumatic phase, while blood loss is still compensated and coagulation and other homeostatic parameters are still within normal limits. Arteriography is often asked for when surgery has failed to obtain definite hemostasis or when resuscitation was protracted. Time loss has been significantly decreased in the diagnostic process in some specialized trauma centers by scanning trauma victims on a CT unit that is installed within the emergency environment. Diagnostic efficiency was also increased by the availability of radiologists who are dedicated to trauma and on call around the clock. Despite the general interest of radiologists in trauma, therapeutic angiography is not applied to its full potential (Selby 1992). Reasons for its underemployment are manifold: the absence of an integrated global diagnostic and therapeutic approach to the trauma patient by radiologists is a major limitation. General radiologists who read the CT examination of a trauma patient have a different approach than a trauma dedicated interventional radiologist. Residents who read CT examinations in the emergency room and are not interested in sharing responsibility in therapy are inadequate partners for case discussion on management options with trauma surgeons or intensive care physicians. Due to the dramatic decrease in diagnostic visceral angiographies, it takes now many years to train a radiologist in all aspects of interventional angiography. Besides the intrinsic logistic and functional problems encountered in a radiology department in offering a full range radiological trauma services, still other factors may lead to an untimely implementation of hemostatic angiography or surgical treatment (Ben-Menachem et al. 1979, 1981; Ben-Menachem 1988):

- Over-reliance on a technically inadequate CT examination or declaring that injuries recognized on CT are not at risk of bleeding.
- Miscalculation of the severity of injury: a shock status should not be attributed to brain injury alone, unless proved otherwise. Children compensate for considerable blood loss by maintaining normal blood pressure for a longer period of time than adults. Clinical examination and laboratory findings are not reliable predictive factors of need for hemostatic intervention in children or adults. Absence of contrast medium extravasation on a positive CT for injuries is not a sign of definite hemostasis. A patient may rebleed when arterial pressure has increased again and vasoconstriction has ceased or after endogenous clot lysis. The most severe injury seen on CT is not necessarily one that will rebleed: a severe hepatic contusion might have stopped bleeding, while an injured lumbar artery goes on bleeding profusely.
- Inadequate assessment of the mechanism of injury: in blunt trauma, right, left, and midline package abdominal injury must be understood

to extrapolate all potential organs that might be involved together in the same anatomical area. Injuries created by contra-coup are located on the side opposite the impact, and can be a concomitant source of bleeding (Rao et al. 1997).

- Inadequate assessment of postoperative hemorrhage: a missed or an inadequately treated vascular injury rather than a wash-out coagulopathy should be searched for when hemorrhage persists or recurs after operation. A marginally stable patient who is transferred to a specialized trauma center after a damage control laparotomy should undergo systematic arteriography before reintervention, to disclose either a missed or an additional iatrogenic vascular injury created during the first intervention. CT alone may not be sufficient, as selective arteriography is still able to show more small vascular injuries than CT.
- A classic adage recommends that one "never put an unstable patient on the X-ray table": CT and angiography can be obtained in the emergency room environment while resuscitation is ongoing. Unnecessary patient transfer can be avoided by the use of a combined CT-angio room (Capasso et al. 1996; Kos et al. 1999). Unstable patients with retroperitoneal hemorrhage, which is best treated by selective embolization, should be deliberately moved to the angiography suite, provided that medical and paramedical radiological expertise is available to the same degree as in the operating room.

22.5.2 Technique

22.5.2.1 Principles

After having localized the source of hemorrhage angiographically, hemostasis is obtained by catheter embolization. The hemostatic endovascular embolization technique is different in principle from (chemo)embolization for tumor mass or organ function reduction or vaso-occlusion of a vascular malformation. In trauma, spontaneous hemostasis of a visceral or extravisceral artery is usually induced by vasoconstriction and formation of a clot at the site of vascular tear and subsequent scar formation by granulation tissue or vessel lumen recanalization. Catheter-mediated treatment should be diverted from the physiological process of hemostasis:

- A temporary arterial occlusion with resorbable material may be sufficient to initiate local thrombus formation. Late vessel lumen recanalization is not a concern.
- Vaso-occlusion should take place exclusively at the site of vascular injury.
- No or minimal tissue loss should be induced by embolization.
- Furthermore, recurrent bleeding should be avoided by formation of a stable clot.

22.5.2.2 Percutaneous Arterial Access

Percutaneous access is gained in general by a right or left femoral approach. When major pelvic bone fractures or severe tissue damage is present at the inguinal region, the opposite femoral side or a left brachial or axillary arterial puncture is chosen. In a hypotensive patient with a faint pulse, ultrasound Doppler guidance or bone landmarks may be helpful with fluoroscopy monitoring to guide vessel puncture. When the femoral vein was inadvertently punctured, venous access should be preserved and a hemostatic valve sheath should be placed. The sheath can serve as a landmark for the arterial puncture and as an additional large-flow infusion line. A 5F valve sheath is adequate for diagnosis and embolization in all cases and is particularly useful in trauma angiography, allowing for rapid catheter exchange or immediate withdrawal of a catheter blocked with plugged embolization agents or a partially delivered coil.

22.5.2.3 Catheterization Technique for Diagnostic Arteriography

Even though 90% of angiographies are based on contrast extravasation, shown on CT, a midstream thoracic or abdominal and pelvic aortogram should always be obtained before selective catheterization (Sclafani 1985). An aortogram shows the mapping of aortic collaterals, anatomical variants, and unsuspected traumatic or nontraumatic preexisting lesions. It also establishes priorities in selective catheterization, when several bleeding sites coexist. Selective arteriography is based on CT and midstream aortography findings. Preshaped sidewinder Simmons type or Cobra-shaped 4F or 5F catheters are usually adequate for most catheterizations. Catheter manipulation should be carried out rapidly, but gently, avoiding creation of endothelial injury, which makes further catheterization impossible. Vasoconstriction in a shocked patient favors arterial dissection by the catheter tip and thrombosis. Hydrophilic catheters and guidewires are helpful. A negative midstream aortogram does not eliminate the possibility of extravasation, as concentration of contrast medium, as well as flow and pressure conditions are different at the site of vascular injury during an aortic or a selective arterial injection. Care must be applied to obtain a selective arteriogram of the hepatic, splenic, or renal artery, for instance, with a proximal position of the catheter tip. A too distal catheterization may miss significant branches such as an upper pole splenic artery or a proximal division of a renal or common hepatic artery.

22.5.2.4 Carbon Dioxide Arteriography

Carbon dioxide digital subtraction angiography (CO_2-DSA) was introduced in the early 1980s and thereafter applied to the diagnosis of vascular injury in a limited number of reports (Sato et al. 1991; Hashimoto et al. 1997; Hawkins et al. 1997). The assumption was that the lower viscosity of CO_2 compared to iodinated contrast medium would make even minute bleeding through a minimal tear in the vascular wall visible. In one series, intra-arterial CO_2-DSA demonstrated extravasation in 52% of the cases, whereas iodinated contrast extravasation was seen in only 13% of the same patients (Hashimoto et al. 1997). It has not been proven whether extravasation shown by CO_2-DSA that was not evidenced on iodine DSA requires hemostasis in all cases. Injection in the hepatic artery shows arterioportal shunting in normal liver, and CO_2 may still pass in the gastrointestinal lumen after embolization, despite demonstration by iodine angiography of complete vaso-occlusion. Therefore, CO_2-DSA is at risk of overdiagnosing extravasation or arterioportal fistula, and when used alone, without iodine angiography, it may lead to overtreatment. CO_2-DSA is too sensitive to determine significance of bleeding and to appreciate the endpoint of embolization (Hawkins et al. 1997). Advantages of CO_2-DSA are absence of allergic reaction, nephrotoxicity and other significant side effects, low cost, unlimited permissible volume, and easy passage through the smallest catheter. However, due to the possible gas embolism in the brain or myocardium, intra-arterial injection is contraindicated in arteries located above the diaphragm.

22.5.2.5 Implementation of an Integrated CT-Angiography Unit

The use of an integrated CT-angiography unit has undeniable advantages in urgent angiographic management of posttraumatic hemorrhage (Capasso et al. 1996; Kos et al. 1999). Both devices are preferably installed in the emergency department environment and are linked with a common patient support. The table may be shifted or turned from the CT to the angiography position and vice-versa, as in the prototype unit that we have designed (Fig. 22.2). Other room configurations have been envisioned such as an

a 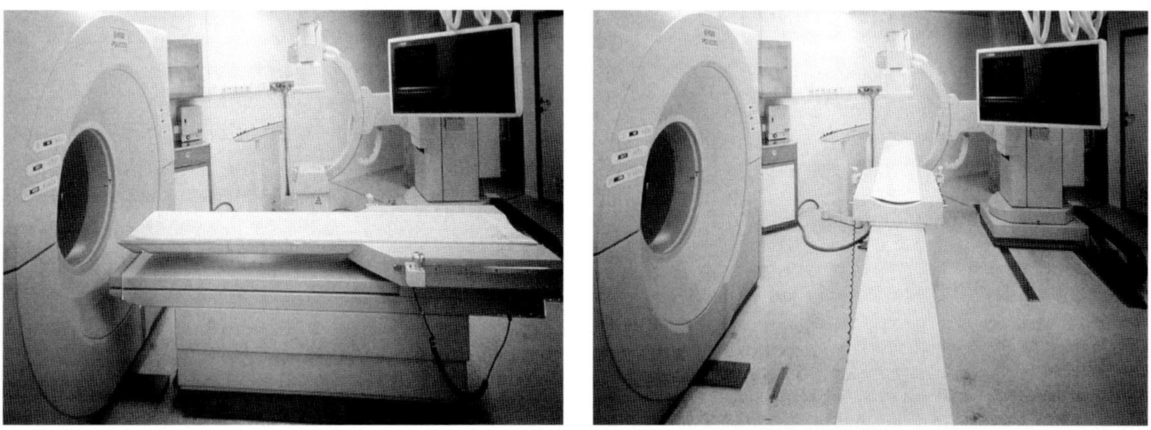 b

Fig. 22.2a, b. Computed tomography equipment and an angiography unit with a mobile C-arm are installed together in the emergency environment. Both units are served by a common patient support, avoiding patient transfer and time loss between CT examination and hemostatic arteriographic embolization. A prototype unit presented with a movable patient support, pivoting between the CT (**a**) and angiography position (**b**) alignment of the CT gantry and the C-arm, making pivoting of the table unnecessary, or a mobile angiography C-arm and/or a mobile CT gantry. The CT and angiography unit can also be installed separately in adjacent rooms for independent use and are brought together on rails when needed. No mobilization of the patient or of the anesthesiology team or ancillary equipment is required. Prolonged transit time of the trauma patient in the radiology suite and the risk of severe hypothermia is avoided. Absence of patient mobilization minimizes creation or increase in damage in hypotensive patients or those presenting with spinal or pelvic bone fractures.

A radiologist who is an expert in trauma imaging, including CT and vascular diagnostic and interventional procedures, should be on duty to ensure the full potential of such an integrated CT-angiography suite. Reading the CT examinations is now done exclusively on the console, using the cine mode, and the decision to treat arterial hemorrhage by embolization should be made immediately at the end of the CT examination by the multidisciplinary trauma team.

22.5.2.6 Embolization Agents

The principal agents used for vaso-occlusion in trauma include Gelfoam, coils, and particles (Ayella et al. 1978; Probst et al. 1978; Panetta et al. 1985b; Klein et al. 1990).

- Gelfoam pledgets of variable size are cut and injected with a syringe containing contrast medium (Fig. 22.3a). Small fragments of Gelfoam pass through the lumen of a 3F catheter. Gelfoam powder should be avoided, as it may result in too distal embolization, carrying the risk of tissue infarction or late abscess formation.
- Particulate material of small size (100–500 μm) is used during flow directed embolization of a bleeding source that is located in a small vessel (Fig. 22.3b). Polygonal particles should be preferred to spherical particles, to avoid too distal embolization. The risk of fan-embolization in adjacent territories is higher with particles than with Gelfoam pledgets.
- Coils come in different shapes, lengths, and diameters (Fig. 22.3c). Their main advantage is a precise targeted delivery. When properly selected, secondary coil migration after delivery almost never occurs. Coils with a tornado configuration allow for immediate luminal occlusion by a compact coiling.
- Vaso-occlusion can also be simply achieved by an occlusive catheterization of an end-artery such as in the kidney or spleen. Iatrogenic posttraumatic intrarenal pseudoaneurysm or arteriovenous fistula may thrombose, by simply stopping the flow for several minutes, while the tip of the catheter is maintained in an occluded position. In noniatrogenic injury, however, this technique is not recommended, as several potentially hemorrhaging injuries might coexist on the same artery, or the ability of the patient to coagulate may be impaired, resulting in rebleeding.

22.5.2.7 Catheterization Technique for Therapeutic Occlusion

Selective catheterization is directed without time loss to the bleeding artery, but an overview angiographic run, demonstrating the entire organ or region is mandatory before selective catheterization, to recognize all

a
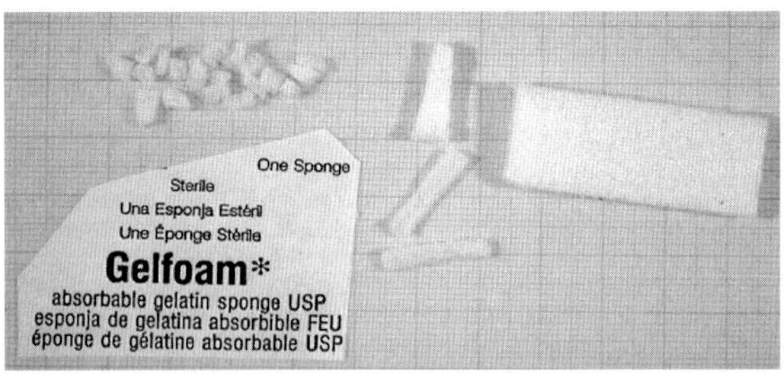

b
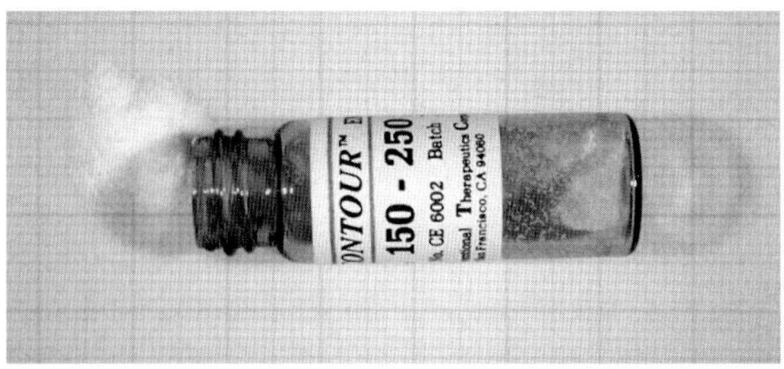

c
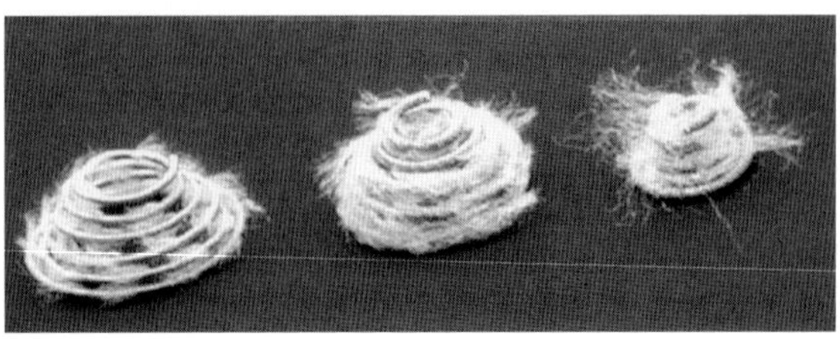

Fig. 22.3. **a** Gelfoam strips, cut into small pledgets pass through an 3F microcatheter and give a temporary hemostatic vaso-occlusion. **b** Polyvinyl alcohol particles with a diameter of 100–500 μm pass through a microcatheter and are suitable for selective embolization of end arterioles. **c** Macrocoils or microcoils with cotton strands are available in various configurations, lengths, and diameters and are most suitable for elective placement, giving a permanent vaso-occlusion

arteries feeding the bleeding site. The bleeding arterial branch should be catheterized as selectively as possible to avoid undesirable tissue infarction, or amputation of organ function. Injection of the embolizing agent is thus precisely targeted, the tip of the catheter being placed proximal to the site of extravasation. This is the standard technique for intraparenchymal end arteries such as in the splenic or renal parenchyma. Five-French catheters are usually too large for a selective catheterization of the site of hemorrhage; 3F or 2F catheters that are introduced coaxially, are best suited for a targeted deposition of embolization material. Selective angiograms by manual injection of several milliliters of contrast are sufficient to check the catheter position and flow conditions before embolization. The road mapping technique, multiple projections, and direct magnification are useful.

22.5.2.8
Vaso-Occlusive Technique

- When an arterial rupture with discontinuous flow is evidenced in a lobar liver artery, for instance, a sandwich embolization technique is used, placing coils distal and proximal to the arterial interruption.
- When a pseudoaneurysm is present, a similar sandwich technique should be used, and never intrasaccular filling with coils. Indeed, the pseudowall of a recent posttraumatic pseudoaneurysm is extremely fragile and may rupture at the contact of the guidewire or catheter tip. Intrasaccular filling with coils increases the pressure in the sac, which may result in acute or delayed rupture and fatal hemorrhage if the parent vessel remains patent.
- Embolization with coils in the splenic artery proximal to the hilar branching was described as an equivalent to the surgical Keramidas procedure. The intervention consists in ligation of the splenic artery at the splenic hilum, without creating necrosis to the spleen, which remains vascularized through epiploic, short gastric, and transcapsular arteries (Keramidas 1979). This technique might be used in high-grade splenic injury, without extravasation seen, as a preventive treatment of rebleeding. Proximal embolization of the renal and hepatic artery is contraindicated, as irreversible renal ischemia would follow and severe disturbances of the liver function, particularly in a patient with traumatic shock.
- A large artery that shows a cut-off on arteriography, should be embolized systematically with coils, proximal to the complete vessel interruption, even in the absence of contrast medium extravasation, to avoid rebleeding after resolution of vasospasm and endogenous thrombolysis. High-pressure injection of contrast medium through a catheter placed close to a large thrombosed artery (iliac artery for instance) should be avoided, as a primary hemostatic thrombus may be fragmented by pressure and the ruptured vessel open again to extravasation. The burst effect of injection of CO_2 may have similar effects.
- A tangential vascular wall rupture in a large-caliber patent artery (iliac, subclavian artery) can be treated by urgent placement of a covered metal stent. Posttraumatic rupture of the thoracic aorta at the level of the isthmus or descending portion were treated in semi-urgent conditions by placement of a stent graft (Rousseau et al. 1999).

22.6
Organ-Specific Hemostatic Embolization

22.6.1
Splenic Injuries

In the spleen, transcatheter hemostatic arterial embolization is carried out in selected patients as an alternative to surgical spleen-preserving interventions (Chuang and Reuter 1975). Indications are based on focal intra- or extrasplenic contrast medium extravasation seen on CT. In the spleen, helical CT confidently predicts extravasation observed on splenic arteriography and the need for hemostatic arterial embolization (Shanmuganathan et al. 2000). However, treatment was obtained in stable patients. Some of the vascular lesions observed may have regressed and thrombosed spontaneously. Splenic arteriography precisely localizes a pseudoaneurysm or an arteriovenous fistula or thrombosis of a disrupted arterial branch. The systematic use of microcatheters that are introduced coaxially through a guiding catheter, placed in the proximal part of the splenic artery, allows a selective catheterization of a bleeding intrasplenic branch. Technical failures caused by tortuosity of the splenic artery are thus limited. As intrasplenic arteries are terminal vessels, selective embolization of the branch, proximal to the site of extravasation, gives a definitive vaso-occlusion, without risk of recanalization by collateral or retrograde flow. When several intrasplenic bleeding sites are documented, each branch feeding an extravasation should be selectively catheterized and embolized close to the vascular injury, to limit the extent of splenic tissue infarction. Minicoils or particulate agents are most often used in the smallest arterial branches. Placement of macrocoils or large Gelfoam fragments in the main splenic artery at the hilar bifurcation, as an equivalent to arterial ligation (Keramidas intervention), should be avoided except in a shattered spleen as a prevention of rebleeding, when no extravasation is seen (Keramidas 1979) (Fig. 22.4). Reducing the pressure in the intrasplenic arteries by a proximal embolization in the main splenic artery might not be sufficient to obtain a permanent hemostasis, and massive splenic gastric wall or pancreatic infarction is a potential complication when a too proximal embolization has been performed.

Selective embolization, without the need for subsequent splenic surgery, being part of the initial management protocol and based on extravasation seen on CT or angiography, is successful in 87%–95% of patients (Sclafani et al. 1991; Hagiwara et al. 1996). In another study, an intrasplenic blush of contrast was seen on CT in 8% of patients with blunt splenic injury and confirmed to be a pseudoaneurysm on arteriography; 20 of 26 patients were successfully embolized, and 6 underwent splenectomy for technical failure of embolization (Davis et al. 1998). In a personal experience of 19 patients managed with arterial splenic embolization at admission, bleeding was stopped in 17 without requiring splenectomy. CT shows on postembolization examinations splenic infarcts in two-thirds of the patients after proximal embolization and in all cases after distal vaso-occlusion. Gas in the embolized splenic area or in small arterial branches may be seen, particularly after Gelfoam embolization. Necrotic areas, liquefaction, and air fluid level are suggestive of abscess formation (Killeen et al. 2001).

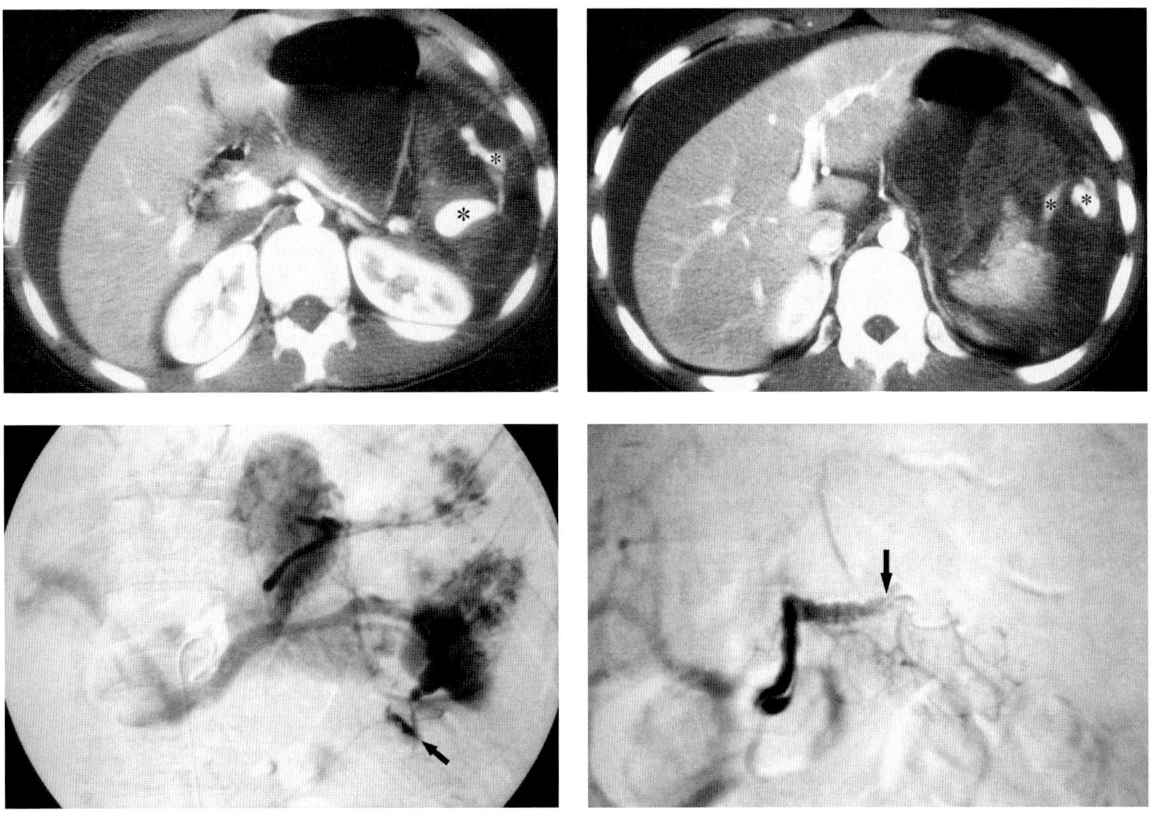

Fig. 24.4a–d. This patient was admitted in shock after blunt abdominal trauma. **a, b** CT at admission showed a shattered spleen with multiple sites of contrast extravasation (*asterisk*), an intra- and perisplenic hematoma, and perihepatic hemoperitoneum. **c** Splenic arteriography was obtained on an integrated CT-angiography unit, without patient transfer. The parenchymal phase showed a fragmented spleen and contrast extravasation at the lower pole of the spleen (*arrow*). **d** Embolization of the splenic artery with large Gelfoam fragments was obtained at the level of the hilar bifurcation (*arrow*) for immediate and definitive hemostasis

22.6.2 Hepatic Injuries

Hepatic artery embolization was shown to be a valuable adjunct in the management of posttraumatic hepatic hemorrhage (Boijsen et al. 1966; Bass and Crosier 1977; Allison et al. 1985). Embolization on an emergency basis and as a primary hemostatic treatment was reported in small series of patients (Bass and Crosier 1977; Allison et al. 1985; Jander et al. 1977; Rubin and Katzen 1977; Hashimoto et al. 1990; Yitzhak et al. 2001) (Fig. 22.5). Emergency arterial liver embolization can be performed in marginally stable patients with complex liver injury in specialized centers. Other reports illustrated the value of arterial embolization for ongoing or recurrent hemorrhage, despite laparotomy (Bass and Crosier 1977; Wagner et al. 1985; Fandrich et al. 1989; De Toma et al. 1994; Yitzhak et al. 2001). General indications for angiography and arterial hepatic embolization are evidence of continuous hemorrhage or patients who remain borderline after resuscitation and in whom contrast medium extravasation or intraparenchymal blush or contrast staining is seen on CT (Sherman 1996; Carillo et al. 1999; Gorich et al. 1999; Harper and Maull 2000). Such management requires optimal organization and skills in the radiology department (Sugimoto et al. 1994). Patients with early ongoing hepatic bleeding after primary surgical hemostasis and patients who

a b c d

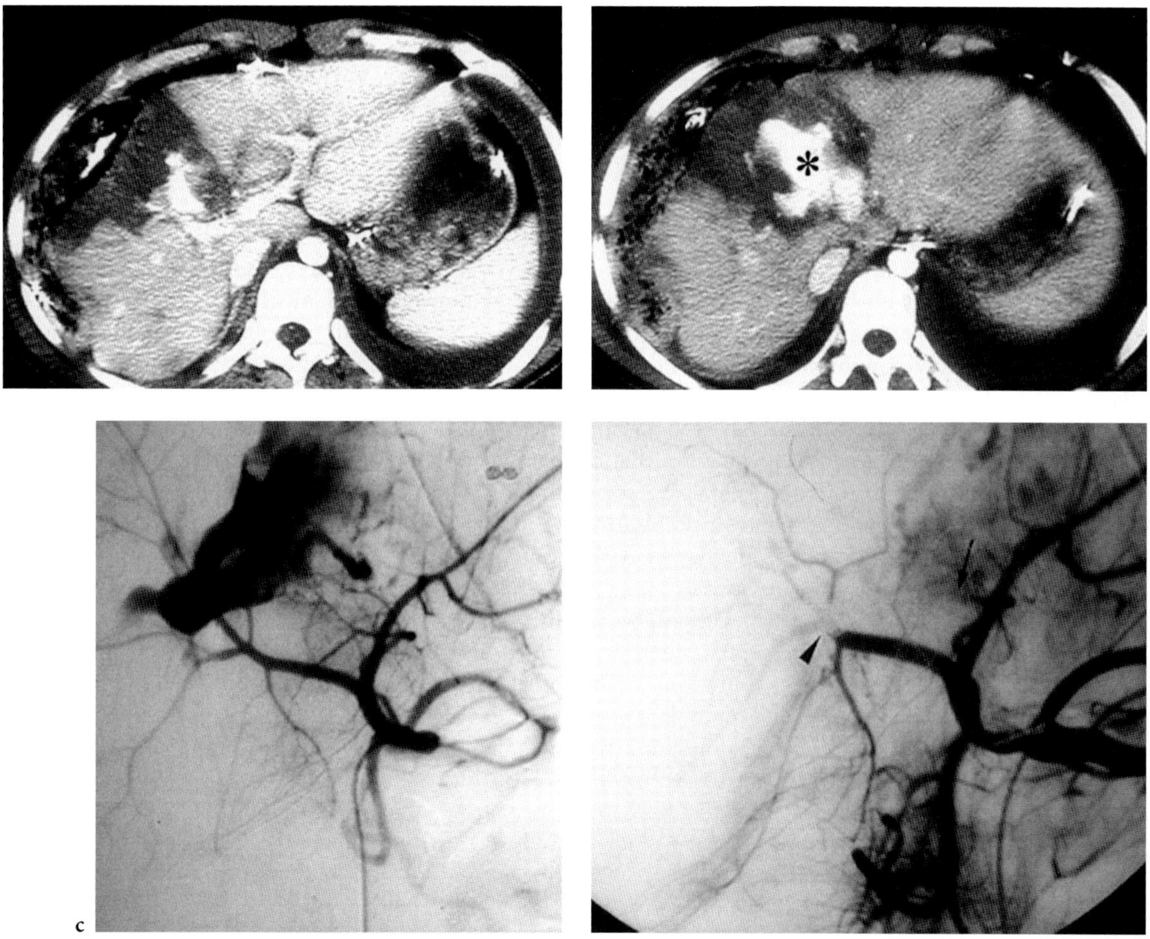

Fig. 22.5a–d. A 42-year-old male was transferred from another hospital after emergency laparotomy for abdominal trauma. At admission, the patient was marginally stable, blood oozing through the surgical drains. **a, b** CT repeated at admission showed massive contrast extravasation at arterial phase within the right hepatic contusion (*asterisk*). Note perihepatic packing. **c** Hepatic arteriography was immediately obtained on a combined CT-angiography unit, which reproduced massive intrahepatic contrast extravasation from the right and left hepatic artery. Hemostatic embolization was achieved with Gelfoam pledgets. **d** Postembolization arteriography showed effective vaso-occlusion of the right hepatic artery (*arrowhead*) and of medial branches (*arrow*) of the left hepatic artery. Definitive hemostasis required an additional embolization of the left hepatic artery 24 h later

are referred after a crash laparotomy should also undergo arteriography and when necessary, embolization, avoiding reoperation (De Toma et al. 1994). Patients who rebleed after an initially successful embolization should be treated again angiographically. Arterial embolization is said to be contributive to the overall better outcome of liver injuries, which is also explained by a relative decrease in major liver injuries and improved surgical results for major injury (Richardson et al. 2000).

In a recent study, arterial embolization was shown 100% effective in treating extravasation of contrast medium in the liver following blunt hepatic injury in a cohort of hemodynamically stabilized patients with 52% grade 3 and 4 injury. Fifty-four percent of patients submitted to angiography showed contrast extravasation. Following embolization, CT was repeated for 3 weeks, once a week. A pseudoaneurysm was detected during follow-up in 6% of patients and treated by embolization. Overall mortality was 0%. However, two patients developed severe hepatic hemorrhage at 2 and 3 weeks following admission, requiring a second emergency embolization of a bleeding pseudoaneurysm (Hagiwara et al. 1997). In another study, 16 of 30 patients with blunt liver injury underwent arterial hemostatic embolization. Patients were markedly unstable and had hemoperitoneum, deep liver laceration (grade III), and contrast extravasation on angiography in 14 of 16. Patients were stabilized after embolization and no major complication was observed (Murakami et al. 1993). In another study of 24 patients with posttraumatic vascular lesions, transcatheter occlusion was successful in 88%. Cause of failure was inability to catheterize the lesion with the catheter, persistent flow in an arteriovenous fistula after embolization, and late recurrence (Schwartz et al. 1993). Patients with grade IV and V hepatic injury who remain hemodynamically stable with continued resuscitation, could undergo hepatic arteriography and embolization, bridging the therapeutic option of nonoperative intervention and surgery. Treatment was effective in 10 of 11 patients (Giraulo et al. 1998).

Recent experience in high-grade liver injury (grades IV and V) managed with a surgical, angiographic, and endoscopic biliary approach showed an overall mortality of 14% and hepatic surgery-related mortality of 9% (8% for grade IV and 22% for grade V) (Asensio et al. 2000).

Complications of arterial hepatic embolization mainly include rebleeding due to incomplete vaso-occlusion or coagulopathy and later hepatic infarction or abscess, bile duct or gallbladder necrosis or biloma-hematoma. Hepatic infarct is most likely to occur when the portal vein or a lobar branch is occluded concomitantly to arterial embolization (Takukawa et al. 1993). Delayed rebleeding after embolization is reported only in a small percentage of patients, and also occurs in a few percent after surgical hemostasis. Emphasis is put on the possible relation between a biloma and formation of a pseudoaneurysm that is responsible for secondary hemorrhage, despite initially successful embolization (Hagiwara 1993).

22.6.3 Renal Injuries

Renal contusions are accessible to conservative management in the majority of cases; however, avulsion of the vascular pedicle must be treated surgically in the first hours following injury to preserve renal function. Renal arteriography is indicated, based on CT findings, when extravasation of contrast is seen in or around the kidney. Extravasation should not be confused with extravasated opaque urine, resulting from a previous contrast injection (brain CT, IVP, or others). In some hemodynamically unstable patients with evidence of a flank impact and suspicion of massive renal and/or retroperitoneal hemorrhage, urgent arteriography may be obtained without a previous CT examination. Renal arteriography must include a midstream aortogram, to confirm the presence of a normal contralateral kidney and display the number and origin of renal arteries (Fig. 22.6). Embolization should be carried out rapidly, before a subcapsular hematoma severely compresses the underlying renal parenchyma and makes selective intrarenal catheterization difficult or impossible. The number and location of the bleeding sites must be precisely identified by serial angiographic runs during and after embolization. The use of 3F catheters for selective distal intraparenchymal catheterization is standard (Fig. 22.7). When multiple intraparenchymal arteries bleed, requiring total nephrectomy, complete vaso-occlusion is an alternative, making it possible to control other associated injuries first and perform nephrectomy later in a stabilized patient.

Hemostatic embolization in the kidney is successful in 82%–100% as a primary treatment (Uflacker et al. 1984; Fisher and Ben-Menachem 1985; Fisher et al. 1989; De Bock and Verhagen 1989; Kramer et al. 1998). When hematuria persists or recurs, renal arteriography should be repeated and when posi-

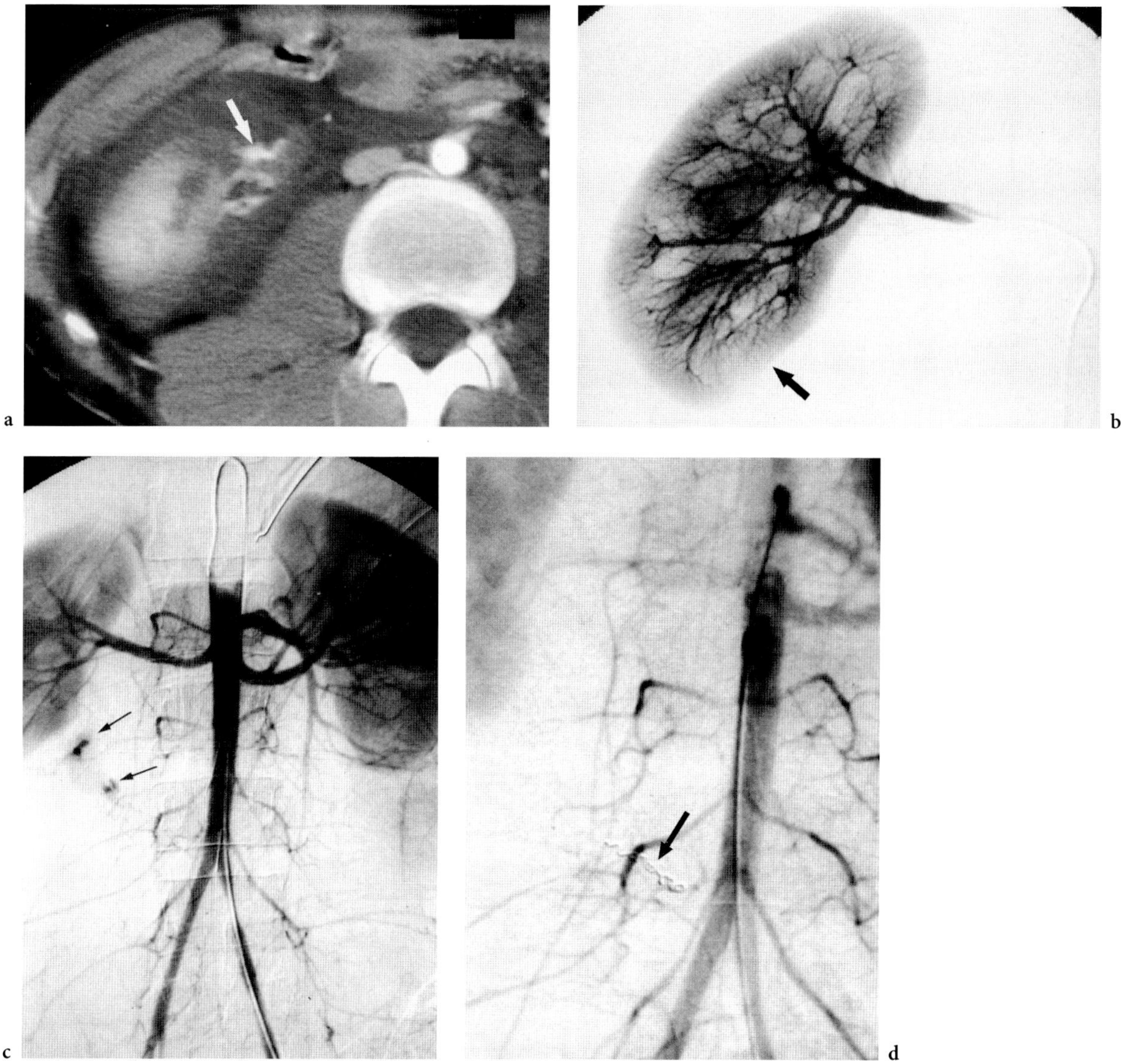

Fig. 22.6a–d. A 22-year-old patient was admitted after a blunt impact to the right flank. **a** CT at admission showed, at the arterial phase, contrast extravasation (*arrow*) around the lower pole of the right kidney, a limited renal parenchymal contusion, and perirenal and retroperitoneal hematoma. **b** Selective arteriography of the right kidney was normal but the flattened medial contour of the lower pole (arrow) suggested the presence of an inferior polar renal artery. **c** Abdominal aortography showed two foci of contrast extravasation (*arrows*), probably from a small lower pole renal artery, originating from the distal abdominal aorta. **d** After catheterization of the angiographically invisible lower pole renal artery and embolization with microcoils (*arrow*), no extravasation was seen on abdominal aortography

tive, a persistent or new vascular injury should be re-embolized. Less than 10% of severe complications are noted following embolization, including sepsis, urinary fistula, or renal infarction (Fisher and Ben-Menachem 1985; Larsen and Pentecost 1992). When conservative treatment is applied, serial cross-section imaging must ensure that no vascular injury persists or develops, which may lead to significant delayed hemorrhage (Teigen et al. 1992).

22.6.4 Retroperitoneal Injuries

Posttraumatic retroperitoneal bleeding is primarily investigated and treated angiographically. Often, surgery carries the risk of cataclysmic hemorrhage by dissection of the retroperitoneal space and loss of passive tamponade of a hematoma. Classically, one or several lumbar arteries bleed, and giant pseudoaneurysms

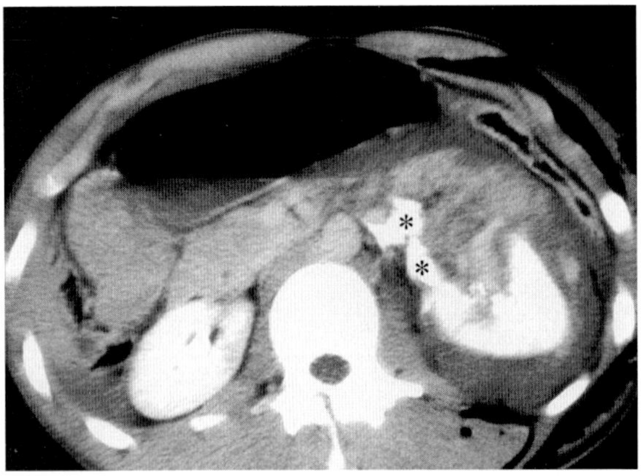

a

Fig. 24.7a–d. This 42-year-old male was admitted in shock after a blunt impact to the left flank. **a** CT showed contrast extravasation at the arterial phase, accumulating at the hilum of the left kidney. Extravasated high-density arterial contrast (*asterisk*) should not be mistaken for extravasated urine at the late phase, after IV contrast medium injection. **b** Midstream abdominal aortography and left renal arteriography were obtained immediately after CT on combined CT-angiography equipment. Contrast extravasation (*arrow*) is better seen on selective renal arteriography than on aortography. Note diffuse arterial vasoconstriction due to massive retroperitoneal hemorrhage. **c** Several bleeding sites were evidenced angiographically (*asterisk*) and treated by selective embolization with microcoils using a coaxial catheterization technique. **d** Left renal arteriography after embolization (*arrows*) showed limited vascular amputation of the lower pole renal parenchyma

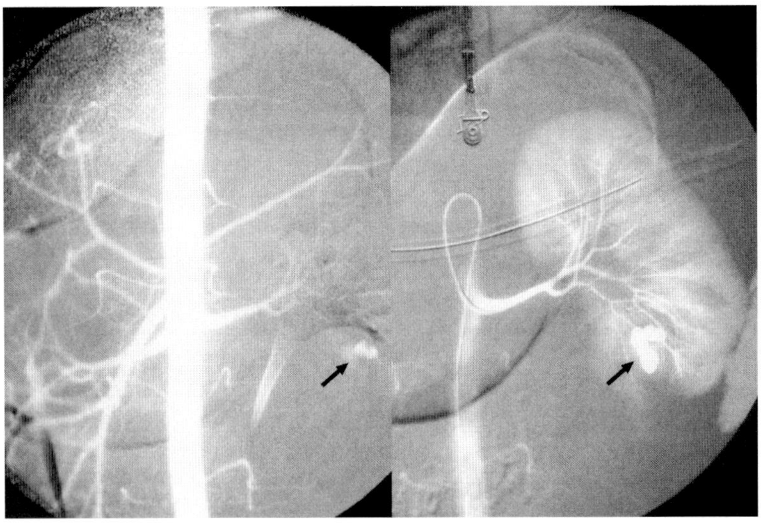

b

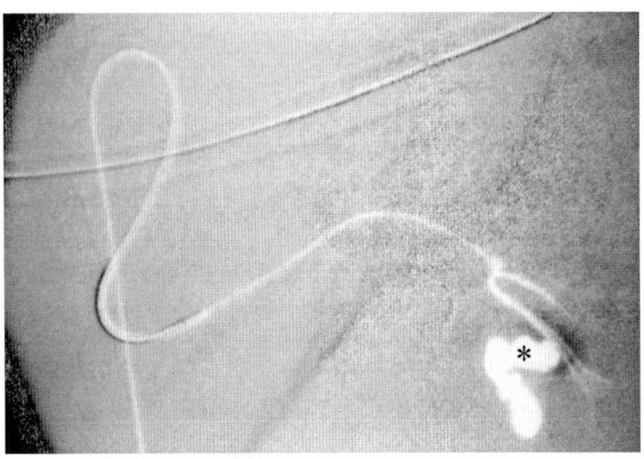

c

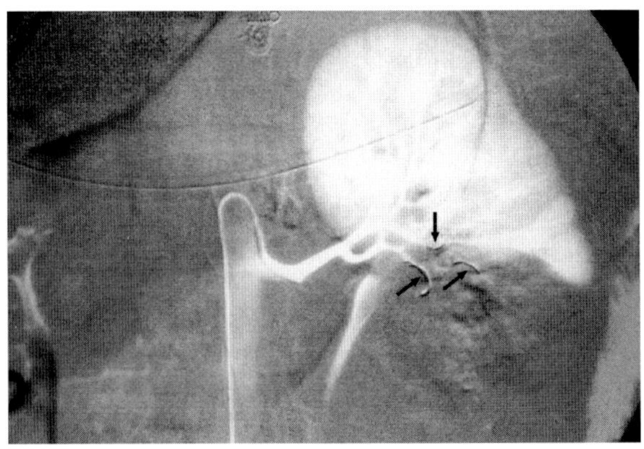

d

can be found. Other arterial branches such as those originating from intercostal, inferior phrenic, adrenal, pancreaticoduodenal and other arteries may participate in feeding a retroperitoneal hemorrhage (Chang et al. 1978; Haydu et al. 1978; Fankuchen et al. 1981; Mandel et al. 1987; Sclafani et al. 1987; Ikubo et al. 1993) (Fig. 22.8). These arteries should be catheterized selectively, when a retroperitoneal hematoma increases in size and no extravasation is demonstrated on abdominal aortography and selective lumbar arteriography. In some cases, when selective arteriography and intravenously injected CT are negative for contrast extravasation, a selective arterially enhanced CT may be the only modality that is able to show the bleeding (Kos et al. 1999). When a lumbar or intercostal artery must be embolized at the thoracolumbar level,

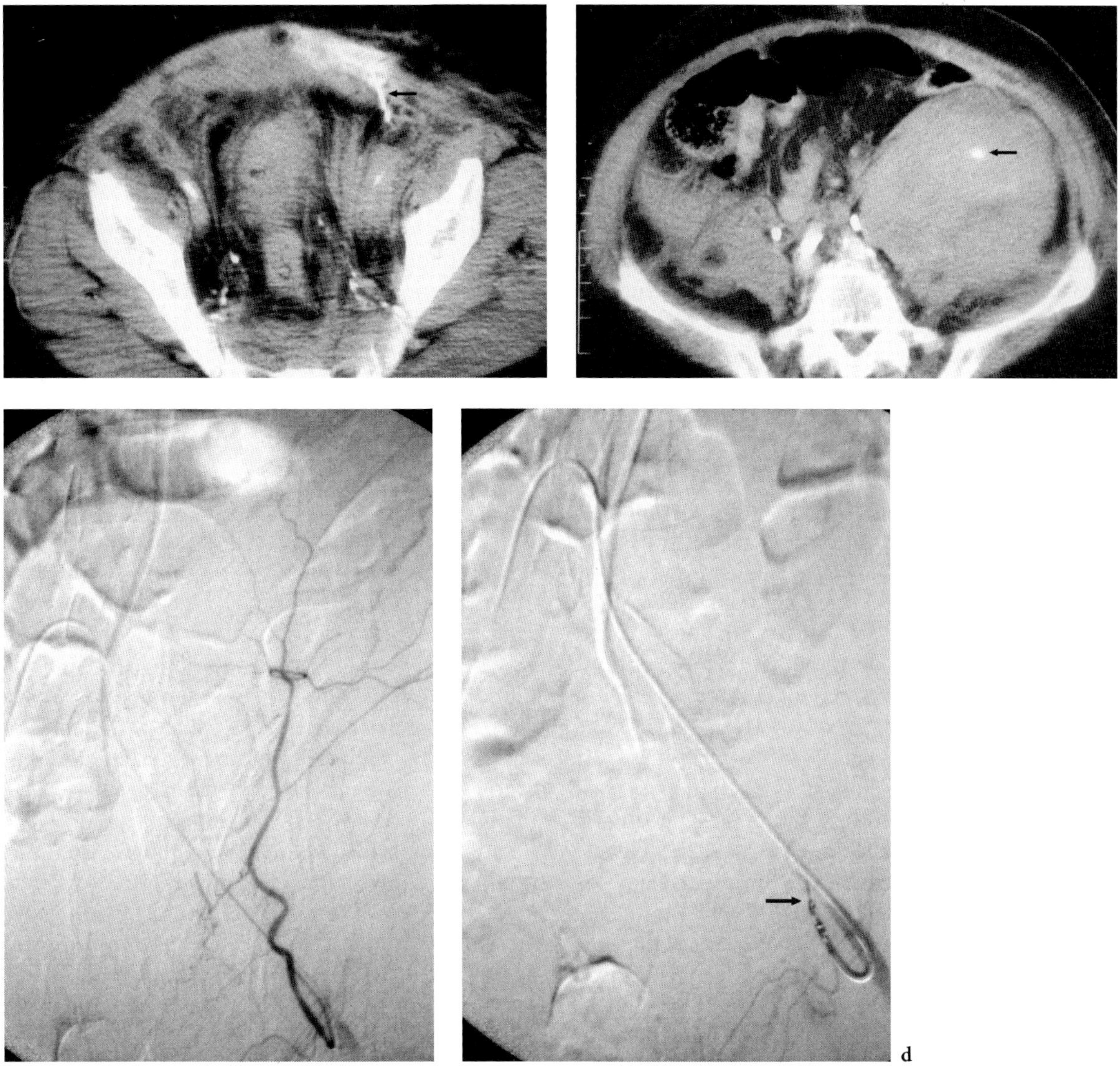

a b c d

Fig. 24.8a–d. An 80-year-old female patient was admitted after blunt abdominal trauma. The patient became unstable after admission and complained of left flank pain. CT showed a large left retroperitoneal hematoma without contrast extravasation (not shown). **a** An arterially enhanced CT examination was obtained on an integrated CT-angiography unit; the catheter was placed selectively in the left inferior epigastric artery (*arrow*). **b** Extravasation was seen (*arrow*) within the left retroperitoneal hematoma. **c** No extravasation was seen on selective DSA of the left inferior epigastric artery. **d** Despite the negative arteriography, but positive CT, the left inferior epigastric artery was embolized with microcoils (*arrow*). The patient was stabilized after hemostatic embolization

the origin of a spinal artery must be recognized, and inadvertent embolization is avoided by distal catheterization and the use of large particles. The metameric levels adjacent to the bleeding lumbar artery should also be occluded, to prevent rebleeding by revascularization through vertical interlumbar connections. In renal injury, when contrast medium extravasation is seen, selective embolization is the treatment of choice in most patients who are stable or marginally stable. Renal vein laceration requires laparotomy to obtain hemostasis (Hagiwara et al. 2001).

22.6.5 Pelvic Injuries

Posttraumatic pelvic bleeding is of arterial, venous, or bone origin. Arterial injuries are the most severe and are predominantly observed in anterior-posterior pelvic compression injuries type 2 and 3, lateral compression injuries type 3, vertical compression injuries, and combined injury mechanisms (Bassam et al. 1998). The instability of pelvic bone fractures and fractures involving the iliosacral region and pelvic symphysis are a good predictor of the need for hemostatic embolization and prompts rapid orthopedic fixation as a first treatment (MAULL and SACHATELLO 1976; MEARS 1980; GYLLING et al. 1985; HORI et al. 1990; BURGESS et al. 1990; BEN-MENACHEM et al. 1991; EASTRIDGE and BURGESS 1997). In one study, the following factors predicted the need for pelvic arterial embolization: older age, high abbreviated injury score for pelvic fractures, number of blood transfusions, and major pelvic ligament rupture (HAMILL et al. 2000). Of patients with pelvic fractures, 2%–5% require arterial embolization (PALMER et al. 1983; MUCHA and WELCH 1988; AGOLINI et al. 1997; GARBUGLIA et al. 1998; PEREIRA et al. 2000). It has been suggested that angiography should be implemented in the unstable patients, when laparotomy was not indicated. If laparotomy is indicated, fixation should be applied intraoperatively, followed by angiography (BASSAM et al. 1998).

As for retroperitoneal bleeding, diagnostic peritoneal lavage and surgical dissection are not indicated to obtain hemostasis, and urological interventions should be postponed after angiographic intervention (BEN-MENACHEM 1988, BEN-MENACHEM et al. 1985; EVERS et al. 1989; GOINS et al. 1992; BEN-MENACHEM 1997). Moreover, spontaneous tamponade, external compression, and blind ligation of the hypogastric artery seem ineffective (PLATZ et al. 1992). Contrast extravasation is seen on CT in patients with fractures in 4.5%, 69% of patients being hemodynamically unstable (PEREIRA et al. 2000). Patients with contrast extravasation had a significantly higher Injury Severity Score, more blood transfusions, and a longer hospital stay. CT was found 80%–92% sensitive and 98% specific in predicting the need for arterial embolization based on contrast extravasation corresponding to significant arterial bleeding (GILLIAND et al. 1982; STEPHEN et al. 1999). A contralateral femoral approach to the suspected side of bleeding is chosen for arteriography. An abdominal and a pelvic aortogram are obtained to demonstrate all potential bleeding sites. The bleeding artery is catheterized by a coaxial crossover technique using a 3F catheter inside a 5F Cobra catheter (Fig. 22.9). Arteries that are involved in posttraumatic pelvic hemorrhage are, in decreasing frequency order: superior gluteal, internal pudendal, (lateral) sacral, iliolumbar, obturator, urinary bladder, and inferior gluteal arteries (Fig. 22.10). Rarely, bleeding arises from other arteries such as the inferior epigastric artery (SUDARAM et al. 1981; SCLAFANI and BECKER 1982; BOLTER et al. 2000). The treatment of posttraumatic pelvic hemorrhage has raised a considerable interest in the literature. Pelvic trauma is responsible for 6%–8% of death of all trauma patients, rupture of a main pelvic artery carries a mortality of 50%–75% and the main cause of death from pelvic trauma is arterial hemorrhage. Furthermore, pelvic injury is frequently associated with other abdominal, aortic, and neurological injuries, which may be a major source of nonpelvic hemorrhage. Life-threatening hemorrhage may also occur without pelvic bone fracture (BELLEY et al. 1997; BAUMGARTNER et al. 1990; POOLE et al. 1991; KATZ et al. 1992).

A deep selective catheterization of the bleeding artery is obtained for embolization (LANG 1981). Gelfoam powder or liquid embolization agents (alcohol) are avoided because of the risk of nerve damage in the pelvis. Vaso-active drugs should not be injected intra-arterially, as induced vasospasm makes selective catheterization and distal embolization impossible. In the most unstable patients, a unilateral proximal embolization of the internal iliac artery is performed for urgent occlusion of all internal branches. Gelfoam pledgets soaked in an antibiotic solution and coils can be used in combination. Selective of other arterial branches such as the medial sacral artery, inferior epigastric artery, or lumbar arteries may be necessary depending on the type of fractures (HORI et al. 1989; KAWAMATA et al. 1991)

Patients with pelvic hemorrhage may bleed profusely and show a wash-out coagulopathy at time of embolization after multiple blood transfusions. Therefore, embolization and compact coiling are mandatory for a definite mechanical vessel occlusion. In case of laceration of an iliac artery, placement of one or two occlusion balloons before surgery may be a lifesaving procedure (BEN-MENACHEM 1988; BEN-MENACHEM et al. 1985).

Embolization in posttraumatic pelvic hemorrhage is overall successful in 84 to 100%, without significant difference between blunt and penetrating injury (MATALON et al. 1979; JANDER and RUSSINOVICH 1980; GILLILAND et al. 1982; YELLIN et al. 1983; PANETTA et al. 1985a, b; MORENO et al. 1986; YOKOTA et al. 1988; GRABENWOGER et al. 1989; MIRVIS and PAIS 1994; HOFFER 1999; VELMAHOS et al. 2000a, WONG et al. 2000). The time interval from trauma to intervention and the number of blood transfusions (11.3 ± 11 units in patients who died vs 3.2 ± 1.9 units in survivors) was shown to be a significant predictive factor of survival in patients with successful arterial hemostatic embolization (HOLTING et al. 1992; WONG et al. 2000). Potential complications are paraplegia, pelvic visceral necrosis, fistulization, ischemic neuropathy and impotence sensory disturbance, gait

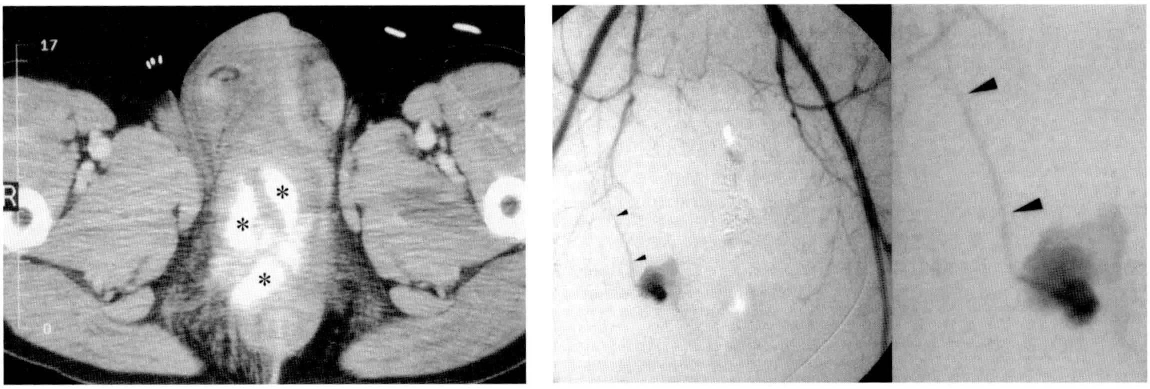

a b

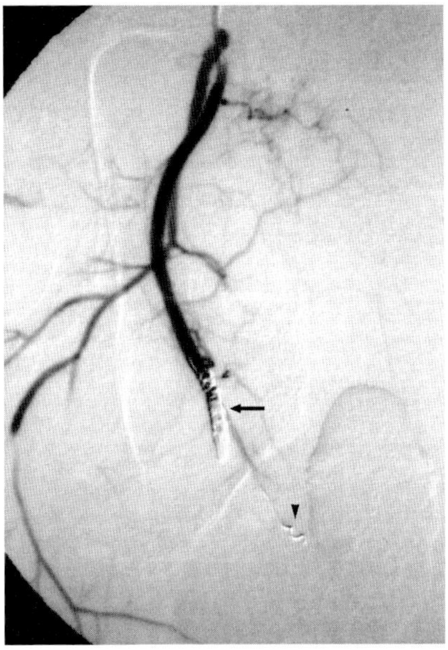

c

Fig. 24.9a–c. CT obtained at admission in a young patient with complex pelvic fractures showed massive perineal contrast extravasation (**a**) (*asterisks*). **b** Pelvic aortography and selective arteriography of the right internal pudendal artery (*arrowheads*) showed distal contrast extravasation. **c** Distal embolization with small microcoils (*arrowhead*) was ineffective due to impaired coagulation after multiple blood transfusions. Hemostasis was achieved after placement of a dozen coils in the trunk of the internal pudendal artery (*arrow*)

disturbance, dysuria, and difficulty in defecation due to an overly massive embolization or vaso-occlusion of overlapping arterial territories (Hietala 1978; Weingrad et al. 1979; Hori 1991). Gluteal muscle necrosis was observed in 3.3% of embolized patients (Takahira et al. 2001). Bilateral temporary internal iliac artery embolization did not carry significant complications in 30 consecutive patients (Velmahos et al. 2000b).

When internal fixation of a pelvic ring fracture is applied together with arterial embolization, the risk of sepsis seems increased (Perez et al. 1998).

22.6.6 Posttraumatic High-Flow Priapism

Hemorrhage from penile and testicular arteries is not life-threatening. Perineal work or sport injuries, including straddle injury from impact on the top tube of a bicycle are classical injury mechanisms (De Rose et al. 2001). The resulting arteriocavernous fistula or pseudoaneurysm is usually unilateral but can be occasionally bilateral. US shows the dilated sinusoidal cavernous spaces in almost all patients, color-coded Doppler localizes the fistula, and angiography identifies precisely the arterial feeding branch of the fistula or pseudoaneurysm. Lesions proximal to the symphysis pubis are the most difficult to demonstrate (Kang et al. 1998). Anarterial-cavernous fistula may be missed by Doppler ultrasonography, but is recognized by angiography (Logarakis et al. 2000). Painless priapism and preservations of sexual function contribute to delay in diagnosis (Talic and Al-Damegh 2000).

Posttraumatic pseudoaneurysm or fistula of a cavernosal artery (or deep) penile artery, can be treated by bucrylate, polyvinyl particles, Ethibloc, micro (platinium) coil, autologous clot or gelfoam pledgets (Wear et al. 1977; Alvarez-Gonzales et al. 1994; Kuwahara et al. 1995; Goktas et al. 1996; Numan et

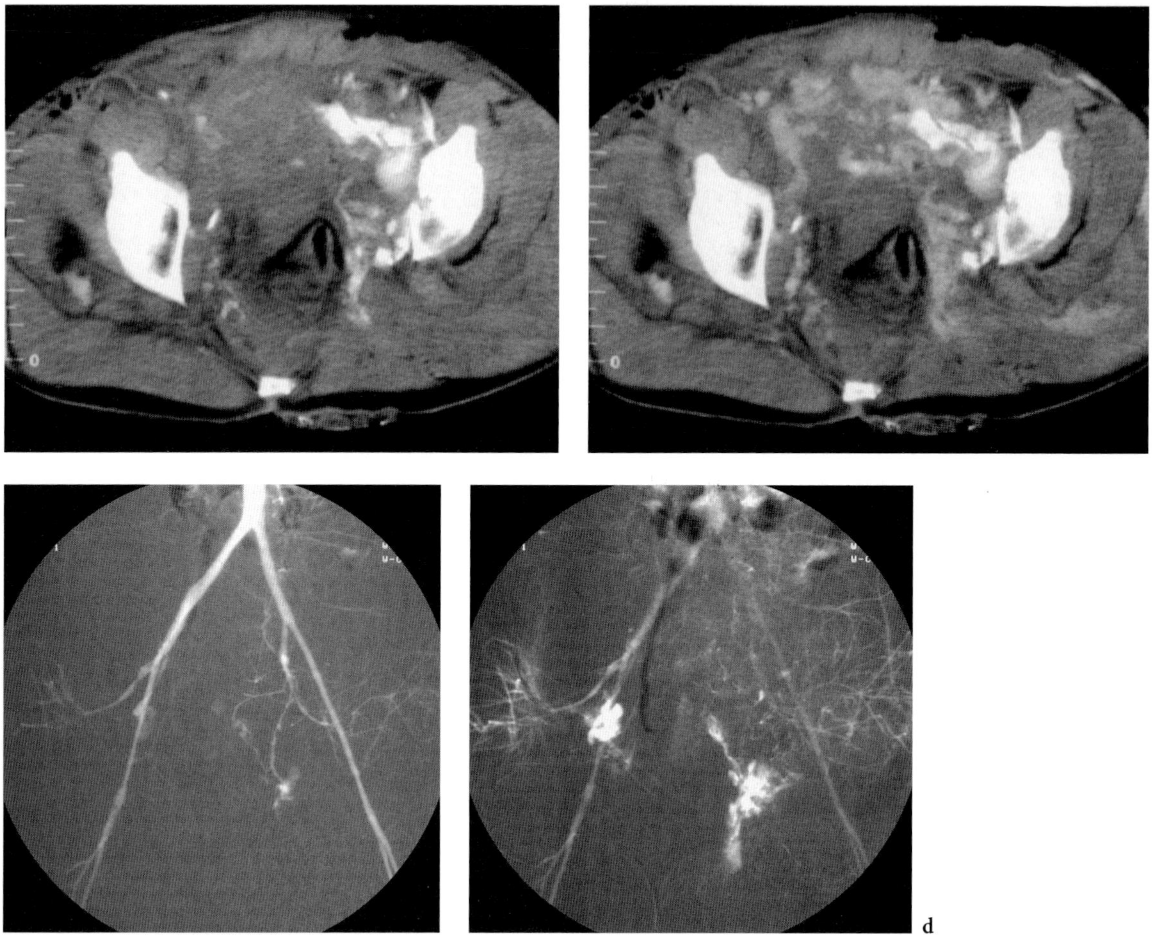

a b c d

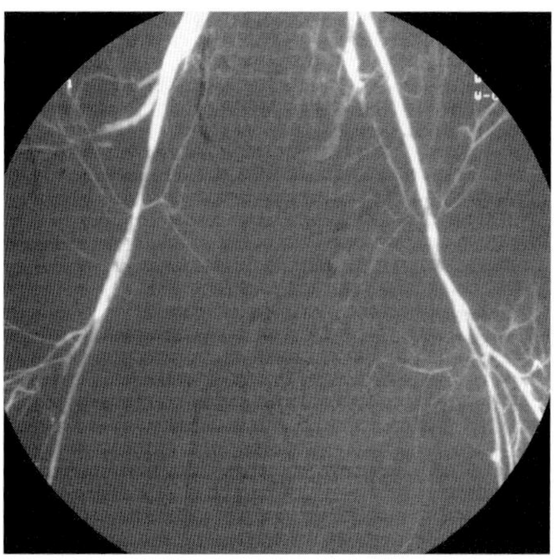

e

Fig. 24.10a–c. A 21-year-old male admitted in shock after a motorcycle accident (**a, b**). Contrast-enhanced CT showed bilateral massive extravasation in the pelvic interstitial tissue. **c, d** Femoral arterial pulses were not palpated. Arteriography obtained via a left axillary approach confirmed extravasation from visceral branches of both internal iliac arteries; severe vasospasm. **e** Hemostasis was achieved by embolization of both internal iliac arteries with polyvinyl alcohol particles (500–700 μm)

al. 1996; Cabezas Checci et al. 1998; Kang et al. 1998; Neubauer et al. 1998; Webber et al. 1998; colombo et al. 1999; Gomez Vegas et al. 1999; Touge et al. 1999; Golash et al. 2000; Goto et al. 2000; Logarakis et al. 2000; Mourikis et al. 2000; Talik and Al-Damegh 2000; Wang et al. 2000; De Rose et al. 2001). Young boys can be included in angiographic treatment (Dewan et al. 1994; Miller et al. 1995; Hierro Garcia et al. 1996; Sperling et al. 1997; Gimbergues et al. 1998; Mathias et al. 1998; Neubauer et al. 1998; Rico Lopez et al. 1998) (Fig. 22.11).

After embolization, detumescence of the penis is obtained and erectile function returns to normal (Wear et al. 1977; Colombo et al. 1999; Golash et

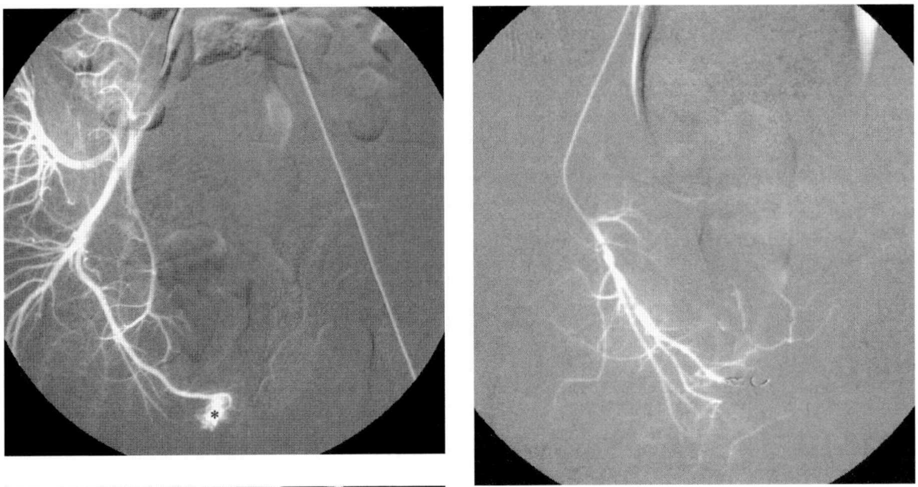

a b

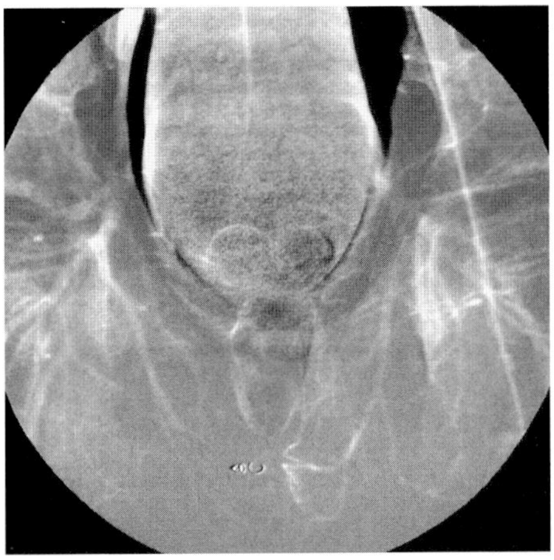

c

Fig. 24.11a–c. A 12-year-old boy presented with priapism 2 weeks after a bicycle accident with blunt perineal injury. Color Doppler examination showed arterial pseudoaneurysm probably located on the distal branches of the right internal pudendal artery (not shown). **a** Selective arteriography of the right internal pudendal artery obtained by cross-over catheterization confirmed the Doppler findings (*asterisk*). **b** Selective embolization of the vascular injury was achieved with two microcoils delivered through a microcatheter. **c** Postembolization nonselective pelvic arteriography showed no persistent filling of the arterial injury and normal left internal pudendal arterial branches

al. 2000; Goto et al. 2000; Logarakis et al. 2000; Mourikis et al. 2000; Wang et al. 2000). Even bilateral superselective embolization of small arterial branches was without effect on erectile function in several case reports (Rilinger et al. 1997; Callewaert et al. 1998; Gujral et al. 2001). The internal pudendal artery itself was also embolized, obtaining cure of priapism (Shankar et al. 2000). Intracavernous irrigation with fibrinolytic agent may be a useful adjunct after embolization, for treatment of incomplete detumescence (Wang et al. 2000). Duplex sonography-guided compression at the site of an arteriocavernous fistula can be added to selective embolization (Sancak and Conkbayir 2001). Among other treatment options, cooling of the penis and puncture of the cavernosal space is inefficient.

Recurrent priapism after embolization should be treated again angiographically (Suzuki et al. 1999). Complications following selective angiographic treatment are rare. An embolized pseudoaneurysm may evolve into an abscess with possible perineal spread (Sandock et al. 1996).

22.6.7 Other Injuries

Urgent hemostatic embolization may also be indicated for treatment of vascular injuries in other territories such as adrenal hemorrhage (Igwilo et al. 1999; Tixedor et al. 1999), ileocolic pseudoaneurysm (Rundback et al. 1999), lateral abdominal wall bleeding, requiring embolization of the deep circumflex iliac artery (Lefere et al. 1999).

A posttraumatic aneurysm of the abdominal aorta can be treated with placement of a covered stent graft in an acute or subacute situation (Fontaine et al. 2001).

22.7 Complications

The long-term behavior of permanent embolization devices such as coils or intravascular stent grafts is unknown in predominantly young patients treated for posttraumatic hemorrhage and should be assessed by follow-up studies (Weiss and Chaikoff 1999). Potential complications that may follow embolization in specific territories were described in detail above: the most feared are neurological damage, tissue necrosis, and infection. Recently, no significant morbidity was noted in 102 patients who underwent hemostatic embolization in the pelvis, liver, spleen, and kidney (Velmahos et al. 2000a).

References

Agolini SF, Shah K, Jaffe J, Newsomb J, Rhodes M, Reed JF III (1997) Arterial embolization is a rapid and effective technique for controlling pelvic fracture hemorrhage. J Trauma 43:395–399

Allison DJ, Jordan H, Hennessy O (1985) Therapeutic embolization of the hepatic artery: a review of 75 procedures. Lancet 1:595–599

Alvarez Gonzalez E, Pamplona M, Rodriguez A, Garcia-Hidalgo E, Nunez V, Leiva O (1994) High flow priapism after blunt perineal trauma: resolution with bucrylate embolization (review). J Urol 151:426–428

Anderson R, Alwmark A, Gullstrand P, Offerbarti K, Bengmark S (1986) Nonoperative treatment of blunt trauma to liver and spleen. Acta Chir Scand 152:739–741

Asensio JA, Demetriades D, Chahwan S et al (2000) Approach to the management of complex hepatic injuries. J Trauma 48:66–69

Ayella RY, Dupriest RW Jr, Khaneja SC et al (1978) Transcatheter embolization of autologous clot in the management of bleeding associated with fractures of the pelvis. Surg Gynaecol Obstet 147:849–852

Bass EM, Crosier JH (1977) Percutaneous control of post-traumatic hepatic hemorrhage by Gelfoam embolization. J Trauma 17:61–63

Bassam D, Cephas GA, Ferguson KA, Beard LN, Young JS (1998) A protocol for the initial management of unstable pelvic fractures. Am Surg 64:862–867

Baum S, Roy R, Finkelstein AK, Blakemore WS (1965) Clinical applications of selective cardiac and superior mesenteric arteriography. Radiology 84:279–294

Baumgartner F, White GH, White RA et al (1990) Delayed exsanguinating pelvic hemorrhage after blunt trauma without bony fracture: case report. J Trauma 30:1603–1605

Beal SL (1990) Fatal hepatic hemorrhage: an unsolved problem in the management of complex liver injuries. J Trauma 30: 163–169

Belley G, Gallix BP, Derossis AM, Mulder DS, Brown RA (1997) Profound hypotension in blunt trauma associated with superior gluteal artery rupture without pelvic fracture. J Trauma 43:703–705

Ben-Menachem Y (1988) Pelvic fractures: diagnostic and therapeutic angiography. In: Bassett FH (ed) Instructional course lectures. American Academy of Orthopaedic Surgeons, Park Ridge, IL 37:139–141

Ben-Menachem Y, Bahramipour P (1997) Interventional radiologic damage control. Semin Intervent Radiol 14:151–162

Ben-Menachem Y, Handel SF, Thaggard A 3rd, Carnovale RL, Katrogadda C, Glass TF (1979) Therapeutic arterial embolization in trauma. J Trauma 19:944–952

Ben-Menachem Y, Fisher RG, Ward RE (1981) Are "occult" intra-abdominal and extraperitoneal injuries really occult. Radiol Clin North Am 19:125–140

Ben-Menachem Y, Handel SF, Ray RD, Childs TL (1985) Embolization procedures in trauma: a matter of urgency. Semin Intervent Radiol 2:107–117

Ben-Menachem Y, Coldwell DM, Young JW, Burgess AR (1991) Hemorrhage associated with pelvic fractures: causes, diagnosis, and emergent management. AJR 157:1005–1014

Boijsen E, Judkins MP, Simay A (1966) Angiographic diagnosis of hepatic rupture. Radiology 86:66–72

Bolter S, Haueisen H, Renner N, Roeren T (2000) Inferior epigastric artery. An atypical source of bleeding in pelvic fracture. Unfallchirurg 103:318–321

Burgess AR, Eastridge BJ, Young JWR et al (1990) Pelvic ring disruptions: effective classification system and treatment protocols. J Trauma 30:848–856

Cabezas Checci C, Farina L, Martinez Carrancio L et al (1998) High-flow priapism after perineal trauma. Actas Urol Esp 22:359–361

Callewaert P, Stockx L, Bogaert G, Baert L (1998) Post-traumatic high-flow priapism in a 6-year-old boy: management by percutaneous placement of bilateral vascular coils. Urology 52:134–137

Capasso P, Trotteur G, Flandroy P, Dondelinger RF (1996) A combined CT and angiography suite with a pivoting table. Radiology199:561–563

Carillo EH, Spain DA, Wohltmann CD et al (1999) Interventional techniques are useful adjuncts in nonoperative management of hepatic injuries. J Trauma 46:619–622

Catalano O, Lobianco R, Esposito M, Sandomenico F, Siani A (1999) Contrast medium extravasation in upper abdominal injuries: detection with spiral computerized tomography. Radiol Med (Torino) 97:138–143

Chang J, Katzen BT, Sullivan KP (1978) Transcatheter Gelfoam embolization of posttraumatic bleeding pseudoaneurysms. AJR 131:645–650

Chiu WC, Cushing BM, Rodriguez A et al (1997) Abdominal injuries without hemoperitoneum: a potential limitation of focused abdominal sonography for trauma (FAST). J Trauma 42:817–822

Chuang VP, Reuter SR (1975) Selective arterial embolization for the control of traumatic splenic bleeding. Invest Radiol 10:18–24

Colombo F, Lovaria A, Saccheri S, Pozzoni F, Montanaris E (1999) Arterial embolization in the treatment of post-traumatic priapism. Ann Urol (Paris) 33:210–218

Davis KA, Fabian TC, Croce MA et al (1998) Improved success in nonoperative management of blunt splenic injuries: embolization of splenic artery pseudoaneurysms. J Trauma 44:1008–1013

De Bock L, Verhagen PF (1989) Selective embolization in the treatment of severe blunt renal injury. Neth J Surg 41: 31–34

De Rose AF, Giglio M, De Caro G, Corbu C, Traverso P, Carmignani G (2001) Arterial priapism and cycling: a new worrisome reality? Urology 58:462

De Toma G, Mingoli A, Modini C, Cavallaro A, Stipa S (1994) The value of angiography and selective hepatic artery embolization for continuous bleeding after surgery in liver trauma: case reports. J Trauma 37:508–511

Dewan PA, Lorenz C, Davies RP (1994) Posttraumatic priapism in a 7-year-old boy. Eur Urol 25:85–87

Dondelinger RF, Kurdziel JC (1991) A plea for conservative nonoperative management of hepatic contusion. Ann Chir 45:863–876

Eastbridge BJ, Burgess AR (1997) Pedestrian pelvic fractures: 5-year experience of a major urban trauma center. J Trauma 42:695–700

Evers BM, Cryer HM, Miller FB (1989) Pelvic fracture hemorrhage. Priorities in management. Arch Surg 124:422–424

Fandrich BL, Gnanadev DA, Jaecks R, Boyle W (1989) Selective hepatic artery embolization as an adjunct to liver packing in severe hepatic trauma: case report. J Trauma 29: 1716–1718

Fankuchen EI, Martin EC, Karlson KB, Mattern RF, Casarella WJ (1981) Small coils for large hemorrhages. AJR 136: 816–818

Federle MP (1983) Computed tomography of blunt abdominal trauma. Radiol Clin North Am 21:461–475

Federle MP, Crass RA, Jeffrey RB, Trunkey DD (1982) Computed tomography in blunt abdominal trauma. Arch Surg 117:645–650

Federle MP, Courcoulas AP, Powell M, Ferris JV, Peitzman AB (1998) Blunt splenic injury in adults: clinical and CT criteria for management, with emphasis on active extravasation. Radiology 206:137–142

Fisher RG, Ben-Menachem Y (1985) Embolization procedures in trauma: the abdomen: extraperitoneal. Semin Intervent Radiol 2:148–157

Fisher RG, Foucar K, Estrada B, Ben-Menchem Y (1981) Splenic rupture in blunt trauma – correlation of angiographic and pathological records. Radiol Clin North Am 19:141–146

Fisher RG, Ben-Menachem Y, Wigham C (1989) Stab wounds of the renal artery branches: angiographic diagnosis and treatment by embolization. AJR 152:1231–1235

Fontaine AB, Nicholls SC, Borsa JJ, Hoffer E, Bloch RD, Kohler T (2001) Seat belt aorta: endovascular management with a stent graft. J Endovasc Ther 8:83–86

Freeark RJ, Love L, Baker RJ (1968) The role of aortography in the management of blunt abdominal trauma. J Trauma 8:557–571

Freeman T, Fischer RP (1976) The inadequacy of peritoneal lavage in diagnosing acute diaphragmatic rupture. J Trauma 16:538–540

Garbuglia A, Bossi E, Ronzani C et al (1998) Severe pelvic injuries: indications and techniques of skeletal fixation. Chir Ital 50:61–71

Gavant ML, Schurr M, Frick PA et al (1997) Predicting clinical outcome of nonsurgical management of blunt splenic injury: using CT to reveal abnormalities of splenic vasculature. AJR 168:207–211

Gilliland MG, Ward RE, Flynn TC, Miller PW, Ben-Menachem Y, Duke JH Jr (1982) Peritoneal lavage and angiography in the management of patients with pelvic fractures. Am J Surg 144:744–747

Gimbergues P, Raynaud F, Ravel A (1998) Treatment using percutaneous arterial embolization of post-traumatic priapism in children. Prog Urol 8:258–261

Giraulo DL, Luk S, Palter M et al (1998) Selective hepatic arterial embolization of grade IV and V blunt hepatic injuries: an extension of resuscitation in the nonoperative management of traumatic hepatic injuries. J Trauma 45:353–359

Goins WA, Rodriguez A, Lewis J, Brathwaite CE, James E (1992) Retroperitoneal hematoma after blunt trauma. Surg Gynecol Obstet 174:281–290

Goktas S, Tahmaz L, Atac K, Erduran D, Peker AF, Harmankaya C (1996) Embolization therapy in two subtypes of priapism. Int Urol Nephrol 28:723–727

Golash A, Gray R, Ruttley MS, Jenkins BJ (2000) Traumatic priapism: an unusual cycling injury. Br J Sports Med 34: 310–311

Gomez Vegas A, Delgado Martin JA, Blazquez Izquierdo J, Silmi Moyano A, Resel Estevez L (1999) Arterial priapism. Resolution following embolization with autologous thrombus. Arch Esp Urol 52:285–289

Gorich J, Rilinger N, Brado M et al (1999) Non-operative management of arterial liver hemorrhages. Eur Radiol 9:85–88

Goto T, Noguchi A, Hamamato Y et al (2000) A case of traumatic priapism. Hinyokika Kiyo 46:907–910

Grabenwoger F, Dock W, Ittner G (1989) Percutaneous embolization of retroperitoneal hemorrhage in pelvic fractures. ROFO 150:335–338

Gujral S, MacDonagh RP, Cavanagh PM (2001) Bilateral superselective arterial microcoil embolization in delayed posttraumatic high flow priapism. Postgrad Med J 77:193–194

Gylling SF, Ward RF, Holcroft JW et al (1985) Immediate external fixation of unstable pelvic fractures. Am J Surg 150: 721–724

Hagiwara A, Yukioka T, Shimazaki S, Megawa T, Matuda H (1993) Delayed hemorrhage following catheter arterial embolization for blunt hepatic injury. Cardiovasc Intervent Radiol 16:380–383

Hagiwara A, Yukioka T, Ohta S, Nitatori T, Matsuda N, Shimazaki S (1996) Nonsurgical management of patients with blunt splenic injury: efficacy of transcatheter arterial embolization. AJR 167:159–166

Hagiwara A, Yukioka T, Ohta S et al (1997) Nonsurgical management of patients with blunt hepatic injury: efficacy of transcatheter arterial embolization. AJR 169:1151–1156

Hagiwara A, Sakaki S, Goto H et al (2001) The role of interventional radiology in the management of blunt renal injury: a practical protocol. J Trauma 51:526–531

Hamill J, Holden A, Paice R, Civil I (2000) Pelvic fracture pattern predicts pelvic arterial hemorrhage. Aust N Z J Surg 70:338–343

Harper HC III, Maull KI (2000) Transcatheter arterial embolization in blunt hepatic trauma. South Med J 93:663–665

Hashimoto S, Ido K, Hiramatsu K et al (1990) Expanding role of emergency embolization in the management of severe blunt hepatic trauma. Cardiovasc Intervent Radiol 13:193–197

Hashimoto S, Hiramatsu K, Sato M (1997) CO_2 as an intraarterial digital subtraction angiography (IADSA) agent in the management of trauma. Seminars Intervent Radiol 14: 163–173

Hawkins IF, Caridi JG, Wiechmann BN, Kerns SR (1997) Carbon dioxide (CO_2), digital subtraction angiography in trauma patients. Seminars Intervent Radiol 14:175–180

Haydu P, Chang J, Knox G, Nealson TF Jr (1978) Transcatheter arterial embolization of a traumatic lumbar artery false aneurysm. Surgery 84:288–291

Hierro Garcia D, Silveira Paez U, Sarmentero Ortiz E (1996) Remission of post-traumatic high flow priapism with embolization with self-coagulum. Actas Urol Esp 20:471–473

Hietala SO (1978) Urinary bladder necrosis following selective embolization of the internal iliac artery. Acta Radiol Diagn (Stockh) 19:316–320

Hoffer EK (1999) Interventional angiography for treatment of hemorrhage in pelvic trauma. Emerg Radiol 6:216–226
Holting T, Buhr HJ, Richter GM, Roeren T, Friedl W, Herfarth C (1992) Diagnosis and treatment of retroperitoneal hematoma in multiple trauma patients. Arch Orthop Trauma Surg 111:323–326
Hori A, Nagata Y, Hanashiro Y et al (1989) Embolization of the lumbar artery for pelvic fracture. Rinsho Hoshasen 34: 1047–1050
Hori A, Nagata Y, Shimabukuro K, Ohshiro K, Yasutani T, Makita O (1990) Diagnosis of the pelvic fracture which requires TAE on plain pelvic radiograph. Rinsho Hoshasen 35:935–938
Hori A (1991) Complications following transcatheter arterial embolization for massive hemorrhage associated with pelvic fracture. Nippon Igaku Hoshasen Gakkai Zasshi 51: 365–374
Hubbard SG, Bivins BA, Sachatello CR, Griffen WO Jr (1979) Diagnostic errors with peritoneal lavage in patients with pelvic fractures. Arch Surg 114:844–846
Igwilo OC, Sulkowski RJ, Shah MR, Messink WF, Kinnas NC (1999) Embolization of traumatic adrenal hemorrhage. J Trauma 47:1153–1155
Ikubo A, Komura M, Matoba N et al (1993) Lumbar artery pseudoaneurysm: an unusual cause of a retroperitoneal hematoma: report of a case. Surg Today 23:635–638
Jander HP, Laws HL, Kogutt MS, Mihas AA (1977) Emergency embolization in blunt hepatic trauma. AJR 129:249–252
Jander HP, Russinovich AE (1980) Transcatheter Gelfoam embolization in abdominal, retroperitoneal and pelvic hemorrhage. Radiology 136:337–344
Jeffrey RB Jr, Cardoza JD, Olcott EW (1991) Detection of active intraabdominal arterial hemorrhage: value of dynamic contrast-enhanced CT. AJR 156:725–729
Kang BC, Lee DY, Byun JY, Baek SY, Lee SW, Kim KW (1998) Post-traumatic arterial priapism: colour Doppler examination and superselective arterial embolization. Clin Radiol 53:830–834
Katz MD, Teitelbaum GP, Pentecosdt MJ (1992) Diagnostic arteriography and therapeutic transcatheter embolization for posttraumatic pelvic hemorrhage. Seminars Intervent Radiol 9:4–12
Kawamata H, Kumazaki T, Tajima H, Gemma K, Ito K, Ebata K (1991) Value of "additional arterial embolization" to bilateral internal iliac TAE in patients with severe pelvic fractures. Nippon Igaku Hoshasen Gakkai Zasshi 25:649–655
Keramidas DC (1979) The ligation of the splenic artery in the treatment of traumatic rupture of the spleen. Surgery 85: 530–533
Killeen KL, Shanmuganathan K, Boydkranis R, Scalea TM, Mirvis SE (2001) CT findings after embolization for blunt splenic trauma. J Vasc Interv Radiol 12:209–214
Klein SR, Mehringer CM, Bongard FS (1990) Endovascular occlusive intervention in the management of trauma. Ann Vasc Surg 4:424–430
Kos X, Fanchamps JM, Trotteur G, Dondelinger RF (1999) Radiologic damage control: evaluation of a combined CT and angiography suite with a pivoting table. Cardiovasc Intervent Radiol 22:124–129
Kramer SC, Gorich J, Rilinger N, Gottfried HW, Mattes R, Aschof AJ (1998) The perentaneous transarterial embolization therapy of traumatic kidney hemorrhages, ROFO 169: 297–301
Kurdziel JC, Dondelinger RF, Hemmer M (1987) Radiological management of blunt polytrauma with computed tomography and angiography: an integrated approach. Ann Radiol 30:121–124
Kuwahara M, Fujisaki N, Nakamura K, Ohta K, Nishitani M, Takagi N (1995) High flow priapism after perineal trauma, successfully treated by unilateral embolization of the internal pudendal artery: a case report (review). Nippon Hinyokika Gakkai Zasshi 86:333–336
Lang EK (1976) The role of arteriography in trauma. Radiol Clin North Am 14:353–370
Lang EK (1981) Transcatheter embolization of pelvic vessels for control of intractable hemorrhage. Radiology 140:331–339
Lang EK (1990) Intra-abdominal and retroperitoneal organ injuries diagnosed on computed tomograms obtained for assessment of renal trauma. J Trauma 30:1161–1168
Larsen DW, Pentecost MJ (1992) Embolotherapy in renal trauma. Semin Intervent Radiol 9:13–18
Lefere P, Gryspeerdt S, Van Holsbeeck B, Baekelandt M (1999) Diagnosis and treatment of expanding haematoma of the lateral abdominal wall after blunt abdominal trauma. Eur Radiol 9:1553–1555
Logarakis NF, Simons ME, Hassouna M (2000) Selective arterial embolization for post-traumatic high flow priapism. Can J Urol 7:1051–1054
Love L, Greenfield GB, Braun TW, Moncada R, Freeark RJ, Baker RJ (1968) Arteriography in splenic trauma. Radiology 91:96–102
Mandel SR, Jaques PF, Sanofsky S, Mauro MA (1987) Nonoperative management of peripancreatic arterial aneurysms. A 10-year experience. Ann Surg 205:126–128
Matalon TSA, Athanasoulis CA, Margolies NM et al (1979) Hemorrhage with pelvic fractures: efficacy of transcatheter embolization. AJR 133:859–864
Mathias K, Jager H, Witkowski M, Aspiotis A, Schulze H, Albrecht M (1998) High-flow priapism following blunt perineal trauma. Interventional therapy. Radiologe 38:710–713
Maull KI, Sachatello CR (1976) Current management of pelvic fractures: a combined surgical-angiographic approach to hemorrhage. South Med J 69:1285–1289
Mears D (1980) External fixation of pelvic fractures. Orthop Clin North Am 11:465–479
Miller SF, Chait PG, Burrows PE et al (1995) Posttraumatic arterial priapism in children: management with embolization. Radiology 196:59–62
Mirvis SE, Pais SO (1994) Trauma radiology: part III. Diagnostic an therapeutic angiography in trauma. J. Intensive Care Med, 9:244–256
Moore EE (1984) Critical decision making in the management of hepatic trauma. Am J Surg 6:712–716
Moreno C, Moore EE, Rosenberger A, Cleveland HC (1986) Hemorrhage associated with major pelvic fracture: a multispecialty challenge. J Trauma 26:987–994
Mourikis D, Chatziioannou AN, Konstantinidis P, Panourgias E, Antoniou A, Vlachos L (2000) Superselective microcoil embolization of a traumatic pseudoaneurysm of the cavernosal artery. Urol Int 64:220–222
Mucha P Jr, Welch TJ (1988) Hemorrhage in major pelvic fractures. Surg Clin North Am 68:757–773
Murakami R, Tajima H, Kumazaki T (1993) Transcatheter hepatic arterial embolization for the treatment of blunt hepatic injury. Nippon Igaku Hoshasen Gakkai Zasshi 53: 395–402

Mutabagani KH, Coley BD, Zumberge N et al (1999) Preliminary experience with focused abdominal sonography for trauma (FAST) in children: is it useful? J Pediatr Surg 34: 48–52
Neubauer S, Derakhshani P, Krug B, Lackner K, Heidenreich A, Engelmann U (1998) Posttraumatic high-flow priapism in a 10-year-old boy: superselective embolization of the arteriovenous fistula. Eur Urol 33:337–339
Norell HG (1957) Traumatic rupture of the spleen diagnosed by abdominal aortography. Acta Radiol 48:449–452
Numan F, Cakirer S, Islak C et al (1996) Posttraumatic high-flow priapism treated by N-butyl-cyanoacrylate embolization (review). Cardiovasc Intervent Radiol 19:278–280
Nunez LW, Simmons S, Kozar R, Kinback R, Hallowell MJ, Mulhern C Jr (2001) Feasibility and profitability of a radiology department providing trauma US as a part of a trauma alert team. Acad Radiol 8:88–95
Ochsner MG, Knudson MM, Pachter HL et al (2000) Significance of minimal or no intraperitoneal fluid visible on CT scan associated with blunt liver and splenic injuries: a multicenter analysis. J Trauma 49:505–510
Omert LA, Salyer D, Dunham CM, Porter J, Silva A, Protetch J (2001) Implications of the "contrast blush" finding on computed tomography scan of the spleen in trauma. J Trauma 51:272–277
Palmer JK, Bensons GS, Corriere JN jr. (1983) Diagnosis and initial management of urological injuries associated with 200 consecutive pelvic fractures. J Urol 130:712–714
Panetta T, Sclafani SJA, Goldstein AS et al (1985a) Percutaneous transcatheter embolization for massive bleeding from pelvic fractures. J Trauma 25:1021–1029
Panetta T, Sclafani SJ, Goldstein AS, Philips TF (1985b) Percutaneous transcatheter embolization for arterial trauma. J Vasc Surg 2:54–64
Pereira SJ, O'Brien DP, Luchette FA et al (2000) Dynamic helical computed tomography scan accurately detects hemorrhage in patients with pelvic fracture. Surgery 128:678–685
Perez JV, Hughes TM, Bowers K (1998) Angiographic embolisation in pelvic fracture. Injury 29:187–191
Platz A, Friedl HP, Kohler A, Trentz O (1992) Surgical management of severe pelvic crush injuries. Helv Chir Acta 58: 925–929
Poole GV, Ward EF, Muakkassa FF, Hsu HS, Griswold JA, Thodes RS (1991) Pelvic fracture from major blunt trauma. Outcome is determined by associated injuries. Ann Surg 213:532–539
Probst P, Castaneda-Zuniga WR, Gomes AS, Amplatz K (1978) Which embolic material is best suited for which embolization procedure ? ROFO 129:447–454
Rao PM, Rhea JT, Novelline RA (1997) CT diagnosis of acute abdominal trauma. Semin Intervent Radiol 14:111–124
Richardson DJ, Franklin GA, Lukan JK et al (2000) Evolution in the management of hepatic trauma: a 25-year perspective. Ann Surg 232:324–330
Rico Lopez J, Amaya Gutierrez J, Blasco Hernandez P et al (1998) Posttraumatic high-flow priapism in prepubertal age. Actas Urol Esp 22:531–537
Rilinger N, Kramer S, De Petriconi R, Luther A, Tomczak R, Gorich J (1997) Percutaneous superselective bilateral embolization for the therapy of traumatic juvenile arterial priapism (review). ROFO 166:263–265
Rose SC, Moore EE (1987) Emergency trauma angiography: accuracy, safety and pitfalls. AJR 148:1243–1246
Rousseau H, Soula P, Perreault P et al (1999) Delayed treatment of traumatic rupture of the thoracic aorta with endoluminal covered stent. Circulation 99:498–504
Rozycki GS, Ballard RB, Feliciano DV, Schmidt JA, Pennington SD (1998) Surgeon-performed ultrasound for the assessment of truncal injuries: lessons learned from 1540 patients. Ann Surg 228:557–567
Rubin BE, Katzen BT (1977) Selective hepatic artery embolization to control massive hepatic hemorrhage after trauma. AJR 129:253–256
Rundback JH, Chughtai S, Rozenblit G, Panageas E, Poplausky M (1999) Traumatic ileocolic pseudoaneurysm: diagnosis and transcatheter treatment. Catheter Cardiovasc Interv 48:217–219
Sancak T, Conkbayir I (2001) Post-traumatic high-flow priapism: management by superselective transcatheter autologous clot embolization and duplex sonography-guided compression. J Clin Ultrasound 29:349–353
Sandock DS, Seftel AD, Herbener TE, Goldstein I, Greenfield AJ (1996) Perineal abscess after embolization for high-flow priapism. Urology 48:308–311
Sato M, Fujisawa H, Hagiwara A et al (1991) Traumatic hemorrhage of the spleen diagnosed by CO_2 DSA. JJAAM 2: 728–732
Scalea TM, Rodriguez A, Chiu WC et al (1999) Focused Assessment with Sonography for Trauma (FAST): results from an international consensus conference. J Trauma 46:466–472
Schwartz RA, Teitelbaum GP, Katz MD, Pentecost MJ (1993) Effectiveness of transcatheter embolization in the control of hepatic vascular injuries. J Vasc Interv Radiol 4:359–365
Sclafani SJA (1985) Angiographic control of intraperitoneal hemorrhage caused by injuries to the liver and spleen. Semin Intervent Radiol 2:139–147
Sclafani SJ, Becker JA (1982) Traumatic presacral hemorrhage: angiographic diagnosis and therapy. AJR 138:123–126
Sclafani SJ, Shaftan GW, McAuley et al (1984) Interventional radiology in the management of hepatic trauma. J Trauma 24:256–262
Sclafani SJ, Florence LO, Phillips TF et al. (1987) Lumbar arterial injury: radiologic diagnosis and management. Radiology 165:709–714
Sclafani SJA, Weisberg A, Scalea TM, Philips TF, Duncan AO (1991) Blunt splenic injuries: nonsurgical treatment with CT, arteriography and transcatheter arterial embolization of the splenic artery. Radiology 181:189–196
Sclafani SJA, Shaftan GW, Scalea TM et al (1995) Nonoperative salvage of computed tomography – diagnosed splenic injuries: utilization of angiography for triage and embolization for hemostasis. J Trauma 39:818–825
Selby JB Jr (1992) Interventional radiology of trauma. Radiol Clin North Am 30:427–439
Shankar KR, Babar S, Rowlands P, Jones MO (2000) Posttraumatic high-flow priapism: treatment with selective embolisation. Pediatr Surg Int 16:454–456
Shanmuganathan K, Mirvis SE, Sover ER (1993) Value of contrast-enhanced CT in detecting active hemorrhage in patients with blunt abdominal or pelvic trauma. AJR 161: 65–69
Shanmuganathan K, Mirvis SE, Boyd-Kranis R, Takada T, Scalea T (2000) Nonsurgical management of blunt splenic injury: use of CT criteria to select patients for splenic arteriography and potential endovascular therapy. Radiology 217:75–82

Sherman HF (1996) Failure of nonoperative treatment of a gunshot wound to the liver predicted by computed tomography. J Trauma 41:171
Sperling H, Goepel M, Lummen G, Stoblen F, Rubben H (1997) Post-traumatic priapism in a 10-year-old boy. Urologe A 36:162–164
Stephen DJ, Kreder HJ, Day AC et al (1999) Early detection of arterial bleeding in acute pelvic trauma. J Trauma 47: 638–642
Sugimoto K, Horiike S, Hirata M, Ohwada T, Maekawa K (1994) The role of angiography in the assessment of blunt liver injury. Injury 25:283–287
Sundaram M, Patel B, Wolverson MK, Riaz MA (1981) Superior gluteal artery haemorrhage following pelvic features controlled by embolization. Clin Radiol 32:187–190
Suzuki N, Sato Y, Tsukamoto T, Koito K, Maruta H, Hisasue S (1999) Post-traumatic arterial priapism evaluation with color Doppler ultrasonography: a case report. Hinyokika Kiyo 45:65–68
Takahira N, Shindo M, Tanaka K, Nishimaki H, Ohwada T, Itoman M (2001) Gluteal muscle necrosis following transcatheter angiographic embolisation for retroperitoneal haemorrhage associated with pelvic fracture. Injury 32: 27–32
Takakuwa T, Yokota J, Sugimoto T (1993) Liver infarction produced by dual vessel occlusion due to trauma and TAE: long follow-up using CT, US and MRI. Med J Osaka Univ 41/42:23–27
Talic RF, Al-Damegh SA (2000) Posttraumatic high-flow arterial priapism. The need for increased awareness among health care professionals. Saudi Med J 21:382–385
Taylor GA, Sivit CJ (1995) Posttraumatic peritoneal fluid: is it a reliable indicator of intraabdominal injury in children? J Pediatr Surg 30:1644–1648
Teigen CL, Venbrux AC, Quinlan DM, Jeffs RD (1992) Late massive hematuria as a complication of conservative management of blunt renal trauma in children. J Urol 147: 1333–1336
Tixedor N, Lesnik A, Vernhet H, Drianno N, Bousquet C, Senac JP (1999) Embolization treatment of a traumatic adrenal hemorrhage. J Radiol 80:733–735
Touge H, Watanabe T, Fujinaga T, Kawabata M (1999) Posttraumatic high flow priapism: a case report. Int J Urol 6: 623–626
Trunkey DD (1983) Trauma. Sci Am 249:28–35
Udekwu PO, Gurkin B, Oller DW (1996) The use of computed tomography in blunt abdominal injuries. Am Surg 62: 56–59
Ulflacker R, Paolini RM, Lima S (1984) Management of traumatic hematuria by selective renal artery embolization. J Urol 132:662–667
Velmahos GC, Chawan S, Falabella A, Hanks SE, Demetriades D (2000a) Angiographic embolization for intraperitoneal and retroperitoneal injuries. World J Surg 24:539–545
Velmahos GC, Chahwan S, Hanks SE et al (2000b) Angiographic embolization of bilateral internal iliac arteries to control life-threatening hemorrhage after blunt trauma to the pelvis. Am Surg 66:858–862
Vogler E, Bergmann M (1963) Angiography in blunt kidney trauma. ROFO 98:675–685
Wagner WH, Lundell CJ, Donovan AJ (1985) Percutaneous angiographic embolization for hepatic arterial hemorrhage. Arch Surg 120:1241–1249
Walt AJ (1969) The surgical management of hepatic trauma and its complications. Ann R Coll Surg Engl 45:319–339
Wang CC, Chen JH, Liu SP, Hung JJ, Liang PC, Hsieh JT (2000) Post-traumatic, high-flow priapism treated with selective cavernous artery embolization and intracavernous streptokinase irrigation: a case report. J Formos Med Assoc 99: 952–954
Wear JB Jr, Crummy AB, Munson BO (1977) A new approach to the treatment of priapism. J Urol 117:252–254
Webber RJ, Thirsk I, Moffat LE, Hussey J (1998) Selective arterial embolization in the treatment of arterial priapism. J R Coll Surg Edinb 43:61
Weingrad DN, Doppman JL, Chretien PB, Di Chiro G (1979) Paraplegia due to posttraumatic pelvic arteriovenous fistula treated by surgery and embolization. Case report. J Neurosurg 50:805–810
Weiss VJ, Chaikoff EL (1999) Endovascular treatment of vascular injuries. Surg Clin North Am 79:653–655
Wong YC, Wang LJ, Ng CJ, Tseng IC, See LC (2000) Mortality after successful transcatheter arterial embolization in patients with unstable pelvic fractures: rate of blood transfusion as a predictive factor. J Trauma 49:71–75
Yellin AE, Lundell CJ, Finck EJ (1983) Diagnosis and control of posttraumatic pelvic hemorrhage. Transcatheter angiographic embolization techniques. Arch Surg 118:1378–1383
Yitzhak A, Shaked G, Lupu L, Mizrahi S, Kluger Y (2001) Selective embolization of hepatic arteries – an additional precaution to control hemorrhage in the management of severe liver trauma. Harefuah 140:193–196
Yokota J, Kawakami M, Iwai A et al (1988) Efficacy of transcatheter embolization for massive bleeding from pelvic fracture. Nippon Geka Gakkai Zasshi 89:757–762

23 Imaging and Intervention of Posttraumatic Abdominal Complications

P. Goffette and P.-F. Laterre

CONTENTS

P. Goffette, MD
Professor, Angiography and Interventional Radiology Unit, Department of Medical Imaging, Saint-Luc University Hospital, Louvain Medical School, 10, avenue Hippocrate, 1200 Brussels, Belgium
P.-F. Laterre, MD
Professor, Emergency and Critical Care Department, Saint-Luc University Hospital, Louvain Medical School, 10, avenue Hippocrate, 1200 Brussels, Belgium

- The nonsurgical treatment of delayed complications after abdominal trauma can be considered nowadays as the first therapeutic option.
- The success of this approach is conditioned by early recognition of these complications, which are primarily expected in the highest-grade severe trauma.
- Interventional radiology has a key role in the multidisciplinary and complementary management of delayed complications occurring after an abdominal injury.

23.1 Introduction

During the past decade, nonoperative management of abdominal trauma, in the absence of hollow viscus rupture, has become the standard care in children (MacGillivray and Valentine 1989; Sjövall and Hirsh 1997). Based on the excellent success rate in children (90%–95%), this approach has been extended to adult trauma patients (rate 65%–90%) (Heller et al. 1994; Brasel et al. 1997; Goan et al. 1998; Malhotra et al. 2000). Nonoperative management may also be indicated in patients regaining hemodynamic stability after trauma, regardless of the extent or grade of solid organs injuries (Pachter and Hofstetter 1995; Ciraulo et al. 1998; Carrillo et al. 1998). Recent work has suggested that carefully selected patients with abdominal gunshot wounds can also be safely managed nonoperatively (Demetriades et al. 1997, 1999; Velmahos et al. 2000a). Several factors have promoted the use of conservative therapy, including the widespread use of new-generation CT, which provides precise evaluation and grading of solid organ injuries and reduces the risk of unrecognized hollow viscus injuries (Yoo et al. 1996; Cuff et al. 2000), the high success rate and clinical benefits of angiographic embolization in the treatment of intra- or retroperitoneal bleeding (Sclafani et al. 1984b, 1995b; Hagiwara et al. 1996, 1997; Velmahos et al. 2000b), and a better understanding of the natural history and pathophysiology of organ injuries and associated complications. The improvement in resuscitation allows conservative management of what have been historically called “surgical candidates”. This trend is reinforced by the requirement for cost-effective care, as physicians and administrators look for ways to reduce costs without impairing the quality of care.

As more patients with complex abdominal injuries are now treated nonoperatively, uncommon delayed complications not encountered after surgery are coming to the forefront (Bynoe et al. 1992; Carrillo et al. 1998; Frumiento et al. 2000). Causes of delayed complications are multiple and include abnormal or insufficient injury healing process, retention of necrotic tissue, secondary infection of initially sterile collections, and underestimation of injury severity. Unrecognized hollow viscus and diaphragmatic injuries may also complicate the conservative management of abdominal trauma (Yoo et al. 1996). Historically, most of these complications have been treated surgically. Nowadays recent advanced technologies detect them noninvasively and manage them by minimally invasive techniques including interventional radiology, endoscopy, and laparoscopy.

The purpose of this chapter is to identify, for every traumatized abdominal organ or structure, the type, incidence and optimal treatment modalities of complications attributable to nonoperative management or surgery in adults and children.

23.2 Liver and Bile Ducts

23.2.1 Types and Incidence of Complications

Complications secondary to liver trauma are reported in up to 64% of patients (Cogbill et al. 1988; Knudson et al. 1990; Hammond et al. 1992). After initial surgery, the predominant factors predisposing to postoperative complications are the extent of liver trauma and associated injuries (Fabian et al. 1991; Boone et al. 1995; Pachter et al. 1996). As the conservative management of blunt hepatic trauma is becoming the initial approach, even for high-grade injuries, complications previously not encountered after surgery are now more commonly described (MacGillivray and Valentine 1989; Ciraulo et al. 1998; Goan et al. 1998; Carrillo et al. 1999; Asensio et al. 2000).

A variety of delayed complications involving the liver and biliary system are observed after abdominal trauma, arising either as a result of direct liver trauma such as bile duct disruption, bile peritonitis, biloma, intra-abdominal abscess formation, delayed hemorrhage, nonbleeding vascular malformations, hemobilia and bilhemia or occurring in the course of posttraumatic critical care such as acute acalculous cholecystitis (MacGillivray and Valentine 1989; Bynoe et al. 1992; Carles et al. 1994; Boone et al. 1995; Pachter and Hofstetter 1995; Hagiwara et al. 1996; Pachter et al. 1996; Brasel et al. 1997; Krige et al. 1997; Carrillo et al. 1999; Parks et al. 1999; Letoublon et al. 1999; Cuff et al. 2000). These complications are predictable, consequences of the successful nonoperative management of complex liver injuries. Over 60% of patients with grade IV or V liver laceration treated nonoperatively will require some type of interventional procedures to treat a variety of complications resulting from the conservative approach (Carrillo et al. 1999). Complications can occur weeks to months after injury and often after discharge of the patient. In the past, most of these complications were treated surgically (PARKS et al. 1999).

Liver-related complications appear to be less frequent in patients managed without operation than in those managed surgically (BYNOE et al. 1992). Overall complication rates in patients undergoing nonoperative treatment are reported in 12%–24% in adults (BYNOE et al. 1992; CARRILLO et al. 1999) and in 7%–10% in children (MACGILLIVRAY and VALENTINE 1989). The type and timing of complications may be explained by the different mechanisms of liver blunt injury and the healing process. Superficial liver injuries, in the absence of capsular disruption, most frequently require no intervention. Deep liver injuries are more likely to disrupt major blood vessels and bile ducts. Blood clots may obstruct regional bile ducts and lead to formation of a parenchymal cavity. Persistent bleeding or accumulation of bile increase intracavitary pressure and may lead to hepatic necrosis (CARRILLO et al. 1999). After control of bleeding from the hepatic artery by initial embolization or hepatic artery ligation, bile leakage and bleeding from the portal vein may continue (BOONE et al. 1995; LAU and DIAMOND 1997; SHILYANSKY et al. 1999). Delayed complications associated with nonoperative management of liver trauma and detailed by the most important series between 1990 and 2000 are summarized in Tables 23.1 and 23.2.

Table 23.1. Delayed complications after nonoperative management of blunt liver trauma (1990–2000)

Reference	No. of patients	Grade of liver injury	Complications							
			No. of patients	Rebleeding	Biliary	Abscess	Missed enteric injury	Successful radiological intervention or observation	Surgery	Success NOM
KNUDSON et al. (1990)	52	I–II 65% III–V 35%	1 (2%)	1	0	0	0	0	1	98%
BYNOE et al. (1992)	26	I–II 62% III–V 38%	5 (19%)	0	Leak 2 Biloma 3	0	0	Biloma 3	2	92%
CARLES et al. (1994)	142	NA	6 (4%)	1	Leak 1 Biloma 1	2	1	Biloma 1 Abscess 2	3	94%
MEREDITH et al. (1994)	72	I–II 54% III–V 46%	2 (3%)	2 (pseudoaneurysm)	0	0	0	0	2	97%
SHERMAN et al. (1994)	30	I–II 34% III–V 66%	1 (3%)	1	0	0	0	1	0	100%
BOONE et al. (1995)	46	I–II 30% III–V 70%	7 (15%)	2	Leak 2 Biloma 1	2	0	Biliary 2 Abscess 2	4	91%
PACHTER et al. (1996)	404	I–II 50% III–V 50%	21 (5%)	14	Biloma 2	3	2	Drainage 4 Embolization 4	6	93%
BRASEL et al. (1997)	50	I–II 76% III–V 28%	3 (6%)	2 (pseudoaneurysm)	Leak 1	0	0	Drainage 1 Embolization 2	0	96%
HAGIWARA et al. (1997)	54 (15E)	I–II 48% III–V 52%	4 (7%)	3 (pseudoaneurysm)	Biloma 4 (3 with pseudoaneurysm)	0	0	Drainage 1 Embolization 3	0	100%
CARRILLO et al. (1999)	135	I–II 30% III–V 70%	32 (24%)	12	Leaks 5 Obstruct 2 Bilhemia 1	0	1	Embolization 10 ERCP 7 Drain 10	1	96%
CUFF et al. (2000)	52	I–II 30% III–V 70%	3 (6%)	1 (AVF)	Biloma and leak 1	0	1	Embolization 1 Drainage 1	1	98%

NOM, nonoperative management; *E*, embolization at admission; *AVF*, arteriovenous fistula; *NA*, not available.

Table 23.2. Delayed complications after nonoperative management (NOM) of splenic trauma

Reference	No. of patients	CT grade of injury	Delayed complications				NOM success
			No. of patients	Type	Treatment	Mortality	
Cogbill et al. (1989)	112	I–II 71% III–IV 29%	13	Bleeding 12 Pancreatic cyst 1	Splenectomy 13	0	99 (88%)
Sclafani et al. (1995b)	150 90 60 (E)	I–II 71% III–IV 29% I–II 37% III–IV 63%	9	Bleeding 4 Abscess 3 Hematoma 2	Splenectomy 4 Drainage 2 Conservative 3	4	143 (95%)
Hagiwara et al. (1996)	28 13 15 (E)	I–II 77% III–IV 23% I–II 27% III–IV 73%	0	0	0	0	26 (93%)
Cocanour et al. (1998)	87	NA	7	Bleeding 5 Abscess 1 Cyst 1	Splenectomy 5 Embolization 2 (pseudoaneurysm)	0	82 (94%)
Davis et al. (1998)	332 312 20 (E)	I–II 62% III–IV 38%	16	Bleeding 16	Splenectomy 16	0	310 (93%)
Pachter et al. (1998)	102	I–II 66% III–IV 34%	2	Bleeding 2	Splenectomy 2	0	100 (98%)
Frumiento et al. (100%)	40 (children)	I–II 60% III–IV 40%	3	Pseudo-aneurysm 2 Abscess 1	Spontaneous resolution 2 Drainage 1	0	40 (2000)

E, embolization at admission; *NOM*, nonoperative management, *NA*, not available.

23.2.2 Vascular Complications

23.2.2.1 Clinical Presentation and Imaging

Vascular complications after nonoperative management of liver blunt injuries are suspected in the presence of recurrent abdominal pain, hypotension, impaired liver function tests, or findings on routine noninvasive diagnostic procedures such as abdominal US or CT, MRI, nuclear imaging studies or angiography (Haney et al. 1982; Yamamoto et al. 1993; Zeman et al. 1984; Hatten and Hamrick-Turner 1996; Terk and Rozenberg 1998; Balci et al. 1999; Carrillo et al. 1999; Parks et al. 1999; Cuff et al. 2000; Malhotra et al. 2000).

Delayed Hemorrhage

Delayed or recurrent hemorrhage is the most common complication of nonoperative management of hepatic injuries, with an overall incidence of 2.4%–5% and has been shown to be the most commonly reported indication of delayed surgery in patients in whom nonoperative management has failed (Meredith et al. 1994; Croce et al. 1995; Pachter and Hofstetter 1995; Brasel et al. 1997; Carrillo et al. 1998). The exact prevalence of bleeding in patients with blunt hepatic injuries managed nonoperatively is unknown. In selected series, where strict guidelines for nonoperative management were applied, the incidence of delayed hemorrhage ranged from 0% (Hammond et al. 1992) to less than 3.5% (Farnell et al. 1988; Sherman et al. 1994; Pachter et al. 1996) with only 0.7%–1.7% of patients requiring surgery. An incidence of 1%–3% has been reported in children (Oldham et al. 1986; Bond et al. 1996; Sjövall and Hirsh 1997; Shilyansky et al. 1999). Deaths related to delayed hemorrhage were reported in both children (Bermann et al. 1992) and adults (Geis et al. 1981; Taff et al. 1990; Pachter et al. 1996; Hagiwara et al. 1997). Delayed hemorrhage should be suspected in patients with ongoing transfusion requirements, a drop in the hemoglobin level or continued blood loss demonstrated by follow-up CT examinations (SCHWEIZER et al. 1993). Persistent complaints in the right upper abdominal quadrant and right shoulder pain after injury can be a sentinel sign suggesting ongoing bleeding within a large central hematoma with capsular distension (SHILYANSKY et al. 1999).

Delayed hemorrhage may be related to either an expanding minimal injury or to a biloma-induced pseudoaneurysm and may result in an expanding hematoma or free intraperitoneal rupture. After surgery, coagulopathy, inadequate initial repair, and missed retrohepatic venous injury may also result in hemorrhage. The incidence of secondary rupture of hepatic hematoma is of 0%–14% and the time elapsed between trauma and rupture ranges from 8 h to 30 days after injury (HAGIWARA et al. 1993; BOONE et al. 1995; CROCE et al. 1995). Common treatment errors in patients with delayed hemorrhage are assuming that the hemorrhage is not related to the liver, treating ongoing liver hemorrhage with multiple blood transfusion and expected bleeding control, misreading the CT and underestimating the amount of hemoperitoneum or active hemorrhage, and overestimating the amount of blood loss from associated injuries (CARRILLO et al. 1998).

A large hematoma was originally an indication for surgical exploration. Inability to define a clear source of bleeding and an increased incidence of infection have led to the expectant management of these injuries. When a delayed hemorrhage is suspected in patients initially managed without operation, either an immediate laparotomy or an abdominal CT should be performed, depending on hemodynamic stability. Indeed this complication may be safely treated nonsurgically.

Vascular Abnormalities

Posttraumatic pseudoaneurysms (PPA), associated or not with an arteriovenous fistula (AVF) are rare and an often delayed vascular complication of liver trauma. Their frequency varies between 1% and 2% in penetrating trauma and is below 1% in blunt trauma, and is even less in children (MACGILLIVRAY and VALENTINE 1992; GOW et al. 1996; PACHTER et al. 1996; BASILE et al. 1999; SIDHU et al. 1999). An incidence of 1.2% of PPA presenting with hemobilia was reported in a series of 482 patients with hepatic trauma (CROCE et al. 1995). Potential complications of a hepatic PPA include rupture and associated hemorrhage, rupture into the biliary system causing hemobilia and subsequent hematemesis or melena, or direct enteric fistulization into the duodenum (KESTENBERG and MITTAL 1992; CROCE et al. 1994; GOW et al. 1996; ABOUJAOUDE et al. 1996) (Fig. 23.1). Many hepatic PPAs do not present with bleeding, but are discovered during evaluation for other reasons, including abdominal pain, jaundice, or anemia. In contrast to splenic pseudoaneurysms, hepatic aneurysms have a high rupture rate, up to 44% (OWINGS and LENGLE 1995; GOW et al. 1996; SIDHU et al. 1999), which dictates a more aggressive management. Although their presence can sometimes be demonstrated by CT, the detection of PPA usually requires angiography, which is the most sensitive diagnostic modality. Reasons for the high false-negative rate of CT (35%) and US (40%–50%) include small size PPA and suboptimal contrast enhancement. Multislice helical CT angiography seems of particular interest in detecting small size vascular lesions noninvasively. In sequential scanning, misregistration from section to section may cause omission of structures or lesions and degradation in the quality of multiplanar reconstructions. Biphasic acquisition is performed, allowing for a temporal resolution with selective study of arteries and veins (GALEON et al. 1997).

Intrahepatic arteriovenous fistulae are rare and most commonly related to trauma. The majority of these fistulae are located between the hepatic artery and a portal vein branch. Hepatic artery-to-hepatic vein fistulae are much less common. Traumatic arterioportal fistulae may form from direct laceration of adjacent arteries and veins or via a connection with a pseudoaneurysm (SALVAT et al. 1980; SCLAFANI et al. 1981; SHENOY et al. 1981; REDMOND and KUMPE 1988; TANAKA et al. 1991; LERUT et al. 1992; KAYSER et al. 1996) (Fig. 23.2). Patients with an arterioportal fistulae may develop cramps and abdominal pain, several days to years after injury, or gastrointestinal bleeding and ascites resulting from portal hypertension and mucosal hyperemia due to mesenteric venous congestion (SCHMIDT et al. 1980; SCLAFANI et al. 1995a; KAYSER et al. 1996; KIRCHGATTERER et al. 1998). In case of communication between the hepatic artery and a hepatic vein, cardiac failure caused by high out-put may develop, depending on the size of the shunt. Portohepatic fistula is rarely observed and may be combined with a portal pseudoaneurysm and requires technical refinements for treatment (STROZ et al. 1996).

Hemobilia

Hemobilia is a feared complication of the nonoperative management of hepatic trauma. Before 1990, it had only been reported twice in a review of 22 series

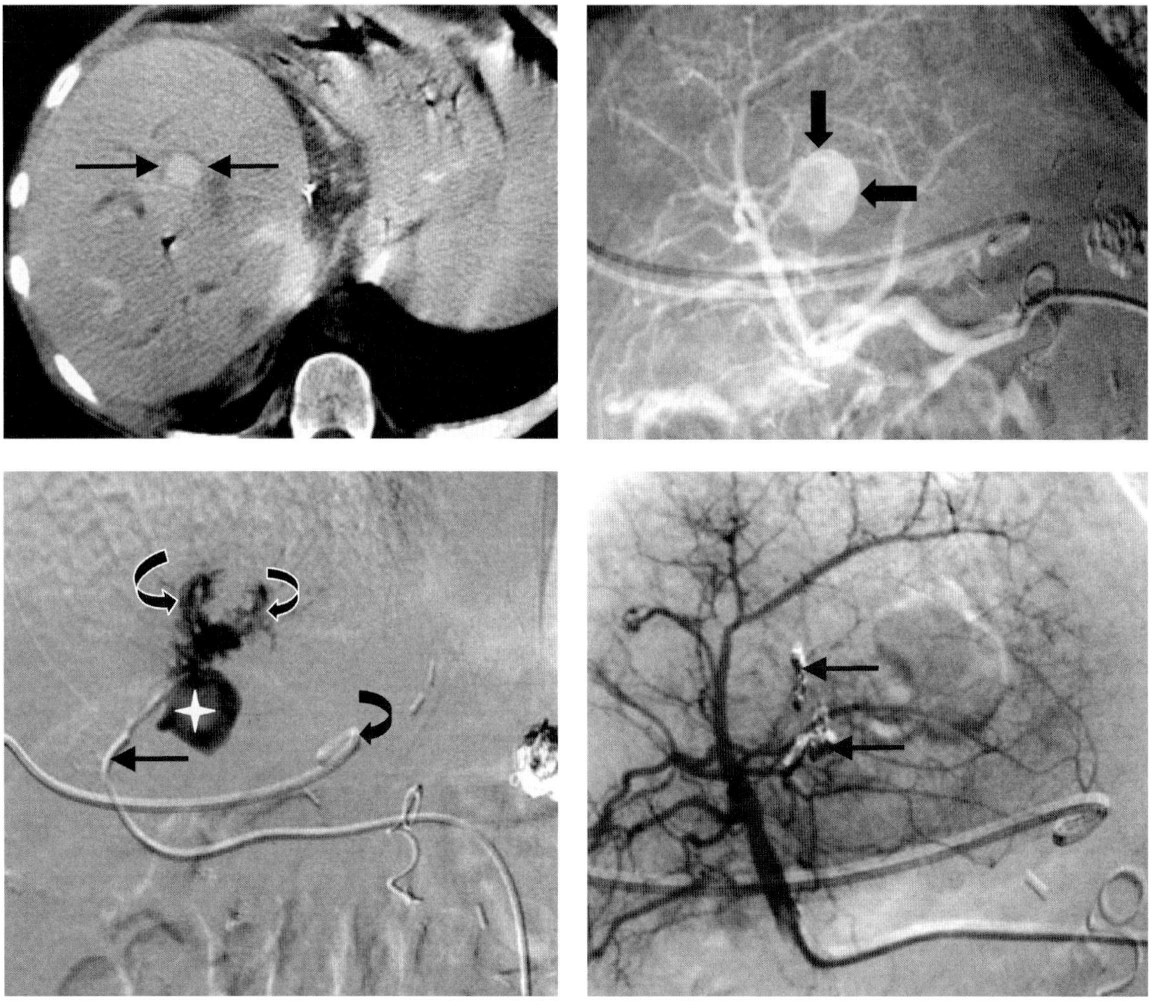

Fig. 23.1a–d. A 29-year-old man sustained severe blunt abdominal trauma following a high-speed motorcycle accident. CT at admission showed grade IV left lobe hepatic injury and several areas of contusion in the right lobe. Persistent hypovolemic shock indicated emergent left hepatectomy. On day 12, intra- and extrahepatic bilomas were drained percutaneously. The patient presented with continuous melena and three episodes of massive hematemesis requiring blood transfusions. Upper GI endoscopy showed blood seeping from the papilla and clots in the common bile duct, confirming the clinical suspicion of hemobilia. **a** CT of the upper abdomen shows a focal, rounded, enhancing lesion (*arrows*) located at the site of the drained biloma and moderate intrahepatic bile duct dilation. **b** Right hepatic angiography confirms a 12-mm pseudoaneurysm (*arrows*) supplied by a small anterior segmental hepatic artery. **c** After selective catheterization of the feeding artery with a 4-F catheter (*arrow*), wedged contrast injection clearly demonstrates rapid bleeding (*black and white curved arrows*) from the pseudoaneurysm (*star*) in the surrounding biloma. A transhepatic pig-tail catheter draining an extrahepatic biloma is still present (*black curved arrow*). **d** After superselective catheterization of the subsegmental arterial feeder beyond the aneurysmal neck with a 3-F microcatheter (Leggerio-Terumo Corporation, Japan), the pseudoaneurysm is completely excluded by deposition of five Hilal microcoils (Cook, Denmark) distal and proximal (*arrows*) to the neck. No recurrence of the pseudoaneurysm was observed on serial CTs and clinical outcome was uneventful

of nonoperative management of liver trauma (Knudson et al. 1990). Traumatic hemobilia, first described as "an hemorrhage into the biliary tract", has been noted after surgical repair of liver injuries and may be more frequently associated with central liver injuries (Sandblom 1948). The most common causes of hemobilia are percutaneous diagnostic or therapeutic procedures performed in the hepatobiliary system (Savader et al. 1992; Croce et al. 1994). The incidence of hemobilia after conservative management of hepatic injury is about 1%, with most cases being secondary to blunt liver trauma (Croce et al. 1994). Hemobilia is suspected when melena or hematemesis follow hepatic trauma. A history of abdominal

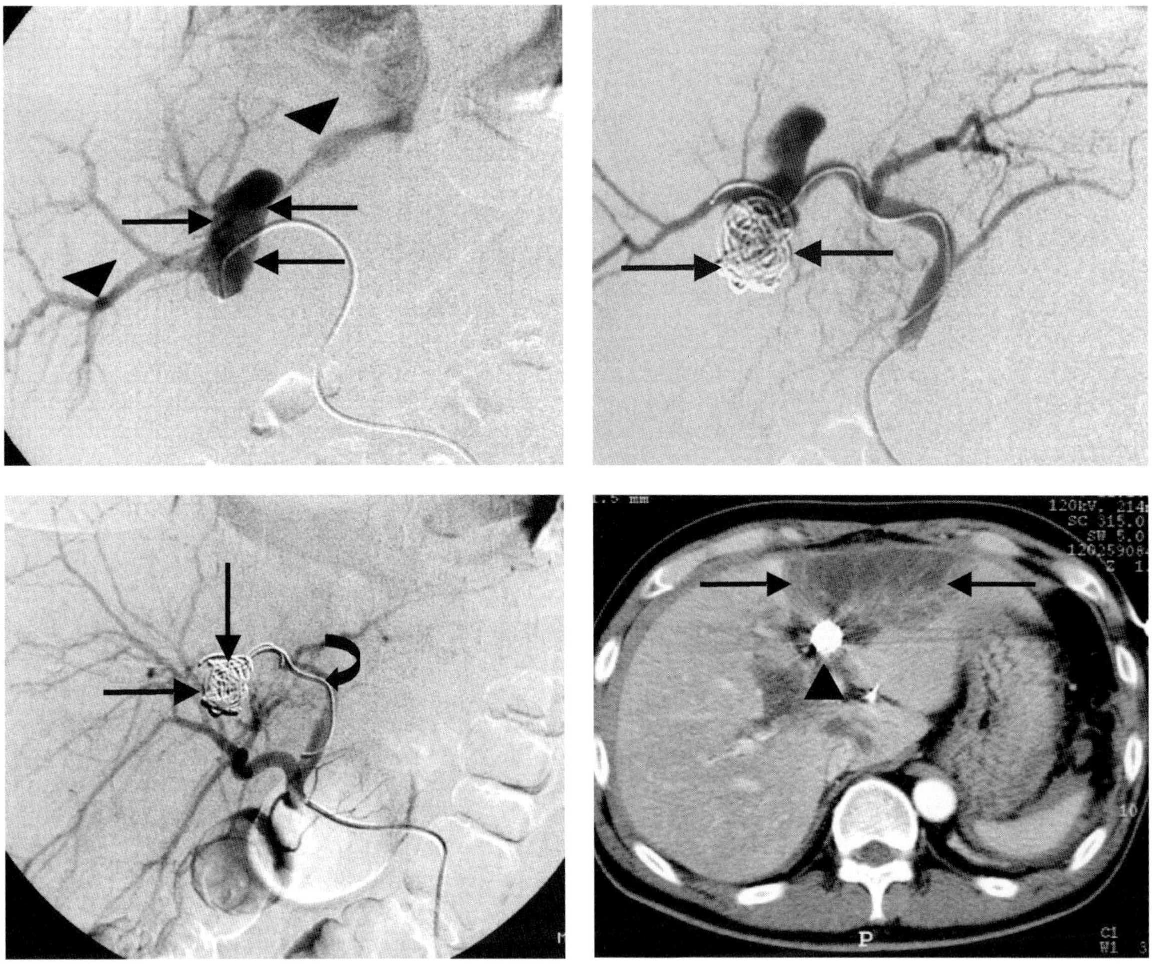

Fig. 23.2a–d. A 27-year-old woman had sustained grade III liver injury after a motorcycle accident and was managed conservatively. On routine follow-up CT at day 7, a vascular malformation was suspected in the injured area of the liver. Increasing hemoperitoneum was also observed. **a** Selective left hepatic arteriography shows a 20×8-mm pseudoaneurysm (*arrows*) located in segment IV and filling of an arterioportal fistula (*arrowheads*). **b** After packing of eight Gianturco coils in the lower portion of the aneurysm (*arrows*), the arterioportal fistula was occluded. **c** A complete obliteration of the pseudoaneurysm was obtained after placement of three additional coils inside the aneurysmal sac (*arrows*) and in the injured artery of segment IV. Misplacement of one coil extending far in the feeding artery (*curved arrow*) was secondary to retrograde catheter dislodgment during coil delivery. Multiple attempts to snare and retrieve the coil by lasso technique failed. **d** Follow-up CT shows a partial infarction of the left liver lobe (*arrows*) secondary to combined segmental arterial and portal occlusion. The aneurysmal sack is completely filled by coils (*arrowhead*). Clinical follow-up was uneventful

trauma, obstructive jaundice, right upper-quadrant colicky pain and hematemesis or melena should point to this diagnosis, but the complete triad occurs in a minority of patients (Fig. 23.1) (Cleveland et al. 1970; Savader et al. 1992; Clancy and Warren 1997). Hemobilia usually develops within 4 weeks of liver injury (Dunlop et al. 1977; Franklin et al. 1980; Pilla et al. 1987; Croce et al. 1994; Hidalgo et al. 1995), but may occur later than 1 month (MacGillivray and Valentine 1989). Direct endoscopic visualization of blood oozing from the papilla or angiographic demonstration of bleeding into the bile ducts or gallbladder confirms the diagnosis (Katz and Meng 1970). Extravasation of contrast into the biliary tree is rarely observed (Sclafani et al. 1984b; Hidalgo et al. 1995). The presence of high-density material (>50 Hounsfield units) within the gallbladder or filling defects within biliary system on CT may suggest hemobilia (Hidalgo et al. 1995; Sidhu et al. 1999).

Angiographic embolization is the first-line treatment of hemobilia (Franklin et al. 1980; Shenoy et al. 1981; Vadon et al. 1984; Pilla et al. 1987; Steiner et al. 1994). Surgery, including selective artery ligation and/or hepatectomy, is indicated only in cases of embolization failure or for large intrahepatic cavities with suspected superinfection (Croce et al. 1994). If surgery is considered, preoperative embolization should be performed to avoid catastrophic intraoperative bleeding (Croce et al. 1994).

23.2.2.2 Endovascular Management

Technique

Transcatheter embolization has been proven a safe and effective primary procedure that can be applied to true or false hepatic aneurysm (Baker et al. 1987; Salam et al. 1992). Superselective embolization preserves other intrahepatic vascular branches. This is important for the resorption of the hematoma and local contusion (Galeon et al. 1997). Ideally, embolization should be done as close as possible to the injury to decrease the risk of liver ischemia and avoid retrograde collateral flow from branches distal to the site of embolization (Schwartz et al. 1993; Hidalgo et al. 1995) (Fig. 23.1). The use of a coaxial microcatheter system (mainly Tracker-18 and Tracker-325, Target Therapeutics, Fremont, Calif. or 3-F Focus microcatheter, Terumo, Japan), inserted coaxially through a 5- or 6-F guiding catheter or 0.038-in. inner lumen diagnostic catheters, allows vessel occlusion close to the vascular lesion. A variety of embolic agents, including fibrilled or nonfibrilled complex helical or straight platinum microcoils, gelatin sponge particles, alcohol, and isobutyl-2-cyanoacrylate can be delivered through such microcatheters. Minimal vaso-occlusion minimizes the amount of tissue necrosis in end-organ embolization and the risk of lesion recurrence due to the recruitment of collateral vessels distal to the site of coil deployment (Schwartz et al. 1993; Teitelbaum et al. 1993a; Hidalgo et al. 1995). In the right hepatic artery, selective embolization reduces the risk of gallbladder infarction (Takayasu et al. 1985). Besides facilitating specific distal vascular occlusion in injured vessels prone to spasm, a coaxial microcatheter system also allows for easier and more rapid cannulation of the target vessel. An open-ended guidewire may also be used together with either 0.025-in. coils or particulate materials such as gelatin sponge (Kaufman et al. 1992). Embolization with glue is useful for occluding a pseudoaneurysm, which is difficult to control by coils alone, especially those located in a small or severely affected vessel or when multiple efferent arteries originate from the pseudoaneurysm (Yamakado et al. 2000). For a pseudoaneurysm arising from a large, proximal branch of the hepatic artery, both distal and proximal embolization should be performed to reduce the risk of PPA reconstitution by retrograde collateral filling (Hidalgo et al. 1995). This technique may not be feasible despite the use of a variety of miniaturized guidewires and catheters. If distal embolization is not possible because of vessel or aneurysm size or location, a single proximal coil may provide a sufficient blood flow reduction, inducing secondary thrombosis (Gow et al. 1996; Sidhu et al. 1999). Nonselective distal embolization with polyvinyl alcohol particles (PVA) is an alternative technique to distal coil deposition when selective catheterization has failed (Fig. 23.3). This technique should be applied with caution, especially in patients with compromised portal flow, because of an increased risk of liver ischemia.

AVFs are technically more challenging since a high flow state may result in non-target embolization of occlusive material to the pulmonary arteries. As the first goal of fistula occlusion is the blockage of the feeding artery as close as possible to the nidus of the fistula, an effective method is the careful deposition of a large fibrilled coil, which then may provide a matrix for the nesting of smaller coils in order to produce complete vaso-occlusion. Nonfibrilled coils provide adequate arterial blockade if deployed in a tightly packed fashion (Redmond and Kumpe 1988; Teitelbaum et al. 1993a; Eastridge and Minei 1997; Kirchgatterer et al. 1998). When superselective occlusion of the artery feeding an AVF is not feasible, the siphoning effect of the lesion may allow proximal injection of large particulate material because of preferential migration to the appropriate site (Schwartz et al. 1993). A large AVF may be difficult to occlude and may require repeat embolizations (Lerut et al. 1992).

Results

The technical success rate of embolization of post-traumatic hepatic vascular lesions with microcatheter systems is 88%–94%, without clinically significant complications (Kaufman et al. 1992; Schwartz et al. 1993; Teitelbaum et al. 1993b). Tissue necrosis in the liver is uncommon due to the dual hepatic blood supply (Schwartz et al. 1993). Technical failures are due to the erroneous selection of the appropriate vessel for embolization and a persistent high-flow AVF (Fig. 23.4). Recurrences may usually

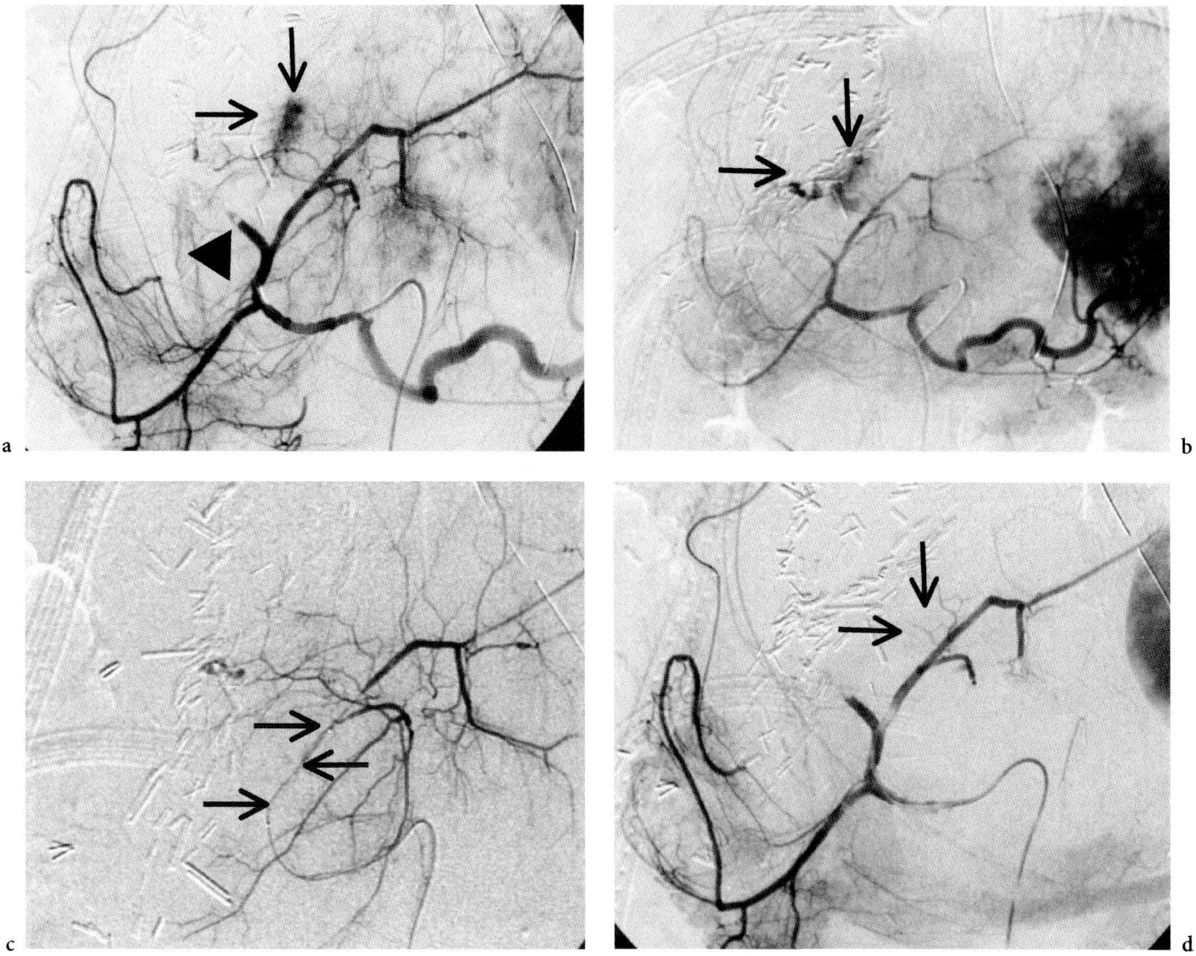

Fig. 23.3a–d. A 45-year-old female developed shock secondary to massive bleeding through the surgical drains, 3 days after a right hepatectomy done for grade IV liver injury following a traffic accident. **a, b** Hepatic arteriography shows active arterial bleeding from small liver surface branches (*arrows*). No leak on the stump of the ligated right hepatic artery is observed (*arrowhead*). The inhomogeneous left lobe parenchymography is due to diffuse areas of contusion. **c** After selective catheterization of the proximal left hepatic artery with a 0.018-in. microcatheter, severe spasm occurred (*arrows*), precluding further distal catheterization. **d** Embolization performed with 250–350 calibrated polyvinyl alcohol microparticles, allowed definitive control of the bleeding (*arrows*). Transient liver failure, probably due to peripheral ischemia of the residual left lobe, was noted during early follow-up

be controlled by re-embolization (Lukancic et al. 1991; Lerut et al. 1992; Garby et al. 1997). Occlusion of difficult lesions such as large pseudoaneurysms sometimes requires a combination of occluding agents, i.e., multiple coils and ultimately thrombin. Alcohol or phenol should not be used, because of the risk of hepatic necrosis and biliary fibrosis.

Complications

Complications of embolization include hepatic necrosis, abscess formation, nontargeted embolization, gallbladder infarction and catheter-induced vascular damage. A few cases of complications, occurring after embolization for hemobilia or PPA, such as hepatic necrosis, rebleeding, coil misplacement or migration, have been reported (Garby et al. 1997; Bokhari et al. 1999). Migrated coils from a cystic artery PPA into the common bile duct were successfully removed endoscopically using papillotomy and a balloon, without complication (Bokhari et al. 1999). Misplacement or retrograde coil migration may be related to the catheter delivery, placement of the coil, likelihood of reflux and coil size. Coil migration is often the result of subtle catheter displacement or movement during coil delivery. A crucial

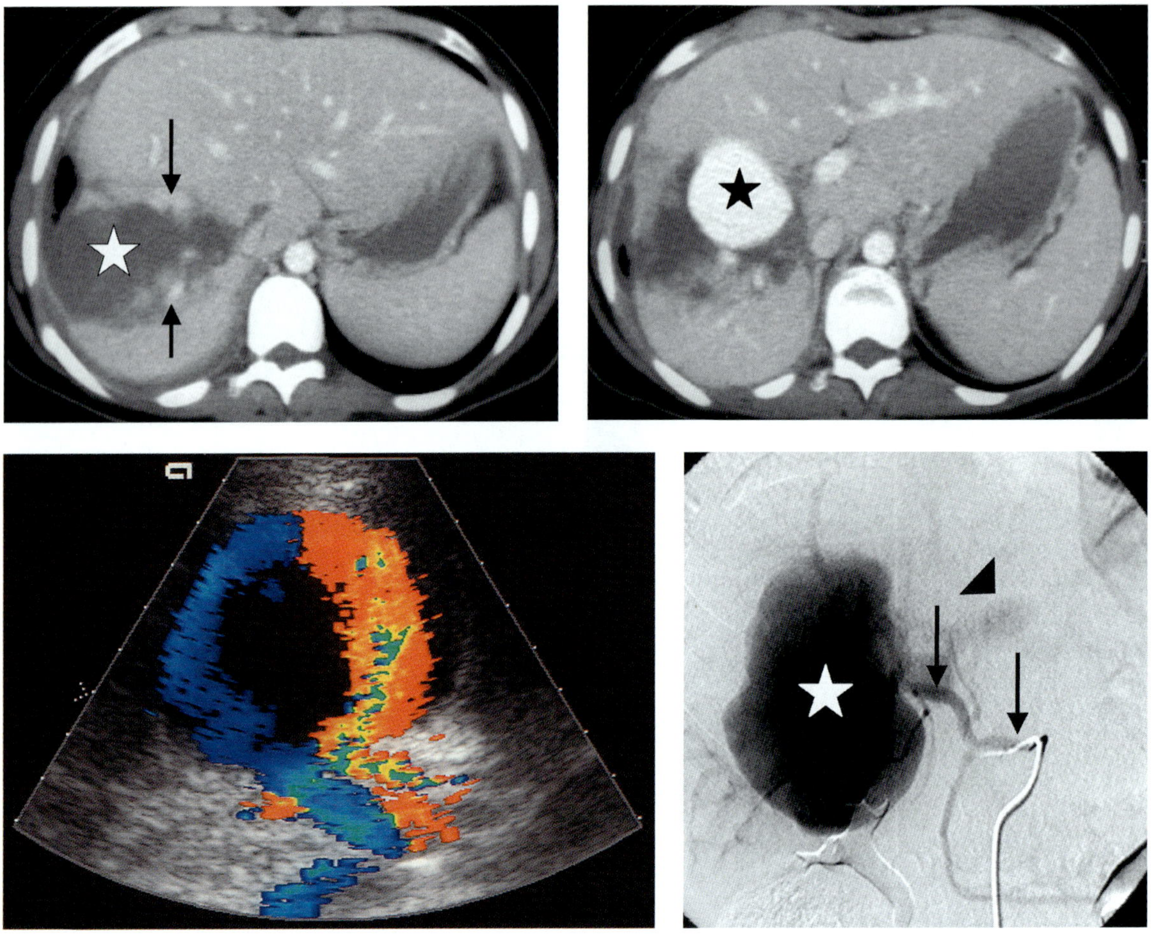

a b c d

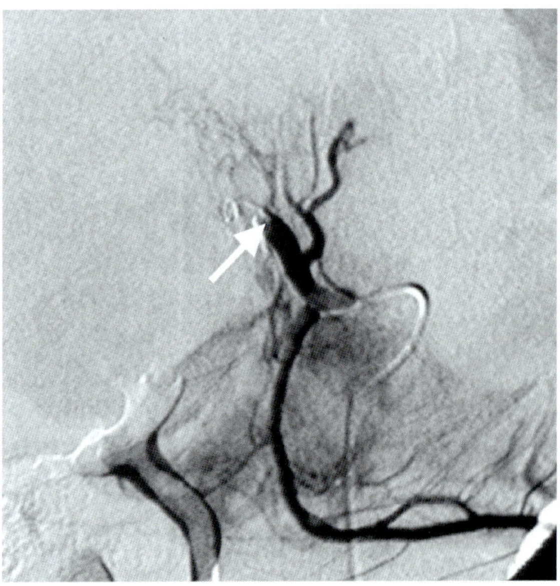

e

Fig. 23.4a–j. A 22-year-old woman presented with grade IV right liver laceration with massive hemoperitoneum after a skiing injury. She underwent an emergent laparotomy and hepatorrhaphy. **a** Early postoperative CT shows a large right posterior hepatic contusion area (*star*). Notice apparently normal adjacent vascular structures (*arrows*). **b** CT at 2 weeks demonstrates a large pseudoaneurysm (*star*) developed within the area of hepatic contusion. **c** Color-Doppler also shows an arterial pseudoaneurysm and demonstrates arterialized flow within the right portal branches, suggesting a combined arterioportal fistula. **d** Hepatic angiography shows a large pseudoaneurysm (*star*), supplied by the right hepatic artery (*arrows*), with early filling of the right portal vein (*arrowhead*). **e** Embolization of the right hepatic artery with Gianturco coils (*arrow*) is performed. **f** Embolization of the pseudoaneurysm was only partially, successful as shown on CT. Persistent flow (*arrow*) in the aneurysmal sac is seen. *Curved arrow* points to the arterial coils. **g** The residual pseudoaneurysm (*star*) is supplied by multiple small branches arising from the gastroduodenal, left hepatic, and intrahepatic arteries (*arrows*).The right hepatic artery is occluded. **h** Embolization of all remain-

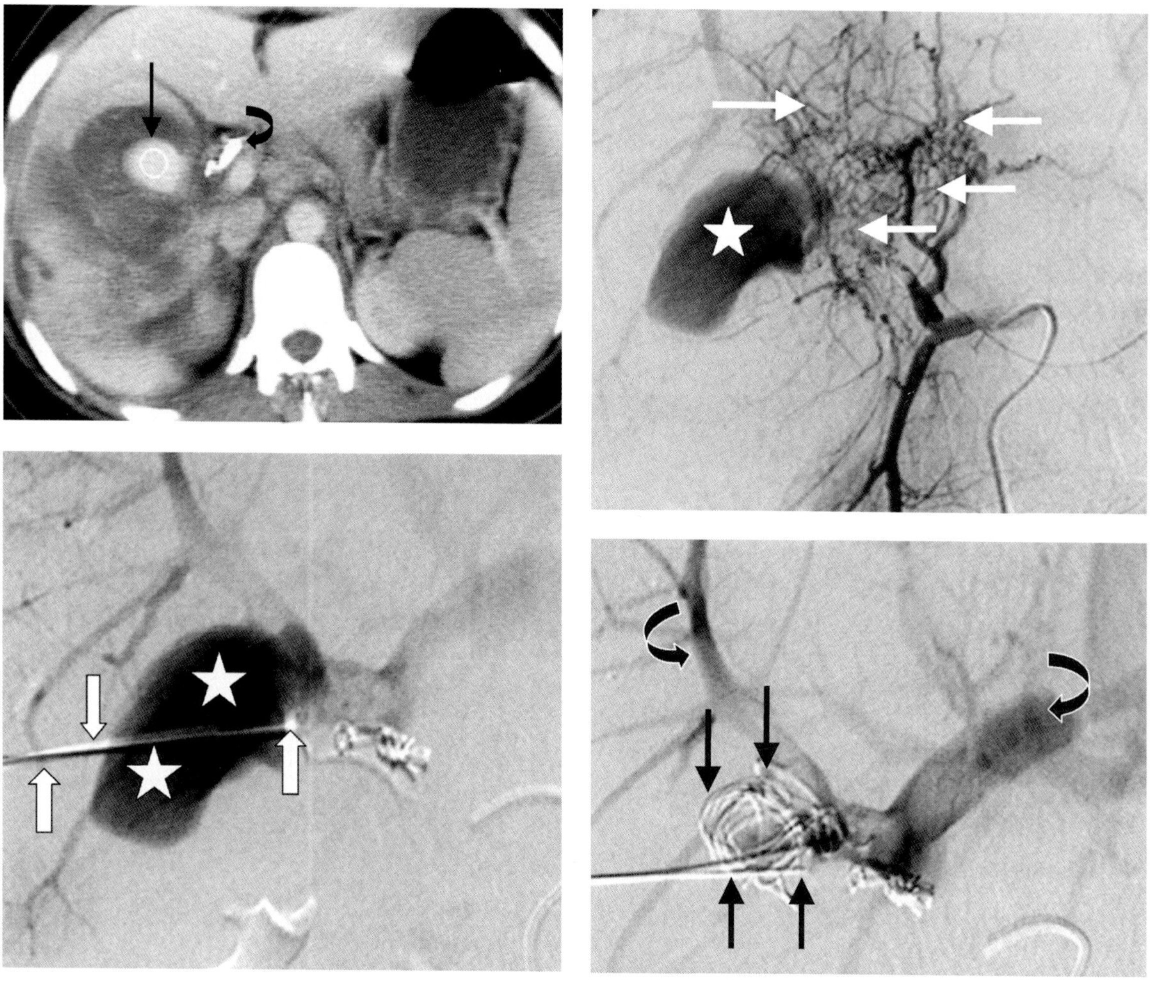

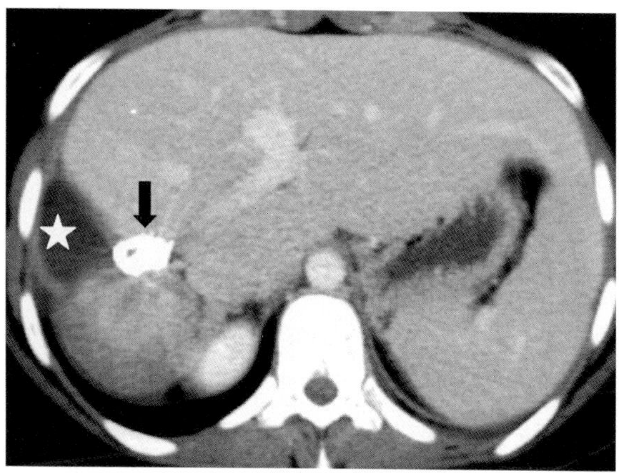

ing arterial feeders could not be considered because of the risk of massive liver necrosis due to fistula-related persistent hepatofugal portal flow. Direct percutaneous transhepatic puncture of the aneurysmal sac (*star*) with a 5-Fr Teflon sheathed needle (*arrows*) under sonographic guidance is performed to obtain complete thrombosis of the sac. **i** The aneurysmal sac is filled with twelve 15- to 20-mm steel macrocoils (*arrows*) and several large gelatin sponge torpedoes. The intrahepatic portal branches (*curved arrows*) remain patent except the right posterolateral branch. **j** CT obtained 5 weeks after the percutaneous procedure confirms complete obliteration of the pseudoaneurysm, which is retracted around the steel coils (*arrow*). A small residual biloma (*star*) and a marked left liver lobe hypertrophy, due to right posterior portal branch occlusion, are observed

consideration is selecting a coil size that will occlude the aneurysm completely without hampering intrahepatic collateral flow development.

Spontaneous hepatic abscess formation after blunt hepatic trauma is common, making it difficult to assess the specific incidence of embolization-induced necrosis or abscess formation after interventional radiology (Savader et al. 1992; Schwartz et al. 1993). Gallbladder infarction may be avoided by precisely localizing the origin of the cystic artery before embolization of the right liver lobe, in order to inject the embolic material beyond the ostium of the cystic artery (Takayasu et al. 1985).

23.2.2.3 Percutaneous Approach

Previous interventions, such as arterial embolization or ligation, atherosclerosis, intimal dissection or anatomical variants may preclude selective catheterization, rendering the pseudoaneurysm inaccessible to transcatheter embolization. In these cases, a direct percutaneous approach is an alternative (Cope and Zeit 1986; Rothbarth et al. 1989; Lukancic et al. 1991; Vauthey et al. 1997; Araoz and Andrews 2000) (Fig. 23.5). Direct puncture of the pseudoaneurysm is ideally performed with color Doppler. However, in case of a small size or a deeply located lesion, color Doppler may be inadequate. In this situation, the precise localization offered by C-arm fluoroscopy is essential for exact needle placement and for limiting the number of needle passes, thereby reducing potential hemorrhagic or biliary complications (Lukancic et al. 1991). To minimize both, possible aneurysmal rupture and damage to the surrounding tissue, small-gauge Teflon needles are used. Different

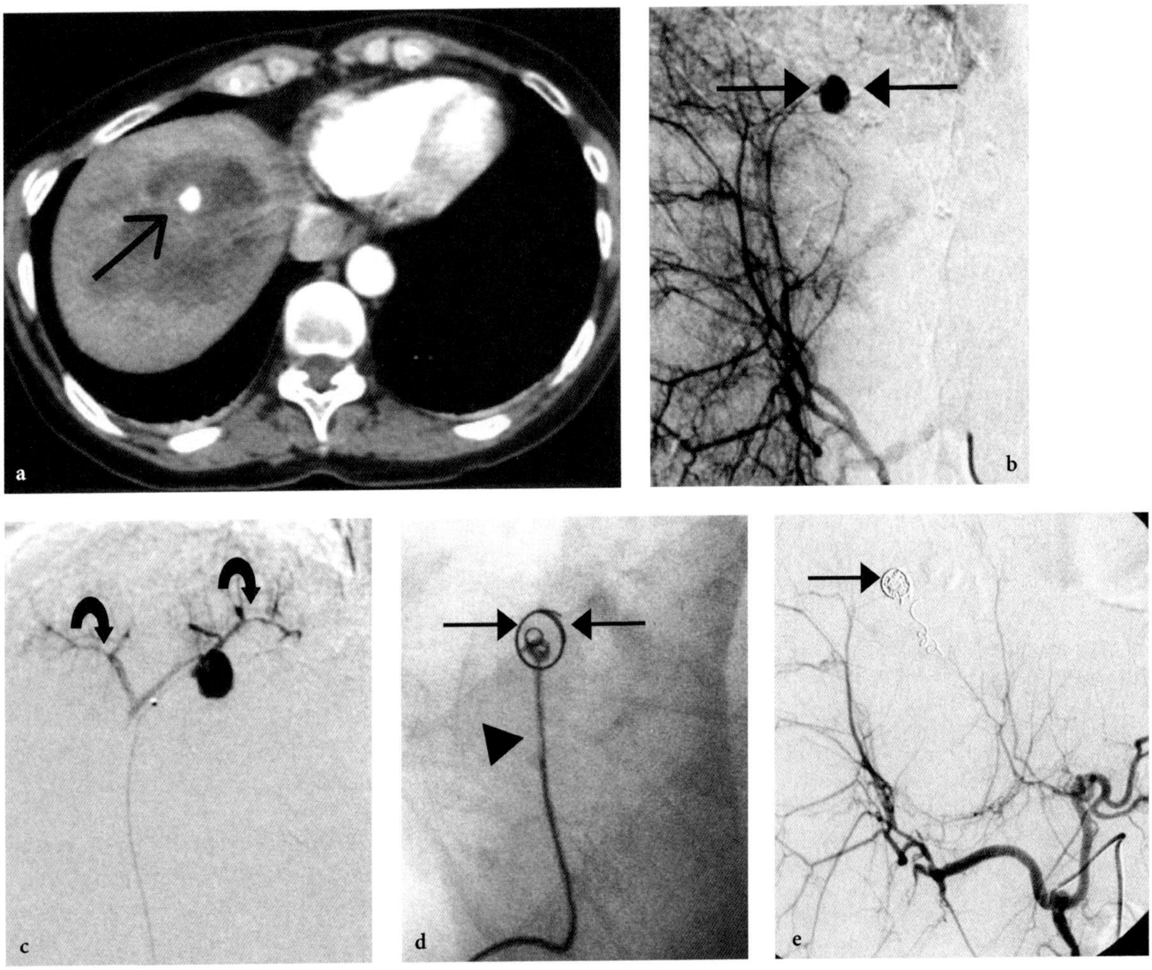

Fig. 23.5a–e. A 48-year-old polytraumatized patient was treated conservatively for grade III liver injury. CT at admission showed a large nonenhancing intrahepatic fluid collection with no hepatic vascular abnormality. **a** Routine control helical CT at day 7 demonstrates a small focal hyperdense lesion (*arrow*) with arterial enhancement, highly suggestive of a posttraumatic pseudoaneurysm. **b** A pseudoaneurysm (*arrows*) is confirmed by selective right hepatic angiography in segment VIII and is surrounded by a hypovascular area of contusion. **c** Superselective angiography of the feeding artery through a 0.018-in. Fast-Tracker microcatheter (Target Therapeutics, California) shows an arterioportal fistula with opacification of distal portal vein branches (*curved arrows*). **d** After placement of circular Hilal microcoil (Cook) inside the pseudoaneurysm (*black arrows*), the microcatheter was dislodged due to spasm, precluding further embolization. A direct percutaneous puncture (*arrowhead*) under sonographic guidance was performed, using a 5-F Teflon-sheathed needle to fill the residual cavity with standard Gianturco coils (*white arrow*). **e** During removal of the needle, the hepatic tract was embolized by two additional coils to avoid bleeding or a bile fistula. Hepatic arteriography demonstrates complete exclusion of the pseudoaneurysm (*arrow*) and preservation of the peripheral intrahepatic arterial branches

embolic agents have been injected, including stainless steel coils (Capek et al. 1992; Vauthey et al. 1997; Lukancic et al. 1991), thrombin or thrombin-soaked gelatin sponge pledgets (Cope and Zeit 1986; Uflacker et al. 1989), alcohol (Kuno et al. 1995) or a combination of different materials with gelatin sponge (Rothbarth et al. 1989) (Fig. 23.4).

The successful use of a nonarterial route was reported through an existing transhepatic drainage catheter tract for embolization of a hepatic artery pseudoaneurysm developed adjacent to a biliary drainage catheter (Rosen and Rothberg 1982). A biliary T-tube tract may also be considered as an alternative route for the embolization of a false aneurysm or with an arterioportal fistula located on an intrahepatic arterial branch when the conventional angiographic approach has failed (Beningfield et al. 1991). Endoscopic retrograde cholangiographic guidance may also be feasible for embolization of an external biliary fistula by using a technique similar to that described above (Krige et al. 1997). Potential procedural complications include coil migration, especially in case of biliary-arterial fistula (Araoz and Andrews 2000), abscess formation, that can be treated by percutaneous drainage (Rothbarth et al. 1989), and tract bleeding after needle removal. This last complication may be avoided by placing coils or gelatin sponge pledgets inside the tract after completion of the procedure. Aneurysm rupture has not been reported in a direct percutaneous embolization procedure. In case of persistent flow inside the lesion or delayed recurrence, repeated endovascular treatments are effective in most cases (Schwartz et al. 1993; Hidalgo et al. 1995).

23.2.3 Biliary Complications

23.2.3.1 Bilhemia

Clinical Presentation and Imaging

The bilhemia syndrome is an extremely rare complication, usually consecutive to blunt hepatic injury with severe deceleration. It may also result from either iatrogenic or gunshot liver injury. It is caused by a pathological communication between an intrahepatic bile duct and a hepatic vein, followed by the formation of an extensive liver hematoma within necrotic tissue, leading to excessive serum bilirubin levels, but a moderate rise of serum liver enzymes. Passage of bile from a disrupted bile duct into an hepatic vein is due to an increased biliary-venous pressure gradient of 15–20 cm H_2O and occurs during the reabsorption of the cavity. A few cases have been reported in the literature (Inberg and Ahonen 1977; Struyven et al. 1982; Blum et al. 1993). Posttraumatic bilhemia is clinically characterized by the rapid development of jaundice after blunt hepatic trauma, with a marked increase of the total and conjugated serum bilirubin level, generally without hepatic failure (Blum et al. 1993). The precise localization of the biliovenous fistula requires a direct opacification of the bile duct by either an endoscopic retrograde cholangiography (ERCP), a cholangiography via a T-tube, or a fine needle percutaneous transhepatic cholangiography (PTC).

Management

The classic management has been surgical by either resection of the fistula or drainage of the collection and T-tube suction drainage (Glazer et al. 1994) or percutaneous either by direct occlusion of the fistula with a catheter (Struyven et al. 1982) or by insertion of a drainage catheter in the causative biloma in order to decrease the pressure and allow closure of the shunt (Blum et al. 1993). The actual ideal treatment of posttraumatic bilhemia is combined endoscopic sphincterotomy and biliary stenting (Blum et al. 1993; Glazer et al. 1994; Gable et al. 1997). The mortality rate is high without specific treatment or after surgery. The outcome of patients treated percutaneously or endoscopically seems to be more favorable.

23.2.3.2 Biliary Leakage

Leakage of bile from a liver laceration is common but in most cases of small volume and transient, without sequelae. Nonoperative management of abdominal trauma results in a delayed recognition of significant bile leaks (Hollands and Little 1991; Sugimoto et al. 1993). Persistent bile leaks will develop in 4% of children or adults (Hollands and Little 1991; Scioscia et al. 1994; Sugiyama et al. 2000). ERCP is rarely indicated in the first few days after hepatic trauma but should be performed in case of persistent bile leaks or bilhemia (Bynoe et al. 1992; Scioscia et al. 1994; Jenkins and Ponsky 1995; Eid et al. 1996; Clancy and Warren 1997; Sugiyama et al. 2000). Depending on the criteria and the method used to diagnose a bile leakage, the incidence of significant bile leaks resulting in biloma or biliary fistula in patients treated conservatively after liver injury ranges from 0.5% to 20% (HOLLANDS and LITTLE 1991; CROCE et al. 1995; PACHTER et al. 1996; CARRILLO et al. 1998). A higher incidence, up to 22.5%, was observed following major liver trauma or after extended resection following hepatic injuries (SHAHRUDIN and NOORI 1997; ASENSIO et al. 2000; D'AMOURS et al. 2000). The exact incidence of intrahepatic bile duct injuries after blunt abdominal trauma is unknown. Indeed, many peripheral bile ducts injuries go unrecognized, as most are below the threshold of current imaging techniques and heal without complications (D'AMOURS et al. 2000). Persistent biliary fistulae prolong hospitalization and may result in abscess, bile peritonitis, or hemobilia. Factors responsible for prolonged bile drainage are distal obstruction or infection and foreign body material. If the bile leaks continuously discharge through a drain, maintenance of drainage is required while awaiting spontaneous resolution, which occurs in most cases (COGBILL et al. 1988; HOLLANDS and LITTLE 1991; PACHTER et al. 1996).

Biloma

Intra- or extrahepatic bilomas are reported with a frequency ranging from 2% to 12% (CROCE et al. 1995; PACHTER et al. 1996; ASENSIO et al. 2000). Biloma may be asymptomatic or may present with right upper quadrant fullness or pain. Delayed infection or hemorrhage into a bile collection may occur, prompting clinical recognition. Persistence or continued growth of an intra- or perihepatic collection after hepatic trauma suggests the diagnosis of biloma. Bilomas are identified with increasing frequency by using cross-sectional imaging techniques and bile nuclear medicine studies (WEISSMANN et al. 1979; ZEMAN et al. 1984). Bilomas appear on CT as low-attenuation collections in or around the liver that may mimic resolving hematomas or abscesses. Biloma is diagnosed from 11 days to 2.5 years following trauma (FABIAN et al. 1991; PACHTER et al. 1996). Confirmation of suspected biloma requires percutaneous aspiration of bile or demonstration of a communication with the biliary tree by 99 m Tc-PIPIDA cholescintigraphy (ZEMAN et al. 1984).

Small bilomas, of less than 3 cm in diameter, usually do not require treatment and resolve with conservative management unless they become infected. Non-drainage of such bilomas does not result in an increased rate of septic complications but secondary infection of a large intrahepatic hematoma or bile collection may be responsible of pyogenic liver abscesses (FABIAN et al. 1991; MALHOTRA et al. 2000). Pseudoaneurysm formation may also be induced by a large bile collection.

A biloma larger than 3 cm should systematically be treated, preferentially by percutaneous drainage or surgically (BOONE et al. 1995; HAGIWARA et al. 1997). The presence of bile delays liver wound healing by the inflammatory reaction induced in nearby the vessels. This process could lead to rupture of a blood vessel wall with formation of a pseudoaneurysm (CARRILLO et al. 1999). A systematic assessment of the bile ducts after delayed hemorrhage in patients with complex hepatic injuries has been proposed. Conversely, when a large biloma is detected, angiography should be performed to detect an asymptomatic vascular injury that may result in delayed hemorrhage. Percutaneous catheter drainage, performed to treat a symptomatic, expanding or infected biloma, should remain in place until communication with the biliary system is no longer demonstrated by contrast opacification (MASSON et al. 1993; BOONE et al. 1995; DE BACKER et al. 1998; CARRILLO et al. 1999).

Biliary Fistula

A bile fistula may originate from either a peripheral intrahepatic biliary radical or a major hepatic duct. Nuclear medicine studies (HIDA) and ERCP are mainly used (ZEMAN et al. 1984; SCIOSCIA et al. 1994). Hepatobiliary nuclear scanning with technetium 99m-dimethyl iminodiacetic acid (HIDA) is a sensitive test for studying the hepatic parenchyma and documenting the presence or absence of biliary leaks, because the tracing agent is concentrated and excreted into the bile ducts (GARTMAN et al. 1985). However, scintigraphy is not precise enough to pinpoint injuries to the extrahepatic bile ducts. Once a biliary fistula is diagnosed, a cholangiogram, either by a percutaneous transhepatic approach or preferentially by ERCP is required to localize the fistula (JENKINS and PONSKY 1995; ASENSIO et al. 2000; SUGIYAMA et al. 2000; D'AMOURS et al. 2000).

Conventional therapy is surgical intervention with débridement, ductal repair, and controlled drainage to seal the fistula (BYNOE et al. 1992; OLDHAM et al. 1986). Because of adhesions and inflammation in the damaged liver parenchyma, surgery is often difficult, as shown by the mortality rate of reintervention for control of a biliary fistula after hepatobiliary surgery, ranging from 5% to 8%. Direct surgical exploration and ligation of the extra- or intrahepatic duct, hepatic resection or a Roux-en-Y hepaticojejunostomy is an option, when conservative means have failed (Hollands and Little 1991).

Several types of nonoperative management have been described. Endoscopic treatment, including combined sphincterotomy, nasobiliary drainage or biliary stent insertion, are effective to treat posttraumatic bile leakage (Scioscia et al. 1994; Jenkins and Ponsky 1995; Poli et al. 1995; De Backer et al. 1998; D'Amours et al. 2000; Sugiyama et al. 2000) (Fig. 23.6). For leaks from branches of either the right or left main hepatic ducts, a temporary stent should be placed to bridge the duct laceration with subsequent healing of the fistula, which is confirmed by ERCP and/or radionuclide scan before stent removal (Ponchon et al. 1989; Eid et al. 1996; Krige et al. 1997; De Backer et al. 1998; Asensio et al. 2000). Biliary stent placement may also be used to bridge or bypass a defect of the common bile duct (Ponchon et al. 1989; Jenkins and Ponsky 1995; Sugiyama et al. 2000).

Endoscopic sphincterotomy contributes to reducing the output of the fistula by decreasing the intrabiliary pressure (Scioscia et al. 1994) (Fig. 23.6). Reducing the pressure gradient within the common bile duct diverts the flow of bile away from the fistula into the duodenum. Peripheral biliary fistulae are best treated by combined percutaneous drainage of the biloma and endoscopic sphincterotomy. This approach appears to allow the site of leakage to seal via the biliary decompression effect (Fig. 23.7). Although endoscopic sphincterotomy alone may result in closure of a peripheral biliary fistula in some patients (Scioscia et al. 1994), it does not guarantee complete elimination of the choledochoduodenal pressure gradient, unlike endoscopic stent insertion (Jenkins and Ponsky 1995; Poli et al. 1995; Griffen et al. 2000; Sugiyama et al. 2000). Therefore, biliary stent placement without sphincterotomy has been mainly recommended (Jenkins and Ponsky 1995; Sugiyama et al. 2000). If the distal bile duct is stenosed, balloon dilatation or the insertion of a large stent through the stenosis will be required. Nasobiliary drainage may also be effective for treating a biliary fistula and allows for serial cholangiographies (Poli et al. 1995). However, a protruding catheter is less comfortable for the patient than an internal stent. The effect of endoscopic treatment is limited when ERCP does not detect a biliary fistula because of sequestration (Sugiyama et al. 2000). When the distal part of the injured bile duct is closed, bile continues to leak from the upper part of the injured portion (Ponchon et al. 1989). In such a condition, percutaneous transhepatic biliary drainage may allow the fistula to heal, but catheter placement is often difficult in posttraumatic patients who generally have nondilated intrahepatic bile ducts. The use of percutaneous drainage may be beneficial if an active bile leak is not detected, but the risk of secondary infection restricts this treatment to a relatively short period. Percutaneous microcoil embolization of an intrahepatic or extrahepatic biliary fistula may be a therapeutic option in cases where conservative treatment has failed and other techniques are contraindicated (Hunt et al. 1997).

Thoracobiliary fistulae, including pleurobiliary and bronchobiliary communications, are rare, but represent severe complications of synchronous diaphragmatic and hepatic injuries (Oparah and Mandal 1978; Sheik-Gafoor et al. 1998). Secure closure of all diaphragmatic perforations and adequate drainage of all bile collections are essential in successful management of these biliary fistulae. Thoracotomy should not be delayed beyond 3 weeks in case of complicated fistulae (Oparah and Mandal 1978). Choledochocaval fistula after trauma is exceedingly rare. One case, resulting from a right flank stab wound and presenting by repeated hematochezia, has been reported (Cocanour et al. 2000).

Bile Peritonitis

The diagnosis of bile peritonitis after nonoperative management of blunt liver injury requires a high level of suspicion (Griffen et al. 2000). Patients without evidence of associated injury and who subsequently develop fever, persistent abdominal pain, and leukocytosis a few days after hepatic trauma should be highly suspected of developing bile peritonitis (Bynoe et al. 1992). Repeated CT identifies a fluid collection and possibly detects missed liver injuries. However, intrahepatic bile duct injury is not evident on CT (Sugimoto et al. 1993). Biliary nuclear scan is the key to the diagnosis of bile peritonitis (Zeman et al. 1984; Poli et al. 1995). The formation of a large bile leak with secondary bile ascites and bile peritonitis has generally mandated laparotomy, which is aimed at the evacuation and irrigation of the peritoneal cavity, localization of the bile leak, possible repair of the duct and finally drainage (Griffen et al. 2000). A percutaneous transhepatic biliary catheterization combined with percutaneous drainage of bile ascites may be an alternative to surgery in poor surgical candidates (Fig. 23.8). The combination of laparoscopic surgery and percutaneous or endoscopic biliary stenting provides a minimally invasive alternative to

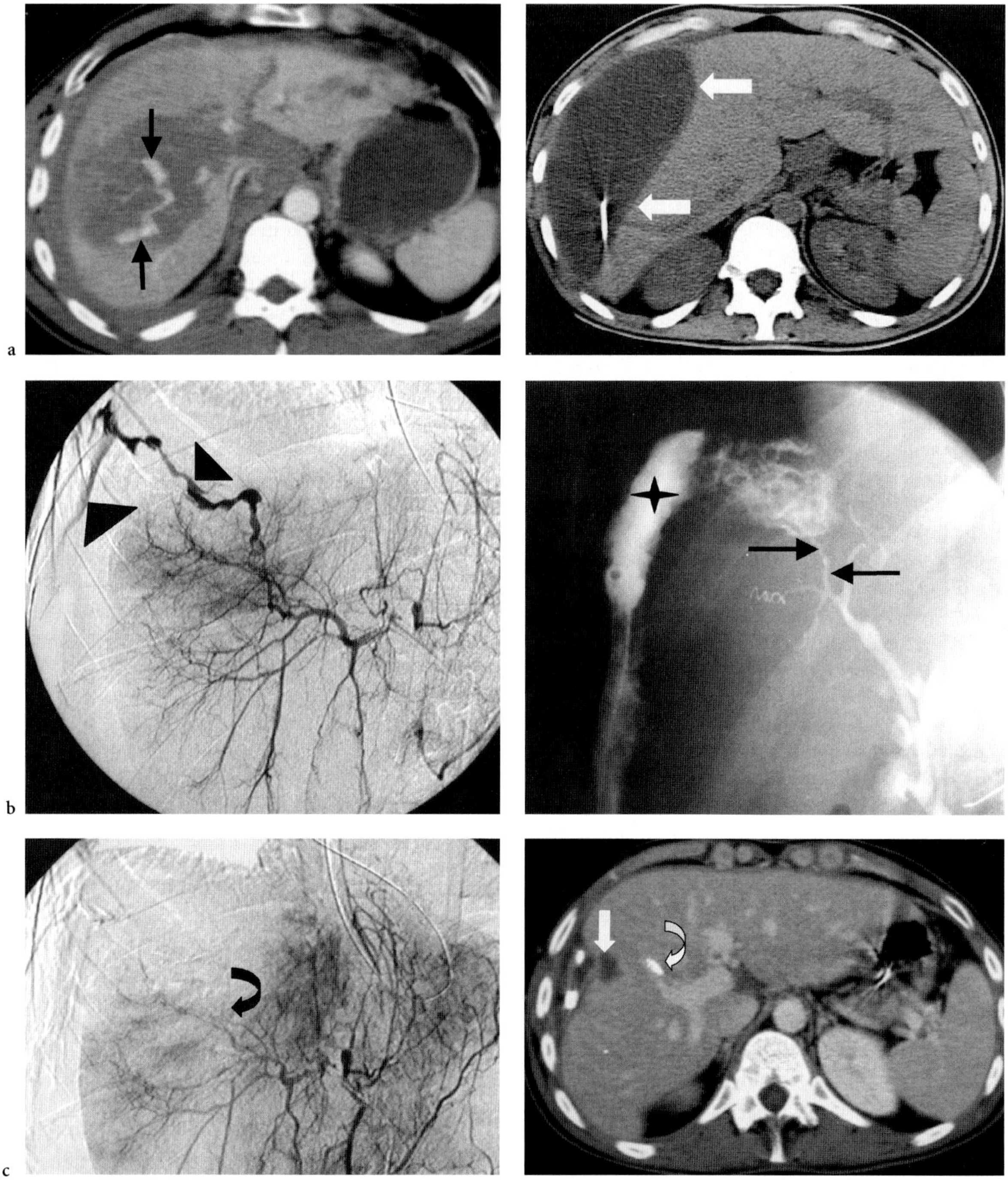

Fig. 23.6a–f. Hepatic injury in a 26-year-old polytraumatized male after a fall. **a** CT at admission shows grade IV hepatic injury with a massive central hematoma. High-density contrast extravasation (*arrows*) is seen within the liver contusion. **b** Selective hepatic arteriography performed at admission shows massive contrast extravasation extending from the hepatic parenchyma to the peritoneal cavity (*arrowheads*) **c** Selective hepatic arteriography after embolization by two gelatin sponge pledgets and one fibered coil shows complete occlusion of segment VII artery (*curved arrow*) without residual bleeding. The other segmental hepatic branches and the cystic artery are preserved. **d** On day 8 after injury, follow-up CT shows a large subcapsular and perihepatic biliohematoma (*arrows*), which was drained percutaneously. **e** Endoscopic retrograde cholangiography was obtained due to the persistence of a large collection despite prolonged external catheter drainage. ERCP showed peripheral biliary fistulas (*arrows*) communicating with the biloma (*star*). Sphincterotomy, without stenting, was performed to improve sealing of the bile fistula. **f** Prolonged drainage of the biloma for 24 days, combined with endoscopic sphincterotomy, allowed nonoperative management of the bile fistula complication. CT obtained on day 45 showed almost complete resolution of the biloma (*arrow*). Small high-density area (*curved arrow*) corresponds to the deployed coil in the artery of segment VII

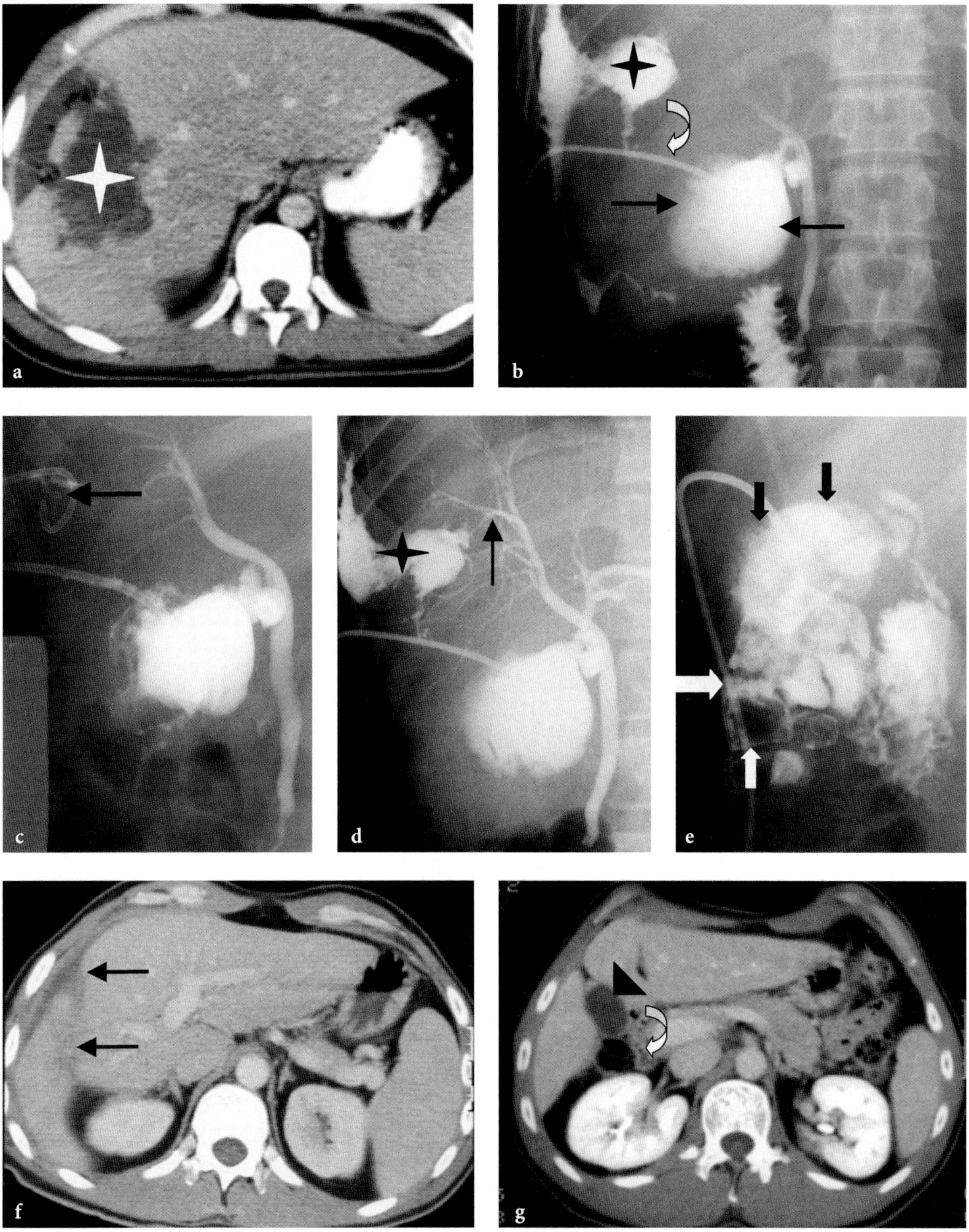

Fig. 23.7a–g. A 45-year-old male had sustained a right flank gunshot injury requiring emergent hepatorrhaphy and suture of a right colon injury. **a,b** During the postoperative period, intra- and perihepatic bilomas had formed (*star*) and an acalculous cholecystitis (*arrows*) was drained percutaneously (*curved arrow*). **c** A second percutaneous drain was placed in the biloma (*arrow*). **d** Cholangiography performed via the cholecystostomy catheter demonstrates biliary fistulae (*arrow*) communicating with the biloma (*star*). An endoscopic sphincterotomy was performed to facilitate sealing of the fistulous tracts by decreasing pressure in the common bile duct. **e** A fistula between the gallbladder and the right colon, which was suspected on CT, is confirmed by a cholangiogram showing passage of contrast from the gallbladder (*black arrows*) to the colon (*white arrows*). **f, g** The cholecystocolic fistula healed after prolonged gallbladder drainage and total parenteral nutrition for 3 additional weeks. CT obtained at 3 months shows complete healing of the hepatic injury with local scar (**f**, *arrows*) and normal gallbladder (**g**, *arrowhead*) and right colon (**g**, *curved arrow*)

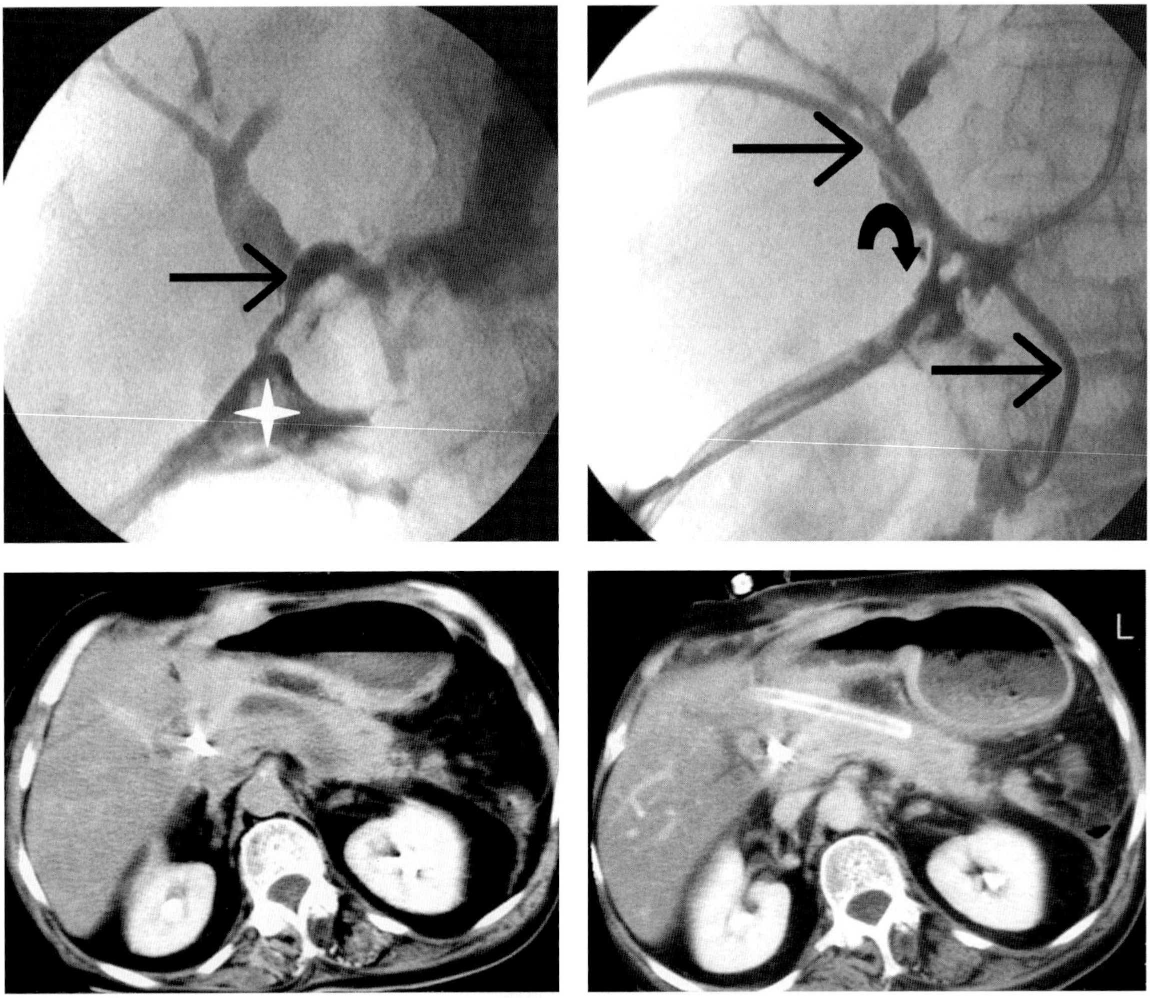

a b c d

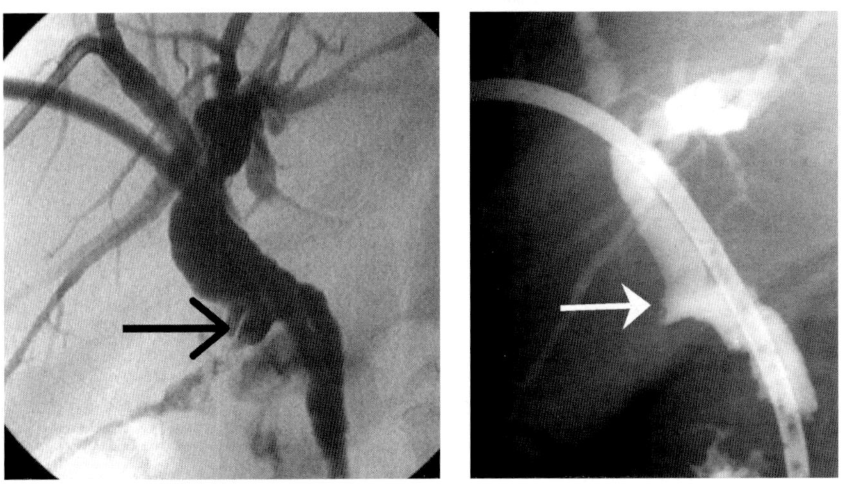

e, f

Fig. 23.8a–f. A 62-year-old female developed massive bile ascites and jaundice 9 days after a blunt liver injury managed conservatively. Percutaneous drains were initially placed in both flanks in order to evacuate the bile and perform peritoneal lavage. **a** Percutaneous transhepatic external biliary drainage was performed for bile derivation from the site of leakage. Transcatheter biliary opacification demonstrates complete common bile duct rupture (*arrow*) and massive free peritoneal bile leakage (*star*). **b** Seven days later, transhepatic catheterization of the distal common bile duct stump is performed, and a 12-F catheter was placed in a transpapillary position (*arrows*). The injured bile duct is catheterized via a percutaneous extrahepatic approach in a retrograde fashion (*curved arrow*) in order to create an external controlled fistula. **c,d** A peripancreatic bile fistula (*star*) responsible of edematous pancreatitis is treated by transperitoneal insertion of a large-bore 16-F sump catheter, which was maintained for 21 days. **e,f** After complete disappearance of the bile collections and jaundice (day 38), all extrahepatic drains were removed, leaving a small biliocutaneous fistula. A transhepatic biliary drain was inserted to improve complete duct healing (*arrow*) and is combined with endoscopic sphincterotomy to lower the intraductal bile duct pressure conventional laparotomy in patients with delayed bile peritonitis (Griffen et al. 2000). Laparoscopy is useful for evacuating bile and/or blood to place a drain for adequate irrigation and drainage of the peritoneal cavity and assess the extent of the liver injury, the gallbladder and the extrahepatic tree, thereby obviating the need for celiotomy (Pachter and Hofstetter 1995; Carrillo et al. 1998). ERCP should be performed for several reasons: to precisely delineate the source of the bile leak, to exclude obstruction in the distal biliary tree by, for example, a blood clot, incidental stricture or choledocholithiasis, which could interfere with closure of the bile leak, and to bridge the bile leak with a stent if possible (Poli et al. 1995; Carrillo et al. 1998; Griffen et al. 2000) (Fig. 23.9).

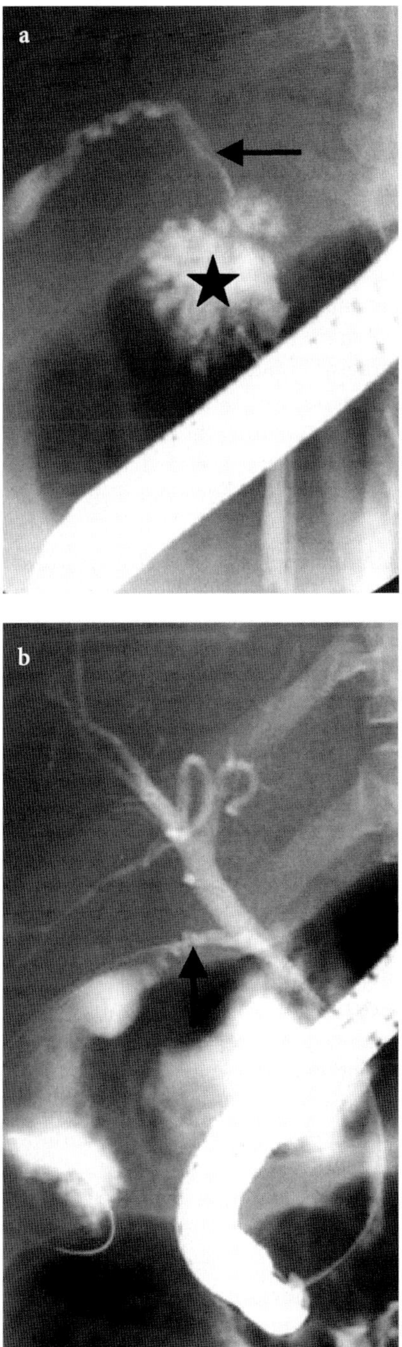

Fig. 23.9a–e. A 56-year-old woman complained of upper abdominal pain after a motor vehicle accident in the absence of direct trauma (seat-belt injury). **a** In the following days, choleperitoneum developed, but abdominal CT showed no intrahepatic biliary abnormality. Endoscopic retrograde cholangiography (ERCP) demonstrates partial common bile duct rupture below the cystic duct level (*arrow*) with formation of a biloma (*star*). **b** A catheter was positioned endoscopically in the gallbladder (*arrow*) and in the main hepatic duct demonstrating normal intrahepatic bile ducts. **c** A naso-gallbladder catheter drainage (*arrows*) is performed to avoid cholecystitis and a plastic endoprosthesis is successfully positioned to by-pass the choledochal leak. **d** ERCP performed 4 months later discloses a tight posttraumatic focal bile duct stricture (*arrow*). **e** The stricture is successfully managed by balloon dilation and long-term large biliary stent implantation (*arrows*)

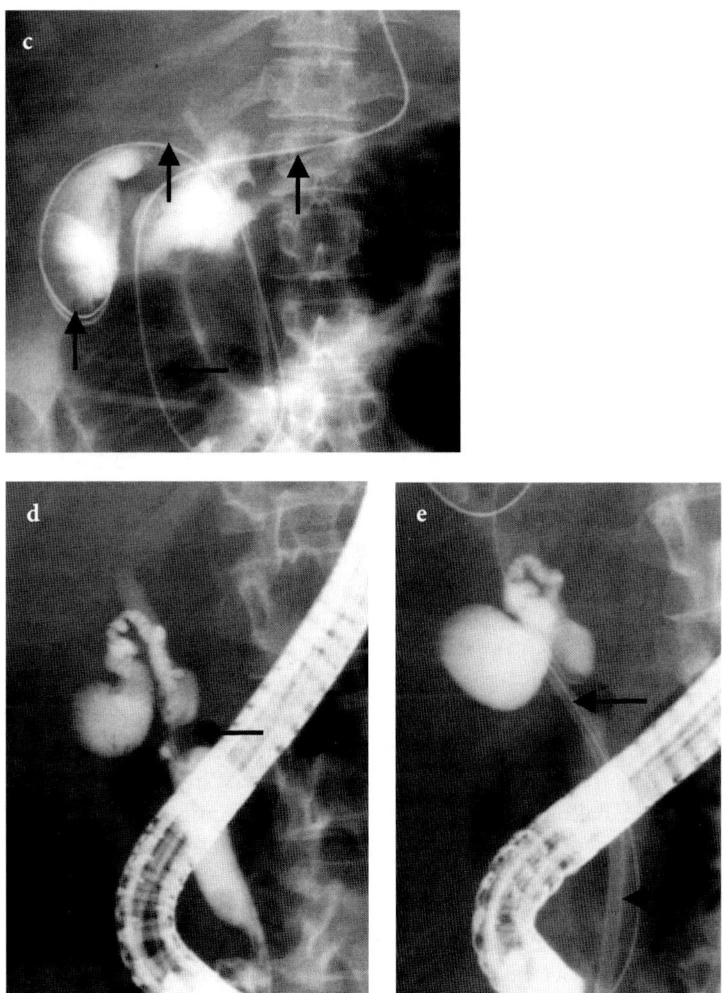

23.2.3.3
Biliary Stricture

Most penetrating injuries of the bile ducts are easily diagnosed immediately after trauma and managed with emergency laparotomy. Conversely, in blunt traumatic injuries, diagnosis is often delayed until the appearance of clinical manifestations such as jaundice or abnormal laboratory results (IVATURY et al. 1985; YOON et al. 1998). Extra and intrabiliary strictures or occlusions that occur as a delayed complication of blunt abdominal trauma have been reported in only a few cases (SHERMAN et al. 1992; HALME et al. 1994; YOON et al. 1998). Late diagnosis can result in permanent damage to the bile duct and cause liver cirrhosis (IVATURY et al. 1985; SHERMAN et al. 1992). Biliary strictures that develop after blunt abdominal trauma may result either from traumatic pancreatitis or as a sequela of bile duct injury. CT findings, such as diffuse bile duct dilatation or abrupt narrowing of the dilated duct and ERCP findings, including concentric narrowing or abrupt termination of the common bile duct with proximal ductal dilatation, are nonspecific and can mimic a malignant stricture. An intramural bile duct hematoma may be observed on CT (YOON et al. 1998). A correct diagnosis may be difficult with CT or ERCP findings alone without clinical history or evidence of sequelae of other injuries (HALME et al. 1994; YOON et al. 1998). Regardless of the mechanism of injury, stricture formation is induced by a minute leakage of bile causing inflammation and fibrosis of the bile duct and periductal tissue (SKOW and LONGMIRE 1974).

Surgery has been used traditionally to treat benign biliary strictures with a long-term postoperative recurrence rate of about 18% (IVATURY et al. 1985). Nowadays permanent or temporary endoscopic plastic stent placement should be considered a possible therapeutic option for both biliary decompression and bile duct stricture management (YOON et al. 1998) (Fig. 23.9). Percutaneous transhepatic biliary diversion and balloon cholangioplasty may be useful in case of hilar stricture, which is inaccessible by a retrograde endoscopic approach (CITRON and MARTIN 1991). When bile duct balloon dilatation and stenting cannot be performed using ERCP or via a percutaneous transhepatic route, surgical reconstructions such as primary repair or biliary-enteric anastomosis, depending on the location of the injury, should be performed (IVATURY et al. 1985; HALME et al. 1994; YOON et al. 1998).

23.2.3.4
Acalculous Cholecystitis

Although acalculous cholecystitis (AC) is not a direct result of hepatobiliary trauma, it is a complication that is associated with multiple injuries and prolonged critical illness. AC results from a gradual increase in bile viscosity due to prolonged stasis of bile flow, leading to a functional obstruction of the cystic duct. Other potential causes include gastrointestinal ileus, gallbladder ischemia due to hypotension or vasoconstrictive drugs, positive pressure ventilation, and use of morphine (CORNWELL et al. 1989; MIRVIS et al. 1987). US or CT demonstration of a gallbladder wall thickness greater than 3 mm, a rim of low-attenuation edema within the gallbladder wall, a pericholecystic fluid collection, and poor delineation between the gallbladder wall and the liver parenchyma are suggestive signs of gallbladder inflammation. US and CT are accurate tests, especially when other sources of intraabdominal sepsis are anticipated (MIRVIS et al. 1987). US-guided percutaneous aspiration of bile may be a valuable method for confirming the diagnosis of AC. Percutaneous transhepatic catheter drainage may serve as a temporizing measure or definitive treatment in selected patients (MCGAHAN and LINDFORS 1989). A transcatheter cholecystography should be performed to exclude a gallbladder perforation and detect stone-induced cystic duct obstruction.

23.2.4
Fluid Collections and Sepsis

23.2.4.1
Clinical Presentation and Imaging

Occasionally a subcapsular or intraparenchymal hematoma does not resolve. In this case, a posttraumatic cyst may develop (KRIGE et al. 1997). With CT bile cysts are recognized with increasing frequency (CHUANG and HUANG 1996). As bile cysts may sometimes resolve spontaneously, they should not be drained unless the patient is symptomatic or febrile or the cyst is seen to expand on serial scans (CHUANG and HUANG 1996).

Sepsis related to liver injury, most commonly pneumonia, intra-abdominal abscess, or wound infection, accounts for up to 15% of deaths and is the second cause of mortality after hemorrhage in liver trauma (HANEY et al. 1982). Six percent of patients with a liver injury will develop an intra-abdominal abscess and 7% of patients with abscess after penetrating trauma die. Intra-abdominal or intrahepatic abscesses occur frequently in major hepatic trauma with a frequency of 15%–27.5% (Eng et al. 1981; Cywes et al. 1991; Asensio et al. 2000). Abscesses tend to develop in patients requiring liver hemostasis, multiple surgical repairs, or GI perforation (Malhotra et al. 2000). Factors that may increase the likelihood of infectious complications after liver trauma include failure to adequately resect or débride devitalized tissue, failure to provide adequate external drainage, and superficial surgical closure or packing of deep central hepatic injuries with residual devitalized liver tissue, bile, blood and bacteria (Boone et al. 1995; Pachter et al. 1996; Malhotra et al. 2000). Intrahepatic abscess can be difficult to distinguish from hematoma or biloma. The appearance of gas bubbles within a fluid collection may indicate infection but has also been reported to result from liver necrosis, liver rupture, penetrating trauma and posttraumatic herniation of lung into the liver. Perihepatic packing to control hemorrhage following trauma has been associated with a 3%–33% incidence of intra-abdominal abscess (Feliciano et al. 1986; Pachter et al. 1996). The rate of intra-abdominal abscesses is not increased with nonoperative management: the incidence was lower in the nonoperative cohort (2%–4%) versus the operative cohort (7%) in a comparative series (Malhotra et al. 2000).

23.2.4.2 Percutaneous Drainage

CT-guided percutaneous drainage for the management of fluid collections is widely accepted as the mainstay of treatment and is successful in 78%–100% of patients (Carles et al. 1994; Boone et al. 1995; Owings and Lengele 1995; Yoo et al. 1996; Pachter et al. 1996). CT or US-guided percutaneous aspiration of a suspected infected collection should be performed, followed by Gram stain of the aspirate. If negative, no drainage should be done. Indeed, percutaneous placement of a catheter into a noninfected liver hematoma commits the patient to potentially prolonged drainage as blood clot dissolves slowly when admixed with bile. Removal of the drainage catheter prior to complete evacuation of the hematoma is at risk of leaving an undrained contaminated collection. Patients with a well-organized intrahepatic abscess should undergo a trial of medical treatment with percutaneous drainage. If there is no improvement, or if fungi are isolated from the circulating blood or the abscess, more aggressive treatment should be considered. Association between hepatic abscess and multiple hepatic PPA following blunt hepatic trauma has been reported (Owings and Lengle 1995; Basile et al. 1999). In this setting, it is postulated that the hepatic vessels were damaged by the trauma, then further weakened by the inflammatory process accompanying the abscess. The PPA should be controlled before drainage to prevent hemorrhage into the abscess cavity when drainage is performed (Owings and Lengle 1995).

23.2.5 Postoperative Complications

Complications following surgery for liver trauma are of respiratory nature in up to 40% of patients, wound sepsis in up to 29%, liver failure, or hyperpyrexia, which occurs in up to 64% of cases, and may be due to resorption of devitalized parenchyma and hepatocellular regeneration and acalculous cholecystitis (Hammond et al. 1992; Krige et al. 1997). Pancreatic, duodenal, or small bowel fistulae may also develop (Krige et al. 1997).

23.3 Spleen

Patients with splenic injury, treated either surgically or nonoperatively, have the potential for developing life-threatening delayed complications such as delayed rebleeding, vascular lesions, intraparenchymal or subcapsular pseudocysts, and intrasplenic or subphrenic abscesses (Sclafani et al. 1995b; Cocanour et al. 1998; Davis et al. 1998; Frumiento et al. 2000). The incidence of delayed complications after nonoperative management of splenic injuries is up to 8% in adults (Schurr et al. 1995; Cocanour et al. 1998; Davis et al. 1998) and from 0% to 7.5% in children (Giacomantonio et al. 1984; Sjövall and Hirsh 1997; Frumiento et al. 2000). Complications are factors that may lead to failure of nonoperative management of blunt splenic injuries in both children and adults (Heller et al. 1994; Sjövall and Hirsh 1997; Davis et al. 1998). Indiscriminate discharge of patients with blunt splenic injury may be potentially harmful. Table 23.2 summarizes the delayed complications after nonoperative management reported in six recently published series.

23.3.1 Vascular Complications

23.3.1.1 Clinical Presentation and Imaging

During the course of nonoperative management of splenic trauma, rupture of a subcapsular hematoma has been recognized as the cause of most delayed splenic bleeding. However, a subcapsular hematoma is neither a predictor for delayed splenic rupture nor an indicator for operative treatment (Black et al. 1992). The sudden onset of delayed bleeding is the result of either lysis of a subcapsular clot that had sealed a tear or rupture of a posttraumatic false aneurysm or arteriovenous fistula (Olsen and Polley 1977). In 70% of patients, hemorrhage occurs within 2 weeks of the injury, but hemorrhage in rare instances can occur months after injury (Olsen and Polley 1977). As 75%–90% of adult pseudoaneurysms or arteriovenous fistulas (Davis et al. 1998) and all such lesions in the pediatric population are noted on delayed imaging studies after 24 h or more in patients with grade III or IV injury, follow-up CT is mandatory in patients with such high-grade injury (Hiraide et al. 1994; Gow et al. 1996; James et al. 1996; Oguzkurt et al. 1996; Sarioglu et al. 1996; Nagar et al. 1997; Maloo et al. 1999).

Delayed Rupture

The so-called delayed splenic rupture is a progressive injury including both missed primary ruptures and true secondary rupture, due to either clot lysis in the injured arterial wall or increasing hematoma by osmotic pressure changes (Hertzanu and Mendelsohn 1984; Farhat et al. 1992; Kluger et al. 1994). The true incidence of delayed rupture seems to be less than 1%. Until CT became available, the incidence of delayed splenic rupture was estimated to be as high as 5%–40% of all splenic injuries (McIndoe 1931). In the late 1970s, incidence was reevaluated and considered to be around 1% (Olsen and Polley 1977). Indeed, a distinction should be made between delayed ruptures (normal initial CT) and delayed recognition of rupture (no initial or misread initial CT) (Farhat et al. 1992). If strict criteria are used, only a few case reports can be considered as true delayed splenic rupture (Pappas et al. 1987; Leppaniemi et al. 1988b; Farhat et al. 1992). The true clinical entity of delayed rupture is defined as bleeding occurring more than 48 h after blunt trauma in a previously hemodynamically stable patient following an initially normal CT (Pappas et al. 1987; Kluger et al. 1994) (Fig 23.10). During the so-called 48-h period of Baudet, no clinical symptom or finding or predisposing factor can correctly predict delayed splenic rupture (Baudet 1907; Olsen and Polley 1977; Leppaniemi et al. 1988b; Farhat et al. 1992). Delayed rupture can occur days to weeks after an initially normal CT and after both minor or major injury treated conservatively (Farhat et al. 1992; Kluger et al. 1994). Minor trauma seems more prone to complication (Farhat et al. 1992). One theory suggests elevated capsular pressure secondary to clot lysis, causing increased pressure and subsequent rupture. Another theory suggests that a perisplenic hematoma is contained by surrounding organs and later ruptures. Inflammatory reaction from omentum adherent to the splenic capsule can result in maceration of the capsule with secondary free intraperitoneal bleeding.

Secondary rupture has a higher mortality rate compared with primary splenic injury (5%–15% vs 1%–3 %) (Cogbill et al. 1989). Besides enlarging subcapsular hematoma, delayed pseudoaneurysm formation can be the cause of late splenic rupture. A CT too soon after trauma, obtained before a subcapsular hematoma has grown enough to be visible, may be the reason for the delay in the detection of some splenic injuries (Black et al. 1992; Pappas et al. 1987).

A classification system to assess splenic injury has been suggested, differentiating true delayed splenic rupture (category 1) from delayed diagnosis (category 2) or failure of nonsurgical or conservative surgical management of splenic injury (categories 3 and 4) (Kluger et al. 1994). The remarkable decrease in the incidence of delayed diagnosis of splenic rupture may be attributed to a wider use of abdominal CT in blunt abdominal trauma. Repeated imaging may be helpful in detecting splenic rupture at a early stage in a patient at risk (Farhat et al. 1992). Isolated posttraumatic enlargement of the spleen could be a possible sign of delayed rupture (Blocker et al. 1998). The only consistent sign of impending rupture is an increase in size of a subcapsular hematoma.

Splenectomy has been the standard treatment for delayed splenic rupture. More conservative surgical procedures, observation without surgery or endovascular embolization are gaining acceptance (Leppaniemi et al. 1988b; Farhat et al. 1992; Kluger et al. 1994). Failure to demonstrate reabsorption of intraperitoneal hemorrhage by CT at day 5 after splenic trauma or persistent intraperitoneal fluid collection at follow-up CT should lead to the search for

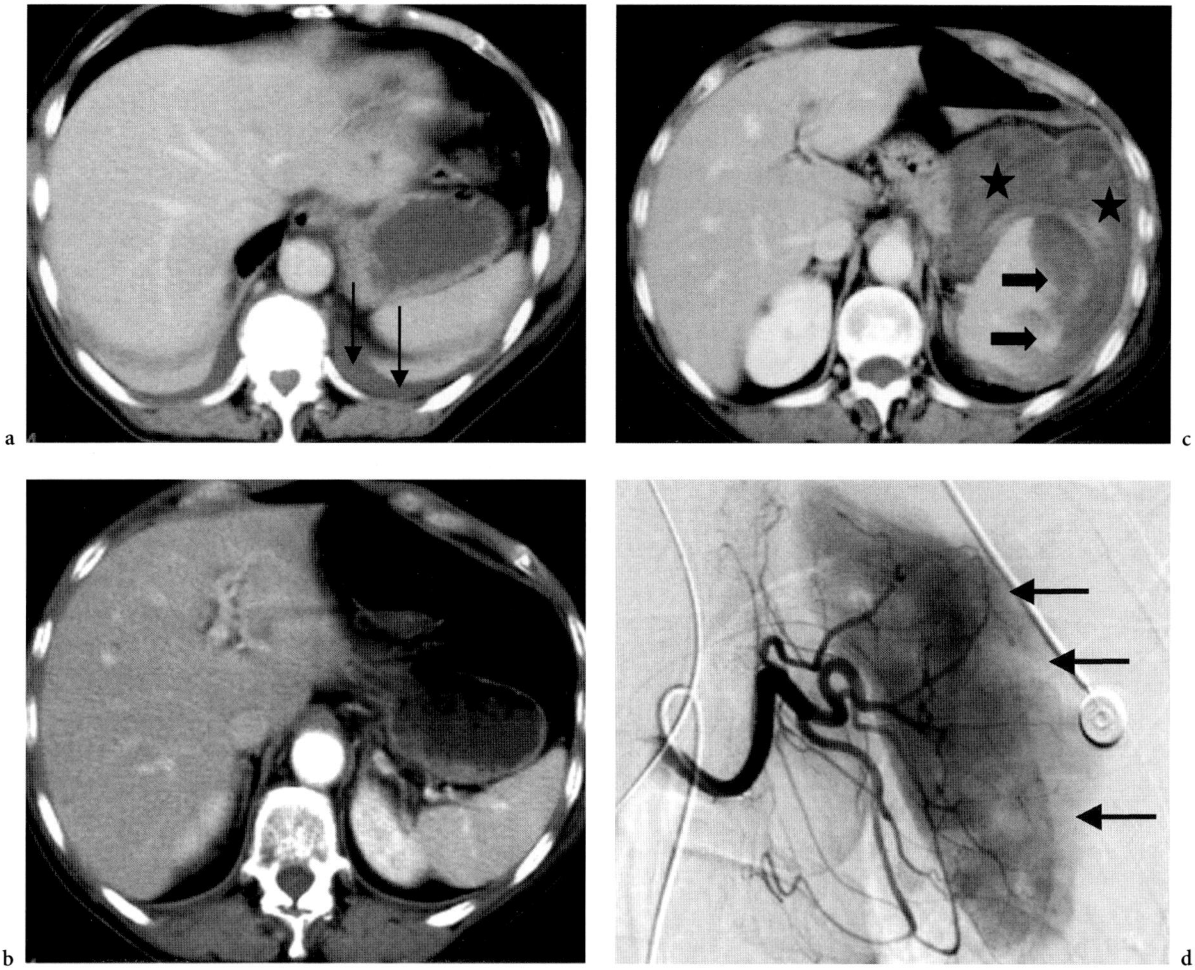

Fig. 23.10a–d. A 51-year-old woman was admitted after being involved in a motor vehicle accident. Chest X-ray showed a small left pleural effusion and fractures of the left lower ribs. **a,b** Contrast-enhanced CT shows normal spleen and liver and a left pleural effusion (*arrows*). No hemoperitoneum is seen. The patient remained asymptomatic for 4 days. **c** Sudden severe abdominal pain and in the left shoulder with a concomitant drop in the hemoglobin level led to suspicion of a delayed splenic rupture. Contrast-enhanced CT shows a rupture of the spleen and a hyperdense subcapsular (*arrows*) and perisplenic (*stars*) hematoma. **d** Splenic arteriography showed no vascular lesion, but an irregular patchy parenchyma (*arrows*) due to the compressive hematoma. No catheter embolization was performed. The patient was treated conservatively without further complication

other missed intra-abdominal injuries (Cogbill et al. 1989; Knudson et al. 1990).

Pseudoaneurysm

Traumatic pseudoaneurysm is a complication of vascular injury and has been described in arteries of various organs. The mechanism for the development of traumatic splenic artery pseudoaneurysm has been related to intimal trauma and disruption of elastic fibers associated with deceleration injury, with intimal fragmentation and weakening of the arterial wall (Hiraide et al. 1994; Norotsky et al. 1995; Sugg et al. 1995; Davis et al. 1998). Vascular blushes on CT were proven to be false aneurysm of intraparenchymal branches of the splenic artery (Schurr et al. 1995). From intraoperative inspection of the spleen, it was found that the CT contrast blush is a contained intrasplenic hematoma with active hemorrhage that slowly enlarges and ruptures finally in most cases (Hiraide et al. 1994; Norotsky et al. 1995; James et al. 1996; Kennedy et al. 1999). Rapidly enlarging posttraumatic intrasplenic pseudoaneurysms may develop from pulpar laceration and hematoma continuously supplied with blood from injured intrasplenic arteries. The natural history of false splenic aneurysm is unclear, but they have been implicated as the source of secondary delayed splenic hemorrhage (3%–42%) in both children and adults (Smith et al. 1989; Nance and Nance 1995; Schurr et al. 1995; Gow et al. 1996; Cocanour et al. 1998; Davis et al. 1998; Kennedy et al. 1999; Fitoz et al. 2001). Delayed presentation may be due to clot lysis at the site of injury of the wall or to an inadequate timing of contrast bolus on CT, leading to non-visualization of the pseudoaneurysm (Davis et al. 1998). The most simple and reliable means of diagnosis of posttraumatic pseudoaneurysm is US-Doppler, which accurately detects the presence of arterial blood flow within hypo- or anechoic lesions of the spleen (Goletti et al. 1996). Color flow Doppler shows a jet of arterial flow into the pseudoaneurysm and turbulent flow within the cystic lesion (Goletti et al. 1996; Kennedy et al. 1999; Fitoz et al. 2001). Bolus-enhanced CT with rapid imaging at the arterial phase after iodine injection is required to diagnose a vascular lesion (Goletti et al. 1996; Oguzkurt et al. 1996; Patel et al. 1996; Kennedy et al. 1999; Fitoz et al. 2001). Contrast-enhanced CT may fail to demonstrate small areas of enhancement that are only identifiable using high-resolution US (Norotsky et al. 1995). Although more costly and less suitable than US-color Doppler, abdominal MRI is effective for the diagnosis of intrasplenic pseudoaneurysm by demonstrating a flow void within a pseudoaneurysm (Goletti et al. 1996; James et al. 1996; Kennedy et al. 1999).

The incidence of false aneurysm appears to be lower in children and progression is less predictable than in adults (Hiraide et al. 1994; Gow et al. 1996; Frumiento et al. 2000). Only eight cases occurring in children have been reported (Hiraide et al. 1994; Gow et al. 1996; Nagar et al. 1997; Frumiento et al. 2000; Henry et al. 1998; Fitoz et al. 2001). Seven asymptomatic pediatric pseudoaneurysms were noted on CT or US imaging studies obtained 48 h after injury, either as routine follow-up or because of abdominal pain. One patient presented with delayed rupture of a hematoma. Such lesions in children are more likely to resolve spontaneously and are less likely to bleed than in adults (Gow et al. 1996; Nagar et al. 1997; Frumiento et al. 2000). Spontaneous resolution of splenic pseudoaneurysm has been attributed to self-tamponade with resultant thrombosis (Schurr et al. 1995; Frumiento et al. 2000). The thicker capsule and more elastic parenchyma of the pediatric spleen may contribute to spontaneous pseudoaneurysm thrombosis. It seems justified to follow-up stable pediatric patients with splenic pseudoaneurysm with repeated color Doppler examinations, expecting spontaneous resolution of the lesion. In adults, pseudoaneurysm formation occurs more likely in higher-grade (grade III or IV) splenic injuries and is associated with intraparenchymal hematoma that is actively bleeding as shown by a vascular blush on CT (Davis et al. 1998; Frumiento et al. 2000). These lesions progress over time, as demonstrated by their absence on CT at admission (Sugg et al. 1995), and a significant proportion are thought to increase in size and ultimately rupture days, months, or even years after the trauma (Schurr et al. 1995; Davis et al. 1998; Pachter 1998). In our series, 67% of adults who did not respond to nonoperative management of splenic injury had splenic artery pseudoaneurysm (Schurr et al. 1995). (Fig. 23.11). As all pediatric cases and a large majority of pseudoaneurysms in adults are noted on delayed imaging studies, the need for follow-up studies to document healing is obvious, especially in grade III or IV injuries (Fig. 23.12).

Arteriovenous Fistula

Posttraumatic splenic arteriovenous fistulae are rare and are mostly seen in adults. They are often extrasplenic and may complicate prognosis because of the formation of a high-flow portal hypertension (Gartside and Gamelli 1987; Campbell et al. 1991; Sarioglu et al. 1996; Salis et al. 1999). This complication is unusual in the pediatric age group (Oguzkurt et al. 1996; Henry et al. 1998; Maloo et al. 1999) and may be observed after blunt or penetrating trauma, most commonly following gunshot injuries or after splenectomy (Thiele et al. 1980; Gartside and Gamelli 1987) (Fig. 23.13), from either a preexisting arterial splenic aneurysm or a newly developed pseudoaneurysm rupture into the adjacent vein. Splenic arteriovenous fistulae may be asymptomatic for an extended interval and are often diagnosed by follow-up US or by auscultation of a continuous systolic bruit in the left upper quadrant (Campbell et al. 1991; Oguzkurt et al. 1996; Henry et al. 1998). The clinical features of chronic splenic arteriovenous fistula are a continuous thrill, abdominal pain, diarrhea due to the congestion of the mesenteric veins, and rarely ascites. Diarrhea and chronic abdominal pain from bowel ischemia secondary to a mesenteric steal syndrome have also been described (Maloo et al. 1999). In long-standing fistulae, splenomegaly and portal hypertension or high-output cardiac failure may result from high flow. Occasionally, the diagnosis is heralded by hypovolemic shock secondary to rupture of an associated false aneurysm (Salis et al. 1999). Late spontaneous disappearance of an arteriovenous fistula may be observed (Henry et al. 1998).

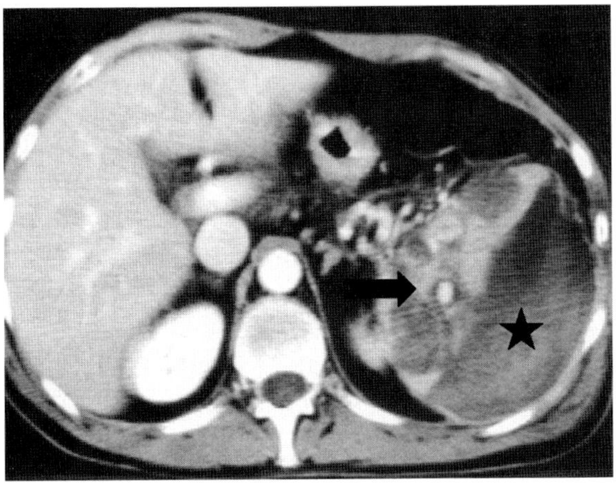
a

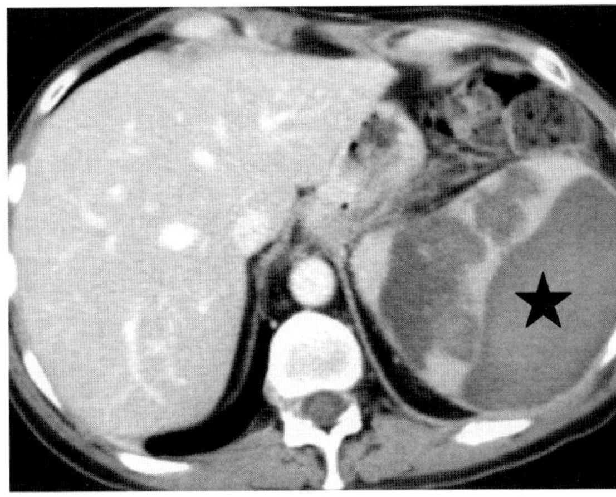
d

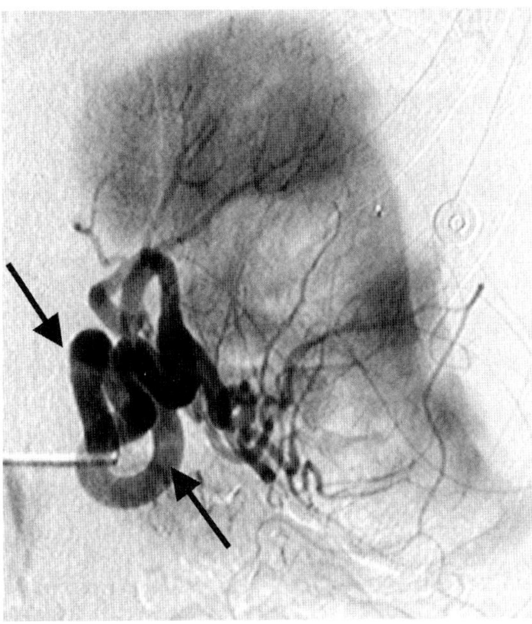
b

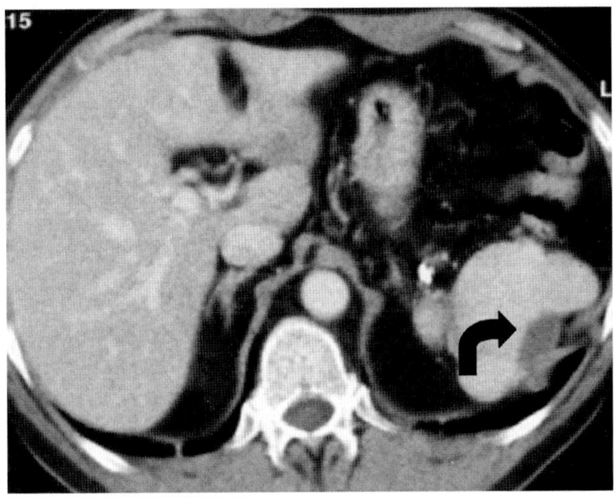

e

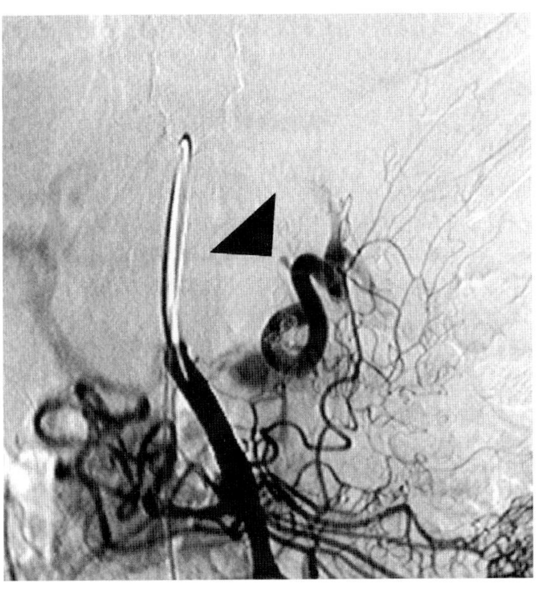
c

Fig. 23.11a–e. A 51-year-old male presented with sudden recurrent pain in the left upper quadrant and drop of hemoglobin level on day 9 after conservative management of grade III blunt splenic trauma. **a** The early arterial phase of contrast-enhanced CT shows an intrasplenic nodule (*arrows*) with strong contrast enhancement and other hyperdense areas in the subcapsular hematoma (*star*). These findings suggest a bleeding pseudoaneurysm. **b,c** Because of marked tortuosity of the splenic artery (*arrows*), superselective catheterization of the artery feeding the vascular lesion failed. Therefore, the proximal part of the splenic artery was occluded with coils with the intention to induce spontaneous thrombosis of the pseudoaneurysm by decreased perfusion pressure. Superior mesenteric vein (SMA) angiography demonstrates preserved patency of the splenic artery by collateral filling (*arrowhead*). **d** CT obtained 3 days later shows an enlarging subcapsular hematoma (**star**) due to osmotic changes. The hematoma was treated by two needle aspirations at days 4 and 8 to avoid delayed free peritoneal splenic rupture and to reduce persistent pain by capsular distension. **e** A marked parenchymal retraction (*curved arrow*) and almost complete resorption of the hematoma is observed at 4 months

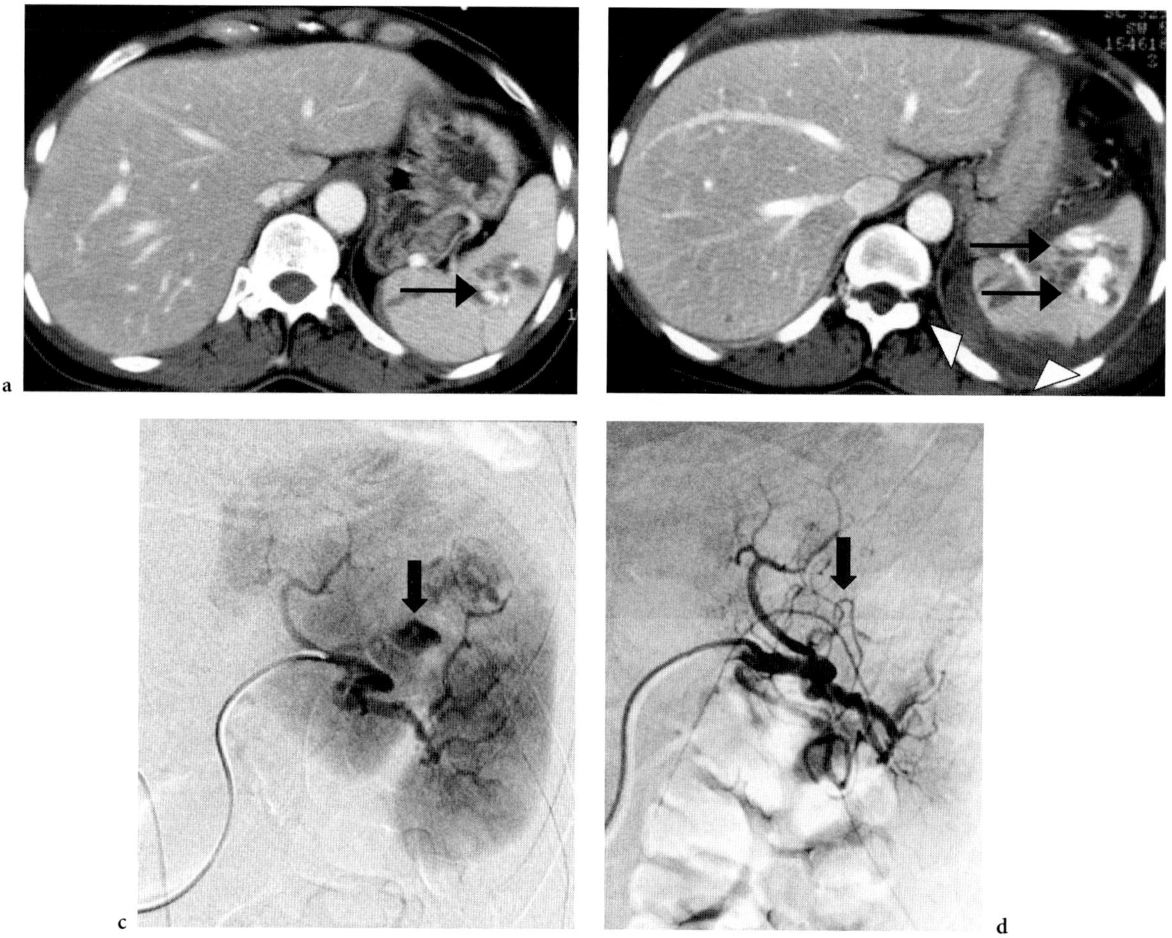

Fig. 23.12a–d. Isolated grade III blunt splenic injury in a 52-year-old female, which was managed conservatively. **a** Despite small intraparenchymatous areas (*arrow*) of abnormal contrast blush on initial CT, angiography was not performed because the patient remained hemodynamically stable. **b** Drop in hemoglobin level and increased abdominal pain in the left upper quadrant, led to early CT, which showed two large intrasplenic pseudoaneurysms (*arrows*) and a perisplenic hematoma increasing in size (*white arrowheads*). **c** Selective splenic arteriography confirms the posttraumatic pseudoaneurysms (*arrow*). Selective embolization of two intrasplenic arteries with large polyvinyl alcohol particles were performed with a 0.018-in. Transit microcatheter (Cordis). **d** Angiography shows complete exclusion of the pseudoaneurysms. The proximal arterial feeders are still patent (*arrow*), and perfusion of the remaining spleen is preserved

23.3.1.2
Endovascular Management

Treatment options include observation, angiographic embolization, splenectomy, or surgery with splenic preservation if angiographic embolization is found not to be technically feasible. In adults, a liberal use of embolization seems mandatory to decrease the failure rate of nonoperative management due to late rebleeding caused by rupture of a false aneurysm (Cocanour et al. 1998; Davis et al. 1998; Frumiento et al. 2000) (Figs. 23.13, 23.14).

Technique

In the acute setting of splenic rupture with free intraperitoneal bleeding, the most common technique of arterial embolization is superselective injection of gelatin sponge combined with placement of steel coils in the proximal trunk of the splenic artery (Sclafani et al. 1995b; Hagiwara et al. 1996). When extravasation is documented within the splenic parenchyma, isolated coil occlusion of the proximal splenic artery is preferred. The theory behind these techniques is that occluding the proximal splenic artery will decrease blood pressure to the organ, therefore promoting

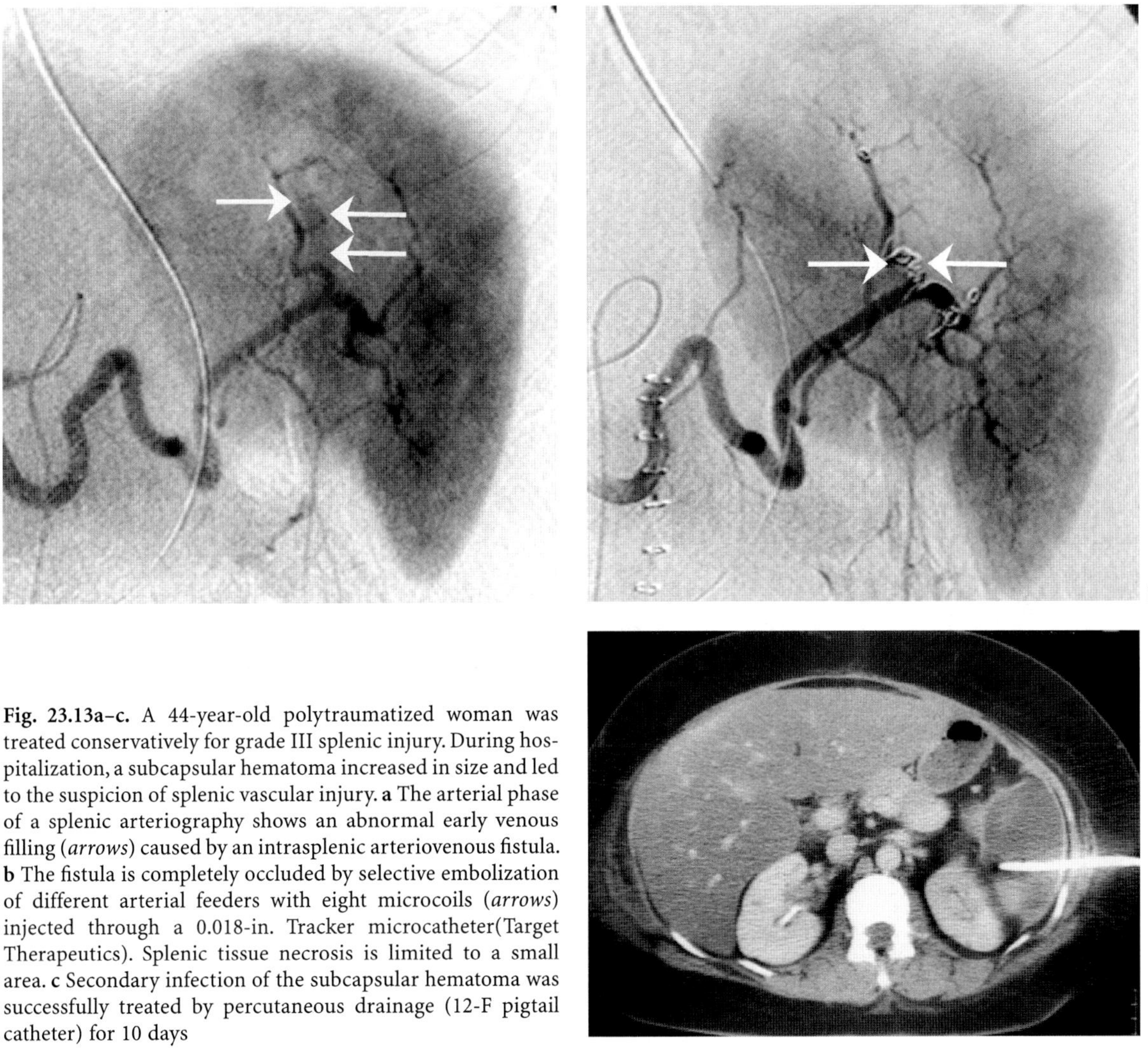

Fig. 23.13a–c. A 44-year-old polytraumatized woman was treated conservatively for grade III splenic injury. During hospitalization, a subcapsular hematoma increased in size and led to the suspicion of splenic vascular injury. **a** The arterial phase of a splenic arteriography shows an abnormal early venous filling (*arrows*) caused by an intrasplenic arteriovenous fistula. **b** The fistula is completely occluded by selective embolization of different arterial feeders with eight microcoils (*arrows*) injected through a 0.018-in. Tracker microcatheter(Target Therapeutics). Splenic tissue necrosis is limited to a small area. **c** Secondary infection of the subcapsular hematoma was successfully treated by percutaneous drainage (12-F pigtail catheter) for 10 days

thrombosis of the visualized area of extravasation. Collateral flow through the short gastric arteries and branches of the left gastric and gastroepiploic arteries creates continuous perfusion, resulting in low risk of tissue infarction (Hagiwara et al. 1996; Firstenberg et al. 1998) (Fig. 23.11). This technique may be applied as an alternative to splenectomy in case of delayed bleeding without angiographic demonstration of a true vascular lesion (Firstenberg et al. 1998). However, a pseudoaneurysm or an arteriovenous fistula can remain patent after proximal splenic arterial occlusion only (Salis et al. 1999). Moreover, both sepsis and splenic abscess have complicated this technique. It has been shown that the risk of sepsis is reduced when only a segmental branch is occluded (Baker et al. 1987; Davis et al. 1998). The most efficient means to definitively occlude a pseudoaneurysm or arteriovenous fistula, without risk of sepsis, is to perform a superselective embolization (MacDermott et al. 1994; Goletti et al. 1996; James et al. 1996; Patel et al. 1996; Davis et al. 1998; Kennedy et al. 1999; Maloo et al. 1999; Salis et al. 1999) (Fig. 23.12). As most splenic pseudoaneurysms occur either in the distal main trunk or mostly in the intraparenchymal branches, selective distal catheterization is necessary for sparing collateral vessels in order to preserve the spleen. Catheterization of the distal splenic artery or branches may be difficult and requires use of a microcatheter or a flow-directed catheter (MacDermott et al. 1994; Goletti et al. 1996; Patel et al. 1996; Maloo et al. 1999; Salis et al. 1999) (Figs. 23.13, 23.14). As an immediate and permanent occlusion is intended, microcoils or Gianturco coils, depending of the catheter size, are the preferred embolic agents (Goletti et al. 1996; James et al. 1996; Patel et al. 1996; Kennedy et al. 1999; Maloo et al. 1999; Salis et al. 1999). The

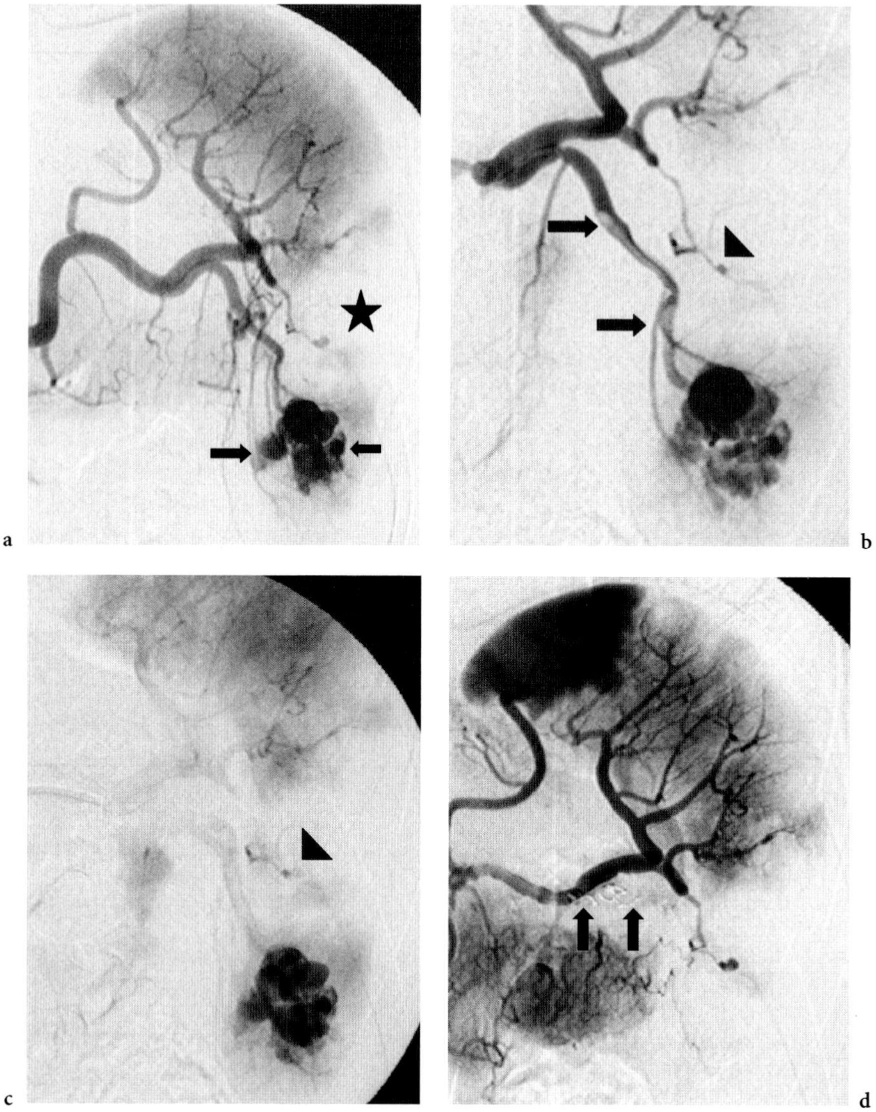

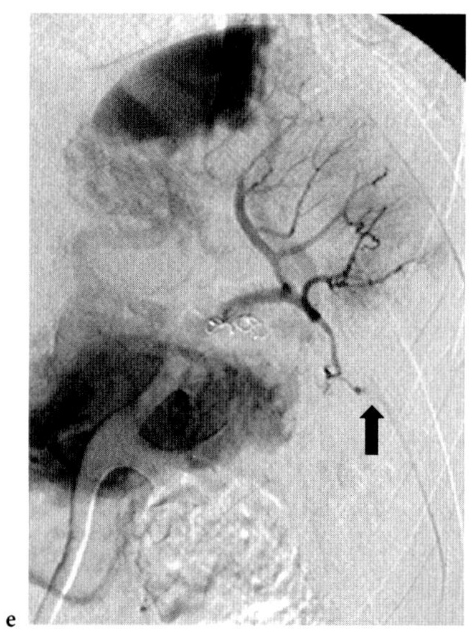

Fig. 23.14a–e. A 25-year-old woman was treated conservatively for an isolated grade III splenic injury following a fall from a horse. No abnormal vascular blush was seen on the enhanced CT obtained at admission. Routine follow-up CT before discharge (day 13) revealed a grape-like enhanced area in the lower pole of the spleen. **a** Splenic arteriography shows a large multiloculated pseudoaneurysm (*arrows*) in the lower pole of the spleen and surrounded by a devascularized area of contusion (*star*). **b,c** Arterial (**b**) and venous (**c**) phase of selective distal splenic injection identify the main arterial feeder of the large vascular lesion (*arrows*) and a small pseudoaneurysm located on a spastic lower polar arterial branch (*arrowhead*). **d** The large pseudoaneurysm is selectively embolized by occlusion of the arterial feeder with four flower platinum microcoils (Target Therapeutics) (*arrows*) deposited through a 0.018-in. microcatheter. **e** The small pseudoaneurysm was occluded (*arrow*) by selective injection of few small gelatin sponge particles in order to avoid complete devascularization of the lower pole of the spleen. The patient was placed on broad prophylactic intravenous antibiotic therapy for 5 days. Follow-up was uneventful

use of gelatin sponge pledgets or detachable balloons has also been described (BAKER et al. 1987; PIROLLET et al. 1989). The available microcatheters pass coaxially through a 4- or 5-French diagnostic catheter accepting an 0.038-in. guidewire and may be successfully advanced into a small branch with less risk of spasm, thrombotic occlusion, or intimal damage, allowing coil deposition in appropriate relation to the neck of the pseudoaneurysm. Coils need less pressure for deposition than the considerable pressure required to force Gelfoam out of a microcatheter; this force may be transmitted to the fragile pseudoaneurysm wall, which may rupture (LINA et al. 1979; MACDERMOTT et al. 1994). Gelfoam offers few advantages, as it temporarily occludes the vessel, raising the risk of future recanalization of the aneurysm; it may also migrate and occlude small arteries within the spleen, beyond the reach of collateral circulation, causing complications such as pain and infection (MACDERMOTT et al. 1994).

Results

Splenic artery aneurysms and pseudoaneurysms were previously treated with splenectomy, but embolization is reported to be successful in 85% of adult patients (PROBST et al. 1978; MACDERMOTT et al. 1994). The efficacy of this technique as a treatment of delayed posttraumatic splenic vascular lesions has been extensively demonstrated in adults (BAKER et al. 1987; MACDERMOTT et al. 1994; CHIARUGI et al. 1995; PATEL et al. 1996; COCANOUR et al. 1998; DAVIS et al. 1998; KENNEDY et al. 1999). In children, spontaneous resolution of a splenic pseudoaneurysm occurs in most cases (GOW et al. 1996; NAGAR et al. 1997; HENRY et al. 1998). Embolization of a ruptured pseudoaneurysm, with or without associated arteriovenous fistula, was recently described in a few case reports (JAMES et al. 1996; MALOO et al. 1999; FITOZ et al. 2001). Partial or total splenectomy or splenorrhaphy was previously more commonly performed in this population (HIRAIDE et al. 1994; OGUZKURT et al. 1996; SARIOGLU et al. 1996).

Potential complications of embolization include inadvertent occlusion of untargeted vessels, inducing diffuse tissue necrosis and intra-abdominal hemorrhage caused by disruption of the treated vessel (MACDERMOTT et al. 1994; COCANOUR et al. 1998; FRUMIENTO et al. 2000). Continuous extravasation following embolization of the main splenic artery for intrasplenic pseudoaneurysm or arteriovenous fistula and requiring secondary splenectomy has been described (HAGIWARA et al. 1996).

23.3.1.3. Surgical Management

Splenectomy or splenorrhaphy has been performed as a treatment of these vascular injuries (NOROTSKY et al. 1995; SUGG et al. 1995; GOLETTI et al. 1996; OGUZKURT et al. 1996; SARIOGLU et al. 1996; COCANOUR et al. 1998). Splenic artery ligation with preservation of the short gastric branches may result in thrombosis of a pseudoaneurysm. Conservative surgical treatment of an arteriovenous fistula consists in the dissection of the fistula with ligation or repair of the vessels with or without resection of an associated aneurysm. Today these surgical techniques should be considered only when embolization is not technically feasible (SUGG et al. 1995)

23.3.2 Fluid Collection

23.3.2.1 Pseudocyst

Splenic pseudocysts, either subcapsular or intraparenchymal, may occasionally develop and usually result from blunt abdominal trauma. An increased prevalence of such posttraumatic lesions after nonoperative management of splenic injury has been reported (PACHTER et al. 1998). A posttraumatic cyst may form in patients with initially discrete splenic injuries because of delayed development of subcapsular hematoma, even when resolution of the injury was shown on CT (PACHTER et al. 1993). A hematoma leaves behind a fibrous capsule and contents composed of resolving hematoma and pigment from heme breakdown (Fig. 23.15). Clinical signs are local pain or pain referred to the left shoulder as a result of phrenic irritation. Abdominal distention, symptoms associated with splenomegaly such as early satiety, emesis, dysphagia, or left lower-lobe atelectasis may be present (Fig. 23.15). On US, pseudocysts present as an anechoic mass without perceptible wall. Echoes from cholesterol crystals, septations, and calcifications may be observed. On CT, they have the appearance of a low-density, and well-defined fluid collection. Although the natural history of the pseudocyst is not clear, it has been established that 25% will rupture and are associated with significant hemorrhage, peritonitis, abscess formation, or pleural empyema (PACHTER et al. 1993; BRAVO et al. 1998). Cysts continue to grow and treatment should be undertaken if the size is

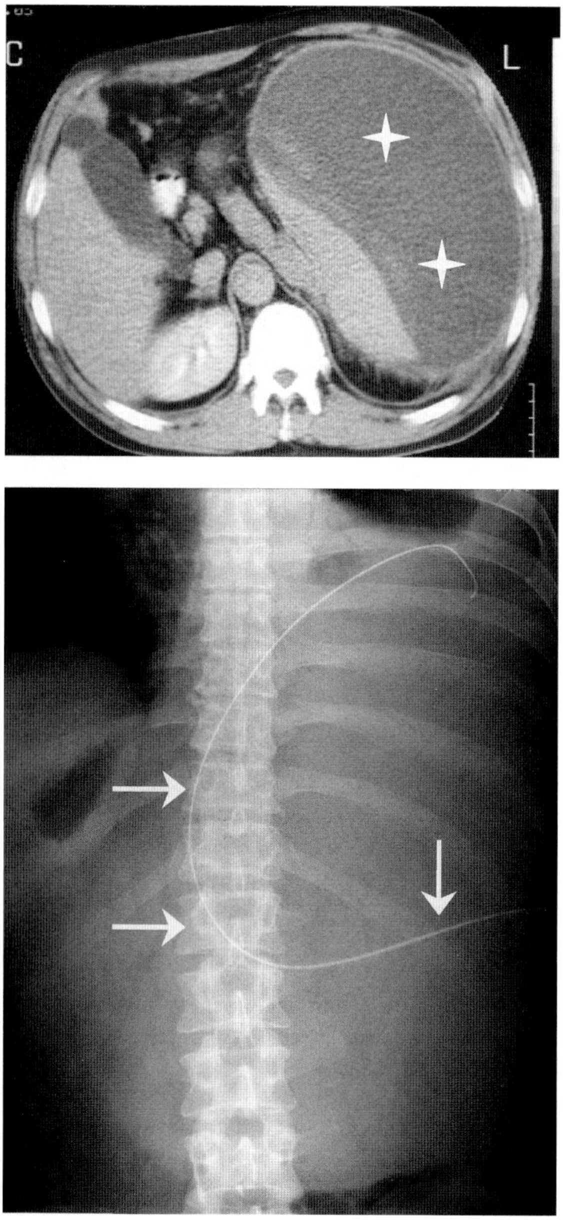

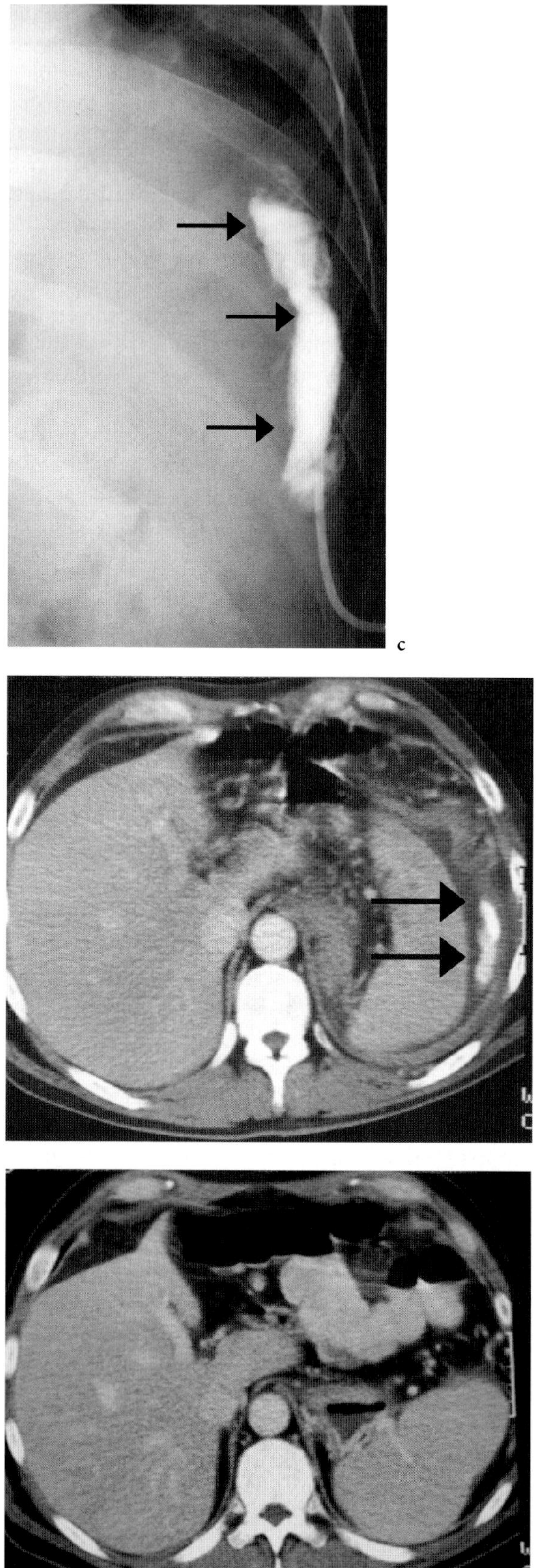

Fig. 23.15a–e. A 42-year-old male complained of progressive left-side abdominal tenderness and early satiety 4 months after a fall from a height of 4 m. No radiological investigation was obtained. **a** Contrast-enhanced CT shows a large subcapsular low-density collection of the spleen (*stars*) with compression of the splenic parenchyma and abnormal viscera. **b** A 12-F pigtail catheter is placed by a left lateral percutaneous approach (*arrows*) allowing drainage of 10.5 l of old blood over an 8-day period. Left pleural effusion is present. **c,d** Abdominal radiograph and contrast-enhanced CT of the residual splenic cavity before removal of the drainage catheter show an irregular small cavity (*arrows*) and a marked thickening of the retracted splenic capsule (*arrowhead*). **e** CT at 1 year follow-up demonstrates complete disappearance of the hematoma

larger than 5 cm. Asymptomatic cysts of less than 5 cm may be managed with observation, since most will regress within 3 months to 3 years (PACHTER et al. 1993). Most authors recommend partial splenectomy, splenorrhaphy, resection of the cyst-bearing portion of the spleen with marsupialization and preservation of the remaining normal parenchyma to avoid delayed abscess formation or rupture (CHRISTINAZ and LE COUTRE 1987; PACHTER et al. 1993; COCANOUR et al. 1998; PACHTER et al. 1998). Laparoscopic decapsulation of the cyst wall with formation of a peritoneal window for decompression has been proposed (LINHARES et al. 1998; VAN DER ZEE et al. 1999). Some authors advocate percutaneous aspiration, followed by the insertion of a pig-tail catheter for infusion sclerotherapy with tetracycline, as an initial approach, in an attempt to collapse the lesion once and for all, proceeding with surgery in case of failure (MOIR et al. 1989; RAVERA and COCOZZA 1999). Percutaneous drainage may result in a dense inflammatory response around the spleen, making subsequent surgery more difficult (PACHTER et al. 1993).

23.3.2.2 Abscess

Clinical Presentation

Splenic abscess is an uncommon complication following nonoperative management of splenic trauma (COCANOUR et al. 1998). Concerns that splenic abscesses would become more frequent with widespread application of nonoperative management has not been confirmed (SANDS et al. 1986; FRUMIENTO et al. 2000). The origin of abscess may be hematogenous or by contiguity. Due to parenchymal disruption, trauma increases the susceptibility of the spleen developing suppuration. Splenic abscess may present within several months or years of trauma (PARIS et al. 1994; TOEVS and BEILMAN 2000). Sepsis development after embolization for hypersplenism is a well-known complication (WHOLEY et al. 1978). Splenic abscess and septicemia within the first week of proximal coil occlusion, with or without selective Gelfoam embolization, of the splenic artery as the primary hemostatic measure after splenic injuries are reported (BAKER et al. 1987; SALAM et al. 1992). Distal embolization of an undercalibrated coil initially placed proximally may be at the origin of delayed infarction (SCLAFANI et al. 1995b). Patients with splenic abscess present with fever, elevated white blood cell count and tenderness in the left upper quadrant.

Management

Because of the high morbidity and mortality rates of posttraumatic splenic abscess despite medical treatment, splenectomy has been the mainstay of treatment (SANDS et al. 1986; DE WIT et al. 1994; OOI and LEONG 1997; COCANOUR et al. 1998). However, CT and US-guided percutaneous drainage of splenic abscesses may be performed in both adults and children with excellent results in selected cases (DE WITT et al. 1994; YOO et al. 1996; OOI and LEONG 1997; FRUMIENTO et al. 2000). The reported success rate is up to 90% in unilocular and 75% in multilocular abscesses. The likelihood of cure by percutaneous drainage is lower in patients with multiloculated or complex splenic abscess, which are frequent (PARIS et al. 1994).

23.3.3 Postoperative Complications

Postoperative complications following splenectomy are various and occur more frequently than with any other abdominal organ injury. Patients undergoing splenectomy or splenorrhaphy are known to be prone to atelectasis, pneumonia and left pleural effusion. The most severe complication is bleeding from short gastric vessels, hilar vessels in the tail of the pancreas or from the spleen itself. Fewer than 2% of survivors of splenic trauma have reoperation for bleeding. Gastric wall injury due to devascularization of the great curvature of the stomach manifests as a subphrenic abscess or a gastric fistula, usually 4–7 days after injury (BEAL and TRUNKEY 1993). Drainage tube-related gastric perforation, clinically diagnosed by a gastrocutaneous fistula, is a rare postoperative complication that can be managed nonoperatively if peritonitis is absent (PARASKEVOPOULOS et al. 2000). Pseudocyst following splenectomy can occur as late as 4–5 weeks after the initial surgery, with an incidence as high as 10%. Pseudocysts are susceptible to superinfection, and may be both diagnosed and treated by needle aspiration, which is preferable to catheter drainage to avoid secondary infection of a sterile fluid collection. Infectious complications are significantly more frequent after splenectomy than after spleen-preserving surgery (BEAL and TRUNKEY 1993; PACHTER et al. 1998). Left subphrenic abscess occurs in 1.3%–13% (PACHTER et al. 1998; SALZANO et al. 1999). CT-guided percutaneous drainage using the trocar technique is the first-line treatment, while surgery is reserved for later stages, when drainage fails or other complications occur (SALZANO et al.

1999). Splenic arteriovenous fistulae or arterial suture leakage can occur after splenectomy for trauma (THIELE et al. 1980; GARTSIDE and GAMELLI 1987). Endovascular occlusion of such postoperative lesions with coils or Fogarty catheter has been successfully performed (ZELCH and HERMANN 1975) (Fig. 23.16).

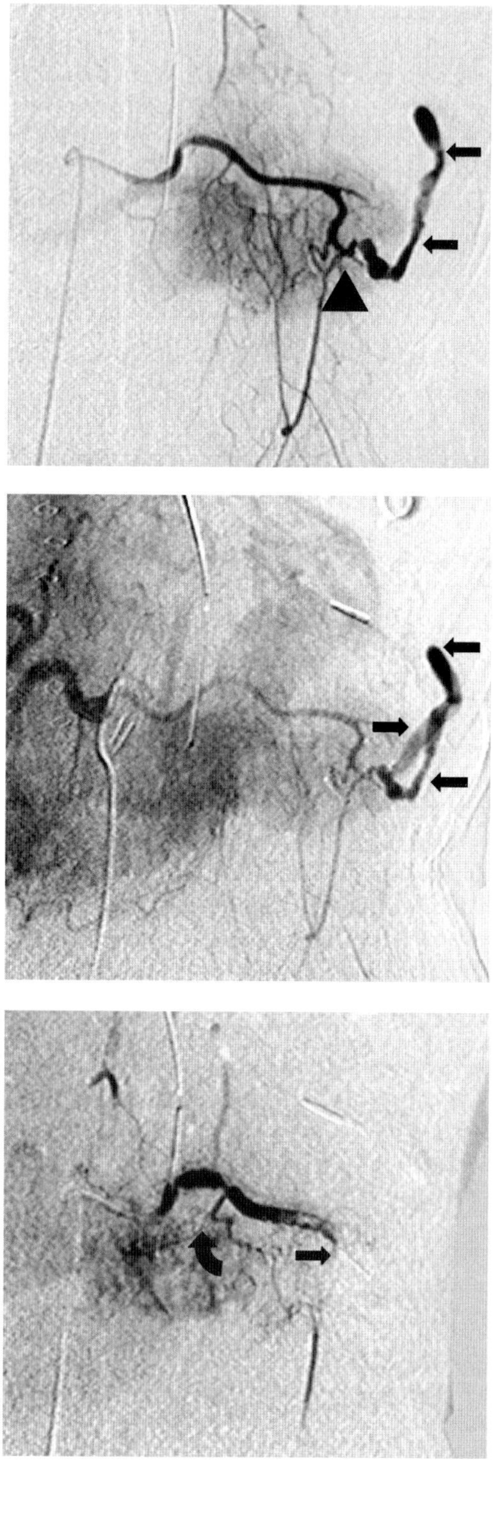
a
b
c

Fig. 23.16a–c. A 58-year-old female presented sudden hypovolemic shock 48 h after splenectomy for trauma (isolated grade IV splenic injury). An urgent angiography is performed. **a,b** Early (**a**) and late (**b**) arterial phases of splenic arteriography demonstrate massive free peritoneal bleeding (*arrows*) arising from the stump of a hilar splenic artery (*arrowhead*). **c** After embolization with gelatin sponge pledgets (immediate hemostasis) and two Gianturco coils (permanent occlusion), bleeding was successfully controlled (*arrow*). Patency of short pancreatic branches is preserved (*curved arrow*). Repeat laparotomy was avoided. The patient recovered without complication

23.4 Pancreas

Complications after pancreatic trauma are observed in one-third of patients. The reported incidence varies from 8% to 45% (COGBILL et al. 1982; JONES 1985). The most common complications include acute pancreatitis, pseudocyst, abscess, internal and external pancreatic fistulae, chronic pancreatitis, late ductal stricture, and hemorrhage (CARR et al. 1989; LEWIS et al. 1993; JURKOVICH and CARRICO 1994; AKHRASS et al. 1997). Injury to the main pancreatic duct with continuous leakage is the principal cause of early significant complications such as pseudocyst, fistula, and abscess (PATTON et al. 1997). Delayed presentation of complications, ranging from 3 months to 21 years after apparent recovery from the original pancreatic injury, has been reported (LEPPANIEMI et al. 1988a; CARR et al. 1989; LEWIS et al. 1993). Stricture of the main pancreatic duct, developing over a period of months as a result of progressive fibrosis at the site of ductal injury and leading to chronic obstructive pancreatitis, has been reported (BRADLEY 1991).

23.4.1 Vascular Complications

23.4.1.1 Clinical Presentation

Posttraumatic pancreatic pseudoaneurysm is rare and usually the result of secondary pancreatitis with enzymatic digestion of the arterial wall. Half of these lesions may rupture into the gastrointestinal (GI) tract via the pancreatic or common bile duct or rupture into a pseudocyst or rarely into the peritoneal cavity. The so-called hemosuccus pancreaticus with hemorrhage in the pancreatic duct is a rare cause of posttraumatic delayed upper GI bleeding. A posttraumatic pseudoaneurysm arising from an anomalous right hepatic artery and bleeding into the pancreatic duct after a gunshot injury has been reported (Kim et al. 2000). Postoperative hemorrhage, occurring in 5%–10% of surgical management of pancreatic trauma, is most often the result of leaking pancreatic enzymes eroding into surrounding vessels, particularly when pancreatic débridement has been required or intra-abdominal infection has occurred (Campbell and Kennedy 1980; Cogbill et al. 1991; Wilson and Moorehead 1991).

23.4.1.2 Management

Angiography is usually required for confirmation of a clinical suspicion of posttraumatic pseudoaneurysm. Selective embolization of pancreatic or peripancreatic pseudoaneurysm, arteriovenous fistula, or bleeding vas-cular injuries is a viable alternative to surgery in patients who are often poor surgical candidates (Fig. 23.17). A success rate between 80% and 95% is reported by most authors (Baker et al. 1987; Mandel et al. 1987; Sato et al. 1998).

a
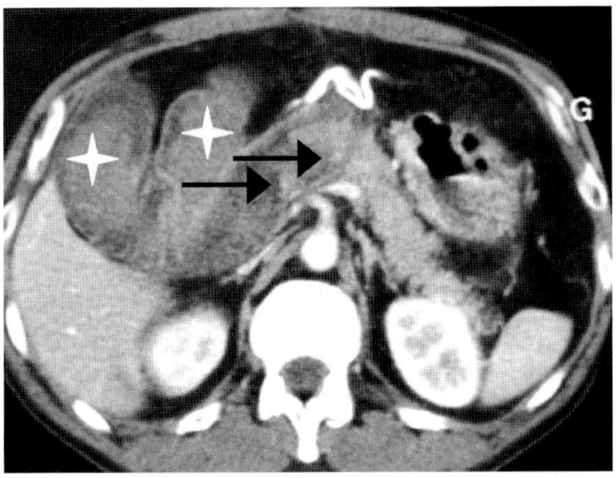

d
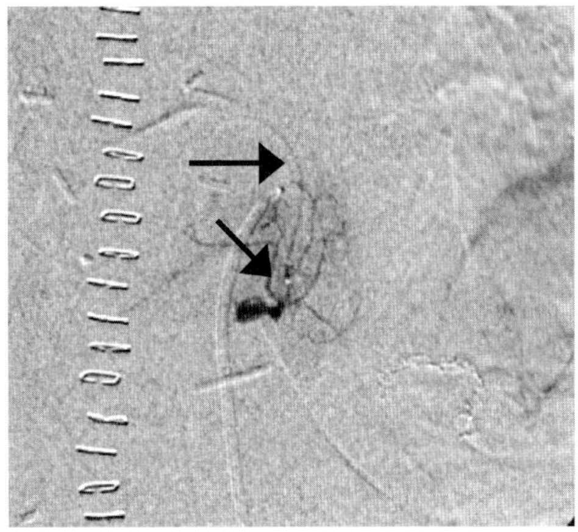

b
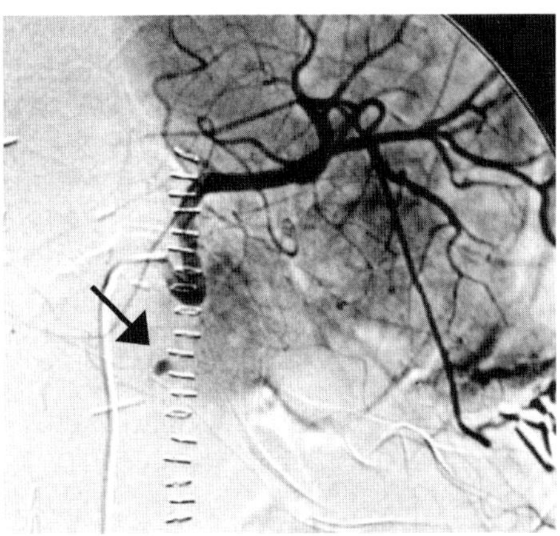

e
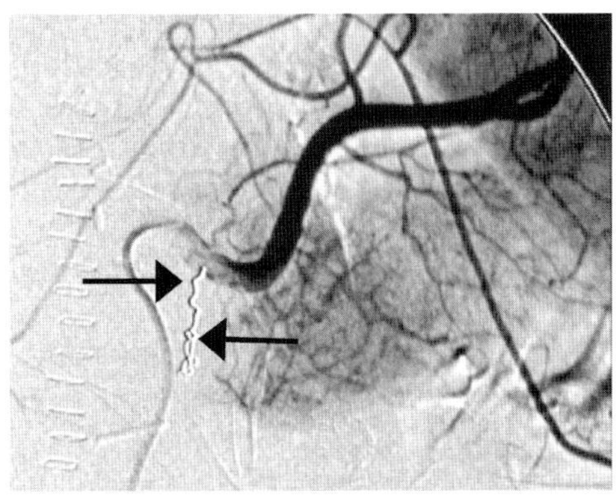

c
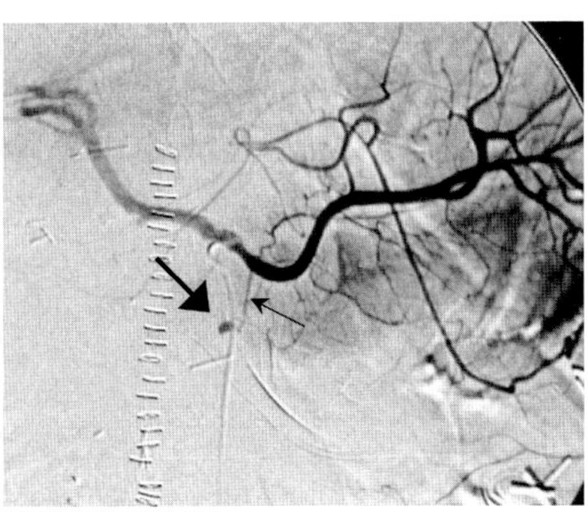

Fig. 23.17a–e. A 48-year-old male presented with massive lower gastrointestinal bleeding 6 days after an emergency Whipple procedure performed for a cephalic pancreatic trauma with complete proximal duct disruption. **a** Contrast-enhanced CT shows hyperdense clots in the efferent loop (*stars*). Two highly attenuating small areas suggestive of vascular lesions are seen near the pancreaticojejunal anastomosis (*arrows*). **b,c** Splenic arteriography demonstrates a 3-mm diameter pseudoaneurysm (*black arrow*) supplied by a short pancreatic arterial branch (*white arrow*). **d** Superselective distal catheterization of the feeding artery was performed with a 0.014-in. Tracker microcatheter (Target Therapeutics) (*arrows*) introduced through a 5-F standard catheter. **e** The pseudoaneurysm was excluded by embolization of the artery with three microcoils, one straight and two flower microcoils (Target Therapeutics) (*arrows*) placed from distal to proximal. Clinical and biological follow-up was uneventful

23.4.2 Ductal Complications and Fluid Collection

23.4.2.1 Clinical Presentation and Imaging

CT and US play a major role in the guidance of percutaneous puncture or drainage of posttraumatic pseudocysts (Siegel and Sivit 1997). They are particularly useful for monitoring changes in size of peripancreatic fluid collections, which may resolve spontaneously or evolve into retroperitoneal or intraperitoneal pseudocysts. Uncomplicated pseudocysts appear anechoic at US and show equal to water density on CT. If complicated by infection or hemorrhage, internal echoes at US and increased attenuation at CT are observed (Bass et al. 1988; Sivit et al. 1992; Siegel and Sivit 1997). Although US is less accurate than CT in determining the severity of the injury, US remains useful in the evaluation and treatment of pancreatic pseudocyst in children (Jaffe et al. 1989; Burnweit et al. 1990; Sivit et al. 1992). ERCP remains the first-line imaging technique when a complete duct transection is suspected (Lewis et al. 1993; Jurkovic and Carrico 1994; Rescorla et al. 1990; Keller et al. 1997).

Magnetic resonance cholangiography (MRCP) seems able to detect or exclude noninvasively pancreatic duct damage and/or pancreas-specific complications following trauma and provides information that may be used to guide management (Fulcher et al. 2000). In addition to delineating the pancreatic duct, MRCP detects pseudocysts that may not be opacified at ERCP. Complementing MRCP with conventional MRI allows the assessment of the pancreatic duct together with the parenchyma (Fulcher et al. 2000). Percutaneous external drainage should be considered as the primary therapeutic procedure for posttraumatic pancreatic collection, if there is no evidence of pancreatic duct transection on MRCP or ERCP.

23.4.2.2 Fistula

Fistulae are the most frequent complication after pancreatic trauma (4.5%–35%) and occur most commonly after blunt trauma (Jurkovich and Carrico 1994; Akhrass et al. 1997). Pancreatic duct discontinuity is the main cause of pancreatic fistula. Despite their relative frequency, low-output fistulae are almost always self-limited and resolve spontaneously in nearly all circumstances within 2 weeks to 3 months of injury (Patton et al. 1997). In case of a high-output fistula or a fistula complicated by an increasing and/or infected collection, sump drainage should be instituted to create a controlled fistula (Cabay et al. 1998). Conservative management involves good percutaneous or endoscopic drainage, protection of the skin, and nutritional support, with careful attention to fluids and electrolyte balance. Intravenous infusion or subcutaneous injection of somatostatin analogue may be used to hasten the closure of external pancreatic fistulae (Prinz et al. 1988). Occasionally, for fistulae from a major pancreatic duct, operation is required to drain the fistula into a Roux-en-Y loop or to resect the pancreatic tail, which is responsible for the intractable leakage (Akhrass et al. 1997; Patton et al. 1997). After failure of conventional medical treatment, endoscopic insertion of a plastic stent in a ruptured main pancreatic duct may be an alternative to conventional surgical technique to deal with a high-output fistula (Fabre et al. 1995; Thanh et al. 1999).

23.4.2.3 Pseudocyst

Pancreatic pseudocyst formation after trauma is reported in 15%–36% of patients, occurring more frequently in the pediatric population, and may be the result of a missed pancreatic injury (40%) (Cogbill et al. 1991; Wilson and Moorehead 1991; Sivit et al. 1992; Akhrass et al. 1997; Sjövall and Hirsh 1997). Pseudocysts are fluid collections without a true epithelial lining, resulting from the accumulation of enzymes secreted by the distal portion of the gland. They arise weeks to months after the initial injury. Posttraumatic pseudocysts and their complications such as secondary infection, spontaneous perforation, and massive hemorrhage can be treated by percutaneous catheter drainage (Jaffe et al. 1989; Akhrass et al. 1997). Depending on the location of the ductal injury, a pseudocyst may require aspiration, external drainage, or surgical resection with partial pancreatectomy, but conservative management has also been successful in selected cases. Most reports of failure of external drainage, due to early recurrence or complications, involve adult patients, but occasionally also involve children (Jurkovich and Carrico 1994; Rescorla et al. 1990).

Pediatric Population

Spontaneous resolution of cysts after medical treatment, including prolonged total parenteral nutrition, is observed in 25%–46% of cases (BASS et al. 1988; CARR et al. 1989; BURNWEIT et al. 1990; FORD et al. 1990; BECMEUR et al. 1993; KELLER et al. 1997; LUCAYA et al. 1998; JOBST et al. 1999). Large or complicated posttraumatic pancreatic pseudocysts in children have been classically treated by surgery. Successful nonoperative management of painful or enlarging pseudocysts are now reported (JAFFE et al. 1989; BURNWEIT et al. 1990). Although simple needle aspiration is a useful diagnostic procedure, it is unsuitable for long-term management of pseudocysts that are refractory to medical treatment. Percutaneous drainage is usually primarily performed under US or CT guidance (BASS et al. 1988; BURNWEIT et al. 1990; YOO et al. 1996; SJÖVALL and HIRSH 1997; LUCAYA et al. 1998; WALES et al. 2001). Direct placement of a drainage catheter into the pseudocyst between the left lobe of the liver and stomach or stomach and spleen seems the preferable approach to avoid catheter dislodgment. Most transgastric catheters become dislodged due to respiratory and gastric motion, needing repositioning or replacement. A transhepatic approach is rarely necessary. Guidewire manipulation through the drainage catheter is able to rupture septations or to drain residual fluid collections (JAFFE et al. 1989). As nearly all posttraumatic pancreatic pseudocysts in children are noninfected, 8.3- to 10-French drainage catheters are usually large enough to provide long-term drainage (SJÖVALL and HIRSH 1997; JAFFE et al. 1989). Potential complications of percutaneous external drainage include sepsis, bleeding, bowel perforation, pneumothorax, empyema, and persistent tract fistula (BURNWEIT et al. 1990; WALES et al. 2001). Before removing the catheter from a pseudocyst, a trial of oral feeding with the drainage catheter clamped is recommended. This trial should be obtained after 3–4 weeks of drainage, when the patient is asymptomatic and drainage nearly ceased (BASS et al. 1988; JAFFE et al. 1989; LUCAYA et al. 1998; WALES et al. 2001). Fluid reaccumulation observed on CT or US, recurrent pain, or a significant rise in the serum amylase level are indicators of a persistent communication between the cyst and the pancreatic duct, which requires prolonged catheter drainage (JAFFE et al. 1989; KELLER et al. 1997; WALES et al. 2001). A pseudocyst that is largely communicating with the pancreatic duct on ERCP takes longer to resolve completely. However, successful percutaneous drainage in such condition has been reported (JAFFE et al. 1989). Pseudocysts that are associated with complete disruption of the main pancreatic duct can sometimes also be managed effectively with prolonged percutaneous drainage (OHNO et al. 1995; WALES et al. 2001). In this condition, the distal pancreatic body and tail usually atrophies. Occasionally, the gland can heal and the duct recanalizes (WALES et al. 2001). Most commonly, complete distal duct injuries are managed by spleen-preserving pancreatectomy and major cephalic duct trauma by endoscopic cystostomy and duct stenting (KELLER et al. 1997; JOBST et al. 1999). Delayed complications of untreated posttraumatic pseudocysts are abscess formation, fistulization or compression of bowel or other adjacent structures (BURNWEIT et al. 1990; LUCAYA et al. 1998).

Adult Population

In adults, the strategy in the management of posttraumatic pancreatic pseudocysts depends on the site and type of ductal injury, the maturity of the cyst wall, and the urgency to treat (LEWIS et al. 1993; AKHRASS et al. 1997; PATTON et al. 1997). If there is a minimal communication with a side branch or distal main duct, conservative treatment or aspiration should be attempted, but external catheter drainage may lead to a prolonged fistula (LEWIS et al. 1993). Pseudocysts due to proximal major duct injury frequently require surgical intervention, using either resection or internal drainage, depending on the maturity of the cyst wall (LEWIS et al. 1993; JURKOVICH and CARRICO 1994). When elective surgical exploration is undertaken, preoperative ERCP allows accurate anatomical delineation of the duct injury and facilitates operative strategy. Pancreatic ascites may occur, when the ductal discontinuity leads to the spillage of pancreatic secretions from the distal pancreas into the abdominal cavity through the ruptured lesser sac. This situation requires urgent distal duct derivation with a Roux-en-Y loop and peritoneal lavage to avoid severe peritonitis.

23.4.2.4 Abscess and Pancreatitis

The development of pancreatitis after pancreatic injury is a common and serious complication with a high mortality rate, especially in patients with hemorrhage (JONES 1985; WILSON and MOOREHEAD 1991; BLEICHNER et al. 1998). Treatment is standard care applicable to any acute severe pancreatitis. The incidence of abscess formation after pancreatic trauma ranges from 10% to 25% (WILSON and MOOREHEAD 1991; JURKOVICH and CARRICO 1994) and carries a high risk of death unless it is diagnosed and drained early (BURNWEIT et al. 1990). Pancreatic abscesses are usually associated with Gram-negative enteric organisms and result from associated intestinal injury. The majority of trauma related abscesses likely represent inadequately drained fluid collections that are secondarily contaminated by the intestinal flora. They are usually characterized as being uniloculated fluid collections with minimal surrounding tissue necrosis and are therefore amenable to simple CT-guided catheter drainage and antibiotic therapy (Patton et al. 1997).

23.4.2.5 Long-Term Complications

Long-term complications of ductal trauma are fibrosis and stricture formation, most commonly encountered when the ductal section has been incomplete. They may cause recurrent episodes of acute pancreatitis (Carr et al. 1989; Bradley 1991). Duct stenosis may induce fibrosis and atrophy of the pancreatic parenchyma with secondary changes of chronic pancreatitis in the obstructed segment of the gland. Symptoms related to ductal strictures are most commonly abdominal pain and recurrent episodes of acute pancreatitis. Pancreaticoenteric drainage or resection of the obstructed segment of pancreas provides prompt and effective relief (Leppaniemi et al. 1988a; Carr et al. 1989; Bradley 1991). Resolution of a main pancreatic duct stricture without endoscopic or surgical treatment has been reported (Apel et al. 2001). Endocrine or exocrine pancreatic dysfunction is rarely reported (Wales et al. 2001). Diabetes mellitus after pancreatic injury is rare, unless necrosis reaches 80%–90% of the gland (Wilson and Moorehead 1991). Exocrine function impairment is unusual, provided that pancreatic fluid has access to the duodenum.

23.4.2.6 Postoperative Complications

Complications following early partial pancreatectomy for ductal rupture are seen in 15%–35% of patients and include intra-abdominal abscesses in 32%, pancreatic fistulae in 14%, pancreatitis in 8%, and pseudocyst formation in 3% after distal pancreatic resection (Campbell and Kennedy 1980; Cogbill et al. 1991).

23.5 Kidney, Adrenal, Urinary Bladder

Long-term sequelae from renal injuries depend on the type and extent of injury, and how long the injury went unrepaired. Complications typically present in a delayed fashion, with hematuria or retroperitoneal bleeding occurring days or weeks following the injury. Major complications sometimes occur in patients who have sustained isolated major renal injuries, but most often result from associated injury and/or the development of sepsis or associated organ failure (Carroll et al. 1990; Knudson et al. 2000). Complications resulting directly from the renal injury or repair occur in less than 10% of patients (Carroll et al. 1990; McAninch 1993).

Early complications, which occur within 4 weeks of trauma, include delayed renal bleeding, persistent urinary extravasation, with eventually urinoma formation and perinephric abscess (McAninch 1993; Knudson et al. 2000). Late complications include pseudoaneurysm and/or arteriovenous fistula formation, hydronephrosis, cyst or stone formation, chronic pyelonephritis, urinary fistulization, and arterial hypertension, which is uncommon and may occur either early or several years after a repaired or untreated injury (McAninch 1993). Follow-up studies with CT and/or US are recommended, especially after grade III or IV injury, to detect and document these potential complications, which are mainly observed after nonsurgical treatment (Carroll et al. 1990; McAninch 1993).

23.5.1 Vascular Complications

Secondary hemorrhage is the most common and most serious delayed complication of renal injury and is usually due to a traumatic pseudoaneurysm or an arteriovenous fistula, bleeding into the pyelocaliceal system or the perinephric area (Uflacker et al. 1984; Teigen et al. 1992; Farrell et al. 1996; Swana et al. 1996; Han et al. 1998; Jebara et al. 1999). Bleeding into the renal collecting system usually causes hematuria and, in rare cases, may produce renal insufficiency from clot retention. This complication occurs in 18%–19% of patients treated conservatively after penetrating injury (Heyns and Van Vollenhoven 1992a; Armenakas et al. 1999) and in 13%–18% of patients with deep cortical lacerations (grade III and IV) due to blunt trauma (Corr and Hacking 1991; Swana et al. 1996; Jebara et al. 1999; KNUDSON et al. 2000). Primary surgical exploration does not necessarily prevent secondary hemorrhage (CARROLL et al. 1990; HEYNS and VAN VOLLENHOVEN 1992a). An incidence of delayed renal bleeding of 3%–15% is reported following primary surgical exploration after trauma (MCANINCH 1993; HEYNS and VAN VOLLENHOVEN 1992a; FARRELL et al. 1996; KNUDSON et al. 2000) (Fig. 23.18). Arterial hypertension and renal failure are observed in 10% of the patients undergoing surgery for major renal trauma (KNUDSON et al. 2000).

23.5.1.1
Pseudoaneurysm and Arteriovenous Fistula

Clinical Presentation and Imaging

Pseudoaneurysm (PSA) and arteriovenous fistula (AVF) are reported mainly following penetrating or iatrogenic injury (HEYNS and VAN VOLLENHOVEN 1992a; HASSANTASH et al. 1995; ARMENAKAS et al. 1999). Pseudoaneurysm, which may cause a mass effect on the collecting system, hematuria or extra-capsular hemorrhage, may be evidenced as a large, enhancing collection within the kidney on CT (SWANA et al. 1996). An AVF may present either in isolation or in combination with a PSA (Fig. 23.19). In rare instances, untreated PSA or AVF may contribute to renal insufficiency (BUI et al. 1994). Isolated AVF, without aneurysm interposition are rare, especially in children, and usually result from percutaneous biopsy, and are rarely observed after blunt or penetrating abdominal trauma of other origin (VAN DER ZEE et al. 1995). The cause of PSA after blunt trauma is not well understood. Penetrating trauma may result in a fistulous communication between adjacent structures. In blunt trauma, the rapid deceleration of solid organs presumably results in shear stress to a visceral artery and unrecognized full-thickness injury, which ultimately presents as delayed bleeding into an adjacent vein or viscus (UFLACKER et al. 1984; KANTOR et al. 1989; HASSANTASH et al. 1995). The danger in not treating these injuries is the risk of delayed rupture, renal loss, cardiac failure and death. In addition to AVF and PSA, the angiographic findings may include arteriocaliceal fistulae, which occur when an arterial injury communicates with

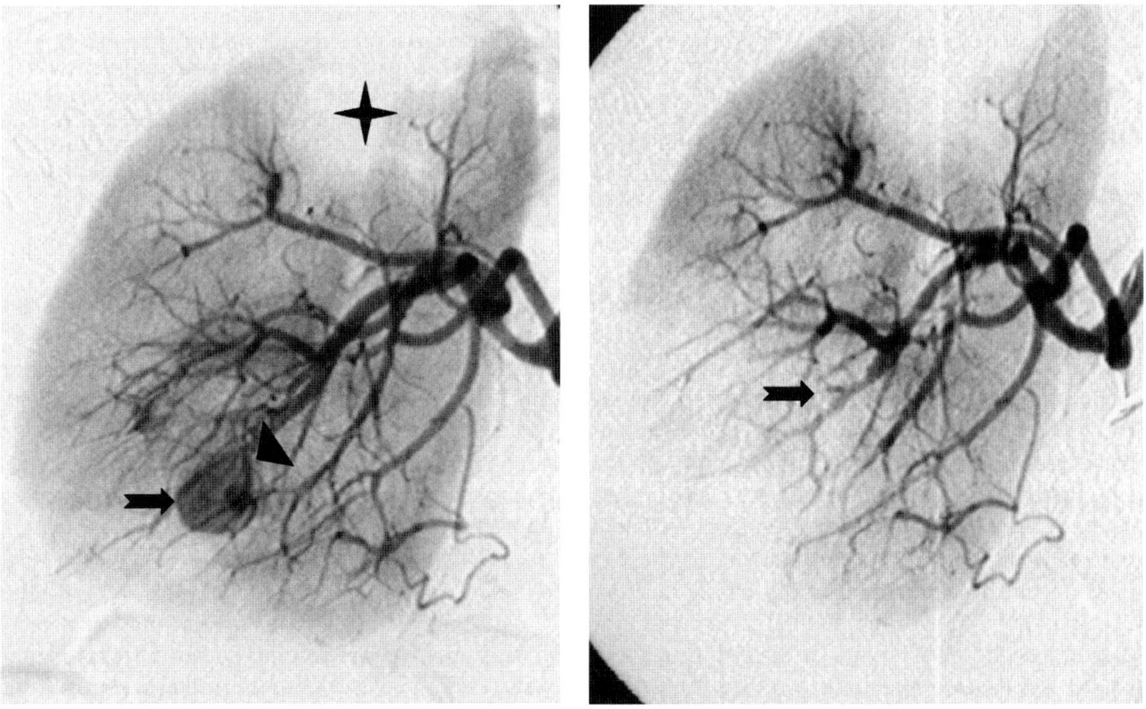

a b

Fig. 23.18a, b. A 61-year-old female presented repeated episodes of gross hematuria following a partial lower pole right nephrectomy for grade III blunt renal trauma. **a** Right renal arteriography demonstrates a 12-mm-diameter pseudoaneurysm (*arrow*), probably arising from a small segmental arterial branch (*arrowhead*). Posttraumatic area of contusion is visible in the upper pole (*star*). **b** Superselective catheterization of the feeding artery with a 3-F catheter and injection of three small gelatin sponge pledgets resulted in an immediate and complete exclusion of the pseudoaneurysm (*arrow*). No bleeding recurred

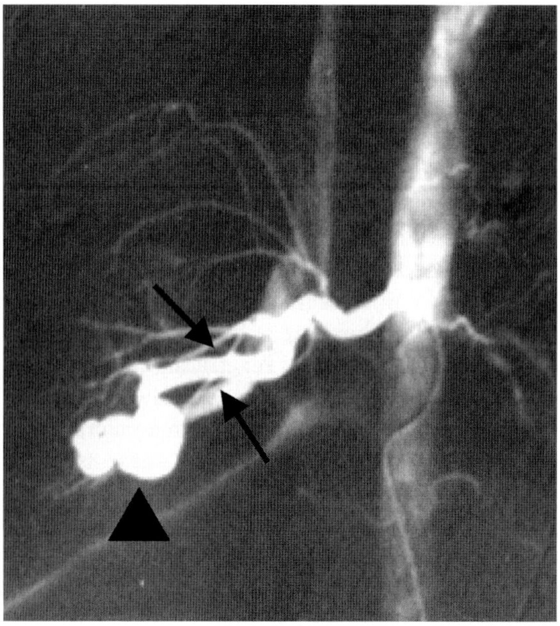

a

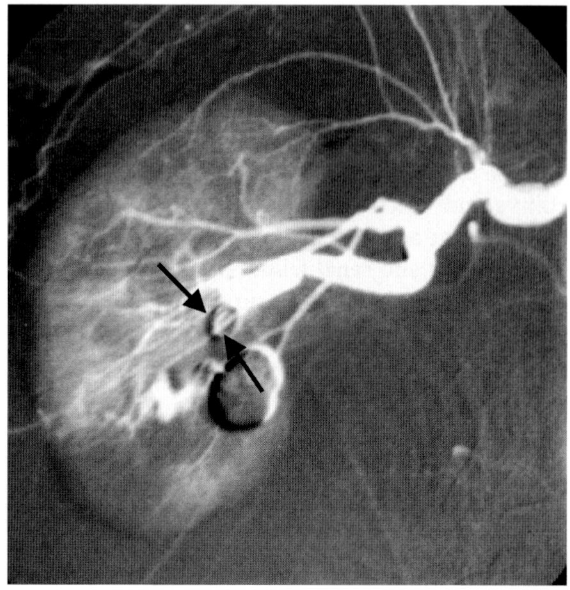

b

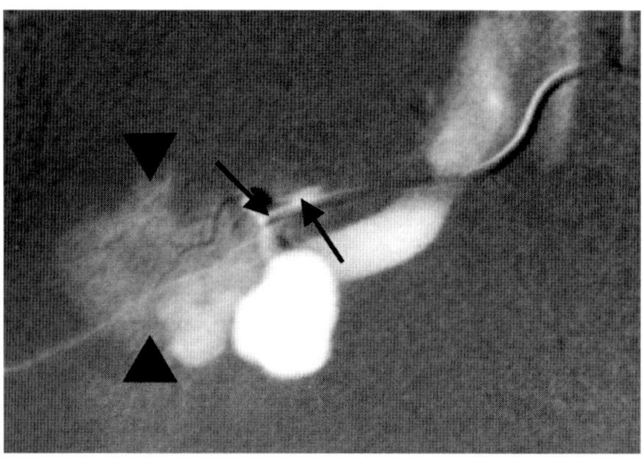

c

Fig. 23.19a–c. A 56-year-old female presented with progressive right cardiac insufficiency, refractory arterial hypertension, and recurrent episodes of moderate hematuria 5 years after blunt right renal injury treated conservatively. **a** Selective right renal arteriogram shows a massive intrarenal arteriovenous fistula (*arrows*) with an interposed pseudoaneurysm (*arrowhead*). Marked decrease in renal perfusion is due to flow steal by the high-flow lesion. **b** Selective catheterization of the dilated arterial branch supplying the fistula is achieved with a 4-F catheter (*arrows*). A limited area of parenchyma is supplied by the same artery (*arrowheads*). **c** Distal selective embolization is performed with three Gianturco coils (4 mm in diameter, 3 cm in length) (*arrows*), resulting in immediate and complete obliteration of the vascular malformation with sparing of the renal parenchyma. Symptoms completely disappeared during follow-up

the renal collecting system and usually results in profuse hematuria (Han et al. 1998; Jebara et al. 1999; Franco de Castro et al. 2001). Extravasation may be apparent on the early and mid arterial phase if there is brisk bleeding. Late arterial and venous phases are required for adequate angiographic lesion demonstration (Kantor et al. 1989). Arteriocaliceal fistula may be difficult to identify on both CT and renal arteriography, because of residual contrast in the collecting system from previous studies such as CT bolus test injection or abdominal aortography (Kantor et al. 1989). In view of the risk that a PSA or AVF will develop after renal trauma, it has been suggested that CT should be performed 3–6 months after any high-grade injury (Guerriero 1988). Renal perfusion scintigraphy may provide a noninvasive method to detect arteriovenous fistulae (Rosen et al. 1986). An angiographic investigation is mandatory in the presence of recurrent gross hematuria, bruit over the kidney, or when de novo arterial hypertension develops after previous renal injury (Uflacker et al. 1984; Bertini et al. 1986; Guerriero 1988; McAninch 1993).

Management

Although spontaneous resolution of PSA or AVF following renal biopsy occurs in 50%–80% of the patients, most arteriovenous fistulae that are detected after major renal trauma do not heal spontaneously (Fischer et al. 1989). Surgical procedures seem much more invasive than an endovascular approach and should be avoided (Bertini et al. 1986). Secondary nephrectomy for delayed renal hemorrhage is required in half of the patients for whom surgery is considered. Alternative surgical procedures, proposed to preserve renal parenchyma and function, include fistula excision, endofistulorrhaphy, ligation of renal branch arteries and occlusion of venous channels (Heyns and Van Vollenhoven 1992a).

Angiography should be considered in any patient who has recurrent or delayed hematuria after the initial episode of bleeding has resolved. Although embolization may result in renal infarction, this technique is justified, because less loss of renal parenchyma is expected from catheter embolization than from operative repair.

Traumatic PSA or AVF treatment requires a careful technique. Usually, embolization is performed through a microcatheter placed within a 5- or 6-F guiding catheter. Various embolic materials may be used, including Gianturco coils or platinum microcoils (Huppert et al. 1993; Triller et al. 1993; Beaujeux et al. 1995; Farrell et al. 1996; Swana et al. 1996), Gelfoam pledgets (Han et al. 1998), detachable balloons (Teigen et al. 1992; Huppert et al. 1993), glue (Huppert et al. 1993; Kerber et al. 1977), and hydrogel particles or Surgicel (Phadke et al. 1997). The choice depends on the site and accessibility of the feeding artery. PSA has a thin wall that may easily rupture, indicating the preferential use of embolic material that can be applied via the catheter without increasing intravascular pressure. Due to the usually peripheral location of PSA, the use of a microcatheter allowing superselective catheterization of segmental and arcuate arteries is warranted in order to induce minimal renal parenchyma loss, especially in patients with a single functioning kidney (Huppert et al. 1993; Triller et al. 1993; Franco de Castro et al. 2001). The kidney differs from other organs in that trapping a PSA or AVF by placing coils distally and proximally or selective catheterization of the PSA neck with packing of the aneurysm is not required because of the end-arterial supply. Retrograde filling of the renal vasculature and subsequent reinjection of the PSA are unlikely to occur. Therefore proximal occlusion of the feeding artery to a PSA with coils usually offers permanent occlusion (Farrell et al. 1996) (Fig. 23.18). Nevertheless, since recanalization of PSA due to intrarenal collateral circulation was reported after coil placement (Uflacker et al. 1984), additional deposition of Gelfoam pledgets may be required to complete the occlusion in case of persistent PSA (Van der Zee et al. 1995). Embolization procedures for AVF or arteriocaliceal fistula are similar to those used to occlude PSA. Coils are the embolic agent of choice since they offer better control of deployment compared to Gelfoam pledgets. Microcoils properly sized to the feeding vessel are less likely to pass through the fistula into the venous system than smaller particles of Gelfoam (Van der Zee et al. 1995) (Fig. 23.19).

In the setting of a posttraumatic complication, control of renal bleeding by embolization is achieved in 80%–100% of cases (Clark et al. 1983; Uflacker et al. 1984; Kantor et al. 1989). Cessation of hematuria is achieved in 88%–100% (Fischer et al. 1989; Corr and Hacking 1991). In most patients, the extent of the renal infarction is lower than 30% (Fischer et al. 1989; Beaujeux et al. 1995). Few patients will require surgery after embolization and long-term sequelae secondary to renal infarction are rare (Corr and Hacking 1991). Furthermore, embolization can be repeated, obviating surgical intervention and possible nephrectomy (Uflacker et al. 1984). Complications due to renal artery embolization and postembolization syndrome are observed in 8%–10% (Clark et al. 1983; Uflacker et al. 1984; Fischer et al. 1989). For patients with a renal stab wound, primary renal angiography with segmental artery embolization is an alternative management strategy that can be performed prior to any surgical exploration (Uflacker et al. 1984; Heyns and Van Vollenhoven 1992b).

23.5.1.2 Arterial Hypertension

Another the long-term complication of renal trauma, observed after both blunt and penetrating injury and probably due to renal infarction, is arterial hypertension. This complication, initially reported with an incidence of 20%–45% after partial embolization, has been largely overestimated. Only 16%–20% of reported cases are documented to be normotensive before injury, many patients having preexisting renal disease (Monstrey et al. 1989). Arterial hypertension or renal failure develops in 10% of the patients after surgery for major renovascular trauma (Knudson et al. 2000). The true incidence and natural history of trauma-induced renovascular hypertension remains elusive. It may result from any type of treatment, including observation. Recent data suggest that the true incidence of posttraumatic hypertension is close to 5%. Hypertension may be transient and observed from 2 weeks to 8 months after injury. Possible mechanisms for the development of posttraumatic hypertension include renal artery occlusion, stenosis or compression, severe renal contusion, arteriovenous fistula or pseudoaneurysm, and a chronic contained subcapsular hematoma with subsequent renal scarring, reducing flow to the kidney and inducing renin-mediated hypertension (Kawashima et al. 2001). Hypertension may resolve spontaneously within 1 year after injury (Bertini et al. 1986). In some cases, nephrectomy of a previously injured kidney may be indicated in patients with refractory hypertension or in order to preserve contralateral renal function (Kawashima et al. 2001). In selected cases, percutaneous embolization of the damaged vessels may be considered to exclude the renal artery injury responsible for hypertension (Cotroneo et al. 1987).

23.5.1.3 Renal Failure

The incidence of posttraumatic renal failure after major renal trauma is around 6.5% (Knudson et al. 2000). In case of bilateral renal artery injuries, every attempt must be made to revascularize at least one kidney. Endovascular stent placement may be considered in cases of intimal tear of the renal artery (Goodman et al. 1998; Paul et al. 1999).

23.5.2 Urinary Tract Complication

23.5.2.1 Urinary Fistula

Persistent extravasation and urinoma are the most frequent complications of expectant management, with a rate of 13%–16% (Matthews et al. 1997). Urinomas following renal trauma form secondary to laceration of the renal collecting system or ureter and subsequent urinary leak into the perirenal or retroperitoneal compartments (Fig. 23.20). Delayed intraperitoneal ureteral rupture, suspected in case of massive urine ascites, is most commonly observed after penetrating trauma and is unusual after blunt trauma (Wilkinson et al. 1989). These complications may be treated successfully with endourological or percutaneous drainage or stenting, thereby avoiding secondary renal exploration (Husmann et al. 1993; Sclafani et al. 1984a; Matthews et al. 1997; Knudson et al. 2000). The vast majority of urinary extravasation will seal spontaneously, while persistent urinomas have to be treated by percutaneous nephrostomy to ensure urine diversion with or without a plastic stent placement (Fig. 23.20). Antegrade ureteral stenting is recommended for the management of a persistent massive ureteral leak after prolonged urine diversion or for treatment of ureteral dehiscence after primary surgical repair (Sclafani et al. 1984a; Knudson et al. 2000). Retrograde stenting may be demanding when the ureter is tortuous or when an interposed urinoma prevents passage across the dehiscence (Lang 1984). Urinary diversion usually allows the laceration to heal and further intervention is rarely necessary. In cases of persistent or large renal pelvic leaks, primary healing may not occur with urinary diversion and further therapy may be warranted. Surgical procedures often include total nephrectomy, because of the extent of retroperitoneal fibrosis and adhesions that may develop in delayed repairs (Matthews et al. 1997). Selective embolization of the renal parenchyma is a less invasive therapeutic approach than surgery, can spare normal renal parenchyma, and has been proven effective in ceasing urine flow into a urinoma (Horikami et al. 1997; Pinto and Chimeno 1998). Posttraumatic nephrobiliary fistula, which is a rare complication of lumbar trauma, may also be treated by selective embolization (Ryu et al. 1998).

23.5.2.2 Ureteral Stenosis

High-pressure balloon catheter angioplasty can be used to dilate a trauma-induced ureteral stenosis or a secondary stricture after primary surgical repair. A success rate of 50% has been reported (Banner and Pollack 1984)

23.5.3 Abscess

Infected urinomas and perinephric abscesses occur more frequently in patients with an unrepaired, devitalized renal segment and bacterial seeding from concomitant pancreatic or bowel injuries (Husmann and Morris 1990; Husmann et al. 1993; Armenakas et al. 1999). Percutaneous drainage is the first line treatment of an infected fluid collection of urine and other trauma-related renal or perirenal abscesses. CT is the preferred imaging guidance, providing an accurate method of detecting abscesses and delineating safe access routes that avoid contamination of uninfected areas (Sclafani et al. 1984a).

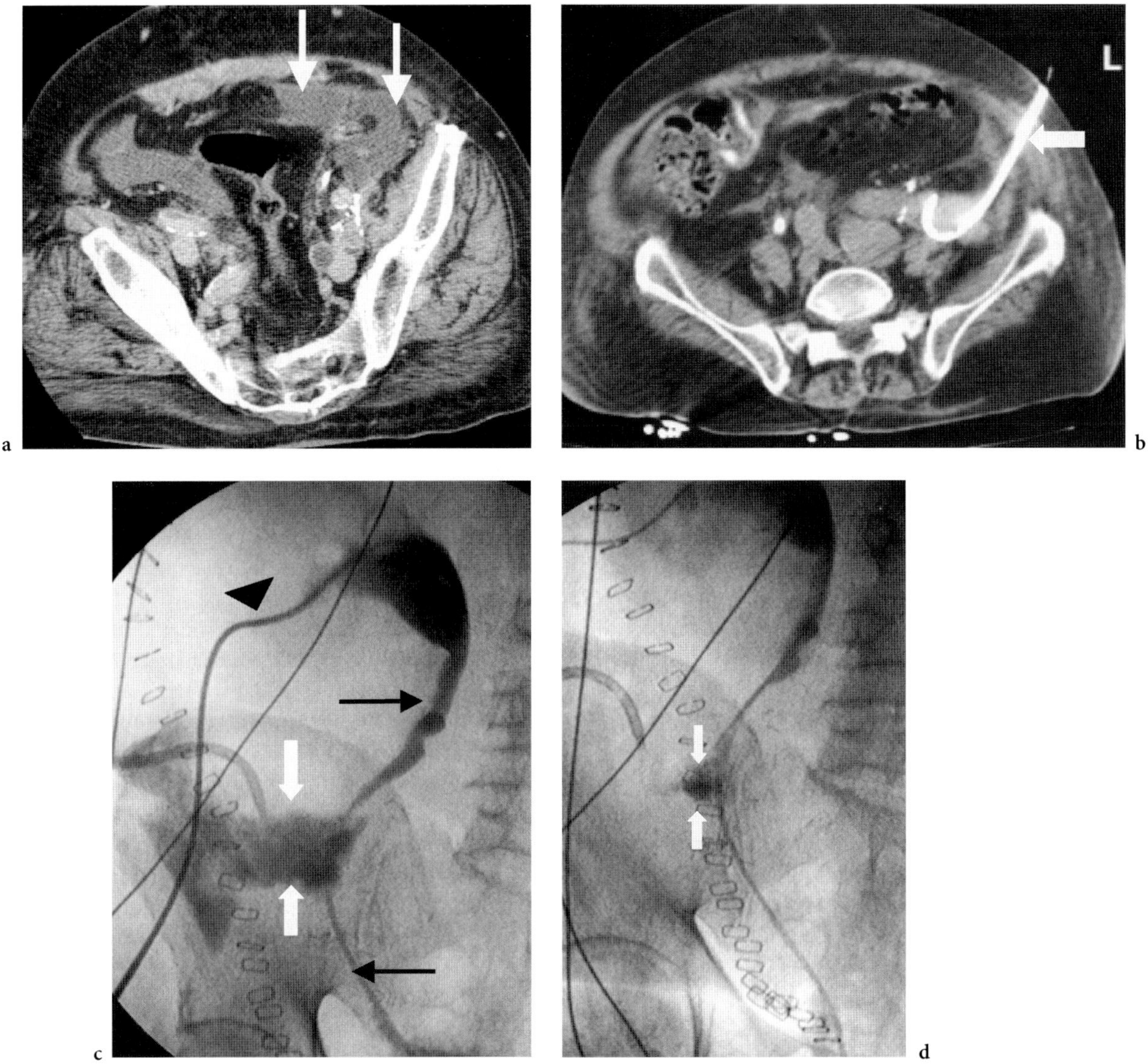

Fig. 23.20a–d. A 81-year-old man had sustained blunt trauma to the back after a fall from a height of 6 m. CT showed a grade II left kidney injury and a small retroperitoneal collection compatible with an urinoma. **a.b** CT at 10 days shows increase in the retroperitoneal fluid collection (*arrows*) (**a**) that is drained percutaneously under CT guidance (*arrow*) (**b**). Fluid analysis confirmed urinoma. **c** A double J stent (*black arrows*) and a nephrostomy catheter (*arrowhead*) were placed percutaneously to seal the urinary leak (*white arrows*). **d** Opacification performed 14 days later showed almost complete healing of the ureteral leak with a small residual blind fistula (*white arrows*) that completely disappeared 2 weeks later

23.5.4 Miscellaneous

A potential hazard of nonoperative management of a renal stab wound is the risk of an unrecognized diaphragmatic laceration. The radiographic findings, even provided by CT, are often nonspecific (Feliciano et al. 1988). Delayed diaphragmatic bowel herniation secondary to a retroperitoneal stab wound occurs predominantly on the left side, since the bulk of the liver prevents herniation through defects on the right side (Feliciano et al. 1988). Delayed posttraumatic adrenal hematoma may occasionally be observed after blunt trauma and should be suspected in traumatized patients with a mild enlargement of the adrenal gland on initial CT and a delayed lumbar pain with a drop of hemoglobin (Oto et al. 2000)

23.5.5 Urinary Bladder

A significant morbidity rate of 25% is observed after nonoperative management of bladder injuries, most commonly extraperitoneal (Kotkin and Koch 1995). Complications include delayed bladder rupture, vesicocutaneous fistula, sepsis and bladder calculi. Patients with multiple pelvic fractures seem to be at high risk of developing complications. Adequate catheter drainage and the use of antibiotic prophylaxis reduces the rate of complications.

23.6 Gastrointestinal Tract

Delayed complications following injury to the gastrointestinal tract include obstruction, perforation, short bowel syndrome, abdominal abscess and wound dehiscence or infection.

23.6.1 Stomach and Duodenum

The two major complications after duodenal trauma are postoperative fistula formation, which is reported with an incidence of 2%–16%, and duodenal obstruction (Cogbill et al. 1990; Jurkovich and Carrico 1994).

23.6.1.1 Fistula

Patients with pyloric exclusion after repair of grade III and grade IV duodenal injuries have an overall incidence of fistula formation of 6%–11% (Cogbill et al. 1990). Most of these duodenal fistulae close spontaneously with nonoperative management. Duodenal fistulae usually present after the 5th postoperative day. In patients with external drainage, the diagnosis is established by the presence of bile at the site of the drainage. The diagnosis is made by opacification of the drain or by gastroduodenal contrast study. The most important aspects in the management of a duodenal fistula are drainage of all intra-abdominal fluid collections, local wound protection to avoid damage from the duodenal secretions, and adequate nutrition of the patient, ideally provided via a distal jejunostomy (Jurkovich and Carrico 1994). Well-diverted duodenal fistulae are managed expectantly, provided good external drainage is present. Most patients without duodenal diversion have lateral duodenal fistulae with a high output requiring further diversion. In such patients or in those where the fistula remains open after a period longer than 2 weeks, operation should be considered to avoid the development of severe malnutrition, intra-abdominal sepsis, or extensive skin necrosis from duodenal contents. Duodenal fistulae have an overall mortality rate of 2% (Cogbill et al. 1990; Carrillo et al. 1996).

23.6.1.2 Obstruction

Duodenal obstruction is seen in 5%–8% of patients after duodenal trauma. After primary surgery, obstruction is more common in patients who have undergone extensive duodenal repair than after gastrojejunostomy and is also observed during follow-up of a large duodenal hematoma. Duodenal hematoma is most commonly seen in children, who are at higher risk than adults because of their weaker abdominal musculature, and usually involves the second portion of the duodenum, but may extend proximally and distally to the first and third portion in 25% of patients (Sidhu et al. 1998). Conservative nonoperative management has become the prevalent treatment of duodenal hematoma. Nonoperative treatment should be tried for at least 3–4 weeks in partial obstruction because of the likelihood of spontaneous resolution of the hematoma and the high postoperative morbidity rate (Maull et al. 1978; Touloukian 1983; Carrillo et al. 1996). Laparotomy may be delayed in some cases of incomplete obstruction, because of a delay in diagnosis, unsatisfactory improvement with nonsurgical treatment, rupture of the hematoma, or late duodenal obstruction (Jewett et al. 1988). Extending duodenal hematoma involving the papilla with subsequent common bile duct and pancreatic duct obstruction has been reported (Takishima et al. 2000). Enlargement of a hematoma may result in obstructive jaundice and hyperamylasemia. Osmotic changes within or subsequent hemorrhage into the hematoma or both conditions may contribute to the delayed expansion of the intramural hematoma of the duodenum. In this setting, surgical drainage should be performed to avoid cholangitis or pancreatitis (Takishima et al. 2000). Intramural duodenal hematoma requires surgical evacuation or local repair only in the presence of uncontrolled hemorrhage, transmural perforation, or hemodynamic instability. In case of continuous bleeding into an intramural duodenal hematoma, embolization using a coaxial catheter system is a possible alternative to surgical evacuation and operative hemostasis (Marra and Sclafani 1999). In patients with complete duodenal obstruction and without improvement after 1 week of nonoperative management, surgical gastrojejunostomy should be considered. Following duodenal hematoma, stricture formation, life-threatening hemorrhage and perforation are rare, especially in children (Jewett et al. 1988).

23.6.2 Small Bowel and Large Bowel

23.6.2.1 Stenosis

Delayed small or large bowel stenosis after conservative management of blunt abdominal trauma may be observed in both adults and children and may result from various pathological mechanisms (Bryner et al. 1980; Hirota et al. 1995; Loberant 1997; Chi and Shin 1998; Konobu et al. 1999). Causes of stenosis include intramural hemorrhage with subsequent narrowing or intussusception, serosa tear resulting in adhesions, unrecognized mesenteric, diaphragmatic, or abdominal wall disruption with subsequent incarceration of the small bowel, or direct bowel contusion (Konobu et al. 1999). The classic features of this entity are an interval of several weeks after trauma before onset of symptoms, clinical and radiological signs of obstruction and a long ileal or colonic stenosis (Bryner et al. 1980; Hirota et al. 1995; Loberant 1997). The time interval between the trauma and the onset of symptoms ranges from 3 days to 11 months but most patients complain of initial symptoms within 5 weeks of trauma (Hirota et al. 1995; Loberant 1997; Konobu et al. 1999; Tsushima et al. 2001). Differences are noted in the clinical manifestations between patients with ileal stenosis (ileus) and those with colonic stenosis (rectal bleeding and diarrhea) (Hirota et al. 1995). Posttraumatic ischemic small bowel stenosis may result from small tears and simple contusion. These lesions may cause partial thickness ischemia of the bowel wall with mucosal ulceration and submucosal inflammation and fibrosis or may cause full-thickness ischemia with fibrosis and scarring of all layers, which leads to stricture formation and obstruction (Hirota et al. 1995; Loberant 1997). The pathological findings may be similar to those of acute intestinal ischemia or spontaneous ischemic jejunoileitis. These findings suggest that intestinal ischemia plays an important role in the pathogenesis of posttraumatic intestinal stenosis (Hirota et al. 1995; Loberant 1997; Konobu et al. 1999). The mechanism is most likely injury to the mesentery and bowel wall producing focal segmental ischemia (Hirota et al. 1995). The stenoses are confined to the proximal and distal ends of the small bowel, where the bowel is relatively constrained by its attachment (Konobu et al. 1999). Few cases report perforation as a complication of stenosis, probably due to ischemic ulceration (Konobu et al. 1999). Radiographic findings consist of a concentric narrowing in the intestinal lumen, of a variable length and associated with mucosal ulcerations (Hirota et al. 1995). US can demonstrate bowel wall thickening and to some extent characterize its nature (Loberant 1997). CT diagnosis of small bowel obstruction is based on the change in caliber of small bowel loops proximal to the site of obstruction compared with the collapse of distal bowel segments (Tsushima et al. 2001). CT is a reliable method for detecting the level and cause of obstruction, but enteroclysis is able to test the distensibility and fixation of the small bowel and therefore provides evaluation of the severity of partial mechanical small bowel obstruction better than CT (Loberant 1997; Chi and Shin 1998). Angiography may show distal mesenteric vessel occlusion and ischemic bowel wall enhancement and thus provides additional information concerning mesenteric injury and subsequent ischemic bowel injury. Delayed large bowel obstruction after a blunt injury may result from a combination of several factors: interference of blood supply by damage to small vessels, edema and hematoma secondary to the injury itself, and the development of fibrosis with gradually increasing obstruction (Vromen et al. 1993). The relatively high rate of involvement of the left colon may be explained by the underdeveloped marginal arterial system, which makes it more susceptible to damage from interference with the blood supply (Mays and Noer 1966; Vromen et al. 1993). Surgery with segmental resection restores normal condition.

23.6.2.2 Perforation

Delayed posttraumatic perforation of the colon and ileum following blunt trauma has been reported (Coats 1991; Mourad et al. 1992; Totte et al. 2000). Perforation usually occurs in patients who have sustained other injuries but can also occur as an isolated event (Chang et al. 2000). Delayed perforation of the sigmoid colon, leading to fecal peritonitis, may be caused by disinsertion of the sigmoid colon mesentery (MOURAD et al. 1992). US may be helpful to detect small bowel perforation after blunt abdominal trauma (CHANG et al. 2000; TOTTE et al. 2000). Seat belt flexion-distraction fracture of the spine, so-called Chance fracture, may be associated with the late development of ileal perforation or enterocolic fistula (COATS 1991; LETTS et al. 1999). Intramural hemorrhage of the intestine, observed after a low-velocity impact, may lead to delayed intestinal perforation (JOHANSSON et al. 1984). In a posttraumatic setting, the association of localized bowel wall thickening combined with intramesenteric hematoma as well as extravasation of contrast material is highly suggestive of trauma-induced vascular compromise of the bowel with perforation and mandates surgical exploration. Penetrating high-velocity trauma to the abdomen may lead to a delayed small bowel injury by a mechanism similar to low-pressure explosive blast injury (VELITCHKOV et al. 2000).

23.7 Vascular Complications

23.7.1 Superior Mesenteric Artery

Blunt and penetrating abdominal trauma, especially stab wounds, are a recognized cause of superior mesenteric arterial (SMA) pseudoaneurysm or arteriovenous fistula. Post-traumatic SMA arteriovenous fistulae or aneurysms are usually due to penetrating trauma and may be occult for a prolonged period (UFLACKER and SAADI 1982; HENNESSY et al. 1986; SAUNDERS et al. 1992). Mesenteric arteriovenous fistula may also result from previous abdominal surgery with bowel resection (UFLACKER and SAADI 1982). A few cases of posttraumatic intraluminal rupture of intramural jejunal or duodenal pseudoaneurysms are reported (WEST et al. 1968; BLEICHRODT et al. 1984). Delayed presentation of mesenteric pseudoaneurysm may be revealed by massive gastrointestinal hemorrhage due to erosion or perforation into an adjacent hollow viscus or delayed intraperitoneal rupture (FERRELLA 1992; KESTENBERG and MITTAL 1992). Late hemorrhage after trauma can be explained by a weakened arterial medial layer resulting in a subsequent delayed dissection and rupture (FERRELLA 1992; HASSANTASH et al. 1995). A traumatic SMA fistula is caused by simultaneous injury to contiguous artery and vein in the mesentery, usually resulting from blunt trauma or stab wounds (SAUNDERS et al. 1992). Immediately after injury, the affected area is usually surrounded by a hematoma, which becomes a false aneurysmal sac, communicating with the injured artery and vein. Untreated SMA arteriovenous fistula can result in portal hypertension and bowel ischemia (UFLACKER and SAADI 1982; HENNESSY et al. 1986; DESAI et al. 1987; REPASKY et al. 1993; ENGLISH et al. 2001) (Fig. 23.21) and bowel ischemia. Early recognition and treatment of this lesion is mandatory to avoid such complications. Most iatrogenic SMA fistulae produce symptoms more than 1 year after the original surgical procedure, while most posttraumatic SMA fistulae demonstrate symptoms within days or weeks after the injury (SAUNDERS et al. 1992). Symptoms and signs of SMA fistulae are related to bowel ischemia, venous congestion, importance of flow through the fistula, and secondary portal hypertension (DESAI et al. 1987). Symptoms are correlated with the size of the fistula and its duration, and are more pronounced with a proximal location. The most dependable diagnostic signs are the presence of an abdominal bruit or a palpable thrill. Signs of portal hypertension include ascites, esophageal varices, cirrhosis, hepatosplenomegaly, or malnutrition. If the fistula is large and proximal or of long-standing duration, signs of right cardiac failure may also be present (SAUNDERS et al. 1992). If such a lesion is suspected, the best diagnostic test is selective

Fig. 23.21a–h. A 61-year-old man had a history of a motor vehicle accident with rupture of the mesenteric root, requiring emergent surgical repair. Six years later, he presented with massive ascites. Discrete fibrotic changes were observed on liver biopsy. **a,b** Contrast-enhanced CT in axial (**a**) and coronal reconstruction (**b**) show diffuse ascites and a marked enlarged superior mesenteric vein (SMV) (*arrows*). The early enhancement of the dilated SMV is highly suggestive of a chronic mesenteric arterioportal fistula. **c** SMA arteriography confirms a distal mesenteric arterioportal fistula (*arrow*) supplied by a distal branch of the ileocecal artery. **d,e** Superselective catheterization of the ileocecal artery demonstrates a 1-cm-diameter pseudoaneurysm (*arrow*) interposed between two arterial feeders (*arrowhead*) and the dilated mesenteric vein (*curved arrow*). **f** The pseudoaneurysm was selectively occluded by deposition of nine Gianturco coils through a 4-F standard catheter (*arrow*). **g,h** Immediate (**g**) and 6-month follow-up (**h**) SMA arteriography shows complete obliteration of the fistula (*arrows*), preservation of the arterial feeders, and a marked increased perfusion of the peripheral mesenteric arteries (*curved arrows*) due to the suppression of the blood steal phenomenon induced by the fistula. Ascites had completely disappeared at 2-month follow-up

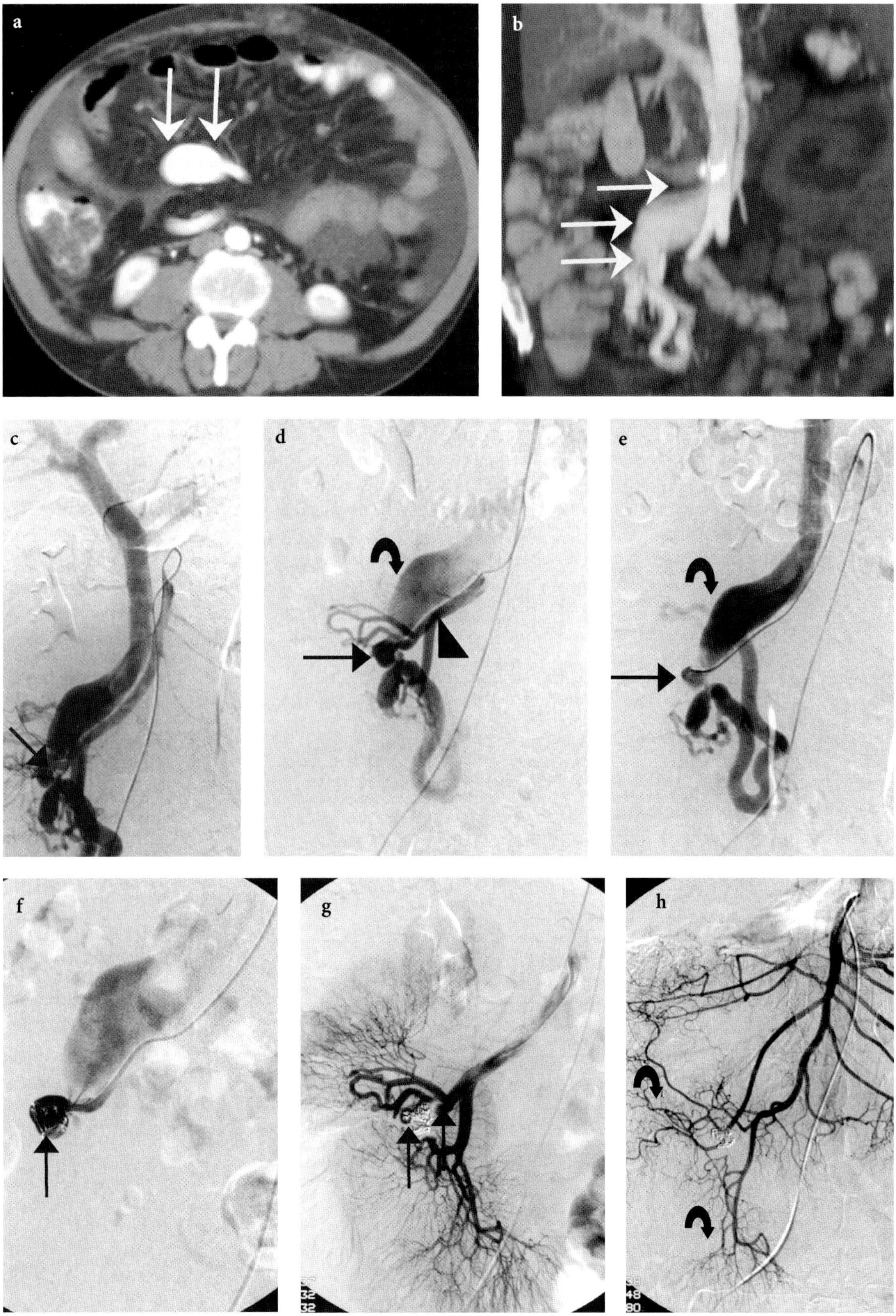
a
b
c
d
e
f
g
h

arteriography delineating the mesenteric and portal circulation, localizing the fistula and allowing a surgical or endovascular treatment. A pseudoaneurysm may be visualized near the fistulous communication (Desai et al. 1987). The fistula may also result from the formation of a postoperative pseudoaneurysm at the proximal end of the SMA that subsequently ruptures into the superior mesenteric vein (SMV). In this setting, both lesions should be treated simultaneously to obtain a successful result and definite cure (Repasky et al. 1993). Despite described spontaneous closure (Smith and Northrop 1987), an overall mortality of 25% is reported in untreated traumatic arteriovenous fistulae of the mesenteric circulation (Repasky et al. 1993; Cekirge et al. 1998). Arteriovenous fistula may be treated by surgical ligation of the arterial and venous communication or resection of the fistula with arterial and venous reconstruction by saphenous vein or an interposition of synthetic graft in the arterial segment (Saunders et al. 1992). An overall operative mortality rate of 18%–28% is reported (Desai et al. 1987).

Endovascular embolization is now an alternative treatment for such arteriovenous fistulae (Uflacker and Saadi 1982; Hennessy et al. 1986; Desai et al. 1987; Repasky et al. 1993). Recent studies have shown that percutaneous embolization of these fistulae is a safe, reliable, and effective treatment, with a low complication rate (Hennessy et al. 1986; Desai et al. 1987; Reparski et al. 1993; Savader et al. 1992) (Table 23.3). The embolization materials of choice are steel coils and detachable balloons (Desai et al. 1987; Savader et al. 1992). Pieces of gelatin sponge, particles, and isobutyl 2-cyanoacrylate are reserved for particularly small fistulae (Uflaker and Saadi 1982). The injection of particulate or liquid embolic material may be hazardous because of the possible passage into the portal circulation. Additional Gelfoam pledget placement after stainless steel coil packing may be necessary to achieve immediate and complete obliteration (Repasky et al. 1993) of high-flow fistula (Rosenthal et al. 1987). Successful embolization of a recurrent SMA fistula using giant steel coils, after initial surgery or after emergent SMA ligation performed to control massive bleeding, has been reported (Hennessy et al. 1986; Deitrick et al. 1990). Risks associated with transcatheter embolization include pseudoaneurysm rupture from

Table 23.3. Posttraumatic superior mesenteric arteriovenous fistulae treated by embolization

Reference	Gender/ age	Type of injury	Interval from injury to symptoms	Location on SMA	Clinical findings	Surgery	Successful emboli-zation (material)	Recur-rence
Uflacker and Saadi (1982)	M/41	Bowel resection (ischemia)	8 years	Distal trunk	Malabsorption, pain bruit	–	Yes (coils)	–
Hennessy et al. (1986)	M/36	Stab wound	18 months	Proximal trunk (with pseudo-aneurysm)	Ascites, GI bleeding diarrhea, pain	Yes (failure)	Yes (coils)	–
Desai et al. (1987)	M/35	Stab wound	4 months	Proximal trunk (with pseudo-aneurysm)	Ascites, pain malabsorption bruit, jaundice	–	Yes (coils)	–
Repasky et al. (1993)	M/22	Gunshot wound	2 weeks	Proximal trunk (with pseudo-aneurysm)	Fever	Yes (failure)	Yes (coils + Gelfoam)	–
Savader et al. (1992)	M/50	Seatbelt injury (+ surgery)	16 years	Distal trunk	Ascites, diarrhea, varices	–	Yes (coils)	Recurrent portal hyper-tension → TIPS
Cekirge et al. (1998)	M/53	Aortobifemoral grafting	5 days	Distal ileal	Bruit	–	Yes (coils, venous approach)	–

catheter manipulation, inadvertent coil deployment in a branch of the SMA resulting in focal intestinal ischemia with possible stricture formation or perforation, and embolization of the coils through the fistula, which could lead to main portal vein or portal vein branch occlusion (Repaski et al. 1993). Prior to treating a main trunk SMA pseudoaneurysm or arteriovenous fistula, it is mandatory to evaluate the potential collateral circulation in case of non-target embolization of the SMA. The transarterial approach to occlude a mesenteric arteriovenous fistula may be technically limited because of the anatomical structure or fistulous communication. A transvenous approach, aiming at occluding the draining vein, may be required in some cases (Cekirge et al. 1998). Recurrence or persistence of portal hypertension despite successful embolization has been reported. This may be due to irreversible liver damage caused by a long-standing arterioportal fistula (Fig. 23.21).

23.7.2 Aorta, Lumbar, and Iliac Arteries

The diagnosis of blunt trauma to the abdominal aorta is delayed in almost one-third of cases (Reisman and Morgan 1990). An occult pseudoaneurysm of the abdominal aorta and iliac arteries usually occurs following gunshot or stab wound injuries (Holland and Ibach 1996; Bardiche et al. 1999), but may be observed after blunt trauma (Israel and Morano 1996). This diagnosis should be suspected in traumatized patients, presenting with persistent back pain, bruit, claudication or decreased peripheral pulses (Reisman and Morgan 1990; Israel and Morano 1996). Delayed clinical manifestation of an aortic stenosis caused by intimal circumferential laceration and eversion secondary to blunt abdominal trauma has also been reported (Shindo et al. 1997). Posttraumatic pelvic arteriovenous fistulae, commonly secondary to penetrating injuries, are suspected in case of lower limb edema, varicosities, pain, audible bruit, or right cardiomegaly. Most of these lesions are currently managed percutaneously either by endovascular stent-graft implantation, allowing vessel patency with isolation of the vascular defect, or by vessel occlusion achievable with various materials including glue, coils, and detachable balloon (Roberts et al. 1996) (Fig. 23.22). For occlusion of a high-flow or wide-neck lesion occlusion, the combined use of a bare self-expandable stent and coils may be used as an alternative to stent-grafting (Roberts et al. 1996).

Lumbar artery pseudoaneurysm formation within an expanding hematoma is a well-known complication of retroperitoneal penetrating trauma (Haydu et al. 1978; Sclafani et al. 1987; Silberzweig 1999). A pulsatile mass, bruit, or thrill may be absent and localized; radiating pain caused by nerve root compression can be the sole symptom (Haydu et al. 1978). Embolization should be performed as close as possible to the aneurysmal neck to avoid both distal reinjection by collaterals from adjacent metameric levels and non-target occlusion of collateral spinal cord supply (Sclafani et al. 1987; Silberzweig 1999). If the endovascular approach is not feasible, pseudoaneurysm occlusion may be performed by a direct posterior percutaneous approach under combined CT and angiographic guidance (Fig. 23.23).

23.7.3 Inferior Vena Cava

Trauma is a rare cause of hepatic venous outflow obstruction (Nagy and Duarte 1990). Secondary thrombosis of the inferior vena cava (IVC) may occur following partial or full thickness injuries of the caval wall at the diaphragmatic hiatus, as this portion is fixed and more vulnerable to shearing forces. Traumatic hepatic venous outflow obstruction (Budd-Chiari syndrome) may also result from compression of the IVC by parenchymal and/or subcapsular liver hematoma producing sufficient mass effect to compress the confluence of the main hepatic veins and/or retrohepatic IVC. Decompression of the IVC and hepatic veins by a percutaneous or surgical drainage of the fluid collection could be curative in most cases (Markert et al. 1997). An asymptomatic nonocclusive IVC thrombus resulting from stasis caused by IVC compression by a large posttraumatic intrahepatic biloma has been reported (Frank et al. 1994).

23.8 Diaphragm

Delayed traumatic diaphragmatic hernia may occur months to years after the causative injury (Maekawa et al. 1997; Slim 1999). Main clinical symptoms are shortness of breath on effort or after meals. The diagnosis is usually made by a chest X-ray that reveals gastrointestinal air in the thorax (Maekawa et al. 1997). Diaphragmatic hernia should be considered as a possible diagnosis in patients with abnormal shadows in the thoracic region and who have recently sustained injury or who have a past history of trauma. A

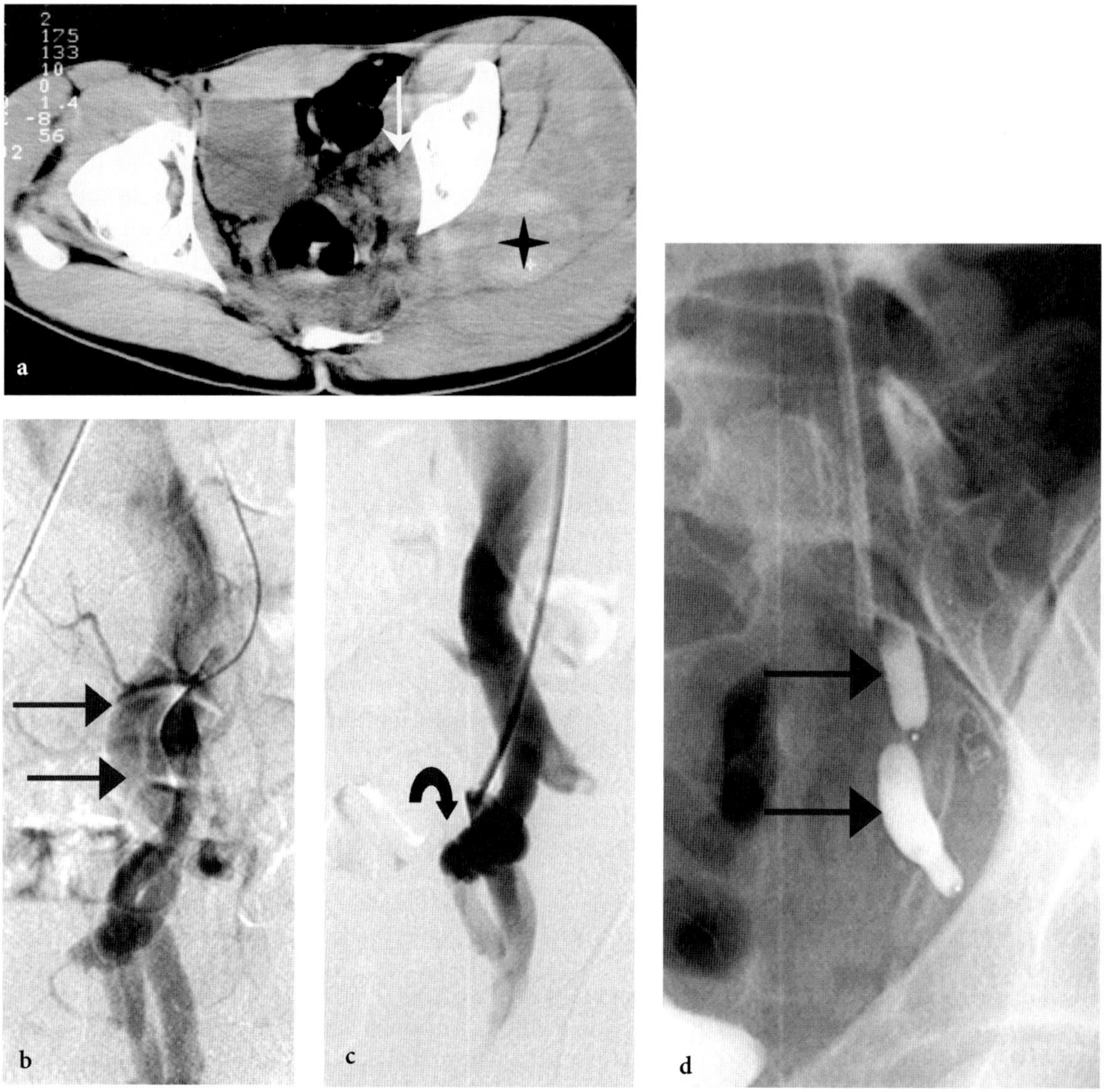

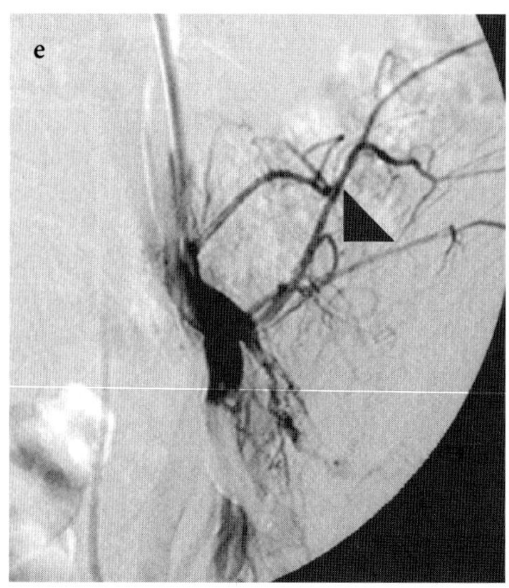

Fig. 23.22a–e. A 20-year-old man, victim of a posterior stab wound to left buttock, was initially treated by gelatin sponge torpedo embolization to control active bleeding from the left superior gluteal artery and by muscle débridement. During the first month of follow-up, the patient complained of persistent pelvic pain and progressive left lower limb edema. A systolo-diastolic bruit was perceptible over the pelvis. **a** Nonenhanced pelvis CT performed 4 weeks after the trauma shows a spontaneously hyperdense area (*star*), corresponding to fresh clot in the left buttock, and dilated left iliac vessels (*arrow*). These findings were highly suggestive of a vascular malformation. **b** Selective left internal iliac (LIIA) arteriography shows an arteriovenous fistula originating from the anterior trunk of the LIIA to a side branch of the left internal iliac vein (*arrows*) with poor visualization of the peripheral arterial branches due to massive flow steal induced by the fistula. **c** A pseudoaneurysm (*curved arrow*) is interposed between the arterial and venous component. **d,e** After placement of two 8+20-mm latex detachable balloons (*arrows*) in the feeding artery using the coaxial technique, no early filling of the fistula and iliac vein is observed. Enhanced-contrast opacification of the peripheral internal iliac arteries (*arrowhead*) is observed immediately after fistula closure. The clinical condition improved dramatically after successful embolization

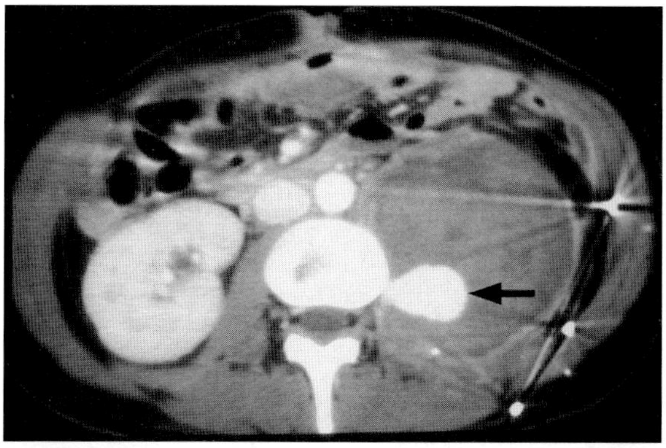
a

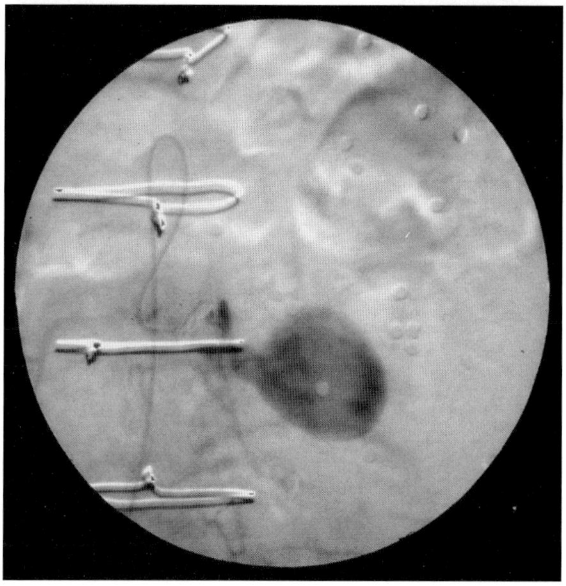
b

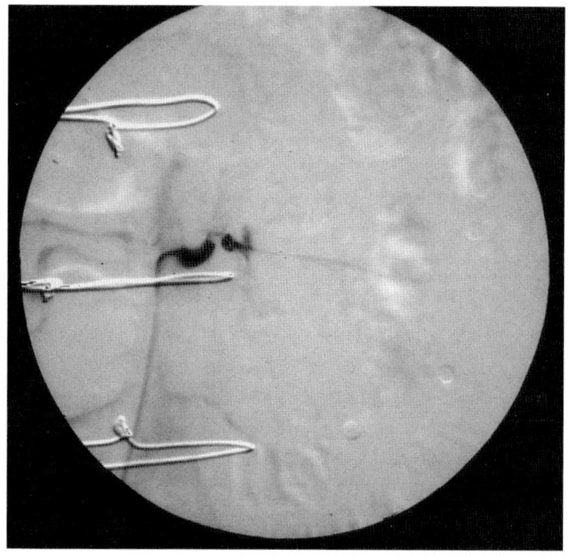
c

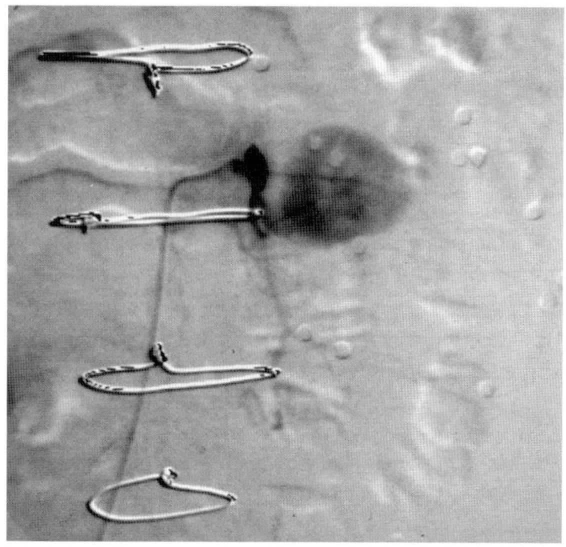
d

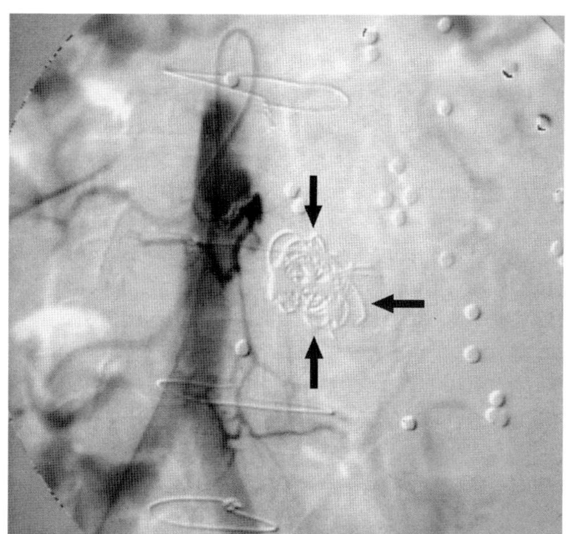
e

Fig. 23.23. A 25-year-old man was shot in the left flank and underwent urgent laparotomy. During the postoperative period, the patient developed persistent pain in the flank. **a** Abdominal contrast-enhanced CT showed at the arterial phase a left retroperitoneal pseudoaneurysm, 9 cm in diameter, with a 3-cm patent blood cavity (*arrow*) and hyperdense fresh peripheral thrombus. **b** Selective arteriography of the 3rd left lumbar artery confirmed posttraumatic pseudoaneurysm. **c** Proximal embolization with microcoils of the 3rd left lumbar artery was obtained. Postembolization arteriography showed occlusion of the pseudoaneurysm. The patient had recurrent left flank pain in the following days. **d** Repeated arteriography showed recanalization of the occluded lumbar artery and persistent filling of the pseudoaneurysm. As the risk of misplacement of additional coils or reflux of particulate embolization material was estimated to be too high, the patent pseudoaneurysm was punctured by a percutaneous posterior approach with CT guidance and macrocoils were placed through the needle in the aneurysmal sac. **e** Semiselective lumbar aortography obtained after completion of percutaneous intra-aneurysmal coil placement (*arrows*) showed complete vaso-occlusion. During follow-up, one coil ulcerated through the percutaneous needle tract and the patient underwent surgical excision of the complete thrombosed pseudoaneurysm (Courtesy of Prof. R.F. Dondelinger) delayed diaphragmatic bleeding into the left pleural space, 4 days after a nonoperative management of a blunt splenic injury has been observed by the authors. Embolization of the inferior phrenic artery was successful (Fig. 23.24). Delayed stenosis of the inferior vena cava induced by a traumatic diaphragmatic hernia has occasionally been reported (Lee et al. 1995). In this condition, the IVC is angulated and markedly narrowed below the right atrium. Herniation of the right lobe of the liver may be associated. The surgical reduction of the herniated viscus and repair of the ruptured diaphragm are definite treatments (Lee et al. 1995; Maekawa et al. 1997).

23.9 Conclusion

The nonoperative management of abdominal trauma and its delayed associated complications has gained success over the last decade. This approach has been extended to severe trauma patients previously considered candidates for surgery. Consequently, the incidence of delayed and uncommonly encountered complications has increased. The application of the nonsurgical approach and interventional radiology to manage delayed complications after abdominal trauma imposes a number of prerequisites: the clinician has to be aware of the natural history of the abdominal trauma and the expected associated complications; an oriented clinical and radiological follow-up has to be performed and the radiologist must have training and skills in the different and complementary techniques required for the diagnosis and treatment of these complications. In addition, the approach and treatment modalities may differ in adults compared to children. Some complications observed in children may resolve spontaneously (i.e., splenic pseudo-aneurysm) while treatment is indicated in adults (rupture and bleeding from the same aneurysm). The knowledge of this different natural history is mandatory in order to provide the most appropriate care to patients. Some post-traumatic lesions are to be treated by surgery (i.e., hollow viscus stenosis, diaphragmatic rupture, late onset distal pancreatic duct stenosis, etc.). Finally, the optimal treatment is a combination of the different complementary techniques in a multidisciplinary fashion, i.e., biliary peritonitis treated by peritoneal laparoscopic lavage, percutaneous drainage of the intrahepatic biloma, and endoscopic stenting of the injured bile duct.

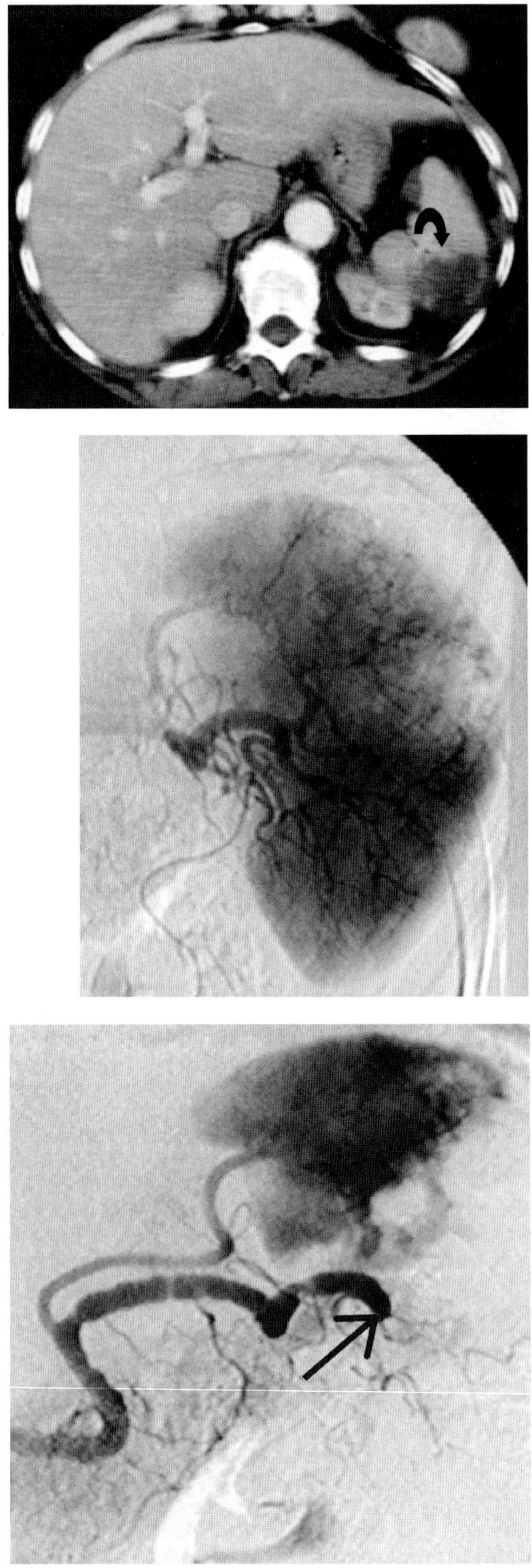
a
b
c ▷

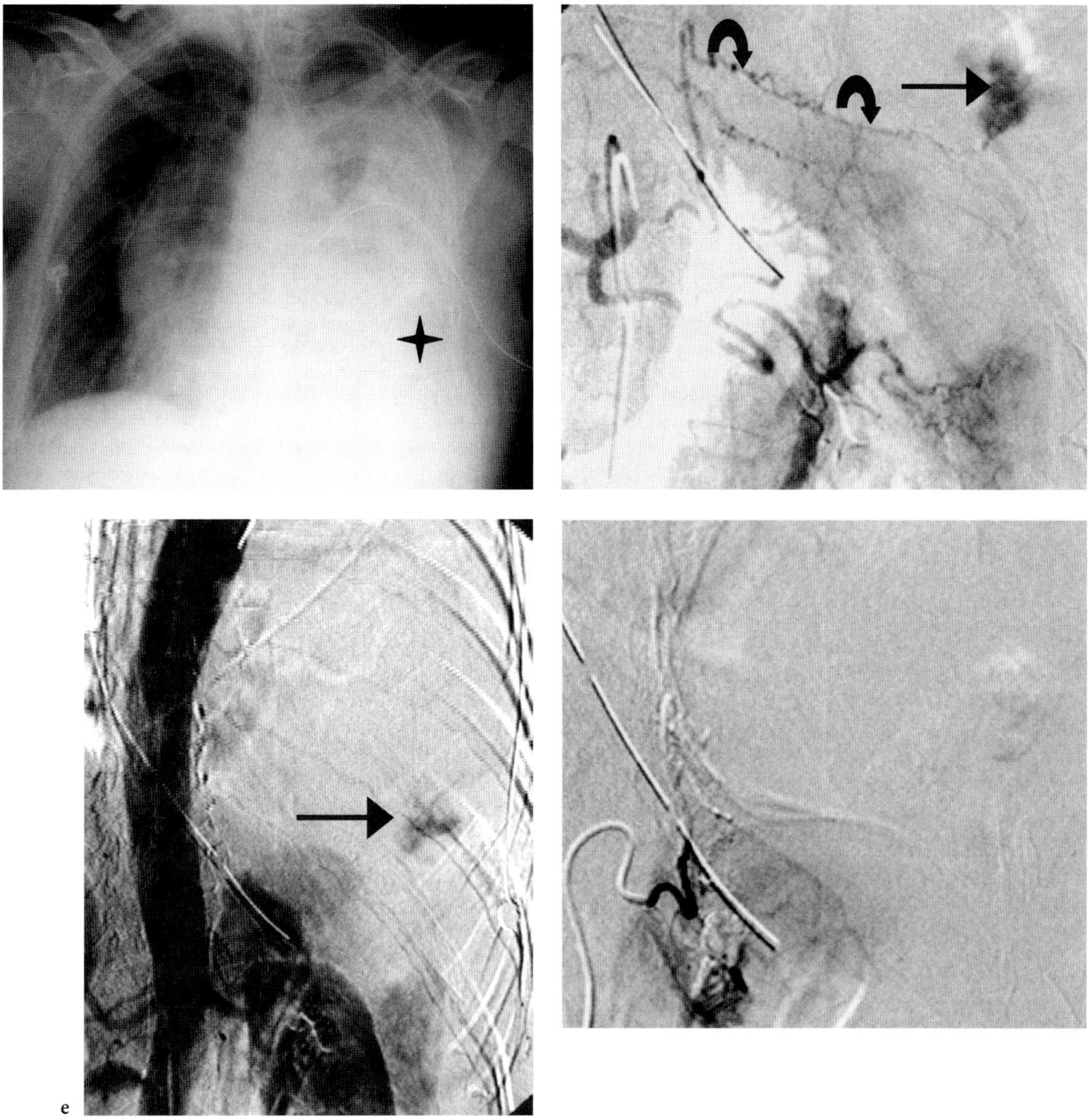

d f e g

Fig. 23.24a–g. A 59-year-old female presented with abdominal tenderness and moderate hemoperitoneum on CT obtained after a motor vehicle accident. Chest radiography showed fractures of the left 6th to 9th ribs without pleural effusion. **a** Contrast-enhanced CT showed grade III splenic injury with capsular tear (*curved arrow*). **b** Selective splenic arteriography shows patchy, irregular intraparenchymal blushes of contrast (Seurat pattern) but without evidence of vascular malformation. **c** Because of persistent need of blood transfusions, selective embolization of the injured arterial splenic branches (*arrow*) was performed with gelatin sponge pledgets, with a good initial clinical result. **d** Four days later, the patient developed a sudden hypovolemic shock and major dyspnea. Chest radiograph showed massive left side pleural effusion (*star*) and color Doppler sonography demonstrated pleural hemorrhage arising from the diaphragmatic area. **e,f** Thoracic aortography confirmed active bleeding located in the left diaphragmatic area (*arrow*) and supplied by a small branch arising from the left inferior diaphragmatic artery (*curved arrow*). **g** Hemorrhage was successfully interrupted by embolization of the left inferior diaphragmatic arterial branches with polyvinyl alcohol particles injected through a 0.018-in. microcatheter positioned far in the truncal diaphragmatic artery. Massive hemothorax was subsequently drained percutaneously. Follow-up was uneventful

References

Aboujaoude M, Noel B, Beaudoin M et al (1996) Pseudoaneurysm of the proper hepatic artery with duodenal fistula appearing as a late complication of blunt abdominal trauma. J Trauma 40:123–125
Akhrass R, Yaffe MB, Brandt CP et al (1997) Pancreatic trauma: a ten-year multi-institutional experience. Am Surg 63: 598–604
Apel D, Jakobs R, Riemann JF (2001) Reversible pancreatic duct stricture after a blunt abdominal trauma. Eur J Gastroenterol Hepatol 13:997–1000
Araoz PA, Andrews JC (2000) Direct percutaneous embolization of visceral artery aneurysms: techniques and pitfalls. J Vasc Interv Radiol 11:1195–1200
Armenakas NA, Duckett CP, McAninch JW (1999) Indications for nonoperative management of renal stab wounds. J Urol 161:768–771
Asensio JA, Demetriades D, Chahwan S et al (2000) Approach to the management of complex hepatic injuries. J Trauma 48:66–69
Baker RS, Tisnado J, Cho S et al (1987) Splanchnic artery aneurysm and pseudoaneurysm: transcatheter embolization. Radiology 163:135–139
Balci NC, Semelka RC, Sandhu JS (1999) Intrahepatic arterioportal fistula: gadolinium-enhanced 3D magnetic resonance angiography findings and angiographic embolization with steel coils. Magn Reson Imaging 17:475–478
Banner MP, Pollack HM (1984) Dilatation of ureteral stenoses: techniques and experience in 44 patients. AJR 143:789–793
Barchiche R, Bove T, Demanet H et al (1999) Traumatic pseudoaneurysm of the abdominal aorta. Acta Chir Belg 99: 174–176
Basile KE, Sivit CJ, Sachs PB et al (1999) Hepatic arterial pseudoaneurysm: a rare complication of blunt abdominal trauma in children. Pediatr Radiol 29:306–308
Bass J, Di Lorenzo M, Desjardins JG et al (1988) Blunt pancreatic injuries in children: the role of percutaneous external drainage in the treatment of pancreatic pseudocysts. J Pediatr Surg 23:721–724
Baudet R (1907) Ruptures de la rate. Med Pratique 3:565–567
Beal SL, Trunkey DD (1993) Splenic injury. In: Blaisdell F, Trunkey DD (eds) Abdominal trauma. Thieme Medical, New York, pp 230–249
Beaujeux R, Saussine C, Al-Fakir et al (1995) Superselective endo-vascular treatment of renal vascular lesions. J Urol 153:14–17
Becmeur F, Dhaoui R, Rousseau R et al (1993) Post-traumatic pancreatic pseudocyst: non-operative conservative management: report on 3 cases. Eur J Pediatr Surg 3:302–305
Beningfield SJ, Bornman PC, Krige JEJ (1991) Control of haemobilia by embolisation of a false aneurysm and arterioportal biliary fistula of the hepatic artery. AJR 156: 1263–1265
Berman SS, Mooney EK, Weireter LJ et al (1992) Late fatal hemorrhage in pediatric liver trauma. J Pediatr Surg 27: 1546–1548
Bertini JE, Flechner SM, Miller P et al (1986) The natural history of traumatic branch renal artery injury. J Urol 135: 228–230
Black JJ, Sinow RM, Wilson SE et al (1992) Subcapsular hematoma as a predictor of delayed splenic rupture. Am Surg 58:732–735
Bleichner JP, Guillou YM, Martin L et al (1998) Pancreatitis after blunt injuries to the abdomen. Ann Fr Anesth Reanim 17:250–253
Bleichrodt RP, Eversdijk Smulders TA, Schreuder F et al (1984) Aneurysms of the jejunal artery. J Cardiovasc Surg 25: 376–380
Blocker C, Brandon JC, Izenberg SD et al (1998) Posttraumatic enlargement of the spleen: a possible sign of delayed rupture. Emerg Radiol 5:263–265
Blum U, Buitrago-Tellez CH, El Seif M et al (1993) Post-traumatic bilhemia: conservative management by percutaneous drainage. Cardio Vasc Intervent Radiol 16:55–57
Bond SJ, Eichelberger MR, Gotschall CS et al (1996) nonoperative management of blunt hepatic and splenic injury in children. Ann Surg 223:286–289
Bokhari F, Nagy K, Roberts R et al (1999) Complications of angiographic embolization for traumatic hemobilia. J Trauma 47:977–978
Boone DC, Federle M, Billiar TR et al (1995) Evolution of management of major hepatic trauma: identification of patterns of injury. J Trauma 39:344–350
Bradley EL (1991) Chronic obstructive pancreatitis as a delayed complication of pancreatic trauma. HPB Surg 5:49–59
Brasel KJ, Delisle CM, Olson CJ et al (1997) Trends in the management of hepatic injury. Am J Surg 174:674–677
Bravo JL, Mangalmurti CS, Kowalak M (1998) Management of a ruptured post-traumatic splenic pseudocyst: case report. J Trauma 45:165–167
Bryner UM, Longerbeam JK, Reeves CD et al (1980) Posttraumatic ischemic stenosis of the small bowel. Arch Surg 115: 1039–1041
Bui BT, Oliva VL, Peloquin F (1994) Correction of deteriorating renal function by superselective embolization of an arcuate renal artery pseudoaneurysm. J Urol 152:2087–2088
Burnweit C, Wesson D, Stringer D et al (1990) Percutaneous drainage of traumatic pancreatic pseudocysts in children. J Trauma 30:1273–1277
Bynoe RP, Bell RM, Miles WS et al (1992) Complications of nonoperative management of blunt hepatic injuries. J Trauma 32:308–315
Cabay JE, Boverie JH, Dondelinger RF (1998) Percutaneous catheter drainage of external fistulas of the pancreatic duct Eur Radiol 8:445–448
Campbell D, Geraghty JG, McNicholas MM et al (1991) Delayed presentation of traumatic splenic arterio-venous fistula. Ir Med J 84:129–130
Campbell R, Kennedy T (1980) The management of pancreatic and pancreaticoduodenal injuries. Br J Surg 67:845–850
Capek P, Rocco M, McGahan et al (1992) Direct aneurysm puncture and coil occlusion: a new approach to peripancreatic pseudoaneurysms. J Vasc Interv Radiol 3:653–656
Carles J, Dubuisson V, Douws C et al (1994) Conservative treatment of hepatic injuries. Management and course. Chirurgie 95:444–450
Carr ND, Cairns SJ, Lees WR et al (1989) Late complications of pancreatic trauma. Br J Surg 76:1244–1246
Carrillo EH, Richardson JD, Miller FB (1996) Evolution in the management of duodenal injuries. J Trauma 40: 1037–1345
Carrillo EH, Platz A, Miller FB et al (1998) Non-operative management of blunt hepatic trauma. Br J Surg 85:461–468

Carrillo EH, Spain DA, Wohltman CD et al (1999) Interventional techniques are useful adjuncts in non-operative management of hepatic injuries. J Trauma 46:619–627
Carroll PR, McAninch JW, Klosterman P et al (1990) Renovascular trauma: risk assessment, surgical management, and outcome. J Trauma 30:547–552
Cekirge S, Özmen M, Akata D et al (1998) Endovascular treatment of a superior mesenteric arteriovenous fistula by a transhepatic portal venous approach. AJR 171:1283–1284
Chang YS, Wang HP, Huang GT et al (2000) Sonographic detection of delayed small bowel perforations after blunt abdominal trauma. J Clin Ultrasound 28:142–145
Chi T, Shin SL (1998) Delayed intestinal stenosis after blunt abdominal trauma: report of a case. Kaohsiung J Med Sci 14:734–737
Chiarugi M, Goletti O, Pucciarelli M et al (1995) Post-traumatic intrasplenic pseudoaneurysm successfully managed by embolization. Injury 26:705–706
Christimaz D, Le Coutre C (1987) Traumatic splenic cysts. Eur J Pediatr Surg 42:193–195
Chuang JH, Huang SC (1996) Posttraumatic hepatic cyst: an unusual sequela of liver injury in the era of imaging. J Pediatr Surg 31:272–274
Ciraulo DL, Luk S, Palter M et al (1998) Selective hepatic arterial embolization of grade IV and V blunt hepatic injuries: an extension of resuscitation in the nonoperative management of traumatic hepatic injuries. J Trauma 45:353–359
Citron SJ, Martin LG (1991) Benign biliary stricture: treatment with percutaneous cholangioplasty. Radiology 178: 339-341
Clancy TE, Warren RL (1997) Endoscopic treatment of biliary colic resulting from hemobilia after nonoperative management of blunt hepatic injury: case report and review of the literature. J Trauma 43:527–529
Clark RA, Gallant TE, Alexander ES (1983) Angiographic management of traumatic arteriovenous fistulas: clinical results. Radiology 147:9–13
Cleveland RJ, Jackson BM, Newman PH et al (1970) Traumatic intrahepatic hepatic artery: portal vein fistula with associated hemobilia. Ann Surg 171:451–454
Coats TJ (1991) Delayed presentation of perforation of the ileum following seat belt trauma. Arch Emerg Med 8:144–146
Cocanour CS, Moore FA, Ware DN et al (1998) Delayed complications of nonoperative management of blunt adult splenic trauma. Arch Surg 133:619–624
Cocanour CS, Middlebrook M, Lopez RM et al (2000) Choledococaval fistula as a result of a right flank stab wound: case report. J Trauma 48:137
Cogbill TH, Moore EE, Kashuk JL (1982) Changing trends in the management of pancreatic trauma. Arch Surg 117: 722–728
Cogbill TH, Moore EE, Jurkovich GJ et al (1988) Severe hepatic trauma: a multicenter experience with 1335 liver injuries. J Trauma 28:1433–1438
Cogbill TH, Moore EE, Jurkovich GJ et al (1989) Nonoperative management of blunt splenic trauma: a multicenter experience. J Trauma 29:1312–1317
Cogbill TH, Moore EE, Feliciano DV et al (1990) Conservative management of duodenal trauma: a multicenter perspective. J Trauma 30:1469–1475
Cogbill TH, Moore EE, Morris JA et al (1991) Distal pancreatectomy for trauma: a multicenter experience. J Trauma 31:1600–1609
Cope C, Zeit R (1986) Coagulation of aneurysms by direct percutaneous thrombin injection. AJR 147:383–387
Cornwell EE, Rodriguez A, Mirvis SE et al (1989) Acute acalculous cholecystitis in critically injured patients. Ann Surg 210:52–55
Corr P, Hacking G (1991) Embolization in traumatic intrarenal vascular injuries. Clin Radiol 43:262–264
Cotroneo AR, Patane D, De Cinque M et al (1987) Therapeutic embolization of renal artery to control severe hypertension due to renal trauma. Eur J Radiol 7:147–148
Croce MO, Fabian TC, Spiers et al (1994) Traumatic hepatic artery pseudoaneurysm with hemobilia. Am J Surg 168: 235–238
Croce MO, Fabian TC, Menke PG et al (1995) Nonoperative management of blunt hepatic trauma is the treatment of choice for hemodynamically stable patients. Results of a prospective trial. Ann Surg 221:744–753
Cuff RF, Cogbill TH, Lambert PJ (2000) Nonoperative management of blunt liver trauma: the value of follow-up abdominal computed tomography scans. Am Surg 66:332–336
Cywes S, Bass DH, Rode H et al (1991) Blunt liver trauma in children. Injury 22:310–314
D'Amours SK, Simons RK, Scudamore CH et al (2000) Major intrahepatic bile duct injuries detected after laparotomy: selective nonoperative management. J Trauma 50:480–484
Davis KA, Fabian TC, Croce MA et al (1998) Improved success in nonoperative management of blunt splenic injuries: embolization of splenic artery pseudoaneurysms. J Trauma 44:1008–1013
De Backer A, Fierens H, De Schepper A et al (1998) Diagnosis and nonsurgical management of bile leak complicated by biloma after blunt liver injury: report of two cases. Eur Radiol 8:1619–1622
Deitrick J, McNeill P, Posner MP et al (1990) Traumatic superior mesenteric artery-portal vein fistula. Ann Vasc Surg 4: 72–76
Demetriades D, Velmahos G, Cornwell E et al (1997) Selective nonoperative management of gunshot wounds of the anterior abdomen. Arch Surg 132:178–183
Demetriades D, Gomez H, Chahwan S et al (1999) Gunshot injuries to the liver: the role of selective nonoperative management. J Am Coll Surg 188:343–348
Desai SB, Modhe JM, Aulakh BG et al (1987) Percutaneous transcatheter steel-coil embolization of a large proximal post-traumatic superior mesenteric arteriovenous fistula. J Trauma 27:1091–1094
De Wit CWM, Bode PJ, van Vugt AB (1994) Splenic abscess following non-operative treatment of a splenic rupture caused by blunt abdominal trauma. Injury 25:405–406
Dunlop W, Lindsay R, Morrish HF et al (1977) Hemobilia associated with a traumatic arteriovenous fistula. Can J Surg 20: 441–443
Eastridge BJ, Minei JP (1997) Intrahepatic arterioportal fistula after hepatic gunshot wound: a case report and review of the literature. J Trauma 43:523–526
Eid A, Almogy G, Pikarsky AJ et al (1996) Conservative treatment of a traumatic tear of the left hepatic duct: case report. J Trauma 41:912–913
Eng RH, Tecson-Tumang F, Corrado ML (1981) Blunt trauma and liver abscess. Am J Gastroenterol 76:252–255
English WP, Johnson MB, Borman KR et al (2001) Mesenteric ischemia: an unusual presentation of traumatic intrahepatic arterioportal fistula. Am Surg 67:865–867

Fabian TC, Croce MA, Stanford GG et al (1991) Factors affecting morbidity following hepatic trauma: a prospective analysis of 482 liver injuries. Ann Surg 213:540–547
Fabre JM, Bauret P, Prudhomme M et al (1995) Posttraumatic pancreatic fistula cured by endoprosthesis in the pancreatic duct. Am J Gastroenterol 90:804–806
Farhat GA, Abdu RA, Vanek VN (1992) Delayed splenic rupture: real or imaginary? Am Surg 58:340–348
Farnell MB, Spencer MP, Thompson E et al (1988) Nonoperative management of blunt hepatic trauma in adults. Surgery 104:748–756
Farrell TM, Sutton JE, Burchard KW (1996) Renal artery pseudoaneurysm: a cause of delayed hematuria in blunt trauma. J Trauma 41:1067–1068
Feliciano DV, Mattox KL, Burch JM et al (1986) Packing for control of hepatic hemorrhage. J Trauma 26:738–743
Feliciano DV, Cruse PA, Mattox KL (1988) delayed diagnosis of injuries to the diaphragm after penetrating wounds. J Trauma 28:1135–1144
Ferrella TJ (1992) Delayed rupture of the middle colic artery secondary to blunt abdominal trauma. Ann Emerg Med 21: 428–430
Firstenberg MS, Plaisier B, Newman JS et al (1998) Successful treatment of delayed splenic rupture with splenic artery embolization. Surgery 123:584–586
Fischer RG, Ben-Menachem Y, Whigham C (1989) Stab wounds of the renal artery branches: angiographic diagnosis and treatment by embolization. AJR 152:1231–1235
Fitoz S, Atasoy C, Dusunceli E et al (2001) Post-traumatic intrasplenic pseudoaneurysms with delayed rupture: color Doppler sonographic and CT findings. J Clin Ultrasound 29:102–104
Ford EG, Hardin WD, Mahour GH et al (1990) Pseudocysts of the pancreas in children. Am Surg 56:384–387
Franco de Castro A, Gibanel Garanto R, Real MI et al (2001) Selective embolization of post-traumatic renal pseudoaneurysm in monorenal patient. Actas Urol Esp 25:64–66
Frank MS, Stern EJ, Foy HM (1994) Occult complication of nonoperative treatment of blunt liver injury: detection by CT. AJR 163:333–334
Franklin RH, Bloom WF, Schoffstall RO (1980) Angiographic embolization as the definitive treatment of post-traumatic hemobiliary. J Trauma 20:702–705
Frumiento C, Sartorelli K, Vane D (2000) Complications of splenic injuries: expansion of the nonoperative theorem. J Pediatr Surg 35:788–791
Fulcher AS, Turner MA, Yelon JA et al (2000) Magnetic resonance cholangiopancreatography (MRCP) in the assessment of pancreatic duct trauma and its sequelae: preliminary findings. J Trauma 48:1001–1007
Gable DR, Allen JW, Harrell DJ et al (1997) Endoscopic treatment of posttraumatic "Bilhemia": case report. J Trauma 43:534–536
Galeon M, Goffette P, Van Beers et al (1997) Post-traumatic intra-hepatic pseudoaneurysm: diagnosis with helical CT angiography and management with embolization. J Belge Radiol 80:287–288
Garby KB, King TS, Tsai FY (1997) Recurrence of pseudoaneurysm after successful embolization. J Endovasc Surg 4: 385–388
Gartman DM, Zeman RK, Cahow CE et al (1985) The value of hepatobiliary scanning in complex liver trauma. J Trauma 25:887–891
Gartside R, Gamelli RL (1987) Splenic arteriovenous fistula. J Trauma 27:671–673
Geis WP, Schulz KA, Giacchino JL et al (1981) The fate of unruptured intrahepatic hematomas. Surgery 90:689–697
Giacomantonio M, Filler RM, Rich RH (1984) Blunt hepatic trauma in children: experience with operative and nonoperative management. J Pediatr Surg 19:519–522
Glazer K, Wetscher G, Pointner R et al (1994) Traumatic bilhemia. Surgery 116:24–28
Goan YG, Huang MS, Lin JM (1998) Nonoperative management for extensive hepatic and splenic injuries with significant hemoperitoneum in adults. J Trauma 45:360–364
Goletti O, Ghiselli G, Lippolis PV et al (1996) Intrasplenic posttraumatic pseudoaneurysm: echo color Doppler diagnosis. J Trauma 41:542–545
Goodman DNF, Saibil EA, Kodama RT (1998) Traumatic intimal tear of the renal artery treated by insertion of a Palmaz Stent. Cardiovasc Intervent Radiol 21:69–72
Gow KW, Murphy JJ III, Blair GK et al (1996) Splanchnic artery pseudo-aneurysms secondary to blunt abdominal trauma in children. J Pediatr Surg 31:812–815
Griffen M, Ochoa J, Boulanger BR (2000) A minimally invasive approach to bile peritonitis after blunt liver injury. Am Surg 66:309–312
Guerriero WG (1988) Etiology, classification and management of renal trauma. Surg Clin North Am 68:1071–1084
Hagiwara A, Yukioka T, Shimazaki S et al (1993) Delayed hemorrhage following transcatheter arterial embolization for blunt hepatic injury. Cardiovasc Intervent Radiol 16:380–383
Hagiwara A, Yukioka T, Ohta S et al (1996) Nonsurgical management of patients with blunt splenic injury: efficacy of transcatheter arterial embolization. AJR 167:159–166
Hagiwara A, Yukioka T, Ohta S et al (1997) Nonsurgical management of patients with blunt hepatic injury: efficacy of transcatheter arterial embolization. AJR 169:1151–1156
Halme L, Orko R, Tierala E et al (1994) Late biliary stenosis after conservative management of traumatic liver rupture: case report. J Trauma 36:740–742
Hammond JC, Canal DF, Broadie TA et al (1992) Nonoperative management of adult blunt hepatic trauma in a municipal trauma centre. Am Surg 58:551–555
Han KRK, Goldstein DW, Pantuck AJ et al (1998) Angiographic management of pseudoaneurysm and arteriocalyceal fistula following blunt trauma: case report and review of the literature. Can J Urol 5:654–657
Haney PJ, Whithey NO, Brotman S et al (1982) Liver injury and complication in the postoperative trauma patient: CT evaluation. AJR 139:271–275
Hassantash SA, Mock C, Maier RV (1995) Traumatic visceral artery aneurysm: presentation as massive hemorrhage from perforation into an adjacent hollow viscus. J Trauma 38:357–360
Hatten MT, Hamrick-Turner JE (1996) Segmental hepatic necrosis after blunt abdominal trauma: CT findings. AJR 167:769–770
Haydu P, Chang J, Knox G et al (1978) Transcatheter arterial embolization of a traumatic lumbar artery false aneurysm. Surgery 84:288–291
Heller JA Jr, Papa P, Drugas G et al (1994) Non-operative management of solid organ injuries in children – is it safe? Ann Surg 219:625–631
Hennessy OF, Gibson RN, Allison DJ (1986) Use of giant steel coils in the therapeutic embolization of a superior mesen-

teric artery-portal vein fistula. Cardiovasc Intervent Radiol 9:42–45
Henry C, Dettloff L, Mhiri R et al (1998) Fistule artério-veineuse intrasplénique post-traumatique chez un enfant. J Radiol 79:271–273
Hertzanu Y, Mendelsohn DB (1984) Delayed splenic rupture: a true entity. Clin Radiol 35:393–396
Heyns CF, van Vollenhoven P (1992a) Selective surgical management of renal stab wounds. Br J Urol 69:351–357
Heyns CF, van Vollenhoven P (1992b) Increasing role of angiography and segmental artery embolization in the management of renal stab wounds. J Urol 147:1231–1234
Hidalgo F, Narvaez JA, Rene M et al (1995) Treatment of hemobilia with selective hepatic artery embolization. J Vasc Interv Radiol 6:793–798
Hiraide A, Yamamoto H, Yahata K et al (1994) Delayed rupture of the spleen caused by an intrasplenic pseudoaneurysm following blunt trauma: a case report. J Trauma 36: 743–744
Hirota C, Iida M, Aoyagi K et al (1995) Posttraumatic intestinal stenosis: clinical and radiographic features in four patients. Radiology 194:813–815
Holland AJ, Ibach EG (1996) False aneurysm of the inferior gluteal artery following penetrating buttock trauma: case report and review of the literature. Cardiovasc Surg 4: 841–843
Hollands B, Little J (1991) Post-traumatic bile fistulae. J Trauma 31:117–120
Horikami K, Matsuoka Y, Nagaoki K et al (1997) Treatment of post-traumatic urinoma by means of selective arterial embolization. J Vasc Interv Radiol 8:221–224
Hunt JA, Gallagher PJ, Heintze SW et al (1997) Percutaneous microcoil embolization of intraperitoneal intrahepatic and extrahepatic biliary fistulas. Aust N Z J Surg 67:424–427
Huppert PE, Duda SH, Erley CM et al (1993) Embolization of renal vascular lesions: clinical experience with microcoils and tracker catheters. Cardiovasc Intervent Radiol 16:361–367
Husmann DA, Morris JS (1990) Attempted nonoperative management of blunt renal lacerations extending through the corticomedullary junction: the short-term and long-term sequelae. J Urol 143:682–684
Husmann DA, Gilling PJ, Perry MO et al (1993) Major renal lacerations with a devitalized fragment following blunt abdominal trauma: a comparison between nonoperative (expectant) versus surgical management. J Urol 150:1774–1777
Inberg MV, Ahonen J (1971) Blunt trauma to the liver and hepatic vein. A special reference to the intense postoperative conjugated hyperbilirubinemia: a case report. Acta Chir Scand 137:93–96
Israel LJ, Morano JU (1996) Abdominal aortic injury in blunt abdominal trauma. Emerg Radiol 3:296–297
Ivatury RR, Rohman M, Nallathambi M et al (1985) The morbidity of injuries of the extrahepatic biliary system. J Trauma 25:967–973
Jaffe RB, Arata JA, Matlak ME (1989) Percutaneous drainage of traumatic pancreatic pseudocysts in childhood. AJR 152: 591–595
James CA, Emanuel PG, Vasquez WD et al (1996) Embolization of splenic artery branch pseudoaneurysm after blunt abdominal trauma. J Trauma 40:835–837
Jebara VA, El Rassi I, Achouh PE et al (1999) Renal artery pseudoaneurysm after blunt abdominal trauma. J Vasc Surg 27: 362–365
Jenkins MA, Ponsky JL (1995) Endoscopic retrograde cholangiopancreatography and endobiliary stenting in the treatment of biliary injury resulting from liver trauma. Surg Laparosc Endosc 5:118–120
Jewett TC, Caldarola V, Karp MP et al (1988) Intramural hematoma of the duodenum. Arch Surg 123:54–58
Jobst MA, Canty TG, Lynch FP (1999) Management of pancreatic injury in pediatric blunt abdominal trauma. J Pediatr Surg 34:818–823
Johansson L, Jonsson A, Norrby K et al (1984) Intestinal intramural haemorrhage after blunt abdominal trauma. Acta Chir Scand 150:165–171
Jones RC (1985) Management of pancreatic trauma. Am J Surg 150:698–704
Jurkovich GJ, Carrico CJ (1994) Pancreatic trauma. Surg Clin North Am 70:575–593
Kantor A, Sclafani SJA, Scalea T et al (1989) The role of interventional radiology in the management of genitourinary trauma. Urol Clin North Am 16:255–265
Katz MC, Meng CH (1970) Angiographic evaluation of traumatic intrahepatic pseudoaneurysm and hemobilia. Radiology 94:95–99
Kaufman SL, Martin LG, Zuckermann AL (1992) Peripheral transcatheter embolization with platinum coils. Radiology 184:369–372
Kawashima A, Sandler CM, Franck MC et al (2001) Imaging of renal trauma: a comprehensive review. Radiographics 21: 557–574
Kayser S, Marincek B, Schlumpf R et al (1996) Rapidly progressive portal hypertension 23 years after post-traumatic arterioportal fistula of the liver. Am J Gastroenterol 91: 1442–1446
Keller MS, Stafford PW, Vane DW (1997) Conservative management of pancreatic trauma in children. J Trauma 42: 1097–1100
Kennedy JA, Majury C, Kelly I et al (1999) Post traumatic pseudoaneurysm of an intrasplenic segmental artery; a mechanism of delayed splenic rupture. Injury 30:535–536
Kerber CW, Freeny PC, Cromwell L et al (1977) Cyanoacrylate occlusion of a renal arteriovenous fistula. AJR 128:663–665
Kestenberg WL, Mittal VK (1992) Post-traumatic pseudoaneurysm of the left hepatic artery initially appearing as gastrointestinal hemorrhage secondary to hepatic artery-duodenal fistula. A case study. Am Surg 58:451–455
Kim SS, Roberts RR, Nagy KK et al (2000) Hemosuccus pancreaticus after penetrating trauma to the abdomen. J Trauma 49:948–950
Kirchgatterer A, Baldinger C, Lenglinger F et al (1998) Portal hypertension due to traumatic hepatic arterioportal fistula: report of successful embolization. Eur J Gastroenterol Hepatol 10:1057–1059
Kluger Y, Paul DS, Raves JJ et al (1994) Delayed rupture of the spleen: myths, facts, and their importance: case reports and literature review. J Trauma 36:568–571
Knudson MM, Lim RC, Oakes DD et al (1990) Nonoperative management of blunt liver injuries in adults: the need for continued surveillance. J Trauma 30:1494–1500
Knudson MM, Harrisson PB, Hoyt DB et al (2000) Outcome after major renovascular injuries: a Western Trauma Association Multicenter Report. J Trauma 49:1116–1122
Konobu T, Murao Y, Miyamoto S et al (1999) Posttraumatic intestinal stenosis presenting as a perforation: report of a case. Surg Today Jpn J Surg 29:564–567

Kotkin I, Koch MO (1995) Morbidity associated with nonoperative management of extraperitoneal bladder injuries. J Trauma 38:895–898
Krige JE, Bornman PC, Terblanche J (1997) Liver trauma in 446 patients. South Afr J Surg 35:10–15
Kuno RC, Althaus SJ, Glickerman DJ (1995) Direct percutaneous coil and ethanol embolization of a celiac artery pseudoaneurysm. J Vasc Interv Radiol 6:357–360
Lang EK (1984) Antegrade ureteral stenting for dehiscence, strictures and fistulae. AJR 143:795–801
Lau LL, Diamond T (1997) Delayed presentation of porta hepatis injury following blunt abdominal trauma. HPB Surg 10: 249–252
Lee HK, Kim IO, Kim WS et al (1995) Stenosis of the inferior vena cava caused by a traumatic diaphragmatic hernia: case report. Pediatr Radiol 25:S175–S177
Leppaniemi A, Haapiainen R, Kiviluoto T et al (1988a) Pancreatic trauma: acute and late manifestations. Br J Surg 75: 165–167
Leppaniemi A, Haapiainen R, Standertskjold-Nordenstam CG et al (1988b) Delayed presentation of blunt splenic injury. Am J Surg 155:745–749
Lerut J, Vauthey N, Triller J et al (1992) Intrahepatic arterioportal fistula following conservative treatment of a traumatic liver rupture: case report. J Trauma 33:760–764
Letoublon C, Lachachi F, Arvieux C et al (1999) Current treatment of closed injuries of the liver: benefits and pitfalls. Chirurgie 124:20–30
Letts M, Davidson D, Fleuriau-Chateau P et al (1999) Seat belt fracture with late development of an enterocolic fistula in a child. A case report. Spine 24:1151–1155
Lewis G, Krige JEJ, Bornman PC et al (1993) Traumatic pancreatic pseudocysts. Br J Surg 80:89–93
Lina JR, Jaques P, Mandell V et al (1979) Aneurysm rupture secondary to transcatheter embolisation. AJR 132:553–556
Linhares MM, Caetano EM Jr, Louzano R et al (1998) Surgical resection of traumatic spleen cysts by laparoscopy. Int Surg 83:308–310
Loberant N (1997) Post-traumatic intestinal stenosis: radiographic and sonographic appearance. Eur Radiol 7:524
Lucaya J, Vazquez E, Caballero F et al (1998) Non-operative management of traumatic pancreatic pseudocysts associated with pancreatic duct laceration in children. Pediatr Radiol 28:5–8
Lukancic SP, Nemcek AA, Vogelzang RL (1991) Post-traumatic intra-hepatic arterial pseudo-aneurysm: treatment with direct percutaneous puncture. J Vasc Interv Radiol 2: 335–337
MacDermott VG, Shlansky-Goldberg R, Cope C (1994) Endovascular management of splenic artery aneurysms and pseudoaneurysms. Cardiovasc Intervent Radiol 17: 179–184
MacGillivray DC, Valentine RJ (1989) Nonoperative management of blunt pediatric liver injury – late complications: case report. J Trauma 29:251–254
Maekawa T, Yabuki K, Satou K et al (1997) A patient with a traumatic right diaphragmatic hernia occurring 4 years after sustaining injury – statistical observations of a delayed diaphragmatic hernia caused by uncomplicated injury in Japan. Nippon Geka Hokan 66:116–125
Malhotra AK, Fabian TC, Croce MA et al (2000) Blunt hepatic injury: a paradigm shift from operative to nonoperative management in the 1990s. Ann Surg 231:804–813
Maloo MK, Burrows PE, Shamberger RC (1999) Traumatic splenic arteriovenous fistula: splenic conservation by embolization. J Trauma 47:173–175
Mandel SR, Jaques PF, Sanofsky S et al (1987) Nonoperative management of peripancreatic arterial aneurysms. Ann Surg 205:126–128
Markert DJ, Shanmuganathan K, Mirvis SE et al (1997) Budd-Chiari syndrome resulting from intrahepatic IVC compression secondary to blunt hepatic trauma. Clin Radiol 52:384–387
Marra JM, Sclafani SJ (1999) Embolotherapy for expanding duodenal hematoma. Emerg Radiol 6:193–196
Masson D, Soyer P, Sihassen C et al (1993) Collection intrahépatique communiquant avec les voies biliaires: apport du drainage percutané temporaire. Rev Im Med 5:45–48
Matthews LA, Smith EM, Spirnak JP (1997) Nonoperative treatment of major blunt renal lacerations with urinary extravasation. J Urol 157:2056–2058
Maull KI, Fallahzadeh H, Mays ET (1978) Selective management of post-traumatic obstructing intramural hematoma of the duodenum. Surg Gynecol Obstet 146:221–224
Mays ET, Noer RJ (1966) Colonic stenosis after trauma. J Trauma 6:316–331
McAninch JW (1993) Editorial: renal trauma. J Urol 150:1778
McGahan JP, Lindfors KK (1989) Percutaneous cholecystostomy: an alternative to surgical cholecystostomy for acute cholecystitis. Radiology 173:481–485
McIndoe AH (1931) Delayed hemorrhage following traumatic rupture of the spleen. Br J Surg 20:249–268
Meredith JW, Young JS, Bowling J et al (1994) Nonoperative management of blunt hepatic trauma: the exception or the rule? J Trauma 36:529–534
Mirvis SE, Whitley NO, Miller JW et al (1987) CT diagnosis of acalculous cholecystitis. J Comput Assist Tomogr 11:83–87
Moir C, Guttman F, Jequier S et al (1989) Splenic cysts: aspiration, sclerosis, or resection. J Pediatr Surg 24:646–650
Monstrey SJ, Beerthuizen GI, van der Werken C et al (1989) Renal trauma and hypertension. J Trauma 29:65–70
Mourad M, Desrousseaux B, Atat I et al (1992) Delayed perforation of the sigmoid colon following closed abdominal trauma. A propos of a case report. Acta Chir Belg 92: 172–175
Nagar H, Kessler A, Weiss J (1997) Traumatic intraparenchymal splenic pseudoaneurysms in a child: nonoperative management. J Trauma 43:552–555
Nagy KK, Duarte B (1990) Post-traumatic inferior vena caval thrombosis: case report. J Trauma 30:218–221
Nance FC, Nance ML (1995) Delayed presentation of splenic artery pseudoaneurysms following blunt abdominal trauma. J Trauma 39:620–621
Norotsky MC, Rogers FB, Shackford SR (1995) Delayed presentation of splenic artery pseudoaneurysms following blunt abdominal trauma: case reports. J Trauma 38:444–447
Oguzkurt L, Balkanci F, Ariyurek M et al (1996) Traumatic aneurysm and arteriovenous fistula of the splenic artery. Pediatr Radiol 26:195–197
Ohno Y, Ohgami H, Nagasaki A et al (1995) Complete disruption of the main pancreatic duct: a case successfully managed by percutaneous drainage. J Pediatr Surg 30:1741–1742
Oldham KT, Guice KS, Ryckman F et al (1986) Blunt liver injury in childhood: evolution of therapy and current perspective. Surgery 100:542–549
Olsen WR, Polley TZ (1977) A second look at delayed splenic rupture. Arch Surg 112:422–425

Oparah SS, Mandal AK (1978) Traumatic thoracobiliary (pleurobiliary and bronchobiliary) fistulas: clinical and review study. J Trauma 18:539–544
Ooi LLPG, Leong SS (1997) Splenic abscess from 1987 to 1995. Am J Surg 174:87–92
Oto A, Özgen B, Akhan O et al (2000) Delayed posttraumatic adrenal hematoma. Eur Radiol 10:903–905
Owings JT, Lengle SJ (1995) Combined hepatic abscess and arterial pseudoaneurysms from blunt trauma: a case report and management strategy. J Trauma 38:634–638
Pachter HL (1998) The usefulness of remote CT scanning in blunt splenic injuries. Surgery 124:941–942
Pachter HL, Hofstetter SR (1995) The current status of nonoperative management of adult blunt hepatic injuries. Am J Surg 169:442–454
Pachter HL, Hofsletter SR, Elkowitz A et al (1993) Traumatic cysts of the spleen – the role of cystectomy and splenic preservation: experience with seven conservative patients. J Trauma 35:430–436
Pachter HL, Knudson MM, Esrig B et al (1996) Status of nonoperative management of blunt hepatic injuries in 1995: a multicenter experience with 404 patients. J Trauma 40:31–38
Pachter HL, Guth AA, Hofstetter SR et al (1998) Changing patterns in the management of splenic trauma: the impact of nonoperative management. Ann Surg 227:708–717
Pappas D, Mirvis SE, Crepps JT et al (1987) Splenic trauma: false-negative CT diagnosis in cases of delayed rupture. AJR 149:727–728
Paraskevopoulos JA, Samoilis S, Papadakis G et al (2000) Drainage tube perforation of the stomach: an exceptionally rare complication. J Trauma Injury Inf Crit Care 48:330–331
Paris S, Weiss SM, Ayers VVH et al (1994) Splenic abscess. Am J Surg 60:358–361
Parks RW, Chrysos E, Diamond T (1999) Management of liver trauma. Br J Surg 86:1121–1135
Patel NY, Cogbill TH, Gundersen LF (1996) Angioembolization of multiple intrasplenic pseudoaneurysms as a result of blunt trauma. J Vasc Surg 24:299–301
Patton JH, Lyden SP, Croce MA et al (1997) Pancreatic trauma: a simplified management guideline. J Trauma 43:234–239
Paul JL, Otal P, Perreault P et al (1999) Treatment of posttraumatic dissection of the renal artery with endoprosthesis in a 15-year-old girl. J Trauma 47:169–172
Phadke RV, Sawlani V, Rastogi H et al (1997) Iatrogenic renal vascular injuries and their radiological management. Clin Radiol 52:119–123
Pilla TJ, Tantana S, Schilds JB (1987) Embolization of blunt trauma in the pediatric patient. Cardiovasc Intervent Radiol 10:153–156
Pinto IT, Chimeno PC (1998) Treatment of an urinoma and a post-traumatic pseudo-aneurysm using selective arterial embolisation. Cardiovasc Intervent Radiol 21:506–508
Pirollet P, Picard L, Bracard S et al (1989) Anevrysme de l'artère splénique. Traitement par radiologie interventionnelle. Gastroenterol Clin Biol 13:849–850
Poli ML, Lefèbvre F, Ludot H et al (1995) Nonoperative management of biliary tract fistulas after blunt abdominal trauma in a child. J Pediatr Surg 30:1719–1721
Ponchon T,Gallez J-F, Valette P-J et al (1989) Endoscopic treatment of biliary tract fistula. Gastrointest Endosc 35:490–498
Prinz RA, Pickelman J, Hoffman JP (1988) Treatment of pancreatic cutaneous fistulas with a somatostatin analog. Am J Surg 155:36–42
Probst P, Castaneda-Zuniga WR, Gomes AS et al (1978) Nonsurgical treatment of splenic artery aneurysm. Radiology 128:619–625
Ravera M, Cocozza E (1999) Post-traumatic pseudocyst of the spleen: case report on a conservative management through percutaneous drainage. G Chir 20:471–473
Redmond PL, Kumpe DA (1988) Embolization of an intrahepatic arterioportal fistula: case report and review of the literature. Cardiovasc Intervent Radiol 11:274–279
Reisman JD, Morgan AS (1990) Analysis of 46 intra-abdominal aortic injuries from blunt trauma: case reports and literature review. J Trauma 30:1294–1297
Repasky RG, Tisnado J, Freedman AM (1993) Transcatheter embolization of a superior mesenteric artery pseudoaneurysm and arteriovenous fistula. J Vasc Interv Radiol 4:241–244
Rescorla FJ, Cory D, Vane DW et al (1990) Failure of percutaneous drainage in children with traumatic pancreatic pseudocysts. J Pediatr Surg 25:1038–1042
Roberts A, Hays DA, McFarland DR (1996) Coil embolization of an internal iliac artery arteriovenous fistula with a Wallstent. J Vasc Interv Radiol 7:611–613
Rosen JM, Binkert BL, Seldin DW et al (1986) Scintigraphic criteria for the diagnosis of renal arteriovenous fistulas. Clin Nucl Med 11:847–852
Rosen RJ, Rothberg (1982) Transhepatic embolisation of hepatic artery pseudoaneurysm following biliary drainage. Radiology 145:532–533
Rosenthal D, Ellison RG, Luke JP et al (1987) Traumatic superior mesenteric arteriovenous fistula: report of a case and review of the literature. J Vasc Surg 5:486–490
Rothbarth LJ, Redmond PL, Kumpe DA (1989) Percutaneous transhepatic treatment of a large intrahepatic aneurysm. AJR 153:1077–1078
Ryu R, Novak Z, Coldwell D (1998) Percutaneous embolization of a posttraumatic nephrobiliary fistula. J Trauma 44: 389–391
Salam TA, Lumsden A, Martin L (1992) nonoperative management of visceral aneurysms and pseudoaneurysms. Am J Surg 164:215–219
Salis A, Pais SO, Vennos A et al (1999) Superselective embolization of a traumatic intrasplenic arteriovenous fistula. J Trauma 46:186–188
Salvat F, Burelle H, Bohe D et al (1980) Fistule artério-portale extra-hépatique, post-traumatique. J Radiol 61:185–187
Salzano A, Rossi E, de Rosa A et al (1999) The role of computed tomography in assessing subphrenic abscesses after posttraumatic splenectomy. Radiol Med (Torino) 98:173–177
Sandblom P (1948) Hemorrhage into the biliary tract following trauma – "Traumatic hemobilia". Surgery 24:571–586
Sands M, Page D, Brown RB (1986) Splenic abscess following non-operative management of splenic rupture. J Pediatr Surg 21:900–901
Sarioglu A, Tanyel FC, Ariyurek M et al (1996) Aneurysmatic arteriovenous fistula complicating splenic injury. Eur J Pediatr Surg 6:183–185
Sato N, Yamaguchi K, Shimizu S et al (1998) Coil embolization of bleeding visceral pseudoaneurysms following pancreatectomy. Arch Surg 133:1099–1102
Saunders MS, Riberi A, Massullo EA (1992) Delayed traumatic superior mesenteric arteriovenous fistula after a stab wound: case report. J Trauma 32:101–106
Savader SJ, Trerotola SO, Merine DS et al (1992) Hemobilia after percutaneous transhepatic biliary drainage: treatment

with transcatheter embolotherapy. J Vasc Interv Radiol 3: 345–352

Schmidt B, Bhatt GM, Abo MN (1980) Management of post-traumatic vascular malformations of the liver by catheter embolization. Am J Surg 140:332–335

Schurr MJ, Fabian TC, Gavant M et al (1995) Management of blunt splenic trauma: computed tomographic contrast blush predicts failure of non-operative management. J Trauma 39:507–513

Schwartz RA, Teitelbaum GP, Katz MD et al (1993) Effectiveness of transcatheter embolization in the control of hepatic vascular injuries. J Vasc Interv Radiol 4:359–365

Schweizer W, Tanner S, Baer HU et al (1993) Management of traumatic liver injuries. Br J Surg 80:86–88

Scioscia PJ, Dillon PW, Cilley RE et al (1994) Endoscopic sphincterotomy in the management of posttraumatic biliary fistula. J Pediatr Surg 29:3–6

Sclafani SJA, Nayaranaswamy T, Mitchell WG (1981) Radiologic management of traumatic hepatic artery-portal vein arteriovenous fistulae. J Trauma 21:576–580

Sclafani SJA, Goldstein AS, Lipkowitz GS (1984a) Radiologic management of disrupted ureteral anastomosis and infected urinoma after gunshot wound. J Trauma 24:1060–1062

Sclafani SJA, Shaftan GW, McAuley J et al (1984b) Interventional radiology in the management of hepatic trauma. J Trauma 24:256–262

Sclafani JA, Florence LO, Phillips TF et al (1987) Lumbar arterial injury: radiologic diagnosis and management. Radiology 165:709–714

Sclafani SJA, Herskowitz M, Rachlin S et al (1995a) Intestinal plethora: an early sign of acute posttraumatic hepatic artery–portal vein arteriovenous fistula. Emerg Radiol 2:380–383

Sclafani SJA, Shaftan GW, Scalea TM et al (1995b) Nonoperative salvage of computed tomography-diagnosed splenic injuries: utilization of angiography for triage and embolization for hemostasis. J Trauma 39:818–827

Shahrudin MD, Noori SM (1997) Biloma and biliary fistula associated with hepatorrhaphy for liver injury. Hepatogastroenterology 44:519–521

Sheik-Gafoor MH, Singh B, Moodley J (1998) Traumatic thoracobiliary fistula: report of a case successfully managed conservatively, with an overview of current diagnostic and therapeutic options. J Trauma 45:819–821

Shenoy SS, Bergsland J, Cerra FB (1981) Arterial embolization for traumatic hemobilia with hepato-portal fistula. Cardiovasc Intervent Radiol 4:206–208

Sherman HF, Higler JS, Jones LM et al (1992) Delayed diagnosis of extrahepatic biliary injury. Eur J Surg 158:575–578

Sherman HF, Savage BA, Jones LM et al (1994) Nonoperative management of blunt hepatic injuries: safe at any grade? J Trauma 37:616–621

Shilyansky J, Navarro O, Superina RA et al (1999) Delayed hemorrhage after nonoperative management of blunt hepatic trauma in children: a rare but significant event. J Pediatr Surg 34:60–64

Shindo S, Ogata K, Katahira S et al (1997) Delayed manifestation of aortic stenosis after blunt abdominal trauma: report of a case. Surg Today 27:76–79

Sidhu MK, Weinberger E, Healey P (1998) Intramural duodenal hematoma after blunt abdominal trauma. AJR 170:38

Sidhu MK, Shaw DWW, Daly CP et al (1999) Post-traumatic hepatic pseudoaneurysms in children. Pediatr Radiol 29: 46–52

Siegel MJ, Sivit CJ (1997) Pancreatic emergencies. Radiol Clin North Am 35:815–830

Silberzweig JE (1999) Ruptured lumbar artery pseudoaneurysm: a diagnostic dilemma in retroperitoneal hemorrhage after abdominal trauma. J Trauma 46:531–532

Sivit CJ, Eicheberger MR, Taylor GA et al (1992) Blunt pancreatic trauma in children: CT diagnosis. AJR 158:1097–11O0

Sjövall A, Hirsch K (1997) Blunt abdominal trauma in children: risks of nonoperative treatment. J Pediatr Surg 32: 1169–1174

Skow JR, Longmire WP (1974) Common duct strictures secondary to abdominal trauma. Am Surg 40:576–578

Slim K (1999) Ruptures and injuries to the diaphragm. J Chir 136:67–75

Smith GR, Northrop CH (1987) Stab wound causing mesenteric-portal arteriovenous fistula: an unusual case with a spontaneous closure. J Trauma 16:408–411

Smith JA, MacLeish DG, Collier NA (1989) Aneurysms of the visceral arteries. Aust N Z J Surg. 59:329–344

Steiner Z, Brown RA, Jamieson DH et al (1994) Management of hemobilia and persistent biliary fistula after blunt liver trauma. J Pediatr Surg 29:1575–1577

Stroz P, Asch M, Salem S et al (1996) Transhepatic embolization of a portohepatic venous fistula. J Vasc Interv Radiol 7:705–707

Struyven J, Cremer M, Pirson P et al (1982) Posttraumatic bilhemia: diagnosis and catheter therapy. AJR 138:746–747

Sugg SL, Gerndt SJ, Hamilton BJ et al (1995) Pseudoaneurysms of the intraparenchymal splenic artery after blunt abdominal trauma: a complication of nonoperative therapy and its management. J Trauma 39:593–595

Sugimoto K, Asari Y, Sakagushi T et al (1993) Endoscopic retrograde cholangiography in the nonsurgical management of blunt liver injury. J Trauma 35:192–199

Sugiyama M, Atomi Y, Matsuoka T et al (2000) Endoscopic biliary stenting for treatment of persistent biliary fistula after blunt hepatic injury. Gastrointest Endosc 51:42–44

Swana HS, Cohn SM, Burns GA et al (1996) Renal artery pseudoaneurysm after blunt abdominal trauma: case report and literature review. J Trauma 40:459–461

Taff ML, Wolodzko AA, Boglioli LR (1990) Sudden death due to delayed rupture of hepatic subcapsular hematoma following blunt abdominal trauma. Am J Forensic Med Pathol 11:270–274

Takayasu K, Moriyama N, Muramatsu J et al (1985) Gallbladder infarction after hepatic artery embolization. AJR 144: 135–138

Takishima T, Hirata M, Kataoka Y et al (2000) Delayed development of obstructive jaundice and pancreatitis resulting from traumatic intramural hematoma of the duodenum: report of a case requiring deferred laparotomy. J Trauma 49:160–162

Tanaka H, Iwai A, Sugimoto H et al (1991) Intrahepatic arterioportal fistula after blunt hepatic trauma: case reports. J Trauma 31:143–146

Teigen CL, Venbrux AC, Quinlan DM et al (1992) Late massive hematuria as a complication of conservative management of blunt renal trauma in children. J Urol 147:1333–1336

Teitelbaum GP, Reed RA, Larsen D et al (1993a) Microcatheter embolization of non-neurologic traumatic vascular lesions. J Vasc Interv Radiol 4:149–154

Teitelbaum GP, Katz MD, Pentecost MJ et al (1993b) Effectiveness of transcatheter embolization in the control of hepatic vascular injuries. J Vasc Interv Radiol 4:359

Terk MR, Rozenberg D (1998) Gadolinium-enhanced MR imaging of traumatic hepatic injury. AJR 171:665–669
Thanh LN, Duchmann JC, Latrive JP et al (1999) Conservation of the left pancreas after rupture of the pancreatic isthmus. A propos of 3 cases. Chirurgie 124:165–170
Thiele BL, Royle JP, Thomas D (1980) Splenic arteriovenous fistula: a report of two cases. Vasc Surg 14:4–8
Toevs CC, Beilman GJ (2000) Splenic abscess 10 years after splenic trauma: a case report. Am Surg 66:204–205
Totte E, van Hee R, Discart H et al (2000) Isolated colonic injury following blunt abdominal trauma. Acta Chir Belg 100:71–73
Touloukian RJ (1983) Protocol for the nonoperative treatment of obstructing intramural duodenum hematoma during childhood. Am J Surg 145:330–334
Triller J, Krebs T, Ackermann D (1993) Superselective embolisation of traumatic renal pseudoaneurysm with a Tracker-18 catheter and microcoils. Eur Radiol 3:261–263
Tsushima Y, Yamada S, Aoki J et al (2001) Ischaemic ileal stenosis following blunt abdominal trauma and demonstrated by CT. Br J Radiol 74:277–279
Uflacker R, Saadi J (1982) Transcatheter embolization of superior mesenteric arteriovenous fistula. AJR 139:1212–1214
Uflacker R, Paolini RM, Lima S (1984) Management of traumatic hematuria by selective renal artery embolization. J Urol 132:662–667
Uflacker R, Mourao GS, Piske RL et al (1989) Hemobilia: transcatheter occlusive therapy and long-term follow-up. Cardiovasc Intervent Radiol 12:136–141
Vadon G, Karacsonyi S, Engloner L (1984) Transcatheter embolization for the control of posttraumatic hemobilia. Eur J Radiol 4:190–192
Van der Zee JA, van den Hoek J, Weerts JGE (1995) Traumatic renal arteriovenous fistula in a 3-year-old girl, successfully treated by percutaneous transluminal embolization. J Pediatr Surg 30:1513–1514
Van der Zee DC, Kramer WL, Ure BM et al (1999) Laparoscopic management of a large posttraumatic splenic cyst in a child. Surg Endosc 13:1241–1242
Vauthey JN, Tomczak RJ, Helmberger T et al (1997) The arterioportal fistula syndrome: clinicopathologic features, diagnosis, and therapy. Gastroenterology 113:1390–1401
Velitchkov NG, Losanoff JE, Kjossev KT et al (2000) Delayed small bowel injury as a result of penetrating extraperitoneal high-velocity ballistic trauma to the abdomen. J Trauma 48:169
Velmahos GC, Chan LS, Kamel E et al (2000a) Non-operative management of splenic injuries: have we gone too far? Arch Surg 135:674–679
Velmahos GC, Chahwan S, Falabella A et al (2000b) Angiographic embolization for intraperitoneal and retroperitoneal injuries. World J Surg 24:539–545
Vromen A, Beglaibter N, Feigen E et al (1993) Delayed large bowel obstruction after blunt abdominal injury. Eur J Surg 159:447–448
Wales PW, Shuckett B, Kim PC (2001) Long-term outcome after nonoperative management of complete traumatic pancreatic transection in children. J Pediatr Surg 36:823–827
Weissmann HS, Chun KJ, Frank M et al (1979) Demonstration of traumatic bile leakage and cholescintigraphy and ultrasonography. AJR 133:843–847
West JE, Bernhardt H, Bowers RF (1968) Aneurysms of the pancreaticoduodenal artery. Am Surg 115:835–839
Wholey MH, Chamorro HA, Rao G et al (1978) Splenic infarction and spontaneous rupture of the spleen after therapeutic embolisation. Cardiovasc Radiol 1:249–253
Wilkinson S, Loughhead MG, Holmes AB et al (1989) Delayed intraperitoneal ureteric rupture following blunt abdominal trauma: case report. J Trauma 29:1292–1294
Wilson RH, Moorehead RJ (1991) Current management of trauma to the pancreas. Br J Surg 78:1196–1202
Yamakado K, Nakatsuka A, Tanaka N et al (2000) Transcatheter arterial embolisation of ruptured pseudoaneurysms with coils and n-butyl cyanoacrylate. J Vasc Interv Radiol 11:66–72
Yamamoto F, Pu Y, Igimi H et al (1993) MR imaging of traumatic hepatic laceration: evaluation and course of healing after surgery. Abdom Imaging 18:253–257
Yoo SY, Lim KS, Kang SJ (1996) Pitfalls of nonoperative management of blunt abdominal trauma in children in Korea. J Pediatr Surg 31:263–266
Yoon KH, Ha HK, Kim MH et al (1998) Biliary stricture caused by blunt abdominal trauma: clinical and radiologic features in five patients. Radiology 207:737–741
Zeman RK, Lee CH, Stahl R et al (1984) Strategy for the use of biliary scintigraphy in non-iatrogenic biliary trauma. Radiology 151:771–777
Zelch JV, Hermann RE (1975) Control of arteriovenous fistula of splenic vessels by Fogarty catheter. Arch Surg 110:329–331

24 Embolization of Posttraumatic and Postsurgical Lower Gastrointestinal Bleeding

N. Bulakbasi

CONTENTS

N. Bulakbasi, MD
Assistant Professor of Radiology, Department of Radiology, Gülhane Military Medical Academy, 06018 Ankara, Turkey

- When diagnostic angiography is positive for active lower gastrointestinal bleeding, embolization must be performed to protect poor surgical candidates against the risks of surgery by achieving immediate homeostasis.
- Embolization following superselective catheterization is essential with the first target being the vasa recta, following marginal artery or distal intestinal arcade when the first is not possible.
- Even if embolization fails to control bleeding or ischemic complications occur, it can be repeated to provide more time to stabilize poor surgical candidates for elective surgery in better conditions. Alternatively, directed segmental resection of the ischemic area allows lesser magnitude than blind surgical resection.

24.1 History

In the early 1960s Nusbaum and Baum first described selective visceral angiography in the investigation of patients with gastrointestinal bleeding (Nusbaum and Baum 1963; Baum et al. 1965). In 1972 Rosch et al., using autologous clot, were the first to use embolization for the treatment of gastrointestinal bleeding (Rosch et al. 1972). Transcatheter arterial embolization for lower gastrointestinal bleeding was first reported in 1975 (Goldstein et al. 1975).

24.2 Incidence

Simultaneous injury to three major abdominal organs presents a mortality rate of 70%, half of this from bleeding (Carmona et al. 1982). Acute lower gastrointestinal bleeding is one of the most frequently encountered bleeding sources in postoperative patients with multiorgan trauma (Carmona et al. 1982; Dertinger et al. 1996). The mortality rate of 14%–19% in patients with lower gastrointestinal bleeding reaches up to 35% in the postoperative period (Carmona et al. 1982; Kouraklis et al. 1995; Dertinger et al. 1996). Most of gastrointestinal bleeding stops spontaneously and does not recur, but it can persist or recur in 10%–15%, requiring urgent diagnostic and therapeutic procedures, with 8%–21% mortality rate (Rahn et al. 1982; Kadir and Ernest 1983; Leitman et al. 1989; Billingham 1997).

24.3 Mechanism

Lower gastrointestinal injuries following blunt abdominal trauma have been characterized by disruption of the bowel, with or without perforation and damage to the adjacent mesentery, with the advent of seatbelts (McBoyle et al. 1984). Penetrating missile wounds and blunt forces can cause bleeding within the intestinal wall or into intestinal lumen. Such bleeding often occurs at multiple sites. Macroscopic progression can occur during the observation time in 64% of these lesions of primarily innocent appearance, with perforation in 5.4% (Johansson et al. 1984). Formation of visceral aneurysm or pseudoaneurysms, which is associated with a high rate of rupture, is the late complication of abdominal trauma (Salam et al. 1992). Postoperative abdominal bleeding is possibly related to the operative anastomosis sites and to medium-to-small-sized arteries of the gastrointestinal system that are not noticeable under emergent surgical conditions (Bulakbasi et al. 1999).

24.4 Clinical Symptoms and Findings

Massive or recurrent rectal bleeding is the major clinical sign of lower gastrointestinal bleeding. Other clinical findings of massive bleeding are tachycardia, orthostatic hypotension, peripheral vasoconstriction, hypovolemic shock, and change in consciousness status, usually encountered after loss of 20% of circulating blood volume (approximately 1000 ml for an adult). These patients usually require blood transfusion of more than 5 packs of red blood cells in 24 h. Laboratory findings such as a decrease in thrombocytes as well as prothrombin and partial prothrombin time usually become prominent before changes in hemoglobin concentration and hematocrit values.

24.5 Imaging

24.5.1 Radionuclide Studies

24.5.1.1 Technique

Tc-99m sulfur colloid scintigraphy is usually used for active bleeding and can detect bleeding rates as low as 0.05–0.1 ml/min, but the imaging time is markedly limited (probably no more than 10 min). Tc-99m-labeled red blood cell scintigraphy is the main scintigraphic approach, because of long-standing labeled red blood cells (up to 48 h) in the intravascular space that allow excellent imaging for intermittent or slow bleeding. This technique can demonstrate active bleeding at a rate of 0.1–0.5 ml/min (Williams et al. 2000). Scintigraphic images must be obtained 2–5 min after the injection of Tc-99m-labeled red blood cells and repeated at every 2–5 min during a 60- to 90-min period. Longer imaging times can be used if patients can tolerate it. The positive criteria for active bleeding are increased activity detected outside of great arteries, changing activity in positional images, and delayed increased activity that had not been detected previously (Fig. 24.1).

24.5.1.2 Pitfalls

Normally increased activity can be detected in the liver, spleen, great arteries, and penis. The major pitfall of Tc-99m-labeled red blood cell scintigraphy is the movement of extravasated blood in the bowel lumen, which can cause incorrect localization of bleeding site (Fig. 24.1c). This can be eliminated by pharmacological inhibition of bowel movements. Other potential false positive results are vascular neoplasms, splenosis, varices, vascular grafts, and inflammation (Williams et al. 2000).

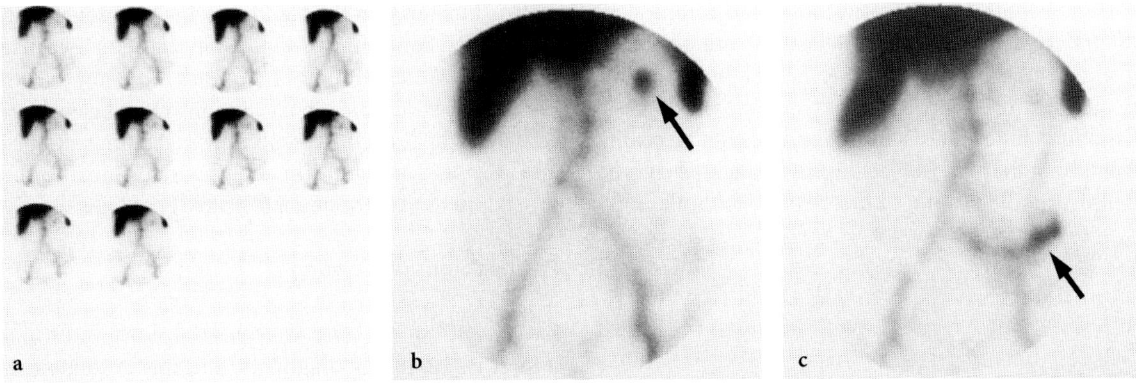

Fig. 24.1a–c. A 23-year-old man with active rectal bleeding due to gunshot injury. **a** Positive Tc-99m-labeled red blood cell scintigraphy shows focal collection of increased activity in the left upper quadrant on the initial dynamic images. **b** Bleeding (*arrow*) is more prominent on 10-min image. **c** Subsequent intraluminal passage of radionuclide material (*arrow*) is seen in distal colonic segments. (Courtesy of S. Ilgan, MD)

24.5.1.3 Results

The sensitivity of Tc-99m sulfur colloid scintigraphy in the detection of gastrointestinal bleeding is about 30% of the labeled red blood cell technique, which is 51%–96% with 43%–97% of true localizing rate to a specific anatomical site (Leitman et al. 1989; Imdahl et al. 1991; Linnet and Abrahamsen 1995; Schwab et al. 1995; Suzman et al. 1996; Gutierrez et al. 1998; Williams et al. 2000).

In the evaluation of traumatic and postoperative patients with gastrointestinal bleeding, Tc-99m-labeled red blood cell scintigraphy is recommended as the first choice imaging modality unless free bleeding or shock is present (Suzman et al. 1996; Ng et al. 1997; Bulakbasi et al. 1999), because a negative Tc-99m-labeled red blood cell scintigraphy can only exclude ongoing gastrointestinal bleeding (Linnet and Abrahamsen 1995). Angiography will more likely be positive in patients with immediate blush on Tc-99m-labeled red blood cell scintigraphy rather than patients with delayed blush (Ng et al. 1997).

24.5.2 Angiography

Angiography is the method of choice in the evaluation of traumatic or postoperative patients with acute gastrointestinal bleeding and is usually performed in emergency conditions. Logically it will be most effective when the patient is actively bleeding. It must be reserved for patients who are treated by embolization or surgery, because 95% of lower gastrointestinal bleeding settles with conservative measures (Nicholson et al. 1998).

24.5.2.1 Iodinated Contrast Angiography

Technique

Selective catheter angiography is performed using the Seldinger method from the common femoral artery (Seldinger 1953). Angiography of abdominal aorta is obtained by a 20- to 25-ml bolus injection of contrast material (300–350 mg iodine/ml) for assessing the anatomical variations and major traumatic pathologies such as aortoenteric fistula, intestinal angina, or ischemia due to hypovolemic status of the patient. The superior (SMA) and inferior (IMA) mesenteric arteries as well as the coeliac trunk and its branches have to be evaluated for the detection of possible lower gastrointestinal bleeding by selective catheterization. The caliber of examined mesenteric vessel should be matched by injection volume and rate of contrast material for proper visualization of the bleeding. For this purpose, 9- to 12-ml/s injection rates for coeliac trunk, 6- to 9-ml/s for the SMA, and 3- to 6-ml/s for the IMA are usually used for a 6- to 10-s period. Rapid filming (1–2 frame/s) should be preferred during the arterial phase, and slowed to a rate of 1 frame/3–5 s for capillary and venous phases. Imaging should be carried out to at least 30 s, to detect the late slow extravasation of the blood. Angiographic examination of the pelvic vessels should be added in traumatic patients for the evaluation of coexisting femoroenteric or femorogenital fistulas (Fig. 24.2).

Digital subtraction or conventional techniques can be preferred for imaging. Selective catheterization of a suspected bleeding vessel has higher probability of diagnosis and treatment (Wojtowycz 1990). Although clinical and scintigraphic results give some clues about the level of bleeding, in suspicious patients the IMA should be imaged first before accumulation of contrast material in the bladder or the bladder should be emptied continuously by a Foley catheter. Because of the high total amount of contrast injection during mesenteric study, the renal functions must be evaluated before the procedure, especially in trauma patients, and the patient should be well-hydrated during the procedure to prevent possible acute renal failure.

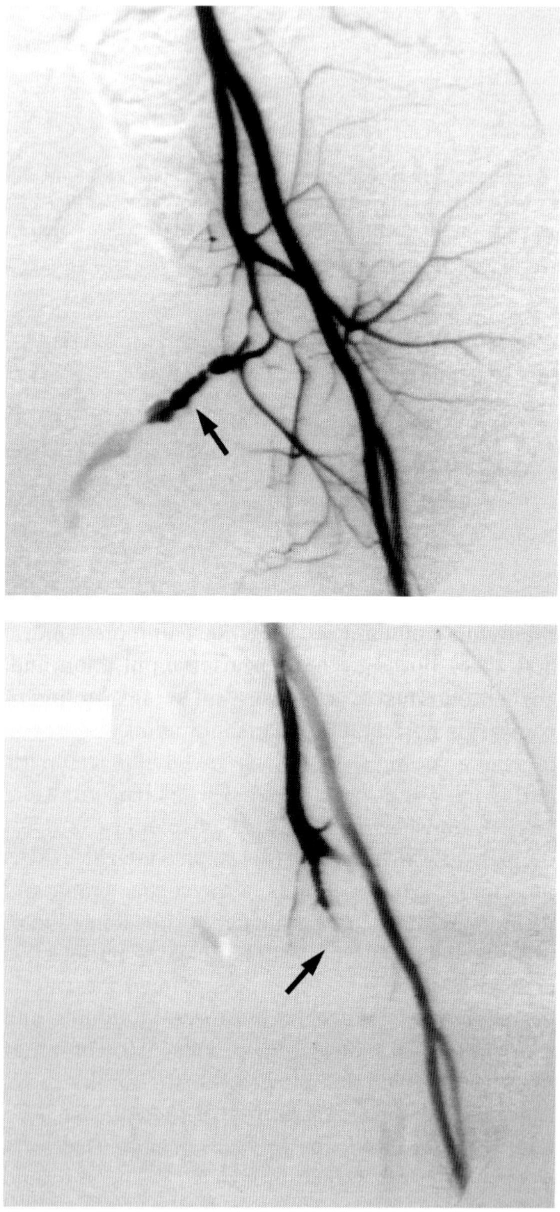

a b

Fig. 24.2a,b. A 38-year-old woman presented with massive rectal and vaginal bleeding after a traffic accident with multiple pelvic fractures. **a** Left internal iliac arteriography shows contrast extravasation (*arrow*) into vagina from anterior trunk of left internal iliac artery. No evident gastrointestinal bleeding can be demonstrated. **b** After selective embolization by PVA and microcoil, bleeding is controlled successfully. (Courtesy of N. Bulakbasi, MD)

Positive Signs of Bleeding

Extravasation of contrast material into intestinal lumen is the major diagnostic finding in angiography. This appearance can be changed due to rate of bleeding. It can be immediate pooling of blood in bowel lumen, as in frank bleeding, or small linear contrast collection between mucosal folding, as in small leakage (Fig. 24.3). The staining of intestinal folds or demonstration of contrast collection in the intestinal lumen is clearly shown in the arterial phase and becomes more prominent in delayed images (Fig. 24.4). Although the bleeding less than 0.5 ml/min can be detected by angiography using the proper technique, the diagnosis of small leakage is still problematic (Peterson 1988; Frezza et al. 1996).

Pitfalls

In postoperative patients, the major pitfall lies in the distorted anatomical structures. Other major technical difficulties are uncontrolled breathing motions and bowel peristalsis, insufficient cooperation of the patient, and rebound collection of excessive intestinal gas in posttraumatic and postoperative patients. Especially in digital subtraction studies, these motion artifacts and intestinal gas can cause false images interpreted as active bleeding, which are usually unrelated to vascular structures and disappear or change their shapes and locations in time. These can be diminished using the conventional angiographic technique, bowel cleaning, which is usually not possible in emergent cases, and adequate conscious sedation, which can be problematic in patients with hypotension or hypovolemic shock.

24.5.2.2 Carbon Dioxide Angiography

Technique

Intraarterial CO_2 gas can cause radiographic density between the gas and the surrounding soft tissue using digital subtraction and electronic enhancement. CO_2 gas is 400 times less viscous than iodinated contrast material and this allows the passage of gas through

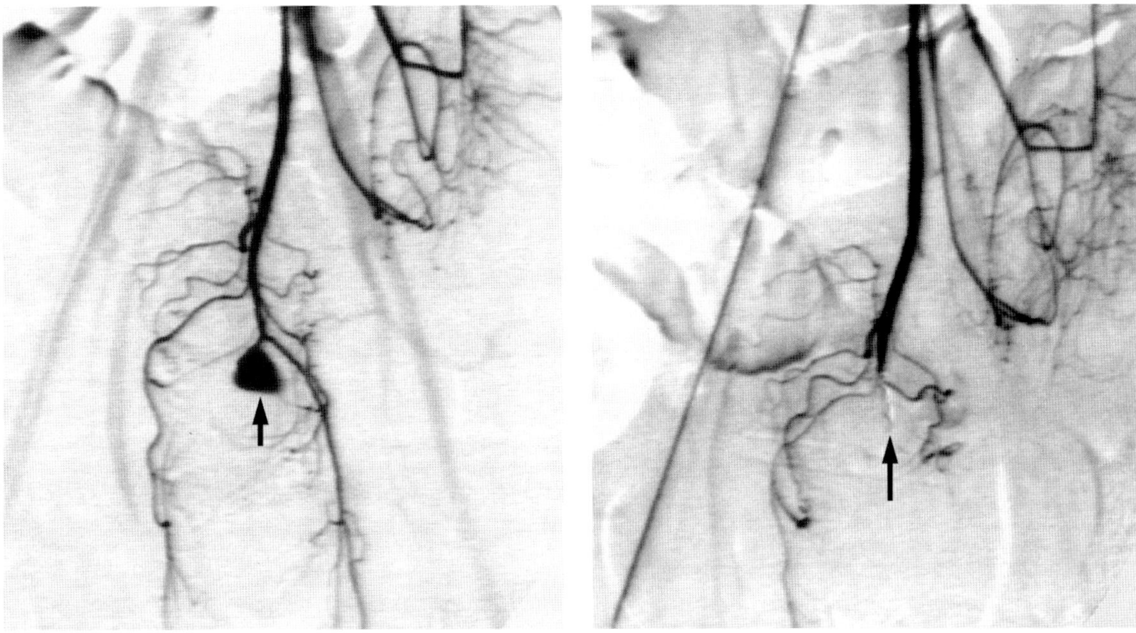

Fig. 24.3a, b. A 41-year-old woman in a coagulopathic state presented in shock with massive rectal bleeding after partial colon resection and left nephrectomy. After her first embolization with PVA, she had recurrent bleeding after 48 h. **a** Inferior mesenteric arteriography shows contrast extravasation (*arrow*) into the rectum from the bifurcation of the superior rectal artery. **b** After the second unsuccessful embolization with PVA, GI bleeding was controlled with microcoil (*arrow*) embolization. (Courtesy of N. Bulakbasi, MD; from Bulakbasi et al. 1999)

small diameters (Back et al. 1998). A dedicated CO_2 injector and a closed plastic bag delivery system can deliver noncompressed controlled volumes of pure medical grade CO_2 gas. Special software programs are needed to overcome fragmentation of CO_2 by flowing blood. In vessels with less than 10 mm inner diameter, annular flow can be achieved relatively easily with injection rates above 20–30 ml/s. When imaging a 2-cm artery, the best that can be realized clinically is intermittent flow with large bubbles (Lang et al. 1999). While 20–40 ml of CO_2 gas at a rate of 40 ml/s is used initially for abdominal aorta run-off imaging, imaging of mesenteric arteries can be performed by selective injection of 10–30 ml of CO_2 gas delivered over 0.5–2.0 s.

Pitfalls and Benefits

Intraarterial injection of CO_2 can cause ischemic injury to peripheral organs by trapping gas bubbles within small arteries or the microvasculature. Although small CO_2 bubbles are likely to pass through capillary beds, the buoyancy of larger bubbles could lead to gas trapping within larger vessels in nondependent portions of organs, or in any nonhorizontal vessels in which the buoyant force of bubbles equals the momentum force of antegrade blood flow (Back et al. 1998). Bowel gas motion, arterial pulsation, and patient movement can degrade the resolution of images. CO_2 angiography has no allergic potential, no renal toxicity and it is extremely inexpensive compared to nonionic iodinated contrast material. The only contraindication of CO_2 angiography is chronic obstructive pulmonary disease because of severe CO_2 retention (Weaver et al. 1991; Frankhouse et al. 1995).

24.5.2.3 Results

Diagnostic accuracy of emergent angiography in acute gastrointestinal bleeding can change depending on the experience of the radiologist. Expert visceral angiography is strongly recommended before surgery and after laparotomy when no cause has been found (Thompson et al. 1987). Its sensitivity usually changes 34%–86.5%, but this is still better than blind surgery, which finds the source of bleeding in only 30% (Rahn et al. 1982; Kadir and Ernest 1983; Thompson et al. 1987; Ng et al. 1987; Leitman et al. 1989; Imdahl et al. 1991; Schwab et al. 1995). A source of bleeding is identified in only 20% of patients

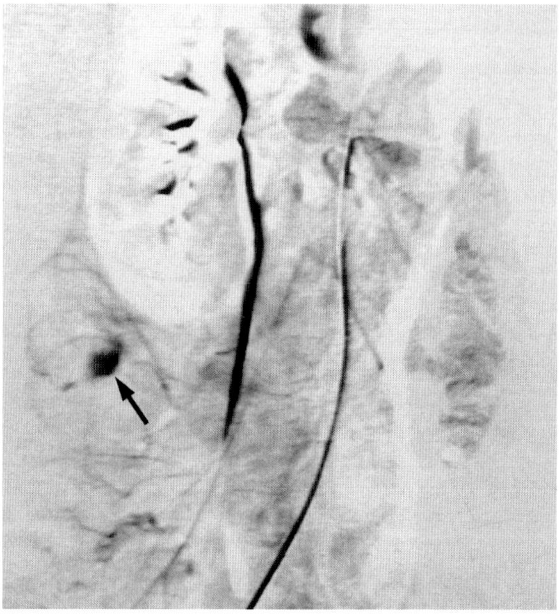
a

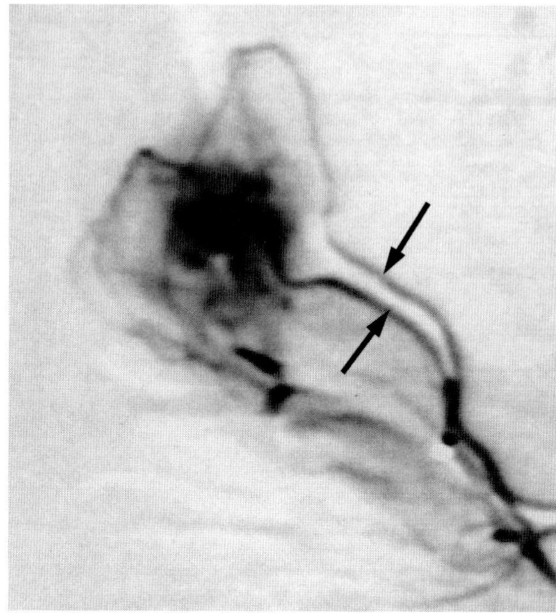
b

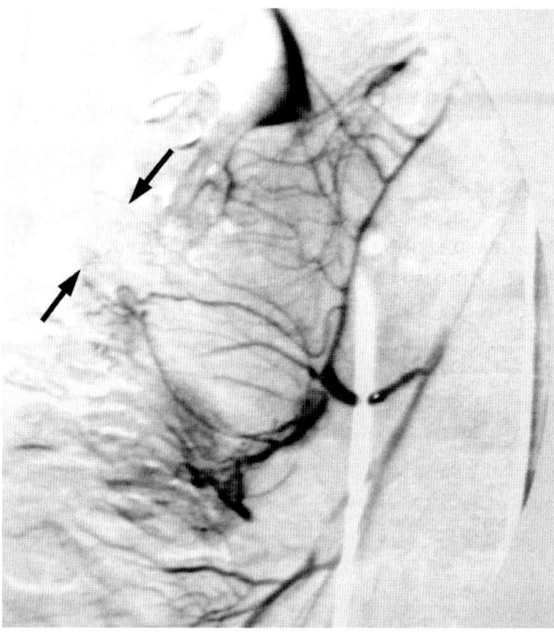
c

Fig. 24.4a–c. A 22-year-old man presented on postoperative day 4 in shock with massive lower GI bleeding after surgical primary repair of the liver, splenectomy, and ileal resection due to gunshot injury. **a** Superior mesenteric angiography shows active late arterial contrast extravasation (*arrow*) in the fresh ileoileal anastomosis region. **b** Superselective ileocolic artery catheterization shows the bleeding branch (*arrows*). **c** Late phase of the postembolization demonstrates occlusion of the ileocolic branch and control of bleeding (*arrows*). (Courtesy of N. Bulakbasi, MD; from Bulakbasi et al. 1999)

who are not actively bleeding (Whittaker and Gregson 1993). In recent years, the yield of positive findings is improved by the advances in angiographic equipment both in high-resolution image capability and in sophisticated catheter and guidewire systems. Although higher detection rates (44%) of CO_2 over iodinated contrast material (14%) were reported in the diagnosis of suspected gastrointestinal bleeding (Seeger et al. 1993; Textor et al. 1997), recent study shows no advantage of CO_2 in the demonstration of active bleeding (Sandhu et al. 1999).

24.5.3 Endoscopy

Endoscopic techniques such as rectoscopy, flexible sigmoidoscopy, or fiber optic colonoscopy can be used for diagnostic and therapeutic purposes in lower gastrointestinal bleeding. The positive diagnostic yield of endoscopic techniques ranges from 68% to 90% in nontraumatic gastrointestinal bleeding and provides the opportunity for successful therapy up to 69% of patients (Salem et al. 1985; IMDAHL et al. 1991; GUPTA et al. 1995; LEWIS et al. 1995; RICHTER et al. 1995; SCHWAB et al. 1995; FREZZA et al. 1996; VERNAVA et al. 1997). In traumatic patients, endoscopic procedures are usually used during surgery to avoid extensive surgical excision and to evaluate ischemic complications after embolization.

24.6 Management

After positive mesenteric angiography for massive lower gastrointestinal bleeding, one is faced with a localized bleeding site and the therapeutic options of observation, vasopressin infusion, embolization or operation (PENNOYER et al. 1996). The least invasive effective solution in the management of gastrointestinal bleeding is the best, as in diagnosis.

24.6.1 Conservative Management

Conservative management is preferred in most patients because bleeding usually stops spontaneously (WAGNER et al. 1992; BILLINGHAM 1997; NICHOLSON et al. 1998). Observation is recommended unless there are significant clinical findings such as peritoneal signs, hemodynamic instability, gross hematuria or rectal bleeding (VELMAHOS et al. 1998). The initial success rate of this type of management is about 17%–40.5% (WAGNER et al. 1992; VELMAHOS et al. 1998). Close clinical observation and laboratory follow-up with proper medical treatment are mandatory. The decision of conservative management should be navigated properly, because it can cause excessive blood loss, predisposing to hypovolemic shock, which makes transcatheter interventions more difficult.

24.6.2 Arterial Vasopressor Infusion

In the literature, arterial infusion of vasopressor substances such as vasopressin, prostaglandin F2a, and octreotide has been reported, usually for the treatment of gastrointestinal bleeding from nontraumatic causes such as gastroesophageal varices, peptic ulcer, and colonic angiodysplasia or diverticular disease (ATHANASOULIS et al. 1975; FARA et al. 1979; WALTMAN 1980).

24.6.2.1 Technique

After proper catheterization, intraarterial vasopressin should be infused at a rate of 0.2 IU/min and the infusion site should be checked at every 20 min for successful bleeding control. If bleeding cannot be controlled successfully, the infusion dose can be increased to a maximum of 0.4 IU/min. The infusion dose should be tapered gradually over several hours and saline must be infused for some time to avoid a rebound hyperemia (Fig. 24.5) (WALKER et al. 1980; KADIR and ERNEST 1983; UFLACKER 1987).

24.6.2.2 Contraindications

Vasopressor therapy must be avoided in patients with cardiac, mesenteric, and acral ischemia because it can cause serious complications (CLARK et al. 1981; ECKSTEIN et al. 1984; UFLACKER 1987; CHEN et al. 1998). Dosages over 0.4 IU/min may cause bowel infarction (WALKER et al. 1980). Long-term placement of an infusion catheter at the femoral artery is not recommended in atherosclerotic old patients (UFLACKER 1987; DUBOIS et al. 1989).

24.6.2.3 Results

Subselective intraarterial injection of vasoconstrictor substances has been found to be 52%–90% effective in controlling nontraumatic lower gastrointestinal bleeding, with an 18%–50% recurrent bleeding rate after discontinuation of perfusion (ATHANASOULIS et al. 1975; CLARK et al. 1981; RAHN et al. 1982; BROWDER et al. 1986; GOMES et al. 1986; UFLACKER 1987; CHEN et al. 1998). The average overall success is about 52%, but can reach up to 88% when combined with embolization (GOMES et al. 1986). It is also less successful in controlling bleeding from large arteries because, unlike peripheral arterioles and capillaries, large vessels do not constrict in response to vasopressin (RAHN et al. 1982). In traumatic or postoperative patients, excessive blood loss and large amounts of packed blood transfusion cause hemodynamic instability and abnormal bleeding parameters which do not allow normal coagulation. These factors usually prevent the usage of vasopressor infusion in such patients with predisposing ischemic state either due to surgery or trauma.

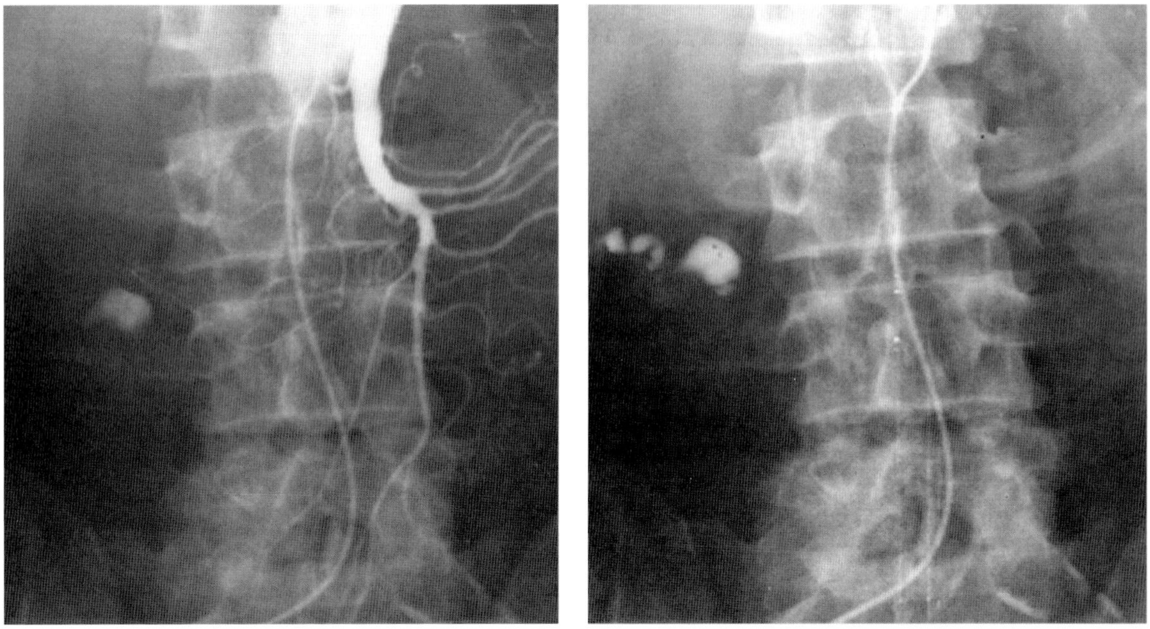

a b

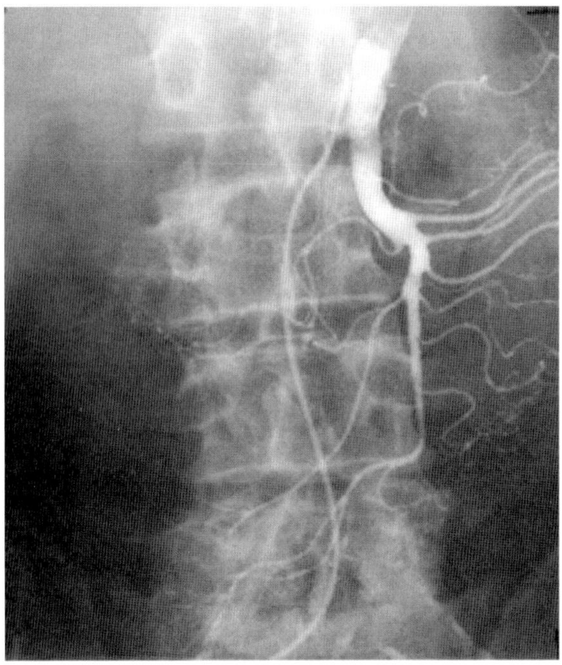

c

Fig. 24.5a–c. A 67-year-old woman presented with lower gastrointestinal bleeding in the postoperative period. **a** Superior mesenteric angiography shows active contrast extravasation into ascending colon from a branch of the right colic artery. **b** Because of unsuccessful control of bleeding after 20 min infusion of 0.2 IU/min pitressin, the dose was increased to 0.4 IU/min. **c** After 6 h infusion of pitressin, bleeding was controlled sufficiently and the dose tapered gradually with no complications. (Courtesy of R. Uflacker, MD)

24.6.2.4 Complications

Although vasopressin infusion is relatively simple and requires less selective positioning of the infusion catheter, it requires potentially extended catheterization with increased risk of potential morbidity (DuBois et al. 1989). Abdominal cramping is a common side effect due to bowel contraction induced by the vasopressin. The complication rate for pressor infusion has been reported to be as high as 43% and controlling these adverse effects usually requires expensive monitoring in intensive care units. These side effects are:

- Cardiac complications such as arrhythmia, bradycardia, hypertension, cardiac or respiratory arrest, myocardial infarctions (Conn et al. 1975).
- Visceral infarctions due to thrombosis of nonbleeding visceral arteries and veins as well as

constriction of collateral circulation (RENERT et al. 1972; SIRINEK et al. 1977; DUBOIS et al. 1989);

- Acral infarctions due to long-term indwelling of an infusion catheter at the femoral artery (ROBERTS and MADDISON 1976; TWIFORD et al. 1978);
- Hyponatremia and excessive water retention resulting in cerebral edema due to the water reabsorption effect of vasopressin, causing sodium and urea reabsorption (HAYS 1976).

24.6.3 Embolization

Selective arterial embolization has been found to be effective in controlling lower gastrointestinal bleeding, which otherwise would not be controlled by conservative management in poor surgical candidates (GUY et al. 1992; VELMAHOS et al. 1999; KRAMER et al. 2000; EVANGELISTA and HALLISEY 2000; LUCHTEFELD et al. 2000; NEMCEK 2000).

24.6.3.1 Vascular Anatomy

Anatomical variations between arterial supply and collateral circulation of small and large intestines are very important for successful and safe embolization.

Macroanatomical Connections and Variations

The arterial supply of the jejunum and ileum is mainly from the jejunal and ileal branches of SMA. Ileocolic, right, and middle colic branches of the SMA also supply the terminal ileum, caecum, appendix, and the ascending and transverse colon. The left colic, sigmoid, rectosigmoid, and superior rectal branches of the IMA supply the rest of the colon except the distal rectum, which is supplied by the middle and inferior rectal branches of the internal iliac artery.

Collateral circulation is also possible from the coeliac trunk by anastomosis between the inferior and superior pancreaticoduodenal arteries, from the marginal artery of Drummond which anastomoses between the branches of the SMA and IMA, and from the internal iliac artery by anastomosis between the superior and middle-inferior colic arteries. The marginal artery is the most important of them, because it can provide adequate collateral supply to a number of critical points (APRIL 1984). These are the ileocecal region due to the lack of sufficient anastomosis between the ileal and ileocolic branches of the SMA; the splenic flexure due to the lack of sufficient anastomosis between the middle colic branches of the SMA and the left colic branches of the IMA and the lack of the Riolan arc, which provides strong collateral circulation between the middle colic artery and the IMA. Simultaneous embolization of two mesenteric branches, especially including these anatomical regions, should be avoided because of possible ischemic complications (UFLACKER 1987).

There are also anatomical variations that provide potential collateral circulation when they exist (KADIR et al. 1991). They must be investigated during angiography for possible sources of lower gastrointestinal bleeding. They are:

- The SMA originating from the celiac trunk.
- Jejunal branches originating from the dorsal pancreatic or gastroduodenal artery.
- The middle colic or accessory middle colic artery originating from dorsal pancreatic or rarely from right hepatic, splenic, or coeliac arteries.
- An absent or aberrant right colic artery originating from or with ileocolic artery.
- The middle mesenteric artery is a rare congenital variant, which supplies the transverse and descending colon and may anastomose with the left and middle colic arteries.
- The arc of Bühler is a communication between the coeliac trunk and the SMA.
- The arc of Barkow is an epiploic arc lying in the omentum and provides small branches to the transverse colon.

Microanatomical Connections and Variations

The jejunal and ileal branches of the SMA form up to three of six arcades parallel to the intestine, which provide abundant collateral circulation during the peristaltic movement of the intestine. While these arcades are small in number and form large loops in jejunal segments, they are numerous and form short loops in ileal segments (NOER 1943; CHO et al. 1979; APRIL 1984). The closest arcades to the intestine give off numerous individual straight branches (vasa recta) oriented perpendicular to the long axis of the intestines. They divide into anterior and posterior branches when they enter the intestinal wall (Fig. 24.6a). The branches on the mesenteric site form an intramural plexus, providing anastomotic pathways, which are sufficient to sustain several centimeters of intestine in the event of disruption of direct blood flow. The mural anastomoses in the jejunum are greater than in the ileum (PALMAZ et al. 1984). On the other hand, the branches on antimesenteric site are

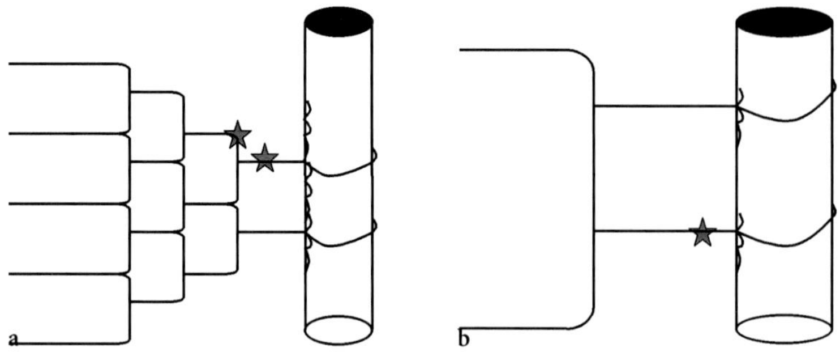

Fig. 24.6. Most suitable locations for superselective embolization in small **a** and large **b** intestines are marked on schematic representation of arterial distribution of small and large intestine

end arteries with no significant anastomosis (Ross 1952; April 1984; Kadir et al. 1991).

Colonic segments are usually supplied from end arteries (vasa recta) originating directly from marginal artery with poor anastomotic connections (Fig. 24.6b) (Griffiths 1961). For this reason, colonic segments are more vulnerable to ischemia than jejunal or ileal segments (Ross 1952).

24.6.3.2 Technique

The aim of embolization in traumatic bleeding is to diminish perfusion to the point where endogenous homeostatic mechanisms stop bleeding without causing significant ischemia or infraction.

Delivery System

For the demonstration of the bleeding source, standard catheter systems are usually sufficient, but the embolization procedure always needs superselective catheterization by the usage of coaxial microcatheter systems. These systems usually include flow-directed or microguiding 135- to 150-cm-long 2.7–3.2 F semirigid highly torquable microcatheters tapered to a flexible tip, via 0.012- to 0.018-in. hydrophilic guidewires. They are easily placed through 5- to 6-F standard catheters and also capable of delivering small Gelfoam and PVA particles. Flow-directed or microguiding catheters can be used depending on the preference or experience of the radiologist or the type and tortuosity of the catheterized vessel.

Choice of Embolic Material

While small embolic materials cause too distal embolization at the level of vasa recta or more distally can more likely produce ischemic complications, larger ones, which produce proximal occlusion of the feeding artery, cannot be effective because of insufficient control of bleeding from collateral vessels. For these reasons it is very important to chose a proper size of embolic material, which should be appropriate to the size of the bleeding vessel and must make an occlusion precisely to the arcade just proximal to the vasa recta supplying the bleeding segment (Uflacker 1987; Okazaki et al. 1992). The material should be deposited as selectively and closely to the site of bleeding as possible. Ideally, the occlusion must be long enough to allow sufficient hemostasis and short enough to prevent ischemia and provide optimal tissue perfusion by recanalization for the long term.

Frequently used embolic materials for control of lower gastrointestinal bleeding are Gelatin sponge (Gelfoam), polyvinyl alcohol (PVA) particles (Ivalon) and microcoils (Goldberger and Bookstein 1977; Jander and Russinovich 1980; Clark et al. 1981; Rahn et al. 1982; Gomes et al. 1986; Uflacker 1987; Leitman et al. 1989; Encarnacion et al. 1992; Guy et al. 1992; Okazaki et al. 1992; Pennoyer et al. 1996; Suzman et al. 1996; Gordon et al. 1997; Ledermann et al. 1998; Nicholson et al. 1998; Peck et al. 1998; Bulakbasi et al. 1999; Velmahos et al. 1999; Kramer et al. 2000; Evangelista and Hallisey 2000; Luchtefeld et al. 2000).

Gelfoam is a very suitable and widely used embolic material for this purpose because it can cause temporary occlusion and be obtained in the desired size. Also, it is quite thrombogenic and usually recanalizes in 1–2 weeks to allow sufficient reperfusion. Gelfoam is very suitable for temporary occlusion of larger vessels (Ledermann et al. 1998). It should be soaked in contrast material to provide sufficient visualization. It can be delivered from standard catheter systems easily but great care must be taken to avoid forceful catheter flushing or selective injection of contrast material into the vessel because particle reflux can result. The combination with proximal coil occlusion can provide permanent occlusion in insufficient bleeding control and also avoid reflux of Gelfoam particles (Fig. 24.7).

Polyvinyl alcohol (PVA) particles (Ivalon) are usually available in powder form in different sizes:

150–250 µm, 250–355 µm, 355–500 µm, 500–710 µm, and 710–1000 µm. Usually the 355- to 500-µm size is suitable for an appropriate match to bleeding mesenteric vessel size and allows the use of PVA from coaxial microcatheter systems. PVA particles smaller than 300 µm can cause ischemic complications by the embolization of smaller arterioles in the peripheral mural circulation (LEDERMANN et al. 1998) and larger than 500 µm can cause inadvertent occlusion of coaxial microcatheter systems for superselective embolization. PVA is a permanent agent and makes a complete occlusion in vessel lumen without defragmentation causing more distal embolization (GUY et al. 1992). It can be recanalized in 3–6 months following resolution of vasospasm surrounding embolic material rather than fragmentation of the embolic material itself (NAKSTAD et al. 1992; PURDY et al. 1992). For this reason it can be used safely in the control of lower gastrointestinal bleeding (KUSANO et al. 1987; GUY et al. 1992; BULAKBASI et al. 1999). It should also be mixed well with contrast material for sufficient visualization and to avoid inadvertent aggregation of poorly mixed particles in the catheter lumen (Fig. 24.4).

Another embolic material used for lower gastrointestinal bleeding is microcoils (GORDON et al. 1997; LEDERMANN et al. 1998). They are permanent and highly radiopaque agents and make proximal occlusion of the feeding artery. They are usually combined with Gelfoam or PVA when others fail to control active bleeding (Figs. 24.2, 24.3, 24.8). Microcoil has to be matched in size and length to the vessel lumen. If it is too large elongated coil can project into the feeding artery and erode the artery wall, resulting in perforation or pseudoaneurysm formation. If it is too small it can migrate more distally or cause unintended embolization by reflux to another vessel lumen (WOJTOWYCZ 1990).

Pitfalls and Their Solutions

The major problem of embolization is technical failure in placing the coaxial catheter distally enough to allow safe embolization of bleeding arteries. This occurs more often in postoperative patients because of distorted anatomy from surgery, vascular tortuosity, vessel spasm, or spontaneous cessation of bleeding. Technical failure has been reported to be 3%–20% in the literature (Table 24.1) (UFLACKER 1987; GORDON et al. 1997; LEDERMANN et al. 1998; PECK et al. 1998; BULAKBASI et al. 1999). By using a coaxial microcatheter system and hydrophilic guidewires, it is usually

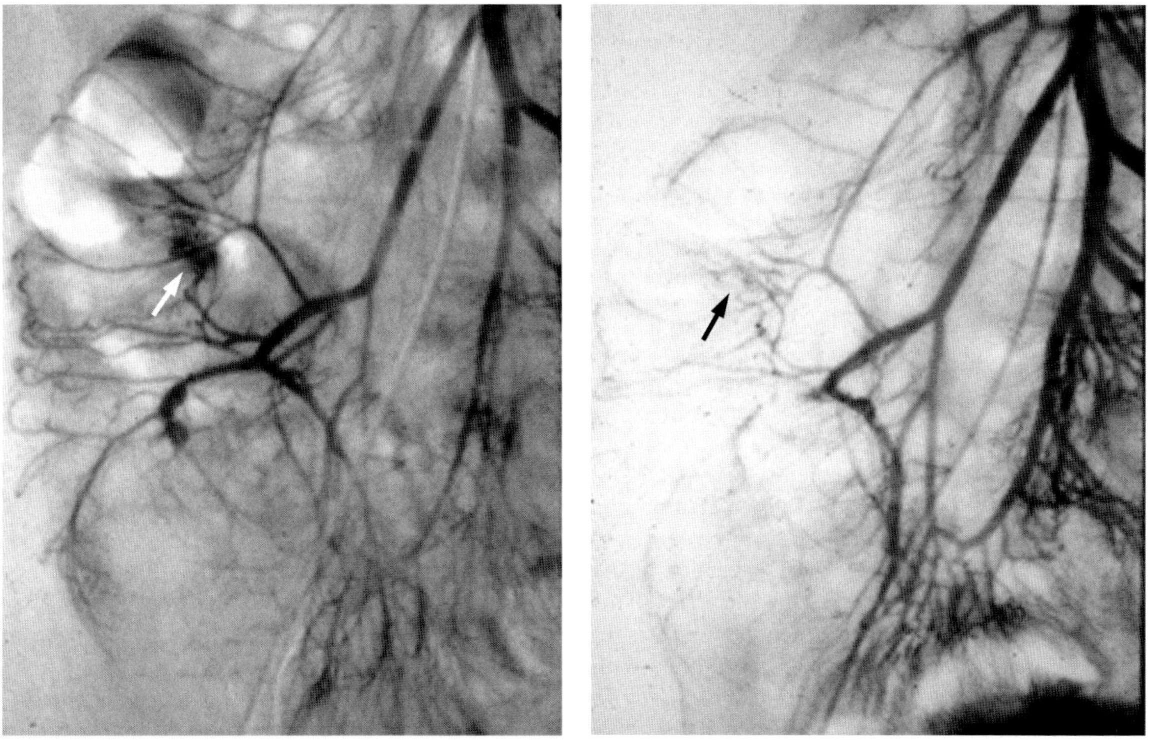

a b

Fig. 24.7a, b. A 14-year-old boy presented with rectal bleeding after appendectomy. **a** Superior mesenteric angiography shows active bleeding (*arrow*) from the ileocolic branch of SMA. **b** After Gelfoam embolization bleeding (*arrow*) was successfully controlled. (Courtesy of R. Uflacker, MD)

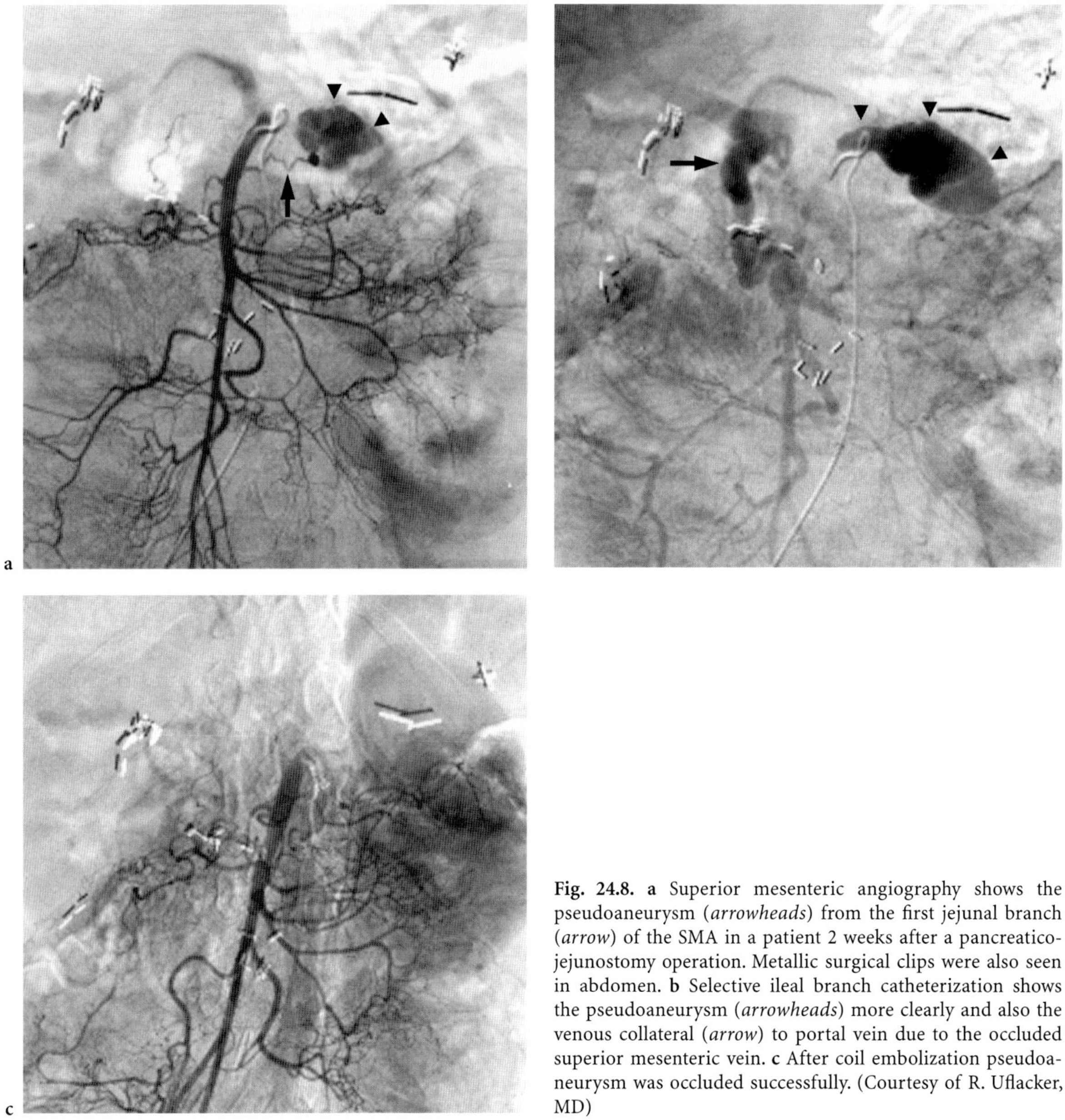

Fig. 24.8. **a** Superior mesenteric angiography shows the pseudoaneurysm (*arrowheads*) from the first jejunal branch (*arrow*) of the SMA in a patient 2 weeks after a pancreatico-jejunostomy operation. Metallic surgical clips were also seen in abdomen. **b** Selective ileal branch catheterization shows the pseudoaneurysm (*arrowheads*) more clearly and also the venous collateral (*arrow*) to portal vein due to the occluded superior mesenteric vein. **c** After coil embolization pseudoaneurysm was occluded successfully. (Courtesy of R. Uflacker, MD)

possible to manipulate the catheters into small and tortuous vessels, which has greatly increased the safety and efficacy of the method.

Another problem is inadvertent occlusion of the microcatheter system by embolic material. This can be avoided by preparing a good mixture of embolic agents with contrast material diluted with saline. Usually a mixture of 40%–50% saline with 50%–60% iodinated contrast material (350 mg/ml) is sufficient. Also, catheter system-embolic material compatibility should be checked in vitro before the procedure.

24.6.3.3
Contraindications

There are no absolute contraindications of embolotherapy unless technical failure occurs. If proper catheterization is achieved, embolization can be safely performed. Predisposing factors such as coagulopathy, shock, diabetes, cirrhosis, malignancy, and infection are not contraindications, but they can effect the success of embolotherapy (Wilson et al. 1987; Encarnacion et al. 1992; Bulakbasi et al. 1999).

Table 24.1. Comparison of the results of large series[a]

Study	EM (number of uses)	Number of					
		Pts	E	CS	R/FC	IC	TF
Walker et al. (1980)	VP (9) G (5)	11	9/11 5/11	6 (66%) 5 (100%)	3 (33%) 0	 1 (20%)	NA
Jander and Russinovich(1980)	G (4)	4/55	4	4 (100%)	0	1 (25%)	NA
Clarck et al. (1981)	VP G+C	63	62/65 18/65	47 (75%) 10 (55%)	15 (25%) 8 (45%)	0	NA
Gomes et al. (1986)	VP G, P, C	47	23/47 24/47	12 (52%) 21 (88%)	4 (17%) 4 (16%)	2 (8.5%) 3 (12.5%)	NA
Uflacker (1987)	V (3) G (12)	13	3 12	0 11 (85%)	3 2 (15%)	0 2 (15%)	 1 (7.7%)
Guy et al. (1992)	P (10)	9	10	7+2 (77%–100%)	3 (33%)	2 (22%)	NA
Encarnacion et al. (1992)	G (30), G+C (2), C(2),) P (2)	29	36	18/29 (62%)	11/29 (38%)	0	NA
Okazaki et al. (1992)	G (2), G+C (2), C (2)	6	6	6/6 (100%)	0	0	0
Pennoyer et al. (1996)	VP (10) E (7)	17	10 7	9/10 (90%) 7/7 (100%)	1/10 (10%) 1/7 (14%)	0	NA
Gordon et al. (1997)	C (14), G (3), P (1)	17	14	13/17 (76.6%)	1/17 (6%)	0	3/17 (17%)
Ledermann et al. (1998)	C (5), P+C (4), G+C (1)	10	10	8/10 (80%)	NA	0	2/10 (20%)
Nicholson et al. (1998)	C (14)	14/48	14	12/14 (86%)	2/14 (14%)	3/14 (21.4%)	NA
Peck et al. (1998)	G (11), C (5), G+C (1)	21	17	15 (71%)	3 (14%)	0	4 (19%)
Bulakbasi et al. (1999)	P (9), P+C (3)	10	12	6+3 (60%–100%)	3/10 (30%)	0	1/10 (10%)
Luchtefeld et al. (2000)	-	16	17	14 (82%)	3 (18%)	1 (6%)	NA
Evangelista and Hallisey(2000)	C (11), P+C (4), P (2), G+C (1)	17	18	13/17 (76%)	4/17 (24%)	0	NA

[a]Modified and updated from Bulakbasi et al. (1999).
EM, embolic material; *Pts*, patients; *E*, embolization; *CS*, clinical success; *R/FC*, rebleeding/failure of control; *IS*, ischemic complications; *TF*, technical failure; *VP*, vasopressin; *G*, Gelfoam; *C*, coil; *P*, polyvinyl alcohol particles; *NA*, not available.

24.6.3.4 Results

Achieving immediate hemostasis, embolization provides an attractive alternative in the management of lower gastrointestinal bleeding, especially when surgery has failed. The overall success of embolization ranges from 55% to 100%, as shown in Table 24.1. It was effective in controlling 73.3%–90% of postoperative intraabdominal bleeding (Panetta et al. 1985; Bulakbasi et al. 1999). While clinical success with Gelfoam is about 36%–100% with an average rate of 70%–88% (Goldberger and Bookstein 1977; Jander and Russinovich 1980; Clark et al. 1981; Rahn et al. 1982; Gomes et al. 1986; Uflacker 1987; Leitman et al. 1989; Encarnacion et al. 1992; Guy et al. 1992; Okazaki et al. 1992; Suzman et al. 1996; Pennoyer et al. 1996; Gordon et al. 1997; Ledermann et al. 1998; Nicholson et al. 1998; Peck et al. 1998; Velmahos et al. 1999; Kramer et al. 2000; Evangelista and Hallisey 2000; Luchtefeld et al. 2000), it ranges from 60% to 77% for PVA and microcoil combinations (Guy et al. 1992; Bulakbasi et al. 1999).

As shown in Table 24.1, unsuccessful clinical results of embolization such as rebleeding or insufficient control of bleeding is reported about 17% (range, 0%–45%), but it can be improved by repeated sessions of embolization (Bulakbasi et al. 1999). Embolization is also ideal for control of late vascular complications when reoperation is not desirable (Velmahos et al. 1999; Bulakbasi et al. 1999). It is the primary treatment modality for posttraumatic visceral artery aneurysms with a low risk and high success rates, and may obviate but not preclude the difficult surgical procedure (Fig. 24.8) (Salam et al. 1992).

24.6.3.5
Complications and Their Solutions

The major risk of embolization for control of lower GI bleeding is irreversible intestinal ischemia in the short term and ischemic bowel strictures in the long term (Fig. 24.9). When ischemic damage is severe enough to become clinically prominent, it can cause postembolization syndrome, which includes pain, fever, leukocytosis, nausea and vomiting, rush, abdominal tenderness and peritoneal signs, and marked change in bowel sounds. The ischemic segment can be best demonstrated on CT by irregular thickening of bowel wall with or without gas collection (Fig. 24.10). If it is perforated it can cause pneumoperitoneum. The origin of the gas is partly from porous embolic materials such as PVA or Gelfoam but mostly from necrotic tissue itself (Wojtowycz 1990). Gas resorption can take several weeks because of hypoperfusion of the ischemic area. The prevalence of postembolic intestinal infarction in reported series ranged from 0% to 25%, with the collective rate approximating 15% (Table 24.1) (Walker et al. 1980; Jander and Russinovich 1980; Clark et al. 1981; Rosenkrantz et al. 1982; Gomes et al. 1986; Encarnacion et al. 1992; Okazaki et al. 1992; Pennoyer et al. 1996; Gordon et al. 1997; Ledermann et al. 1998; Nicholson et al. 1998; Peck et al. 1998; Bulakbasi et al. 1999; Kramer et al. 2000; Luchtefeld et al. 2000).

High complication rates in early studies are probably due to use of larger catheters (7 F) and nonsteerable guidewires that only allowed embolization of marginal arteries, which rendered large areas ischemic (Nicholson et al. 1998). Significant improvement of embolic agents, hydrophilic coaxial microcatheter and guidewire systems, and refinement in technique and imaging equipment allowing superselective embolization may be the most efficacious in reducing the frequency of complication in recent studies (Encarnacion et al. 1992; Okazaki et al. 1992; Pennoyer et al. 1996; Gordon et al. 1997; Ledermann et al. 1998; Nicholson et al. 1998; Peck et al. 1998; Bulakbasi et al. 1999; Kramer et al. 2000; Luchtefeld et al. 2000).

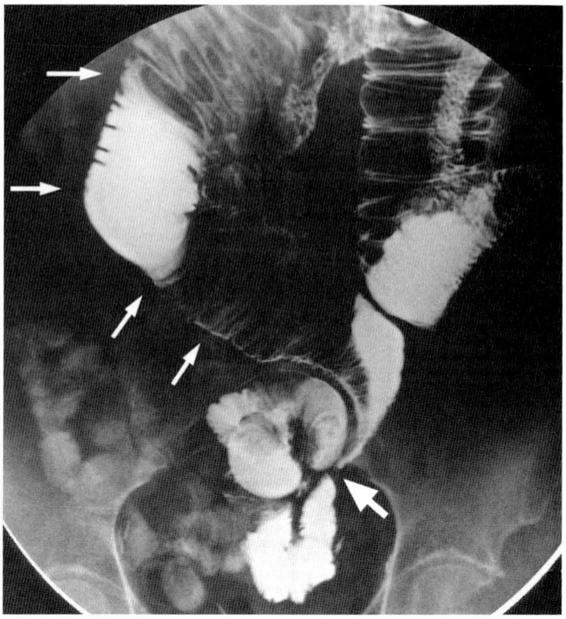

Fig. 24.9. A 31-year-old man after proximal ileal embolization due to traumatic gastrointestinal bleeding. Late-phase barium study shows intestinal ischemic stricture of proximal ileum (*thick arrow*) with dilatation of jejunal segments (*thin arrows*). (Courtesy of N. Bulakbasi, MD)

Ischemic complications are more prominent in the colon than in the small intestines and in the ileum than in the jejunum. Significant ischemia in small intestine embolization may be avoided if the embolic agent is delivered precisely to the distal arcade just proximal or into vasa recta supplying the bleeding segment (Fig. 24.5a) (Walker et al. 1980; Rosenkrantz et al. 1982; Uflacker 1987; Dubois et al. 1989; Guy et al. 1992; Okazaki et al. 1992; Gordon et al. 1997; Ledermann et al. 1998; Peck et al. 1998). This will reduce the intraarterial pressure to the affected segment, without completely occluding the vasa recta, and allow the preservation of the intramural collateral circulation, preventing ischemia or infarction (Guy et al. 1992; Caldwell et al. 1994; Kerns 1994). In colonic embolization, early experiments advised relatively more proximal placement of temporary embolic material, where distal occlusion of the poorly anastomosing vasa recta beyond the marginal artery is more liable to produce infarction after embolization (Chuang et al. 1979; Walker et al. 1980; Jander and Russinovich 1980; Rosenkrantz et al. 1982; Palmaz et al. 1984; Uflacker 1987). However, recent studies show that significant

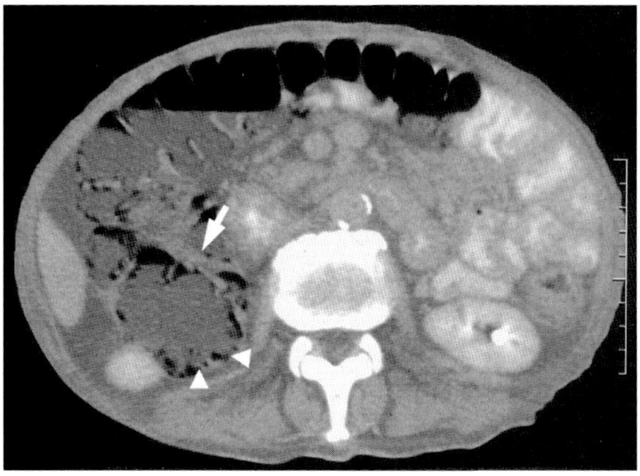

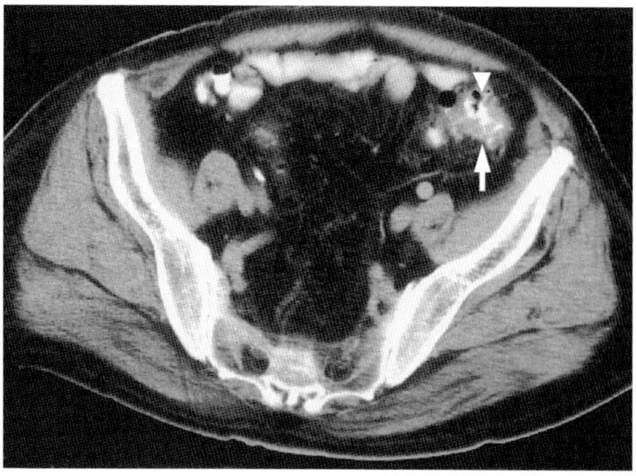

Fig. 24.10. a A 45-year-old woman with massive rectal bleeding from the ileocolonic branch of the superior mesenteric artery due to an abdominal gunshot injury was embolized by a Gelfoam + coil combination. 24 h later, the patient presented with abdominal pain and tenderness. Axial abdominal computed tomography of the patient shows air/fluid level in distended colon and irregular increased thickness (*arrows*) of bowel segment with gas collection (*arrowhead*) within bowel wall resulting from ischemic infarction after embolization. **b** A 31-year-old man with massive rectal bleeding embolized by PVA. Axial abdominal CT 6 days later after embolotherapy shows irregular wall thickness (*arrow*) with gas collection (*arrowhead*) within the ischemic bowel wall. (Courtesy of N. Bulakbasi, MD)

ischemia can only be avoided by superselective embolization of arteria recta supplying the bleeding site (Fig. 24.5b) (Guy et al. 1992; Nicholson et al. 1998; Bulakbasi et al. 1999). In all conditions, meticulous attention is necessary for selective embolization to sufficiently minimize the extent of the devascularized area. Slower infusion of low-dose larger PVA particles or Gelfoam powder (>300 μm) can provide sufficient arterial occlusion, without impairment of intramural collateral microcirculation, and selective distal catheterization produces a very limited area of potential ischemia (Kusano et al. 1987; Choe et al. 1997; Ledermann et al. 1998; Bulakbasi et al. 1999). Infection can be superimposed on infarcted tissue. Besides these complications, there are others that can arise from angiography such as bleeding at the puncture site, acute renal failure, especially in patients with previous diminished renal function, and anaphylactic shock or idiosyncratic reactions due to contrast media (Wojtowycz 1990). CO_2 angiography is a safe solution to overcome these problems related to iodinated contrast materials.

24.6.4 Surgery

In traumatic and postoperative patients, the aim of therapy is to keep the patients from surgery as much as possible because of their poor clinical conditions. Mandatory exploration as a standard procedure for managing patients with penetrating abdominal trauma is associated with a high incidence of unnecessary laparotomies and significant morbidity (Velmahos et al. 1998). But if the source of bleeding cannot be found and cured by other therapeutic options, surgery is inevitable, even for these poor surgical candidates.

24.6.4.1 Technique

The aim of the surgery is maximizing therapeutic benefit while minimizing morbidity and mortality (Billingham 1997). Surgical procedures mainly range from partial bowel resection to subtotal colectomy. Laparotomy, with enteroscopy on the table where indicated, elucidated the cause of bleeding in up to 83% of patients (Lewis et al. 1995). The best way is elective partial resection with accurate detection of the bleeding site. Segmental bowel resection may be confidently performed on the basis of scintigraphic or angiographic findings, with the little risk for bleeding and decreased complications (Browder et al. 1986).

24.6.4.2 Results

Mandatory exploration laparotomy has perioperative mortality rates around 25% (0%–50%) for hemicolectomy and 10% (0%–25%) for partial bowel resection (Carmona et al. 1982; Browder et al. 1986; Leitman et al. 1989; Bender et al. 1991; Guy et al. 1992; Setya et al. 1992; Wagner et al. 1992; Kouraklis et al. 1995; Dertinger et al. 1996; Klas and Madoff 1997). These rates are higher in patients with repeated operation or trauma. Rebleeding can occur in 7%–26% after appropriate surgery (Lewis et al. 1995; Schwab et al. 1995). Although exploratory laparotomy is the final diagnostic modality, there is a controversy as to whether to perform a blind colonic resection if a source has not been identified (Setya et al. 1992; Wagner et al. 1992), but approximately 50% of those treated with empiric left hemicolectomies for severe gastrointestinal bleeding later had clinically significant rebleeding (Jensen and Machicado 1997).

24.7 Conclusion

When the diagnostic angiography is positive for active lower gastrointestinal bleeding, embolization is a logical extension of diagnostic angiography given the desirability of avoiding emergent surgery. It is a life-saving procedure for patients who are poor candidates for surgery. Superselective catheterization must be performed with the first target being the vasa recta, following the marginal artery or distal intestinal arcade when the first is not possible. If the patient with active bleeding in the postoperative or posttraumatic period has received large volumes of replaced blood and the clinical condition is rapidly deteriorating, emergent embolization must be preferred regardless of the size or type of blood vessel involved, or even the technical success of superselective catheterization. Even if embolization fails to control bleeding or rebleeding occurs, it can be repeated safely and it provides more time for stabilization and preparation of poor surgical candidates for elective surgical procedures in better conditions than emergent situations offer. With evidence of ischemic complications, the presence of a focal grossly apparent identifiable lesion will be a benefit at the time of surgery, allowing directed segmental resection. It is likely that this operation will be of lesser magnitude than blind surgery in a patient actively bleeding form an unidentified source.

References

April EW (1984) Anatomy. Wiley Medical, New York

Athanasoulis CA, Baum S, Rosch J et al (1975) Mesenteric arterial infusions of vasopressin for bleeding from colonic diverticulosis. Am J Surg 129:212–216

Back MR, Caridi JG, Hawkins IF et al (1998) Angiography with carbon dioxide (CO_2). Surg Clin North Am 78:575–591

Baum S, Nusbaum M, Blakemore WS et al (1965) The preoperative radiographic demonstration of intra-abdominal bleeding from undetermined sites by percutaneous selective celiac and superior mesenteric angiography. Surgery 58:797–805

Bender JS, Wiencek RG, Bowman DL (1991) Morbidity and mortality following total abdominal colectomy for massive lower gastrointestinal bleeding. Am Surg 57:536–541

Billingham RP (1997) The conundrum of lower gastrointestinal bleeding. Surg Clin North Am 77:241–252

Browder W, Cerise EJ, Litwin MS (1986) Impact of emergency angiography in massive lower gastrointestinal bleeding. Ann Surg 204:530–536

Bulakbasi N, Kurtaran K, Ustunsoz B et al (1999) Massive lower gastrointestinal bleeding from the surgical anastomosis in patients with multiorgan trauma: treatment by subselective embolization with polyvinyl alcohol particles. Cardiovasc Intervent Radiol 22:461–467

Caldwell D, Stokes K, Yakes W (1994) Embolotherapy: agents, clinical applications and techniques. Radiographics 14: 623–643

Carmona RH, Lim RC Jr, Clark GC (1982) Morbidity and mortality in hepatic trauma: a five-year study. Am J Surg 144: 88–94

Chen HM, Jan YY, Chen MF (1998) Intra-arterial infusion of octreotide to stop gastrointestinal tract bleeding that is difficult to manage surgically: a case report. Hepatogastroenterology 45:128–132

Cho KJ, Schmidt RW, Lenz J (1979) Effects of experimental embolization of superior mesenteric artery branch on the intestine. Invest Radiol 14:207–212

Choe DH, Han MH, Kang GH et al (1997) An experimental study of embolic effect according to infusion rate and concentration of suspension in transarterial particulate embolization. Invest Radiol 32:260–267

Chuang VP, Wallace S, Zornoza J et al (1979) Transcatheter arterial occlusion in the management of rectosigmoid bleeding. Radiology 133:605–609

Clark RA, Colley DP, Eggers FM (1981) Acute arterial gastrointestinal hemorrhage: efficacy of transcatheter control. AJR 136:1185–1189

Conn HO, Ramsby GR, Storer EH et al (1975) Intraarterial vasopressin in the treatment of upper gastrointestinal hemorrhage: a prospective, controlled clinical trial. Gastroenterology 68:211–221

Dertinger SH, Vestner H, Muller K et al (1996) Prospective study of diagnosis, therapy and follow-up of acute gastrointestinal hemorrhage in 397 patients. Wien Klin Wochenschr 108:717–721

Dubois JJ, Ostrow LB, Smith GB et al (1989) Transcatheter embolization of small bowel anastomosis: a case report and review of the literature. Mil Med 154:505–507

Eckstein MR, Kelemouridis V, Athanasoulis CA et al (1984) Gastric bleeding: therapy with intraarterial vasopressin and transcatheter embolization. Radiology 152:643–646

Encarnacion CE, Kadir S, Beam CA et al (1992) Gastrointestinal bleeding: treatment with gastrointestinal arterial embolization. Radiology 183:505–508
Evangelista PT, Hallisey MJ (2000) Transcatheter embolization for acute lower gastrointestinal hemorrhage. J Vasc Interv Radiol 11:601–606
Fara JW, Barth KH, White RI Jr et al (1979) Mesenteric vascular effects of prostaglandins F2 alpha and B2: possible advantages over vasopressin in control of gastrointestinal bleeding. Radiology 133:317–320
Frankhouse JH, Ryan MG, Papanicolaou G et al (1995) Carbon dioxide/digital subtraction arteriography-assisted transluminal angioplasty. Ann Vasc Surg 9:448–452
Frezza M, Buri L, Peri A et al (1996) Emergencies in colorectal diseases: role of the endoscopist. Ann Ital Chir 67:161–169
Goldberger LE, Bookstein JJ (1977) Transcatheter embolization for treatment of diverticular hemorrhage. Radiology 122:613–617
Goldstein HM, Medellin H, Ben-Menachem Y et al (1975) Transarterial embolization in the management of bleeding in the cancer patients. Radiology 115:603–608
Gomes AS, Lois JF, McCoy RD (1986) Angiographic treatment of gastrointestinal hemorrhage: comparison of vasopressin infusion and embolization. AJR 146:1031–1037
Gordon RL, Ahl KL, Kerlan RK et al (1997) Selective arterial embolization for the control of lower gastrointestinal bleeding. Am J Surg 174:24–28
Griffiths JD (1961) Extramural and intramural blood supply of the colon. Br Med J 1:323–326
Gupta N, Longo WE, Vernava AM III (1995) Angiodysplasia of the lower gastrointestinal tract: an entity readily diagnosed by colonoscopy and primarily managed nonoperatively. Dis Colon Rectum 38:979–982
Gutierrez C, Mariano M, Vander Laan T et al (1998) The use of technetium-labeled erythrocyte scintigraphy in the evaluation and treatment of lower gastrointestinal hemorrhage. Am Surg 64:989–992
Guy GE, Shetty PC, Sharma RP et al (1992) Acute lower gastrointestinal hemorrhage: treatment by superselective embolization with polyvinyl alcohol particles. AJR 159:521–526
Hays RM (1976) Antidiuretic hormone and water transfer. Kidney Int 9:223–230
Imdahl A, Salm R, Ruckauer K et al (1991) Diagnosis and management of lower gastrointestinal hemorrhage. Retrospective analysis of 233 cases. Langenbecks Arch Chir 376:152–157
Jander HP, Russinovich NAE (1980) Transcatheter gelfoam embolization in abdominal, retroperitoneal and pelvic hemorrhage. Radiology 136:337–344
Jensen DM, Machicado GA (1997) Colonoscopy for diagnosis and treatment of severe lower gastrointestinal bleeding: routine outcomes and cost analysis. Gastrointest Endosc Clin North Am 7:477–498
Johansson L, Norrby K, Nystrom PO, Lennquist S (1984) Intestinal intramural haemorrhage after abdominal missile trauma – clinical classification and prognosis. Acta Chir Scand 150:51–56
Kadir S, Ernest CB (1983) Current concepts in angiographic management of gastrointestinal bleeding. Curr Prob Surg 20:281–343
Kadir S, Lundell C, Saeed M (1991) Celiac, superior and inferior mesenteric arteries. In: Kadir S (ed) Atlas of normal and variant angiographic anatomy. Saunders, Philadelphia, pp 297–364
Kerns SR (1994) How safe is the use of platinum microcoils for embolization of small mesenteric arteries in patients with gastrointestinal bleeding? AJR 162:1497
Klas JV, Madoff RD (1997) Surgical options in lower gastrointestinal bleeding. Semin Colon Rectal Surg 8:172–177
Kouraklis G, Misiakos E, Karatzas G et al (1995) Diagnostic approach and management of active lower gastrointestinal hemorrhage. Int Surg 80:138–140
Kramer SC, Gorich J, Rilinger N et al (2000) Embolization for gastrointestinal hemorrhages. Eur Radiol 10:802–805
Kusano S, Murata K, Ohuchi H et al (1987) Low-dose particulate polyvinyl alcohol embolization in massive small artery intestinal hemorrhage: experimental and clinical results. Invest Radiol 22:388–392
Lang EV, Gossler AA, Fick LJ et al (1999) Carbon dioxide angiography: effect of injection parameters on bolus configuration. J Vasc Interv Radiol 10:41–49
Ledermann HP, Schoch E, Jost R et al (1998) Superselective coil embolization in acute gastrointestinal hemorrhage: personal experience in 10 patients and review of the literature. J Vasc Interv Radiol 9:753–760
Leitman IM, Paull DE, Shires GT III (1989) Evaluation and management of massive lower gastrointestinal hemorrhage. Ann Surg 209:175–180
Lewis MP, Khoo DE, Spencer J (1995) Value of laparotomy in the diagnosis of obscure gastrointestinal haemorrhage. Gut 37:187–190
Linnet J, Abrahamsen J (1995) Scintigraphy of bleeding. The diagnostic value based on a 10-year period. Ugeskr Laeger 157:5373–5377
Luchtefeld MA, Senagore AJ, Szomstein M et al (2000) Evaluation of transarterial embolization for lower gastrointestinal bleeding. Dis Colon Rectum 43:532–534
McBoyle MF, Schiller WR, Hurt AV (1984) Massive gastrointestinal bleeding following blunt abdominal trauma: an unusual case presentation. J Trauma 24:1057–1059
Nakstad PH, Bakke SJ, Halid JK (1992) Embolization of intracranial arteriovenous malformations and fistulas with polyvinyl alcohol and platinum fibre coils. Neuroradiology 34:348–351
Nemcek AA Jr (2000) Transcatheter therapy for lower gastrointestinal bleeding. Techn Vasc Interv Radiol 3:139–146
Ng BL, Thompson JN, Adam A et al (1987) Selective visceral angiography in obscure postoperative gastrointestinal bleeding. Ann R Coll Surg Engl 69:237–240
Ng DA, Opelka FG, Beck DE et al (1997) Predictive value of technetium Tc 99m-labeled red blood cell scintigraphy for positive angiogram in massive lower gastrointestinal hemorrhage. Dis Colon Rectum 40:471–477
Nicholson AA, Ettles DF, Hartley JE et al (1998) Transcatheter coil embolotherapy: a safe and effective option for major colonic haemorrhage. Gut 43:79–84
Noer RJ (1943) The blood vessels of the jejunum and ileum: a comparative study of man and certain laboratory animals. Am J Anat 73:293–334
Nusbaum M, Baum S (1963) Radiographic demonstration of unknown sites of gastrointestinal bleeding. Surg Forum 14: 374–375
Okazaki M, Furui S, Higashihara H et al (1992) Emergent embolotherapy of small intestine hemorrhage. Gastrointest Radiol 17:223–228
Palmaz JC, Walter JF, Cho KJ (1984) Therapeutic embolization of the small bowel arteries. Radiology 152:377–382

Panetta T, Sclafani SJ, Goldstein AS et al (1985) Percutaneous transcatheter embolization for arterial trauma. J Vasc Surg 2:54–64
Peck DJ, McLoughlin RF, Hughson MN et al (1998) Percutaneous embolotherapy of lower gastrointestinal hemorrhage. J Vasc Interv Radiol 9:747–751
Pennoyer WP, Vignati PV, Cohen JL (1996) Management of angiogram-positive lower gastrointestinal hemorrhage: long-term follow-up of non-operative treatments. Int J Colorectal Dis 11:279–282
Peterson WL (1988) Obscure gastrointestinal bleeding. Med Clin North Am 72:1169–1176
Purdy PD, Batjer HH, Risser RC et al (1992) Arteriovenous malformations of the brain: choosing embolic materials to enhance safety and ease of excision. J Neurosurg 77:212–217
Rahn NH III, Tishler JM, Han SY et al (1982) Diagnostic and interventional angiography in acute gastrointestinal hemorrhage. Radiology 143:361–366
Renert WA, Button KF, Fuld SI et al (1972) Mesenteric venous thrombosis and small bowel infarction following infusion of vasopressin into superior mesenteric artery. Radiology 102:299–302
Richter JM, Christensen MR, Kaplan LM et al (1995) Effectiveness of current technology in the diagnosis and management of lower gastrointestinal hemorrhage. Gastrointest Endosc 41:93–98
Roberts C, Maddison FE (1976) Partial mesenteric arterial occlusion with subsequent ischemic bowel damage due to pitressin infusion. AJR 126:829–831
Rosch J, Dotter CT, Brown MJ (1972) Selective arterial embolization: new method for control of acute gastrointestinal bleeding. Radiology 102:303–306
Rosenkrantz H, Bookstein JJ, Rosen RJ et al (1982) Postembolic colonic infarction. Radiology 142:47–51
Ross JA (1952) Vascular patterns of small and large intestine compared. Br J Surg 39:330–333
Salam TA, Lumsden AB, Martin LG et al (1992) Nonoperative management of visceral aneurysms and pseudoaneurysms. Am J Surg 164:215–219
Salem RR, Wood CB, Rees HC et al (1985) A comparison of colonoscopy and selective visceral angiography in the diagnosis of colonic angiodysplasia. Ann R Coll Surg Engl 67:225–226
Sandhu C, Buckenham TM, Belli AM (1999) Using CO_2-enhanced arteriography to investigate acute gastrointestinal hemorrhage. AJR 173:1399–1401
Schwab M, Richter A, Tubergen D et al (1995) Diagnostic and therapeutic problems of acute lower gastrointestinal hemorrhage. Zentralbl Chir 120:59–62
Seeger JM, Self S, Harward TR et al (1993) Carbon dioxide gas as an arterial contrast agent. Ann Surg 217:688–697
Seldinger SI (1953) Catheter replacement of the needle in percutaneous arteriography. Acta Radiol 39:368–376
Setya V, Singer JA, Minken SL (1992) Subtotal colectomy as a last resort for unrelenting, unlocalized, lower gastrointestinal hemorrhage: experience with 12 cases. Am Surg 58: 295–299
Sirinek KR, Thomford NR, Pace WG (1977) Adverse cardiodynamic effect of vasopressin not avoided by selective intraarterial administration. Surgery 81:723–728
Suzman MS, Talmor M, Jennis R et al (1996) Accurate localization and surgical management of active lower gastrointestinal hemorrhage with technetium-labeled erythrocyte scintigraphy. Ann Surg 224:29–36
Textor HJ, Wilhelm K, Strunk H et al (1997) The diagnosis of intra-abdominal hemorrhages with CO_2 as the contrast medium. ROFO Fortschr Geb Rontgenstr Neuen Bildgeb Verfahr 166:51–53
Thompson JN, Salem RR, Hemingway AP et al (1987) Specialist investigation of obscure gastrointestinal bleeding. Gut 28:47–51
Twiford TW Jr, Granmayeh M, Tucker MJ (1978) Gangrene of the feet associated with mesenteric intraarterial vasopressin. AJR 130:558–560
Uflacker R (1987) Transcatheter embolization for treatment of acute lower gastrointestinal bleeding. Acta Radiol 28: 425–430
Velmahos GC, Demetriades D, Cornwell EE III (1998) Transpelvic gunshot wounds: routine laparotomy or selective management? World J Surg 22:1034–1038
Velmahos GC, Demetriades D, Chahwan S et al (1999) Angiographic embolization for arrest of bleeding after penetrating trauma to the abdomen. Am J Surg 178:367–373
Vernava AM III, Moore BA, Longo WE et al (1997) Lower gastrointestinal bleeding. Dis Colon Rectum 40:846–858
Wagner HE, Stain SC, Gilg M et al (1992) Systematic assessment of massive bleeding of the lower part of the gastrointestinal tract. Surg Gynecol Obstet 175:445–449
Walker WJ, Goldin AR, Shaff MI et al (1980) Per catheter control of haemorrhage from superior and inferior mesenteric arteries. Clin Radiol 31:71–80
Waltman AC (1980) Transcatheter embolization versus vasopressin infusion for the control of arteriocapillary gastrointestinal bleeding. Cardiovasc Intervent Radiol 3: 289–295
Weaver FA, Pentecost MJ, Yellin AE et al (1991) Clinical applications of carbon dioxide/digital subtraction angiography. J Vasc Surg 13:266–272
Williams SC, Tulchinski M, Allen TW et al (2000) Nuclear medicine. Online textbook of Madigan Army Medical Center Radiology Department
Wilson RF, Dulchausky SA, Soulier G et al (1987) Problems with 20 units or more blood transfusions in 24 hours. Am Surg 53:410–417
Whittaker SC, Gregson RHS (1993) The role of angiography in the investigation of acute or chronic GI haemorrhage. Clin Radiol 47:382–388
Wojtowycz M (1990) Handbooks in radiology. Interventional radiology and angiography. Year Book Medical Publishers, Chicago

25 Relevance of Imaging to Surgical Management of Abdominal Injuries

N. Zügel, K. Breitschaft, E. Mayr, H. Häuser

CONTENTS

- Ultrasonography is the standard examination in blunt abdominal trauma.
- Computed tomography should be performed in stable patients.
- Diagnostic peritoneal lavage to clarify free fluid has been replaced by ultrasonography and computed tomography.
- Early recognition of intraabdominal traumas is extremely significant for prognosis.

N. Zügel, MD
Klinik für Allgemein- und Abdominalchirurgie, Klinikum Augsburg, Stenglinstrasse 2, 86156 Augsburg, Germany
K. Breitschaft, MD
Klinik für Allgemein- und Viszeralchirurgie, Klinikum Augsburg, Stenglinstrasse 2, 86156 Augsburg, Germany
E. Mayr, MD
Klinik für Diagnostische Radiologie und Neuroradiologie, Klinikum Augsburg, Stenglinstrasse 2, 86156 Augsburg, Germany
H. Häuser, MD
Klinik für Diagnostische Radiologie und Neuroradiologie, Klinikum Augsburg, Stenglinstrasse 2, 86156 Augsburg, Germany

25.1 Introduction

Abdominal and retroperitoneal traumas occur as a result of blunt or penetrating force or are deceleration injuries sustained in accidents, a fall from a great height, or high-speed traumas. Blunt abdominal traumas are usually the result of traffic or leisure accidents, whereas penetrating traumas are largely caused by bullet or stab wounds. Blunt abdominal injury is considerably more common than penetrating trauma in Central Europe and rarely occurs on its own (Bardenheuer et al. 2000). It is usually seen in multiple-system injuries. Blunt trauma often causes injury to several abdominal organs and is highly lethal. In addition to craniocerebral traumas, massive abdominal hemorrhage, as might occur with hepatic, splenic, or mesenteric injuries, is a major cause of early death, whereby the principal causes of morbidity and mortality in abdominal trauma are associated with delays in diagnosis or treatment. They have been identified as secondary inflammatory injury, sepsis, and multiple organ failure (MOF) syndromes, as may occur with bowel, pancreas, or biliary tract injuries (Enderson and Maull 1991; Davis et al. 1992; Shackford et al. 1993; Nast-Kolb et al. 1998). Delayed diagnosis or treatment of abdominal injuries is one of the most common causes of preventable mortality and is therefore a critical area of trauma management. The clinical findings in blunt abdominal trauma patients are of only limited use, even if the patient is awake and cooperative. Injuries to the adjoining areas of the trunk, i.e., the thorax and the pelvis, also need to be reliably recorded. Imaging procedures are therefore of high diagnostic value. Direct blunt force often causes hollow viscera to rupture or parenchymal organs to burst. Ideally, after performing a physical examination and imaging by the radiologist and obtaining an overview of the vital signs by the anesthesiologist, the surgeon has all the necessary information within a short space of time to develop a treatment strategy.

The following three current issues are of great significance from the surgeon's point of view for the tactical and therapeutic approach in abdominal trauma patients:

- What imaging information is crucial for planning treatment?
- When is a precise diagnosis required?
- What are the limitations of imaging?

25.2 Blunt Abdominal Trauma

The term "blunt abdominal trauma" refers to the effect of force on the abdomen, either directly through the abdominal wall or indirectly as a result of deceleration forces. The term does not include open abdominal trauma, i.e., the traumatic opening of the abdominal wall, or penetrating abdominal trauma, in which a circumscribed area of the abdominal wall has been penetrated by an object. In the presence of associated neurological injuries or other painful distracting injuries, physical examination of the abdomen is even less reliable (ANDERSON and IRVING 1990; SCHURINK et al. 1997). Physical examination is a subjective measure; the sensitivity reported in previous studies varies greatly and is often not much greater than 60%.

Contusion marks indicate the area that was subject to the greatest force. In contusion of organs or the mesentery, visceral pain in the affected part of the abdominal wall predominates. Hemorrhage causes delayed somatic pain as a result of peritoneal irritation.

Despite the unremarkable clinical findings, intraabdominal injuries have often been sustained. It should be noted, however, that even in the presence of intestinal perforation or major hemoperitoneum, initial physical findings are often minimal or absent. Diagnostic imaging procedures are therefore important. If the history of the trauma leads to suspicion of a blunt abdominal trauma, abdominal organ injury needs to be ruled out. This also applies if the adjoining areas of the trunk have been injured, e.g., pelvic ring fracture or fracture of ribs close to the diaphragm. This is because early recognition of intraabdominal traumas is extremely significant in terms of the prognosis (Fig. 25.1).

25.2.1 Free Fluid

Diagnostic peritoneal lavage to clarify free fluid has been replaced in Europe by ultrasonography (US) and computed tomography (CT). In hemodynamically unstable patients, the abdominal status is clarified by US (NAST-KOLB et al. 1994; ERTEL and TRENTZ 1996). If a large amount of free fluid is found, an emergency laparotomy is performed. If the patient is hemodynamically stable, abdominal CT is performed (FEUSSNER et al. 1999).

25.2.1.1 Ultrasonography

US is the method of choice. It allows intraabdominal fluid, hemothorax, or hemopericardium to be quickly visualized and has been associated with good sensitivity as experience has accumulated (SINGH

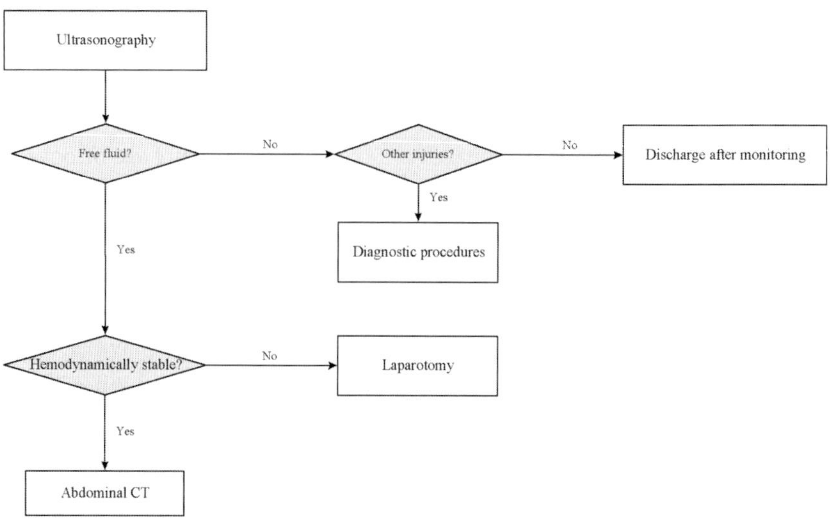

Fig. 25.1. Algorithm for imaging blunt abdominal trauma

et al. 1997; Yoshii et al. 1998). It is not difficult to demonstrate large amounts of free fluid (McKenney et al. 1998; Smith et al. 1998). The problem is to identify small amounts of free fluid as an indirect sign of organ injury or perforation of a cavity. Typical sites where this is likely to occur are the hepatorenal sinus (Morison's pouch), the perisplenic region (Koller's pouch), Douglas' space, and the gaps between the intestinal loops. The examination has to be performed swiftly using a strictly standardized technique. In multiple-trauma patients who have to be operated on without delay due to another life-threatening injury and in whom CT therefore cannot be performed, US should also be performed in the operating room, if appropriate.

US has several advantages. US equipment and experienced operators are available in practically every hospital. US is quick, noninvasive, and inexpensive. The equipment can be brought to the patient any time, thus obviating the need for transporting patients.

Limitations and pitfalls are the operator dependence of image interpretation and a higher subjectivity compared with CT. Sensitivity of US is poor in penetrating injuries. Fluid-filled organs may be misinterpreted as free fluid, e.g., fluid-filled right flexure, renal cysts, ovarian cysts, or retroperitoneal fluid. Subcutaneous emphysema makes it impossible to interpret the images reliably. The shape of the patient's body, flatus, open wounds, and the patient's position limit the usefulness of US. A low-echo transverse abdominal muscle can be misinterpreted as free fluid (Wachsberg 1999).

25.2.1.2 Computed Tomography

If free fluid or pathological findings are demonstrated by US, or are inadequately assessed, intraabdominal organs, contrast-enhanced CT should be added to the diagnostic procedures performed in hemodynamically stable patients. Contrast-enhanced CT can be used to differentiate between blood (>30 Hounsfield Units) and watertight fluids (0–10 HU). In addition, blood (30–45 HU), clotted blood (40–60 HU), and active hemorrhage (blood and contrast medium, 80–300 HU) can be distinguished. Determination of the HU is recommended to diagnose free fluid without organ injury. Watertight values suggest a rupture of the urinary bladder or gallbladder, chyloperitoneum, or preexisting ascites. If the HU values are between 30 and 45 HU, denoting the presence of a small, self-limiting injury to a parenchymal organ, a conservative approach or less urgent surgery, enterorrhexis, or mesenteric laceration should be considered. Enterorrhexis has to be surgically treated immediately, as it is associated with a high mortality rate, up to 50%, if the operation is delayed (Schumpelick et al. 1999).

In case of doubt, CT is repeated, using oral and rectal contrast medium. If there is still any doubt and if the patient is hemodynamically stable, CT is repeated later. The principal pitfalls of CT scanning for blunt abdominal trauma are the possibility of missing small amounts of free intraperitoneal fluid associated with blunt intestinal injury and a relatively poor sensitivity for these injuries (Sherck et al. 1994; Udekwu et al. 1996).

25.2.2 Free Air

Free intraabdominal and/or retroperitoneal air is usually an indirect sign of a hollow viscus perforation. Secondary accumulation of air, either by urinary bladder catheterization and opacification in bladder rupture or by pneumothorax, where the air enters the retroperitoneal space via the mediastinum or directly escapes into the intraabdominal space through an injury to the diaphragm, should be ruled out. Free intraabdominal air is always an indication for surgery.

25.2.3 Injury to Abdominal Organs

US often allows an initial assessment to be made of parenchymal organ injury. A hypoechoic area with no clear delimitation suggests intraparenchymal hemorrhage, while a hyperechoic area is caused by hematoma or a parenchymal rupture; a heterogeneous ultrasound pattern suggests an extensive injury. In a study performed by Bühne et al., CT led to modification of the treatment that was originally decided on in 41.4% of patients with conspicuous US results (Bühne et al. 2001). CT should therefore always be performed in stable patients with conspicuous US findings. Interestingly, CT also provided information that led to modification of treatment in 6.6% of patients with unremarkable US findings. In view of the high morbidity and mortality rates of abdominal traumas if treatment is delayed, the efficiency of the routine use of CT in stable patients with unremarkable US findings needs to be further evaluated in prospective studies.

25.2.3.1 Liver

Of organ injuries associated with a blunt abdominal trauma, 20% involve the liver (NOVELLINE et al. 1999). Possible types of injury include subcapsular hematoma, contusion, laceration, hepatic artery injury, hepatic vein injury, injury to the biliary tree, or injury to the portal system. Hepatic injuries may be graded (grades I–VI) according to size, location, and involvement of vascular structures (MOORE et al. 1995). Injuries to the bare area of the liver lead to hemorrhage in the retroperitoneal space. A total of 70%–80% of all traumatic liver injuries are grade I or II traumas (FELICIANO et al. 1986; BRASEL et al. 1997). These can in principle be treated conservatively. For nonoperative treatment to be successful, hemodynamic stability, the absence of coagulopathy, and maximum transfusion requirements of two erythrocyte concentrates in 24 h are required. In addition, peritoneal irritation and secondary abdominal traumas should not be present. Intensive monitoring by US and, if appropriate, CT in the intensive care unit is mandatory. If bleeding activity or the amount of intraabdominal fluid increases, or if signs of infection become apparent, a laparotomy has to be performed. The patient should be monitored for at least 10 days, as most complications occur 1 week after the trauma. The long-term history of nonoperative management is relatively benign, and the usefulness of routine follow-up CT scans for this group has been questioned (ALLINS et al. 1996; CIRAULO et al. 1996).

However, if a patient has to undergo laparotomy for other reasons, grade I and II traumas can be adequately repaired, without using special techniques of liver surgery, by temporary compression of superficial lacerations or capsular defects, by capsulorrhaphy, or by applying hemostatic agents such as collagen fleece or fibrin glue. In hemorrhage from grade III–V traumas, occlusion of the hepatoduodenal ligament or a Pringle's maneuver can be used to achieve temporary control of hemorrhage (≤60 min) and hence to obtain an overview of the situation. Bleeding can then be brought under control by targeted suturing or coagulation with infrared argon beamer. Partial hepatectomy may be indicated. If bleeding is difficult to arrest, the technically easiest and often the most effective measure is application of a perihepatic tamponade or liver packing. Care should be taken when inserting the abdominal pads that neither the vena cava nor the portal vein is constricted, to avoid venous congestion and parenchymal necrosis. In case of doubt, this complication can be seen on CT. The advantage of a liver tamponade is that even heavy bleeding from the liver can be stopped quickly and effectively; in addition, primary resection of an unnecessary amount of liver tissue can be avoided. During a second-look procedure after 48–74 h, liver necrosis has then become apparent. The necrotic tissue can be resected in a targeted way, sparing the vital hepatic parenchyma (DENTON et al. 1997).

In the event of hemorrhage from the retrohepatic vena cava or from injuries to central hepatic veins, the suprahepatic and infrahepatic vena cava need to be clamped before treatment (KREMER and HENNE-BRUNS 1993). Hepatectomy with liver transplantation is only possible at a few centers and is associated with a high mortality rate (>80%) (RINGE and PICHLMAYR 1995). Right hepatic artery ligation is also associated with a mortality rate of more than 80% and therefore no longer plays any role. This is because of the development of extensive liver necrosis with septic complications. In contrast, selective embolization of hepatic arteries offers the advantage that the formation of liver necrosis is minimized. It is not yet clear what role it will play as a routine procedure in the conservative treatment of liver traumas (DENTON et al. 1997; CIRAULO et al. 1998). In patients who do not undergo an emergency laparotomy and who have higher-grade injuries (grades III and IV) in Moore's classification, in terms of CT morphology, angiographic visualization of the hepatic arteries is indicated. If extravasation of contrast medium is seen, primary hemostasis by embolization is a promising approach (SUGIMOTO et al. 1994; HAGIWARA et al. 1997; HARPER and MAULL 2000).

25.2.3.2 Spleen

In patients with splenic injuries, spleen-preserving methods of treatment have become increasingly important not only in children, but also in adults. The advantages are that the immune function of the spleen is maintained, overwhelming post-splenectomy infection (OPSI) is avoided, and there are fewer exploratory laparotomies and fewer complications caused by surgery. The risk of OPSI following splenectomy for trauma has been estimated at 0.026% and 0.8% for adults and children, respectively, with an estimated mortality rate of between 50% and 70%. Organ-preserving surgical methods have been developed. Splenic injuries are typically graded I–V as a function of size and location (MOORE et al. 1995). In superficial splenic lesions, parenchymal or capsular sutures, fibrin glue, and coagulation methods are used. Deeper injuries can be repaired by partial resection or by parenchymal wrapping. The technical results obtained with splenorrhaphy have been good, with a low incidence of reoperation of 2%–3% and an estimated intraoperative success rate of 70%–90%. The spleen-preserving resection methods are time-consuming. In patients with protracted shock, heavily bleeding hilar injuries, burst injuries of the entire organ, and in harmful delay in treating other abdominal or extraabdominal injuries, emergency splenectomy is therefore the method of choice. Asher et al. (1976) drew up criteria for diagnosis of splenic rupture by US: enlarged organ size, irregular contours, change in position, and free intraperitoneal fluid. An inhomogeneous echo pattern and the left butterfly sign corresponding to minimal amounts of free fluid on both sides of the vessels of the hilus of spleen have been described as signs of spleen trauma (Froelich et al. 1982; Weill et al. 1988). El Mouaaouy et al. (1991) mention physiological splenic lobulation for differential diagnosis by US. It usually occurs at the anterior extremity of the spleen and can be demonstrated by US as soon as the organ is surrounded by free fluid. A splenic lesion can often be diagnosed by US, but the extent of parenchymal damage unfortunately cannot be sufficiently determined. In particular, US does not provide a definitive answer as to whether the spleen can be preserved and whether this can be achieved by surgical or interventional treatment in order to help the physician decide which form of treatment to use. The extent of lesions can be seen much better on CT. In unstable patients, further differentiation according to morphological criteria on CT is of secondary importance, as a splenectomy is usually indicated for the aforementioned reasons. In patients with isolated splenic trauma, CT can help to decide which form of treatment to use if the splenic injury is classified according to CT criteria, paying particular attention to the involvement of the hilum (Moore et al. 1995). Grade I and II traumas can be treated conservatively. Intensive monitoring by US at 12-h intervals to monitor the course is recommended for the first 2 days after the trauma. From day 3 onward, the patient can be transferred to the ward and US performed every 2 days if the course is unremarkable. Patients with isolated abdominal traumas should remain in hospital for 8–10 days.

Grade III traumas may also be treated conservatively as described above unless a trabecular vessel is involved. In such cases, active hemorrhage is visible on CT and the intraparenchymal hematoma increases in size. Parenchymal wrapping is a suitable form of surgical, spleen-preserving treatment here (Fig. 25.2). If the segment concerned shows extensive parenchymal fragmentation, resection of the segment is necessary. Grade IV traumas are treated surgically, and organ-preserving treatment is rarely possible. In grade V traumas, the spleen is removed. This method is the current standard. Conservative treatment is costly, and the risk of a secondary rupture remains. This is because CT does not provide any direct information about vascular injuries within the organ. This means that the risk of secondary bleeding by progressive hematoma development cannot be reliably identified (Mirvis et al. 1989). Occasionally, in less than 5%, even grade I or II splenic injuries bear a risk of delayed rupture (Shanmuganathan et al. 2000). Classification of spleen traumas according to CT morphology alone is thus to some extent unreliable for a conservative approach. Angiographic examination of the vascular architecture is useful here (Table 25.1). It primarily offers the possibility of simultaneous interventional hemostasis. Even after embolization of the main branch of the splenic artery, splenic function is retained as a result of the

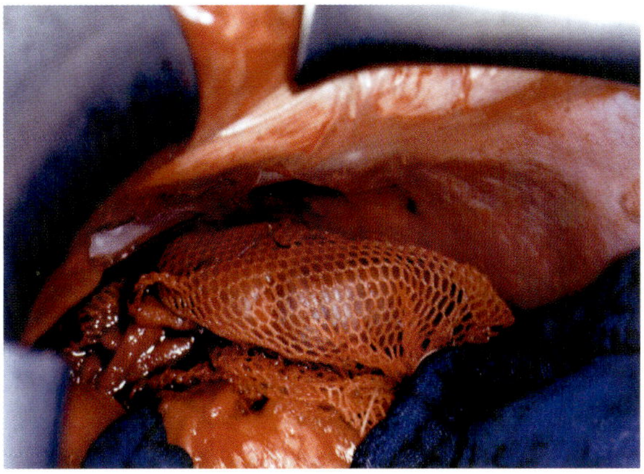

Fig. 25.2. Parenchymal wrapping is a suitable form of surgical, spleen-preserving treatment for grade III injuries

Table 25.1. Angiographic signs of parenchymal trauma and criteria for embolization

1	Extravasation of contrast medium, particularly beyond the organ boundaries
2	Extravasation in the parenchyma
3	Abnormal vascular architecture without detectable extravasation (as in laceration of terminal arteries of the superior, inferior, or middle segment) or fairly large arteriovenous fistulas
4	Irregular avascular areas or inhomogeneous contrast medium, e.g., Seurat pattern (dots of contrast medium)
5	Indirect signs of a subcapsular hematoma (vascular obstruction)

collateral vessels via the gastroepiploic and left gastric arteries. This procedure increases the safety of nonoperative management, allows intrasplenic vascular injuries to be diagnosed, and shows bleeding activity. The rate of conservative spleen-preserving operations might also be able to be further increased using this interventional technique (Cocanour et al. 1998; Davis et al. 1998). Even patients who have to undergo laparotomy due to other injuries should benefit from this preoperative embolization. Hagiwara et al. reported successful angiographic treatment in 93% of patients for whom this form of treatment was chosen (Hagiwara et al. 1996). The duration of hospitalization and the length of time that patients are unfit for work are also decreased. However, prospective studies are required to show whether this procedure can establish itself as a widespread method in the first stage of treatment.

It would be desirable to have a classification system that shows whether a spleen injury has to be monitored using imaging procedures, whether embolization of a segmental artery or the main branch of the splenic artery is indicated, or whether surgical treatment is the safest form of therapy. In future, multislice CT with three-dimensional reconstruction might make this possible.

25.2.3.3 Pancreas and Duodenum

The incidence of traumatic pancreas injury as part of an abdominal trauma is reported as being 3%–12% (Glancy 1989; Nelson et al. 1994; Jurkovich 1996). In a comprehensive patient register, 67% of the pancreatic injuries were caused by penetrating traumas, and 37% occurred in a blunt abdominal trauma. The mortality rate was 16.6%, and the complication rate 42% (Akhrass et al. 1997).

Injury to the pancreas by blunt force rarely occurs alone. Concomitant injuries such as hepatic, splenic, gastric, vascular, renal, or thoracic occur in approximately 70% of the patients. Pancreatic injury is usually due to the effect of sagittal, blunt force against the abdomen and frequently occurs in conjunction with duodenal, bile duct, and liver injuries for the proximal pancreas or with splenic lesions for the distal pancreas. In patients with renal injuries, a concomitant pancreatic injury should also be considered. In most cases, the mechanism of injury is massive blunt force directed against the epigastric region. The pancreas is pressed against the spine and is lacerated at the level of the superior mesenteric vessels. Children and adolescents more frequently sustain this type of injury. The fact that they have less peripancreatic fatty tissue may play a role, as this tissue protects adults against injury. The high morbidity and mortality rate in patients with pancreatic trauma is due to the concomitant injuries and late septic complications. Thus patients with pancreas trauma often die within the first 48 h as a result of the blood loss caused by extrapancreatic injuries. Injuries to the major pancreatic duct and pancreas injuries that are not initially recognized are the cause of secondary morbidity and mortality. Severe septic complications play a central role here. Early recognition of this type of injury is therefore decisive. Serum amylase assay is not suitable for showing the presence of a pancreas trauma. It has a sensitivity of only 50% and the amylase value does not correlate with the size of the injury. CT scanning remains the diagnostic method of choice for blunt pancreatic and duodenal injuries because of its sensitivity in detecting retroperitoneal fluid or free air and in visualizing the pancreas. A classification system was proposed (Moore et al. 1990). However, the sensitivity of the examination is only 62.5%, as shown by Bigattini et al. (1999) in a retrospective study. The authors looked through their CT images again and were able to recognize two-thirds of the injuries that were not initially diagnosed, thus showing that the sensitivity can be increased by using good CT protocols and by accurately interpreting the images. CT does not provide reliable evidence of injury to the major pancreatic duct, particularly when used soon after the injury. Scans should be performed using both oral and i.v. contrast. In a study conducted by Bradley et al. (1998), a significant correlation was found between pancreas-specific morbidity and injury to the duct of Wirsung. If a grade I or II injury is shown on CT or if a pancreas trauma is suspected, the integrity of the main pancreatic duct should be verified by endoscopic retrograde pancreatography (ERP). In certain patients, a stent can be placed over the injured portion of the duct during the same session (Canty and Weinman 2001). The specific treatment of pancreatic injuries primarily depends on two factors: the presence or absence of major pancreatic duct injury and the anatomical location of the injury (Bradley et al. 1998). If a pancreatic injury is suspected on CT, conservative treatment approaches are rare and surgical exploration is usually indicated because the extent of injury cannot be reliably estimated using CT and also due to the high incidence of concomitant injuries. Pancreatic contusion and minor superficial lacerations without duct injury can be treated by drainage alone, which is left in place until the secretion stops. Complications include pancreatic fistulas, pancreatic pseudocysts, and pancreatitis. Other surgical procedures include distal pancreatectomy for major pancreatic duct laceration at or to the left of the superior mesenteric vessels, pancreatorrhaphy, internal drainage, and proximal resection. The procedure depends on the intraoperative findings. Classification according to CT morphology is therefore of secondary importance. If, in the future, precise evaluation of pancreas trauma becomes possible using new imaging procedures such as multislice CT, three-dimensional reconstruction, or magnetic resonance pancreatography (MRP), it is conceivable that minor organ injuries can be treated conservatively more safely.

25.2.3.4 Gallbladder

Gallbladder trauma is rare. It often occurs in conjunction with liver or duodenal injury. The mechanism of injury is the effect of force on the full gallbladder and responsible for gallbladder contusion, rupture, or avulsion. Here, surgical treatment by cholecystectomy with ligature of the cystic duct is always necessary (Parks and Diamond 1995).

25.2.3.5 Intestine and Mesentery

Contusions or traction injuries to the bowel may occur in blunt abdominal trauma patients, causing full-thickness tears or perforations, devascularizing mesenteric injuries, or full-thickness bowel wall ischemic injury. It is difficult to establish a reliable diagnosis of intestinal or mesenteric injury in patients with blunt abdominal trauma. Early diagnosis and treatment are important in order to reduce morbidity and mortality in these patients. Due to septic complications, enterorrhexis that is initially overlooked is associated with a high mortality rate of over 60% in multiple-trauma patients (Nast-Kolb et al. 1993). In the emergency room, CT is the imaging method of choice to assess the gastrointestinal tract. The sensitivity of CT for blunt intestinal injuries may be improved by closing scrutinizing scans for what may be more subtle signs of injury. These include unexplained free peritoneal fluid, mesenteric "streaking" or "stranding" consistent with blood, unexplained thickening in the intestinal wall, free air, and gastrointestinal contrast extravasation. Butela et al. (2001) report a sensitivity of 64%, an accuracy of 82%, and a specificity of 97% for CT in recognizing intestinal injuries after blunt trauma. An intestinal or mesenteric injury is present in 5% of patients who undergo laparotomy due to blunt abdominal trauma (Novelline et al. 1999). Small-bowel injuries are known to occur more frequently in the vicinity of the retroperitoneal ligament attachments at the duodenojejunal or ileocecal transition. If colon injuries occur, the cecum, transverse colon, and sigmoid colon are often involved. In diagnostic terms, this means that particular attention needs to be paid to the aforementioned regions so as not to overlook injuries. Mesenteric injuries are caused by compression or shearing forces. Such lesions are usually small and not able to be diagnosed by CT. However, such injuries may certainly be relevant, as persistent bleeding into the mesentery results in the formation of large hematomas, which compromise intestinal perfusion and lead to intestinal ischemia. Monitoring the course by CT helps to recognize erosive mesenteric bleeding in time, i.e., before it leads to intestinal perforation.

As new indications for nonoperative management of blunt abdominal trauma are continually being added, there needs to be a strong suspicion of rare concomitant injuries. Nance et al. (1997), in a large patient population, pointed out the concomitant hollow viscus injuries in patients with injuries to the solid organs, namely the liver, spleen, pancreas, and kidneys. Thus, in patients with injuries to the parenchymal organs, a hollow viscus perforation was also present in 7.3%. If two organs were involved, this increased to 15.4%, and if three were involved to 34.4%. The authors concluded that injury to several parenchymal organs, particularly if the pancreas was involved, or a single injury with an Abbreviated Injury Scale score of 6 or higher was associated with an increased rate of hollow viscus perforation. They advocate early surgical intervention in patients with injuries such as these. Due to local contusion, segmental resection is usually necessary in traumatic intestinal perforation that is initially recognized. Direct suture is only used in exceptional cases, such as in duodenal perforation recognized initially. Later, the risk of suture breakdown is too high, and a bypass procedure is therefore also indicated in patients with duodenal injuries (Lucas and Legerwood 1975).

In order to avoid putting patients at risk, reliable determination of the absence or presence of hollow viscus injury would be desirable. If there are CT signs suggesting the presence of intestinal injury, such as intestinal discontinuity, extraluminal oral contrast medium, intraabdominal air, retroperitoneal air, or free fluid, surgery is clearly indicated. Intestinal injuries that can be treated conservatively, such as intestinal contusion or shearing off of mucus, cannot be reliably identified by CT (Brody et al. 2000). In patients with unreliable signs of intestinal injury, such as intramural air, thickening of the intestinal wall, and little free fluid, which cannot be identified as signs of other entities, the course should be monitored within the space of a few hours. The indication for surgical exploration should be interpreted broadly.

25.2.3.6 Kidneys

Progress has been made in the diagnosis and management of kidney trauma in recent years. Thus, in the past, minor kidney injuries were treated conservatively, whereas higher-grade injuries were usually treated surgically. Progress in the assessment of injuries by the use of imaging procedures, particularly CT, has changed the procedure followed in patients with higher-grade kidney trauma. These injuries are now often treated conservatively also.

Imaging is indicated in all trauma patients with micro- and macrohematuria, after blunt force to the abdomen, and in severe deceleration injuries. US is the method of choice here. The reliability of US in the primary diagnosis of blunt kidney traumas was confirmed by Jakse and Madersbacher (1977), among others. The injury may involve the renal parenchyma, the excretory system, and/or vascular supply. The criteria for the classification of kidney injury are based on morphological and radiological signs. The classification initially proposed by Moore et al. (1989) is in widespread use. Some 90% of all kidney traumas are caused by blunt force (Miller and McAninch 1995). CT is the most sensitive method for accurate diagnosis and classification of renal injuries. After administration of contrast medium, images are taken during the arterial phase, the tubular phase, and finally the excretory phase. A conventional plain abdominal radiograph is then taken to obtain an excretory urogram. Rupture of the renal arteries is usually the result of an anteroposterior or cephalocaudal deceleration trauma. The artery is overstretched or twisted. This results in intimal tears with arterial thrombosis. The right renal artery is less vulnerable, as it is stabilized by the duodenum and the inferior vena cava. Two-thirds of injuries to the renal arteries are to the left renal artery (Letsou and Gusberg 1990). In patients with injuries to the renal arteries, no or only minimal renal perfusion is seen on CT. This may be due to arterial thrombosis, arterial avulsion, or severe angiospasm after arterial contusion. The treatment recommendations, which are based on the severity of the kidney injury, can only be applied without limitation in patients with isolated trauma. Treatment of kidney polytrauma is determined by the overall picture and the priorities of the injuries in each case. Less severe kidney injuries graded I, II, and III do not require surgical treatment. Even grade IV injuries may be treated conservatively if the patient is hemodynamically stable (Matthews et al. 1997). Conservative treatment includes bed rest, creatinine and blood count monitoring, monitoring of vital signs, and repeated examinations by US and, where necessary, CT. Altman et al. (2000) published their experience with the conservative treatment of grade V injuries. Precise additional information about the type of kidney injury is necessary here, including the extent of parenchymal injury, the proportion of devascularized parenchyma, the presence of an injury to the renal pelvis with extravasation, and the size of the retroperitoneal hematoma. If there is more than 25% devascularized parenchyma, reasons to suspect urinary extravasation, extensive parenchymal injury, or a large retroperitoneal hematoma, surgical treatment is recommended (McAninch 1993; Carroll et al. 1994). Generally speaking, a conservative approach can only be used in isolated patients.

The question as to what type of injury and therapeutic approach encourage the development of hypertension cannot be answered with certainty. However, Cass et al. emphasize the considerable risk of secondary hypertension after the nonsurgical management of deep parenchymal lacerations (Cass et al. 1987).

The contralateral kidney should always be assessed before surgery is performed. This once again emphasizes the significance of CT as a diagnostic tool. Patients are operated on if there is persistent bleeding, if the patient is hemodynamically unstable, or if injury to the vascular stalk is suspected. In such cases, angiography provides information about the localization of the lesion for the purposes of preoperative planning. Injuries to renal parenchyma with urinary extravasation do not necessarily need to be repaired by open surgery. Urinary drainage via a double J-stent ensures that urine is discharged and reduces the urinoma and the risk of secondary infection. Matthews et al. (1997) showed that leakage ceased spontaneously in 90% of such injuries. Conservative treatment is therefore a safe treatment option even in patients with severe kidney injury. If concomitant injuries to the abdominal hollow viscera or the pancreas are present, there is an increased risk that an infected urinoma will develop. In patients with intestinal injury, surgery is unavoidable. ROSEN and MCANINCH (1994) reported on successful conservative treatment in patients with combined kidney and pancreas injuries.

Selective embolization has been described as a treatment option in patients with intrarenal arterial injury (CALARN et al. 1996; STEFFENS et al. 1996; KRAMER et al. 1998; PINTO and CHIMENO 1998). Surgery can thus very probably be avoided.

Concerning surgical technique, a transperitoneal approach and an early search for the vascular pedicle together with temporary clamping make it easier to control bleeding. This increases the likelihood of being able to preserve the organ. During débridement, care should be taken to spare the fibrous capsule. Peritoneum or greater omentum can be used to cover the defect. Good results have been obtained by encasing the kidneys with a Vicryl net. In conjunction with fibrin glue, even multiple ruptures can thus be repaired without parenchymal sutures.

25.2.3.7
Urinary Bladder

The bladder is involved in about 5% of cases of blunt abdominal trauma. As a result of sudden blunt force, intraperitoneal ruptures occur when the bladder is full, the most common site being the roof or the posterior wall of the bladder. If there is a concomitant pelvic fracture, the risk of injury increases to 10%. In such cases, extraperitoneal perforation is most common, caused by penetrating fragments of the pubic bone. Imaging can be performed to distinguish between an extraperitoneal rupture, which accounts for 80%–90% of urinary bladder injuries, an intraperitoneal rupture seen in 15%–20% of cases, and a combined injury which occurs in up to 12% (NOVELLINE et al. 1999).

Before a plain radiograph or CT scan is taken, the urinary bladder is filled retrogradely with contrast medium. If contrast medium enters the Retzius space, a definite diagnosis of extraperitoneal rupture can be made. It may also spread between the rectum and the sacrum. If it spreads into the abdominal wall, this may be misinterpreted as a rupture of the abdominal wall. If the diagnosis is made by plain radiography, a post voiding radiograph must also be obtained, as a small amount of extravasation may be concealed behind the contrast medium-filled urinary bladder and might thus be overlooked. Intraperitoneal bladder rupture constitutes an absolute indication for surgery. After débridement of the bladder flaps, the bladder wall is closed using single button sutures in two rows. Involvement of the ureter should in principle be ruled out intraoperatively.

Small extraperitoneal injuries to the bladder can be treated conservatively after urinary drainage by a urinary catheter which has been inserted. Larger injuries require surgical repair.

25.3
Retroperitoneal Hematomas and Vascular Injuries

Traumatic retroperitoneal hematomas, while not strictly intraabdominal injuries, may be associated with major hemorrhage, with and without surgically repairable lesions. The most frequent cause of such hematomas are spinal and pelvic injuries. Other mechanisms include compression and laceration of retroperitoneal organs by blunt force. Opinion differs as to the optimal treatment strategy. An important criterion in the decision between surgical and conservative treatment is the localization of the retroperitoneal hematoma. The retroperitoneal space is divided into a central, flank, and pelvic region (SELIVANOV et al. 1984; SCHUMPELICK et al. 1999):

- Central region:
  All hematomas that develop in this region have to be explored, as they are caused by injury to the aorta, the vena cava, the hepatic veins, the pancreas, or the duodenum.
- Flank region:
  Retroperitoneal hematomas of the flank region are usually caused by kidney injuries. The indication for surgery depends on the extent of the kidney injury. Most kidney injuries are treated conservatively.
- Pelvic region:
  Pelvic hematomas are usually the result of venous hemorrhage due to a pelvic and/or spinal injury. Operative exploration should be avoided if possible, as the tamponade of the compartment falls off after opening, surgical control is rarely possible, and exploratory decompression of the hematoma may exacerbate hemorrhage leading to early, potentially preventable mortality. Stabilization of the pelvis using a pelvic clamp or an external fixator leads to compression of the sources of venous hemorrhage and hence usually to cessation of bleeding. If bleeding cannot be arrested by this method, angiography can be performed to obtain

information about the source of bleeding. In rare cases, there is isolated arterial bleeding, which can be embolized after superselective visualization (AGOLINI et al. 1997).

As the risk of bleeding increases after the retroperitoneal space has been opened due to the tamponade being removed, conservative treatment should be preferred. This only applies to patients in whom laparotomy is not otherwise indicated. If the retroperitoneal hematomas penetrate intraperitoneally, this leads to the problem that free intraperitoneal fluid imitates an intraperitoneal source of bleeding. The main objective of primary extirpation of retroperitoneal hepatomas is to rule out the presence of injuries to larger vessels and retroperitoneal organs. Particularly at central sites and in the renal area, fairly large amounts of blood may be lost during the procedure.

25.4 Combined Injuries

25.4.1 Combined Abdominopelvic Injuries

As a result of the large amount of energy involved in such accidents, pelvic ring fractures are often associated with injuries to intraabdominal organs. Due to the complex anatomical structure of the pelvis, pelvic injuries present a challenge in terms of diagnosis and treatment. This applies both to pelvic ring fractures and acetabular fractures. From a traumatological point of view, the main focus is always on the fracture localization, the stability of the anatomical unit, and the fragment dislocation. However, concomitant injuries also have to be adequately recorded and assessed. Both conventional X-ray and tomography can be used for this purpose.

In patients with pelvic ring injury, the issue of stability, in particular, has the highest priority. In principle, a distinction can be made between stable and unstable injuries, and unstable injuries can be further divided into injuries with rotatory and translatory instability. In rotatory instability injuries, at least half of the pelvis can rotate externally or internally as a result of the injury. However, the pelvis is stable in the vertical, i.e., craniocaudal direction. In contrast, in translatory instability injuries, both the bones and the ligaments of half of the pelvis are almost completely separated from the rest of the pelvis and dislocation is therefore possible in all directions. If, in addition, the neurovascular bundle of the affected limb is lacerated at the level of the pelvis, this is referred to as a traumatic hemipelvectomy.

In addition to a plain anteroposterior pelvic radiograph, conventional radiographs of pelvic ring injuries also include special views such as inlet and outlet views. The plain pelvic radiograph is the primary standard examination. It provides an initial overview of the injury. However, the pelvis is tipped in relation to the imaging plane, which leads to considerable overlapping and artifacts, and this considerably limits the usefulness of the radiograph, particularly in the area of the posterior pelvic ring. Special pelvic inlet and outlet views may fill a diagnostic gap here. Both types of image are particularly used to assess the course of a fracture and fragment dislocation in the dorsal parts of the pelvis. The inlet view provides information about the dorsoventral, and the outlet view about the craniocaudal displacement of fragments. Since the X-ray tube has to be tipped by 45° to the imaging plane in both views and hence the thickness of the imaged tissue considerably increases, these views soon come up against limits, particularly in corpulent patients, but also in multiple-system injuries. This is one of the reasons why they have increasingly been replaced by CT in recent years. This method not only allows the bony injuries to the pelvic ring to be visualized precisely, it also provides reliable information about any concomitant injuries including penetrating perineal injuries, rectal tears, or subprostatic urethral disruption. This is the only way to avoid septic complications as a result of severe concomitant injuries to the perineum or rectum in time by performing discontinuity surgery by a Hartmann procedure. With good anatomical knowledge and by paying attention to the symmetry of bone structures that exists under normal circumstances, CT can be used to obtain a precise idea of stability, fragment location, and fragment dislocation. In many cases, even the mechanism of injury can be reconstructed without anamnestic details. Other tomographic methods, such as magnetic resonance imaging (MRI), currently offer little additional information for the assessment of pelvic ring injuries, even though they allow the ligamentous structures of the pelvis to be clearly visualized.

25.4.2 Combined Thoracoabdominal Injuries

Injuries to the diaphragm occur in nearly 3% of blunt abdominal injuries. The size of the injury varies between clinically insignificant lacerations to the right half of the diaphragm and complete laceration of the diaphragm. In patients with rupture of the left diaphragm, the loosely fixed organs such as the stomach, colon, spleen, and small bowel may be displaced into the pectoral cavity. Progressive respiratory compromise may occur as a result of progressive herniation of the viscera into the chest caused by the negative thoracoabdominal pressure gradient. For this reason, and because there are often associated intraabdominal injuries, diaphragmatic rupture should be regarded as a true surgical emergency requiring immediate operation under most circumstances. If the pericardial part is lacerated, cardiac hernias have been described (Van Loenhout et al. 1986; Van Brussel et al. 2000). If abdominal organs are displaced into the thorax, a diaphragmatic rupture may be suspected even on a plain thorax radiograph, but radiographs may be completely normal in as many as 50% of patients. A definitive diagnosis can be made if the chest X-ray shows a gastric bubble in the left chest or a nasogastric tube positioned above the left diaphragm. CT reinforces the diagnosis here. On the other hand, if there is no herniation of abdominal organs into the thorax, the diaphragmatic rupture is quite often overlooked even with spiral CT (Scaglione et al. 2000). If the clinical findings suggest an acute diaphragmatic rupture, the injury is repaired using a transabdominal approach due to the frequency of associated intraabdominal injuries. In exceptional cases of hemodynamically stable patients with no concomitant injuries, laparoscopy may be useful (Murray et al. 1998; Meyer et al. 2000).

25.5 Conclusion

Blunt abdominal trauma is the main cause of abdominal trauma seen in Europe. It often occurs in polytrauma patients. In addition to severe craniocerebral traumas, massive abdominal hemorrhage is the most common cause of death within the first few hours. In unstable patients, priority should therefore be given to immediate blood transfusion and rapid diagnosis of the free intraperitoneal fluid by US. Laparotomy is subsequently performed without any further diagnostic imaging tools. US is the standard examination in blunt abdominal trauma. In patients with a stable circulation, it is supplemented by CT for diagnostic purposes. In order to obtain reliable results, oral, rectal, and intravenous administration of contrast medium is absolutely necessary. Angiography may be indicated in special cases. In patients with isolated injury to parenchymal organs, a conservative approach is reasonable if the patient's circulation remains stable and the need for transfusion does not increase. Hollow viscus injuries require surgical repair. If little free fluid is found without this being shown to be due to an organ injury, an intestinal and/or mesenteric injury that was not established by CT should be considered. Monitoring of the course is recommended within 6 h in all cases. However, the indication for laparotomy should be interpreted broadly in multiple system injuries or unstable patients. Hollow viscus and pancreas injuries present a diagnostic problem. If they are initially recognized, surgical treatment is usually unproblematic and few complications occur.

References

Agolini SF, Shah K, Jaffe J et al (1997) Arterial embolization is a rapid and effective technique for controlling pelvic fracture hemorrhage. J Trauma 43:395–399

Akhrass R, Yaffe MB, Brandt CP et al (1997) Pancreatic trauma: a ten-year multi-institutional experience. Am Surg 63:598–604

Allins A, Ho T, Nguyen TH et al (1996) Limited value of routine follow-up CT scans in nonoperative management of blunt liver and splenic injuries. Am Surg 62:883–886

Altman AL, Haas C, Dinchman KH et al (2000) Selective nonoperative treatment of blunt grade 5 renal injury. J Urol 164:27–31

Anderson ID, Irving MH (1990) The investigation of abdominal trauma. Arch Emerg Med 7:1–8

Asher W, Parvin S, Virgilio R et al (1976) Echographic evaluation of splenic injury after blunt trauma. Radiology 118: 411–415

Bardenheuer M, Obertacke U, Waydhas C, Nast-Kolb D (2000) Epidemiology of the severely injured patient. A prospective assessment of preclinical and clinical management. AG polytrauma of DGU. Unfallchirurg 103:355–363

Bigattini D, Boverie JH, Dondelinger RF (1999) CT of blunt trauma of the pancreas in adults. Eur Radiol 9:244–249

Bradley EL III, Young PR, Chang MC (1998) Diagnosis and initial treatment of blunt pancreatic trauma: a multi-institutional review. Ann Surg 227:861–869

Brasel KJ, Delisle CM, Olson CJ et al (1997) Trends in the management of hepatic injury. Am J Surg 174:674–677

Brody JM, Leighton DB, Murphy BL et al (2000) CT of blunt trauma bowel and mesenteric injury: typical findings and pitfalls in diagnosis. Radiographics 20:1525–1536

Bühne KH, Zügel N, Mayr E, Häuser H (2001) Routine abdominal sonography and computed tomography in multiple trauma patients. Chirurg 72:43–48

Butela ST, Federle MP, Chang PJ et al (2001) Performance of CT in detection of bowel injury. AJR 176:129–135

Calarn P, Nonent M, Fournier G et al (1996) Endovascular treatment of traumatic and iatrogenic intrarenal arterial lesions by microcoil embolization. Ann Radiol 39:234–239

Canty TG, Weinman G (2001) Treatment of pancreatic duct disruption in children by an endoscopically placed stent. J Pediatr Surg 36:345–348
Carroll PR, McAninch JW, Wong A et al (1994) Outcome after temporary vascular occlusion for the management of renal trauma. J Urol 141:1171–1173
Cass AS, Luxenberg M, Gleich P (1987) Long-term results of conservative and surgical management of blunt renal lacerations. Br J Urol 59:17–20
Ciraulo DL, Nikkanen HE, Palter M et al (1996) Clinical analysis of the utility of repeat computed tomographic scan before discharge in blunt hepatic injury. J Trauma 41:821–824
Ciraulo DL, Luk S, Palter M et al (1998) Selective hepatic arterial embolization of grade IV and V blunt hepatic injuries: an extension of resuscitation in the nonoperative management of traumatic hepatic injuries. J Trauma 45:353–358
Cocanour CS, Moore FA, Ware DN et al (1998) Delayed complications of nonoperative management of blunt adult splenic trauma. Arch Surg 133:619–624
Davis JW, Hoyt DB, McArdle MS et al (1992) An analysis of errors causing morbidity and mortality in a trauma system: a guide for quality improvement. J Trauma 32:660–665
Davis KA, Fabian TC, Croce MA et al (1998) Improved success in nonoperative management of blunt splenic injuries: embolization of splenic artery pseudoaneurysms. J Trauma 44:1008–1013
Denton JR, Moore G, Coldwell DM et al (1997) Multimodality treatment for grade V hepatic injuries: perihepatic packing, arterial embolization, and venous stenting. J Trauma 42:964–967
El Mouaaouy A, Zittel TT, Becker D (1991) Blunt abdominal trauma: differential diagnosis of splenic lobulation and splenic rupture. Ultraschall Med 12:91–94
Enderson BL, Maull KI (1991) Missed injuries. The trauma surgeon's nemesis. Surg Clin North Am 71:399–418
Ertel W, Trentz O (1996) Blunt and penetrating abdominal trauma. Patient assessment algorithm and principles for management. Unfallchirurg 99:288–303
Feliciano DV, Mattox KL, Burch JM et al (1986) Packing for control of hepatic hemorrhage. J Trauma 26:738–743
Feussner H, Papaziogas W, Siewert JR (1999) Modern diagnostic workup of blunt abdominal trauma. Chirurg 70:1246–1254
Froelich W, Simeone J, McKusick K et al (1982) Radionuclide imaging and ultrasound in liver and spleen trauma – a prospective comparison. Radiology 145:457–461
Glancy KE (1989) Review of pancreatic trauma. West J Med 151:45–51
Hagiwara A, Yukioka T, Ohta S et al (1996) Nonsurgical management of patients with blunt splenic injury: efficacy of transcatheter arterial embolization. AJR 167:159–166
Hagiwara A, Yukioka T, Ohta S et al (1997) Nonsurgical management of patients with blunt hepatic injury: efficacy of transcatheter arterial embolization. AJR 169:1151–1156
Harper HC, Maull KI (2000) Transcatheter arterial embolization in blunt hepatic trauma. South Med J 93:663–665
Jakse G, Madersbacher H (1977) Winter sports injuries of the urogenital tract. Urologe A 16:315–319
Jurkovich GJ (1996) Injuries to the duodenum and pancreas. In: Feliciano DV, Moore EE, Mattox KL (eds) Trauma, 3rd edn. Appleton and Lange, Stamford, pp 573–594
Kramer SC, Gorich J, Rilinger N et al (1998) The percutaneous transarterial embolization therapy of traumatic kidney hemorrhages. ROFO 169:297–301
Kremer B, Henne-Bruns D (1993) Value of various techniques in liver rupture. Chirurg 64:852–859
Letsou GV, Gusberg R (1990) Isolated bilateral renal artery thrombosis: an unusual consequence of blunt abdominal trauma. J Trauma 30:509–511
Lucas CE, Legerwood AM (1975) Factors influencing outcome after blunt duodenal injury. J Trauma 15:839–846
Matthews LA, Smith EM, Spirnak JP (1997) Nonoperative treatment of major blunt renal lacerations with urinary extravasation. J Urol 157:2056–2058
McAninch JW (1993) Editorial: renal trauma. J Urol 150:1778
McKenney MG, McKenney KL, Compton RP et al (1998) Can surgeons evaluate emergency ultrasound scans for blunt abdominal trauma? J Trauma 44:649–653
Meyer G, Huttl TP, Hatz RA et al (2000) Laparoscopic repair of traumatic diaphragmatic hernias. Surg Endosc 14:1010–1014
Miller KS, McAninch JW (1995) Radiographic assessment of renal trauma: our 15-year experience. J Urol 154:352–355
Mirvis SE, Whitley NO, Gens DR (1989) Blunt splenic trauma in adults: CT-based classification and correlation with prognosis and treatment. Radiology 171:33–39
Moore EE, Shackford SR, Pachter HL et al (1989) Organ injury scaling: spleen, liver and kidney. J Trauma 29:1664
Moore EE, Cogbill TH, Malagoni MA et al (1990) Organ injury scaling. II. Pancreas, duodenum, small bowel, colon, and rectum. J Trauma 30:1427–1429
Moore EE, Cogbill TH, Jurkovich GJ et al (1995) Organ injury scaling: spleen and liver (1994 revision). J Trauma 38: 323–324
Murray JA, Demetriades D, Asensio JA et al (1998) Occult injuries to the diaphragm: prospective evaluation of laparoscopy in penetrating injuries to the left lower chest. J Am Coll Surg 187:626–630
Nance ML, Peden GW, Shapiro MB et al (1997) Solid viscus injury predicts hollow viscus injury in blunt abdominal trauma. J Trauma 43:618–622
Nast-Kolb D, Waydhas C, Kastl S et al (1993) The role of an abdominal injury in follow-up of polytrauma patients. Chirurg 64:552–559
Nast-Kolb D, Waydhas C, Kanz KG et al (1994) An algorithm for management of shock in polytrauma. Unfallchirurg 97: 292–302
Nast-Kolb D, Trupka A, Ruchholtz S, Schweiberer L (1998) Abdominal trauma. Unfallchirurg 101:82–91
Nelson MG, Jones DR, Vasilakis A et al (1994) Computed tomographic diagnosis of acute blunt pancreatic transection. W V Med J 90:274–278
Novelline RA, Rhea JT, Bell T (1999) Helical CT of abdominal trauma. Radiol Clin North Am 37:591–612
Parks RW, Diamond T (1995) Non-surgical trauma to extrahepatic biliary tract. Br J Surg 82:1303–1310
Pinto IT, Chimeno PC (1998) Treatment of a urinoma and a post-traumatic pseudoaneurysm using selective arterial embolization. Cardiovasc Intervent Radiol 21:506–508
Ringe P, Pichlmayr R (1995) Total hepatectomy and liver transplantation: a life-saving procedure in patients with severe hepatic trauma. Br J Surg 82:837–839
Rosen MA, McAninch JW (1994) Management of combined renal and pancreatic trauma. J Urol 152:22–25
Scaglione M, Pinto F, Grasi R et al (2000) Diagnostic sensitivity of computerized tomography in closed trauma of the diaphragm. Retrospective study of 35 consecutive cases. Radiol Med (Torino) 99:46–50

Schumpelick V, Ambacher T, Riesener KP (1999) Current therapy of injuries of the colon and retroperitoneum. Chirurg 70:1269–1277

Schurink GW, Bode PJ, van Luijt PA et al (1997) The value of physical examination in the diagnosis of patients with blunt abdominal trauma: a retrospective study. Injury 28:261–265

Selivanov V, Chi HS, Alverdy JC et al (1984) Mortality in retroperitoneal hematoma. J Trauma 24:1022–1027

Shackford SR, MacKersie RC, Holbroock T et al (1993) The epidemiology of trauma death: a population-based analysis. Arch Surg 128:571–575

Shanmuganathan K, Mirvis SE, Boyd-Kranis R et al (2000) Nonsurgical management of blunt splenic injury: use of CT criteria to select patients for splenic arteriography and potential endovascular therapy. Radiology 217:75–82

Sherck J, Shatney C, Sensaki K, Selivanov V (1994) The accuracy of computed tomography in the diagnosis of blunt small-bowel perforation. Am J Surg 168:670–675

Singh G, Arya N, Safaya R et al (1997) Role of ultrasonography in blunt abdominal trauma. Injury 28:667–670

Smith RS, Kern SJ, Fry WR et al (1998) Institutional learning curve of surgeon-performed trauma ultrasound. Arch Surg 133:530–535

Steffens MG, Bode PJ, Lycklama A, Nijeholt AA et al (1996) Selective embolization of pseudo-aneurysms of the renal artery after blunt abdominal injury in a patient with a single kidney. Injury 27:219–220

Sugimoto K, Horiike S, Hirata M et al (1994) The role of angiography in the assessment of blunt liver injury. Injury 25: 283–287

Udekwu PO, Gurkin B, Oller DW (1996) The use of computed tomography in blunt abdominal injuries. Am Surg 62:56–59

Van Brussel JP, Vlees WJ, Leenen LP (2000) Luxatio cordis in blunt-trauma thoraco-abdominal injuries. Ned Tijdschr Geneeskd 144:1073–1075

Van Loenhout RM, Schiphorst TJ, Wittens CH (1986) Traumatic intrapericardial diaphragmatic hernia. J Trauma 26:271–275

Wachsberg RH (1999) The right transversus abdominis muscle: an ultrasonographic mimic of free peritoneal fluid. Emerg Radiol 6:81–84

Weill F, Rohmer P, Didier D et al (1988) Ultrasound of the traumatized spleen – left butterfly sign in lesions masked by echogenic blood clots. Gastrointest Radiol 13:169–172

Yoshii H, Sato M, Yamamoto S et al (1998) Usefulness and limitations of ultrasonography in the initial evaluation of blunt abdominal trauma. J Trauma 45:45–50

26 Medicolegal Aspects in Trauma Imaging

A. K. Dixon

CONTENTS

- Look at all CT images, at all settings, on an electronic workstation.
- Discuss all serious findings urgently with clinical colleagues.
- Keep a close check on quality control in imaging for trauma.

26.1 Introduction

All aspects of medicine are now open to enquiry from both within and without the profession; emergency medicine is no exception. Indeed, because of the increased power of journalism, patients admitted with abdominal trauma are frequently reported in local and even national newspapers, which then expect daily official bulletins about progress. Thus the outcome of the patient, favorable and unfavorable, is very much in the public eye.

A. K. Dixon, MD
Department of Radiology, Addenbrooke's Hospital and the University of Cambridge, Hills Road, Cambridge CB2 2QQ, UK

Against this background, the increasing questioning of standards within the medical profession offers little comfort. There have been numerous recent scandals in every country where some aspect of medical care has been found below acceptable standards. The medical profession can no longer hide in complex technical jargon and secrecy. Patients, journalists, and lawyers can all search for reports of optimal practice, for example by searching the Internet or reading this book, and come to some opinion as to whether the care delivered was adequate or not.

Because abdominal trauma warranting hospital admission is usually serious, and often associated with other trauma such as cranial or musculoskeletal, the long-term consequences for the patient and society can be enormous. A patient in an automobile accident who is off work for 6 months and can then only return to work in a less well paid job might be able to claim large sums in compensation, much of which will be met from insurance of some kind.

And lawyers will be there to assist and maximize or, for the defense, minimize those claims. Because the sums involved are large, there will be attempts to pass on some of the costs to the medical system, either the hospital or practitioner, wherever possible. Hence the need for all those involved in the care of the patient to be aware these aspects. In any event, it is important to deliver the best possible care to every patient. Consideration and awareness of likely problems go a long way to deliver to the best possible care.

26.1.1 Differences in Various Countries

It is beyond the scope of this chapter to detail all possible variations in health and legal care for the inhabitants of every country. However, it is worth considering various options which may influence management at different moments in the care of the patient.

There is wide variation in the way in which countries view the so-called Good Samaritan act of helping a patient with abdominal trauma before admission to hospital – and all doctors should make sure that their cover for this type of help is sound so that they are free to offer advice and help. Radiologists are not usually well trained in resuscitation and, in industrialized countries, it may be better to leave things to well-trained paramedical emergency personnel, especially when help is close at hand.

Even when ambulances are readily available, there are occasional and somewhat apocryphal stories of staff checking that the insurance of the patient is valid before taking them to certain hospitals! Thankfully, it is now easier for a hospital to treat and then claim reimbursement, where appropriate, later. But this need to claim reimbursement is an important issue because the total care of a patient with trauma may cost tens of thousands of euros. And lifetime care can run into the millions. Even in countries where health care is state funded, e.g., the UK, there are now methods whereby these costs can be recouped, for example, from automobile insurance agencies.

Some counties have enlightened attitudes as to the complex relationships between ill health, accidents and, even, medical misadventure. Their argument is that no one purposefully set out to inflict this damage and thus no individual is at fault. Hence the culture of "no fault compensation," which is set by an independent tribunal on the basis of long-term disability and reduced earning power. Of course, if it can be proved that there was medical negligence, then the doctor in question may face disciplinary measures from the agencies that govern medical standards. New Zealand was one of the first countries to explore such a policy, although some aspects of such policies have had to be revised in recent years.

26.1.2 Standards

The best defense against possible claims for inadequate medical or radiological care is to have agreed protocols and standards for all routine procedures. A regular audit should then be performed to ensure that the protocols are being adhered to and that the standards are being met. In many areas of radiology there are well-developed standards and quality is then assured; for example, many developed countries have well-established breast screening programs where there are known standards including overall accuracy, sensitivity, benign to malignant biopsy rates, etc. For trauma, some of the examinations have to be tailored according to the particular injuries and thus may be one-off procedures. Nevertheless, there are several routine examinations in abdominal trauma, e.g., abdominal CT, where each hospital should have established protocols and the images subjected to audit. In a study from our own hospital, which reviewed CT examinations in liver trauma, there was wide variation in image quality (Padhani et al. 1992); the reasons included machine specification, body habitus, associated injuries, etc. Nevertheless the results from that study led to certain recommendations for subsequent examinations. Ultimately, the individual radiologist's reports should be checked against the gold standard and overall accuracy checked. Problems here relate to the fact that the ultimate gold standard – surgical proof – is rarely available in trauma due to the increasing propensity for conservative management. Surrogate checks on an individual radiologist's reports can be made by dual reporting exercises, but there can be wide variation in radiological opinion even amongst experts (Wakeley et al. 1995; Robinson et al. 1999).

The introduction in Europe of more stringent directives on the use of ionizing radiation (EU Council Directive 1997) also imposes greater imperative for all hospitals to have agreed protocols for all radiological procedures. The new laws, which have been variously adapted by member states, demand considerable responsibility from the institution/employer, the referrer, the practitioner, and the operator. The primary objective is to ensure that ionizing radiation is used with care and in an appropriate fashion. Thus the choice of radiological investigation should be made in accordance with agreed referral criteria/guidelines and knowledge of the associated radiation dose (Royal College of Radiologists 1998). Someone who has been trained in the interpretation of such procedures should document a report of each investigation in the patient's case notes. To take an example, it may not be appropriate to perform CT under sedation/general anesthesia in a child with minor abdominal trauma when the particular clinical question could have been answered by ultrasound; not only is there the potential risk of sedation/anesthesia in an injured child, there is also the theoretical risk of the radiation.

26.2 The Choice of Radiological Investigations

The respective merits of each of the various radiological investigations have been considered in detail in previous chapters. Inevitably there will be some local variation according to expertise, availability of equipment, and funding constraints.

Because of the theoretical risk of ionizing radiation there is likely to be more ultrasound expertise available in centers, which are used to deal with large number of pediatric trauma referrals. Conversely, a center with an extensive adult trauma practice may be so familiar with a protocol for trauma based on CT findings that the pediatric patient is better served by a high-quality CT examination rather than a less sophisticated ultrasound examination, despite the radiation dose. An adult patient may be so obese that ultrasound is unlikely to be rewarding and CT preferred. The patient may have to undergo magnetic resonance (MR)for the spine; it may be sensible to also examine the abdomen by MR at the same time, thereby saving the injured patient yet another move around the hospital site. In all these situations, the reason for the choice of a particular investigation should be recorded in the patient's notes.

A more worrying aspect is when the choice of investigation is influenced by the lack of suitable equipment. All centers handling traumatized patients should have CT equipment on site. However, not all CT systems have equal technical specifications. For example, not all European centers yet have spiral CT facilities, let alone multidetector systems. Clearly there are considerable advantages for the injured patient to have access to the latest technology: the procedure will be quicker and this may be associated with reduced morbidity; the images will be more likely to be obtained during optimal organ opacification.

There may be delays for the patient in getting access to the appropriate imaging investigation. With regards to ultrasound, the expert in assessing the pediatric abdomen may not be immediately at hand; ultrasound is, par excellence, an operator-dependent investigation. Is it better for the patient to undergo an immediate ultrasound investigation by a less experienced operator or to wait for the definitive examination by the expert? And what would a court of law say about the two options?

With regards to CT and MRI, there is often a curious anomaly that it may be quicker to get access during the night or weekend, rather than during the working day when the machines are being used intensively. Relatively few trauma centers enjoy the luxury of an empty CT machine waiting for a patient with abdominal trauma to appear! In well-organized centers, the routine work is temporarily suspended when a patient with major trauma requires access to CT. However, for obvious reasons, such mani of the workload has to be fully justifiable a be impossible (a case under general anesthet have just started). There have been legal case cerning delays before CT following trauma, particularly concerning postoperative complications. In the UK, there have also been several high-profile cases of patients having to be moved in order to get CT at a larger hospital with 24-h CT/MRI cover. Although the smaller hospital may have CT on site, the funding may be insufficient to cover the staffing costs needed to provide a full 24-h, 7-day-a-week service.

It is interesting to speculate who should be liable for the potential complications described above. Is it the health provider for not having 24-h CT available in every hospital and clinic in every town or village: surely not. Is it the hospital for not having a multidetector system: surely not. Is it the competent but relatively inexperienced radiologist for performing an immediate abdominal ultrasound in the knowledge that his pediatric expert colleague will not be available for at least 6 h? What if this obliging radiologist makes a mistake? This leads to the question as to whether the perceived expert should be the only radiologist issuing reports! And in terms of accuracy, 50% of all radiologists will have skills below the median! Will lawyers eventually only support radiologists with proven performance in the top 10%, 25%, 33%, 50% or 75%?

Just occasionally it may be impossible to use the optimal investigation because of particular complexities of the case. The patient may have experienced cardiac damage and required pacing, which is a contraindication to MRI. The patient may then undergo CT or even myelography in order to investigate the spine. The patient may be too obese for the CT gantry or aperture. In all such cases it is important to document the reasons for the alternative investigations and to assess how they may compromise the diagnostic information provided.

26.3 Radiological Techniques and Interpretation

Again the recommended techniques for imaging the various parts of the abdomen and related anatomy have been covered in the preceding individual chapters. Only a few pertinent points will be made relating to the various sections, mainly with respect to problem areas where medicolegal issues could arise.

26.3.1 Plain Radiography

It goes without saying that radiographic technique is paramount here. However, in the stress of the trauma room, with numerous doctors trying to get at various parts of the patient's anatomy simultaneously, it may be extremely difficult for the radiographer to obtain optimal images. And, because of time pressures, mistakes, e.g. right/left mislabeling, are more likely to occur. Furthermore, there is unlikely to be a radiologist in attendance when the images are obtained; therefore the radiographers have to provide their own quality control.

Some radiologists might argue that if the patient is going on to more sophisticated imaging anyway, e.g., CT, there is little point in wasting time with plain radiographs. But if the readily available chest or abdominopelvic radiographs show a life-threatening event, e.g., pneumothorax, it can be promptly dealt with (McLellan et al. 1996). And what would the lawyer say about a system where such conventional radiographs were not obtained and there was a delay before digital views were obtained on the CT system?

26.3.2 Ultrasound

The problems about the operator dependence of ultrasound have already been aired in "The Choice of Radiological Investigations." Also, only those images, which are recorded on hard copy, can be used for subsequent reinterrogation. Even these hard copy images may be difficult to interpret by anyone other than the operator who performed the examination; the operator is the only person who gets a feel for the whole examination, even when a video recording is made. Thus the competence of the operator is paramount and easier to monitor in countries where the majority of abdominal ultrasound examinations are performed under the auspices of a radiology department. In many countries, ultrasound, particularly for trauma, is carried out by a variety of personnel with a range of training and expertise. Although such personnel may become highly skilled in the recognition of the presence of free fluid and some of the more obvious lacerations, it is unlikely that they will become so expert as the full-time ultrasonographer who may be able to recognize subtle signs suggesting duodenal trauma (Shackford et al. 1999).

For the above reasons, there have been relatively few legal claims about erroneous ultrasound reports; they are difficult to prove without clear hard copy images and the defendant can usually claim that good views were not possible because of various reasons such as overlying bowel gas, body habitus, etc.

26.3.3 Computed Tomography

Here the images are available for all to see and comment on in retrospect. This may be a contributing factor to the relatively frequent number of claims concerning CT. By and large, problems with technique are relatively rare. Despite what may be written in leading articles, it is rare that the technique itself will lead to a lesion being missed. One obvious exception relates to opacification of bowel; lesions will generally be easier to identify with good preparation – either with contrast medium (positive) or water (negative); some anesthesiologists are reluctant to distend the stomach and small bowel in patients who might aspirate or need urgent surgery. Another source of error can arise if the liver, or spleen, is not imaged during optimal parenchymal opacification during intravenous enhancement with contrast medium. Perhaps the greatest problems with technique revolve around whether unenhanced images should be performed and how much of the chest should be included for problems related to abdominal trauma and vice versa. A pneumothorax may be evident on CT, which is not apparent on the chest radiograph.

Problems with interpretation are much more common (Cook et al. 1986). Even amongst experts, there will be numerous areas of disagreement. It is important that radiologists look at all images at all settings on the monitor. This is especially important in trauma where a subtle pneumothorax may only be discerned at the lung base at rather bizarre settings of window width and level. Likewise the skeleton must be formally reviewed at bony windows. Most experienced radiologists find all this much easier on a workstation where images can be viewed in cine mode with real-time manipulation of the windows; this is even more relevant in these days of multidetector CT, where the large data sets make photography of every image impractical. It will be interesting to see how the courts will respond to cases where a perceived error is made on electronic rather than hard copy reporting.

26.3.4 Magnetic Resonance Imaging

MRI is rarely used as the first-line investigation for abdominal trauma except for associated lumbar spine problems. Again, technique will rarely be the cause of an error in diagnosis. However, technical problems can lead to litigation: e.g., burns from the heating induced in ECG wires.

The likeliest area for litigation is again the missed diagnosis (Cook et al. 1986; Bloom et al. 1996; Sung and Kim 1996). Like CT, MR images are available for retrospective interrogation. Again the radiologist is well advised to view all images on the workstation. The conscientious radiographer may well have coned magnified images down to show just the lumbar spine free from artifacts from the vessels or the moving anterior abdominal wall. However, in so doing, the key part of the image showing the retroperitoneal hemorrhage may have been coned off; hence the advantage of reviewing the source images rather than just the hard copy highlights.

26.3.5 Individual Organs

Injury to the diaphragm is frequently overlooked at axial CT; recognition is much easier at US or MRI because of the improved multiplanar capabilities. Awareness of this potential error should make the radiologist circumspect about calling a diaphragm normal on axial imaging alone, especially when there are other abnormalities in this region, e.g., pleural effusion. Medicolegal claims have been successful with regard to missed diagnosis.

Significant trauma to the liver is usually readily recognized by all cross-sectional techniques. CT is the most widely used investigation (Matsubara et al. 1990). Claims here will tend to be made for perceived inadequate management by the clinician rather than diagnostic errors by the radiologist. Of course, it is very much up to the radiologist to comment on those lesions which are serious on account of their anatomical site, e.g., running close to the inferior vena cava. Serious errors of diagnosis can occur with respect to biliary damage. The fact that the biliary system has been ruptured means that there will usually be no distension; free bile in the peritoneum cannot be distinguished from blood in the acute stages; the scene is set for a delay in diagnosis which can prove fatal and thereby costly in medicolegal terms. Hence the renewed interest in nuclear medicine (HIDA) techniques and even intravenous cholangiography, to prevent such problems being overlooked.

The spleen is usually best demonstrated by CT. Indeed, the CT findings are now increasingly being used to determine whether or not conservative management is appropriate. This is in order to try to leave some functioning splenic tissue to protect against subsequent pneumococcal sepsis. Arterial embolization is also being used to control splenic hemorrhage. Because of these factors, it is likely that radiologists will be sued for information contributing to the decision to withhold surgery. However, delayed rupture is rare and, so long as the CT evidence and the long-term risks of splenectomy are carefully explained to the patient, the radiologist and clinician should be able to withstand a claim. Of course the clinician is always in a better position to discuss things with patients and may, inadvertently, suggest to the patient that the radiologist "'got it wrong", thereby triggering a claim.

Trauma to the pancreas may not be immediately apparent (Sivit et al. 1992). Thus the initial US or CT may appear normal. Even if there is a trace of peripancreatic fluid, this may not seem very significant among other intraperitoneal or retroperitoneal blood. The diagnosis may only become apparent later, often in the light of a rising amylase level, when fluid accumulates in the lesser sac and the rent in the pancreas becomes apparent. Radiologists should be aware of this relatively common sequence of events and should not be culpable of a missed diagnosis on the initial examination.

Radiologists should be aware that failure to recognize trauma to the bowel, particularly the second or third part of the duodenum, is one of the more common serious errors that they can make (Barandica and Patel 1997; Bloom et al. 1996). Thus it is sensible to comment on any free fluid in this region and interrogate the images carefully on the workstation, maybe close to lung window levels, to exclude all-important flecks of gas in this region. They should also be open to performing early follow-up CT to exclude an enlarging collection when the history is suggestive of bowel injury, e.g., lap belt injury with bruising.

Trauma to the urinary tract is usually managed conservatively. Only occasionally is radiology implicated in legal claims. However, it is incumbent on the radiologist to help the clinician by identifying sites of leakage, maybe by performing appropriate nephrostograms and nephrostomies and by raising the possibility of and excluding urethral damage before attempts at catheterization.

Trauma to the pelvis should be readily recognized by CT viewed at bony settings. Thin CT sections are needed to allow subsequent multiplanar display of complex fractures, which may help the clinician. Careful viewing on the workstation is needed to identify small detached fragments of bone, e.g., in the hip joint. More difficult is the diagnosis of sacroiliac diastasis and the identification of bleeding points around the gluteal vessels for which embolization might be appropriate. The identification of bleeding points during peak concentration of arterial contrast medium should be easier using multidetector CT systems; indeed all trauma centers should have access to this technology as soon as possible. It is interesting to speculate whether a claim would be successful against a center if it could be proved that an error had occurred partly because of old technology.

Medicolegal issues are more frequent in relation to lumbar spine trauma; the fracture may be overlooked, the seriousness of a fracture may not be recognized at the initial abdominal CT – there should therefore be a low threshold to proceed to urgent MRI. Medicolegal claims may follow many years after relatively minor trauma, especially if the accident happened at work. At this late stage, the radiologist may have to defend old reports on which the presence or absence of trauma was equivocal at the time of injury. There may have been mild deformity of a lumbar vertebra because of adolescent end plate change (Schmorl node, Scheuermann's disease, etc.); plain radiographs may have shown marked degenerative changes around a vertebral body. Against this background, the claimant may also be suffering from coincidental lumbar spine disease. Despite all these confounding factors, lawyers may still claim that large sums of compensation should still be attributed to the original trauma!

26.4 Iatrogenic Complications

26.4.1 Nonradiological Problems

Inevitably, the seriously injured patient, with trauma often affecting numerous organs, poses serious management issues. The best possible care for the abdomen, e.g., conservative treatment of splenic hemorrhage with transfusion, may not be optimal for the care of coexistent neurological problems, etc. Furthermore, in many medical centers, confusion may exist as to which group of doctors is in overall charge of the patient (anesthesiologists, neurosurgeon, abdominal surgeon, or orthopedic team). Against this background, there is considerable scope for communication issues. Even in the best hands, some aspects of management will go wrong: a drain may fall out, a pneumothorax drain may inserted incorrectly, etc.

The job of radiologists is to offer prompt and sympathetic support to their clinical colleagues when such problems do occur. For example, if a patient is shown to have an intraabdominal collection following surgery for splenic trauma, it is incumbent on the radiologist to enter into urgent dialogue with the clinician to see whether percutaneous drainage is required. And if an extraneous structure is seen in an inappropriate position, e.g., a chest drain traversing the diaphragm, the radiological report should comment factually without suggesting that an error has occurred. It is far better to discuss this sort of problem with the clinician personally, e.g., on the telephone, than in the written report. The report should, however, state "these findings were discussed with the (named) clinician."

26.4.2 Radiological Problems

Only in the field of interventional radiology is it likely that direct harm will come to the patient. Coils used to try to block the flow to feeding vessels in pelvic trauma may inadvertently enter the wrong vessel or an attempt to drain intraabdominal collections might perforate bowel. All these procedures may be considerably more difficult in the setting of trauma than when being done electively, e.g., embolization of an arteriovenous fistula. Firstly, the patient may be restless and surrounded by paraphernalia relating to other injuries such as orthopaedic traction devices. Secondly, many procedures for trauma are needed at night or weekends when the usual team may not be available. It is a matter of clinical governance and risk management to balance the hours worked and the out-of-hours staffing. And who should perform such procedures? If the radiologist in question does not regularly carry out these procedures during their routine work, should they be advised to make a one-time attempt during the night? But the patient may not survive the move to a larger center where a more experienced radiologist might be available. Again, the balance is a matter of fine judgment, but not beyond legal scrutiny. Sadly, increasing legal activity is likely to make radiologists less enthusiastic to help their clinical colleagues in these difficult cases, especially when they are at the margin of their clinical expertise.

A more common problem is that an error is made on the radiological report. These may range from the trivial: a coincidental gallstone is not commented on – to the serious – renal trauma is incorrectly ascribed to the right instead of the left. Ultimately, the latter example, which may only be a momentary lapse of concentration by the radiologist or typist, could lead to inappropriate surgery with devastating consequences. Hence the need for a meticulous approach to reporting and checking reports. In larger centers, where reports are often issued with colleagues in attendance, there is often a form of double reporting, which minimizes risk (Robinson 1997).

There is also pressure to deliver the report in a timely fashion. However, complex trauma cases, with over 100 CT images, are difficult to report without due care and attention. It is probably better to offer an immediate provisional report stating that a formal final report will follow, and subsequently to analyze the images in detail in peace and quiet. If a new feature is then seen between the provisional short report and the issuing of the formal report, it is essential to communicate this with the clinical team and to record the fact that this new feature on the formal report has been discussed with the clinician. Otherwise, inappropriate action might be assumed on the basis of the inaccurate provisional short report.

26.4.3 Errors and Conclusion

The real problem for radiology is that the images are there for all to interrogate and thus radiologists are frequently open to legal challenges. Of course, it is often easier to see a lesion in retrospect when further clinical details emerge. All of us will have missed a rib or similar fracture only for it to become glaringly obvious when the clinician provides the secondary information that the patient has pain at a particular spot! Rib fractures may be very difficult to identify on the initial radiographs; the presence of callus a few weeks later reveals the initial observational error. Apart from errors of observation, there are also errors of interpretation (Robinson 1997). The splenic tear may have been assumed to be an artifact caused by beam hardening and movement of an adjacent rib; if this is the case the report should at least describe the abnormality and then offer an explanation for the final conclusion. Given that such errors are inevitable, it is perhaps reasonable to describe them as discrepancies.

Even in the best departments, such discrepancies will occur. They must be openly acknowledged and a secondary report with the new observation and interpretation added as an addendum. They should be audited to see whether a recurring theme is present. It is tempting to use them to show that fewer discrepancies occur in one particular part of a department, but doctors who report a lot of discrepancies may be doing the most difficult work or carrying out the most work, or they may be the most conscientious about auditing their work.

Of course, to gain substantial damages, it has to be proven that the patient's clinical condition suffered directly as a result of the misleading information provided by the radiological report and that the radiologist's report and actions were below the standard expected from that in a similar institution. It is unusual that such deterioration in a patient's clinical condition occurs if a discrepancy is recognized while the patient is in hospital when there is close contact between the clinical and radiological teams. Clinico-radiological meetings provide a good forum for such exchange of clinical information (Leung and Dixon 1992). The law recognizes that no doctor is infallible and that radiological interpretation is not an exact science. In most countries, the onus is on the claimant to prove that the radiological care was below that which might reasonably be expected in that institution. Radiologists have to be able to prove that they keep up to date and that their work is subjected to audit (Godwin et al. 1996). This is the best route to successful defense. It is also the best method of providing optimal care to the patient.

References

Barandica R, Patel M (1997) Pediatric duodenal perforation missed on computed tomography. Ann Emerg Med 30: 545–547

Bloom AI, Rivkind A, Zamir G et al (1996) Blunt injury of the small intestine and mesentery – the trauma surgeon's Achilles heel? Eur J Emerg Med 3:85–91

Cook DE, Walsh JW, Vick CW, Brewer WH (1986) Upper abdominal trauma: pitfalls in CT diagnosis. Radiology 159: 65–69

EU Council Directive (1997) Health protection of individuals against the dangers of ionising radiation in relation to medical exposure. EU Directive 1997/43/Euratom, 30 June 1997

Godwin R, De Lacey G, Manhire A (1996) Clinical audit in radiology. Royal College of Radiologists, London

Leung DPY, Dixon AK (1992) Clinicoradiological meetings: are they worthwhile? Clin Radiol 46:279–280

Matsubara TK, Fong HM, Burns CM (1990) Computed tomography of abdomen (CTA) in management of blunt abdominal trauma. J Trauma 30:410–414

McLellan BA, Ali J, Towers MJ, Sharkey W (1996) Role of the trauma-room chest X-ray film in assessing the patient with severe blunt traumatic injury. Can J Surg 39:36–41

Padhani AR, Watson CJE, Clements L, Calne RY, Dixon AK (1992) Computed tomography in abdominal trauma: an audit of usage and image quality. Br J Radiol 65: 397–402

Robinson PJ (1997) Radiology's Achilles' heel: error and variation in the interpretation of the Rontgen image. Br J Radiol 70:1085–1098

Robinson PJ, Wilson D, Coral A, Murphy A, Verow P (1999) Variation between experienced observers in the interpretation of accident and emergency radiographs. Br J Radiol 72:323–330

Royal College of Radiologists (1998) Making the best use of a department of clinical radiology: guidelines for doctors, 4th edn. Royal College of Radiologists, London

Shackford SR, Rogers FB, Osler TM, Trabulsy ME, Clauss DW, Vane DW (1999) Focused abdominal sonogram for trauma: the learning curve of nonradiologist clinicians in detecting hemoperitoneum. J Trauma 46:553–562

Sivit CJ, Eichelberger MR, Taylor GA, Bulas DI, Gotschall CS, Kushner DC (1992) Blunt pancreatic trauma in children: CT diagnosis. AJR 158:1097–1100

Sung CK, Kim KH (1996) Missed injuries in abdominal trauma. J Trauma 41:276–282

Wakeley CJ, Jones AM, Kabala JE, Prince D, Goddard PR (1995) Audit of the value of double reading magnetic resonance imaging films. Br J Radiol 68:358–360

27 A Selection of Published Surgical and Radiological Classifications of Abdominal Injuries

O. Cornet and R. F. Dondelinger

CONTENTS

- Classifications of injuries are a useful tool for comparison of diagnostic and therapeutic results and formulation of prognosis of a trauma victim population on a statistical basis.
- Classifications of injuries are less useful to guide management of an individual patient, when they are used as a sole criterion.
- Radiological classifications do not necessarily correlate well with surgical findings.
- In blunt hepatic and splenic injuries, grading systems based on CT findings give equivocal results on predicting the need for intervention, the presence of vascular injuries responsible for rebleeding and other delayed complications.

O. Cornet, MD
Resident, Deptartment of Medical Imaging, University Hospital Sart Tilman, Domaine du Sart Tilman B35, 4000 Liège, Belgium
R. F. Dondelinger, MD
Professor and Chairman, Department of Medical Imaging, University Hospital Sart Tilman, Domaine Universitaire du Sart Tilman B35, 4000 Liège, Belgium

In this chapter, a selection of published abdominal injuries is presented, including lumbar spine and pelvic fractures. Surgical and radiological injury classifications are given for each organ, in chronological order, as they appeared in the literature. For some organs, the Organ Injury Scaling (OIS) was the only grading system available. Comments are mainly extracted from the original publications, including correlations with management options, when available. Overlap between publications is unavoidable. The chronological order best reflects evolution of trends in therapy and refinement in diagnostic techniques.

27.1 Hemoperitoneum

Reference

Federle MP, Jeffrey RB (1983) Hemoperitoneum studied by computed tomography. Radiology 148:187–192
Mirvis SE, Whitley MO, Vainwright JR, Gens DR (1989) Blunt hepatic trauma in adults: CT-based classification and correlation with prognosis and treatment. Radiology 171: 27–32

Grade	Volume of hemoperitoneum	Description of anatomical location of hemoperitoneum
0	–	None detected
1	Small: 100–200 ml	Confined to a single anatomical area such as Morison's pouch, perihepatic space, perisplenic space, or either the left or right paracolic gutter
2	Moderate: 250–500 ml	In two or more anatomical spaces in addition to collections in the pelvis
3	Large: >500 ml	Loculations in the pelvis and other locations

Three hundred patients who had sustained blunt abdominal injury were evaluated with CT. The presence, location and amount of hemoperitoneum were recorded in 56 patients. The images showed areas of hemorrhage by varying attenuation coefficients (average, 45 HU; exceeding 30 HU in all cases except in those patients with bleeding more than 48 h before). Small hematomas tended to accumulate near the site of origin, while free intraperitoneal bleeding most frequently accumulated in Morison's pouch, the paracolic gutters, and pelvis. CT estimates of the extent of hemoperitoneum (small, moderate, or large) correlated well with clinical assessments and surgical findings. Only one false-negative and two false-positive CT interpretations occurred, and each was potentially avoidable in retrospect.

Reference

Huang MS, Liu M, Wu JK, Shih HC, Ko TJ, Lee CH (1994) Ultrasonography for the evaluation of hemoperitoneum during resuscitation: a simple scoring system. J Trauma 36:173–177

Location of hemoperitoneum	Points
Morison's pouch	
Significant[a]	2
Minimal[b]	1
Douglas' pouch	
Significant[a]	2
Minimal[b]	1
Perisplenic space	1
Paracolic gutter	1
Floating intestinal loops	2

[a] More than 2 mm of free fluid
[b] Less than or equal to 2 mm of free fluid

To assess the need for therapeutic laparotomy in patients with blunt abdominal trauma (BAT), ultrasonography (US) and a simple US scoring system were used to estimate the amount of hemoperitoneum during resuscitation. According to the location and US image, 1 or 2 points were assigned. The points were summed to obtain the US score, which ranged from 0 to 8. 442 patients with BAT were admitted to the emergency room and hemoperitoneum was revealed in 49 patients by the initial US examination. These patients were divided into two groups according to the US score. For patients with a US score of 3 or higher (group I), laparotomy was performed as soon possible; for a US score less than 3 (group II), but patients still in shock, laparotomy was also indicated; for a US score less than 3 (group II) and stable vital signs, further diagnostic studies were arranged and the patient was closely observed with repeated US studies. In group I (BAT with a US score ≤3), 24 of 25 patients (96%) required therapeutic laparotomy. In group II (BAT with a US score <3), therapeutic laparotomy was required in 9 of 24 patients (38%); nonsurgical treatment may be justified in hemodynamically stable patients. Appropriate decisions can be made to perform urgent laparotomy when intra-abdominal bleeding is the culprit in BAT patients. Unnecessary laparotomy can be avoided when the major site of blood loss is not in the abdomen. US, an initial rapid screening procedure in BAT patients, is useful for trauma surgeons in decision-making during resuscitation.

Reference

McKenney KL, McKenney MG, Nunez DB, McDowell L, Martin L (1996) Interpreting the trauma ultrasound: observations in 62 positive cases. Emerg Radiol 3:113–117

The subphrenic spaces, the subhepatic space (Morison's pouch) and the free edge of liver, the perisplenic area and splenic tip, both parcolic gutters and the pelvis were imaged with ultrasound (US). The location in which the largest amount of fluid occurred was determined from hardcopy images. The depth of this fluid collection was measured in centimeters. To obtain this measurement, a line was drawn from the most anterior aspect of the collection to the posterior extent using either the longitudinal or transverse image. In Morison's pouch, however, owing to its configuration, this number was obtained by measuring a line drawn between the liver and kidney. This number for the maximum depth of fluid was then added to the total number of additional areas positive for fluid to arrive at a total hemoperitoneum score. All 62 positive trauma abdominal ultrasound examinations over a 17-month period were reviewed. A US examination was considered positive if free intraperitoneal fluid was identified or if an injury was directly visualized, with or without associate free fluid. Results of the scoring system were correlated with the need for laparotomy. Free fluid was found in all areas; however, four areas (the right subphrenic, subhepatic, and perisplenic areas and the pelvis) were diagnostic when a positive examination resulted from fluid found in only one site. Eighteen parenchymal injuries were identified during sonography. Patients with a score of 2 or more were found to have a significantly higher incidence of operation requirement.

27.2 Liver

Reference

Flint LM, Mays ET, Aaron WS, Fulton RL, Polk HC (1977) Selectivity in the management of hepatic trauma. Ann Surg 185:613–618

Grade	Description of injury
I	Capsular tears
II	Non-bleeding (<5 cm) Through and through missile tracts (non-bleeding)
III	Small actively bleeding lacerations Bleeding missile tracts Subsegmental tissue destruction (non-bleeding)
IV	Large fractures Lobar tissue destruction
V	Extensive parenchymal disruption with hepatic arterial or venous injury

This retrospective review of 178 consecutive patients who sustained hepatic injuries claimed to show that selective application of hepatic artery ligation is an efficient means of definitive hemostasis. Only 2 of 20 immediate deaths resulted from hepatic parenchymal hemorrhage. Hepatic wounds were managed by drainage, suture, resectional debridement, selective hepatic artery ligation (SHAL), and formal lobectomy, or a combination thereof. As injury grade increased, SHAL was employed more frequently. Hepatic artery interruption was successful in controlling arterial bleeding from the hepatic parenchyma in all patients in whom it was employed. The operative records of 59 patients undergoing hepatic artery ligation disclosed that in 82%, the decision to employ SHAL followed the failure of conventional modalities to control arterial bleeding. Hepatic artery interruption and subsequent hepatic parenchymal ischemia are potentially dangerous. The effects of SHAL on mortality and development of perihepatic sepsis were analyzed in the 59 patients who underwent SHAL. Mortality among these patients was 31% compared to an overall mortality for all other treatment modalities of 22%. Similarly, the incidence of perihepatic sepsis following hepatic artery interruption was not significantly increased when compared to other modalities. The frequency with which patients presented in shock increased with grade of injury. Septic complications and deaths also became more frequent as grade of injury increased.

Reference

Fuchs K, Castrup HJ, Hölscher M (1978) Choice of management in operative treatment of liver injury. Chirurg 49:419–423

Type	Description of injury
I[a]	Superficial rupture
II[b]	Deep, uncomplicated trisegmental rupture
III[c]	Deep, horizontal rupture
IV[d]	Deep, complicated rupture

[a] Type I injuries are treated by parenchymal or capsular suture and drainage
[b] Type II injuries are treated by debridement, segment resection (left lateral sector) or right or left lobectomy or trisegmentectomy
[c] Type III injuries are treated by parenchymal sutures, vascular ligation, and drainage
[d] Type IV injuries are treated by an attempts of vascular reconstruction at the hepatic vein-caval junction or porta hepatis

Reference

Guiset J, Combemale B, Lagache G (1978) Correlation of posttraumatic liver injury and prognosis. Proposal of a classification. Lille Chir 33:113–116

Capsule	I[a]	II[b]	III[c]	
A: not ruptured	Erosion	Subcapsular hematoma	Central hematoma	
B: ruptured	Cleft	Fracture	Burst	
Type A and B Capsular injury	I[a] Contusion, erosion, cleft	II[b] Avulsion, fracture, subcapsular hematoma	III[c] Burst, stellar fracture, central hematoma	IV[d] Major vascular injury (portal vein or hepatic veins)
Lesion	Superficial		Deep	Deep
Fracture	0	1	Several	Several
Progression	Relatively benign	Critical	Most severe	Most severe
Treatment	No treatment or superficial suture	Treatment by tamponade, suture, or resection	Resection	Suture

[a] Type I shows no fracture. Progression is usually benign. No treatment or superficial suture
[b] Type II is a surgical emergency. Treatment is obtained by tamponade, suture or resection. Only one fracture is present. Blood and bile are oozing
[c] Type III. Deep injury. Several fractures are present. Treatment is done by resection
[d] Type IV. Deep injury. Several fractures of the liver parenchyma are present. Suture and/or resection are recommended

For 49 patients admitted with liver injury, there were no mortalities in type I, a mortality rate of 52% and 50% in type II and type III, respectively, and more than 80% mortality in type IV.

Reference

Calne RY, Wells FC, Forty J (1982) Twenty-six cases of liver trauma. Br J Surg 69:365–368

Grade	Description of injury
I	Capsular tear with minor bleeding, which stops spontaneously or after a few simple sutures: parenchyma not damaged
II	Parenchymal damage of the liver, where careful suturing to secure local hemostasis will stop bleeding at the time of the operation, without any major surgical procedure
III	Parenchymal damage of the liver, with major hemorrhage from intrahepatic arteries and/or veins, threatening life and producing shock
IV	The damage described in grade III together with a tear of the inferior vena cava or major hepatic vessels

Twenty-six patients were admitted to the hospital during a 10-year period with grade II to IV damage to the liver. There were nine grade II injuries, with a 0% mortality rate and an 11% rate for operative management. In the group of 11 grade III injuries, the mortality rate was 9% and 45% required surgical intervention. For the six grade IV injuries, the mortality rate reached 50%, with 100% surgical intervention.

Reference

Mirvis SE, Whitley NO, Vainwright JR, Gens DR (1989) Blunt hepatic trauma in adults: CT-based classification and correlation with prognosis and treatment. Radiology 171:27–32

Grade	Description of injury
1	Capsular avulsion, superficial laceration(s) <1 cm deep, subcapsular hematoma <1 cm maximal thickness, periportal blood tracking only
2	Laceration(s) 1–3 cm deep, central or subcapsular hematoma(s) 1–3 cm in diameter
3	Laceration(s) >3 cm deep, central or subcapsular hematoma(s) >3 cm in diameter
4	Massive central or subcapsular hematoma >10 cm, lobar tissue destruction (maceration) or devascularization
5	Bilobar tissue destruction (maceration) or devascularization

A CT-based hepatic injury classification system partly derived from similar systems established with surgical assessment was devised to grade the severity of hepatic injury. CT-based injury scores ranging from grade 1 to 5 were compared with the clinical outcome in patients treated surgically and nonsurgically. In addition, the presence and quantity of intraperitoneal hemorrhage were determined by means of the semiquantitative method of Federle and Jeffrey (see 27.1, “Hemoperitoneum”). In the 37 patients of the study, 31 (83.7%) with injury graded 1 to 3 were successfully treated without surgery, including 21 of the 24 patients with grade 3 injury and all three patients with grade 4 injury, as verified with CT. Furthermore, four patients (10%) had findings at celiotomy that did not require further surgery. No patient initially treated without surgery required delayed celiotomy due to hepatic injury. Only two complications were encountered in the group of patients treated without surgery and they were successfully treated with percutaneous methods. The results indicated that even major hepatic injury, up to and including grade 4 severity, assessed with preoperative CT, can usually be managed without surgery in hemodynamically stable patients. The quantity of intra-abdominal hemorrhage determined with preoperative CT before peritoneal lavage, although roughly correlated with the injury-severity score, does not by itself suggest the need for laparotomy in hemodynamically stable patients.

Reference

Yamamoto S, Kasai T, Maekawa K et al (1989) Liver injury of the Japanese Association of Surgery for Trauma (in Japanese). J Jpn Assoc Surg Trauma 3:118–119

Type	Description of injury
I	Subcapsular injury
Ia	Subcapsular hematoma
Ib	Central rupture
II	Superficial injury (<3 cm parenchyma depth)
III	Deep injury (>3 cm parenchymal depth)
IIIa	Simple type (without tissue necrosis)
IIIb	Complex type (with tissue necrosis)

Reference

Buechter KJ, Zeppa R, Gomez G (1990) The use of segmental anatomy for an operative classification of liver injuries. Ann Surg 211:669–675

Grade	Description of injury
I	Injuries requiring no operative intervention, or any injury that requires operative intervention limited to a segment or less
II	Any injury that requires operative intervention, involving two or more segments
III	Any injury with an associated juxta- or retrohepatic vein injury

This classification was based on segmental anatomy. Patients with grade I injury had a 1% death rate, patients with grade II injury had a 46% death rate, and patients with grade III had a 69% death rate. Postoperative morbidity was 7% for grade I, 57% for grade II, and 50% for grade III. Morbidity and mortality from liver injury were directly related to the volume of parenchyma involved, based on segmental anatomy. Mortality from retrohepatic vein injuries was dependent on associated parenchymal injury. Such involvement is either the result of the initial injury or the operative intervention used to manage the injury. Thus mortality will be determined by the amount of parenchyma involved at the end of the operation.

Reference

Croce MA, Fabian TC, Kudsk KA et al (1991) AAST organ injury scale: correlation of CT-graded liver injuries and operative findings. J Trauma 31:806–812

Grade[a]	Type of injury	Description of injury
I	Hematoma	Subcapsular, nonexpanding, <10% surface area
	Laceration	Capsular tear, nonbleeding, <1 cm parenchymal depth
II	Hematoma	Subcapsular, nonexpanding, 10%–50% surface area
	Laceration	Capsular tear, active bleeding; 1–3 cm parenchymal depth, <10 cm in length
III	Hematoma	Subcapsular, >50% surface area or expanding; ruptured subcapsular hematoma with active bleeding; intraparenchymal hematoma >2 cm or expanding
	Laceration	>3 cm parenchymal depth
IV	Hematoma	Ruptured intraparenchymal hematoma with active bleeding
	Laceration	Parenchymal disruption involving 25%–50% of hepatic lobe
V	Hematoma	Parenchymal disruption involving >50% of hepatic lobe
	Vascular	Juxtahepatic venous injuries, i.e., retrohepatic vena cava/major hepatic veins
VI	Vascular	Hepatic avulsion

[a] Advance one grade for multiple injuries to the same organ

This classification is based on CT and operative findings. The hepatic injury scale (HIS), based on parenchymal laceration and intrahepatic hematoma, includes grade I–VI, representing the least to most severe injury. This study classifies liver injury by findings at celiotomy, correlates operative findings with transfusion requirements and method of management of liver injury, and relates preoperative CT to anatomical findings at laparotomy. This classification is based upon the classification given by Moore et al. and considers several additional parameters such as nonexpanding or expanding hematoma and nonbleeding or actively bleeding laceration. Thirty-seven patients with blunt liver injury were evaluated by abdominal CT with and without intravenous contrast and then underwent celiotomy. Increasing operative HIS correlated well with increasing severity of injury as measured by transfusions and operative management. Thirty-one CT grades did not correlate with operative findings (84%). Four patients had intrahepatic hematomas that were not discovered at operation. Twelve lacerations were graded too high by CT and 15 too low. The CT findings overestimated operative findings by two or more grades in five cases and underestimated operative findings by two or more grades in 10 cases. Injuries around the falciform ligament occurred in three of the low misclassifications. One patient with intrahepatic hematoma developed hepatic artery pseudoaneurysm. In conclusion, the HIS readily characterizes operative findings of hepatic lacerations and showed that increasing operative grade correlates well with transfusion requirements and operative management. CT can define intrahepatic hematomas, but does not correlate well with hepatic lacerations. Extreme caution is required when using CT alone to define "minimal" liver injury for prospective management of blunt trauma victims.

Reference

Namieno T, Hata Y, Uchino JI, Matsubara I, Tedo I (1994) Blunt liver trauma: a new concept for classification of liver trauma based on vessel injury. Int Surg 79:52–59

Type	Subtype	Description of injury
I		Subcapsular Glissonian vessel injury
	Ia	Subcapsular hematoma
	Ib	Central hematoma
II		Transcapsular Glissonian vessel injury
	IIa	Superficial injury with simple laceration and minimal contusion
	IIb	Deep injury with complicated laceration and massive contusion
III		In-/out-flow vessel injury
	IIIa	Juxtahepaticocaval injury with rupture of hepatic vein and/or inferior vena cava
	IIIb	Hilar injury with rupture of hepatic artery and/or portal vein

The authors reviewed a consecutive series of 143 cases of blunt liver trauma, 43 children and 100 adults, to reasonably select treatment, either nonoperative or operative. The primary determinant in the prognosis of liver trauma was hemorrhage, due to vessel injuries and its main treatment was hemostasis. The authors developed a new concept for the classification of blunt liver trauma based on vessel injuries: 20%–30% of patients needed control of hemorrhage. The difference in urgency among such cases probably depends more on the extent and site of the vessel injuries than on hepatic parenchymal damage. Distribution of liver trauma according to the present classification was as follows: type I, 23% in pediatric cases and 22% in adult cases; type II, 65% and 64%; and type III, 12% and 14%, respectively. The main management was nonoperative for type I, minor or major surgery for type II, and extended surgery for type III. The analysis of mortality showed the following results: type I, 0% in pediatric cases and 6% in adults; type II, 60% and 55%; type III, 40% and 39%, respectively. The direct cause of mortality was hemorrhage: 60% in pediatric cases and 49% in adults.

Reference

Vade A, Demos TC, Salvino C, Korach JL (1994) Periportal tracking in pediatric blunt abdominal trauma. Correlation with liver enzymes and liver injury. Clin Imaging 18: 189–194

Grade	Description of periportal tracking
0	No zone of decreased attenuation adjacent to the portal vessels
1	Zone of decreased attenuation only on one side of the main portal vein and its proximal branches
2	Zone of decreased attenuation on both sides of the main portal vein and its proximal branches
3	Zone of decreased attenuation on both sides of the portal vessels extending to the periphery of the liver

A retrospective study of the computed tomography (CT) examinations and medical records of 243 consecutive pediatric patients sent for CT studies after blunt abdominal trauma was conducted. Periportal tracking (PPT) was divided into four grades (0–3), depending upon the distribution of decreased attenuation adjacent to the portal vessels. Circumferential PPT extending to the periphery of the liver (grade 3) was found in 20 of 243 children. They had a higher incidence of liver parenchyma injury seen on CT: 20% vs 0.5% in combined PPT grades 0–2. Sixteen children with grade 3 PPT and no liver injury had significantly elevated liver enzymes as compared to children with combined 0–2 grade PPT. Eleven of the 20 children with grade 3 PPT had no other CT evidence of intra-abdominal injury and none of these patients developed intra-abdominal hemorrhage. Isolated grade 3 PPT in children with blunt abdominal trauma may represent a subclinical liver injury, as evidenced by elevated serum glutamic-oxaloacetic transaminase (SGOT) and serum glutamic-pyruvic transaminase (SGPT). The finding of PPT in the absence of any other CT abnormality, however, was not found to be a clinically significant lesion based on liver enzyme levels and clinical follow-up. When PPT is an isolated finding, this study showed that further evaluation by CT was not indicated, since no patient showed evidence of delayed intra-abdominal hemorrhage.

Reference

Moore EE, Cogbill TH, Jurkovich GJ et al (1995) Organ injury scaling: spleen and liver (1994 revision). J Trauma 38: 323–324

Grade[a]	Type of injury	Description of injury
I	Hematoma	Subcapsular, <10% surface area
	Laceration	Capsular tear, <1 cm parenchyma depth
II	Hematoma	Subcapsular, 10%–50% surface area; intraparenchymal, <10 cm in diameter
	Laceration	1–3 cm parenchymal depth, <10 cm in length
III	Hematoma	Subcapsular, >50% surface area or expanding; ruptured subcapsular or parenchymal hematoma Intraparenchymal hematoma >10 cm or expanding
	Laceration	>3 cm parenchymal depth
IV	Laceration	Parenchymal disruption involving 25%–75% of hepatic lobe or 1–3 Couinaud segments within a single lobe
V	Laceration	Parenchymal disruption involving >75% of hepatic lobe or >3 Couinaud segments within a single lobe
	Vascular	Juxtahepatic venous injuries; i.e., retrohepatic vena cava/central major hepatic veins
VI	Vascular	Hepatic avulsion

[a] Advance one grade for multiple injuries, up to grade III

The fundamental purpose of this classification was to devise injury severity scores for individual organs, to facilitate clinical investigation and outcomes research. The Organ Injury Scaling (OIS) is a classification scheme based on the anatomical disruption of an individual organ scaled I–VI, representing the least to most severe injury. Grades I–V represent increasingly complex injuries encountered in salvageable patients, while grade VI is a destructive lesion incompatible with survival.

Reference

Ruess L, Sivit CJ, Eichelberger MR, Taylor GA, Bond SJ (1995) Blunt hepatic and splenic trauma in children: correlation of a CT injury severity scale with clinical outcome. Pediatr Radiol 25:321–325

Grade	Description of injury
1	Laceration involving <25% (of lobar volume)
2	Laceration involving 25%–50% (of lobar volume)
3	Laceration involving >50% (of lobar volume) or bilobar injury

Sixty-nine children with isolated hepatic injury and 53 with isolated splenic injury were prospectively classified at CT, according to extent of parenchymal involvement. Hepatic injury was classified according to volume of involved lobe and not the entire liver. Isolated subcapsular hematoma was classified as a grade 1 injury. Clinical records were reviewed to determine clinical outcome. A majority of children with hepatic and splenic injury were managed nonoperatively, without requiring blood transfusion. The severity of injury graded by CT did not correlate with the need for surgery. Increasing grade of hepatic injury at CT was associated with increasing frequency of blood transfusion. CT staging was not discriminatory in predicting transfusion requirement in splenic injury.

Reference

Becker CD, Gal I, Baer HU, Vock P (1996) Blunt hepatic trauma in adults: correlation of CT injury grading with outcome. Radiology 201:215–220

Grade	Description of injury	Lesion size
1	Capsular disruption/parenchymal laceration	1 cm
2	Subcapsular hematoma, capsular disruption Parenchymal laceration or intrahepatic hematoma	3 cm
3	Subcapsular hematoma, parenchymal laceration, or intrahepatic hematoma	>3 cm
4	Parenchymal laceration in more than two segments; Intrahepatic hematoma or devascularization in more than one segment	
5	Tissue destruction or devascularization that involves both lobes	

Forty-eight patients with proved blunt hepatic injuries underwent dynamic CT with contrast enhancement before treatment. The injuries were classified with a five-point CT-based grading system. The CT injury grades and the amount of hemoperitoneum seen on CT scans were compared with the clinical and surgical findings, radiological follow-up, and outcome. Hepatic injuries were classified as CT grade 1 in 2 patients, grade 2 in 15 patients, grade 3 in 21 patients, and grade 4 in 10 patients. Conservative treatment was performed in 38 patients, including 2 patients with CT grade 1 hepatic injuries, 11 patients with grade 2 injuries, 15 patients with grade 3 injuries, and all 10 patients with grade 4 injuries. Of these patients, 10 also had major hemoperitoneum (>500 ml), but the amount of free intraperitoneal fluid did not correlate well with the CT injury grades. Conservative treatment was successful in 37 patients, but was complicated in 2 patients by development of an arteriovenous fistula or a biloma and failed in 1 patient because of delayed hepatic rupture. In these three patients with CT grade 4 injuries, complications were recognized at follow-up CT, but at retrospective analysis, the initial CT scans revealed no signs that enabled early detection. Exploratory laparotomy was performed in 10 patients but revealed marked active hepatic bleeding in only 1 patient. Injury grading with CT may reflect the degree of hepatic parenchymal damage, but does not indicate patients in whom complications may develop or surgery is necessary. Furthermore, the degree of hemoperitoneum seen on CT scans at admission examination cannot be used to assess the need for surgical repair of hepatic injuries. Monitoring of conservative treatment with CT allows detection of resultant clinically occult complications.

27.3 Bile Ducts

Reference

Bismuth H (1982) Postoperative strictures of the bile duct. In: Blumgart LH (ed) The biliary tract. Churchill Livingstone, Edinburgh, pp 209–218

Type	Description of stricture
1	Low common hepatic duct stricture: the hepatic stump is longer than 2 cm
2	Middle common hepatic duct stricture: the hepatic stump is less than 2 cm
3	High stricture or hilar stricture preserving the biliary confluence: the hepatic duct no longer exists. The stricture reaches the confluence of the right and left hepatic ducts, but communication between the two branches is preserved across the confluence
4	Hilar stricture interrupts the confluence: communication between the left and right branches no longer exists. If the fibrotic scar joining the two branches is thin, then they may remain in continuity, but if the process has destroyed an important part of the ductal tissue, the right and left hepatic ducts may be separated by 1–2 cm
5	When the trauma has involved an anomalous distribution of the segmental right branches ("convergence étagée"[a]), one of these two ducts can be separated from the biliary tract by the stricture

[a] Separate junction of posterior right sectorial duct below the major confluence

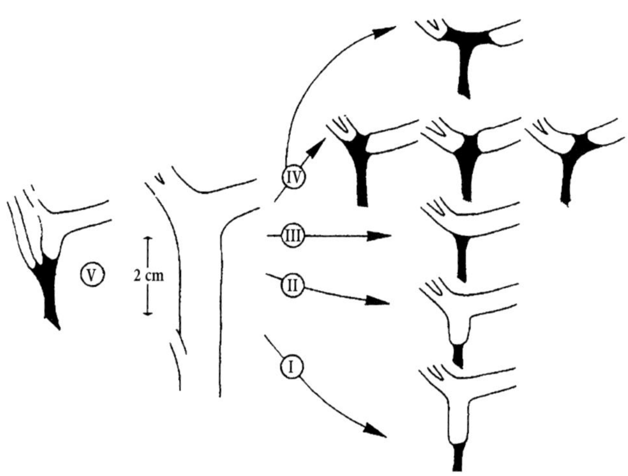

In benign strictures of the common bile duct, 90% are secondary to previous surgery. The cicatricial process, which characterizes the postoperative biliary stricture, comprises three main features: sclerosis of the duct wall at the level of the trauma, retraction of the biliary stump, and dilatation of the upper part of the bile duct. Since the length of the superior biliary stump is a determining factor assessing the difficulty and the outcome of the subsequent biliary repair, a classification of postoperative biliary strictures, according to the level where healthy biliary mucosa can be found, may be proposed. Cholangiography is indispensable for precise knowledge of the level of the stricture. The authors classified postoperative strictures of the common bile duct into five types. Jaundice and cholangitis are the main and usually the only symptoms. The most important factors of the preoperative investigations are: a) the level of the biliary stenosis; b) the degree of dilatation of the hepatic stump and of the hepatic branches; and c) the influence of cholestasis on the liver and the presence of liver hypertrophy or of secondary biliary cirrhosis. The basic principle of the operation of biliary repair is to reestablish mucosal continuity between the biliary tract and the digestive mucosa. This mucosa-to-mucosa, "bord à bord", approach is the best approach to prevent recurrence of the stricture and requires both normal biliary mucosa and close contact with this biliary mucosa and another healthy mucosal surface.

Reference

Chartrand-Lefèbvre C, Dufresne MP, Lafortune M, Lapointe R, Dagenais M, Roy A (1994) Iatrogenic injury to the bile duct: a working classification for radiologists. Radiology 193:523–526

Type	Description of injury
I	Injury of the main bile duct, located more than 2 cm distal from the biliary confluence
II	Injury of the main bile duct, situated less than 2 cm distal to the biliary confluence
III	Injury that completely destroys the hepatic stump distal to the confluence, but leaves the confluence intact
IV	Complete or partial destruction of the biliary confluence
V	Injury to a right variant segmentary branch with or without injury to the main duct

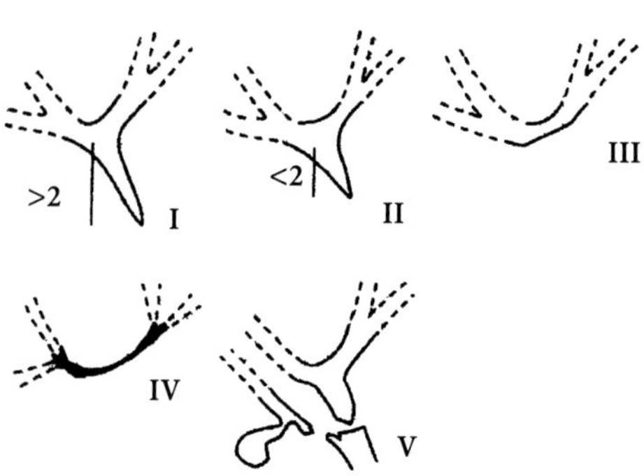

The records of 33 patients who underwent open or laparoscopic cholecystectomy and who sustained injuries to the biliary tract during the course of these procedures were reviewed retrospectively. The accuracy of the predominantly percutaneous transhepatic cholangiographic localization of bile duct injury was assessed with the Bismuth classification method, which is based on the localization of the traumatic lesion according to the distance from the biliary confluence. An exact correspondence between cholangiographic and surgical findings was found in 85% of the subjects. A minimal discrepancy was found in the remainder. There was no interobserver variation. The use of the Bismuth classification method appears to be an accurate and practical method for the grading of postoperative bile duct lesions with percutaneous transhepatic cholangiography, not only suggesting the strategy for bile duct repair but also assessing the rate of success or failure and the risk of morbidity and mortality.

Reference

Strasberg SM, Hertl M, Soper NJ (1995) An analysis of the problem of biliary injury during laparoscopic cholecystectomy. J Am Coll Surg 180:101–125

Class	Description of injury
A	Injury to small ducts in continuity with the biliary system with a leak in the duct of Luschka or the cystic duct
B	Injury to a sectorial duct, with resultant obstruction of part of the biliary system
C	Injury to a sectorial duct with the bile leak; bile leakage occurs from a duct noncontinuous with the biliary system
D	Lateral injury to the extrahepatic biliary duct
E1	Stricture more than 2 cm from the bifurcation of the right and left bile ducts
E2	Stricture less than 2 cm from the bifurcation of the right and left bile ducts
E3	Stricture at the bifurcation of the right and left bile ducts
E4	Stricture involving the right and left bile ducts; the right and left ducts are not continuous
E5	Complete occlusion of all bile ducts, including sectorial ducts

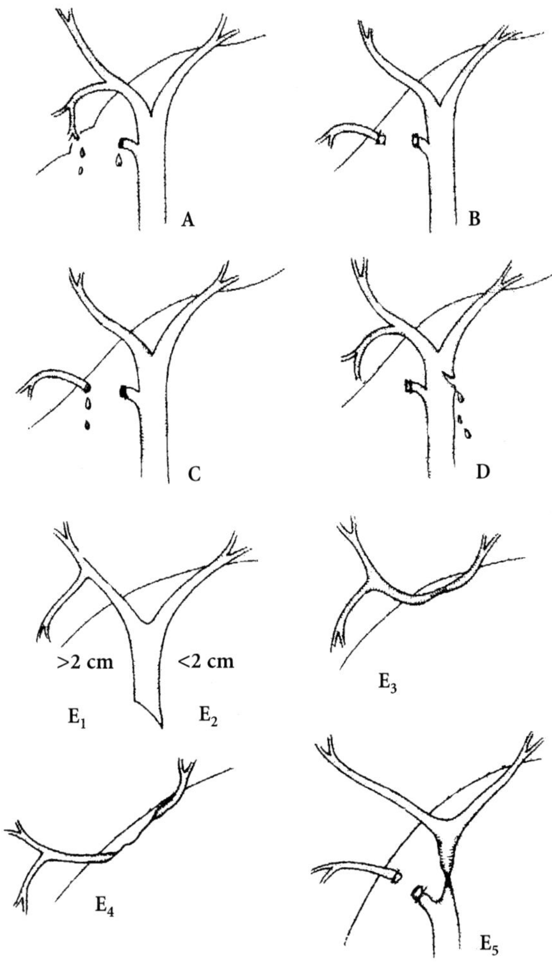

The authors answered eight questions about incidence, classification, risk factors, direct causes, prevention, clinical presentation, correct management, and long-term outcome of biliary iatrogenic laparoscopic injuries. The incidence of reported biliary injuries, according to the proposed classification, shows that type E injuries predominate in surgical series and type A injuries are more prominent in the radiological and endoscopic literature. Of 270 patients who could be classified, 23% had type A injuries, 0.4% had type B injuries, 3% had type C injuries, 9% had type D injuries, and 65% had type E injuries. About 85% of type A injuries were cystic duct leaks. The 97 type E injuries that could be classified were fairly evenly distributed among the first four Bismuth types. The immediate causes of biliary injury may be classified as either misidentification of an anatomical structure or technical. The clinical presentation of type A and type E injuries have been characterized; the important differences in presentation can be helpful in diagnosis. Patients with the classic type A injury present early in the postoperative period with pain, fever, and sepsis or with a bile leak, and elevated alkaline phosphatase and bilirubin, but without jaundice. The patients with a classic type E injury present with jaundice and pain. The type C and D injuries are less well characterized, but when patients with those injuries are not diagnosed by intraoperative bile leak, they present much like type A injuries. Type B injuries are often asymptomatic or the patient presents later with pain or cholangitis in the occluded segment.

Reference

Moore EE, Jurkovich GJ, Knudson MM et al (1995) Organ injury scaling VI: extrahepatic biliary, esophagus, stomach, vulva, vagina, uterus (nonpregnant), uterus (pregnant), fallopian tube, and ovary. J Trauma 39:1069–1070

Grade[a]	Description of injury
I	Gallbladder contusion Portal triad contusion
II	Partial gallbladder avulsion from liver bed; cystic duct intact Laceration or perforation of the gallbladder
III	Complete gallbladder avulsion from liver bed Cystic duct laceration/transection
IV	Partial or complete right hepatic duct laceration Partial or complete left hepatic duct laceration Partial common hepatic duct laceration (≤50%) Partial common bile duct laceration (≤50%)
V	>50% transection of common hepatic duct >50% transection of common bile duct Combined right and left hepatic duct injuries Intraduodenal or intrapancreatic bile duct injuries

[a] Advance one grade for multiple injuries up to grade III.

The fundamental purpose of this classification was to devise injury severity scores for individual organs to facilitate clinical investigation and outcomes research. The OIS is a classification scheme based on the anatomical disruption of an individual organ scaled I–V, representing the least to most severe injury. Grades I–V represent increasingly complex injuries encountered in salvageable patients, whereas grade VI is a destructive lesion incompatible with survival.

27.4 Spleen

Reference

Fisher RG, Foucar K, Estrada R, Ben-Menachem Y (1981) Splenic rupture in blunt trauma: correlation of angiographic and pathologic records. Radiol Clin North Am 19:141–165

Type	Class	Angiographic criteria
Massive (A)	A1	Fragmentation
	A2	Transection of major arterial branches
Major (B)	B1	Large extrasplenic extravasations
	B2	Large intrasplenic extravasations
	B3	Extrasplenic hematoma
	B4	Subcapsular hematoma
	B5	Large avascular areas
Minor (C)	C1	Small avascular areas
	C2	Small widespread extravasations with a snowstorm appearance
	C3	Small regional extravasations with snowstorm appearance
	C4	Small extravasations, Seurat pattern

This classification considers angiographic signs of splenic injury. Only 53% of the splenic injuries confirmed by pathology were observed on splenic arteriograms. Negative arteriography was reliable in only 76% of the cases and 24 patients with a positive splenic arteriogram, including 13 injuries classified as major, required no therapy.

Reference

Shackford SR, Sise MJ, Virgilio RW, Peters RM (1981) Evaluation of splenorrhaphy: a grading system for splenic trauma. J Trauma 21:538–542

Grade	Type of splenorrhaphy
I	Capsular injuries not actively bleeding at the time of laparotomy and not requiring treatment
II	Capsular or parenchymal injuries requiring topical hemostatic agent only
III	Parenchymal injuries requiring suture ligation or suture approximation with or without a topical agent
IV	Parenchymal injuries requiring partial splenic resection
V	Total splenic devascularization or uncontrollable bleeding from the splenic pedicle requiring splenectomy

To evaluate the efficacy of splenorrhaphy as the considered procedure of choice for splenic trauma, the authors graded splenic injury based upon the extent of splenic repair in 77 patients with blunt abdominal trauma and eight from stab wounds. Of these, 51% were found to have grade I–IV injuries and underwent splenorrhaphy, 49% had a grade V injury and underwent splenectomy. Operative time and total blood loss increased with the severity of injury in the splenorrhaphy group, but were not significantly different between the splenorrhaphy and the splenectomy group. Complication rates were not related to the degree of splenic injury.

Reference

Barrett J, Sheaff C, Abuabara S, Jonasson O (1983) Splenic preservation in adults after blunt and penetrating trauma. Am J Surg 145:313–317

Type	Description of injury
I	Capsular disruption without significant parenchymal injury
II	Capsular disruption with parenchymal injury, without extension into the hilum
III	Deep laceration extending into the hilum
IV	Shattered spleen or avulsed from its pedicle

This study evaluated the possibility and safety of splenic preservation in adults based upon the classification to both blunt and penetrating trauma. A total of 36 splenic injuries were studied, 18 due to blunt trauma, 11 due to gunshot wounds, and 7 due to stab wounds. A total of 18 spleens were repaired, eight (45%) in the blunt trauma group, four (36%) in the gunshot group, and six (85%) in the stab wound group. In types I, II, III, and IV of blunt injury 1/1, 2/3, 5/6, and 0/8 injured spleens were preserved. There were no deaths in the entire group nor were there any complications associated with splenic salvage.

Reference

Buntain WL, Gould HR, Maull KI (1988) Predictability of splenic salvage by computed tomography. J Trauma 28:24–34

Class	Criteria
I	Localized capsular disruption or subcapsular hematoma, without significant parenchymal injury
II	Single or multiple capsular and parenchymal disruptions, transverse or longitudinal, that do not extend into the hilum or involve major vessels. Intraparenchymal hematoma may or may not coexist
III	Deep fractures, single or multiple, transverse or longitudinal, extending into the hilum and involving major blood vessels
IV	Completely shattered or fragmented spleen, or separated from its normal blood supply at the pedicle
A	Without other intra-abdominal injury
B	With other associated intra-abdominal injury
B1	Solid viscus
B2	Hollow viscus
E	With associated extra-abdominal injury

CT is an accurate technique to determine the extent of splenic injury. CT classification of splenic trauma has a high correlation with anatomical findings and need for operation. Early operation in patients with severe class II and all class III injuries affords optimal conditions for splenic salvage. Early definitive management of splenic trauma significantly reduces late splenectomy and shortens hospitalization. The authors developed and reported a classification of severity for splenic injuries based on CT and applicable quantitatively as well as qualitatively to help address this problem. Ten pediatric patients (15 years of age and under) and 36 adults comprised the series of splenic injuries. There were 4 class I injuries (9%), 24 class II injuries (52%), 17 class III injuries (37%), and 1 class IV injury (2%). Sixteen of the patients, 6 of the children and 10 of the adults, were managed nonoperatively, 15 with class II injuries and 1 with class III injury. Of the 30 who underwent abdominal operation, there were 12 splenectomies (only 1 in a child) and 18 splenorrhaphies accomplished. Operative splenic salvage was 60% overall, 75% for the children, and 58% for the adults. Patients with class I or class II injuries were then directly admitted to the appropriate critical care unit for observation and monitoring. Patients with class III or class IV injuries and those with class II injuries, accompanied by what appeared to be significant intra-abdominal bleeding or associated with other severe intra-abdominal injuries, were taken directly from CT to the operating room for celiotomy and confirmation of the splenic injury. Splenic salvage was accomplished when possible.

Reference

Resciniti A, Fink MP, Raptopoulos V, Davidoff A, Silva WE (1988) Nonoperative treatment of adult splenic trauma: development of a computed tomographic scoring system that detects appropriate candidates for expectant management. J Trauma 28:828–831

Region	Score	Description of injury
Splenic parenchyma	0	Intact
	1	Laceration (linear defects)
	2	Fracture (thick, irregular defects)
	3	Shattered
Splenic capsule	0	Intact
	1	Perisplenic fluid present
Abdominal fluid	0	None
	1	Any intraperitoneal fluid except perisplenic
Pelvic fluid	0	None
	1	Any intraperitoneal pelvic fluid

Total splenic trauma score (maximum 6) is calculated by addition of all points. Half a point is added when the description of splenic injury falls between two grades. Questionable observations of fluid are assigned half a point.

The authors describe a CT scoring system, based on the degree and pattern of splenic parenchymal and capsular injury and the amount of fluid in the perisplenic space, abdomen, and pelvis. Splenic salvage was achieved in 54 patients (60%), 33 (61%) were successfully managed nonoperatively and 21 (39%) underwent successful splenorrhaphy. Splenic salvage was more common in children (83%) than in adults (52%). The data support the idea that conservative management of splenic trauma is safer in children than in adults. Nevertheless, CT can be used to select a subset of adults with splenic trauma who are excellent candidates for a trial of nonoperative management. Patients with a total CT score of less than 2.5 have a very low probability of requiring delayed operation.

Reference

Mirvis SE, Whitley NO, Gens DR (1989) Blunt splenic trauma in adults: CT-based classification and correlation with prognosis and treatment. Radiology 171:33–39

Grade	Criteria
1	Capsular avulsion, superficial laceration(s), or subcapsular hematoma <1 cm
2	Parenchymal laceration(s) 1–3 cm deep, central or subcapsular hematoma(s) <3 cm
3	Laceration(s) >3 cm deep, central or subcapsular hematoma(s) >3 cm
4	Fragmentation of 3 or more sections, devascularized (nonenhanced) spleen

A CT-based injury-severity score consisting of four grades was devised and applied in 39 adult patients with blunt splenic injury, as the sole or predominant intraperitoneal injury detected with preoperative CT. Results show that CT cannot reliably help predict the outcome of blunt splenic injury in adults. Treatment choices should therefore be based on the hemodynamic status of the patient and results of serial laboratory and bedside assessments. Eight (35%) of 23 patients with initial grade 3 or 4 injury were treated successfully without surgery and 4 (29%) of 15 patients with grade 1 or 2 injury initially treated nonsurgically required delayed celiotomy or emergency rehospitalization. In addition, while the quantity of intraperitoneal hemorrhage tends to increase with the severity of splenic injury, this factor provided no additional guidance in selecting patients for nonsurgical treatment.

Reference

Sugrue M, Knox A, Sarre R, McIntosh N, Toouli J (1991) Management of splenic trauma: a new CT-guided splenic injury grading system. Aust N Z J Surg 61:349–353

Grade	Criteria
1	Capsular avulsion, superficial laceration, or subcapsular hematoma <1 cm
2	Parenchymal laceration(s) 1–3 cm deep Central or subcapsular hematoma(s) <3 cm
3	Laceration(s) >3 cm deep Central or subcapsular hematoma(s) >3 cm
4	Fragmentation into three or more pieces Devascularized (nonenhancing) spleen

This study assesses a newly developed CT-based splenic injury index in predicting the outcome of splenic injury. The splenic injury index was obtained by multiplying the parenchymal score according to the grading system given by Mirvis et al. (see 27.4, "Spleen"). by the volume of hemoperitoneum, which was measured on CT and divided by 10. The results show a significant statistical difference between the mean splenic injury index of 475 in the three patients who failed conservative management and the mean index of 99.5 in the nine patients treated conservatively. This CT-based splenic injury index allows morphological assessment of splenic injury and may predict the outcome of splenic trauma.

Reference

Gay SB, Sistrom CL (1992) Computed tomographic evaluation of blunt abdominal trauma. Radiol Clin North Am 30: 367–388

Type	Criteria
I	Localized capsular disruption Small subcapsular hematoma
II	Small peripheral laceration Parenchymal hematoma <3 cm
III	Fracture extending to hilum Parenchymal hematoma >3 cm
IV	Shattered spleen Vascular disruption

Type I and less severe type II injuries often can be safely managed with an initial trial of bed rest and close observation, including serial hematocrit determinations. More severe type II and all type III disruptions seem to do well with splenorrhaphy. Type IV often requires splenectomy.

Reference

Schweizer W, Böhlen L, Dennison A, Blumgart LH (1992) Prospective study in adults of splenic preservation after traumatic rupture. Br J Surg 79:1330–1333

Grade	Description of injury
I	Subcapsular hematoma
II	Capsular tear
IIIa	Superficial parenchymal tear (<1 cm)
IIIb	Deep parenchymal tear (>1 cm) without involvement of hilum
IV	Parenchymal tear with involvement of hilum
V	Fragmentation

Stable patients received nonoperative treatment regardless of the grade of splenic injury determined by US and CT. Blunt splenic injury was grade I–V. Of the 75 traumatized patients, 37 required splenectomy. A total of 38 spleens were preserved, 18 without operation and 20 following surgery. Of 22 patients initially receiving nonoperative treatment, there were 4 secondary hemorrhages which made surgery necessary. The present study demonstrates the ability to preserve an increasing number of traumatized spleens in adults by surgical preservation or nonoperative therapy. No firm correlation between injury grading and type of management is established.

Reference

Becker CD, Spring P, Glättli A, Schweizer W (1994) Blunt splenic trauma in adults: can CT findings be used to determine the need for surgery. AJR 162:343–347

Grade	Finding
I	Subcapsular or intrasplenic hematoma
II	Capsular disruption or superficial parenchymal tears (≤1 cm)
III	Deep parenchymal tears (>1 cm) without hilar involvement
IV	Parenchymal tears with hilar involvement
V	Fragmentation of spleen

The grading system is adapted from the surgical classification by Schweizer et al. The CT scans of 45 patients with blunt splenic injuries were analyzed retrospectively and the CT findings were correlated with the need for surgery. The authors used a CT scale (I–V) for splenic parenchymal injuries that also allowed a comparison with the surgical findings in patients who underwent laparotomy and the classification given by Resciniti et al., which refers to both the extent of parenchymal injuries and the amount of hemoperitoneum. All 5 patients who required delayed laparotomy initially had only minor injuries (grade I or II), whereas 11 patients (58%) with injuries of grade III, IV, or V were successfully treated conservatively. Twelve patients had CT-based score below 2.5 and 2 patients (17%) needed delayed surgery. Twenty (69%) patients with initial scores of 2.5 or higher and eight patients (57%) with initial scores higher than 4 were successfully managed without surgery. The results show that CT findings cannot be used to determine reliably which patients require surgery and which can be treated conservatively. The choice between operative and nonoperative management of splenic trauma should be mainly based on clinical findings rather than CT findings. In this retrospective study, the Resciniti CT score (1–6) correlated better with the need for surgery than did the CT scale (I–V). CT should be used to delineate the presence or absence of splenic injury.

Reference

Olivero G, Franchello A, Adduci A, Orlando E, Cotogni P (1994) Lesions of the spleen caused by blunt trauma. Proposal of a classification based on CT and correlation with prognosis and treatment. Minerva Chir 49:751–757

Criteria	Point	Description of injury
A. Free intra-peritoneal fluid	0	Absent
	1	Perisplenic
	2	Any other compartment except perisplenic or pelvic
	3	Perivesical compartments
	4	Superior to 500 ml
B. Associated abdominal injury	0	Absent
	1	Nonsignificant (moderate)
	2	Significant, but requiring no intervention
	5	Surgery required
C. Type of splenic injury	0	No injury
	1	Linear laceration, hematoma ≤3 cm
	2	Deep and irregular fracture Hematoma >3 cm
	3	Ruptured subcapsular or intraparenchymal hematoma
	5	Shattered spleen or severe vascular lesion
D. Location of splenic injury	0	Polar
	1	Central
	2	Parahilar

A scoring system was elaborated on the basis of data obtained from CT by evaluating four parameters: extent of free intraperitoneal effusion, concomitant lesions to other abdominal organs, severity and site of splenic lesion. This classification gives a high degree of prognostic accuracy and provides a useful guideline in the choice of the most appropriate treatment. Stable patients with a total score inferior or equal to 5 could be selected for conservative treatment; patients with a higher score should undergo laparotomy. Absolute indication for surgery is required for class A4, B5, and C5.

Reference

Moore EE, Cogbill TH, Jurkovich GJ, Shackford SR, Malangoni MA, Champion HR (1995) Organ injury scaling: spleen and liver (1994 revision). J Trauma 38:323–324

Grade[a]	Type of injury	Description of injury
I	Hematoma	Subcapsular, <10% surface area
	Laceration	Capsular tear, <1 cm parenchymal depth
II	Hematoma	Subcapsular, 10%–50% surface area;
		Intraparenchymal, <5 cm in diameter
	Laceration	1–3 cm parenchymal depth, which does not involve a trabecular vessel
III	Hematoma	Subcapsular, >50% surface area or expanding
		Ruptured subcapsular or parenchymal hematoma
		Intraparenchymal hematoma >5 cm or expanding
	Laceration	>3 cm parenchymal depth or involving trabecular vessels
IV	Laceration	Laceration involving segmental or hilar vessels producing major devascularization (>25% of spleen)
V	Laceration	Completely shattered spleen
	Vascular	Hilar vascular injury which devascularizes spleen

[a]Advance one grade for multiple injuries, up to grade III.

The fundamental purpose of this classification was to devise injury severity scores for individual organs to facilitate clinical investigation and outcomes research. The OIS is a classification scheme based on the anatomical disruption of an individual organ scaled I–V, representing the least to most severe injury. Grades I–V represent increasingly complex injuries encountered in salvageable patients, whereas grade VI is a destructive lesion incompatible with survival.

Reference

Ruess L, Sivit CJ, Eichelberger MR, Taylor GA, Bond SJ (1995) Blunt hepatic and splenic trauma in children: correlation of a CT injury severity scale with clinical outcome. Pediatr Radiol 25:321–325

Grade	Description
1	Laceration involving <25% (of splenic volume)
2	Laceration involving 25%–50% (of splenic volume)
3	Shattered spleen

Sixty-nine children with isolated hepatic injury and 53 with isolated splenic injury were prospectively classified at CT according to extent of parenchymal involvement. Isolated subcapsular hematoma was classified as a grade 1 injury. Clinical records were reviewed to determine clinical outcome. A majority of children with hepatic and splenic injury were managed nonoperatively without requiring blood transfusion. The severity of injury graded by CT did not correlate with the need for surgery. Increasing grade of hepatic injury at CT was associated with increasing frequency of blood transfusion. CT staging was not discriminatory in predicting transfusion requirement in splenic injury.

Reference

Williams RA, Black JJ, Sinow RM, Wilson SE (1997) Computed tomography-assisted management of splenic trauma. Am J Surg 174:276–279

Grade	Description of injury
A	Subcapsular hematoma and capsular disruption
B	Parenchymal injury not extending into hilum
C	Parenchymal injury extending into hilum

The severity of splenic trauma evidenced on CT guides safe nonoperative management. Hemodynamically stable patients, not suffering injury to the splenic hilum (A and B scores), can be managed without operation, resulting in shorter hospital stays and fewer blood products used. The frequency of celiotomy has fallen with 27% fewer grade A patients and 27% fewer grade B patients undergoing laparotomy, when discussion was based on the CT grading system vs the surgeon's choice. The formation of a subcapsular hematoma is not a good predictor of delayed splenic rupture.

27.5 Diaphragm

Reference

Moore EE, Malagoni MA, Cogbill TH et al. (1994) Organ injury scaling. IV: Thoracic vascular, lung, cardiac, and diaphragm. J Trauma 36:299–300

Grade[a]	Description of injury
I	Contusion
II	Laceration ≤ 2 cm
III	Laceration 2–10 cm
IV	Laceration > 10 cm with tissue loss ≤ 25 cm^2
V	Laceration with tissue loss > 25 cm^2

[a]Advance one grade for bilateral injuries

The fundamental purpose of this classification was to devise injury severity scores for individual organs to facilitate clincal investigations and outcomes research. The Organ Injury Scaling (OIS) is a classification scheme based on the anatomic disruption of an individual organ scaled I to V, representing the least to most severe injury. Grades I to V represent increasingly complex injuries encountered in salvageable patients.

This classification is anatomic but, does not include pericardiophrenic ruptures. No attempt in the current literature has been made to correlate this classification to the severity of trauma and outcome.

27.6 Pancreas

Reference

Lucas CE (1977) Diagnosis and treatment of pancreatic and duodenal injury. Surg Clin North Am 57:49–65

Class	Description of injury
I	Contusion, peripheral laceration, intact ductal system
II	Distal laceration, transection, disruption, suspected ductal disruption; no duodenal injury
III	Proximal laceration, transection, disruption, suspected ductal injury; no duodenal injury
IV	Severe combined pancreaticoduodenal disruption

Morbidity and mortality are directly related to the severity of both pancreatic and duodenal injury and the presence of combined pancreaticoduodenal injury. Minor pancreatic injury such as contusion, hematoma, or small laceration (class I injury) of the body and tail of the pancreas, obviously not involving the main pancreatic duct, is best treated by obtaining hemostasis followed by drainage. Major lacerations, fractures, or intraparenchymal hematomas (class II injury) of the body and tail of the pancreas are best treated by distal pancreatectomy with splenectomy. Following distal pancreatectomy, several options are available, including Roux-en-Y pancreaticojejunostomy or simple closure of the resected margin in a "fish mouth" manner. Class III pancreatic injury in the absence of duodenal injury is best treated by the duodenal diverticulization procedure if the main pancreatic duct is uninvolved. Involvement of the main pancreatic duct at this level requires completion of the pancreatic transection to the right of the superior mesenteric vein. Class IV pancreatic injuries are severe pancreaticoduodenal injuries; the selection of treatment is based upon the integrity of the main pancreatic duct.

Reference

Jurkovich J, Carrico J (1990) Pancreatic trauma. Surg Clin North Am 70:575–593

Grade	Description of injury	Treatment[a]
1	Contusion and laceration without duct injury	External drainage, infrequent distal pancreatectomy
2	Distal transection or parenchymal injury with duct injury	Distal pancreatectomy
3	Proximal transection or parenchymal injury with probable duct injury	Distal pancreatectomy or Roux-en-Y pancreaticojejunostomy
4	Combined pancreatic and duodenal injury, ampulla and blood supply intact	Repair/exclude duodenum; treat pancreas as per 1, 2, 3
	Massive injury, ampulla destroyed, devascularization	Pancreatico-duodenectomy

[a]External drainage is necessary following any pancreatic resection, debridement or repair.

The management of specific pancreatic injury depends on the status of the main pancreatic duct, the degree of parenchymal damage and the anatomical location of the injury. Complete visualization of the gland and accurate determination of the duct status are key intraoperative maneuvers. Failure to recognize significant pancreatic duct and parenchymal injury is the major cause of postoperative morbidity. The vast majority of pancreatic injuries can be managed by simple drainage with or without debridement or suture. However, the occasional major transection or pancreatic duct injury warrants rigorous efforts to determine the status of the major ducts.

Reference

Moore EE, Cogbill TH, Malangoni MA et al (1995) Organ injury scaling. Surg Clin North Am 75:293–303

Grade[a]	Type of injury	Description of injury
I	Hematoma	Minor contusion without duct injury
	Laceration	Superficial laceration without duct injury
II	Hematoma	Major contusion without duct injury or tissue loss
	Laceration	Major laceration without duct injury or tissue loss
III	Laceration	Distal transection or parenchymal injury with duct injury
IV	Laceration	Proximal[b] transection or parenchymal injury involving ampulla
V	Laceration	Massive disruption of pancreatic head

[a]Advance one grade for multiple injuries up to grade III.

[b]Proximal pancreas is to the patient's right of the superior mesenteric vein.

The fundamental purpose of this classification was to devise injury severity scores for individual organs to facilitate clinical investigation and outcomes research. The OIS is a classification scheme based on the anatomical disruption of an individual organ scaled I–V, representing the least to most severe injury. Grades I–V represent increasingly complex injuries encountered in salvageable patients.

Reference

Takishima T, Sugimoto K, Hirata M, Asari Y, Ohwada T, Kakita A (1997) Serum amylase level on admission in the diagnosis of blunt injury to the pancreas. Its significance and limitations. Ann Surg 226:70–76

Type	Description of injury
I	Contusion
	A mild pancreatic injury without any laceration of the retroperitoneal fascia that allows the pancreatic fluid to spread into the peritoneal cavity
II	Laceration
	Various parenchymal injuries without injury to the main pancreatic ducts
III	Ductal injury
IIIa[a]	Injury to the main pancreatic duct in the body or the tail of the pancreas
IIIb[a]	Injury to the main pancreatic duct in the head of the pancreas, injury to the accessory pancreatic duct, or injury to the intrapancreatic bile duct

[a]The borderline used to discriminate between type IIIa and IIIb is the right margin of the superior mesenteric vein.

Pancreatic injury is graded by reference to the classification of pancreatic injuries provided by the Japanese Association for the Surgery of Trauma. Determination of the serum amylase level is not diagnostic within 3 h or less of trauma, irrespective of the type of injury.

Reference

Wong YC, Wang LJ, Lin BC, Chen CJ, Lim KE, Chen RJ (1997) CT grading of blunt pancreatic injuries: prediction of ductal disruption and surgical correlation. J Comput Assist Tomogr 21:246–250

Grade	CT Description of injury
A	Pancreatitis and/or superficial lacerations at any site
BI	Deep lacerations at distal pancreas
BII	Transections at distal pancreas
CI	Deep lacerations at proximal pancreas
CII	Transections at proximal pancreas

The authors retrospectively reviewed CT scans of 22 patients with proven blunt pancreatic injuries. They graded injuries on CT, based on the presence or absence of pancreatic lacerations, site, and depth (superficial, <50% of thickness; deep, >50% of thickness). CT grading was correlated with surgical findings for glandular and ductal injuries based on the modified OIS for the pancreas. CT grading of blunt pancreatic injuries was useful in predicting ductal integrity or disruption. Ductal disruption was likely present if the pancreas appeared to have a transection or deep laceration on CT. Grading was accurate in grade A and B injuries, overestimation could occur in grade CI and CII injuries. There were 2 normal scans, 10 grade A, 5 grade B (1 BI, 4 BII), and 5 grade C (1 CI, 4 CII) blunt pancreatic injuries on the CT grading scheme.

Reference

Shilyansky J, Sena LM, Kreller M, Chait P, Babyn PS, Filler RM (1998) Nonoperative management of pancreatic injuries in children. J Pediatr Surg 33:343–349

Group (clinical)	Type (CT)	Pancreatic injury	Description of injury
I	1	Contusion	Diffuse or focal swelling of the pancreas
II	2	Stellate fragmentation	Fluid or blood dissecting within pancreatic parenchyma
	3	Partial fracture	Incomplete separation of two portions of the pancreas
	4	Complete transection	Complete separation of two portions of the pancreas
III	5	Pseudocyst	Persistent peripancreatic fluid collection

Thirty-five consecutive children with pancreatic injuries treated over the past 10 years were reviewed. Twenty-eight children (80%) sustaining pancreatic injuries were treated nonoperatively. Abdominal imaging in these children demonstrated pancreatic contusion in 14, transection in 11, and pseudocyst in 3. Children with types 2, 3, and 4 (group II) pancreatic injuries had a significantly higher incidence of pseudocysts, compared with children with type 1 (14% vs 45%) injury and only children in group II required percutaneous drainage (0% vs 36%). Nonoperative management of pancreatic contusion and transection diagnosed radiologically is effective and safe. Pseudocysts may form after pancreatic injury and if large or symptomatic, can be managed successfully by percutaneous drainage.

Reference

Jobst MA, Canty TG, Lynch FP (1999) Management of pancreatic injury in pediatric blunt abdominal trauma. J Pediatr Surg 34:818–824

Class	Description of injury
I	Contusion or laceration without duct injury
II	Distal transection or parenchymal injury with probable duct injury
III	Proximal transection or parenchymal injury with probable duct injury
IV	Combined pancreatic and duodenal injury

Pancreatic injury was documented in 56 children, aged 2 months to 14 years, with blunt mechanisms of injury. The majority of pancreatic injuries can be managed nonoperatively. Initial nonoperative management of injuries of the proximal pancreatic duct allows for the formation and uneventful delayed drainage of a pseudocyst, rather than the risks of early radical interventions. Distal duct injuries are best managed by prompt spleen-sparing distal pancreatectomy. There is no benefit of closed drainage for management of minor pancreatic injuries discovered at laparotomy. The study shows that CT imaging obtained at admission is a valuable tool, when positive for pancreatic injury, because it identified injury location consistently and rarely overgraded injuries. However, CT should not be used as a study of exclusion, because many patients with normal initial CT scans were later found to have pancreatic injury on repeat imaging or laparotomy.

Reference

Takishima T, Hirata M, Kataoka Y et al (2000) Pancreatographic classification of pancreatic ductal injuries caused by blunt injury to the pancreas. J Trauma 48:745–751

Class	Description of injury
1	Radiographically normal pancreatic ductal system
2a	Injury to branches of the pancreatic duct without contrast extravasation outside the pancreatic parenchyma
2b	Injury to branches of the pancreatic duct with contrast extravasation into the retroperitoneal space
3a	Main duct injury in the body or tail of the pancreas
3b	Main duct injury in the head of the pancreas

The authors developed a classification system for pancreatic ductal injuries, based on a retrospective analysis of blunt pancreatic injuries in 40 patients. They assessed the relationship between findings on pancreatography (36 endoscopic retrograde procedures and 4 transduodenal procedures), the treatment modality, and the clinical course. The results of pancreatography that indicated injury to the pancreatic duct included extravasation of contrast medium from the pancreatic ductal system, obstruction of this system, or both. Patients with class 1 injuries (radiographically normal ducts, n=13) could be treated nonsurgically without major complications. Patients with class 2 injuries (branch injuries, n=7), in whom contrast medium from ductal branches did not leak from the pancreatic parenchyma (class 2a, n=3), could be treated nonsurgically. Patients with leaks into the retroperitoneal space (class 2b, n=4) required at least a drainage laparotomy. Patients with class 3 injuries (main duct injuries, n=20), including two patients in whom conservative treatment resulted in severe complications, required laparotomy. Early use of endoscopic retrograde pancreatography (ERP) to detect injury to the pancreatic ductal system, including branches of the pancreatic duct, is determinant for management and this classification system may facilitate the selection of appropriate therapeutic modalities for patients with blunt pancreatic injury.

27.7 Kidney

Reference

Sargent JC, Marquardt CR (1950) Renal injuries. J Urol 63:1–8

Type	Description of injury
I	Minor fracture
II	Major fracture
III	Shattered kidney

The authors studied over 200 patients and established three major categories of injuries. The most common type of renal injury is contusion or minor parenchymal fracture (120 cases), characterized by more or less pain, a brief spell of gross hematuria, and essentially negative X-ray findings. There were 72 cases of major parenchymal fracture. Patients had localized pain and rigidity, with gross bleeding lasting several to many days, and presented either pyelographic evidence of parenchymal fracture or soft tissue shadows, indicating perirenal hematoma. There were 14 cases of shattered kidney. Patients usually shot or severely injured otherwise, with massive perirenal hemorrhage and with complete loss of normal pelvic architecture in the pyelogram. All of the cases of renal injury known to be of minor degree were treated conservatively and there was no recorded complication related to the renal injury. Of the 72 cases suffering from major parenchymal fracture, but with pyelic architecture reasonably preserved, only two were subject to prompt surgery (2.7%). Nine of the 70 cases (13%) of major parenchymal fractures treated conservatively are known to have suffered from important sequelae. Six of the 14 cases of shattered kidney were diagnosed at autopsy and six were operated upon at once. There were two other cases that were treated expectantly and finally nephrectomized.

Reference

Vermillion CD, McLaughlin AP, Pfister RC (1971) Management of blunt renal trauma. J Urol 106:478–484

Group	Description of injury
1	Renal parenchymal contusions – no radiographic abnormality
2	Renal parenchymal injuries with intact renal capsule and collecting system
3	Renal parenchymal injuries with disrupted renal capsule and intact collecting system
4	Renal parenchymal injuries involving renal collecting system
5	Renal pedicle injuries

Ninety-two cases of blunt renal trauma were seen, in 88 cases excretory urograms (IVPs) were obtained when the patient was admitted to the hospital. Five retrograde pyelograms and nine selective renal angiograms were necessary for definitive diagnosis. Patients were grouped into five categories based on radiographic and surgical findings. Experience of the authors with blunt renal trauma suggests that most patients fall into two categories. The larger category (groups 1 and 2) included 65 patients (71%) with contusions or relatively mild intrarenal injuries. All these patients have done well and have had no long-term complications. Only one patient required operation for a congenital anomaly. Twenty-four patients (25%) in groups 3 and 4 sustained major renal injuries accompanied by retroperitoneal extravasation of blood or urine. Ultimately, 14 general surgical procedures were performed, 8 of which were urological, with 3 immediate, 2 delayed and 1 partial nephrectomy. The remaining 16 were treated conservatively; these patients are symptomatic and have had normal IVPs for 1–5 years after trauma. Three patients with renal pedicle injuries were seen and all were operated upon shortly after admission. Despite early surgical intervention, only one of these kidneys was salvaged.

Reference

Wein AJ, Murphy JJ, Mulholland SG, Chait AW, Arger PH (1977) A conservative approach to the management of blunt renal trauma. J Urol 117:425–427

Group	Radiological abnormality
I	None
II	Intrarenal distortion, incomplete visualization, intrarenal or extrarenal extravasation, parenchymal fracture, caliceal or pelvic clots, perirenal hematoma
III	Extensive fragmentation, pedicle injury
Subgroup of II	Finding in patients managed conservatively
IIa	Intrarenal hematoma, extravasation or distortion
IIb	Poor or incomplete visualization
IIc	Extrarenal extravasation, no definite evidence of fracture
IId	Parenchymal fracture with extravasation
IIe	Collecting system, pelvic or ureteral clots
IIf	Perirenal hematoma

Eighty-five cases of blunt renal trauma studied with intravenous pyelography were evaluated. Injuries were retrospectively grouped on the basis of findings present on the initial radiological examination. Further early evaluation and subsequent management were guided primarily by close clinical observation and frequent reevaluation of signs and symptoms rather than by the initial radiological appearance of the kidney alone. Indications for more aggressive evaluation and surgical intervention included clinical or laboratory evidence of persistent blood loss, an expanding flank mass, and the development of increasing or persistent pain and fever. Patients with group I injuries will rarely, if ever, require angiography or an operation for reasons related to kidney injury alone. Of the 38 patients in group I, all were initially clinically stable and remained so. All patients were treated with bed rest alone until the symptoms and signs disappeared. None has had complications. Early operative intervention in group II patients can be shown statistically to have resulted in nephrectomy rates as high as 35%. Conservative management has resulted in nephrectomy rates as low as 4%–6%. Only six surgical procedures were ultimately performed for reasons related to renal trauma in 42 patients in group II, who were managed conservatively. Delayed complications, which eventually require treatment, such as hemorrhage, infection, hypertension, hydronephrosis, and segmental or total nonfunction or atrophy, are uncommon. Patients with group III injuries can be expected to produce clinical instability or deterioration and require an immediate or delayed operation, usually nephrectomy. A conservative nonoperative approach is advocated in all clinically stable patients, if renal pedicle injury can be ruled out.

Reference

Ney C, Friedenberg M (1981) Trauma to the kidney. In: Ney C (ed) Radiographic atlas of the genitourinary system. Lippincott, Philadelphia, pp 457–514

Grade	Description of injury
1	Simple contusion without extensive parenchymal destruction
2	Minor fractures communicating with one or two calyces
3	Major parenchymal ruptures
4	Major vascular injury

This classification is particularly related to plain radiographs and intravenous pyelography. Simple contusion (grade 1) is the most frequent renal injury (>50%), usually consisting of minor parenchymal infarctions, not communicating with the calyces, and associated with an intact renal capsule. There may be areas of subcapsular hemorrhage. Transient hematuria is present. Usually there will be no significant radiographic findings. Conservative therapy is sufficient. Minor fractures (grade 2) communicate with one or two calyces (30% of injuries). The renal capsule is frequently intact. Extravasation of contrast material may be seen on the urogram, but not uncommonly, the examination will appear to be normal. Gross hematuria is usually present. Pyelography is not indicated because of the possibility of increasing bleeding or introducing infection. Significant perirenal or retroperitoneal hematoma is usually not present. Conservative therapy usually suffices. Major parenchymal ruptures (grade 3) may vary from multiple ruptures communicating with many of the calyces to a split kidney, transected in the midportion, to a shattered kidney that may show little recognizable renal structure. The renal capsule usually is torn and an extrarenal hematoma is present. If function is present, extravasation is often seen on the intravenous urogram. Aside from split or shattered kidneys, the majority of major injuries, which represent about 10% of cases, may still be treated conservatively. Major vascular injury (grade 4) includes twisting, stretching, or puncture wounds, which occasionally may damage the vascular pedicle, producing renal artery or less commonly renal vein occlusion or hemorrhage. Thrombosis usually occurs at the junction of the fixed and mobile portions (junction of proximal and middle third) of the artery. Sudden stretching may tear the intima, which protrudes as a flap into the artery, leading to thrombosis. Angiography should be performed promptly. Sudden complete occlusion is a surgical emergency, and must be operated on as soon as possible, certainly within 24 h, to ensure return of renal function. Angioplasty may become an important treatment modality. Management is best guided by clinical findings and not solely by radiologic demonstration of renal injury

Reference

Federle MP, Kaiser JA, McAninch JW, Jeffrey RB, Mall JC (1981) The role of computed tomography in renal trauma. Radiology 141:455–460

Grade	Description of injury
I minor	Contusion and minor cortical laceration without disruption of the caliceal system
II major	Cortical lesions which communicate with the collecting system (complete laceration and renal fracture)
III catastrophic	Shattered kidney and injuries to the renal pedicle

CT and excretory urography were performed in 15 patients, thought to have major renal trauma, which was blunt in 11 and penetrating in 4. In four cases, CT demonstrated extravasation of urine not detected by urography and in all cases parenchymal injuries and extrarenal hematomas were depicted more accurately by CT. CT also proved to be superior to excretory urography in distinguishing relatively minor renal injuries (contusion, incomplete laceration, intrarenal hematoma, small extrarenal hematoma) from major or catastrophic injuries (complete laceration, fracture, shattered kidney), which significantly influenced the choice of surgical or medical therapy. There is general agreement among urologists that category I lesions (minor, 75%–85% of injuries) are best managed conservatively, while category III lesions (catastrophic, 5% of injuries) require urgent surgery. Though opinion is divided over proper management of category II lesions (major, 10% of injuries), virtually all authors stress the need for more accurate evaluation of the type and extent of injury, so that therapy can be planned. CT also detected concurrent injuries of the spleen, liver and/or pancreas in four cases. The authors feel that CT is valuable in the assessment of major renal trauma.

Reference

Guerriero WG (1982) Trauma to the kidneys, ureters, bladder, and urethra. Surg Clin North Am 62:1047–1074

Grade	Description of injury
Minor	Contusion Shallow cortical laceration Forniceal disruption
Major	Renal pedicle injury Deep parenchymal injury with an intact capsule Deep parenchymal injury with a disrupted capsule Shattered kidney with an intact capsule Shattered kidney with a disrupted capsule Ureteral or renal pelvis injury

This classification divides patients into those who have suffered either major or minor renal trauma. All patients with minor injury (85%) may be managed expectantly, while the major injuries (15%) demand surgical exploration in most cases. Deep parenchymal injury with an intact capsule and shattered kidney with an intact capsule are considered intermediate. In these two subgroups, management may be either expectant or surgical, depending on the clinical status of the patient.

Reference

Bretan PN, McAninch JW, Federle MP, Jeffrey RB Jr (1986) Computerized tomographic staging of renal trauma: 85 consecutive cases. J Urol 136:561–565

Grade	Description of injury
A	Minor laceration
B	Renal contusion
C	Major laceration (deep medullary laceration)
D	Major laceration (fractured kidney)
E	Major laceration (laceration into collecting system)
F	Vascular injury

In 85 patients with renal trauma, the authors compared the findings on CT with those of excretory urography, renal or intra-abdominal surgery, and angiography. Blunt trauma accounted for 87.1% of the renal injuries and penetrating trauma for 12.9%. There was no correlation between the severity of injury found on CT staging and the grade of hematuria. It is concluded that CT is rapid and noninvasive, and can stage renal trauma more sensitively and specifically than intravenous pyelography (IVP), nephrotomography, or arteriography. It can differentiate major from minor renal lacerations, assess concomitant retroperitoneal and abdominal injuries, and enable physiological functional assessment of the renal parenchyma. CT allowed for precise staging of renal trauma, thus, enabling a more accurate assessment of the need for surgery. The subdivision of major laceration in grade C and D is probably not relevant to treatment, since in both cases there is no involvement of the collecting system.

Reference

Karp MP, Jewett TC Jr, Kuhn JP, Allen JE, Dokler ML, Cooney DR (1986) The impact of computed tomography scanning on the child with renal trauma. J Pediatr Surg 21:617–623

Grade	Description of injury
I	Small parenchymal injury
	No subcapsular or perirenal fluid
	Uninjured anomaly
II	Incomplete renal laceration
	Subcapsular or small perirenal fluid
III	Extensive laceration or fracture
	Large perirenal collection
IV	Multiple fragments (shattered)
V	Vascular injury

One hundred seventy-six consecutive patients with suspected renal trauma were reviewed. One hundred thirty-eight were evaluated by CT and IVP, the other 38 by excretory urogram alone. A radiologist, unaware of the clinical course, graded each of the CT scans according to injury severity and the treatment decision; the decision as to operative vs nonoperative management was made based on injury severity and the patient's hemodynamic stability following initial resuscitation. Forty-four renal injuries were identified, 36 (77%) resolved without operation. Four patients underwent immediate surgery. Two cases had nephrectomies for unrepairable grade V vascular injuries. One nephrectomy and one nephrorrhaphy were performed on grade IV kidneys. No immediate surgical procedure was necessary on grades I, II, and III injuries. Of the four delayed operations, two (grade I) were performed for ureteropelvic junction obstruction, diagnosed during the renal trauma workup. An additional patient underwent a delayed renal exploration to differentiate a grade III lesion from a suspected renal tumor. A perirenal hematoma was found and drained. The fourth patient underwent retrograde placement of a ureteral catheter due to transient ureteral obstruction. CT provides better definition of the injury for making the decision to operate or place the patient in nonoperative management. The extravasation seen on CT is frequently exaggerated and should not be an absolute indication for exploration.

Reference

Marberger H (1988) Blunt injuries of the kidney. In: Cass AS (ed) Genitourinary trauma. Blackwell Scientific, Boston, pp 11–35

Grade	Description of injury
I	Minor injuries: hematuria, minor changes on IVP, limited-localized hematoma, good general condition
II	Major injuries: visible rupture, extrarenal hematoma, severe symptoms
III	Complex injuries: rupture of solitary or malformed kidney, significant vascular lesions, rupture of renal pelvis or ureter.

This classification includes morphological and clinical parameters, which can be used as prognostic factors.

Reference

Federle M (1989) Evaluation of renal trauma. In: Pollack HM (ed) Clinical urography. Saunders, Philadelphia, pp 1472–1494

Grade	Description of injury
I	Minor: contusion, small corticomedullary lacerations that do not communicate with the collecting system, and small perinephric hematoma
II	Major: deep corticomedullary lacerations that communicate with the collecting system (complete laceration and renal "fracture")
III	Catastrophic: shattered kidney, main vascular pedicle injury
IV	Ureteropelvic junction avulsion and/or lacerations of the renal pelvis

A special category is assigned to the relatively uncommon entity of ureteropelvic junction avulsion and/or laceration of the renal pelvis (category IV).

Reference

Moore EE, Shackford SR, Pachter HL et al (1989) Organ injury scaling: spleen, liver, and kidney. J Trauma 29:1664–1666

Grade[a]	Type of injury	Description of injury
I	Contusion	Microscopic or gross hematuria; urological studies normal
	Hematoma	Subcapsular, nonexpanding without parenchymal laceration
II	Hematoma	Nonexpanding perirenal hematoma confined to renal retroperitoneum
	Laceration	<1 cm parenchymal depth of renal cortex without urinary extravasation
III	Laceration	>1 cm parenchymal depth of renal cortex without collecting system rupture or urinary extravasation
IV	Laceration	Parenchymal laceration extending through the renal cortex, medulla, and collecting system
	Vascular	Main renal artery or vein injury with contained hemorrhage
V	Laceration	Completely shattered kidney
	Vascular	Avulsion of renal hilum which devascularizes kidney

[a]Advance one grade for bilateral injury up to grade III.

The fundamental purpose of this classification was to devise injury severity scores for individual organs to facilitate clinical investigation and outcomes research. The OIS is a classification scheme based on the anatomical disruption of an individual organ scaled I–V, representing the least to most severe injury. Grades I–V represent increasingly complex injuries encountered in salvageable patients, whereas grade VI is a destructive lesion incompatible with survival.

Reference

Mee SL, McAninch JW (1989) Indications for radiographic assessment in suspected renal trauma. Urol Clin North Am 16:187–192

Mee SL, McAninch JW, Robinson AL, Auerbach PS, Carroll PR (1989) Radiographic assessment of renal trauma: a 10-year prospective study of patient selection. J Urol 141:1095–1098

Grade	Description of injury
1	Contusions: bruises or subcapsular hematomas with an intact renal capsule
2	Minor lacerations: superficial cortical parenchymal disruption that does not involve the collecting system or the deep renal medulla
3	Major lacerations: parenchymal disruptions extending through the cortex, deep medulla or collecting system
4	Vascular injuries: occlusions or tears of the renal artery or vein or their segmental branches

This classification is similar to the American Association for the Surgery of Trauma classification; however, it gathers in one group (grade 3) lacerations that do not involve the collecting system and laceration with urinary extravasation. This is probably incorrect, since management of these two types of tears is different: conservative for major tears without expanding hematomas and more often surgical for tears with significant urine leakage. In hemodynamically stable patients in whom renal injury alone is suspected, intravenous urography with nephrotomography is recommended as the first imaging study. This study will adequately stage 60%–85% of renal injuries. CT is more sensitive and specific and should be performed if the urography results are equivocal and as a primary staging modality when multiple injuries are suspected. Arteriography can be reserved for patients with suspected renovascular injuries in whom CT scans are inconclusive. Patients who undergo emergency laparotomy for associated injuries without complete urological evaluation need and intravenous urogram on the operating table before renal exploration is undertaken.

Reference

Fanney DR, Casillas J, Murphy BJ (1990) CT in the diagnosis of renal trauma. Radiographics 10:29–40

Category	Description of injury
1	Renal contusion Intrarenal hematoma Segmental infarction Small subcapsular hematoma
2	Large subcapsular hematoma Corticomedullary laceration Complete renal laceration Renal fracture Disruption of ureteropelvic junction Shattered kidney with contained fragments Renal vein injury
3	Shattered kidney with disrupted fragments Renal artery occlusion Renal artery avulsion

This classification relies only on CT findings in grading renal injuries to give an indication for surgical treatment. Renal injuries are classified into three categories. Category 1 lesions (75%–85%) are relatively minor and are treated conservatively. Category 2 lesions are more serious injuries, for which the type of therapy used depends on the amount of nonviable tissue, the extent of hemorrhage, and the presence or absence of extravasated urine. These lesions may be treated conservatively or surgically, depending on the clinical status of the patient and radiological assessment. CT has greatly influenced the management of these lesions, since it can accurately depict the extent of injury. Category 3 lesions (5%) are catastrophic injuries that require urgent surgery. Prompt diagnosis by means of CT allows successful reconstruction in some cases.

Reference

Lent V (1995) What management for renal injuries? Chirurg 66:708–714

Lent V (1996) What classification is appropriate in renal trauma? Eur Urol 30:327–334

Grade	Description of injury
P – Pathogenesis	1 Blunt injury 2 Perforating injury
LA – Parenchymal injuries	x Not appraisable 0 Not detectable 1 Contusion without rupture 2 Partial rupture 3 Complete rupture 4 Partial dislocation 5 Complete dislocation 6 Partial sequestration 7 Complete sequestration
LB – Renal pelvis injuries	x Not appraisable 0 Not detectable 1 Complete rupture 2 Complete detachment
LC – Vascular injuries	x Not appraisable 0 Not detectable 1 Partial arterial (intimal) rupture 2 Partial venous occlusion 3 Partial arterial occlusion 4 Complete venous occlusion 5 Complete arterial occlusion 6 Complete venous rupture 7 Complete arterial rupture 8 Complete venous detachment 9 Complete arterial detachment
SA – Symptoms of hemorrhage	x Not appraisable 0 Not detectable 1 Irrelevant hematuria/hematoma 2 Compensatable hematuria/hematoma 3 Progressive/potentially/fatal hemorrhage
SB – Symptoms of urinary extravasation	x Not appraisable 0 Not detectable 1 Intracapsular/intrafascial extravasation 2 Extrafascial/retroperitoneal extravasation 3 Progressive extravasation, urinoma
SC – Symptoms of kidney damage	x Not appraisable 0 Not detectable 1 Loss of function 0%–30% 2 Loss of function 31%–60% 3 Loss of function 61%–100%

To take into consideration all criteria which may be important for the outcome of renal trauma, a differentiated PLS classification is proposed comprising the following elements: the pathogenesis P1 (blunt injuries), P2 (perforating injuries); the locations of the injuries LA (parenchyma), LB (renal pelvis), LC (vascular system); with their degrees of injuries LA 0–7, LB 0–2, LC 0–9; and the symptoms of injury SA (hemorrhage), SB (extravasation of urine), SC (kidney damage); with their degrees of severity SA 0–3, SB 0–3, SC 0–3 as prognostic factors. In making clinical decisions, injuries with a defined trauma formula can be treated according to alternative concepts, e.g., LA 1–4, LC 1–3, SA–C 1–2 with conservative methods, LA 5–7, LB 1–2, LC 4–9, SA–C 3 with surgical methods.

Reference

Kawashima A, Sandler CM, Corl FM et al (2001) Imaging of renal trauma: a comprehensive review. Radiographics 21: 557–574

Category	Description of injury
I	Minor injury: renal contusion, intrarenal and subcapsular hematoma, minor laceration with limited perinephric hematoma without extension to the collecting system or medulla, small subsegmental cortical infarct
II	Major injury: major renal laceration through the cortex extending to the medulla or collecting system with or without urine extravasation, segmental renal infarct
III	Catastrophic injury: multiple renal lacerations, vascular injury involving the renal pedicle
IV	Ureteropelvic junction injury: avulsion (complete transection), or laceration (incomplete tear)

Renal injuries can be classified into four large categories based on imaging findings. Category I renal injuries constitute 75%–85% of all renal injuries in most series and are generally managed conservatively. Lesions in category II comprise approximately 10% of renal injuries, their management is variable. Affected patients are usually treated conservatively, but occasionally require surgical exploration, depending on hemodynamic status and the evolution of the injury. Lesions in category III are catastrophic injuries; they account for approximately 5% of cases and generally require surgical exploration, often nephrectomy. Category IV injuries are uncommon ureteropelvic junction injuries. Avulsion is usually treated with surgical repair, whereas laceration may be treated conservatively or with stent placement.

27.8 Adrenal

Reference

Moore EE, Malangoni MA, Cogbill TH et al (1996) Organ injury scaling VII: cervical vascular, peripheral vascular, adrenal, penis, testis, and scrotum. J Trauma 41:523–524

Grade[a]	Description of injury
I	Contusion
II	Laceration involving only cortex (<2 cm)
III	Laceration extending into medulla (≥2 cm)
IV	>50% parenchymal destruction
V	Total parenchymal destruction (including massive intraparenchymal hemorrhage)
	Avulsion from blood supply

[a]Advance one grade for bilateral lesions up to grade V.

The fundamental purpose was to devise injury severity scores for individual organs to facilitate clinical investigation and outcomes research. The OIS is a classification scheme based on the anatomical disruption of an individual organ scaled I–V, representing the least to most severe injury. Grades I–V represent increasingly complex injuries encountered in salvageable patients.

27.9 Ureter

Reference

Moore EE, Cogbill TH, Malangoni MA et al (1995) Organ injury scaling. Surg Clin North Am 75:293–303

Grade[a]	Type of injury	Description of injury
I	Hematoma	Contusion or hematoma without devascularization
II	Laceration	<50% transection
III	Laceration	>50% transection
IV	Laceration	Complete transection with <2 cm devascularization
V	Laceration	Avulsion with >2 cm of devascularization

[a]Advance one grade for bilateral lesions up to grade III.

The fundamental purpose was to devise injury severity scores for individual organs to facilitate clinical investigation and outcomes research. The OIS is a classification scheme based on the anatomical disruption of an individual organ scaled I–V, representing the least to most severe injury. Grades I–V represent increasingly complex injuries encountered in salvageable patients.

27.10 Urinary Bladder

Reference

Sandler CM, Hall JT, Rodriguez MB, Corriere JN (1986) Bladder injury in blunt pelvic trauma. Radiology 158:633–638
Vaccaro JP, Brody JM (2000) CT cystography in the evaluation of major bladder trauma. Radiographics 20:1373–1381

Type	Description of injury
1	Bladder contusion
2	Intraperitoneal rupture
3	Interstitial rupture
4a	Simple extraperitoneal rupture
4b	Complex extraperitoneal rupture
5	Combined rupture

A classification of bladder injury based on cystographic patterns of extravasation is proposed. Bladder contusion is defined as an incomplete or nonperforating tear of the bladder mucosa following blunt trauma to the pelvis. Hematuria will be present, but cystograms appear normal. Bladder contusion (type 1) is self-limiting and requires no specific therapy. Intraperitoneal bladder rupture (type 2) occurs in approximately 10%–20% of major bladder injuries, as a result of blows to the lower abdomen, in a patient with a distended bladder. This results in a nearly horizontal tear along the peritoneal portion of the bladder wall and thus intraperitoneal extravasation. Interstitial bladder rupture (type 3) is rare and is defined on cystograms as a mural defect in the contrast material-filled bladder adjacent to the bony pelvis but without frank perivesical extravasation. It describes a dissecting rupture of the bladder without a complete perforation. Simple extraperitoneal rupture (type 4a) is defined as extravasation of contrast material limited to the perivesical space. In complex extraperitoneal injury (type 4b), extravasation outside the confines of the perivesical space is present. Combined bladder rupture (type 5) associates intraperitoneal and extraperitoneal extravasation. Ninety-seven patients with bladder injury secondary to blunt pelvic trauma were reviewed. Fifty-five patients had extraperitoneal bladder rupture, 35 intraperitoneal rupture, 2 interstitial bladder injury, and 5 combined intraperitoneal and extraperitoneal bladder rupture. Of the 61 of 97 patients with film studies available for review, 2 patients with surgically proved intraperitoneal rupture had false-negative cystograms. In two other cases of intraperitoneal rupture, the diagnosis was established with cystography but was not demonstrated with urography. All cases of extraperitoneal rupture were demonstrated cystographically; in 15 cases from this group, injury was complex. In three of the cases of simple extraperitoneal bladder rupture, the diagnosis could only be made on the postdrainage film. In two additional patients, incomplete bladder injury termed interstitial bladder rupture was identified.

Accurate classification of injury in the clinical setting is critical for proper treatment. Intraperitoneal bladder ruptures (type 2) and combined intraperitoneal and extraperitoneal ruptures (type 5) require laparotomy with surgical repair of the bladder defect and diverting vesicostomy. Contusions (type 1) and interstitial injuries (type 3) are managed conservatively with Foley catheterization. Most extraperitoneal ruptures (type 4) may be treated with catheter drainage if the urine clears of blood, the catheter functions well, and the bladder neck is not injured; otherwise, formal surgical repair is necessary. Prognosis for clinical recovery is excellent if these diagnostic criteria are used.

Reference

Moore EE, Cogbill TH, Malangoni MA et al (1995) Organ injury scaling. Surg Clin North Am 75:293–303

Grade[a]	Type of injury	Description of injury
I	Hematoma	Contusion, intramural hematoma
	Laceration	Partial thickness
II	Laceration	Extraperitoneal bladder wall laceration <2 cm
III	Laceration	Extraperitoneal (>2 cm) or intraperitoneal (<2 cm) bladder wall laceration
IV	Laceration	Intraperitoneal bladder wall laceration >2 cm
V	Laceration	Intraperitoneal or extraperitoneal bladder wall laceration extending into the bladder neck or ureteral orifice (trigone)

[a]Advance one grade for multiple lesions up to grade III.

The fundamental purpose of this classification was to devise injury severity scores for individual organs to facilitate clinical investigation and outcomes research. The OIS is a classification scheme based on the anatomical disruption of an individual organ scaled I–V, representing the least to most severe injury. Grades I–V represent increasingly complex injuries encountered in salvageable patients.

27.11 Urethra

Reference

Colapinto V, McCallum RW (1977) Injury to the male posterior urethra in fractured pelvis: a new classification. J Urol 118: 575–580

Type	Description of injury
I	The prostate or the urogenital diaphragm is dislocated, causing elongation and tension of the bulbomembranous urethra. There may be urethral contusion or laceration (not full thickness)
II	The membranous urethra is ruptured above the urogenital diaphragm, with or without prostatic injury. The bulbous urethra is intact. The rupture may be partial or complete
III	The membranous urethra is disrupted above and below the urogenital diaphragm. The rupture usually is complete and may be associated with rupture of the urogenital diaphragm and/or rupture of the bulbous urethra

Clinical criteria used to diagnose a ruptured posterior urethra in case of fractured pelvis do not provide accurate information on the degree and site of the urethral injury. The results obtained by retrograde urethrography are reported in 15 cases. On the basis of these results, a new classification of membranous urethral rupture in cases of fractured pelvis is proposed.

Reference

Moore EE, Cogbill TH, Malangoni MA et al (1995) Organ injury scaling. Surg Clin North Am 75:293–303

Grade[a]	Type of injury	Description of injury
I	Contusion	Blood at urethral meatus, urethrography normal
II	Stretch injury	Elongation of urethra without extravasation on urethrography
III	Partial disruption	Extravasation of urethrography contrast at injury site with contrast visualized in the bladder
IV	Complete disruption	Extravasation of urethrography contrast at injury site without visualization in the bladder, <2 cm of urethral separation
V	Complete disruption	Complete transection with >2 cm urethral separation, or extension into the prostate or vagina

[a]Advance one grade for bilateral injuries up to grade III.

The fundamental purpose of this classification was to devise injury severity scores for individual organs to facilitate clinical investigation and outcomes research. The OIS is a classification scheme based on the anatomical disruption of an individual organ scaled I–V, representing the least to most severe injury. Grades I–V represent increasingly complex injuries encountered in salvageable patients.

Reference

Goldman SM, Sandler CM, Corriere JN, McGuire EJ (1997) Blunt urethral trauma: a unified, anatomical mechanical classification. J Urol 157:85–89

Type	Description of injury
I	Posterior urethra intact but stretched
II	Partial or complete pure posterior injury with tear of membranous urethra above the urogenital diaphragm
III	Partial or complete combined anterior/posterior urethral injury with disruption of the urogenital diaphragm
IV	Bladder neck injury with extension into the urethra
IVa	Injury of the base of the bladder with periurethral extravasation simulating a true type IV urethral injury
V	Partial or complete pure anterior urethral injury

A simple, anatomically based classification of blunt urethral injury is given. Most importantly the type III injury, which involves a tear of the membranous urethra and disruption of the urogenital diaphragm, and which was believed to be the most common of the three types, is not isolated to the posterior urethra, but extends into the adjacent bulbous urethra. Therefore, type III injury is not a pure posterior urethral injury, but a combined anterior and posterior urethral injury. This classification includes injuries of the bladder neck, that extend into the proximal urethra. Such injuries require special attention, because, if not properly repaired, they may result in incontinence or stricture. Injuries of the anterior urethra are also considered.

27.12 Scrotum and Testis

Reference

Couvelaire R, Schimmel F (1976) Scrotal contusions. Concours Med 98:6785–6794

Type	Description of injury
1	Contusion of scrotal soft tissues with intact vaginalis and tunica albuginea
2	Intratesticular hematoma without rupture of tunica albuginea and hematocele
3	Testicular fracture with ruptured tunica albuginea and protrusion of testicular parenchyma

Isolated contusion of the scrotum, without hemorrhage in the vaginalis and with an intact tunica albuginea, will have a favorable course without treatment, but clinical diagnosis is difficult. The intratesticular hematoma without hematocele and intact tunica albuginea compresses the testis and the hematoma may evolve into fibrous scar tissue. Testicular fracture associated with ruptured tunica albuginea and protrusion of testicular parenchyma usually results in a transverse fracture. The protruded parenchyma will rapidly undergo necrosis. Without treatment, testicular hematocele and fracture induce atrophy. These lesions must be explored surgically.

Reference

Sauvage P, Geiss S, Leculee R, Hideux S (1988) Pediatric testicular injuries. Chir Ped 22:136–141

Grade	Description
I	Testicular contusion without rupture of the tunica albuginea
II	Rupture and retraction of the tunica albuginea
III	Complete testicular fracture
IV	Fragmentation of the testicle

Thirty-three blunt testicular trauma cases with 17 grade I, 10 grade II, 4 grade III, and 2 grade IV injuries were analyzed. Only six patients (18%) were treated nonsurgically. Conservative treatment for grade I consists in removal of nonviable testicular parenchyma and for grades II and III in evacuation of the hematocele, excision of the contused testicular parenchyma, and suture of the tunica albuginea. Orchidectomy was the only treatment for grade IV. After surgical treatment, results show 9% of orchidectomy (1 case in grades I, III and IV) and 25% of testicular atrophy (6% of grade I, 40% of grade II, and 50% of grades III and IV).

Reference

Moore EE, Malangoni MA, Cogbill TH et al (1996) Organ injury scaling VII: cervical, vascular, peripheral vascular, adrenal, penis, testis and scrotum. J Trauma 41:523–524

Grade	Description of injury (scrotal)
I	Contusion
II	Laceration <25% of scrotal diameter
III	Laceration ≥25% of scrotal diameter or stellate
IV	Avulsion <50%
V	Avulsion ≥50%

Grade[a]	Description of injury (testicular)
I	Contusion/hematoma
II	Subclinical laceration of tunica albuginea
III	Laceration of tunica albuginea with <50% parenchymal loss
IV	Major laceration of tunica albuginea with ≥50% parenchymal loss
V	Total testicular destruction or avulsion

[a]Advance one grade for bilateral lesions up to grade V.

The fundamental purpose was to devise injury severity scores for individual organs to facilitate clinical investigation and outcomes research. The OIS is a classification scheme based on the anatomical disruption of an individual organ scaled I–V, representing the least to most severe injury. Grades I–V represent increasingly complex injuries encountered in salvageable patients.

Reference

El Kamel R, Atallah R, Rouis M, Mosbah AT (1997) Proposal of a classification of scrotal contusions. J Urol 103:17–19

Type of injury	Description of injury
Simple contusion	Superficial scrotal hematoma without rupture of the tunica albuginea
Testicular fracture	Ruptured tunica albuginea and testicular protrusion
Severe contusion	Complex testicular fracture or fragmentation and spermatic cord injury

A classification of scrotal contusions and the results of a survey involving 50 closed scrotal traumas are reported. Simple contusion will evolve favorably without treatment. Testicular fracture must be explored surgically, in emergency, with a conservative approach. Orchidectomy is justified only for severe contusion with complete testicular destruction.

27.13 Vulva, Vagina, Uterus (Nonpregnant), Uterus (Pregnant), Fallopian Tube, Ovary, Penis

Reference

Moore EE, Jurkovich GJ, Knudson MM et al (1995) Organ injury scaling VI: extrahepatic biliary, esophagus, stomach, vulva, vagina, uterus (nonpregnant), uterus (pregnant), fallopian tube, and ovary. J Trauma 39:1069–1070

Grade[a]	Description of injury (vulva)
I	Contusion/hematoma
II	Laceration – superficial (skin only)
III	Laceration – deep (into fat/muscle)
IV	Avulsion – skin/fat/muscle
V	Injury into adjacent organs (anus/rectum/urethra/bladder)

[a]Advance one grade for multiple injuries up to grade III.

Grade[a]	Description of injury (vagina)
I	Contusion/hematoma
II	Laceration – superficial (mucosa only)
III	Laceration – deep into fat/muscle
IV	Laceration – complex, into cervix or peritoneum
V	Injury into adjacent organs (anus/rectum/urethra/bladder)

[a]Advance one grade for multiple injuries up to grade III.

Grade[a]	Description of injury (uterus non pregnant)
I	Contusion/hematoma
II	Superficial laceration (≤1 cm)
III	Deep laceration (>1 cm)
IV	Laceration involving uterine artery
V	Avulsion, devascularized

[a]Advance one grade for multiple injuries up to grade III.

Grade[a]	Description of injury (uterus pregnant)
I	Contusion/hematoma (without placental abruption)
II	Superficial laceration (≤1 cm) or partial placental abruption <25%
III	Deep laceration (>1 cm) occurring in second trimester or placental abruption >25% but <50% Deep laceration (>1 cm) in third trimester
IV	Laceration involving uterine artery Deep laceration (>1 cm) with >50% placental abruption
V	Uterine rupture – Second trimester – Third trimester Complete placental abruption

[a]Advance one grade for multiple injuries up to grade III.

Grade[a]	Description of injury (fallopian tube)
I	Contusion/hematoma
II	Laceration ≤50% circumference
III	Laceration >50% circumference
IV	Transection
V	Vascular, devascularized segment

[a]Advance one grade for bilateral injuries up to grade III.

Grade[a]	Description of injury (ovary)
I	Contusion/hematoma
II	Superficial laceration (depth ≤0.5 cm)
III	Deep laceration (depth >0.5 cm)
IV	Partial disruption of blood supply
V	Avulsion or complete parenchymal destruction

[a]Advance one grade for bilateral injuries up to grade III.

Grade[a]	Description of injury (penis)
I	Cutaneous laceration/contusion
II	Buck's fascia (cavernosum) laceration without tissue loss
III	Cutaneous avulsion Laceration through glans/meatus Cavernosal or urethral defect <2 cm
IV	Partial penectomy Cavernosal or urethral defect ≥2 cm
V	Total penectomy

[a]Advance one grade for multiple injuries up to grade III.

The fundamental purpose of this classification was to devise injury severity scores for individual organs to facilitate clinical investigation and outcomes research. The OIS is a classification scheme based on the anatomical disruption of an individual organ scaled I–VI, representing the least to most severe injury. Grades I–V represent increasingly complex injuries encountered in salvageable patients.

27.14 Esophagus, Stomach

Reference

Moore EE, Jurkovich GJ, Knudson MM et al (1995) Organ injury scaling VI: extrahepatic biliary, esophagus, stomach, vulva, vagina, uterus (nonpregnant), uterus (pregnant), fallopian tube, and ovary. J Trauma 39:1069–1070

Grade[a]	Description of injury (esophagus)
I	Contusion/hematoma Partial thickness laceration
II	Laceration ≤50% circumference
III	Laceration >50% circumference
IV	Segmental loss or devascularization ≤2 cm
V	Segmental loss or devascularization >2 cm

[a]Advance one grade for multiple lesions up to grade III.

Grade[a]	Description of injury (stomach)
I	Contusion/hematoma Partial-thickness laceration
II	Laceration ≤2 cm in GE junction or pylorus ≤5 cm in proximal 1/3 stomach ≤10 cm in distal 2/3 stomach
III	Laceration >2 cm in GE junction or pylorus >5 cm in proximal 1/3 stomach >10 cm in distal 2/3 stomach
IV	Tissue loss or devascularization ≤2/3 stomach
V	Tissue loss or devascularization >2/3 stomach

[a]Advance one grade for multiple lesions up to grade III.

The fundamental purpose of this classification was to devise injury severity scores for individual organs to facilitate clinical investigation and outcomes research. The OIS is a classification scheme based on the anatomical disruption of an individual organ scaled I–VI, representing the least to most severe injury. Grades I–V represent increasingly complex injuries encountered in salvageable patients.

27.15 Duodenum

Reference

Lucas CE (1977) Diagnosis and treatment of pancreatic and duodenal injury. Surg Clin North Am 57:49–65

Class	Description of injury
I	Serosal tear, contusion, intramural hematoma; no pancreatic injury
II	Complete perforation; no pancreatic injury
III	Duodenal contusion or perforation; pancreatic contusion, small peripheral laceration
IV	Severe combined pancreaticoduodenal disruption

Morbidity and mortality are directly related to the severity of both pancreatic and duodenal injury and the presence of combined pancreaticoduodenal injury. Repair of duodenal injury varies with the extent of injury. Intramural duodenal hematoma or serosal tear (class I injury) diagnosed is best treated by evacuation of the hematoma with careful serosal reapproximation. Intramural duodenal hematoma diagnosed later because of duodenal obstruction may be observed nonoperatively for 1–3 weeks with reasonably good expectation of resolution of the hematoma with alleviation of the obstruction. Class II duodenal injury (complete perforation without pancreatic injury) is usually best treated by simple transverse closure in two layers. Complete circumferential duodenal transection can usually be treated by an end-to-end anastomosis when the transected margins appear viable. Duodenal injury in combination with contusion, hematoma, or peripheral laceration of the pancreas (class III injury) is best treated by primary repair of the duodenal injury and drainage of the pancreatic injury if operated upon within the first 24 h. Severe combined pancreaticoduodenal injury (class IV injury) requires either the duodenal diverticulization procedure or pancreaticoduodenectomy. The decision rests on suspected involvement of the main pancreatic duct. Resection of the injured pancreas and duodenum is indicated for severe lacerations or disruptions of the head of the pancreas with obvious ductal injury.

Reference

Moore EE, Cogbill TH, Malangoni MA et al (1995) Organ injury scaling. Surg Clin North Am 75:293–303

Grade[a]	Type of injury	Description of injury
I	Hematoma	Involving single portion of duodenum
	Laceration	Partial thickness, no perforation
II	Hematoma	Involving more than one portion
	Laceration	Disruption <50% of circumference
III	Laceration	Disruption 50%–75% circumference of D2
		Disruption of 50%–100% circumference of D1, D3, D4
IV	Laceration	Disruption >75% circumference of D2
		Involving ampulla or distal common bile duct
V	Laceration	Massive disruption of duodenopancreatic complex
	Vascular	Devascularization of duodenum

[a]Advance one grade for multiple injuries up to grade III. D1, first portion of duodenum; D2, second portion of duodenum; D3, third portion of duodenum; D4, fourth portion of duodenum

The fundamental purpose of this classification was to devise injury severity scores for individual organs to facilitate clinical investigation and outcomes research. The OIS is a classification scheme based on the anatomical disruption of an individual organ scaled I–VI, representing the least to most severe injury. Grades I–V represent increasingly complex injuries encountered in salvageable patients.

27.16 Small Bowel, Colon, Rectum, Abdominal Vascular

Reference

Moore EE, Cogbill TH, Malangoni MA et al (1995) Organ injury scaling. Surg Clin North Am 75:293–303

Grade[a]	Type of injury	Description of injury (small bowel)
I	Hematoma	Contusion or hematoma without devascularization
	Laceration	Partial thickness, no perforation
II	Laceration	Laceration <50% of circumference
III	Laceration	Laceration ≥50% of circumference without transection
IV	Laceration	Transection of the small bowel
V	Laceration	Transection of the small bowel with segmental tissue loss
	Vascular	Devascularized segment

[a]Advance one grade for multiple injuries up to grade III.

Grade[a]	Type of injury	Description of injury (colon)
I	Hematoma	Contusion or hematoma, without devascularization
	Laceration	Partial thickness, no perforation
II	Laceration	Laceration <50% of circumference
III	Laceration	Laceration ≥50% of circumference without transection
IV	Laceration	Transection of the colon
V	Laceration	Transection of the colon with segmental tissue loss

[a]Advance one grade for multiple injuries up to grade III.

Grade[a]	Type of injury	Description of injury (rectum)
I	Hematoma	Contusion or hematoma, without devascularization
	Laceration	Partial thickness laceration
II	Laceration	Laceration <50% of circumference
III	Laceration	Laceration ≥50% of circumference
IV	Laceration	Full-thickness laceration with extension into the perineum
V	Vascular	Devascularized segment

[a]Advance one grade for multiple injuries up to grade III.

Grade[a]	Description of injury (abdominal vascular)
I	Unnamed superior mesenteric artery or superior mesenteric vein branches Unnamed inferior mesenteric artery or inferior mesenteric vein branches Phrenic artery/vein Lumbar artery/vein Gonadal artery/vein Ovarian artery/vein Other unnamed small arterial or venous structures requiring ligation
II	Right, left or common hepatic artery Splenic artery/vein Right or left gastric arteries Gastroduodenal artery Inferior mesenteric artery, trunk or inferior mesenteric vein, trunk Primary named branches of mesenteric artery (e.g., ileocolic artery) or mesenteric vein Other named abdominal vessels requiring ligation/repair
III	Superior mesenteric vein, trunk Renal artery/vein Iliac artery/vein Hypogastric artery/vein Vena cava, infra-renal
IV	Superior mesenteric artery, trunk Celiac axis proper Vena cava, suprarenal, and infra-hepatic Aorta, infra-renal
V	Portal vein Extraparenchymal hepatic vein Vena cava, retrohepatic or suprahepatic Aorta, suprarenal, subdiaphragmatic

[a]Increase one grade for multiple grade III or IV injuries involving >50% vessel circumference. Downgrade one grade if <25% vessels circumference laceration for grade IV or V.

The fundamental purpose of this classification was to devise injury severity scores for individual organs to facilitate clinical investigation and outcomes research. The OIS is a classification scheme based on the anatomical disruption of an individual organ scaled I–VI, representing the least to most severe injury. Grades I–V represent increasingly complex injuries encountered in salvageable patients, whereas grade VI is a destructive lesion incompatible with survival.

The last classification system is applicable for extraparenchymal vascular injuries. If the vessel injury is within 2 cm of the organ parenchyma, refer to specific organ injury scale.

27.17 Lumbar Spine

Reference

Holdsworth F (1963) Fractures, dislocations and fracture/dislocations of the spine. J Bone Joint Surg Br 45B:6–20

Stable Injuries

Wedge compression fracture
Compression burst fracture

Unstable Injuries

Dislocations
Extension fractures and dislocations
Rotational fracture-dislocations

	Flexion	Flexion and rotation	Extension	Compression
Wedge compression	Yes			
Compression burst				Yes
Dislocations		Yes		
Extension fractures and dislocations			Yes	
Rotational fracture dislocations		Yes		

In Holdsworth's concept, stability is proposed as being dependent on integrity of the posterior ligament complex, composed of the capsule of the apophysial joints, the intraspinous and supraspinous ligaments and the ligaments flava. This description is flawed, because Holdsworth describes an extension injury as unstable, but also states that the anterior ligament complex is disrupted rather than the posterior one and flexion distraction injury is not included (see Chapt. 15, "Injuries of the Lumbar Spine").

Reference

Kelly RP, Whitesides TE (1968) Treatment of lumbodorsal fracture-dislocations. Ann Surg 167:705–717

Type	Description of injury
I	Stable fractures A. Wedging fractures 1. Anterior wedging (flexion injuries) 2. Lateral wedging B. Stable burst injuries
II	Unstable injuries, dislocation either persists or has been reduced A. Recent injuries 1. Flexion dislocation. Fracture generally accompanies 2. Flexion-rotation fracture; dislocation ("slice" injuries) 3. Others Unstable burst? B. Old injuries 1. Stability restored 2. Instability persists

The spine functions not as one column but as two; one of solid bone, one composed of neural arches. While not primarily weight-bearing, the column of neural arches has great strength and is capable of weight-bearing. Working together, these two columns support the body weight. When stability of the posterior column is lost, the surgical techniques developed for anterior surgical attack may be applied.

Reference

Denis F (1983) The three-column spine and its significance in the classification of acute thoracolumbar spinal injuries. Spine 8:817–831
Denis F (1984) Spinal instability as defined by the three-column spine concept in acute spinal trauma. Clin Orthop 189:65–76

Type of fracture	Column		
	Anterior	Middle	Posterior
Compression	Compression	None	None or distraction (severe)
Burst	Compression	Compression	None
Seat-belt type	None or compression	Distraction	Distraction
Fracture dislocation	Compression Rotation shear	Distraction Rotation shear	Distraction Rotation shear

Type	Mechanism
Compression	**Flexion**
Anterior	Anterior flexion
Lateral	Lateral flexion
Burst	**Axial load**
Type A	Axial load
Type B	Axial load and flexion
Type C	Axial load and flexion
Type D	Axial load and rotation
Type E	Axial load and lateral flexion
Seat-belt type	Flexion distraction
Fracture dislocation	
Flexion rotation	**Flexion rotation**
Shear	**Shear**
	AP shear
	PA shear
Flexion Distraction	**Flexion distraction**

Types

Compression

Type A[a]	Anterior compression affecting both end-plates
Type B[a]	Anterior compression affecting the superior end-plate
Type C[a]	Anterior compression affecting the inferior end-plate
Type D[b]	Lateral compression

Burst

Type A[a]	Fracture of both end-plates
Type B[a]	Fracture of superior end-plate
Type C[a]	Fracture of inferior end-plate
Type D[b]	Burst rotation
Type E[b]	Burst lateral flexion

[a]Types A to C are diagnosed on the lateral radiograph.

[b]Types D and E are diagnosed on the AP radiograph, type D looking like a type A on the lateral and type E looking like a type A, B, or C on the lateral radiograph.

Seat-belt type

Type A	One-level bone injury
Type B	One-level ligamentous injury
Type C	Two-level through bone middle column
Type D	Two-level through ligamentous middle column

Fracture dislocation

Type A	Flexion rotation
Type B	Shear
Type C	Flexion distraction

From a retrospective study of 412 thoracolumbar injuries, the author introduces the concept of middle column or middle osteoligamentous complex between the traditionally recognized posterior ligamentous complex and the anterior longitudinal ligament. This middle column is formed by the posterior wall of the vertebral body, the posterior longitudinal ligament, and posterior annulus fibrosus. The third column appears crucial, as the mode of its failure correlates both with the type of spinal fracture and with its neurological injury. Spinal injuries were subdivided into minor and major. Minor injuries are represented by fractures of transverse processes, facets, pars interarticularis, and spinous process. Major spinal injuries are classified into four different categories: compression fractures, burst fractures, seat-belt-type injuries, and fracture dislocations. These four well-recognized injuries have been studied carefully in clinical terms as well as on roentgenograms and computerized axial tomograms. They were then subdivided into subtypes demonstrating the very wide spectrums of these four entities. The correlation between the three-column system, the classification, the stability, and the therapeutic indications are presented (see also comments in Chapt. 15, "Injuries of the Lumbar Spine").

Reference

McAfee PC, Yuan HA, Fredrickson BE, Lubicky JP (1983) The value of computed tomography in thoracolumbar fractures. An analysis of one hundred consecutive cases and a new classification. J Bone Joint Surg Am 65:461–473

Type of fracture	Column		
	Anterior	Middle	Posterior
Wedge compression	Yes	No	No
Stable burst	Yes	Yes	No
Unstable burst	Yes	Yes	Yes
Chance	Probable	Probable	Yes
Flexion-distraction	Yes	Yes	Yes
Translational injuries	Yes	Yes	Yes

Mechanisms involved are classified according to the type of fracture.

Fracture	Hyper-flexion	Hyper-extension	Rotation/ shearing	Axial compression	Distraction
Wedge	Yes			Yes	
Stable burst	Probable			Yes	
Unstable burst	Probable			Yes	
Chance	Yes if severe				Yes
Flexion-distraction	Yes			Yes	Yes
Translational	Yes		Yes	Yes	

A simplified classification was developed using the forces on the middle column, namely axial compression, axial distraction and translation within the transverse plane. The authors studied 100 consecutive patients with potentially unstable fractures and fracture-dislocations by multiplane computed tomography. The mechanism of failure of the middle osteoligamentous complex of the spine (posterior longitudinal ligament, posterior part of the vertebral body, and posterior annulus fibrosus) was determined by three-dimensional analysis. Three modes of middle-column failure were used to classify the injuries: axial compression (73 patients), axial distraction (15 patients), and translation within the transverse plane (12 patients). Fifty of 86 patients who were evaluated in the acute phase of injury underwent operative stabilization and the mechanism of middle-column disruption determined the type of instrumentation that was used. Compression and distraction injuries of the middle complex could be appropriately treated by Harrington distraction and compression instrumentation, respectively. However, in translational injuries (torn posterior longitudinal ligament), routine Harrington instrumentation was contraindicated due to the risk of overdistraction. Translational injuries were associated with the greatest degree of instability and often had complete ligament discontinuity at the level of the affected vertebrae. Patients with a translational injury had the most severe neural deficits (6 of 11 patients studied acutely having a complete spinal cord lesion). Translational injuries of the middle column were treated by segmental spinal instrumentation to provide strong fixation with minimum risk of neural sequelae from passing sublaminar wires. Moreover, postoperative use of a cast over insensate skin was not required.

Computed tomography was more sensitive than any other modality in the diagnosis of disruption of the posterior elements in unstable burst fractures and computer-reconstructed sagittal images were accurate in evaluating the nature of facet-joint failure in distraction injuries. Computed tomography with metrizamide proved superior to either conventional tomography or myelography alone in localizing the site of neural canal compromise in acute thoracolumbar injuries.

The mode of failure of the middle osteoligamentous complex as visualized by computed tomography determined the pattern of spinal injury, the severity of the neural deficit, the degree of instability, and the type of instrumentation required (see also comments in Chap. 15, "Injuries of the Lumbar Spine").

Reference

Magerl F, Aebi M, Gertzbein SD, Harms J, Nazarian S (1994) A comprehensive classification of thoracic and lumbar injuries. Eur Spine J 3:184–201

Type A. Vertebral body compression

A1. Impaction fractures
- A1.1. End-plate impaction
- A1.2. Wedge impaction fractures
  1. Superior wedge impaction fracture
  2. Lateral wedge impaction fracture
  3. Inferior wedge impaction fracture
- A1.3. Vertebral body collapse

A2. Split fractures
- A2.1. Sagittal split fracture
- A2.2. Coronal split fracture
- A2.3. Pincer fracture

A3. Burst fractures
- A3.1. Incomplete burst fracture
  1. Superior incomplete burst fracture
  2. Lateral incomplete burst fracture
  3. Inferior incomplete burst fracture
- A3.2. Burst-split fracture
  1. Superior burst-split fracture
  2. Lateral burst-split fracture
  3. Inferior burst-split fracture
- A3.3 Complete burst fracture
  1. Pincer burst fracture
  2. Complete flexion burst fracture
  3. Complete axial burst fracture

Type B. Anterior and posterior element injury with distraction

B1. Posterior disruption predominantly ligamentous (flexion-distraction injury)
- B1.1. With transverse disruption of the disc
  1. Flexion-subluxation
  2. Anterior dislocation
  3. Flexion-subluxation/anterior dislocation with fracture of the articular processes
- B1.2. With type A fracture of the vertebral body
  1. Flexion-subluxation + type A fracture
  2. Anterior dislocation + type A fracture
  3. Flexion-subluxation/anterior dislocation with fracture of the articular processes + type A fracture

B2. Posterior disruption predominantly osseous (flexion-distraction injury)
- B2.1. Transverse bicolumn fracture
- B2.2. With transverse disruption of the disc
  1. Disruption through the pedicle and disc
  2. Disruption through the pars interarticularis and disc (flexion-spondylolysis)
- B2.3. With type A fracture of the vertebral body
  1. Fracture through the pedicle + type A fracture
  2. Fracture through the pars interarticularis (flexion-spondylolysis) + type A fracture >>>

B3. Anterior disruption through the disc (hyperextension-shear injury)
- B3.1. Hyperextension-subluxations
  1. Without injury of the posterior column
  2. With injury of the posterior column
- B3.2. Hyperextension-spondylolysis
- B3.3. Posterior dislocation

Type C. Anterior and posterior element injury with rotation

C1. Type A injuries with rotation (compression injuries with rotation)
- C1.1. Rotational wedge fracture
- C1.2. Rotational split fractures
  1. Rotational sagittal split fracture
  2. Rotational coronal split fracture
  3. Rotational pincer fracture
  4. Vertebral body separation
- C1.3. Rotational burst fractures
  1. Incomplete rotational burst fracture
  2. Rotational burst-split fracture
  3. Complete rotational burst fracture

C2. Type B injuries with rotation
- C2.1.-B1. Injuries with rotation (flexion-distraction injuries with rotation)
  1. Rotational flexion subluxation
  2. Rotational flexion subluxation with unilateral articular process fracture
  3. Unilateral dislocation
  4. Rotational anterior dislocation without/with fracture of articular processes
  5. Rotational flexion subluxation without/with unilateral articular process fracture + type A fracture
  6. Unilateral dislocation + type A fracture
  7. Rotational anterior dislocation without/with fracture of articular processes + type A fracture
- C2.2.-B2. Injuries with rotation (flexion distraction injuries with rotation)
  1. Rotational transverse bicolumn fracture
  2. Unilateral flexion spondylolysis with disruption of the disc
  3. Unilateral flexion spondylolysis + type A fracture
- C2.3.-B3. Injuries with rotation (hyperextension-shear injuries with rotation)
  1. Rotational hyperextension-subluxation without/ with fracture of posterior vertebral elements
  2. Unilateral hyperextension-spondylolysis
  3. Posterior dislocation with rotation

C3. Rotational-shear injuries
- C3.1. Slice fracture
- C3.2. Oblique fracture

A comprehensive classification of thoracic and lumbar injuries is proposed. The classification is primarily based on pathomorphological criteria. Categories are established according to the main mechanism of injury, pathomorphological uniformity, and in consideration of prognostic aspects regarding healing potential. The classification reflects a progressive scale of morphological damage, by which the degree of instability is determined. The severity of the injury in terms of instability is expressed by its ranking within the classification system. A simple grid, the 3-3-3 scheme of the ASIF fracture classification, was used in grouping the injuries. This grid consists of three types: A, B, and C. Morphological criteria are predominantly used for further subdivision of the injuries. Severity progresses from type A through type C as well as within the types, groups, and further subdivisions. Most injuries occurred around the thoracolumbar junction. The upper and lower end of the thoracolumbar spine and the T10 level were the most infrequently injured. Type A fractures were found in 66.1%, type B in 14.5%, and type C in 19.4% of the cases. Stable type A1 fractures accounted for 34.7% of the total. The overall incidence of neurological deficit was 22% and increased significantly from type to type: neurological deficit was present in 14% of type A, 32% of type B, and 55% of type C lesions. Only 2% of the A1 and 4% of the A2 fractures showed any neurological deficit.

Reference

Orthopaedic Trauma Association Committee for Coding and Classification (1996) Fracture and dislocation compendium. J Orthop Trauma 10 [Suppl 1]:v–ix

Type A. Compression injuries of the body (compressive forces)

A1. Impaction fractures
- A1.1. Endplate impaction
- A1.2. Wedge impaction
- A1.3. Vertebral body collapse

A2. Split fractures
- A2.1. Sagittal
- A2.2. Coronal
- A2.3. Pincer

A3. Burst fractures
- A3.1. Incomplete burst
- A3.2. Burst-split
- A3.3 Complete burst

Type B. Distraction injuries of the anterior and posterior elements (tensile forces)

B1. Posterior disruption predominantly ligamentous (flexion-distraction injury)
- B1.1. With transverse disruption of the disc
- B1.2. Vertebral body compression fracture

B2. Posterior disruption predominantly osseous (flexion-distraction injury)
- B2.1. Transverse bicolumn fracture
- B2.2. With transverse disruption of the disc
- B2.3. With vertebral body compression

B3. Anterior disruption through the disc (hyperextension-shear injury)
- B3.1. Hyperextension-subluxation
- B3.2. Hyperextension-spondylolysis
- B3.3. Posterior dislocation

Type C. Multidirectional injuries with translation affecting the anterior and posterior elements (axial torque causing rotation injuries)

C1. Rotational wedge, split, and burst fractures
- C1.1. Rotational wedge fractures
- C1.2. Rotational split fractures
- C1.3. Rotational burst fractures

C2. Flexion subluxation with rotation
- C2.1. Flexion-distraction injuries with rotation
- C2.2. B2 with rotation
- C2.3. Hyperextension-shear-rotation of spine

C3. Rotational shear injuries (Holdsworth slice rotation fracture)
- C3.1. Slice
- C3.2. Oblique

The Orthopaedic Trauma Association has defined a systematic classification of fractures in order to allow for standardization of research and communication. The combination of the Comprehensive Long Bone Classification with the classifications of the other bones recorded into the alphanumeric system of the comprehensive classification forms the OTA classifications.

27.18 Bone Pelvis

Reference

Pennal GF, Tile M, Waddell JP, Garside H (1980) Pelvic disruption: assessment and classification. Clin Orthop 151:12–21

Classification of pelvic disruption based on direction of forces
Anteroposterior compression
Lateral compression
A. Ipsilateral anterior and posterior lesion
B. Contralateral anterior and posterior lesion (Bucket-handle)
C. Four-rami and posterior lesion
D. Miscellaneous
Vertical shear

A precise radiological technique for assessing the forces producing pelvic disruption is helpful in arriving at a logical classification of pelvic injury. The radiological examination should include anteroposterior, inlet and outlet views, and CT evaluation. On the basis of this radiological assessment, together with biomechanical studies, a classification of three major forces producing injury is suggested. The anteroposterior and lateral compression types, while vastly different, may both have stable and unstable subtypes associated with them. The vertical shear fracture is always unstable. An accurate history and physical examination in conjunction with the above radiological principles will lead the surgeon to a precise determination of the fracture pattern. A knowledge of the forces necessary to produce this pattern is helpful in the management of the patient with this particular traumatic lesion.

Reference

Young JWR, Burgess AR, Brumbach RJ, Poka A (1986) Pelvic fractures: value of plain radiography in early assessment and management. Radiology 160:445–451

Mechanism	Type	Description of injury
Anteroposterior compression	1	No posterior instability, radiographic or clinical
	2	Separation of the symphysis, with some posterior instability involving the anterior sacroiliac complex
	3	Associated total disruption of the sacroiliac joint
Lateral compression	1	The force is delivered over the posterior aspect of the pelvis, with little resulting pelvic instability, although crush fractures of the sacrum may be seen
	2	The force is more anterior, tending to cause internal displacement of the anterior hemipelvis and thus, potentially, external rotation of the posterior hemipelvis, with the anterior part of the sacroiliac joint acting as a pivot
	3	There is such severe internal rotation of the ipsilateral hemipelvis that contralateral external rotation occurs, with subsequent disruption of the contralateral anterior sacroiliac, sacrotuberous, and sacrospinous ligaments
Vertical shear		
Complex pattern		

Traditional plain-radiographic classifications of the fracture are of limited preoperative value to the surgeon, who must apply corrective force in opposition to the original force vector causing the fracture. In a retrospective analysis of the plain radiographs of 142 cases of pelvic fracture, four patterns of force were identified, presenting distinctive, recognizable radiographic appearances. These patterns are anteroposterior compression (15%), lateral compression (57%), vertical shear (6%), and a complex pattern (22%). The resulting classification of pelvic fracture, based on radiographic and clinical findings, correlates with associated injury to soft-tissue strictures.

Reference

Tile M (1988) Pelvic ring fractures: should they be fixed? J Bone Joint Surg 70B:1–12

Type	Description of injury
A	Stable
A1	Fractures of the pelvis not involving the ring
A2	Stable, minimally displaced fractures of the ring
B	Rotationally unstable, vertically stable
B1	Open book
Stage 1	Disruption of the symphysis pubis <2.5 cm
Stage 2	Disruption of the symphysis pubis >2.5 cm with unilateral posterior lesion
Stage 3	Disruption of the symphysis pubis >2.5 cm with bilateral posterior lesion
B2	Lateral compression: ipsilateral
B3	Lateral compression: contralateral (Bucket handle)
C	Rotationally and vertically unstable
C1	Unilateral
C2	Bilateral
C3	Associated with an acetabular fracture

Disruption of the pelvic ring is a serious injury with a significant mortality and morbidity. Early general management is essential with a concomitant treatment of the musculoskeletal injury. The need for fixation of pelvic fractures depends on many factors and there must be clear reasons for advocating operation. Stabilization is only required for the uncommon type C vertically unstable pelvic disruptions and occasionally for type B rotational instability. Instability is confirmed on radiographic examination: the routine anteroposterior view is less important that the inlet view, which clearly shows posterior displacement, and the outlet view, which shows superior migration or rotation. Radiographic evidence of vertical instability includes posterior or superior displacement of the posterior complex by greater than 1 cm or the presence of a large posterior gap rather than impaction. The best single investigation for determining instability is a CT scan of the sacroiliac complex, while the recent refinement of three-dimensional CT allows clear visualization of the pattern of injury. In the series of the authors of 494 pelvic fractures over 5 years, only about 19% needed stabilization and this was by internal fixation in only 5%.

Reference

Burgess AR, Eastridge BJ, Young JWR et al (1990) Pelvic ring disruptions: effective classification system and treatment protocols. J Trauma 30:848–856

Category	Common characteristic	Differentiating characteristic
Lateral compression I	Anterior transverse fracture (pubic rami)	Sacral compression on side of impact
Lateral compression II	Anterior transverse fracture (pubic rami)	Crescent (iliac wing) fracture
Lateral compression III	Anterior transverse fracture (pubic rami)	Contralateral open-book (anteroposterior compression) injury
Anteroposterior compression I	Symphyseal diastasis	Slight widening of pubic symphysis and/or sacroiliac joint; stretched but intact anterior and posterior ligaments
Anteroposterior compression II	Symphyseal diastasis or anterior vertical fracture	Widened sacroiliac joint; disrupted anterior ligaments; intact posterior ligaments
Anteroposterior compression III	Symphyseal diastasis or anterior vertical fracture	Complete hemipelvis separation, but no vertical displacement; complete sacroiliac joint disruption; complete anterior and posterior ligament disruption
Vertical shear	Symphyseal diastasis or anterior vertical fracture	Vertical displacement anteriorly and posteriorly, usually through sacroiliac joint, occasionally through iliac wing and/or sacrum
Combined mechanical	Anterior and/ or posterior, vertical and/or transverse components	Combination of other injury patterns: lateral compression/vertical shear or lateral compression/ anteroposterior compression.

Two hundred ten consecutive patients with high-energy pelvic ring disruptions were treated per protocol as determined by their injury classification and hemodynamic status; the injury classification system was based on the vector of force involved and the quantification of disruption from that force, lateral compression (LC), anteroposterior compression (APC), vertical shear (VS), and combined mechanical (CM) injury. The 162 pelvic fractures were classified acutely: LC-I, 79 (48.7%); LC-II, 12 (7.4%); LC-III, 15 (9.3%); APC-I, 0 (0%); APC-II, 18 (11.1%); APC-III, 7 (4.3%); VS, 9 (5.6%); CM, 11 (6.8%); and isolated iliac wing fractures, 11 (6.8%). Treatment included the following methods (alone or in combination): acute external fixation (45, 28%), open reduction/internal fixation (22, 13.5%), acute arterial embolization (11, 7%), and bed-rest (68, 42%). Overall mortality was 8.6% (lateral compression, 7%; anteroposterior, 20%; vertical shear, 0%; combined mechanical, 18%). The cause of death was associated with the pelvic fracture in less than 50%. The authors conclude that the predictive value of their classification system (incorporating appreciation of the causative forces and resulting injury patterns) and their classification-based treatment protocols reduce the morbidity and mortality related to pelvic ring disruption.

Reference

Orthopaedic Trauma Association Committee for Coding and Classification (1990) Fracture and dislocation compendium. J Orthop Trauma 10 [Suppl 1]:v–ix

Type A. Lesion sparing (or with no displacement of) posterior arch

A1. Fracture of innominate bone; avulsion
- A1.1. Iliac spine
  - Anterior superior
  - Anterior inferior
  - Pubic spine
- A1.2. Iliac crest
- A1.3. Ischial tuberosity

A2. Fracture of innominate bone; direct blow
- A2.1. Iliac wing
  - One fragment
  - More than one fragment
- A2.2. Unilateral fracture of anterior arch
  - Through pubic bone/rami
  - Through pubic bone involving symphysis pubis
- A2.3. Bifocal fracture of anterior arch
  - Bilateral pubic rami
  - Pubic rami in one side and symphysis pubis

A3. Transverse fracture of sacrum and coccyx
- A3.1. Sacrococcygeal disclocation
- A3.2. Sacrum undisplaced
- A3.3 Sacrum displaced

Type B. Incomplete disruption of posterior arch; partially stable

B1. Unilateral, partial disruption of posterior arch, external rotation (open-book injury)
- B1.1. Sacroiliac joint anterior disruption
- B1.2. Sacral fracture

B2. Unilateral, partial disruption of posterior arch, internal rotation (lateral compression injury)
- B2.1. Anterior compression fracture of sacrum
  - Anterior lesion ipsilateral
  - Anterior lesion contralateral (Bucket-handle)
- B2.2. Partial sacroiliac joint fracture/subluxation
  - Anterior lesion ipsilateral
  - Anterior lesion contralateral (Bucket-handle)
- B2.3. Incomplete posterior iliac fracture
  - Anterior lesion ipsilateral
  - Anterior lesion contralateral (Bucket-handle)

B3. Bilateral, partial lesion of posterior arch
- B3.1. Bilateral B1 (open book, external rotation)
  - Bilateral sacroiliac joint anterior disruption
  - Bilateral sacral fracture
  - Unilateral partial sacroiliac joint disruption/contralateral sacral fracture
- B3.2. B1 and B2
- B3.3. Bilateral B2

Type C. Complete disruption of posterior arch; unstable

C1. Unilateral, complete disruption of posterior arch
- C1.1. Through ilium
- C1.2. Through sacroiliac joint
  - Transiliac fracture dislocation
  - Pure dislocation
  - Transsacral fracture dislocation
- C1.3. Through the sacrum
  - Lateral
  - Foraminal
  - Medial to foramen

C2. Bilateral, ipsilateral complete, contralateral incomplete
- C2.1. Complete through ilium
- C2.2. Complete through sacroiliac joint
  - Transiliac fracture dislocation
  - Pure dislocation
  - Transsacral fracture dislocation
- C2.3. Complete through the sacrum
  - Lateral
  - Foraminal
  - Medial to foramen

C3. Bilateral, complete disruption
- C3.1. Extrasacral on both sides
  - Ilium
  - Sacroiliac joint, transiliac fracture/dislocation
  - Sacroiliac joint, transsacral fracture/dislocation
  - Sacroiliac joint dislocation
- C3.2. Sacral one side, extra sacral other side
  - Sacral alar
  - Sacral foraminal
  - Sacral medial to foramen
- C3.3. Sacral both sides
  - Lateral alar
  - Foraminal
  - Medial

The Orthopaedic Trauma Association has defined a systematic classification of fractures in order to allow for standardization of research and communication. The combination of the Comprehensive Long Bone Classification with the classifications of the other bones recorded into the alphanumeric system of the comprehensive classification forms the OTA classification. The classification of pelvic ring and acetabular fractures is based solely on the work of Pennal and Tile and Judet and Letournel.

27.19. Acetabulum

Reference

Judet R, Judet J, Letournel E (1964) Fractures of the acetabulum: classification and surgical approaches for open reduction. J Bone Joint Surg 46:1615–1646

Anatomical classification		No. of patients
Posterior-lip fracture		57
Fracture of posterior horn of the articular surface	1	
Fracture of posterior lip	3	
Fracture of posterior rim, posterior dislocation	45	
Fracture of posterosuperior portion of the rim, posterosuperior dislocation	8	
Fracture of the ilioischial column		9
Transverse fracture		74
Transverse fracture, posterior-lip fracture, posterior dislocation	23	
Transverse fracture, posterior-lip or posterosuperior fracture, central dislocation	10	
Transverse fracture, central dislocation	25	
Transverse fracture, central dislocation	3	
Transverse fracture, ilioischial-column fracture	6	
Transverse fracture, iliopubic-column fracture	7	
Fracture of iliopubic column		17
Anterior-ridge fracture	1	
Iliopubic-column fracture	16	
Associated fracture of both columns		16

A useful classification of fractures of the acetabulum must be simple and the identification of a fracture must be based on the elementary lesions of the acetabulum, whether they be isolated or in combination.

Reference

Orthopaedic Trauma Association Committee for Coding and Classification (1990) Fracture and dislocation compendium. J Orthop Trauma 10 [Suppl 1]:v–ix

Type A. Partial articular, one column

A1. Posterior wall
- A1.1. Pure fracture dislocation, one fragment
  - Posterior
  - Posterior superior
  - Posterior inferior
- A1.2. Pure fracture dislocation, multifragmentary
  - Posterior
  - Posterior superior
  - Posterior inferior
- A1.3. Fracture dislocation with marginal impaction
  - Posterior
  - Posterior superior
  - Posterior inferior

A2. Posterior column
- A2.1. Through ischium
- A2.2. Through obturator ring
  - Preserving tear drop
  - Involving tear drop
- A2.3. Associated with posterior wall
  - Pure fracture dislocation
  - With marginal impaction

A3. Anterior
- A3.1. Anterior wall
- A3.2. Anterior column, high (fracture to iliac crest)
- A3.3. Low (fracture to anterior border) iliac crest

Type B. Partial articular, transverse

B1. Transverse
- B1.1. Infratectal
- B1.2. Juxtatectal
- B1.3. Transtectal

B2. T-shaped
- B2.1. Infratectal
  - Stem posterior
  - Stem through obturator foramen
  - Stem anterior
- B2.2. Juxtatectal
  - Stem posterior
  - Stem through obturator foramen
  - Stem anterior
- B2.3. Transtectal
  - Stem posterior
  - Stem through obturator foramen
  - Stem anterior

B3. Anterior column, posterior hemitransverse
- B3.1. Anterior wall
- B3.2. Anterior column high
- B3.3. Anterior column low

Type C. Complete articular, both columns

C1. High
- C1.1. Each column simple
- C1.2. Posterior column simple, anterior column multifragmentary
- C1.3. Posterior column and posterior wall

C2. Low
- C2.1. Each column simple
- C2.2. Posterior column simple, anterior column multifragmentary
- C2.3. Posterior column and posterior wall

C3. Involving sacroiliac joint
- C3.1. Anterior wall
  - Anterior column simple, high
  - Anterior column simple, low
  - Anterior column mulitfragmentary, high
  - Anterior column mulitfragmentary, low
- C3.2. Posterior column multifragmentary, anterior column high
- C3.3. Posterior column multifragmentary, anterior column low

The Orthopaedic Trauma Association has defined a systematic classification of fractures in order to allow for standardization of research and communication. The combination of the Comprehensive Long Bone Classification with the classifications of the other bones recorded into the alphanumeric system of the comprehensive classification forms the OTA classification. The classification of pelvic ring and acetabular fractures is based solely on the work of Pennal and Tile and Judet and Letournel.

Subject Index

List of Contributors

GINA M. ALLEN, MD
Consultant Radiologist
Department of Radiology
Nuffield Orthopaedic Centre
Windmill Road
Headington, Oxford OX3 7LD
UK

CHIARA ANDREOLI, MD
Department of Radiology
University of Rome "La Sapienza"
Policlinico Umberto I
Viale Regina Elena n. 324
00161 Rome
Italy

GIANMARCO ANDREOLI, MD
Department of Radiology
University of Rome "La Sapienza"
Policlinico Umberto I
Viale Regina Elena n. 324
00161 Rome
Italy

MARIO BEZZI, MD
Department of Radiology
University of Rome "La Sapienza"
Policlinico Umberto I
Viale Regina Elena n. 324
00161 Rome
Italy

WAQAR A. BHATTI, MD
Professor of Paediatric Radiology
Alder Hey Children's Hospital
Eaton Road
Liverpool L12 2AP
UK

J. H. BOVERIE, MD
Chef de Clinique
Department of Medical Imaging
University Hospital Sart Tilman
Domaine du Sart Tilman B35
4000 Liège
Belgium

KARL BREITSCHAFT, MD
Klinik für Allgemein- und Viszeralchirurgie
Klinikum Augsburg
Stenglinstrasse 2
86156 Augsburg
Germany

NAIL BULAKBASI, MD
Assistant Professor of Radiology
Department of Radiology
Gülhane Military Medical Academy
06018 Ankara
Turkey

HELEN CARTY, MD
Professor of Paediatric Radiology
Alder Hey Children's Hospital
Eaton Road
Liverpool L12 2AP
UK

O. CORNET, MD
Resident, Department of Medical Imaging
University Hospital Sart Tilman
Domaine du Sart Tilman B35
4000 Liège
Belgium

PIERRE DAMAS, MD
General Intensive Care Unit
University Hospital of Liège
Department of Anaesthesia and Intensive Care
Domaine Universitaire du Sart-Tilman
4000 Liège
Belgium

Ph. Deleuse, MD
Department of Medical Imaging
University Hospital Sart Tilman
Domaine du Sart Tilman B35
4000 Liège
Belgium

A. Denys, MD
Service de Radiodiagnostic et
Radiologie interventionelle, CHUV
Rue du Bugnon
1011 Lausanne
Switzerland

Robert F. Dondelinger, MD
Professor and Chairman
Department of Medical Imaging
University Hospital Sart Tilman
Domaine Universitaire du Sart Tilman B35
4000 Liège
Belgium

Adrian K. Dixon, MD
Department of Radiology
Addenbrooke's Hospital
and the University of Cambridge
Hills Road
Cambridge CB2 2QQ
UK

Benoît Ghaye, MD
Department of Medical Imaging
University Hospital Sart Tilman
Domaine du Sart Tilman B35
4000 Liège
Belgium

Pierre Goffette, MD
Professor, Angiography and Interventional
Radiology Unit
Department of Medical Imaging
Saint-Luc University Hospital
Louvain Medical School
10, avenue Hippocrate
1200 Brussels
Belgium

Alison Graham, MD
Hammersmith Hospital
Du Cane Road
London W12 0NN
UK

Hannes Häuser, MD
Klinik für Diagnostische Radiologie und Neuroradiologie
Klinikum Augsburg
Stenglinstrasse 2
86156 Augsburg
Germany

Gary Hartstein, MD
Emergency Unit
University Hospital of Liege
Department of Anaesthesia and Intensive Care
Domaine Universitaire du Sart-Tilman
4000 Liège
Belgium

Peter Huppert, MD
Department of Diagnostic Radiology
Municipal Hospital Darmstadt
Grafenstrasse 9
64283 Darmstadt
Germany

J. Hillier, MD
Department of Radiology
Nuffield Orthopaedic Centre
Windmill Road
Headington, Oxford OX3 7LD
UK

James E. Jackson, MD
Consultant Radiologist
Hammersmith Hospital
Du Cane Road
London W12 0NN
UK

Pierre-François Laterre, MD
Professor, Emergency and Critical Care Department
Saint-Luc University Hospital
Louvain Medical School
10, avenue Hippocrate
1200 Brussels
Belgium

Stephen Ledbetter, MD
Assistant Director of Emergency Radiology
Department of Radiology
Brigham and Women's Hospital
Harvard Medical School
Boston, MA 02115
USA

M. Lewin
Department of Medical Imaging
University Hospital Sart Tilman
Domaine du Sart Tilman B35
4000 Liège
Belgium

Brigitte Martin, MD
Institut de Radiologie de Paris
Scanner - IRM Paris Hoche
31, av. Hoche
75008 Paris
France

Edgar Mayr, MD
Klinik für Diagnostische Radiologie und Neuroradiologie
Klinikum Augsburg
Stenglinstrasse 2
86156 Augsburg
Germany

Vittorio Miele, MD
Department of Radiology
Ospedale S. Camillo
Via Portuense 332
00149 Rome
Italy

E. Mouhsine, MD
Service de Chirurgie Orthopédique, CHUV
Rue du Bugnon
1011 Lausanne
Switzerland

A. Nchimi, MD
Department of Medical Imaging
University Hospital Sart Tilman
Domaine Universitaire du Sart Tilman B35
4000 Liège
Belgium

Diego B. Nunez, Jr., MD
Director of Emergency Radiology
Department of Radiology
Brigham and Women's Hospital
Harvard Medical School
Boston, MA 02115
USA

G. Ponghis, MD
Resident, Department of Medical Imaging
University Hospital Sart Tilman
Domaine du Sart Tilman B35
4000 Liège
Belgium

F. Portier, MD
Service de Radiodiagnostic et
Radiologie interventionelle, CHUV
Rue du Bugnon
1011 Lausanne
Switzerland

David Rickards, FRCR, FFRDSA
University College Hospitals
Imaging Department
The Middlesex Hospital
Mortimer Street
London W1N 8TA
UK

Pierre A. Schnyder, MD
Professor, Service de Radiodiagnostic et
Radiologie interventionelle, CHUV
Rue du Bugnon
1011 Lausanne
Switzerland

Salvatore J. A. Sclafani, MD
Director, Department of Radiology
Kings County Hospital Center
451 Clarkson Avenue
Brooklyn, NY 11203
USA

Sean Sheeran, MD
Department of Radiology
Kings County Hospital
451 Clarkson Ave
Brooklyn, NY 11203
USA

D. Szapiro, MD
Professor and Chairman
Department of Medical Imaging
University Hospital Sart Tilman
Domaine Universitaire du Sart Tilman B35
4000 Liège
Belgium

N. Theumann, MD
Service de Radiodiagnostic et
Radiologie interventionelle, CHUV
Rue du Bugnon
1011 Lausanne
Switzerland

G. Trotteur, MD
Department of Medical Imaging
University Hospital Sart Tilman
Domaine Universitaire du Sart Tilman B35
4000 Liége
Belgium

J. P. Verdon, MD
Service de Radiodiagnostic et
Radiologie interventionelle, CHUV
Rue du Bugnon
1011 Lausanne
Switzerland

V. Willems, MD
Department of Medical Imaging
University Hospital Sart Tilman
Domaine du Sart Tilman B35
4000 Liège
Belgium

David J. Wilson, MD
Consultant Radiologist
Department of Radiology
Nuffield Orthopaedic Centre
Windmill Road
Headington, Oxford OX3 7LD
UK

Nikolaus Zügel, MD
Klinik für Allgemein- und Abdominalchirurgie
Klinikum Augsburg
Stenglinstrasse 2
86156 Augsburg
Germany

Medical Radiology Diagnostic Imaging and Radiation Oncology

Titles in the series already published

Diagnostic Imaging

Innovations in Diagnostic Imaging
Edited by J. H. Anderson

Radiology of the Upper Urinary Tract
Edited by E. K. Lang

The Thymus - Diagnostic Imaging, Functions, and Pathologic Anatomy
Edited by E. Walter, E. Willich, and W. R. Webb

Interventional Neuroradiology
Edited by A. Valavanis

Radiology of the Pancreas
Edited by A. L. Baert, co-edited by G. Delorme

Radiology of the Lower Urinary Tract
Edited by E. K. Lang

Magnetic Resonance Angiography
Edited by I. P. Arlart, G. M. Bongartz, and G. Marchal

Contrast-Enhanced MRI of the Breast
S. Heywang-Köbrunner and R. Beck

Spiral CT of the Chest
Edited by M. Rémy-Jardin and J. Rémy

Radiological Diagnosis of Breast Diseases
Edited by M. Friedrich and E.A. Sickles

Radiology of the Trauma
Edited by M. Heller and A. Fink

Biliary Tract Radiology
Edited by P. Rossi

Radiological Imaging of Sports Injuries
Edited by C. Masciocchi

Modern Imaging of the Alimentary Tube
Edited by A. R. Margulis

Diagnosis and Therapy of Spinal Tumors
Edited by P. R. Algra, J. Valk, and J. J. Heimans

Interventional Magnetic Resonance Imaging
Edited by J. F. Debatin and G. Adam

Abdominal and Pelvic MRI
Edited by A. Heuck and M. Reiser

Orthopedic Imaging
Techniques and Applications
Edited by A. M. Davies and H. Pettersson

Radiology of the Female Pelvic Organs
Edited by E. K.Lang

Magnetic Resonance of the Heart and Great Vessels
Clinical Applications
Edited by J. Bogaert, A. J. Duerinckx, and F. E. Rademakers

Modern Head and Neck Imaging
Edited by S. K. Mukherji and J. A. Castelijns

Radiological Imaging of Endocrine Diseases
Edited by J. N. Bruneton in collaboration with B. Padovani and M.-Y. Mourou

Trends in Contrast Media
Edited by H. S. Thomsen, R. N. Muller, and R. F. Mattrey

Functional MRI
Edited by C. T. W. Moonen and P. A. Bandettini

Radiology of the Pancreas
2nd Revised Edition
Edited by A. L. Baert
Co-edited by G. Delorme and L. Van Hoe

Emergency Pediatric Radiology
Edited by H. Carty

Spiral CT of the Abdomen
Edited by F. Terrier, M. Grossholz, and C. D. Becker

Liver Malignancies
Diagnostic and Interventional Radiology
Edited by C. Bartolozzi and R. Lencioni

Medical Imaging of the Spleen
Edited by A. M. De Schepper and F. Vanhoenacker

Radiology of Peripheral Vascular Diseases
Edited by E. Zeitler

Diagnostic Nuclear Medicine
Edited by C. Schiepers

Radiology of Blunt Trauma of the Chest
P. Schnyder and M. Wintermark

Portal Hypertension
Diagnostic Imaging-Guided Therapy
Edited by P. Rossi
Co-edited by P. Ricci and L. Broglia

Recent Advances in Diagnostic Neuroradiology
Edited by Ph. Demaerel

Virtual Endoscopy and Related 3D Techniques
Edited by P. Rogalla, J. Terwisscha Van Scheltinga, and B. Hamm

Multislice CT
Edited by M. F. Reiser, M. Takahashi, M. Modic, and R. Bruening

Pediatric Uroradiology
Edited by R. Fotter

Transfontanellar Doppler Imaging in Neonates
A. Couture and C. Veyrac

Radiology of AIDS
A Practical Approach
Edited by J.W.A.J. Reeders and P.C. Goodman

CT of the Peritoneum
Armando Rossi and Giorgio Rossi

Magnetic Resonance Angiography
2nd Revised Edition
Edited by I. P. Arlart, G. M. Bongratz, and G. Marchal

Pediatric Chest Imaging
Edited by Javier Lucaya and Janet L. Strife

Applications of Sonography in Head and Neck Pathology
Edited by J. N. Bruneton in collaboration with C. Raffaelli and O. Dassonville

Imaging of the Larynx
Edited by R. Hermans

3D Image Processing
Techniques and Clinical Applications
Edited by D. Caramella and C. Bartolozzi

Imaging of Orbital and Visual Pathway Pathology
Edited by W. S. Müller-Forell

Pediatric ENT Radiology
Edited by S. J. King and A. E. Boothroyd

Radiological Imaging of the Small Intestine
Edited by N. C. Gourtsoyiannis

Imaging of the Knee
Techniques and Applications
Edited by A. M. Davies and V. N. Cassar-Pullicino

Perinatal Imaging
From Ultrasound to MR Imaging
Edited by Fred E. Avni

Radiological Imaging of the Neonatal Chest
Edited by V. Donoghue

Diagnostic and Interventional Radiology in Liver Transplantation
Edited by E. Bücheler, V. Nicolas, C. E. Broelsch, X. Rogiers, and G. Krupski

Radiology of Osteoporosis
Edited by S. Grampp

Imaging and Intervention in Abdominal Trauma
Edited by R. F. Dondelinger

Imaging of the Foot and Ankle
Techniques and Applications
Edited by A. M. Davies, R. W. Whitehouse, and J. P. R. Jenkins

Radiology Imaging of the Ureter
Edited by F. Joffre, Ph. Otal, and M. Soulie

Interventional Radiology in Cancer
Edited by A. Adam, R. F. Dondelinger, and P. R. Mueller

Imaging of the Pancreas
Cystic and Rare Tumors
Edited by C. Procassi and A. J. Megibow

Intracranial Vascular Malformations and Aneurysms
From Diagnostic Work-Up to Endovascular Therapy
Edited by M. Forsting

Imaging Pelvic Floor Disorders
Edited by C. I. Bartram and J. O. L. DeLancey
Associate Editors: S. Halligan, F. M. Kelvin, and J. Stoker

High Resolution Sonography of the Peripheral Nervous System
Edited by S. Peer and G. Bodner

Radiology Imaging of the Ureter
Edited by F. Joffre, Ph. Otal, and M. Soulie

Springer

MEDICAL RADIOLOGY Diagnostic Imaging and Radiation Oncology

Titles in the series already published

RADIATION ONCOLOGY

Lung Cancer
Edited by C.W. Scarantino

Innovations in Radiation Oncology
Edited by H. R. Withers and L. J. Peters

Radiation Therapy of Head and Neck Cancer
Edited by G. E. Laramore

Gastrointestinal Cancer – Radiation Therapy
Edited by R.R. Dobelbower, Jr.

Radiation Exposure and Occupational Risks
Edited by E. Scherer, C. Streffer, and K.-R. Trott

Radiation Therapy of Benign Diseases
A Clinical Guide
S.E. Order and S. S. Donaldson

Interventional Radiation Therapy Techniques – Brachytherapy
Edited by R. Sauer

Radiopathology of Organs and Tissues
Edited by E. Scherer, C. Streffer, and K.-R. Trott

Concomitant Continuous Infusion Chemotherapy and Radiation
Edited by M. Rotman and C. J. Rosenthal

Intraoperative Radiotherapy – Clinical Experiences and Results
Edited by F. A. Calvo, M. Santos, and L.W. Brady

Radiotherapy of Intraocular and Orbital Tumors
Edited by W. E. Alberti and R. H. Sagerman

Interstitial and Intracavitary Thermoradiotherapy
Edited by M. H. Seegenschmiedt and R. Sauer

Non-Disseminated Breast Cancer
Controversial Issues in Management
Edited by G. H. Fletcher and S.H. Levitt

Current Topics in Clinical Radiobiology of Tumors
Edited by H.-P. Beck-Bornholdt

Practical Approaches to Cancer Invasion and Metastases
A Compendium of Radiation Oncologists' Responses to 40 Histories
Edited by A. R. Kagan with the Assistance of R. J. Steckel

Radiation Therapy in Pediatric Oncology
Edited by J. R. Cassady

Radiation Therapy Physics
Edited by A. R. Smith

Late Sequelae in Oncology
Edited by J. Dunst and R. Sauer

Mediastinal Tumors. Update 1995
Edited by D. E. Wood and C. R. Thomas, Jr.

Thermoradiotherapy and Thermochemotherapy

Volume 1:
Biology, Physiology, and Physics

Volume 2:
Clinical Applications
Edited by M.H. Seegenschmiedt, P. Fessenden, and C.C. Vernon

Carcinoma of the Prostate
Innovations in Management
Edited by Z. Petrovich, L. Baert, and L.W. Brady

Radiation Oncology of Gynecological Cancers
Edited by H.W. Vahrson

Carcinoma of the Bladder
Innovations in Management
Edited by Z. Petrovich, L. Baert, and L.W. Brady

Blood Perfusion and Microenvironment of Human Tumors
Implications for Clinical Radiooncology
Edited by M. Molls and P. Vaupel

Radiation Therapy of Benign Diseases
A Clinical Guide
2nd Revised Edition
S. E. Order and S. S. Donaldson

Carcinoma of the Kidney and Testis, and Rare Urologic Malignancies
Innovations in Management
Edited by Z. Petrovich, L. Baert, and L.W. Brady

Progress and Perspectives in the Treatment of Lung Cancer
Edited by P. Van Houtte, J. Klastersky, and P. Rocmans

Combined Modality Therapy of Central Nervous System Tumors
Edited by Z. Petrovich, L. W. Brady, M. L. Apuzzo, and M. Bamberg

Age-Related Macular Degeneration Current Treatment Concepts
Edited by W. A. Alberti, G. Richard, and R. H. Sagerman

Radiotherapy of Intraocular and Orbital Tumors
2nd Revised Edition
Edited by R. H. Sagerman, and W. E. Alberti

Clinical Target Volumes in Conformal and Intensity Modulated Radiation Therapy
A Clinical Guide to Cancer Treatment
Edited by V. Grégoire, P. Scalliet, and K. K. Ang

Biological Modification of Radiation Response
Edited by C. Nieder, L. Milas, and K. K. Ang

Palliative Radiation Oncology
R. G. Parker. N. A. Janjan, and M. T. Selch

Springer